Infectious Diseases Handbook

— *including* —

Antimicrobial Therapy & Laboratory Diagnosis

1995-96

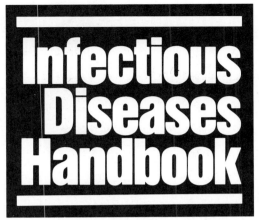

Infectious Diseases Handbook

— including —

Antimicrobial Therapy & Laboratory Diagnosis

Carlos M. Isada, MD
Department of Infectious Disease
Cleveland Clinic Foundation
Cleveland, Ohio

Bernard L. Kasten, Jr, MD
Associate Director
Pathology and Laboratory Services
Bethesda Hospitals
Cincinnati, Ohio

Morton P. Goldman, PharmD
Infectious Disease Pharmacist
Cleveland Clinic Foundation
Cleveland, Ohio

Larry D. Gray, PhD
Director of Microbiology
Bethesda Hospitals
Cincinnati, Ohio

Judith A. Aberg, MD
Fellow
Department of Infectious Disease
Washington University School of Medicine
St. Louis, Missouri

LEXI-COMP INC
Hudson (Cleveland)

AMERICAN
PHARMACEUTICAL
ASSOCIATION APhA

Infectious Diseases Handbook

including

Antimicrobial Therapy
and Laboratory Diagnosis

1995-96

NOTICE

This handbook is intended to serve the user as a handy reference and not as a complete infectious disease resource. The publication covers common diseases with empiric treatment recommendations, common microorganisms, testing procedures necessary for diagnosis, and the majority of anti-infective agents available in the United States. The individual sections of this handbook are specifically designed to present certain important aspects of the disease states, the organisms, laboratory tests, and antimicrobial therapy in a more concise format than is typically found in medical literature or infectious disease texts.

The nature of infectious diseases and their diagnosis and treatment is that it is constantly evolving because of ongoing research and clinical experience and is often subject to interpretation. While great care has been taken to ensure the accuracy of the information presented, the reader is advised that the authors, editors, reviewers, contributors, and publishers cannot be responsible for the continued currency of the information or for any errors or omissions in this book or for any consequences arising therefrom. Because of the dynamic nature of infectious disease as a discipline, readers are advised that decisions regarding the diagnosis and treatment of specific organisms and disease states must be based on the independent judgment of the clinician, changing information regarding drug therapy (eg, as reflected in the literature and drug manufacturer's most current product information), and changing medical practices. The editors are not responsible for any inaccuracy of quotation or for any false or misleading implication that may arise due to the text or formulas used or due to the quotation of revisions no longer official.

The editors, authors, and contributors have written this book in their private capacities. No official support or endorsement by any federal or state agency or pharmaceutical company is intended or inferred.

If you have any suggestions or questions
regarding any information presented in this handbook,
please contact our drug information pharmacist at

1-800-837-LEXI

This manual was produced using the FormuLex™ and Pathfinder™ Programs —
Complete publishing services of Lexi-Comp Inc.

Lexi-Comp Inc.
1100 Terex Road
Hudson, Ohio 44236-3771
(216) 650-6506

TABLE OF CONTENTS

TABLE OF CONTENTS

2

ABOUT THE AUTHORS

Carlos M. Isada, MD

Dr Isada received his undergraduate training and medical degree from the State University of New York at Buffalo. After completing his residency and chief residency in Internal Medicine at the Cleveland Clinic, he stayed on to pursue fellowship training in Infectious Diseases.

Along with his current duties as Staff Physician in the Department of Infectious Disease at the Cleveland Clinic Foundation, Dr Isada also serves as Director of the Infectious Diseases Fellowship Training Program and is Assistant Program Director for the Internal Medicine Residency Training. Dr Isada has developed a special interest in clinical virology and frequently participates in presentations and abstracts on this topic. In addition to these and other presentations and publications, Dr Isada is a major contributor to the *Diagnostic Procedures Handbook* published by Lexi-Comp Inc., and a member of Lexi-Comp's editorial board.

Dr Isada is a member of the Infectious Diseases Society of America, American Society of Microbiology, American College of Physicians, and the American Medical Association.

Bernard L. Kasten, Jr, MD

Dr Kasten is a graduate of Miami University, Oxford, Ohio and the Ohio State University College of Medicine. He interned at the University of Miami, Florida and served his residency in Clinical Pathology at the National Institute of Health Clinical Center followed by a fellowship at the National Cancer Institute Laboratory of Pathology. His staff appointments have included service in the Division of Laboratory Medicine at the Cleveland Clinic. For the last 6 years, he has been Associate Director of Pathology and Laboratory Services at Bethesda Hospitals in Cincinnati. Dr Kasten is active as a fellow in the College of American Pathologists, in which he participates in the Inspection and Accreditation Program, Council on Education and Membership Services, Management Resource Committee, and as Chairman of the Publications Committee and contributor and Chairman of the Editorial Board of *CAP Today* since its inception in 1987. He was the recipient of the 1993 Frank W. Hartman Award in recognition of his service to the College of American Pathologists.

Dr Kasten was a principal author of the first edition of the *Laboratory Test Handbook* and the author of the *Physicians DRG Handbook*. He has written articles on the use of bar codes in the clinical laboratory. He has presented numerous lectures and seminars on the subjects of improving workflow in the laboratory, total quality management, and the appropriate use of laboratory tests, particularly the rational use of screening tests for prostate-specific antigen. He is a member of the editorial board for Lexi-Comp Inc's medical publishing.

Morton P. Goldman, PharmD

Dr Goldman received his bachelor's degree in pharmacy from the University of Pittsburgh, College of Pharmacy and his Doctor of Pharmacy degree from the University of Cincinnati, Division of Graduate Studies and Research. He completed his concurrent 2-year hospital pharmacy residency at the VA Medical Center in Cincinnati. Dr Goldman is presently the Infectious Disease Pharmacist at the Cleveland Clinic Foundation and holds faculty appointments from Case Western Reserve University, College of Medicine, The University of Toledo, College of Pharmacy, and The University of Cincinnati, College of Pharmacy. Dr Goldman is a Board Certified Pharmacotherapy Specialist.

ABOUT THE AUTHORS

In his capacity as Infectious Disease Pharmacist at the Cleveland Clinic Foundation, Dr Goldman is actively involved in patient care and clinical research with the Department of Infectious Disease, as well as the continuing education of the medical and pharmacy staff. He is an editor of the foundation's *Guidelines for Antibiotic Usage* and has coordinated their Renal Dose Monitoring Program. He is a member of the Quality Assurance/Drug Use Evaluation Committee and chairs the Cleveland Clinic's annual Antimicrobial Formulary Review meeting. Dr Goldman has authored numerous journal articles and lectures locally and nationally on infectious diseases topics and current drug therapies. He is currently a reviewer for the *Annals of Pharmacotherapy*, a member of Lexi-Comp's editorial advisory panel, and is an associate editor of the *Drug Information Handbook for the Allied Health Professional* published by Lexi-Comp.

Dr Goldman is an active member of Cleveland's local clinical pharmacy society, as well as the Society of Infectious Disease Pharmacists, and the American College of Clinical Pharmacy.

Larry D. Gray, PhD

Dr Gray received his bachelor's degree from the University of North Carolina at Chapel Hill and his master's and doctorate degrees from Wake Forest University (Bowman Gray School of Medicine). He received his postdoctoral training in Clinical Microbiology and Infectious Diseases at the Mayo Clinic.

Dr Gray has been the Director of Microbiology at Bethesda Hospitals in Cincinnati, Ohio for the last 5 years. He is a Volunteer Associate Professor of Pathology and Laboratory Medicine at the University of Cincinnati College of Medicine, is a Diplomate of the American Board of Medical Microbiology and is on the editorial board of the *Journal of Clinical Microbiology*. In addition, he is an active member of the American Society for Microbiology, the American Board of Medical Microbiology, and the South Central Association for Clinical Microbiology.

Dr Gray's background includes 12 years of research in the pathogenesis of infectious diseases (ocular and pulmonary bacterial infections, electron microscopy) and the publication of many research, review, chapter, and book publications.

Judith A. Aberg, MD

Dr Aberg received a degree in Laboratory Technology from Norfolk General Hospital in 1975 and worked in medical microbiology, where she was responsible for the Mycology Laboratory and curriculum. After 11 years of laboratory experience. Dr Aberg graduated from Millersville University of Pennsylvania, Magna Cum Laude, BSMT. Dr Aberg then graduated from Pennsylvania State University College of Medicine.

During Dr Aberg's medical school training, she was a research technologist in neuroimmunology, resulting in publication of her work with multiple sclerosis. After medical school, Dr Aberg completed her internal medicine residency at the Cleveland Clinic, during which time she had worked as a limited clinical practitioner in the emergency department, and was involved in research projects in the Department of Infectious Disease. Dr Aberg then held a joint position as both Chief Medical Resident and Clinical Associate in Immunology at the Cleveland Clinic. As a clinical associate, she was involved in the HIV Center AIDS education in both the hospital and the community, and clinical trials for HIV-positive individuals.

Dr Aberg is currently a fellow at Washington University School of Medicine in the Department of Infectious Disease. She is active in many professional societies including the American Medical Association. American College of Physicians, American Society for Microbiology, and American Society of Clinical Pathologists.

EDITORIAL ADVISORY PANEL

PREFACE

"All disease is infectious disease". Although that may not be completely accurate, infectious disease crosses every discipline of medicine and surgery. With few exceptions, all physicians will diagnose and/or treat infectious diseases in their day-to-day practices. Infectious diseases are becoming more complicated to diagnose and treat. We are making many of our patients more immunocompromised and are performing more invasive procedures. There are more sophisticated diagnostic tests including serologies, probes, and polymerase chain reaction (PCR). The infecting organisms are becoming smarter -- more resistant to routine therapies; and the number of antimicrobial agents available to us is staggering. Billions of dollars are spent each year on antimicrobial agents in the United States with billions more spent on office visits, hospitalization, and diagnostic procedures related to infection.

It is safe to say, that infectious disease as a discipline is not easy, nor can it be made easy. This handbook is not, therefore, intended as a simplification of infectious disease. Instead, we wish to make the most pertinent aspects of infectious disease readily available to all practitioners as an aid in their infectious disease endeavors. The disease syndromes chapter provides concise, straightforward information on the clinical presentation, differential diagnosis, diagnostic tests, and drug therapy recommended for treatment of the more common diseases. The organism chapter provides descriptions of the microbiology, epidemiology, diagnosis, and treatment of each organism. The laboratory diagnosis chapter describes the performance of specific tests and procedures including preparation of the patient. The antimicrobial therapy chapter provides what we believe are the most important facts and considerations regarding each drug product. In addition, the appendix offers a compilation of tables, guidelines, and conversion information which can be helpful in consideration of patient care. Finally, an alphabetical index offers convenient cross-referencing by page number to each item found in every section of the book.

A unique feature of this handbook is that entries in each of the four sections of the book (disease syndromes, organisms, laboratory diagnosis, and antimicrobial therapy) contain relative information and cross-referencing to one or more of the other three sections. For example, an entry regarding a particular organism will also provide a cross-reference to the appropriate laboratory tests to detect the organism and appropriate antimicrobial agents used against the organism.

The authors envision this handbook to be a useful tool for physicians, residents, students, dentists, nurses, pharmacists, and anyone who has the opportunity to diagnose, treat, or care for patients with infectious diseases.

Accuracy, completeness, and timeliness of each fact or recommendation presented was a major goal of the authors of this handbook. The authors hope this goal has been met. Users of the handbook, however, are strongly encouraged to offer suggestions for improvement, additional entries, and corrections to current entries. Such suggestions will be sincerely welcome and considered for future editions.

ACKNOWLEDGMENTS

This handbook exists in its present form as a result of the concerted efforts of many individuals. The publisher and president of Lexi-Comp Inc, Robert D. Kerscher and the senior director of Programming and Publications, James P. Caro, American Pharmaceutical Association (APhA) deserve much of the credit for bringing the concept of such a book to fruition.

Other members of the Lexi-Comp staff whose contributions were invaluable and whose patience with the editors' enumerable drafts, revisions, deletions, additions, and enhancements was inexhaustible include: Diane Harbart, MT (ASCP), medical editor; Lynn Coppinger, director of product development; Barbara F. Kerscher, production manager; Alexandra Hart, composition specialist; Jeanne Eads, Beth Daulbaugh, Julie Weekes, and Lisa Leukart, project managers; Jil R. Neuman, Julie Kelley, Jacqueline L. Mizer, and Tracey J. Reinecke production assistants; Jeff J. Zaccagnini, Brian B. Vossler, and Jerry Reeves, sales managers; Edmund A. Harbart, vice-president, custom publishing division; and Jack L. Stones, vice-president, reference publishing division. The complex computer programming required for the typesetting of the book was provided by Jay L. Katzen, Dennis P. Smithers, David C. Marcus, Dale Jablonski, and Kenneth J. Hughes, system analysts, under the direction of Thury L. O'Connor, vice-president, and Alan R. Frasz, vice-president, editorial systems.

Other APhA staff members whose contributions were important are Julian I. Graubart, Director Special Projects, and James V. McGinnis, manager of art and production. A special thanks goes to Chris Lomax, PharmD, director of pharmacy, Children's Hospital, Los Angeles, who played a significant role in bringing APhA and Lexi-Comp together.

Much of the material contained in the book was a result of pharmacy contributors throughout the United States and Canada. Lexi-Comp has assisted many medical institutions to develop hospital-specific formulary manuals that contains clinical drug information as well as dosing. Working with these clinical pharmacists, hospital pharmacy and therapeutics committees, and hospital drug information centers, Lexi-Comp has developed an evolutionary drug database that reflects the practice of pharmacy in these major institutions.

In addition, the authors wish to thank their families, friends, and colleagues who supported them in their efforts to complete this handbook.

USE OF THE INFECTIOUS DISEASES HANDBOOK

The *Infectious Diseases Handbook including Antimicrobial Therapy and Laboratory Diagnosis* is organized into four major chapters, an appendix, and an alphabetical index.

Information is presented in a consistent format with extensive cross-referencing between chapters. Each chapter will provide the following.

DISEASE SYNDROMES

Disease Syndrome Name	Common nomenclature for the disease
Synonyms	Other names or abbreviations for the disease state
Clinical Presentation	Signs, symptoms, and findings from physical and laboratory examination
Differential Diagnosis	A wide differential diagnosis of the disease
Likely Pathogens	Possible organisms causing the disease syndrome. Organisms listed in order of probability. Cross-references to the organism chapter.
Diagnostic Tests/Procedures	Appropriate tests necessary for diagnosis. Bulleted tests are more diagnostic. Cross-references to laboratory diagnosis chapter.
Empiric Drug Therapy	Appropriate empiric therapy in the opinion of the authors. Definitive therapy should be used when microbiologic diagnosis is made. Cross-reference to antimicrobial therapy chapter.
Selected Reading	General references are provided

ORGANISMS

Organism Name	Genus and species name
Synonyms	Other names or abbreviations for the organism
Applies To	Other organisms included in the named genus
Microbiology	A description of the organism by morphology, stain, biochemistry, serological differences, etc.
Epidemiology	May include the natural habitat and mode of transmission of the organism. May also include information on outbreaks and transmission prevention.
Clinical Syndromes	Specific disease states that can be caused by the organism
Diagnosis	Methods for determining that the organism is causing disease
Diagnostic Tests/Procedures	Appropriate tests useful for diagnosis. Cross-references to laboratory diagnosis chapter.
Treatment	Description of treatment modalities including nondrug therapies
Drug Therapy	Drugs of choice and alternatives for treatment of disease caused by these organisms. Cross-reference to antimicrobial therapy chapter.
Selected Reading	General references are provided

LABORATORY DIAGNOSIS

Name	Common name for the test
Related Information	Cross-references to other tests or procedures located in this chapter of the book that are related to the named test and may be helpful to the user
Synonyms	Other names or abbreviations for the laboratory test/procedure
Applies To	Refers to various sample sites or specimen types that follow the same procedure
Replaces	Previous test/procedure that has been replaced by this more current test/procedure
Test Includes or Procedure Commonly Includes	All laboratory tests or procedures that may occur when the named test is performed
Abstract	A brief description of the test and its use
Patient Preparation	Any special preparation that the patient must undergo prior to the procedure being performed
Aftercare	Special instructions or warnings for medical personnel for the care of the patient after the procedure is performed
Special Instructions	Specific instructions for the acquisition and handling of specimens
Complications	Problems that may arise for the patient due to testing
Equipment	All equipment needed to perform the named procedure
Technique	Explanation of how procedure is performed
Data Acquired	Data obtained from the performed procedure
Specimen	All possible specimens that can be used for testing
Container	Type of container that specimen must be collected in to acquire and maintain a usable specimen
Sampling Time	The time frame a specimen should be collected
Collection	General and specific collection instructions that should be followed to obtain a proper and usable specimen
Storage Instructions	The appropriate storage of the specimen after collection but prior to testing
Causes for Rejection	Possible reasons why a specimen may be rejected by the laboratory
Turnaround Time	Time it takes for testing to be performed and results to be reported
Normal Range or Normal Findings	Serves as a general guideline. See specific testing facility for their ranges.
Critical Values	Values that alert the medical staff that the patient has reached a value that may be hazardous to the patient
Use	Common uses for the test/procedure
Limitations	Limits of the test/procedure

Contraindications	Reasons why this test should not be performed
Methodology	Testing methodologies available
Additional Information	Additional information about the test/procedure and its uses
Selected Reading	General references are provided

ANTIMICROBIAL THERAPY

Generic Name	U.S. adopted name
Pronunciation Guide	
Related Information	Cross-references to other pertinent drug information found in the Appendix
Brand Names	Common trade names
Synonyms	Other names or accepted abbreviations for the generic drug
Generic Available	Drugs available in generic form
Use	Information pertaining to appropriate indications of the drug
Drug of Choice or Alternate For	Cross-references to organism or disease syndromes chapter
Pregnancy Risk Factor	Five categories established by the FDA to indicate the potential of a systemically absorbed drug for causing birth defects
Contraindications	Information pertaining to inappropriate use of the drug
Warnings/Precautions	Hazardous conditions related to use of the drug and disease states or patient populations in which the drug should be cautiously used
Adverse Reactions	Side effects are grouped by percentage of incidence
Toxicology Drug Interactions Stability	Comments and/or considerations offered when appropriate
Mechanism of Action	How the drug works in the body to elicit a response
Pharmacokinetics	Pharmacokinetics are expressed in terms of absorption, distribution (including appearance in breast milk and crossing of the placenta), metabolism, bioavailability, half-life, time to peak serum concentration, and elimination. Additional pharmacokinetic data can be found in the appendix.
Usual Dosage	The amount of the drug to be typically given or taken during therapy
Overdosage	
Monitoring Parameters	Laboratory tests and patient physical parameters that should be monitored for safety and efficacy of drug therapy are listed when appropriate
Test Interactions	Listing of assay interferences when relevant; (B) = Blood; (S) = Serum; (U) = Urine
Reference Range	Therapeutic and toxic serum concentrations listed when appropriate

Patient Information	Comments and/or considerations are
Nursing Implications	offered when appropriate
Additional Information	Information about sodium content and/or pertinent information about specific brands
Dosage Forms	Information with regard to form, strength, and availability of the drug
Selected Reading	General references are provided

Appendix

The appendix offers a compilation of tables, guidelines, nomograms, and conversion information which can often be helpful when considering patient care.

Alphabetical Index

All disease syndromes, organisms, laboratory diagnosis, and antimicrobial therapy names, brand names, and synonyms are listed alphabetically and the page number on which the monograph may be found is indicated.

FDA PREGNANCY CATEGORIES

Throughout this book there is a field labeled Pregnancy Risk Factor (PRF) and the letter A, B, C, D, or X immediately following which signifies a category. The FDA has established these five categories to indicate the potential of a systemically absorbed drug for causing birth defects. The key differentiation among the categories rests upon the reliability of documentation and the risk:benefit ratio. Pregnancy Category X is particularly notable in that if any data exists that may implicate a drug as a teratogen and the risk:benefit ratio is clearly negative, the drug is contraindicated during pregnancy.

These categories are summarized as follows:

A   Controlled studies in pregnant women fail to demonstrate a risk to the fetus in the first trimester with no evidence of risk in later trimesters. The possibility of fetal harm appears remote.

B   Either animal-reproduction studies have not demonstrated a fetal risk but there are no controlled studies in pregnant women, or animal-reproduction studies have shown an adverse effect (other than a decrease in fertility) that was not confirmed in controlled studies in women in the first trimester and there is no evidence of a risk in later trimesters.

C   Either studies in animals have revealed adverse effects on the fetus (teratogenic or embryocidal effects or other) and there are no controlled studies in women, or studies in women and animals are not available. Drugs should be given only if the potential benefits justify the potential risk to the fetus.

D   There is positive evidence of human fetal risk, but the benefits from use in pregnant women may be acceptable despite the risk (eg, if the drug is needed in a life-threatening situation or for a serious disease for which safer drugs cannot be used or are ineffective).

X   Studies in animals or human beings have demonstrated fetal abnormalities or there is evidence of fetal risk based on human experience, or both, and the risk of the use of the drug in pregnant women clearly outweighs any possible benefit. The drug is contraindicated in women who are or may become pregnant.

SAFE WRITING

Health professionals and their support personnel frequently produce handwritten copies of information they see in print; therefore, such information is subjected to even greater possibilities for error or misinterpretation on the part of others. Thus, particular care must be given to how drug names and strengths are expressed when creating written healthcare documents.

The following are a few examples of safe writing rules suggested by the Institute for Safe Medication Practices, Inc.*

1. There should be a space between a number and its units as it is easier to read. There should be no periods after the abbreviations mg or mL.

Correct	Incorrect
10 mg	10mg
100 mg	100mg

2. Never place a decimal and a zero after a whole number (2 mg is correct and 2.0 mg is incorrect). If the decimal point is not seen because it falls on a line or because individuals are working from copies where the decimal point is not seen, this causes a tenfold overdose.

3. Just the opposite is true for numbers less than one. Always place a zero before a naked decimal (0.5 mL is correct, .5 mL is **in**correct).

4. Never abbreviate the word unit. The handwritten U or u, looks like a 0 (zero), and may cause a tenfold overdose error to be made.

5. Q.D. is not a safe abbreviation for once daily, as when the Q is followed by a sloppy dot, it looks like QID which means four times daily.

6. O.D. is not a safe abbreviation for once daily, as it is properly interpreted as meaning "right eye" and has caused liquid medications such as saturated solution of potassium iodide and lugol's solution to be administered incorrectly. There is no safe abbreviation for once daily. It must be written out in full.

7. Do not use chemical names such as 6-mercaptopurine or 6-thioguanine, as sixfold overdoses have been given when these were not recognized as chemical names. The proper names of these drugs are mercaptopurine or thioguanine.

8. Do not abbreviate drug names (5FC, 6MP, 5-ASA, MTX, HCTZ CPZ, PBZ, etc) as they are misinterpreted and cause error.

9. Do not use the apothecary system or symbols.

10. When writing an outpatient prescription, write a complete prescription. A complete prescription can prevent the prescriber, the pharmacist, and/or the patient from making a mistake and can eliminate the need for further clarification.

The legible prescriptions should contain:

   a. patient's full name
   b. for pediatric or geriatric patients: their age (or weight where applicable)

*From "Safe Writing" by Davis NM, PharmD and Cohen MR, MS, Lecturers and Consultants for Safe Medication Practices, 1143 Wright Drive, Huntingdon Valley, PA 19006. Phone: (215) 947-7566.

    c.   drug name, dosage form and strength; if a drug is new or rarely prescribed, print this information
    d.   number or amount to be dispensed
    e.   complete instructions for the patient, including the purpose of the medication
    f.   when there are recognized contraindications for a prescribed drug, indicate to the pharmacist that you are aware of this fact (ie, when prescribing a potassium salt for a patient receiving an ACE inhibitor, write "K serum leveling being monitored")

SELECTED REFERENCES

AMA Drug Evaluations Subscription, American Medical Association, Department of Drugs, Division of Drugs and Toxicology, Spring, 1990.

Drug Interaction Facts, St Louis, MO: J.B. Lippincott Co (Facts and Comparisons Division), 1994.

Facts and Comparisons, St Louis, MO: J.B. Lippincott Co (Facts and Comparisons Division), 1994.

Handbook of Nonprescription Drugs, 10th ed, Washington, DC: American Pharmaceutical Association, 1993.

Jacobs DS, DeMott WR, Finley PR, et al, *Laboratory Test Handbook with Key Word Index*, 3rd ed, Hudson, OH: Lexi-Comp Inc, 1994.

Lacy CF, Armstrong LL, Lipsy RJ, and Lance LL, *Drug Information Handbook*, 2nd ed, Hudson, OH: Lexi-Comp Inc, 1994.

Lance LL, Lacy CF, and Goldman MP, *Drug Information Handbook for the Allied Health Professional*, Hudson, OH: Lexi-Comp Inc, 1994.

Levin D, *Essentials of Pediatric Intensive Care*, St Louis, MO: Quality Medical Publishing, Inc, 1990.

Mandell GL, Bennett JE, and Dolin R, *Principles and Practice of Infectious Diseases*, 4th ed, New York, NY: Churchill Livingstone, 1995.

Medicus-Bringa M, Hennen CR, Adler RJ, et al, "Selected Adult Intravenous Drug Dosing in Renal Failure," *Hosp Pharm*, 1992, 27:119-21, 124-8, 132.

McEvoy GK and Litvak K, *AHFS Drug Information*, Bethesda, MD: American Society of Hospital Pharmacists, 1994.

Physician's Desk Reference, 48th ed, Oradell, NJ: Medical Economics Books, 1994.

Report of the Committee on Infectious Diseases, American Academy of Pediatrics, 22nd ed, 1991.

Semla TP, Beizer JL, and Higbee MD, *Geriatric Dosage Handbook*, Hudson, OH: Lexi-Comp Inc, 1993.

Taketomo CK, Hodding JH, and Kraus DM, *Pediatric Dosage Handbook*, 2nd ed, Hudson, OH: Lexi-Comp Inc, 1993.

Trissel L, *Handbook of Injectionable Drugs*, 7th ed, Bethesda, MD: American Society of Hospital Pharmacists, 1992.

United States Pharmacopeia Dispensing Information (USP DI), Rockville, MD: United States Pharmacopeial Convention, Inc, 1994.

DISEASE SYNDROMES

Acquired Immunodeficiency Syndrome *see* Human
Immunodeficiency Virus *on page 133*

Actinomycosis *see Actinomyces* Species *on page 51*

Acute Native Valve Infective Endocarditis *see* Endocarditis,
Acute Native Valve *on page 22*

Acute Sinusitis, Community-Acquired *see* Sinusitis, Community-
Acquired, Acute *on page 41*

Acute Suppurative Otitis *see* Otitis Media, Acute
on page 35

Amebiasis *see Entamoeba histolytica on page 102*

Animal and Human Bites Guidelines *see page 736*

Animal Bites *see* Animal and Human Bites Guidelines
on page 736-739

Anthrax *see Bacillus anthracis on page 58*

Antibiotic-Associated Colitis *see Clostridium difficile*
on page 85

Arthritis, Septic
Synonyms Septic Arthritis

Clinical Presentation The onset of septic arthritis is usually abrupt. Symptoms include chills, fever, and a monarthritis with warmth, swelling, erythema, and tenderness. Ten percent present with polyarthritis. Most commonly affects large joints, especially knees, ankles, and wrists. Presentation may be more indolent in patients with rheumatoid arthritis. Gonococcus is the most common cause of septic arthritis in adults.

Differential Diagnosis Crystal induced; palindromic rheumatism; other infections (ie, tubercular, fungal, viral, tendonitis, bursitis, juvenile rheumatoid arthritis)

Likely Pathogens
Neisseria gonorrhoeae on page 161
Staphylococcus aureus, Methicillin-Susceptible *on page 198*

Diagnostic Tests/Procedures
• Aerobic Culture, Body Fluid *on page 244*
• Arthrocentesis *on page 264*
• Biopsy Culture, Routine *on page 270*
• Gram Stain *on page 352*
  Lyme Disease Serology *on page 394*
  Mycobacteria Culture, Biopsy or Body Fluid *on page 404*
  Neisseria gonorrhoeae Culture *on page 412*

Empiric Drug Therapy
Recommended
    Oxacillin Sodium *on page 627*
     or
    Oxacillin Sodium *on page 627*
     used in combination with
    Ceftriaxone Sodium *on page 523*
    Note: Ceftriaxone sodium should be used if there is a high suspicion of gonococcal infection from the clinical setting.

Selected Readings
Goldenberg DL and Reed JI, "Bacterial Arthritis," *N Engl J Med*, 1985, 312(12):764-71.
Mikhail IS and Alarcon GS, "Nongonococcal Bacterial Arthritis," *Rheum Dis Clin North Am*, 1993, 19(2):311-31.
Scopelitis E and Martinez-Osuna P, "Gonococcal Arthritis," *Rheum Dis Clin North Am*, 1993, 19(2):363-77.

Athlete's Foot *see* Dermatophytes *on page 100*

Babesiosis *see Babesia microti on page 57*

Bacillary Angiomatosis *see Bartonella Species on page 62*

Bacterial Vaginosis *see Vaginosis, Bacterial on page 46*

Bilharziasis *see Schistosoma mansoni on page 189*

Blastomycosis *see Blastomyces dermatitidis on page 63*

Blennophthalmia *see Conjunctivitis on page 21*

Botulism *see Clostridium botulinum on page 83*

Bronchitis

Synonyms Tracheobronchitis

Clinical Presentation Chronic bronchitis may be present in as many as 15% of all adults. Characterized by cough, hypersecretion of mucus, and expectoration of sputum for at least 3 months of the year for more than 2 consecutive years. Acute exacerbations may be either bacterial or viral. Bacterial exacerbations are characterized by increased frequency and severity of cough, increased sputum production, purulent sputum, chest discomfort and congestion, dyspnea and wheezing. Acute bacterial exacerbation in chronic bronchitis is the most common cause of hemoptysis. Patients may experience loss of appetite and feelings of fever and chills; however, true fever, rigors, or pleuritic pain suggest pneumonia. Physical exam may be misleading as some patients with chronic bronchitis always have abnormal breath sounds, and it is helpful to know patient's baseline lung exam.

Differential Diagnosis Chronic bronchitis; chronic obstructive pulmonary disease; emphysema; pneumonia; acute bronchitis

Likely Pathogens
Streptococcus pneumoniae on page 206
Haemophilus influenzae on page 119
Moraxella catarrhalis on page 147

Diagnostic Tests/Procedures
Aerobic Culture, Sputum *on page 246*
Gram Stain *on page 352*

Drug Therapy Comment For severe exacerbations of bronchitis in hospitalized patients, intravenous forms of antimicrobial therapy should be used. For mild to moderate recurrent episodes, the various recommended oral antibiotics may be cycled.

Empiric Drug Therapy
  Recommended
    Amoxicillin Trihydrate *on page 491*
    Co-trimoxazole *on page 545*
    Doxycycline *on page 557*
    Cephalosporins, 2nd Generation *on page 527*
    Amoxicillin and Clavulanic Acid *on page 490*

Selected Readings
  Chodosh S, "Acute Bacterial Exacerbations in Bronchitis and Asthma," *Am J Med*, 1987, 82(4A):154-63.
  Isada CM, "Pro: Antibiotics for Chronic Bronchitis With Exacerbations," *Semin Respir Infect*, 1993, 8(4):243-53.
  Isada CM and Stoller JK, "Chronic Bronchitis: The Role of Antibiotics," *Respiratory Infections: A Scientific Basis for Management*, Niederman MS, Sarosi GA, and Glassroth J, eds, Orlando FL: W.B. Saunders, 1994, 621-33.
  Murphy TF and Sethi S, "Bacterial Infection in Chronic Obstructive Pulmonary Disease," *Am Rev Respir Dis*, 1992, 146(4):1067-83.

Brucellosis *see Brucella Species on page 69*

Bubonic Plague *see Yersinia pestis on page 233*

Candidiasis *see Candida Species on page 73*

Catheter Infection, Intravascular

Synonyms Line Sepsis

Clinical Presentation Catheter-related infection refers to an obvious sign of infection at the catheter site such as erythema, induration, or purulence. Catheter-related bacterium refers to isolation of an organism in a catheter segment culture and in the peripheral blood without any clinical signs of sepsis. Less than 1% of patients go on to develop sepsis; however, if sepsis occurs, there is a 10% to 20% mortality rate.

Likely Pathogens

Staphylococcus aureus, Methicillin-Susceptible *on page 198*
Staphylococcus epidermidis, Methicillin-Susceptible *on page 201*
Gram-Negative Bacilli *on page 117*
Enterococcus Species *on page 107*
Candida Species *on page 73*

Diagnostic Tests/Procedures

• Blood Culture, Aerobic and Anaerobic *on page 271*
• Blood Culture, Fungus *on page 275*
• Gram Stain *on page 352*
• Intravenous Line Culture *on page 376*

Empiric Drug Therapy

Recommended

Vancomycin Hydrochloride *on page 691*
used in combination with
Gentamicin Sulfate *on page 575*

Selected Readings

Clarke DE, Raffin TA, "Infectious Complications of Indwelling Long-Term Central Venous Catheters", *Chest*, 1990, 97(4):966-72.

Farkas JC, Liu N, Bleriot JP, "Single-versus Triple-Lumen Central Catheter-Related Sepsis: A Prospective Randomized Study in a Critically Ill Population," *Am J Med*, 1992, 93(3):277-82.

Groeger JS, Lucas AB, Thaler HT, et al, "Infectious Morbidity Associated With Long-Term Use of Venous Access Devices in Patients With Cancer," *Ann Intern Med*, 1993, 119(12):1168-74.

Press OW, Ramsey PG, Larson EB, "Hickman Catheter Infections in Patients With Malignancies," *Medicine (Baltimore)*, 1984, 63(4):189-200.

Cat Scratch Disease *see Bartonella Species on page 62*

Cellulitis *see Skin and Soft Tissue on page 42*

Chancroid *see Haemophilus ducreyi on page 118*

Chickenpox *see Varicella-Zoster Virus on page 227*

Cholera *see Vibrio cholerae on page 230*

Chronic Sinusitis, Community-Acquired *see Sinusitis, Community-Acquired, Chronic on page 41*

Coccidioidomycosis *see Coccidioides immitis on page 89*

Community-Acquired Sinusitis, Acute *see Sinusitis, Community-Acquired, Acute on page 41*

Community-Acquired Sinusitis, Chronic *see Sinusitis, Community-Acquired, Chronic on page 41*

Conjunctivitis
Synonyms Blennophthalmia; Koch-Weeks; Pink Eye; Red Eye

Clinical Presentation Inflammation of the conjunctiva associated with marked hyperemia and mucopurulent or watery discharge. The hyperemia is less intense in the perilimbal region as compared to ciliary flush.

Differential Diagnosis Conjunctivitis – allergic, viral, bacterial, granulomatous; iritis/iridocyclitis; herpes simplex keratitis; acute angle-closure glaucoma; episcleritis; scleritis; subconjunctival hemorrhage; pterygium; foreign body/abrasions

Likely Pathogens
Adenovirus *on page 53*
Chlamydia trachomatis on page 79
Herpes Simplex Virus *on page 128*
Staphylococcus aureus, Methicillin-Susceptible *on page 198*
Neisseria gonorrhoeae on page 161
Haemophilus influenzae on page 119
Streptococcus pneumoniae on page 206

Diagnostic Tests/Procedures
Aerobic Culture, Appropriate Site *on page 244*
Adenovirus Culture *on page 243*
Chlamydia Culture *on page 294*
Gram Stain *on page 352*
Herpes Simplex Virus Culture *on page 364*
Ocular Cytology *on page 416*

Drug Therapy Comment Treatment should be based on suspected organism diagnosed. Many of the ophthalmic anti-infective agents are combined with steroids for their anti-inflammatory activity.

Selected Readings
Gausas RE and Rapoza PA, "Red Eye: Serious or Not?" *Hosp Med*, December, 1992, 63-72.

Croup *see Parainfluenza Virus on page 166*

Cryptococcosis *see Cryptococcus neoformans on page 94*

Cryptosporidiosis *see Cryptosporidium on page 96*

Darling's Disease *see Histoplasma capsulatum on page 130*

Dermatomycoses *see Dermatophytes on page 100*

Desert Rheumatism *see Coccidioides immitis on page 89*

Dysentery *see Shigella Species on page 191*

Ehrlichiosis *see Ehrlichia Species on page 101*

Endocarditis, Acute, I.V. Drug Abuse
Related Information
Prevention of Bacterial Endocarditis *on page 727-730*

Clinical Presentation In acute left-side bacterial endocarditis, patients typically present with high fever and rapid valvular dysfunction resulting in congestive heart failure or arrhythmias. In acute right-sided endocarditis, patients appear ill with fever, have pulmonary infiltrates, and have the murmur of tricuspid or pulmonary insufficiency.

Likely Pathogens
Pseudomonas aeruginosa on page 177
Staphylococcus aureus, Methicillin-Susceptible *on page 198*

Diagnostic Tests/Procedures
• Blood Culture, Aerobic and Anaerobic *on page 271*

(Continued)

21

Endocarditis, Acute, I.V. Drug Abuse *(Continued)*

- Chest Films *on page 293*
- Gram Stain *on page 352*
  Blood Culture, Fungus *on page 275*
  C-Reactive Protein *on page 311*
  Echocardiography, M-Mode *on page 324*
  Sedimentation Rate, Erythrocyte *on page 440*
  Serum Bactericidal Test *on page 441*
  Transesophageal Echocardiography *on page 460*

Empiric Drug Therapy
Recommended
Vancomycin Hydrochloride *on page 691*
used in combination with
Gentamicin Sulfate *on page 575*

Selected Readings
Cherubin CE and Sapira JD, "The Medical Complications of Drug Addiction and the Medical Assessment of the Intravenous Drug User: 25 Years Later," *Ann Intern Med*, 1993, 119(10):1017-28.

Endocarditis, Acute Native Valve
Related Information
Prevention of Bacterial Endocarditis *on page 727-730*

Synonyms Acute Native Valve Infective Endocarditis

Clinical Presentation Between 60% and 80% of patients have a pre-existing cardiac lesion such as rheumatic valvular disease, congenital heart disease, or degenerative heart disease.

In acute left-side bacterial endocarditis, patients typically present with high fever and rapid valvular dysfunction resulting in congestive heart failure or arrhythmias. In acute right-sided endocarditis, patients appear ill with fever, have pulmonary infiltrates, and have the murmur of tricuspid or pulmonary insufficiency.

Likely Pathogens
Staphylococcus aureus, Methicillin-Susceptible *on page 198*
Streptococcus pneumoniae on page 206
Neisseria gonorrhoeae on page 161

Diagnostic Tests/Procedures
- Blood Culture, Aerobic and Anaerobic *on page 271*
- Echocardiography, M-Mode *on page 324*
- Gram Stain *on page 352*
  C-Reactive Protein *on page 311*
  Sedimentation Rate, Erythrocyte *on page 440*
  Serum Bactericidal Test *on page 441*
  Transesophageal Echocardiography *on page 460*

Empiric Drug Therapy
Recommended
Penicillins, Penicillinase-Resistant *on page 637*
used in combination with
Gentamicin Sulfate *on page 575*

Alternate
Vancomycin Hydrochloride *on page 691*
used in combination with
Gentamicin Sulfate *on page 575*

Selected Readings
Keys TF, "Diagnosis and Management of Infective Endocarditis," *Cleve Clin J Med*, 1990, 57(6):558-62.

Longworth DL, "Diagnosing Infective Endocarditis," *Cleve Clin J Med*, 1994, 61(3):172-3.

Endocarditis, Prosthetic Valve, Early
Related Information
Prevention of Bacterial Endocarditis *on page 727-730*

Synonyms Prosthetic Valve Endocarditis, Early; PVE, Early

Clinical Presentation Occurs within 60 days of surgery and is a consequence of valve contamination or bacteremia perioperatively. This usually presents as an acute event. In left sided early prosthetic valve endocarditis, patients typically present with high fever and rapid valvular dysfunction resulting in congestive heart failure or arrhythmias. In right sided disease, patients appear ill with fever, have pulmonary infiltrates, and have insufficiency murmurs.

Likely Pathogens
Staphylococcus epidermidis, Methicillin-Susceptible *on page 201*
Staphylococcus epidermidis, Methicillin-Resistant *on page 200*
Staphylococcus aureus, Methicillin-Susceptible *on page 198*
Staphylococcus aureus, Methicillin-Resistant *on page 195*
Gram-Negative Bacilli *on page 117*
Candida Species *on page 73*

Diagnostic Tests/Procedures
• Blood Culture, Aerobic and Anaerobic *on page 271*
• Gram Stain *on page 352*
  Blood Culture, Fungus *on page 275*
  C-Reactive Protein *on page 311*
  Echocardiography, M-Mode *on page 324*
  Sedimentation Rate, Erythrocyte *on page 440*
  Serum Bactericidal Test *on page 441*
  Transesophageal Echocardiography *on page 460*

Empiric Drug Therapy
Recommended
  Vancomycin Hydrochloride *on page 691*
    used in combination with
  Gentamicin Sulfate *on page 575*

Endocarditis, Prosthetic Valve, Late
Related Information
  Prevention of Bacterial Endocarditis *on page 727-730*
Synonyms Prosthetic Valve Endocarditis, Late; PVE, Late
Clinical Presentation Occurs more than 60 days after valve surgery. This usually presents as an acute event. In left sided late prosthetic valve endocarditis, patients typically present with high fever and rapid valvular dysfunction resulting in congestive heart failure or arrhythmias. In right sided disease, patients appear ill with fever, have pulmonary infiltrates, and have insufficiency murmurs.

Likely Pathogens
Streptococcus, Viridans Group *on page 213*
Staphylococcus epidermidis, Methicillin-Susceptible *on page 201*
Staphylococcus epidermidis, Methicillin-Resistant *on page 200*

Diagnostic Tests/Procedures
• Blood Culture, Aerobic and Anaerobic *on page 271*
• Gram Stain *on page 352*
  C-Reactive Protein *on page 311*
  Echocardiography, M-Mode *on page 324*
  Sedimentation Rate, Erythrocyte *on page 440*
  Serum Bactericidal Test *on page 441*
  Transesophageal Echocardiography *on page 460*

Empiric Drug Therapy
Recommended
  Vancomycin Hydrochloride *on page 691*
    used in combination with
  Gentamicin Sulfate *on page 575*

Endocarditis, Subacute Native Valve
Related Information
  Prevention of Bacterial Endocarditis *on page 727-730*
Clinical Presentation Symptoms generally begin approximately 2 weeks after precipitating event. Onset is gradual with low-grade fever, malaise, and arthralgias. Cardiac murmur is usually present. May present with splenomegaly, petechia, splinter hemorrhages, Roth spots, Osler nodes, Janeway lesions, and clubbing. Embolic events, mycotic aneurysms, brain abscesses, meningitis, and renal disease may occur.

(Continued)
23

Endocarditis, Subacute Native Valve *(Continued)*

Differential Diagnosis Acute rheumatic fever; lupus erythematosus and other collagen vascular diseases; sickle cell; nonbacterial thrombotic endocarditis; malignancy; tuberculosis

Likely Pathogens

Streptococcus, Viridans Group *on page 213*

Enterococcus Species *on page 107*

HACEK Group *on page 117*

Streptococcus bovis *on page 205*

Diagnostic Tests/Procedures

- Blood Culture, Aerobic and Anaerobic *on page 271*
- Gram Stain *on page 352*

Chest Films *on page 293*

C-Reactive Protein *on page 311*

Echocardiography, M-Mode *on page 324*

Q Fever Serology *on page 433*

Sedimentation Rate, Erythrocyte *on page 440*

Serum Bactericidal Test *on page 441*

Transesophageal Echocardiography *on page 460*

Empiric Drug Therapy

Recommended

Gentamicin Sulfate *on page 575*

used in combination with

Penicillin G, Parenteral *on page 633*

Alternate

Vancomycin Hydrochloride *on page 691*

used in combination with

Gentamicin Sulfate *on page 575*

or

Penicillin G, Parenteral *on page 633*

used in combination with

Gentamicin Sulfate *on page 575*

or

Ampicillin *on page 495*

used in combination with

Gentamicin Sulfate *on page 575*

Selected Readings

Bisno AL, Dismukes WE, Durack DT, "Antimicrobial Treatment of Infective Endocarditis Due to Viridans Streptococci, Enterococci, and Staphylococci," *JAMA*, 1989, 261(10):1471-7.

Dajani AS, Bisno AL, Chung KJ, et al, "Prevention of Bacterial Endocarditis: Recommendations by the American Heart Association," *JAMA*, 1990, 264(22):2919-22.

Epiglottitis

Synonyms Supraglottitis

Clinical Presentation Acute epiglottitis is a rapidly progressive inflammation/cellulitis of the epiglottis which may cause airway obstruction. Small children typically present with fever and dysphagia, while older children and adults complain of sore throat. Inspiratory stridor and hoarseness occur frequently, and patients may present with drooling. Diagnosis is confirmed by the presence of an edematous "cherry red" epiglottis which should be visualized in a controlled environment in which one should be able to secure the airway.

Differential Diagnosis Croup; diphtheria; allergic laryngeal edema; foreign body aspiration; abscess – retropharyngeal, peritonsillar

Likely Pathogens

Children:

Haemophilus influenzae *on page 119*

Adults:

Streptococcus pyogenes *on page 207*

Diagnostic Tests/Procedures

Aerobic Culture, Appropriate Site *on page 244*

Group A *Streptococcus* Antigen Test *on page 354*

Throat Culture for Group A Beta-Hemolytic *Streptococcus* *on page 457*

Empiric Drug Therapy
Recommended
Children:

Cephalosporins, 2nd Generation *on page 527*
Cephalosporins, 3rd Generation *on page 528*
Adults:
Cephalosporins, 2nd Generation *on page 527*

Erythema Infectiosum *see* Parvovirus B19
on page 167

European Blastomycosis *see Cryptococcus neoformans*
on page 94

Exanthem Subitum *see* Human Herpesvirus-6
on page 131

Fasciitis *see* Skin and Soft Tissue *on page 42*

Fever, Neutropenic
Clinical Presentation Classically, patients present with absolute neutropenia and fever without evidence of source either by history or physical examination. Generally lack symptoms of sweats and rigors.
Differential Diagnosis Infections – bacterial, viral, fungal, parasitic; drug associated; malignancy, especially lymphoma, leukemia
Likely Pathogens
Gram-Negative Bacilli *on page 117*
Staphylococcus aureus, Methicillin-Susceptible *on page 198*
Staphylococcus epidermidis, Methicillin-Susceptible *on page 201*
Candida Species *on page 73*
Diagnostic Tests/Procedures
• Aerobic Culture, Sputum *on page 246*
• Blood Culture, Aerobic and Anaerobic *on page 271*
• Blood Culture, Fungus *on page 275*
• Intravenous Line Culture *on page 376*
• Gram Stain *on page 352*
• Urine Culture, Clean Catch *on page 470*
Empiric Drug Therapy
Recommended
Penicillins, Extended Spectrum *on page 637*
used in combination with
Aminoglycosides *on page 489*
with or without
Vancomycin Hydrochloride *on page 691*
or
Ceftazidime *on page 520*
used in combination with
Aminoglycosides *on page 489*
with or without
Vancomycin Hydrochloride *on page 691*

Fifth Disease *see* Parvovirus B19 *on page 167*

Food Poisoning *see* Timing of Food Poisoning
on page 723

Gardener's Disease *see Sporothrix schenckii*
on page 193

Gastroenteritis, Bacterial
Clinical Presentation Patients with bacterial gastroenteritis frequently present with lower gastrointestinal symptoms (diarrhea) with or without fever. Patients less likely present with primary upper gastrointestinal symptoms (ie, vomiting). The presence of bloody diarrhea suggests a bacterial pathogen, although *C. difficile* is usually nonhemorrhagic. It is impossible to separate different pathogens based on clinical diagnosis alone.
(Continued)
25

Gastroenteritis, Bacterial *(Continued)*

Differential Diagnosis Gastroenteritis, viral; drug toxicity; inflammatory bowel disease; parasitic gastroenteritis (eg, *Giardia*, cryptosporidia, microsporidia)

Likely Pathogens
Campylobacter jejuni on page 72
Salmonella Species *on page 185*
Escherichia coli, Enterohemorrhagic *on page 112*
Clostridium difficile on page 85

Diagnostic Tests/Procedures
Stool Culture *on page 448*
Stool Culture, Diarrheagenic *E. coli on page 449*
Stool Culture, Uncommon Organisms *on page 451*
Clostridium difficile Toxin Assay *on page 300*

Drug Therapy Comment Drug therapy based on identification of the causative agent.

Selected Readings
Guerrant RL, Shields DA, Thorson SM, et al, "Evaluation and Diagnosis of Acute Infectious Diarrhea," *Am J Med*, 1985, 78(6B):91-8.
Siegel DL, Edelstein PH, Nachamkin I, "Inappropriate Testing for Diarrheal Diseases in the Hospital," *JAMA*, 1990, 263(7):979-82.

Gastroenteritis, Viral

Clinical Presentation Patients with viral gastroenteritis may present with upper gastrointestinal symptoms (vomiting), lower gastrointestinal symptoms (diarrhea), or both. Stools tend to be nonhemorrhagic. Viral gastroenteritis is much more common than bacterial gastroenteritis.

Differential Diagnosis Gastroenteritis, bacterial; drug toxicity; inflammatory bowel disease; parasitic gastroenteritis (eg, *Giardia*, cryptosporidia, microsporidia)

Likely Pathogens
Rotavirus *on page 185*

Diagnostic Tests/Procedures
Viral Culture, Stool *on page 478*
Rotavirus, Direct Detection *on page 437*
Enterovirus Culture *on page 331*

Drug Therapy Comment No antiviral agents have been proven to be effective in the treatment of rotavirus infections. Supportive therapy is recommended.

Genital HSV *see* Herpes Simplex Virus *on page 128*

Gilchrist's Disease *see Blastomyces dermatitidis on page 63*

Granuloma Inguinale *see Calymmatobacterium granulomatis on page 71*

Hepatitis

Clinical Presentation See individual organisms for clinical presentation information.

Likely Pathogens
Hepatitis A Virus *on page 122*
Hepatitis B Virus *on page 122*
Hepatitis C Virus *on page 124*
Hepatitis D Virus *on page 126*
Hepatitis E Virus *on page 127*
Epstein-Barr Virus *on page 110*
Cytomegalovirus *on page 97*

Diagnostic Tests/Procedures
Hepatitis A Profile *on page 358*
Hepatitis B Profile *on page 358*
Hepatitis C Serology *on page 360*
Hepatitis D Serology *on page 361*
Epstein-Barr Virus Serology *on page 332*
Cytomegalovirus Serology *on page 321*

Drug Therapy Comment Drug therapy based on identification of the causative agent.

Histoplasmosis *see Histoplasma capsulatum* *on page 130*

Human Bites *see* Animal and Human Bites Guidelines *on page 736-739*

Impetigo
Clinical Presentation Impetigo is a contagious superficial pyoderma caused by staphylococci and/or streptococci that typically begins as a solitary vesicle ruptures and forms a thick, yellow, honey-colored crust. Patients usually present after multiple lesions occur, most frequently on the face. A superficial glistening base is seen under the crust and no ulcerations are present.

Differential Diagnosis Secondary bacterial infection; ecthyma; herpes simplex, late stage; inflammatory fungal infections

Likely Pathogens
Streptococcus pyogenes on page 207
Staphylococcus aureus, Methicillin-Susceptible *on page 198*

Diagnostic Tests/Procedures
Aerobic Culture, Appropriate Site *on page 244*

Empiric Drug Therapy
  Recommended
    Penicillin V Potassium *on page 638*
    Erythromycin *on page 561*
    Cephalosporins, 1st Generation *on page 527*
    Mupirocin *on page 616*

Influenza *see* Influenza Virus *on page 136*

Jock Itch *see* Dermatophytes *on page 100*

Joint Replacement, Early Infection
Clinical Presentation Most patients present with a long indolent course characterized by progressive increase in joint pain and occasional draining sinuses. May present with acute joint sepsis characterized by high fever, severe joint pain with localized warmth, swelling, and edema.

Differential Diagnosis Hemarthrosis; gout; bland loosening; dislocation

Likely Pathogens
Staphylococcus epidermidis, Methicillin-Resistant *on page 200*
Staphylococcus epidermidis, Methicillin-Susceptible *on page 201*
Staphylococcus aureus, Methicillin-Susceptible *on page 198*
Pseudomonas aeruginosa on page 177

Diagnostic Tests/Procedures
  • Aerobic Culture, Body Fluid *on page 244*
  • Arthrocentesis *on page 264*
  • Biopsy Culture, Routine *on page 270*
  • Blood Culture, Aerobic and Anaerobic *on page 271*
  • Gram Stain *on page 352*
    Arthrogram *on page 267*
    C-Reactive Protein *on page 311*
    Joint Films, Specified Site *on page 379*
    Sedimentation Rate, Erythrocyte *on page 440*

Empiric Drug Therapy
  Recommended
    Vancomycin Hydrochloride *on page 691*

Joint Replacement, Late Infection
Clinical Presentation Most patients present with a long indolent course characterized by progressive increase in joint pain and occasional draining sinuses. May present with acute joint sepsis characterized by high fever, severe joint pain with localized warmth, swelling, and edema.

Differential Diagnosis Hemarthrosis; gout; bland loosening; dislocation

(Continued)

27

Joint Replacement, Late Infection *(Continued)*

Likely Pathogens
Staphylococcus epidermidis, Methicillin-Resistant *on page 200*
Staphylococcus epidermidis, Methicillin-Susceptible *on page 201*
Staphylococcus aureus, Methicillin-Susceptible *on page 198*

Diagnostic Tests/Procedures
• Aerobic Culture, Body Fluid *on page 244*
• Arthrocentesis *on page 264*
• Biopsy Culture, Routine *on page 270*
• Blood Culture, Aerobic and Anaerobic *on page 271*
• Gram Stain *on page 352*
  Arthrogram *on page 267*
  C-Reactive Protein *on page 311*
  Joint Films, Specified Site *on page 379*
  Sedimentation Rate, Erythrocyte *on page 440*

Empiric Drug Therapy
Recommended
Vancomycin Hydrochloride *on page 691*

Selected Readings
Dickinson GM and Bisno A, "Infections Associated With Indwelling Devices: Infections Related to Extravascular Devices," *Antimicrob Agents Chemother*, 1989, 33(5):602-7.

Dougherty SH, "Pathobiology of Infection in Prosthetic Devices," *Rev Infect Dis*, 1988, 10(6):1102-17.

Koch-Weeks *see* Conjunctivitis *on page 21*

Legionellosis *see Legionella pneumophila on page 139*

Legionnaires' Disease *see Legionella pneumophila on page 139*

Leptospirosis *see Leptospira interrogans on page 140*

Line Sepsis *see* Catheter Infection, Intravascular *on page 20*

Listeriosis *see Listeria monocytogenes on page 143*

Lumpy Jaw Syndrome *see Actinomyces* Species *on page 51*

Lyme Disease *see Borrelia burgdorferi on page 68*

Lymphadenitis
Clinical Presentation Can be regional or diffuse depending on the causative organism. Lymph nodes are usually swollen and tender.

Differential Diagnosis Depends on the site of the enlarged node.
Generalized lymphadenopathy: HIV; scarlet fever (group A *Streptococcus*); miliary tuberculosis; brucellosis; syphilis; cat scratch disease; histoplasmosis; lymphogranuloma venereum (LGV); virus (CMV, EBV); toxoplasmosis

Inguinal adenopathy: Syphilis; LGV; chancroid; bacterial

Cervical adenopathy: Bacterial (*Streptococcus*); *Staphylococcus aureus*; tuberculosis; MAI; cat scratch disease; lymphoma; Kawasaki syndrome; others

Likely Pathogens
Toxoplasma gondii on page 217
Mycobacterium Species, Not MTB or MAI *on page 154*
Bartonella Species *on page 62*
Human Immunodeficiency Virus *on page 133*
Staphylococcus aureus, Methicillin-Susceptible *on page 198*
Epstein-Barr Virus *on page 110*

Diagnostic Tests/Procedures Diagnostic tests should be obtained based on clinical suspicion since not all tests are necessary.
Abscess Aerobic and Anaerobic Culture *on page 238*

Epstein-Barr Virus Serology *on page 332*
HIV-1 Serology *on page 368*
Lymph Node Biopsy *on page 395*
Mycobacteria Culture, Biopsy or Body Fluid *on page 404*
Toxoplasma Serology *on page 459*

Drug Therapy Comment Drug therapy based on identification of the causative agent.

Malaria *see Plasmodium Species on page 172*

Measles *see Measles Virus on page 145*

Meningitis, Community Acquired, Adult

Clinical Presentation Patients present with fever, headache, nausea, vomiting, and nuchal rigidity. Focal neurologic abnormalities and papilledema are uncommon.

Differential Diagnosis Bacterial, viral, or other infectious agents; drug-induced; neoplastic; granulomatous; infectious endocarditis; collagen-vascular diseases; subdural hemorrhage; subarachnoid hemorrhage

Likely Pathogens
Haemophilus influenzae on page 119
Neisseria meningitidis on page 163
Streptococcus pneumoniae on page 206

Diagnostic Tests/Procedures
• Blood Culture, Aerobic and Anaerobic *on page 271*
• Cerebrospinal Fluid Analysis *on page 288*
• Gram Stain *on page 352*
• Lumbar Puncture *on page 390*
  Computed Transaxial Tomography, Head Studies *on page 307*
  Cryptococcal Antigen Serology, Serum or Cerebrospinal Fluid *on page 312*
  Enterovirus Culture *on page 331*
  Magnetic Resonance Scan, Brain *on page 397*

Empiric Drug Therapy
Recommended
Ampicillin *on page 495*
used in combination with
Cephalosporins, 3rd Generation *on page 528*
except cefoperazone sodium which does not have reliable CSF penetration and should not be used in meningitis
or
Penicillin G, Parenteral *on page 633*
used in combination with
Cephalosporins, 3rd Generation *on page 528*
except cefoperazone sodium which does not have reliable CSF penetration and should not be used in meningitis

Alternate
Chloramphenicol *on page 531*
Used only in patients with a history of anaphylaxis to penicillin.

Selected Readings
Durand ML, Calderwood SB, Weber DJ, et al, "Acute Bacterial Meningitis in Adults: A Review of 493 Episodes," *N Engl J Med*, 1993, 328(1):21-8.
Pfister HW, Feiden W, and Einhaupl KM, "Spectrum of Complications During Bacterial Meningitis in Adults: Results of a Prospective Clinical Study," *Arch Neurol* 1993, 50(6):575-81.
Quagliarello V and Scheld WM, "Bacterial Meningitis: Pathogenesis, Pathophysiology, and Progress," *N Engl J Med*, 1992, 327(12):864-72.
Roos KL, Tunkel AR, Scheld WM, "Acute Bacterial Meningitis in Children and Adults," *Infections of the Central Nervous System*, Scheld WM, Whitley RJ, and Durack DT, eds, New York, NY: Raven Press, 1991, 335-410.

Meningitis, Neonatal (<2 months of age)

Clinical Presentation Baby is feeding poorly, has fever or is hypothermic, has seizure, sleepiness, irritability, or any other unusual behavior. A full fontanelle indicates progressive disease.

(Continued)

Meningitis, Neonatal (<2 months of age) *(Continued)*

Differential Diagnosis Bacterial, viral, or other infectious agents; neoplasm; metabolic disorders; central nervous system hemorrhage

Likely Pathogens

Escherichia coli, Enterohemorrhagic *on page 112*

Klebsiella Species *on page 137*

Listeria monocytogenes on page 143

Streptococcus agalactiae on page 203

Diagnostic Tests/Procedures

- Blood Culture, Aerobic and Anaerobic *on page 271*
- Cerebrospinal Fluid Analysis *on page 288*
- Gram Stain *on page 352*
- Lumbar Puncture *on page 390*

  Computed Transaxial Tomography, Head Studies *on page 307*

  Cryptococcal Antigen Serology, Serum or Cerebrospinal Fluid *on page 312*

  Enterovirus Culture *on page 331*

  Magnetic Resonance Scan, Brain *on page 397*

Empiric Drug Therapy

Recommended

Ampicillin *on page 495*
  used in combination with
Gentamicin Sulfate *on page 575*
  if hospital acquired add
Vancomycin Hydrochloride *on page 691*

Alternate

Chloramphenicol *on page 531*
  used in combination with
Gentamicin Sulfate *on page 575*
  if hospital acquired add
Vancomycin Hydrochloride *on page 691*

Selected Readings

Roos KL, Tunkel AR, Scheld WM, "Acute Bacterial Meningitis in Children and Adults," *Infections of the Central Nervous System*, Scheld WM, Whitley RJ, and Durack DT, eds, New York, NY: Raven Press, 1991, 335-410.

Meningitis, Pediatric (>2 months of age)

Clinical Presentation Patients present with fever or hypothermia, seizure, sleepiness, irritability, full fontanelle, and stiff neck. Focal neurologic abnormalities and papilledema are uncommon.

Differential Diagnosis Bacterial, viral, or other infectious agents; neoplasm; metabolic disorders; central nervous system hemorrhage

Likely Pathogens

Haemophilus influenzae on page 119

Neisseria meningitidis on page 163

Streptococcus pneumoniae on page 206

Diagnostic Tests/Procedures

- Blood Culture, Aerobic and Anaerobic *on page 271*
- Cerebrospinal Fluid Analysis *on page 288*
- Gram Stain *on page 352*
- Lumbar Puncture *on page 390*

  Computed Transaxial Tomography, Head Studies *on page 307*

  Cryptococcal Antigen Serology, Serum or Cerebrospinal Fluid *on page 312*

  Enterovirus Culture *on page 331*

  Magnetic Resonance Scan, Brain *on page 397*

Empiric Drug Therapy

Recommended

Ceftriaxone Sodium *on page 523*
  used in combination with
Vancomycin Hydrochloride *on page 691*

Alternate

Chloramphenicol *on page 531*
  used in combination with
Vancomycin Hydrochloride *on page 691*

Selected Readings

Odio CM, Faingezicht I, Paris M, et al, "The Beneficial Effects of Early Dexamethasone Administration in Infants and Children With Bacterial Meningitis," *N Engl J Med*, 1991, 324(22):1525-31.

Pfister HW, Fontana A, Tauber MG, "Mechanisms of Brain Injury in Bacterial Meningitis: Workshop Summary," *Clin Infect Dis*, 1994, 19:463-79.

Roos KL, Tunkel AR, Scheld WM, "Acute Bacterial Meningitis in Children and Adults," *Infections of the Central Nervous System*, Scheld WM, Whitley RJ, and Durack DT, eds, New York, NY: Raven Press, 1991, 335-410.

Meningitis, Postsurgical

Clinical Presentation Patients present with fever, headache, nausea, vomiting, and nuchal rigidity. Focal neurologic abnormalities and papilledema are uncommon.

Differential Diagnosis Bacterial, viral, or other infectious agents; drug-induced; neoplastic; granulomatous; infectious endocarditis; collagen-vascular diseases; subdural hemorrhage; subarachnoid hemorrhage

Likely Pathogens

Pseudomonas aeruginosa on page 177

Gram-Negative Bacilli *on page 117*

Staphylococcus aureus, Methicillin-Susceptible *on page 198*

Staphylococcus epidermidis, Methicillin-Susceptible *on page 201*

Diagnostic Tests/Procedures

- Blood Culture, Aerobic and Anaerobic *on page 271*
- Gram Stain *on page 352*
- Lumbar Puncture *on page 390*

  Computed Transaxial Tomography, Head Studies *on page 307*

  Magnetic Resonance Scan, Brain *on page 397*

  Wound Culture *on page 480*

Empiric Drug Therapy

Recommended

Vancomycin Hydrochloride *on page 691*

used in combination with

Ceftazidime *on page 520*

with or without

Tobramycin *on page 685*

Alternate

Vancomycin Hydrochloride *on page 691*

used in combination with

Penicillins, Extended Spectrum *on page 637*

with or without

Tobramycin *on page 685*

Meningitis, Post-Traumatic

Clinical Presentation Patients present with fever, headache, nausea, vomiting, and nuchal rigidity. Focal neurologic abnormalities and papilledema are uncommon.

Differential Diagnosis Bacterial, viral, or other infectious agents; drug-induced; neoplastic; granulomatous; infectious endocarditis; collagen-vascular diseases; subdural hemorrhage; subarachnoid hemorrhage

Likely Pathogens

Haemophilus influenzae on page 119

Staphylococcus aureus, Methicillin-Susceptible *on page 198*

Streptococcus pneumoniae on page 206

Diagnostic Tests/Procedures

- Aerobic Culture, Cerebrospinal Fluid *on page 245*
- Blood Culture, Aerobic and Anaerobic *on page 271*
- Computed Transaxial Tomography, Head Studies *on page 307*
- Gram Stain *on page 352*
- Lumbar Puncture *on page 390*
- Magnetic Resonance Scan, Brain *on page 397*

Empiric Drug Therapy
Recommended

> Vancomycin Hydrochloride *on page 691*
> > *used in combination with*
>
> Cephalosporins, 3rd Generation *on page 528*
> > **except** cefoperazone sodium which does not have reliable CSF pene-
> > tration and should not be used in meningitis.

Alternate

> Vancomycin Hydrochloride *on page 691*
> > *used in combination with*
>
> Penicillins, Extended Spectrum *on page 637*

Microsporidiosis *see Microsporidia on page 146*

Middle Ear Infection *see Otitis Media, Acute on page 35*

Moniliasis *see Candida Species on page 73*

Mononucleosis
Likely Pathogens
Epstein-Barr Virus *on page 110*
Cytomegalovirus *on page 97*
Toxoplasma gondii on page 217

Mucormycosis *see Mucor Species on page 149*

Mumps *see Mumps Virus on page 150*

Mycotic Vulvovaginitis *see Candida Species on page 73*

NGU *see Urethritis, Nongonococcal on page 44*

Nocardiosis *see Nocardia Species on page 164*

Nongonococcal Urethritis *see Urethritis, Nongonococcal on page 44*

"Nonspecific Vaginosis" *see Vaginosis, Bacterial on page 46*

Osteomyelitis, Diabetic Foot
Clinical Presentation Usually involves small bones of the feet and toes. Pa-
tients present with pain, swelling, and/or erythema of the involved bones
with or without presence of ulcer. Most common x-ray finding is mottled
lytic lesions.
Differential Diagnosis Charcot foot; fracture; cellulitis
Likely Pathogens
Staphylococcus aureus, Methicillin-Susceptible *on page 198*
Streptococcus-Related Gram-Positive Cocci *on page 212*
Gram-Negative Bacilli *on page 117*
Diagnostic Tests/Procedures
• Bone Films *on page 277*
• Bone Scan *on page 281*
• C-Reactive Protein *on page 311*
• Gram Stain *on page 352*
• Sedimentation Rate, Erythrocyte *on page 440*
• Biopsy Culture, Routine *on page 270*
  Anaerobic Culture *on page 250*
  Bone Biopsy *on page 276*
  Gallium Scan *on page 347*
  Indium Leukocyte Scan *on page 374*
Empiric Drug Therapy
Recommended
Ticarcillin and Clavulanate Potassium *on page 682*
Ampicillin Sodium and Sulbactam Sodium *on page 497*

Cefoxitin Sodium *on page 518*
Cefotetan Disodium *on page 517*
Alternate
Imipenem/Cilastatin *on page 586*
or
Clindamycin *on page 540*
used in combination with
Cephalosporins, 3rd Generation *on page 528*
Selected Readings
Bamberger DM, Daus GP, and Gerding DN, "Osteomyelitis in the Feet of Diabetic Patients: Long-Term Results, Prognostic Factors, and the Role of Antimicrobial and Surgical Therapy," *Am J Med*, 1987, 83(4):653-60.

Osteomyelitis, Healthy Adult

Clinical Presentation Usually occurs in the face of trauma with surrounding cellulitis; may be hematogenously spread in the face of bacteremia with or without endocarditis (often vertebral) osteomyelitis. Presents with point tenderness, fever, mild leukocytosis, and increased C-reactive protein and erythrocyte sedimentation rate. May be acute or chronic.
Differential Diagnosis Septic arthritis; skin/soft tissue infections; bursitis; tendonitis; fracture; malignancy; diskitis; epidural abscess
Likely Pathogens
Staphylococcus aureus, Methicillin-Susceptible *on page 198*
Diagnostic Tests/Procedures
• Biopsy Culture, Routine *on page 270*
• Bone Films *on page 277*
• Bone Scan *on page 281*
• C-Reactive Protein *on page 311*
• Gram Stain *on page 352*
• Sedimentation Rate, Erythrocyte *on page 440*
Anaerobic Culture *on page 250*
Bone Biopsy *on page 276*
Gallium Scan *on page 347*
Indium Leukocyte Scan *on page 374*
Teichoic Acid Antibody *on page 453*
Empiric Drug Therapy
Recommended
Penicillins, Penicillinase-Resistant *on page 637*
Alternate
Vancomycin Hydrochloride *on page 691*
Cephalosporins, 1st Generation *on page 527*
Clindamycin *on page 540*

Osteomyelitis, Pediatric

Clinical Presentation The child will not be using that extremity, may be limping, etc. Pain, fever, leukocytosis, and increased C-reactive protein and erythrocyte sedimentation rate. Is often hematogenously spread but can also be traumatic. May be acute or chronic.
Differential Diagnosis Septic arthritis; skin/soft tissue infections; bursitis; tendonitis; fracture; malignancy; diskitis; epidural abscess
Likely Pathogens
Staphylococcus aureus, Methicillin-Susceptible *on page 198*
Streptococcus pyogenes on page 207
<2 years old:
Haemophilus influenzae on page 119
Diagnostic Tests/Procedures
• Bone Films *on page 277*
• Bone Scan *on page 281*
• C-Reactive Protein *on page 311*
• Gram Stain *on page 352*
• Sedimentation Rate, Erythrocyte *on page 440*
Biopsy Culture, Routine *on page 270*
Bone Biopsy *on page 276*
Gallium Scan *on page 347*
Indium Leukocyte Scan *on page 374*
Teichoic Acid Antibody *on page 453*

Empiric Drug Therapy
Recommended
Penicillins, Penicillinase-Resistant *on page 637*
Alternate
Vancomycin Hydrochloride *on page 691*
Cephalosporins, 1st Generation *on page 527*
Clindamycin *on page 540*

Otitis Externa, Mild

Synonyms Swimmer's Ear

Clinical Presentation Acute localized otitis externa may present as a pustule, furuncle, or cellulitis within the external auditory canal. Hemorrhagic bullae may be present, as well as localized adenopathy. Gram-positive cocci are usually responsible.

Acute diffuse otitis externa (swimmer's ear) initially presents with itching and becomes painful as the canal swells and reddens. Gram-negative bacilli, particularly *Pseudomonas aeruginosa*, are the most likely pathogens.

Chronic otitis externa is characterized by intense itching secondary to the chronic irritation of drainage from chronic otitis media or granulomatous infections.

Malignant otitis externa is a severe necrotizing infection that spreads to adjacent tissue and bone. Associated with intense pain, tenderness, and pus in the canal.

Likely Pathogens
Pseudomonas aeruginosa on page 177
Diagnostic Tests/Procedures
Aerobic Culture, Appropriate Site *on page 244*
Gram Stain *on page 352*
Empiric Drug Therapy
Recommended
Neomycin Sulfate *on page 619*
Polymyxin B Sulfate *on page 647*

Otitis Externa, Severe (Malignant)

Clinical Presentation Acute localized otitis externa may present as a pustule, furuncle, or cellulitis within the external auditory canal. Hemorrhagic bullae may be present, as well as localized adenopathy. Gram-positive cocci are usually responsible.

Acute diffuse otitis externa (swimmer's ear) initially presents with itching and becomes painful as the canal swells and reddens. Gram-negative bacilli, particularly *Pseudomonas aeruginosa*, are the most likely pathogens.

Chronic otitis externa is characterized by intense itching secondary to the chronic irritation of drainage from chronic otitis media or granulomatous infections.

Malignant otitis externa is a severe necrotizing infection that spreads to adjacent tissue and bone. Associated with intense pain, tenderness, and pus in the canal.

Likely Pathogens
Pseudomonas aeruginosa on page 177
Diagnostic Tests/Procedures
Aerobic Culture, Appropriate Site *on page 244*
Gram Stain *on page 352*
Computed Transaxial Tomography, Paranasal Sinuses
on page 308
Drug Therapy Comment Topical otic suspensions or solutions may also be indicated.
Empiric Drug Therapy
Recommended
Gentamicin Sulfate *on page 575*
used in combination with
Ceftazidime *on page 520*
or
Gentamicin Sulfate *on page 575*
used in combination with
Penicillins, Extended Spectrum *on page 637*

Alternate
Ciprofloxacin Hydrochloride *on page 537*

Otitis Media, Acute
Synonyms Acute Suppurative Otitis; Middle Ear Infection
Clinical Presentation Most commonly occurs in children. Present with otalgia and fever with or without purulent discharge. Infants may present with irritability. Diagnosis is confirmed by examination of the tympanic membrane which is full or bulging, opaque, and has little or no mobility.
Likely Pathogens
Streptococcus pneumoniae on page 206
Haemophilus influenzae on page 119
Moraxella catarrhalis on page 147
Staphylococcus aureus, Methicillin-Susceptible *on page 198*
Diagnostic Tests/Procedures
Aerobic Culture, Body Fluid *on page 244*
Gram Stain *on page 352*
Empiric Drug Therapy
Recommended
Amoxicillin Trihydrate *on page 491*
Co-trimoxazole *on page 545*
Cephalosporins, 2nd Generation *on page 527*
Alternate
Erythromycin and Sulfisoxazole *on page 563*

PCP *see Pneumocystis carinii on page 172*

Pelvic Inflammatory Disease
Synonyms PID
Clinical Presentation Pelvic inflammatory disease (PID) is an infection of the pelvic organs usually by bacteria and its associated inflammatory response. Typically begins as an ascending infection from the vagina or cervix but may occur via hematogenous or lymphatic spread. Patients present with fever, chills, nausea, vomiting, anorexia, vaginal bleeding, and mucopurulent vaginal discharge. Endometritis usually develops postpartum or postabortal, where as salpingo-oophoritis with or without abscess is most associated with sexually transmitted diseases.
Differential Diagnosis Intestinal tract disease; urinary systems disease
Likely Pathogens
Chlamydia trachomatis on page 79
Neisseria gonorrhoeae on page 161
Escherichia coli, Nonenterohemorrhagic *on page 113*
Streptococcus, Viridans Group *on page 213*
Bacteroides Species *on page 61*
Diagnostic Tests/Procedures
Abscess Aerobic and Anaerobic Culture *on page 238*
Aerobic Culture, Body Fluid *on page 244*
Anaerobic Culture *on page 250*
Gram Stain *on page 352*
Empiric Drug Therapy
Recommended
Clindamycin *on page 540*
used in combination with
Gentamicin Sulfate *on page 575*
Alternate
Doxycycline *on page 557*
Selected Readings
Centers for Disease Control, "Sexually Transmitted Diseases Treatment Guidelines," *MMWR Morb Mortal Wkly Rep*, 1993, 42(RR-14):1-102.
Hensell DL, Little BB, Faro S, et al, "Comparison of Three Regimens Recommended by the Centers For Disease Control and Prevention for the Treatment of Women Hospitalized With Acute Pelvic Inflammatory Disease," *Clin Infect Dis*, 1994, 19:720-7.

Perinephric Abscess *see* Urinary Tract Infection, Perinephric Abscess *on page 45*

Peritonitis

Clinical Presentation Patients with primary peritonitis present with abrupt onset of fever, abdominal pain, nausea, vomiting, diarrhea, diffuse abdominal tenderness, rebound tenderness, and hypoactive or absent bowel sounds. Patients with cirrhosis may have an atypical presentation with an insidious onset and lack of peritoneal signs. Most cirrhotics present with fever. Patients with secondary peritonitis present as the primary process with peritoneal signs being the most prominent.

Differential Diagnosis Pneumonia; sickle cell anemia; herpes zoster; diabetic ketoacidosis; tabes dorsalis; porphyria; familial Mediterranean fever; plumbism; lupus erythematosus; uremia; other intra-abdominal infections

Likely Pathogens
Escherichia coli, Nonenterohemorrhagic *on page 113*
Bacteroides Species *on page 61*

Diagnostic Tests/Procedures
Paracentesis *on page 420*
Abscess Aerobic and Anaerobic Culture *on page 238*
Aerobic Culture, Body Fluid *on page 244*
Anaerobic Culture *on page 250*
Gram Stain *on page 352*

Empiric Drug Therapy
Recommended
Gentamicin Sulfate *on page 575*
used in combination with
Clindamycin *on page 540*
or
Gentamicin Sulfate *on page 575*
used in combination with
Metronidazole *on page 610*

Alternate
Cefoxitin Sodium *on page 518*
Cefotetan Disodium *on page 517*
Piperacillin Sodium and Tazobactam Sodium *on page 642*
Ticarcillin and Clavulanate Potassium *on page 682*
Ampicillin Sodium and Sulbactam Sodium *on page 497*

Selected Readings
McClean KL, Sheehan GJ and Harding GM, "Intraabdominal Infection: A Review," *Clin Infect Dis*, 1994, 19:100-16.

Pertussis *see Bordetella pertussis on page 65*

Pharyngitis

Clinical Presentation Acute pharyngitis is an inflammatory syndrome of the pharynx caused by multiple organisms, predominantly viral. Patients complain of soreness, scratching, or irritation of the throat along with signs of congestion, malaise, and headaches. Patients with EBV or strep typically present with fever and an exudative pharyngitis.

Differential Diagnosis Retropharyngeal abscess; epiglottitis; Lemierre's disease

Likely Pathogens
Streptococcus pyogenes on page 207
Respiratory Syncytial Virus *on page 181*
Influenza Virus *on page 136*
Parainfluenza Virus *on page 166*
Adenovirus *on page 53*
Epstein-Barr Virus *on page 110*

Diagnostic Tests/Procedures Viral detection studies indicated for severe or unusual cases and are not routine.
Group A *Streptococcus* Antigen Test *on page 354*

Throat Culture for Group A Beta-Hemolytic *Streptococcus* *on page 457*

Virus, Direct Detection by Fluorescent Antibody *on page 480*

Viral Culture, Throat *on page 479*

Infectious Mononucleosis Serology *on page 374*

Drug Therapy Comment Drug therapy indicated is for *Streptococcus pyogenes* infections only.

Empiric Drug Therapy

Recommended

Penicillin V Potassium *on page 638*

Penicillin G Procaine, Aqueous *on page 636*

Alternate

Erythromycin *on page 561*

Cephalosporins, 1st Generation *on page 527*

Amoxicillin Trihydrate *on page 491*

Phycomycosis *see Mucor* Species *on page 149*

PID *see* Pelvic Inflammatory Disease *on page 35*

Pink Eye *see* Conjunctivitis *on page 21*

Plague *see Yersinia pestis on page 233*

***Pneumocystis carinii* Pneumonia** *see Pneumocystis carinii on page 172*

Pneumonia, Aspiration, Community-Acquired

Clinical Presentation Major symptoms are cough, fever, production of sputum, chest pain, and dyspnea. Although aspiration is a common cause of community-acquired pneumonia, it classically occurs in patients who have difficulty swallowing, no gag reflex, who are at high risk for aspirating.

Differential Diagnosis Congestive heart failure; pulmonary embolism; aspiration of gastric contents; neoplasm; adult respiratory distress syndrome; hypersensitivity pneumonitis; radiation pneumonitis; drug reactions

Likely Pathogens

Streptococcus-Related Gram-Positive Cocci *on page 212*

Streptococcus pneumoniae on page 206

Bacteroides Species *on page 61*

Diagnostic Tests/Procedures

• Aerobic Culture, Sputum *on page 246*

• Blood Culture, Aerobic and Anaerobic *on page 271*

• Chest Films *on page 293*

• Gram Stain *on page 352*

Computed Transaxial Tomography, Thorax *on page 308*

Empiric Drug Therapy

Recommended

Penicillin G, Parenteral *on page 633*

Clindamycin *on page 540*

Alternate

Ampicillin Sodium and Sulbactam Sodium *on page 497*

Selected Readings

Fang GD, Fine M, Orloff J, et al, "New and Emerging Etiologies for Community-Acquired Pneumonia With Implications for Therapy: A Prospective Multicenter Study of 359 Cases," *Medicine (Baltimore)*, 1990, 69(5):307-16.

Pneumonia, Community-Acquired

Clinical Presentation Major symptoms are cough, fever, production of sputum, chest pain, and dyspnea. Viral or *Mycoplasma* pneumonia typically has prodromal upper respiratory tract phase associated with malaise, headache, sore throat, and nonproductive cough.

Differential Diagnosis Congestive heart failure; pulmonary embolism; aspiration of gastric contents; neoplasm; adult respiratory distress syndrome; hypersensitivity pneumonitis; radiation pneumonitis; drug reactions

Likely Pathogens

Streptococcus pneumoniae on page 206

Mycoplasma pneumoniae on page 159

(Continued)

Pneumonia, Community-Acquired *(Continued)*

Legionella pneumophila on page 139
Chlamydia pneumoniae on page 76
Haemophilus influenzae on page 119

Diagnostic Tests/Procedures
Severe Infection
- Aerobic Culture, Sputum *on page 246*
- Blood Culture, Aerobic and Anaerobic *on page 271*
- Chest Films *on page 293*
- Gram Stain *on page 352*
  Legionella Serology on page 384
  Mycoplasma Serology on page 410
  Mycoplasma/Ureaplasma Culture on page 410
Mild Infection
- Aerobic Culture, Sputum *on page 246*
- Gram Stain *on page 352*

Drug Therapy Comment
For severe infections, doxycycline can be substituted for erythromycin for patients that are intolerant.

Empiric Drug Therapy
Recommended
Severe Infection
Erythromycin *on page 561*
used in combination with
Cephalosporins, 3rd Generation *on page 528*
or
Erythromycin *on page 561*
used in combination with
Cefuroxime *on page 524*
or
Erythromycin *on page 561*
used in combination with
Ampicillin Sodium and Sulbactam Sodium *on page 497*
Mild Infection
Amoxicillin Trihydrate *on page 491*
Co-trimoxazole *on page 545*
Amoxicillin and Clavulanic Acid *on page 490*
Cefuroxime *on page 524*

Selected Readings
Bartlett JG, "Anaerobic Bacterial Infections of the Lung," *Chest*, 1987, 91(6):901-9.
Grayston JT, Campbell LA, Kuo CC, et al, "A New Respiratory Tract Pathogen: *Chlamydia pneumoniae* Strain TWAR," *J Infect Dis*, 1990, 161(4):618-25.

Pneumonia, Hospital-Acquired

Clinical Presentation Major symptoms are cough, fever, production of sputum, chest pain, and dyspnea. Although aspiration is a common cause of community-acquired pneumonia, it classically occurs in patients who have difficulty swallowing, no gag reflex, and who are at high risk for aspirating.

Differential Diagnosis Congestive heart failure; pulmonary embolism; aspiration of gastric contents; neoplasm; adult respiratory distress syndrome; hypersensitivity pneumonitis; radiation pneumonitis; drug reactions

Likely Pathogens
Pseudomonas aeruginosa on page 177
Enterobacter Species on page 104
Klebsiella Species on page 137
Serratia Species on page 190
Staphylococcus aureus, Methicillin-Susceptible on page 198

Diagnostic Tests/Procedures
- Aerobic Culture, Sputum *on page 246*
- Chest Films *on page 293*
- Gram Stain *on page 352*

Drug Therapy Comment
Vancomycin hydrochloride added only if evidence of gram-positive infection.

Empiric Drug Therapy
  Recommended
      Vancomycin Hydrochloride *on page 691*
      Ceftazidime *on page 520*
      Gentamicin Sulfate *on page 575*
        all 3 used in combination
         or
      Penicillins, Extended Spectrum *on page 637*
      Aminoglycosides *on page 489*
      Vancomycin Hydrochloride *on page 691*
        all 3 used in combination

Pneumonic Plague *see Yersinia pestis on page 233*

Poliomyelitis *see Poliovirus on page 174*

Pontiac Fever *see Legionella pneumophila on page 139*

Posada-Wernicke's Disease *see Coccidioides immitis on page 89*

Prevention of Bacterial Endocarditis *see page 727*

Primary Atypical Pneumonia
  Likely Pathogens
    Mycoplasma pneumoniae on page 159
    Chlamydia pneumoniae on page 76
    Legionella pneumophila on page 139

Prostatitis
  Clinical Presentation Acute prostatitis typically occurs in young males but may be associated with indwelling urethral catheters. Characterized by fever, chills, dysuria, and a tense or extremely tender prostate on palpation. Chronic form may present as asymptomatic bacteriuria with a normal palpable prostate. May have intermittent symptoms of frequency, urgency, and dysuria.
  Differential Diagnosis Bacterial; nonbacterial; prostatodynia; malignancy
  Likely Pathogens
    Escherichia coli, Nonenterohemorrhagic *on page 113*
    Neisseria gonorrhoeae on page 161
    Chlamydia trachomatis on page 79
    Staphylococcus aureus, Methicillin-Susceptible *on page 198*
  Diagnostic Tests/Procedures
    • Genital Culture *on page 349*
    • Gram Stain *on page 352*
    • *Neisseria gonorrhoeae* Culture *on page 412*
    • Urine Culture, Clean Catch *on page 470*
  Empiric Drug Therapy
  Recommended
      Co-trimoxazole *on page 545*
      Fluoroquinolones *on page 571*
  Selected Readings
  Meares EM Jr, "Acute and Chronic Prostatitis: Diagnosis and Treatment," *Infect Dis Clin North Am*, 1987, 1(4):855-74.
  Lipsky BA, "Urinary Tract Infections in Men: Epidemiology, Pathophysiology, Diagnosis, and Treatment," *Ann Intern Med*, 1989, 110(2):138-50.

Prosthetic Valve Endocarditis, Late *see Endocarditis, Prosthetic Valve, Late on page 23*

Pseudomembranous Colitis *see Clostridium difficile on page 85*

Psittacosis *see Chlamydia psittaci on page 77*

PVE, Early *see Endocarditis, Prosthetic Valve, Early on page 22*

DISEASE SYNDROMES

PVE, Late *see* Endocarditis, Prosthetic Valve, Late
on page 23

Q Fever *see Coxiella burnetii on page 93*

Rabies *see* Rabies Virus *on page 179*

Red Eye *see* Conjunctivitis *on page 21*

Reticuloendotheliosis *see Histoplasma capsulatum*
on page 130

Ringworm *see* Dermatophytes *on page 100*

RMSF *see Rickettsia rickettsii on page 183*

Rocky Mountain Spotted Fever *see Rickettsia rickettsii*
on page 183

Roseola Infantum *see* Human Herpesvirus-6
on page 131

Rubeola *see* Measles Virus *on page 145*

Salmonellosis *see Salmonella* Species *on page 185*

San Joaquin Fever *see Coccidioides immitis*
on page 89

Scabies *see Sarcoptes scabiei on page 188*

Scarlet Fever *see Streptococcus pyogenes on page 207*

Schistosomiasis *see Schistosoma mansoni on page 189*

Sepsis
Clinical Presentation The patient may have fever or hypothermia, may be tachycardiac and tachypneic, may have altered mental status, hypoxia, increased plasma lactate levels, oliguria, or coagulopathy. Septic patients may also go into shock which is characterized by significant drop in blood pressure in the face of fluid challenges.
Likely Pathogens
    Gram-Negative Bacilli *on page 117*
    Staphylococcus aureus, Methicillin-Susceptible *on page 198*
    Candida Species *on page 73*
    Enterococcus Species *on page 107*
Diagnostic Tests/Procedures
    • Aerobic Culture, Sputum *on page 246*
    • Blood Culture, Aerobic and Anaerobic *on page 271*
    • Gram Stain *on page 352*
    • Intravenous Line Culture *on page 376*
    • Urine Culture, Clean Catch *on page 470*
    Computed Transaxial Tomography, Abdomen Studies
    on page 306
Empiric Drug Therapy
  Recommended
    Ceftazidime *on page 520*
    Aminoglycosides *on page 489*
    Vancomycin Hydrochloride *on page 691*
     all 3 used in combination
      or
    Penicillins, Extended Spectrum *on page 637*
    Aminoglycosides *on page 489*
    Vancomycin Hydrochloride *on page 691*
     all 3 used in combination

Septic Arthritis *see* Arthritis, Septic *on page 18*

Septic Thrombophlebitis *see* Thrombophlebitis, Suppurative *on page 43*

Shigellosis *see Shigella* Species *on page 191*

Shingles *see* Varicella-Zoster Virus *on page 227*

Sinusitis, Community-Acquired, Acute
Synonyms Acute Sinusitis, Community-Acquired; Community-Acquired Sinusitis, Acute

Clinical Presentation Symptoms depend on the site of involvement. Patients with maxillary sinusitis typically have pain over the canine/molar teeth and malar area. Patients with anterior ethmoid sinusitis present with temporal or retro-orbital headaches. Posterior ethmoid sinusitis presents with pain in the distribution of the trigeminal nerve and sphenoid sinusitis typically causes pain in the frontal, retro-orbital, or facial area. Patients usually complain of nasal congestion rhinitis, as most often acute sinusitis follows a viral upper respiratory tract infection.

Likely Pathogens
Streptococcus pneumoniae on page 206
Haemophilus influenzae on page 119
Moraxella catarrhalis on page 147
Note: Unusual organisms should be considered in immunosuppressed patients.

Diagnostic Tests/Procedures
Aerobic Culture, Appropriate Site *on page 244*
Gram Stain *on page 352*

Empiric Drug Therapy
Recommended
Co-trimoxazole *on page 545*
Cephalosporins, 2nd Generation *on page 527*
Amoxicillin Trihydrate *on page 491*
Alternate
Amoxicillin and Clavulanic Acid *on page 490*
Azithromycin Dihydrate *on page 500*
Clarithromycin *on page 539*

Sinusitis, Community-Acquired, Chronic
Synonyms Chronic Sinusitis, Community-Acquired; Community-Acquired Sinusitis, Chronic

Clinical Presentation Patients generally complain of intermittent pain, nasal congestion, and rhinitis. Patients frequently have a chronic cough secondary to postnasal drip.

Differential Diagnosis Granulomatous disease

Likely Pathogens
Bacteroides Species *on page 61*
Streptococcus-Related Gram-Positive Cocci *on page 212*

Diagnostic Tests/Procedures
Aerobic Culture, Appropriate Site *on page 244*
Anaerobic Culture *on page 250*
Gram Stain *on page 352*

Drug Therapy Comment Antibiotics are usually not effective.

Empiric Drug Therapy
Recommended
Clindamycin *on page 540*

Sinusitis, Hospital-Acquired
Clinical Presentation Common nosocomial infection in the intensive care units secondary to prolonged intubation with a nasal tracheal or nasal gastric tube. Patients may present with fever and/or leukocytosis. Unexplained fever or leukocytosis with a nasal tube warrants simple CT of the sinuses.
(Continued)

41

Sinusitis, Hospital-Acquired *(Continued)*

Likely Pathogens
Staphylococcus aureus, Methicillin-Resistant *on page 195*
Staphylococcus aureus, Methicillin-Susceptible *on page 198*
Pseudomonas aeruginosa on page 177

Diagnostic Tests/Procedures
Aerobic Culture, Appropriate Site *on page 244*
Gram Stain *on page 352*
Computed Transaxial Tomography, Paranasal Sinuses
on page 308

Empiric Drug Therapy
Recommended
Vancomycin Hydrochloride *on page 691*
Gentamicin Sulfate *on page 575*
Ceftazidime *on page 520*
all 3 used in combination
or
Vancomycin Hydrochloride *on page 691*
Gentamicin Sulfate *on page 575*
Penicillins, Extended Spectrum *on page 637*
all 3 used in combination

Skin and Soft Tissue
Synonyms Cellulitis; Fasciitis
Clinical Presentation Erythema, warmth, and edema around the involved area. Patient may be febrile with leukocytosis. In patients with cellulitis of the extremities, deeper infections must be ruled out. (Patients with necrotizing fasciitis experience hyperesthesia in the face of an unimpressive lesion. Necrotizing disease is a surgical emergency; broad spectrum antimicrobial coverage including anaerobic must be administered.)
Differential Diagnosis Malignancy; osteomyelitis
Likely Pathogens
Staphylococcus aureus, Methicillin-Resistant *on page 195*
Staphylococcus aureus, Methicillin-Susceptible *on page 198*
Streptococcus Species *on page 213*
Clostridium perfringens on page 86
Streptococcus pyogenes on page 207
Diagnostic Tests/Procedures
Anaerobic Culture *on page 250*
Biopsy Culture, Routine *on page 270*
Blood Culture, Aerobic and Anaerobic *on page 271*
Gram Stain *on page 352*
Empiric Drug Therapy
Recommended
Penicillins, Penicillinase-Resistant *on page 637*
Cephalosporins, 1st Generation *on page 527*
Alternate
Clindamycin *on page 540*
Vancomycin Hydrochloride *on page 691*

Slapped Cheek *see Parvovirus B19 on page 167*

Sporotrichosis *see Sporothrix schenckii on page 193*

Strep Throat *see Pharyngitis on page 36*

Strongyloidiasis *see Strongyloides stercoralis on page 215*

Supraglottitis *see Epiglottitis on page 24*

Surgical Wound Infection *see* Wound Infection, Surgical *on page 46*

Swimmer's Ear *see* Otitis Externa, Mild *on page 34*

Syphilis *see Treponema pallidum on page 218*

Tetanus *see Clostridium tetani on page 88*

Thrombophlebitis, Septic *see* Thrombophlebitis, Suppurative *on this page*

Thrombophlebitis, Suppurative
Synonyms Septic Thrombophlebitis; Thrombophlebitis, Septic
Clinical Presentation Frequently associated with thrombosis and bacteremia. Upper extremity suppurative thrombophlebitis usually shows signs of local inflammation and fever. The majority of patients have an implicated catheter left in place for ≥ 5 days. Local inflammation is less prominent in lower extremity disease. Pelvic suppurative thrombophlebitis typically develops 1-2 weeks postpartum or postoperatively presenting with fever, chills, anorexia, nausea, vomiting, and abdominal pain. Majority of pelvic suppurative thrombophlebitis occurs unilaterally.
Differential Diagnosis Septic nonsuppurative thrombophlebitis
Likely Pathogens
Staphylococcus epidermidis, Methicillin-Susceptible *on page 201*
Staphylococcus aureus, Methicillin-Susceptible *on page 198*
Staphylococcus epidermidis, Methicillin-Resistant *on page 200*
Staphylococcus aureus, Methicillin-Resistant *on page 195*
Diagnostic Tests/Procedures
　Blood Culture, Aerobic and Anaerobic *on page 271*
　If deep venous thrombosis is suspected:
　　Ultrasound, Peripheral Arteries and Veins *on page 466*
Empiric Drug Therapy
　Recommended
　　Penicillins, Penicillinase-Resistant *on page 637*
　　Vancomycin Hydrochloride *on page 691*

Thrush *see Candida Species on page 73*

Timing of Food Poisoning *see page 723*

Tinea *see Dermatophytes on page 100*

Toxic Shock Syndrome
Clinical Presentation See individual organisms for clinical presentation information.
Likely Pathogens
Staphylococcus aureus, Methicillin-Resistant *on page 195*
Staphylococcus aureus, Methicillin-Susceptible *on page 198*
Streptococcus pyogenes on page 207
Diagnostic Tests/Procedures
　Blood Culture, Aerobic and Anaerobic *on page 271*
Empiric Drug Therapy
　Recommended
　　Vancomycin Hydrochloride *on page 691*
　　Penicillins, Penicillinase-Resistant *on page 637*

Toxoplasmosis *see Toxoplasma gondii on page 217*

Tracheobronchitis *see* Bronchitis *on page 19*

Trachoma *see Chlamydia trachomatis on page 79*

Trichinosis *see Trichinella spiralis on page 222*

Trichomoniasis *see Trichomonas vaginalis on page 224*

Tuberculosis *see Mycobacterium tuberculosis on page 155*

Uncomplicated Urinary Tract Infection *see* Urinary Tract Infection, Uncomplicated *on next page*

Upper Urinary Tract Infection *see* Urinary Tract Infection, Pyelonephritis *on next page*

Urethritis, Nongonococcal

Synonyms NGU; Nongonococcal Urethritis

Clinical Presentation Urethral discharge is more prominent in men than women and is less seen in NGU than gonococcal urethritis. The discharge may vary from a scant clear mucopurulent to frank pus. Men typically complain of pain at the meatus or distal portion of the penis and may have dysuria. Rarely, men complain of discomfort during ejaculation. Women may complain of dysuria and usually have symptoms of cervicitis although they may be asymptomatic.

Differential Diagnosis Gonococcal urethritis; prostatitis; epididymitis; cervicitis; salpingitis; urinary tract infection, cystitis; noninfectious urethritis

Likely Pathogens
Chlamydia trachomatis on page 79
Trichomonas vaginalis on page 224
Herpes Simplex Virus *on page 128*
Ureaplasma urealyticum on page 225

Diagnostic Tests/Procedures
Chlamydia Culture *on page 294*
Chlamydia trachomatis by DNA Probe *on page 297*
Genital Culture for *Ureaplasma urealyticum on page 350*
Herpes Simplex Virus Culture *on page 364*
Trichomonas Preparation *on page 462*

Empiric Drug Therapy
  Recommended
    Doxycycline *on page 557*
    Tetracycline *on page 679*
    Azithromycin Dihydrate *on page 500*
  Alternate
    Erythromycin *on page 561*

Urinary Tract Infection, Catheter-Associated

Clinical Presentation Patient may have low-grade fever, chills, hematuria, pyuria, and peripheral leukocytosis.

Differential Diagnosis Colonization; trauma; infection – bacterial, fungal

Likely Pathogens
Escherichia coli, Nonenterohemorrhagic *on page 113*
Enterococcus Species *on page 107*
Pseudomonas aeruginosa on page 177
Candida Species *on page 73*

Diagnostic Tests/Procedures
  • Blood Culture, Aerobic and Anaerobic *on page 271*
  • Gram Stain *on page 352*
  • Urine Culture, Clean Catch *on page 470*
  Complete Blood Count *on page 302*
  Fungus Culture, Urine *on page 347*
  Leukocyte Esterase, Urine *on page 386*
  Nitrite, Urine *on page 414*

Empiric Drug Therapy
  Recommended
    Ampicillin *on page 495*
     used in combination with
    Aminoglycosides *on page 489*

Alternate

Vancomycin Hydrochloride *on page 691*
used in combination with
Aminoglycosides *on page 489*

Selected Readings

Stamm WE, "Catheter-Associated Urinary Tract Infections: Epidemiology, Pathogenesis, and Prevention," *Am J Med*, 1991, 91(3B):65S-71S.

Urinary Tract Infection, Perinephric Abscess

Synonyms Perinephric Abscess

Clinical Presentation Often a complication of untreated (or insufficiently treated) urinary tract infection or pyelonephritis. Patient may have fever, flank pain, leukocytosis. Pain may be severe or dull and chronic.

Differential Diagnosis Kidney stones; staghorn calculi; malignancy; infection – bacterial, fungal

Likely Pathogens

Escherichia coli, Nonenterohemorrhagic *on page 113*
Staphylococcus aureus, Methicillin-Susceptible *on page 198*

Diagnostic Tests/Procedures

• Computed Transaxial Tomography, Abdomen Studies
  on page 306
• Ultrasound, Kidneys *on page 466*
• Urine Culture, Clean Catch *on page 470*
  Cystometrogram, Simple *on page 315*

Empiric Drug Therapy
Recommended

Cefazolin Sodium *on page 511*
Co-trimoxazole *on page 545*

Urinary Tract Infection, Pyelonephritis

Synonyms Upper Urinary Tract Infection

Clinical Presentation Most commonly occurs in young females but may occur in any population. Patients may have fever, frequency, dysuria, urgency, hesitancy, plus flank pain. Leukocytosis, pyuria, and hematuria is common.

Differential Diagnosis Kidney stones; staghorn calculi, malignancy, infection – bacterial, fungal.

Likely Pathogens

Escherichia coli, Nonenterohemorrhagic *on page 113*
Proteus Species *on page 176*

Diagnostic Tests/Procedures

• Blood Culture, Aerobic and Anaerobic *on page 271*
• Urine Culture, Clean Catch *on page 470*
  Computed Transaxial Tomography, Abdomen Studies
  on page 306
  Gram Stain *on page 352*

Empiric Drug Therapy
Recommended

Ampicillin *on page 495*
used in combination with
Gentamicin Sulfate *on page 575*
  or
Co-trimoxazole *on page 545*

Alternate

Cephalosporins, 3rd Generation *on page 528*
Fluoroquinolones *on page 571*

Urinary Tract Infection, Uncomplicated

Synonyms Uncomplicated Urinary Tract Infection; UTI, Uncomplicated

Clinical Presentation Patients with only lower tract disease (cystitis) present with dysuria, frequency, urgency, and suprapubic tenderness. Patients with both lower and upper tract disease present with cystitis, fever, and flank pain. Urinalysis reveals pyuria with or without hematuria. Elderly and diabetic patients may be asymptomatic.

Differential Diagnosis Urethritis; pyelonephritis; prostatitis; cervicitis

(Continued)

Urinary Tract Infection, Uncomplicated *(Continued)*

Likely Pathogens
Escherichia coli, Nonenterohemorrhagic *on page 113*
Klebsiella Species *on page 137*
Proteus Species *on page 176*
Staphylococcus saprophyticus on page 203

Diagnostic Tests/Procedures
Urinalysis *on page 467*
Urine Culture, Clean Catch *on page 470*

Empiric Drug Therapy
Recommended
Co-trimoxazole *on page 545*
Alternate
Amoxicillin Trihydrate *on page 491*

Selected Readings
Fang LS, "Urinalysis in the Diagnosis of Urinary Tract Infections," *Clin Lab Med*, 1988, 8(3):567-76.

Johnson JR and Stamm WE, "Diagnosis and Treatment of Acute Urinary Tract Infections," *Infect Dis Clin North Am*, 1987, 1(4):773-91.

Johnson JR and Stamm WE, "Urinary Tract Infections in Women: Diagnosis and Treatment," *Ann Intern Med*, 1989, 111(11):906-17.

Komaroff AL, "Acute Dysuria in Women," *N Engl J Med*, 1984, 310(6):368-75.

Schoolrik GK, "How *Escherichia coli* Infects the Urinary Tract," *N Engl J Med*, 1989, 320(12):804-5.

Stamm WE and Hooton TM, "Management of Urinary Tract Infections in Adults," *N Engl J Med*, 1993, 329(18):1328-34.

Stamm WE, Hooton TM, Johnson JR, et al, "Urinary Tract Infections: From Pathogenesis to Treatment," *J Infect Dis*, 1989, 159(3):400-6.

Vaginosis, Bacterial

Synonyms Bacterial Vaginosis; "Nonspecific Vaginosis"

Clinical Presentation Patients complain of vaginal odor, and a majority note a mild to moderate clear, gray discharge. Patients rarely complain of dysuria or dyspareunia. Physical exam of vagina and cervix are unremarkable except for presence of thin, homogeneous, gray, bubbly discharge.

Differential Diagnosis Other vaginal infections; noninfectious vulvovaginitis

Likely Pathogens
Gardnerella vaginalis on page 114
Bacteroides Species *on page 61*
Streptococcus-Related Gram-Positive Cocci *on page 212*

Diagnostic Tests/Procedures The pH of the vaginal discharge should be tested.
Genital Culture *on page 349*
Trichomonas Preparation *on page 462*

Drug Therapy Comment Clindamycin as a vaginal cream; metronidazole as a vaginal gel.

Empiric Drug Therapy
Recommended
Clindamycin *on page 540*
Metronidazole *on page 610*

Valley Fever *see Coccidioides immitis on page 89*

Vulvovaginitis, Mycotic *see Candida Species on page 73*

Whooping Cough *see Bordetella pertussis on page 65*

Wound Infection, Surgical

Synonyms Surgical Wound Infection

Clinical Presentation The Centers for Disease Control case definition of an incisional surgical wound infection is one that occurs at the incision site within 30 days of surgery and involves skin or subcutaneous tissue above muscle fascia. Infection should not be diagnosed by only the isolation of organisms from the wound site alone as this may represent colonization. The site should show signs of infection as manifested by purulence and breakdown of tissue. A deep surgical wound is one that occurs within 30 days of surgery if no implant is left in place or one that occurs within 1 year of placement of nonhuman derived implantible foreign device. Infection must be related to site and involve tissues at or beneath the muscle fascia. The wound may spontaneously dehisce or require surgical opening especially if the patient has fever, localized pain, or tenderness.

Likely Pathogens
Staphylococcus epidermidis, Methicillin-Susceptible *on page 201*
Staphylococcus aureus, Methicillin-Susceptible *on page 198*
Staphylococcus epidermidis, Methicillin-Resistant *on page 200*
Staphylococcus aureus, Methicillin-Resistant *on page 195*
Gram-Negative Bacilli *on page 117*

Diagnostic Tests/Procedures
Aerobic Culture, Appropriate Site *on page 244*
Anaerobic Culture *on page 250*
Gram Stain *on page 352*

Drug Therapy Comment If gram-negative bacilli seen on Gram stain, use extended spectrum penicillins with or without aminoglycoside.

Empiric Drug Therapy
Recommended
Penicillins, Penicillinase-Resistant *on page 637*
Vancomycin Hydrochloride *on page 691*

Zygomycosis *see Mucor* Species *on page 149*

ORGANISMS

Acinetobacter Species

Microbiology *Acinetobacter* is an aerobic, gram-negative bacillus (or coccobacillus) which has gained importance as a cause of nosocomial infections. Microbiologically, *Acinetobacter* is related to *Neisseria* and *Moraxella* and can sometimes be confused with these organisms on Gram stain, particularly when the *Acinetobacter* is in its coccobacillary form. The organism is readily identified biochemically. Current classification schemes subdivide the single species of *Acinetobacter* (*A. calcoaceticus*) into different biovars (biologically distinct varieties), such as *A. anitratus* and *A. lwoffii*. The majority of significant infections are caused by *A. calcoaceticus* var. *anitratus*.

Epidemiology *Acinetobacter* is ubiquitous in nature and can be isolated in nearly 100% of soil and water samples tested. The organism is commensal in the human respiratory tract, skin, and urinary tract. It is estimated that up to 25% of healthy adults are colonized with *Acinetobacter* on the skin and greater than 5% in the pharynx. Patients requiring tracheostomies for long-term mechanical ventilation have a much higher rate of respiratory colonization. Within the hospital environment, *Acinetobacter* is frequently found in areas of moisture such as humidifiers, bedside commodes, and ventilator tubing. In some series, it is the most common gram-negative organism carried on the hands of hospital workers.

Despite the prevalence of this organism in the environment, *Acinetobacter* is a relatively uncommon cause of bacteremia. The great majority of significant *Acinetobacter* infections are nosocomial and not community acquired. *Acinetobacter* species have been well described as a sporadic cause of hospital outbreaks, frequently in intensive care unit settings. However, in one of the largest studies reported, 52 episodes of *Acinetobacter* bacteremia were examined over a 6-year period and found to occur at a constant rate with no notable outbreaks or clusters.

Risk factors for hospital-acquired *Acinetobacter* bacteremia include the following.

- Malignancies: Some studies suggest a strong association with leukemia and breast cancer, in particular. Neutropenia itself does not seem to be a significant risk factor.
- Trauma patients: Particularly young men in motor vehicle accidents. The source of bacteremia in these cases is more likely from nosocomial pneumonia than from wound infection.
- Burn patients: The portal of entry for *Acinetobacter* is most likely from extensive soft tissue infection. In burn patients, *Acinetobacter* may be present as part of a polymicrobial bacteremia.
- Presence of an intravenous catheter: In some series, the presence of an indwelling central venous catheter appears to be an important risk factor for bacteremia, but in other series, the association is weak or absent. Some authors have speculated that an intravascular catheter should be regarded more as a marker of severity of illness rather than as a risk factor per se for bacteremia.

Clinical Syndromes *Acinetobacter* is an organism of relatively low virulence and is an opportunistic pathogen. However, in the debilitated hospital patient, the severity of infection may range from mild to life-threatening. Common nosocomial infections include:

- sepsis syndrome
- pneumonia, usually ventilator-associated and multilobar
- intravenous catheter-related bacteremias
- urinary tract infections, including cystitis or pyelonephritis associated with indwelling bladder catheters or renal stones
- intra-abdominal sepsis, usually as part of a polymicrobial infection
- soft tissue infections, particularly with postoperative wound dehiscence or extensive burn injuries

Community-acquired *Acinetobacter* infections are unusual but have been reported in certain situations:

- tracheobronchitis in healthy children
- community-acquired pneumonia in alcoholics

Diagnosis The diagnosis of *Acinetobacter* species infections is made by identification of the organism through Gram stain and culture in a patient with a relevant clinical syndrome. No special media or conditions are necessary to grow these organisms.

Diagnostic Tests/Procedures

Aerobic Culture, Appropriate Site *on page 244*

Gram Stain *on page 352*

Treatment *Acinetobacter* has become resistant to several antibiotics due to a variety of mechanisms including plasmid-mediated resistance, production of high levels of beta-lactamase, and production of aminoglycoside inactivating enzymes. This organism is now resistant to the first and second generation cephalosporins, as well as some extended spectrum penicillins. Patients who have received multiple and prolonged courses of antibiotics are at risk for infections caused by *Acinetobacter* isolates which are resistant to third generation cephalosporins and aminoglycosides. Serious infections caused by multiple-drug resistant species are often quite difficult to treat and may require the use of newer, alternative agents.

Acinetobacter species resistant to cephalosporins and extended spectrum penicillins may be susceptible to either imipenem and/or ampicillin/sulbactam, but the clinician must carefully review the antibiogram. One author has described a decreasing susceptibility to ampicillin/sulbactam with only 61% of *Acinetobacter* isolates now susceptible *in vitro*. In addition, *Acinetobacter* species are no longer uniformly susceptible to imipenem, as they once were in many hospitals prior to 1990. Outbreaks of imipenem-resistant *Acinetobacter calcoaceticus* biotype *anitratus* have recently been described (see references). In such cases of imipenem-resistant, beta-lactam resistant *Acinetobacter*, there may be no proven alternative therapy.

Drug Therapy
Recommended
Cephalosporins, 3rd Generation *on page 528*
Penicillins, Extended Spectrum *on page 637*
Alternate
Imipenem/Cilastatin *on page 586*
Ampicillin Sodium and Sulbactam Sodium *on page 497*
Aztreonam *on page 501*

Selected Readings

Bergogne-Berezin E and Joly-Guillou ML, "An Underestimated Nosocomial Pathogen, *Acinetobacter calcoaceticus*," *J Antimicrob Chemother*, 1985, 16(5):535-8.

Hartstein AI, Rashad AL, Liebler JM, et al, "Multiple Intensive Care Unit Outbreak of *Acinetobacter calcoaceticus* Subspecies *anitratus* Respiratory Infection and Colonization Associated With Contaminated, Reusable Ventilator Circuits and Resuscitation Bags," *Am J Med*, 1988, 85(5):624-31.

Ramphal R, Kluge RM, "*Acinetobacter calcoaceticus* Variety *anitratus*: An Increasing Nosocomial Problem," *Am J Med Sci*, 1979, 277(1):57-66.

Rolston KV, Bodey GP, "*In vitro* Susceptibility of *Acinetobacter* Species to Various Antimicrobial Agents," *Antimicrob Agents Chemother*, 1986, 30(5):769-70.

Smego RA Jr, "Endemic Nosocomial *Acinetobacter calcoaceticus* Bacteremia. Clinical Significance, Treatment, and Prognosis," *Arch Intern Med*, 1985, 145(12):2174-9.

Tilley TAG and Roberts FJ, "Bacteremia With *Acinetobacter* Species: Risk Factors and Prognosis in Different Clinical Settings," *Clin Infect Dis*, 1994, 18:896-900.

Traub WH and Spohr M, "Antimicrobial Drug Susceptibility of Clinical Isolates of *Acinetobacter* Species (*A. baumannii*, *A. haemolyticus*, Genospecies 3, and Genospecies 6)," *Antimicrob Agents Chemother*, 1989, 33(9):1617-9.

Urban C, Go E, Mariano N, et al, "Effect of Sulbactam on Infections Caused by Imipenem-Resistant *Acinetobacter calcoaceticus* biotype *anitratus*," *J Infect Dis*, 1993, 167(2):448-51.

Wood CA and Reboli AC, "Infections Caused by Imipenem-Resistant *Acinetobacter calcoaceticus* biotype *anitratus*," *J Infect Dis*, 1993, 168(6):1602-3.

Actinomyces Species

Microbiology *Actinomyces* species are gram-positive, "higher order" bacteria and are related to *Nocardia* species. The most common *Actinomyces* species to cause disease is *Actinomyces israelii*, accounting for about three-fourths of all cases. These organisms are normal residents of the oral flora and are of low virulence. In the laboratory, *Actinomyces* species grow optimally under anaerobic conditions; growth may also occur in a microaerophilic environment (and sometimes aerobically). When stained, the organism appears thin, with filamentous branches, and may be difficult to distinguish from *Nocardia* species. Growth is slow even under optimal conditions, and the laboratory should be notified if *Actinomyces* is suspected. If a patient receives antibiotics, the organism will only rarely grow in culture because of its susceptibility to a number of agents.

In clinical specimens, *Actinomyces israelii* is often found associated with characteristic **sulfur granules**. These granules are irregularly shaped, mineralized masses consisting of calcium phosphate, inflammatory cells, and masses of
(Continued)

Actinomyces Species *(Continued)*

Actinomyces filaments. Occasionally, sulfur granules may be caused by other organisms but are most commonly associated with *Actinomyces israelii*.

Epidemiology *Actinomyces* species are commensal organisms found in the oral cavity and may be cultured from tooth cavities, gingival creases, dental plaque, tonsils, and related areas; they are harmless saprophytes and do not cause disease when mucous membranes are intact. These organisms also may be part of the normal gastrointestinal flora and can be cultured from the female genital region in the absence of disease. The majority of patients who develop *Actinomyces* infections are immunocompetent. Actinomycosis is not considered an opportunistic infection, although it has been reported occasionally with malignancies and AIDS. Infection usually results from breakdown in the normal mucosal barrier with spread of the organism into deeper sites, such as after dental extractions, trauma, etc.

Clinical Syndromes

- **Cervicofacial actinomycosis:** This is the most common syndrome produced by this organism. Also known as the "lumpy jaw syndrome", patients may present with subacute or acute soft tissue swelling in the head or neck. In chronic cases, progression of localized abscesses may lead to draining sinuses and fistulas. Often a history of a preceding dental procedure can be obtained. In some cases, cervicofacial involvement may be dramatic and rapid, with trismus.

- **Pulmonary actinomycosis:** Patients may develop pulmonary *Actinomyces* infection, usually following an aspiration event or as a complication of head and neck actinomycosis. Clinical symptoms may be mild with only a minor cough and no fever. With serious disease, lung cavitation resembling *M. tuberculosis* may be seen. Other potential chest x-ray or CT scan findings include alveolar pneumonia, upper lobe infiltrates, a lung mass with or without invasion into the chest wall, mediastinal mass, rib destruction, and others. Occasionally, a sinus tract may develop from the lung to the chest wall which is highly suggestive of this organism.

- **Abdominal actinomycosis:** Following abdominal surgery or rupture of an abdominal viscus (eg, perforated duodenal ulcer), patients may develop abdominal actinomycosis. This may be a very difficult diagnosis to establish. The development of sinus tracts is suggestive of this organism.

- **Pelvic actinomycosis:** Actinomycosis has been well-known as a potential complication of intrauterine devices (IUDs). There is a wide spectrum of presentations, including pelvic inflammatory disease. It should be noted that since *Actinomyces* species may be harmless residents of the female genital tract, positive cervical cultures or PAP smears for *Actinomyces* species may or may not represent an infectious disease.

- **Brain abscess:** This may occur as a result of direct extension from a cervicofacial site or hematogenously.

- **Human bite wounds:** Local actinomycosis may occur as a complications of a human bite.

- **Disseminated disease:** On rare occasions, *Actinomyces* can disseminate hematogenously and deposit on skin and other organs.

Diagnosis The clinician should consider *Actinomyces* in any patient presenting with a painful subcutaneous swelling in the head and neck. Draining sinus tracts are highly suggestive of actinomycosis, whether in the head and neck, or the thorax. Recurrent infections are the hallmark of this chronic infection, and patients empirically given oral antibiotics for mandibular or neck swelling may show a partial response followed by relapse.

At times, sulfur granules may be found in purulent fluid from abscesses or sinus tracts when the patient is examined at the bedside. These granules are about 2 mm in size and are hard, yellow to white in color, and round in appearance. They should be sent for histopathologic analysis and culture, since other organisms can produce similar-appearing granules. The absence of sulfur granules in no way excludes actinomycosis. Every effort should be made to isolate the organism in the microbiology laboratory. Since *Actinomyces* is fastidious, multiple aspirations or biopsies may be necessary.

As noted above, the finding of a positive culture for *Actinomyces* does not always indicate significant disease since it is part of the normal oral and gastrointestinal flora of many persons.

Treatment Penicillin G remains the drug of choice. For cervicofacial actinomycosis, penicillin G given at 10-20 million units daily I.V. has been effective and well tolerated by most. Surgical debridement may often be necessary in addition to antibiotics and treatment failures with antibiotics alone may occur. After several weeks of parenteral penicillin, oral penicillin at high doses may be substituted, such as penicillin V potassium up to 4 g daily. Some clinicians may use probenecid in combination with oral penicillin. For the penicillin allergic, several antibiotics may be used including erythromycin, tetracycline, and clindamycin. Quinolones and cephalosporins should be avoided.

Drug Therapy
Recommended
Penicillin G, Parenteral *on page 633*
Ampicillin *on page 495*
Alternate
Doxycycline *on page 557*

Selected Readings
Burden P, "*Actinomycosis,*" *J Infect*, 1989, 19(2):95-9.

Russo TA, "Agents of Actinomycosis," *Principles and Practice of Infectious Diseases*, 4th ed, Mandell GL, Bennett JE, and Dolin R, eds, New York, NY: Churchill Livingstone, 1995, 2280-8.

Adenovirus

Microbiology Adenovirus is a double-stranded DNA virus which can cause several infectious syndromes in both adults and children. Exposure to this virus is common, and serologic studies suggest that by 10 years of age most children have experienced either clinical or subclinical infection. The symptoms associated with adenovirus infection are likely due to lysis of infected host cells coupled with a brisk host immune response. Most cases of symptomatic disease are associated with the initial infection in a nonimmune host. However, some evidence suggests that adenovirus can enter a latent (asymptomatic) phase in some individuals and can reactivate later in life, particularly if the host becomes immunosuppressed (organ transplantation, corticosteroids, etc).

Epidemiology With humans providing the only known reservoir for adenoviruses, 5% to 10% of all viral respiratory illnesses in civilians are caused by these viruses. Epidemics are usually restricted to the military with small outbreaks among children. Person-to-person transmission through respiratory and ocular secretions is thought to be the major route of transmission. Adenoviruses associated with infantile gastroenteritis are probably transmitted by the fecal-oral route.

Clinical Syndromes
- **Respiratory tract infection, at all ages:** This is the most common manifestation of adenovirus infection and is responsible for approximately 10% of infant and childhood ambulatory respiratory infections. In boarding schools or military camps, outbreaks of influenza-like respiratory infections have been well described. Adenovirus has also been implicated as a common cause of atypical pneumonia in adults, characterized by low-grade fever, subacute onset, prominent constitutional symptoms (headache, myalgias, malaise), and an absence of purulent sputum.
- **Asymptomatic infection of the tonsils and adenoids (usually adenovirus types 1,2,5) in infants**
- **Pharyngitis in infants**
- **Infantile diarrhea**
- **Pharyngoconjunctival fever in older children:** Especially in summer camps or schools. This is manifested by the acute onset of conjunctivitis, sore throat, fever, and rhinitis, and tends to be a self-limited illness.
- **Hemorrhagic cystitis in adults:** Usually caused by types 11 and 21
- **Keratoconjunctivitis:** Adenovirus is an important cause of epidemic keratoconjunctivitis. Patients present with inflamed conjunctivae (often bilateral) with preauricular adenopathy.
- **Adenovirus and HIV infection:** Persons infected with the human immunodeficiency virus may be carriers of adenovirus. Despite this, there appears to be a very low incidence of recognized adenovirus in persons with AIDS. Case reports have described disseminated adenovirus with hepatic necrosis, adenovirus colitis, and necrotizing adenovirus infection of the renal tubules.
- **Infections in other immunosuppressed patients:** Fatal adenovirus infections due to disseminated disease have been described in transplant recipients (bone marrow, renal transplant), as well as other chronically immunosuppressed patients (see references).

Diagnosis Laboratory studies can confirm suspected cases of adenovirus infection, but the turnaround time can exceed 1 week. Serologic studies demon-

(Continued)

Adenovirus *(Continued)*

strating a fourfold or greater rise in specific IgG titer to adenovirus strongly supports the diagnosis of recent infection. Direct cultures for the virus are available in many laboratories, but the time for viral isolation is variable and highly dependent on the amount of virus in the clinical specimen.

Diagnostic Tests/Procedures

Adenovirus Antibody Titer *on page 243*

Adenovirus Culture *on page 243*

Virus, Direct Detection by Fluorescent Antibody *on page 480*

Treatment No antiviral agents have been proven to be effective in the treatment of adenovirus infections. Supportive care is the treatment of choice.

Selected Readings

Baum SG, "Adenovirus," *Principles and Practice of Infectious Diseases*, 4th ed, Mandell GL, Bennett JE, and Dolin R, eds, New York, NY: Churchill Livingstone, 1995, 1382-7.

Flomenberg P, Babbitt J, Drobyski WR, et al, "Increasing Incidence of Adenovirus Disease in Bone Marrow Transplant Recipients," *J Infect Dis*, 1994, 169(4):775-81.

Green WR, Greaves WL, Frederick WR, et al, "Renal Infection Due to Adenovirus in a Patient With Human Immunodeficiency Virus Infection," *Clin Infect Dis*, 1994, 18:989-91.

Hierholzer JC, "Adenoviruses in the Immunocompromised Host," *Clin Microbiol Rev*, 1992, 5(3):262-74.

Janner D, Petru AM, Belchis D, et al, "Fatal Adenovirus Infection in a Child With Acquired Immunodeficiency Syndrome," *Pediatr Infect Dis J*, 1990, 9(6):434-6.

Krilov LR, Rubin LG, Frogel M, et al, "Disseminated Adenovirus Infection With Hepatic Necrosis in Patients With Human Immunodeficiency Virus Infection and Other Immunodeficiency States," *Rev Infect Dis*, 1990, 12(2):303-7.

Shields AF, Hackman RC, Fife KH, et al, "Adenovirus Infections in Patients Undergoing Bone-Marrow Transplantation," *N Engl J Med*, 1985, 312(9):529-33.

Zahradnik JM, Spencer MJ, and Porter DD, "Adenovirus Infection in the Immunocompromised Patient," *Am J Med*, 1980, 68(5):725-32.

AIDS Virus *see* Human Immunodeficiency Virus *on page 133*

Anaerobic *Streptococcus* *see Streptococcus*-Related Gram-Positive Cocci *on page 212*

Ancylostoma duodenale

Synonyms Hookworm

Applies To *Necator americanus*

Microbiology *Ancylostoma duodenale* is an intestinal roundworm. Often called "Old World hookworm," this parasite is one of two common hookworms causing human disease. The second hookworm, *Necator americanus* ("New World hookworm"), is structurally related to *Ancylostoma duodenale* and differs mainly in geographic distribution. Hookworms have been estimated to infect nearly 25% of the world's population.

Like all other nematodes (roundworms), *Ancylostoma duodenale* is visible to the naked eye, although the adult tends to be only 1 cm long. The infectious cycle begins when filariform larvae penetrate intact skin of the host. The most common portal of entry is the human foot, usually associated with walking barefoot on contaminated soil. Once through the skin, the larvae are carried via the venous circulation into the right heart and pulmonary circulation. The larvae then migrate through the alveoli of the lungs, in a fashion similar to *Ascaris lumbricoides*. Later, the parasites move into the trachea and pharynx and are then swallowed by the host. Within the small bowel, the adult hookworms attach to the mucosa and can remain there for years. The worms suck blood continuously from the intestinal tissue and can ultimately cause an iron deficiency anemia, with an estimated blood loss of 0.2 mL per day. Thousands of eggs are laid each day by the adult worm and are passed into the feces of the host. When contaminated human feces are mixed into the soil, larvae are released. Under the appropriate environmental conditions, these noninfective larvae become infective (filariform larvae), and the cycle begins again.

Epidemiology Hookworm infection is most common in tropical or subtropical regions and has been reported worldwide. Warm climates favor hookworm infection, since the ova do not tolerate cold soil temperatures. Prevalence is highest in areas where sanitation is poor and human feces are mixed with topsoil. Efforts to control hookworm infection in the United States have been generally successful, although cases still occur in the southeastern states.

Clinical Syndromes

- **Iron deficiency anemia:** Caused by the adult hookworm parasitizing blood in the upper small intestine

- **Pneumonitis:** Occurring during the lung migration phase. This is characterized by wheezing, eosinophilia, and diffuse pulmonary infiltrates, resembling Löffler's syndrome.
- **Ground itch:** An allergic reaction to the hookworm localized to the area of initial skin penetration. The individual may present with erythema, pruritus, and a papular rash in the lower extremity.
- **Abdominal pain, diarrhea, weight loss, and malabsorption:** In developing countries, mental retardation can result from chronic nutritional deficiencies caused by the hookworm.

Diagnosis The clinical suspicion of hookworm infection is confirmed by direct examination of stool specimens for the presence of the characteristic eggs.

Diagnostic Tests/Procedures
Ova and Parasites, Stool *on page 416*

Treatment Mebendazole is the drug of choice with cure rates exceeding 90%. The anemia usually responds to standard iron supplementation.

Drug Therapy
Recommended
Mebendazole *on page 604*
Alternate
Thiabendazole *on page 681*
Pyrantel Pamoate *on page 651*

Selected Readings
Mahmoud AA, "Intestinal Nematodes (Roundworms)," *Principles and Practice of Infectious Diseases*, 4th ed, Mandell GL, Bennett JE, and Dolin R, eds, New York, NY: Churchill Livingstone, 1995, 2526-31.
Miller TA, "Hookworm Infection in Man," *Adv Parasitol*, 1979, 17:315-84.
Warren KS, "Hookworm Control," *Lancet*, 1988, 2(8616):897-8.

Animal and Human Bites Guidelines *see page 736*

Ascaris

Microbiology Over 4 million individuals in the United States are infected with the intestinal parasite *Ascaris lumbricoides*, commonly referred to as "the giant roundworm." Ascariasis is the term used to describe human infection with *A. lumbricoides*. With a worldwide prevalence over 1 billion, ascariasis is the single most common worm infection of humans.

Ascaris lumbricoides is a nematode (roundworm) which passes through several developmental stages: egg (ova), larva, and mature adult. The infectious cycle for the human begins with ingestion of *Ascaris* eggs by the host; these eggs are found most often in contaminated food or soil. In the small intestine, the larvae are released from the egg and penetrate through the intestinal mucosa. After entering the venous circulation, the larvae migrate into the pulmonary vessels. For a period of 10-14 days, the larvae grow within the alveoli of the lungs, the so-called "pulmonary phase." The larvae then pass up the trachea and are coughed up and swallowed by the host. The worms return to the jejunum where they mature into adult forms. During this "intestinal phase" which can last several months, the adult worm attains a length of over 15 cm. Thousands of fertilized eggs are passed into the feces of the host and eventually into the environment, where the cycle begins again.

Epidemiology *Ascaris* infections occur worldwide, although more commonly in tropical climates. In the United States, ascariasis is most prevalent in the southeastern states. Poor sanitation is a predisposing factor to infection. The eggs of *Ascaris lumbricoides* are hardy and can survive cold temperatures and dry environments. In communities where human feces contaminate both the food and water supply, ascariasis is endemic because of its fecal-oral transmission. School-age children are at particularly high risk of parasitism.

Clinical Syndromes The clinical presentation depends to some degree on the worm burden and the specific host organ involved.
- **Asymptomatic infection:** This is the most common manifestation, and usually occurs when only a small number of eggs are ingested.
- **Pneumonitis, caused by migration of large numbers of larvae through the lungs:** The individual presents with bronchospasm, pulmonary infiltrates on the chest radiograph, and peripheral blood eosinophilia. This may be mistaken for an asthmatic attack or Löffler's syndrome.
- **Intestinal obstruction, especially when the worm burden is high:** Appendicitis has also been described when a tangled mass of worms obstructs the lumen of the appendix.

(Continued)

Ascaris (Continued)

- **Common bile duct obstruction, usually caused by a single adult worm:** Characteristically, the individual has nausea, vomiting, abdominal pain, and sometimes jaundice.
- **Nutritional deficiencies, particularly in children**

Diagnosis The clinical suspicion of ascariasis is confirmed by direct examination of stool specimens. Because of the enormous numbers of eggs which are shed in the feces each day, in most cases there is little difficulty identifying the fertilized and unfertilized eggs. Less commonly, the adult worm may be passed in the stool as well. In rare cases, the diagnosis of ascariasis may be suspected or confirmed by using radiographic contrast studies of the bowel or biliary tract; the outline of the worm may be seen as a filling defect.

Diagnostic Tests/Procedures
Ova and Parasites, Stool *on page 416*

Treatment Mebendazole is considered the drug of choice for intestinal ascariasis. Piperazine citrate is indicated for cases of intestinal or biliary obstruction. **Note**: In cases of dual or multiple infections with *Ascaris* and other intestinal parasites, *Ascaris* must be treated first. Some antiparasitic agents not directed toward *Ascaris* can antagonize *Ascaris* and cause the large worms to react violently to the point of damaging or even penetrating the bowel.

Drug Therapy
 Recommended
  Mebendazole *on page 604*
 Alternate
  Pyrantel Pamoate *on page 651*

Selected Readings
Khuroo MS, Zargar SA, Mahajan R, et al, "Sonographic Appearances in Biliary Ascariasis," *Gastroenterology*, 1987, 93(2):267-72.

Mahmoud AA, "Intestinal Nematodes (Roundworms)," *Principles and Practice of Infectious Diseases*, 4th ed, Mandell GL, Bennett JE, and Dolin R, eds, New York, NY: Churchill Livingstone, 1995, 2526-31.

Stephenson LS, "The Contribution of *Ascaris lumbricoides* to Malnutrition in Children," *Parasitology*, 1980, 81(1):221-33.

Aspergillus Species

Microbiology *Aspergillus* is a potentially pathogenic fungus found throughout the environment. Aspergillosis is the term used to describe human infection caused by any one of the 900 reported species of this mold. Infection with *Aspergillus* can range from benign colonization of the respiratory tract to lethal blood vessel invasion and remains a major cause of morbidity and mortality in neutropenic patients.

Aspergillus is a mold and is composed of hyphae which grow by extension and branching. The fungus is recognized in tissue specimens by its septate hyphae and its dichotomous, acute angle branching. A definitive diagnosis of *Aspergillus* is quite difficult from histopathologic sections alone unless characteristic sporulation is seen. Confirmation of *Aspergillus* requires growth of the mold on appropriate culture media, but it is well recognized clinically that fungal cultures may still be negative despite positive tissue sections.

Epidemiology *Aspergillus* is ubiquitous in the environment but is not considered part of the normal flora of humans. Although there is no specific reservoir for this fungus, it tends to grow heavily in hay, dung, soil (including the soil of potted plants), grain, and compost piles; occasionally, a history of a massive inhalational exposure can be obtained from individuals with overwhelming infection. Well-documented studies have shown that *Aspergillus* can be recovered from the air of hospital wards, and outbreaks in susceptible patients have been associated with heavily colonized hospital air-ventilation systems. *Aspergillus* outbreaks have also been reported following hospital renovation projects.

Although *Aspergillus* is universally present in the environment, it causes disease in relatively few individuals. Life-threatening acute infection is nearly always limited to immunocompromised patients. *Aspergillus* infections of a more chronic and indolent nature are often seen in individuals with less debilitating underlying diseases (eg, asthma, chronic bronchitis, sarcoidosis). Acquisition of *Aspergillus* is exclusively via inhalation of airborne spores; person-to-person transmission does not occur.

Clinical Syndromes There are three major manifestations of an *Aspergillus* infection which can overlap in an individual patient.

- **Allergic bronchopulmonary aspergillosis (ABPA):** This is a specific form of hypersensitivity pneumonitis. It is characterized by asthma, eosinophilia, immediate skin reactivity to *Aspergillus* antigen, elevated immunoglobulin E (IgE), and positive *Aspergillus* precipitins in the serum. This is considered an allergic response to *Aspergillus* and is not truly infectious in nature. Treatment is with corticosteroids in selected cases, rather than antifungal therapy.

- ***Aspergillus* colonization:** This is the most common scenario, in which *Aspergillus* exists as a fungus ball in a lung cavity such as an old tuberculosis cavity. This fungus ball is a mass of hyphal elements which elicits little inflammatory response. A patient can be colonized for years without symptoms or tissue damage, except for hemoptysis. However, serious complications can occur such as empyema or bronchopleural fistula.

- **Invasive fungal infection:** This occurs almost exclusively as an opportunistic infection in the severely immunocompromised patient. Prolonged neutropenia is a well recognized risk factor. Rarely, invasive disease has been described in otherwise healthy hosts. Systemic aspergillosis is an often lethal infection with fever, progressive pneumonitis with or without cavitation, and widespread dissemination to almost any organ system. *Aspergillus* characteristically invades blood vessels in the lungs and other tissues.

- **Miscellaneous:** Other manifestations of *Aspergillus* have been described, including cerebral infarction, endocarditis, gastrointestinal ulcerations in immunocompromised hosts, necrotizing skin ulcers, and bone lesions. Meningitis has been described rarely.

Diagnosis *Aspergillus* requires identification of the fungus in biopsy samples and/or appropriate body fluids. It should be noted that the recovery of *Aspergillus* from clinical specimens such as expectorated sputum or bronchial lavage fluid does not necessarily imply clinically significant infection. In some cases, *Aspergillus* may be present as a colonizer without damage to surrounding tissues; this does not warrant specific therapy. Demonstration of tissue invasion on histopathologic specimens is the gold standard for diagnosing invasive aspergillosis. In all cases, a positive culture for *Aspergillus* must be viewed in the context of the individual case.

Diagnostic Tests/Procedures
Cytology, Body Fluids *on page 318*
Fungus Culture, Appropriate Site *on page 340*
KOH Preparation *on page 379*

Treatment Surgical excision of sequestered foci of *Aspergillus* infection may be the treatment of choice for diseases such as brain lesions, sinus involvement, infections on prosthetic material, and some lung lesions, with subsequent drug therapy with amphotericin B. As the drug of choice for *Aspergillus* infections, amphotericin B is administered in doses as high as 1 mg/kg/day. Although agents such as flucytosine, rifampin, and clindamycin have been added to amphotericin B in hopes of increasing antifungal activity. These combinations have not been proven to be superior to amphotericin B alone. Itraconazole may be an alternative for long-term maintenance or suppression but has no track record for this or in the treatment of acute *Aspergillus* infection (no intravenous form of itraconazole is available).

Drug Therapy
Recommended
Amphotericin B *on page 493*

Selected Readings
Dar DA, Ahmad M, Weinstein AJ, et al, "Thoracic Aspergillosis," *Cleve Clin Q*, 1984, 51(4):615-30 (Part I), 51(4):631-53 (Part II), 51(4):655-65 (Part III).
Denning DW and Stevens DA, "Antifungal and Surgical Treatment of Invasive Aspergillosis: Review of 2,121 Published Cases," *Rev Infect Dis*, 1990, 12(6):1147-201.
Shirakusa T, Veda H, Saito T, et al, "Surgical Treatment of Pulmonary Aspergilloma and Aspergillus Empyema," *Ann Thorac Surg*, 1989, 48(6):779-82.
Talbot GH, Huang A, and Provencher M, "Invasive *Aspergillus* Rhinosinusitis in Patients With Acute Leukemia," *Rev Infect Dis*, 1991, 13(2):219-32.

Babesia microti

Microbiology *Babesia microti* is an intracellular protozoan which causes a febrile illness in the northeastern United States. The illness, babesiosis, resembles malaria. *Babesia microti* primarily infects animals; humans are incidental hosts. In the United States, rodents are the primary animal reservoir, including the white-footed deer mouse, rats, and field mice. The vector for transmission of the organism from the rodent to the human is the tick *Ixodes dammini*, the hard-shelled tick also responsible for the transmission of Lyme disease. Fol-

(Continued)

Babesia microti (Continued)

lowing the bite of an infected tick, *Babesia microti* invade the human circulation and enter erythrocytes. The trophozoites of *Babesia microti* divide within erythrocytes into two or four daughter cells, sometimes forming a characteristic tetrad ring which can be recognized on a blood smear. The organisms eventually leave the red blood cells, perforating the membrane and causing asynchronous cell lysis. With the merozoites being released, other host erythrocytes are at risk for infection, and the infectious cycle is maintained.

Epidemiology Babesiosis occurs most commonly along the northeastern seaboard of the United States in states such as Massachusetts, New York, and Rhode Island. In particular, Martha's Vineyard, Cape Cod, Shelter Island, Fire Island, and Nantucket Island report a high prevalence. Infections mainly occur from May to September when the nymph form of *Ixodes dammini* is feeding. Epidemiologic studies suggest that most infections with *Babesia microti* are subclinical or asymptomatic. A seroprevalence rate of 3% to 4% was found in endemic areas, with many individuals unaware of past infection. Less commonly, babesiosis has been transmitted by transfusion from an asymptomatic donor.

Clinical Syndromes The incubation period following the bite of the infected tick is 1-3 weeks. The majority of patients are not able to recall a recent tick bite. Most infections with *Babesia microti* are either asymptomatic or mild. In severe cases, symptoms include fever up to 40°C, chills, sweats, myalgias, malaise, and headache. Some individuals may experience photophobia, sore throat, and cough. Hepatosplenomegaly may be observed less commonly, but generalized lymphadenopathy is not seen. The most fulminant cases of babesiosis occur in patients who are asplenic, emphasizing the important role of the spleen in the host defense against this protozoan.

Diagnosis The diagnosis of babesiosis is suspected when there is a characteristic clinical presentation in an individual from an endemic area. The diagnosis is confirmed microbiologically by examination of Wright-Giemsa stained thick and thin blood smears. The parasite is visualized within the erythrocytes. At times it may be difficult to distinguish *Babesia* sp. from other intracellular parasites such as *Plasmodium falciparum* (one of the causative agents of malaria). The finding of intracellular merozoites in a tetrad configuration is pathognomonic for babesiosis but frequently absent. Other laboratory aids include the classic findings of an intravascular hemolytic anemia with hemoglobinuria, elevated reticulocyte count, and depressed haptoglobin level. The diagnosis can also be confirmed by using an indirect immunofluorescent antibody titer against *Babesia microti*, but serum must be sent to the Centers for Disease Control.

Diagnostic Tests/Procedures

Peripheral Blood Smear, Thick and Thin *on page 429*

Treatment Many patients with babesiosis recover without specific therapy. When infection is severe or the patient is known to be asplenic, the drugs of choice are clindamycin intravenously and quinine orally. Chloroquine, which is effective in some cases of malaria, has no efficacy in treating babesiosis; thus, it is important to distinguish babesiosis from malaria on the peripheral blood smear. Life-threatening infections may respond to exchange transfusions in combination with antimicrobial therapy, in an effort to decrease the degree of parasitemia.

Drug Therapy
Recommended

Clindamycin *on page 540*
used in combination with
Quinine Sulfate *on page 658*

Selected Readings

"Babesiosis – Connecticut," *MMWR Morb Mortal Wkly Rep*, 1989, 38(38):649-50.

Rosner F, Zarrabi MH, Benach JL, et al, "Babesiosis in Splenectomized Adults: Review of 22 Reported Cases," *Am J Med*, 1984, 76(4):696-701.

Sun T, Tenenbaum TJ, Greenspan J, et al, "Morphologic and Clinical Observations in Human Infection With *Babesia microti*," *J Infect Dis*, 1983, 148(2):239-48.

White NJ and Breman JG, "Malaria and Babesiosis," *Harrison's Principles of Internal Medicine*, 13th ed, Isselbacher KJ, Braunwald E, Wilson JD, et al, eds, New York, NY: McGraw-Hill, 1994, 887-96.

Bacillus anthracis

Microbiology *Bacillus anthracis* is an aerobic, gram-positive bacillus with a large polypeptide capsule. Some isolates may appear gram-variable rather than gram-positive. On Gram stain, there is a characteristic "box car" appearance to these organisms, a feature common to the genus *Bacillus*. The organism forms spores when grown aerobically in the laboratory, but spores are not seen in clinical specimens. Virulence factors for this organism include anthrax toxin (made up of three components) and a capsule (which protects against host antibodies).

Epidemiology *Bacillus anthracis* causes the disease anthrax. The organism is ubiquitous in the environment, being found in soil and decaying vegetation. The spores of the organism are hardy and survive for years under adverse conditions. These spores contaminate the hide of herbivores such as cattle, sheep, and goats. Animals consume the spores and ultimately expire. In this way, anthrax is a zoonosis. Humans are only incidentally exposed. Direct contact with the contaminated hides or hair of these herbivores leads to human disease. Cases still occur in the United States but are rare. In 1992, there was only one case of anthrax in the United States reported to the Centers for Disease Control. The disease is more common in the Middle East (Iran, Turkey).

Clinical Syndromes

- **Cutaneous anthrax:** This form of human infection results from direct inoculation of *Bacillus anthracis* spores into the skin. Exposure results from handling insulation made from animal hair (usually commercial buildings), infected animal hides, clothing products, or wool. Less commonly, spores come from contaminated soil. Spores enter intact or exposed skin in an extremity such as the forearm. A papule develops locally at the site of inoculation of the spores and later ulcerates and turns into a black eschar. Systemic symptoms of fever, chills, and total body edema can result from the effects of anthrax toxin. The disease is often rapidly fatal if the diagnosis and treatment are delayed.

- **Inhalation anthrax:** Also known as Woolsorter's disease, inhalational anthrax presents as a rapidly progressive pneumonitis. Widening of the mediastinum is a common finding on chest x-ray and may be a clue to the diagnosis. Meningeal involvement is common. Mortality is high.

- **Gastrointestinal anthrax:** This is a rare presentation of the disease in humans.

Diagnosis Because of the rarity of anthrax in the United States, diagnosis is difficult to make in a timely fashion. It is important to obtain an occupational history for all patients who present with an infectious disease, and it is particularly important with anthrax. A history of exposure to animal products may be the only clue to this disease. Patients who present with unusual necrotic ulcerations of the extremities should be questioned along these lines. Notify laboratory of suspected organism.

Diagnostic Tests/Procedures

Aerobic Culture, Appropriate Site *on page 244*
Aerobic Culture, Sputum *on page 246*
Gram Stain *on page 352*

Treatment The antibiotic of choice for *Bacillus anthracis* is penicillin. The organism has remained sensitive to penicillin but may not always be responsive to therapy, particularly if initiated late in the disease course. Adults with cutaneous anthrax can be treated with intravenous penicillin G, 2 million units every 6 hours for several days. Little data is available for inhalation anthrax or gastrointestinal anthrax; high doses of penicillin are recommended since the mortality of inhalation anthrax approaches 100%. Alternative agents include tetracycline or chloramphenicol.

Drug Therapy

Recommended

Penicillin G, Parenteral *on page 633*

Alternate

Tetracycline *on page 679*
Chloramphenicol *on page 531*

Selected Readings

Brachman PS, "Anthrax," *Bacterial Infections of Humans*, 2nd ed, Evans AS and Brachman PS, eds, New York, NY: Plenum Medical Book Company, 1991, 75-86.

Brachman PS, "Inhalation Anthrax," *Ann N Y Acad Sci*, 1980, 353:83-93.

Lew D, "*Bacillus anthracis* (Anthrax)," *Principles and Practice of Infectious Diseases*, 4th ed, Mandell GL, Bennett JE, and Dolin R, eds, New York, NY: Churchill Livingstone, 1995, 1885-9.

"Summary of Notifiable Diseases, United States 1992," *MMWR Morb Mortal Wkly Rep*, 1992, 41:1-73.

Tuazon CU, "Other *Bacillus* Species," *Principles and Practice of Infectious Diseases*, 4th ed, Mandell GL, Bennett JE, and Dolin R, eds, New York, NY: Churchill Livingstone, 1995, 1890-4.

(Continued)

Bacillus anthracis (Continued)

Weber DJ and Rutala WA, "*Bacillus* Species," *Infect Control Hosp Epidemiol*, 1988, 9(8):368-73.

Bacillus cereus

Related Information

Timing of Food Poisoning *on page 723*

Microbiology *Bacillus cereus* is an aerobic, gram-positive bacillus associated with a variety of disease states including food poisoning, ocular infections, bacteremia, and septicemia. *Bacillus cereus* is a spore-forming aerobe which stains gram-positive or gram-variable. It grows readily on standard laboratory media and does not need special culturing techniques.

Epidemiology *Bacillus cereus* is ubiquitous in the environment, growing readily in such diverse areas as soil, water, vegetables, decaying matter, and dust. In certain individuals, it can be part of the normal human flora, explaining in part its tendency to colonize surgical wounds and serious burn injuries. The needles and syringes of heroin addicts in the United States have also been found to be contaminated with this bacterium. *Bacillus cereus* food poisoning, caused by ingestion of a toxin elaborated by this organism, has been reported from several countries around the world, including the United States and Canada.

Clinical Syndromes

- **The "emetic form" of *Bacillus cereus* food poisoning:** This results from the ingestion of a preformed toxin produced by this organism. Nausea, vomiting, and abdominal cramping usually occur soon (1-6 hours) following the ingestion of contaminated foods. In particular, this emetic toxin has been associated with fried rice served in Chinese food restaurants. The spores of *B. cereus* can survive the process of boiling rice followed by quick frying.

- **The "diarrheal form" of *Bacillus cereus* food poisoning:** This results from ingestion of a different, heat-labile enterotoxin. The incubation period is longer than for the emetic form, usually more than 9 hours. Profuse watery diarrhea is the predominant symptom, along with abdominal cramping.

- **Ocular infection, including endophthalmitis:** *Bacillus cereus* is a leading pathogen in post-traumatic endophthalmitis. Other common settings include ophthalmitis in farm workers and intravenous drug users. In the latter case, infection can be fulminant. Several toxins have been identified which may play a role in this often rapidly destructive panophthalmitis: cerelysin, necrotic toxin, and phospholipase C.

- **Bacteremia:** Isolation of *Bacillus cereus* from the blood may have little clinical significance (as in the transient *Bacillus* bacteremia commonly seen in the intravenous drug user or in blood culture contamination) or may represent life-threatening septicemia. Clinically significant bacteremias tend to occur most often in patients with indwelling intravascular catheters and may warrant treatment.

- **Miscellaneous infections:** *Bacillus cereus* can be a cause of pneumonia in the compromised host (rare), endocarditis in the intravenous drug user, necrotizing fasciitis, acute or chronic osteomyelitis, meningitis (often in the setting of disseminated infection), ventricular shunt infection, and can be a part of a polymicrobial wound infection (eg, surgical wounds, tumor, breast prostheses).

Diagnosis *Bacillus cereus* is readily identified in the laboratory from cultures of blood and other sterile body fluids. In cases of suspected *Bacillus* food poisoning, the implicated foods should be cultured for this organism. There is little benefit in culturing the patient's stool since gastrointestinal tract colonization is not uncommon. As mentioned previously, isolation of *Bacillus cereus* from the blood need not be treated in every case, and clinical judgment is required.

Diagnostic Tests/Procedures

Aerobic Culture, Appropriate Site *on page 244*
Gram Stain *on page 352*

Treatment *Bacillus cereus* food poisoning does not respond to antimicrobial therapy. Attention should instead be focused on supportive measures such as hydration and electrolyte balance. Clinically significant infections with this organism should be treated with vancomycin intravenously. Unlike other *Bacillus* species (eg, *Bacillus alvei*, *B. subtilis*, *B. circulans*, etc.), *Bacillus cereus* is often resistant to beta-lactam antibiotics such as the penicillins and cephalosporins. Vancomycin should be used until the antimicrobial susceptibility pattern is finalized; limited data suggests the addition of an aminoglycoside to vancomycin may have some minor benefit in serious infections.

Drug Therapy
Recommended
Vancomycin Hydrochloride *on page 691*

Selected Readings
"*Bacillus cereus* Food Poisoning Associated With Fried Rice at Two Child Day Care Centers – Virginia, 1993," *MMWR Morb Mortal Wkly Rep*, 1994, 43(10):177-8.

Davey RT Jr and Tauber WB, "Post-Traumatic Endophthalmitis: The Emerging Role of *Bacillus cereus* Infection," *Rev Infect Dis*, 1987, 9(1):110-23.

Schricker ME, Thompson GH, and Schreiber JR, "Osteomyelitis Due to *Bacillus cereus* in an Adolescent: Case Report and Review," *Clin Infect Dis*, 1994, 18:863-7.

Sliman R, Rehm S, and Shlaes DM, "Serious Infections Caused by *Bacillus* Species," *Medicine (Baltimore)*, 1987, 66(3):218-23.

Terranova W and Blake PA, "*Bacillus cereus* Food Poisoning," *N Engl J Med*, 1978, 298(3):143-4.

Tuazon CU, "Other *Bacillus* Species," *Principles and Practice of Infectious Diseases*, 4th ed, Mandell GL, Bennett JE, and Dolin R, eds, New York, NY: Churchill Livingstone, 1995, 1890-4.

Bacteroides Species

Microbiology *Bacteroides* species are gram-negative, anaerobic, pleomorphic rods some of which are aerotolerant. Gram staining is pale. The organisms stain irregularly. *B. fragilis* grows as a nonhemolytic glistening colony on blood agar. *B. melaninogenicus* appears as pigmented, brown to black colonies which fluoresce under UV light. *B. fragilis* will grow in 20% bile; *B. melaninogenicus* will not. Catalase positivity and resistance to kanamycin, vancomycin, and colistin are used for preliminary speciation. Biochemical testing utilizing carbohydrate fermentation and gas-liquid chromatography (GLC) are used for definitive speciation. DNA homology has allowed clarification of the taxonomy of the *Bacteroides* species. *Bacteroides* species have a broad spectrum of resistance to antimicrobial agents. *

Epidemiology *Bacteroides* species are normal flora of the oral cavity, gastrointestinal tract, and female genital tract. They are the organism most frequently isolated from suppurative anaerobic infections. Nosocomial colonization by virulent strains of *B. fragilis* may occur. Although *B. fragilis* makes up only a small fraction of the oral and colonic flora, it accounts for a disproportionate percentage of infections due to *Bacteroides* species.

Clinical Syndromes
- **Abscess infection:** *Bacteroides* species infections are associated with closed abscesses and are frequently present in mixed or polymicrobic infections. The most common are intra-abdominal abscesses which result from diverticulitis, rupture of the appendix, surgical procedures, and abdominal trauma or tumor. The liver and subdiaphragmatic space are frequent sites for abscess formation. Splenic, kidney, and perinephric abscesses are also well known. Liver abscess may occur as the result of peritoneal seeding or by spread from the portal or biliary system. *B. fragilis* may be isolated from more than 50% of intra-abdominal abscesses, and anaerobes may be isolated in more than 90%. Most infections are mixed, with aerobic and facultative organisms also being present. Sixty percent to 70% of pelvic abscesses involve *B. fragilis. B. melaninogenicus* is more often implicated in lung abscesses than is *B. fragilis*. In most cases, lung abscesses are polymicrobic.
- **Bacteremia:** Usually heralds a localized site of infection.
- **Endocarditis:** Rare but has been observed in patients without underlying valvular disease.
- **Skin infection:** Often associated with trauma surgery, decubitus ulcers, diabetic foot ulcers, and human bites. Contamination by feces, saliva, and oropharyngeal secretions may allow anaerobic organisms to become established and cause infection.
- **Gangrene, synergistic cellulitis, necrotizing fascitis, and crepitant cellulitis:** May also be frequently attributed to infection with *Bacteroides* species.

Diagnostic Tests/Procedures
Anaerobic Culture *on page 250*
Gram Stain *on page 352*

Duration of Therapy 7-10 days

Treatment Drainage is the treatment of choice for infections with *Bacteroides* species. This can be accomplished either by surgical intervention or by needle
(Continued)

ORGANISMS

Bacteroides Species *(Continued)*

aspiration under ultrasound or CT control. Although there are differences of opinion, coverage for anaerobes is usually included in the therapy of polymicrobic abscesses. Specific therapy for *Bacteroides* infections include metronidazole, clindamycin, cefoxitin, piperacillin, ticarcillin, and imipenem. Cross-reactive resistance to β-lactam antimicrobials has been reported. Metronidazole resistance is rarely encountered. Clindamycin, cefoxitin, and cefotetan are effective alternatives. Selection of an antimicrobial agent may be influenced by susceptibility testing if available.

Drug Therapy
Recommended
Metronidazole *on page 610*
Clindamycin *on page 540*
Alternate
Cefoxitin Sodium *on page 518*
Cefotetan Disodium *on page 517*

Selected Readings
Patrick S, "The Virulence of *Bacteroides fragilis*," *Rev Med Microbiol*, 1993, 4:40-9.
Styrt B and Gorbach SL, "Recent Developments in the Understanding of the Pathogenesis and Treatment of Anaerobic Infections," *N Engl J Med*, 1989, 321(5):298-302.
Wexler HM, "Susceptibility Testing of Anaerobic Bacteria – State of the Art," *Clin Infect Dis*, 1993, 16(Suppl 4):S328-33.

Bartonella Species

Synonyms *Rochalimaea* Species

Microbiology *Bartonella* species are small, pleomorphic gram-negative bacilli which have received considerable attention over recent years because of their role in two important diseases: cat scratch disease and bacillary angiomatosis. Until recently, *Bartonella henselae* and *Bartonella quintana* species were considered *Rochalimaea* species. *Bartonella henselae* was first isolated and described in 1992, when it was cultured from the blood of an HIV-infected individual. *Bartonella* species are slow-growing and difficult to isolate in the laboratory. The organisms have occasionally been recovered from blood cultures, skin biopsies, spleen tissue, and lymph node biopsies. However, because of the fastidious nature of these organisms, clinical specimens may often be culture-negative. Of note, *Bartonella* species are best visualized in clinical specimens (such as lymph nodes) using a Warthin-Starry stain; the finding of Warthin-Starry staining bacteria in lymph node tissue is suggestive of cat scratch disease.

Epidemiology

Cat scratch disease: For years, the cause of cat scratch disease was unknown. Although the epidemiology, clinical manifestations, and therapies of cat scratch disease have been described in the past, only within the past 2 years has *B. henselae* been implicated as the major causative agent of cat scratch disease (CSD). There is some controversy surrounding this because some experts believe that a different organism, *Afipia felis*, is the cause of CSD. Available data suggest that either *B. henselae* or *A. felis* can cause CSD, although the relative importance of each is not known.

The exact distribution of *Bartonella* in the environment is not known, but the organism can be found in soil. Cats appear to be an important reservoir of this organism. In the United States, there are approximately 22,000 cases of cat scratch disease diagnosed each year with about 10% requiring hospitalization. Most cases of CSD occur in children and adolescents who are otherwise healthy (ie, immunocompetent). Family outbreaks have been reported. The majority of cases seem to occur in the fall and winter. Transmission is from direct animal contact. Nearly all patients (90% to 99%) report a recent exposure to a cat, and a history of a cat scratch or bite can be elicited in many (75% to 90%). In some series, kittens appear more likely to transmit disease than older cats. Most animals who transmit CSD are otherwise healthy. Rarely, the picture of CSD has been described in individuals without an animal exposure.

Bacillary angiomatosis: Unlike cat scratch disease, bacillary angiomatosis usually is seen in the immunocompromised, particularly in persons with AIDS. This infection usually occurs late in HIV infection; in one study the average CD4$^+$ cell count was 57/mm^3. Both *B. henselae* and *B. quintana* can cause this disease. A history of a recent cat scratch from a patient with bacillary angiomatosis is uncommon, in some series less than 20%. *B. henselae* has been isolated from the blood of pet cats in some AIDS patients with bacillary angiomatosis. Limited evidence suggests that fleas of infected cats may also become infected with *B. henselae*, although the importance of insect transmission is unknown. Since many cases of bacillary angiomatosis cannot be linked to a feline source, other modes of acquisition are likely and are currently being studied.

Clinical Syndromes

- **Cat scratch disease:** Typically, patients with CSD present with fever and painful lymphadenopathy. In 60% to 90% of cases an "inoculation lesion" is present, consisting of an erythematous pustule or papule at the site of the initial cat scratch or bite. These are most commonly found on the arms, head, and neck. The hallmark of CSD is regional adenopathy which develops within 2 weeks proximal to the initial site of the bite or inoculation lesion. Common nodes involved are the axillary, cervical, and supraclavicular nodes, but others have been described. Other symptoms include headache, malaise, arthralgias, and conjunctivitis. In 1% to 2% of cases, there may be unusual complications such as encephalopathy, Parinaud's oculoglandular syndrome, erythema nodosum, thrombocytopenic purpura, pneumonia, osteomyelitis, hepatosplenomegaly, and others.
- **Bacillary angiomatosis:** Bacillary angiomatosis can be either cutaneous or extracutaneous. Patients with cutaneous bacillary angiomatosis present with bright red round papules on the skin. Often they are multiple but occasionally may be solitary. These lesions are highly vascular and blanch on pressure. Often there are associated constitutional symptoms such as fever and malaise. The lesions may be difficult to distinguish from Kaposi's sarcoma in HIV-infected persons (see references).

Diagnosis A variety of methods are available to help diagnose *Bartonella* infection. The organism can be recovered from blood cultures and from tissue biopsy specimens. However, since the organism is fastidious, other methods may be helpful including:

- histologic examination of tissue (ie, lymph nodes) with Warthin-Starry staining
- serologic methods – indirect fluorescence antibody for *B. henselae* or enzyme immunoassay
- cat scratch skin test (not widely available)
- polymerase chain reaction

Treatment Successful therapy of cat scratch disease has been reported with a variety of antimicrobial agents including co-trimoxazole, ciprofloxacin, gentamicin, and rifampin. No controlled trials are available to determine the most beneficial therapy as each of these agents has also been associated with significant failure rates. The macrolides may also be effective as are the tetracyclines.

Drug Therapy
Recommended
Erythromycin *on page 561*
Doxycycline *on page 557*
Alternate
Co-trimoxazole *on page 545*

Selected Readings
Margileth AM, "Antibiotic Therapy for Cat-Scratch Disease: Clinical Study of Therapeutic Outcome in 268 Patients and a Review of the Literature," *Pediatr Infect Dis J*, 1992, 11:474-8.

Blastomyces dermatitidis

Microbiology *Blastomyces dermatitidis* is a dimorphic fungus uncommonly seen in the immunocompromised population. In the mold form, it has round to pyriform 4-5 μm conidia attached directly on the hyphae or on short stalks. Initially the colony appears yeast-like at room temperature then develops hyphal projections eventually becoming a fluffy white mold. The spores are difficult to isolate from the soil or bird droppings but have been recovered from wet soil.

The yeast form grows as a brown, wrinkled, folded colony at 37°C. Microscopically, the yeasts appear as round, budding, thick-walled yeast cells with a daughter cell forming a single bud that has a broad base 5-15 μm in diameter and which may be found extra- or intracellular in macrophages.

Epidemiology *Blastomyces* usually occurs in healthy hosts and is associated with point-source exposure; more commonly in men than women which may be secondary to more male occupational exposures. Immunosuppressed patients typically develop infection following exposure but may be secondary to

(Continued)

Blastomyces dermatitidis (Continued)

reactivation. It is uncommon in the AIDS population and is not recognized as an AIDS defining illness. When an AIDS patient does develop blastomycosis, it is usually more severe with multiple visceral involvement plus CNS infection and progresses to a fatal course rapidly.

It is endemic in the south-central and midwestern United States. After inhalation of the spores, which are taken up by bronchopulmonary macrophages, there is an approximate 45-day incubation period. The initial response is suppurative and progresses to granuloma formation (also referred to as a pyogranulomatous response). *Blastomyces* most commonly infects the lungs followed by skin, bone, prostate, and CNS.

Clinical Syndromes

- **Subclinical:** Approximately 60% of people living in an endemic area with occupational exposure have laboratory evidence via immune markers of *Blastomyces* but no clinical disease.
- **Acute blastomycosis:** Typically presents as a flu-like illness with fever, malaise, fatigue, weight loss, and pulmonary involvement. Occurs more commonly in men 25-50 years of age with occupational/environmental exposure. Rarely infects children except in epidemics.
- **Acute pneumonia:** Self-limited. Presents with fever, chills, purulent sputum, and sometimes hemoptysis. Chest radiograph reveals alveolar or mass-like infiltrates. May be associated with erythema nodosum.
- **Chronic pneumonia:** Symptoms last 2-6 months, and patient presents with weight loss, night sweats, fever, chest pain, and productive cough.
- **Cutaneous:** Verrucous or ulcerative lesions. Mimics squamous cell cancer and keratoacanthoma. May be found in the brain, skeletal system, prostate, myocardium, pericardium, sinuses, pituitary, or adrenal glands. May invade reticuloendothelial system.
- **Osteomyelitis:** Up to 25% of extrapulmonary cases. Noncaseating granulomas, suppuration or necrosis in the bone may occur. May require surgical debridement as well as antifungal treatment.
- **Genitourinary:** Prostatitis and epididymo-orchitis. Has been isolated in the urine after prostatic massage. Female tract complications have been reported transmitted by male sexual partner with cutaneous form of disease.
- **CNS:** Five percent to 10% disseminated disease may cause epidural or cranial abscesses, as well as meningitis.

No matter where the infection exists, always obtain a chest x-ray because there is almost always a simultaneous pulmonary infection. Infrequent complication is adult respiratory distress syndrome.

Diagnosis Skin test and serological markers are useful epidemiological tools but have too low sensitivity and specificity to be diagnostic. Diagnosis depends on direct examination of tissue or the isolation of *Blastomyces* in culture.

Diagnostic Tests/Procedures

Fungus Culture, Appropriate Site *on page 340*
Fungus Culture, Biopsy *on page 340*
Fungus Culture, Body Fluid *on page 341*
Fungus Culture, Skin *on page 343*
Fungal Serology *on page 337*

Treatment Therapy is determined by the severity of the clinical presentation and presentation and consideration of the toxicities of the antifungal agent. Typically pneumonia is self-limited to 1-2 weeks and does not require therapy. If the pneumonia persists and develops respiratory insufficiency or pleural disease, treatment with ketoconazole, 400-800 mg/day orally is recommended. Amphotericin B, up to 2 g, is recommended in life-threatening systemic disease. There is a 97% cure rate with amphotericin B as opposed to 89% with ketoconazole. Itraconazole, 200-400 mg/day orally may prove to have a higher cure rate then ketoconazole and is still under investigation as is fluconazole. Neither ketoconazole nor itraconazole penetrate the blood-brain barrier so they are not recommended for CNS involvement. Fluconazole, itraconazole, and ketoconazole are all used as suppressive therapy.

Drug Therapy

Recommended
Severe infection:
Amphotericin B *on page 493*
Chronic infection:
Ketoconazole *on page 598*

Alternate
Itraconazole *on page 594*
Fluconazole *on page 569*

Selected Readings
Bradsher RW, "Blastomycosis," *Clin Infect Dis*, 1992, 14(Suppl 1):S82-90.
Pappas PG, Pottage JC, Powderly WG, et al, "Blastomycosis in Patients With the Acquired Immunodeficiency Syndrome," *Ann Intern Med*, 1992, 116(10):847-53.

Blood Fluke *see Schistosoma mansoni on page 189*

Bordetella pertussis

Microbiology *Bordetella pertussis* is a fastidious, nonmotile, gram-negative coccobacillus which tends to arrange itself singly and in pairs. "Pertussis" means violent cough, an appropriate name for the etiologic agent of whooping cough. *B. pertussis* is difficult to grow in culture. The starch-blood-agar medium described by Bordet and Gengou in 1900 was first used to isolate this organism *in vitro*. Some modern microbiology laboratories still use the Bordet and Gengou medium, but others have adopted a synthetic medium with growth factors which supports the growth of this fastidious organism equally well. It is important to notify the microbiology laboratory promptly if infection with *B. pertussis* is suspected since the organism usually cannot grow on routine agar used for planting sputum and other respiratory specimens.

Several virulence factors for *Bordetella pertussis* have been identified.
- Filamentous hemagglutinin – promotes attachment of *Bordetella* to the respiratory epithelium.
- Tracheal cytotoxin – causes ciliostasis in the respiratory epithelium and direct tracheal cell damage. This interferes with the "first line of defense."
- Adenylate cyclase toxin – causes accumulation of cyclic AMP in leukocytes leading to impairment of phagocyte functions such as chemotaxis.
- Dermonecrotic toxin – causes ischemic necrosis of the soft tissue in mice and likely causes local damage to the tracheal mucosa.
- Pertussis toxin – causes a sustained impairment in phagocytosis by a variety of different biological mechanisms and is thought to account for many of the systemic manifestations of pertussis.

Epidemiology Despite the introduction of the pertussis vaccine in many countries, there are still an estimated 51 million cases of pertussis annually worldwide with 600,000 fatalities. In most populations, pertussis is endemic (ie, there is a relatively constant background level of disease), but superimposed epidemics occur at 3- to 4-year intervals. For example, recent peaks in pertussis in the United States occurred in 1983, 1986, and 1990.

The whole-cell pertussis vaccine became available in the United States in the early 1940s. Prior to this, pertussis was most common in children 1-5 years of age. Maternally-acquired antibodies provided passive protection in the first year of life. After the whole-cell pertussis vaccine was licensed as DTP in 1949, there was a steady decrease in the number of pertussis cases in the U.S., reaching a nadir of about 1000 cases in 1976. However, since 1976 there has been a steady increase in the number of pertussis cases in the U.S. with 1990 being a 20-year peak. It is not clear whether this represents a true increase in the incidence of pertussis in the community or whether there is only improved reporting of cases. In addition, there has been a shift in the population at highest risk. Infants younger than 1 year of age now account for half the reported cases; many of these infants were never vaccinated or did not receive vaccinations as recommended (2, 4, 6, and 15-18 months). Vaccination coverage in school-aged children has been relatively broad, accounting for much of the decline in pertussis in this older group.

Pertussis is a highly contagious infection with an attack rate estimated at 50% to 100%. Transmission is via the respiratory route with the organism being carried for several feet in aerosolized droplets. Humans are the only natural reservoir for *B. pertussis*. It is likely that infected adults with undiagnosed pertussis are the major (and perhaps only) reservoir for the organism, which is then transmitted by cough to a susceptible infant.

About 10% to 15% of pertussis cases now involve persons older than 15 years of age. Large outbreaks of pertussis are rare in adolescents and young adults. However, in Massachusetts during 1992, there was an unusual increase in the number of adult pertussis cases. In that year, 78% of reported cases involved people 10-19 years of age, with only 9% involving infants. Many of the cases involved an outbreak in a high school and nearby middle school. A similar outbreak was reported in a Maryland high school the same year. It is clear that

(Continued)

Bordetella pertussis (Continued)

vaccine immunity wanes over time and is estimated to last about 12 years. Thus, pertussis can occur in adolescents and adults, regardless of vaccination status as a child. Adults lacking immunity cannot offer passive immunity to infants, who are at the greatest risk for morbidity and mortality.

Clinical Syndromes

- **Pertussis or whooping cough:** The presentation of pertussis can be divided into three phases, catarrhal phase, paroxysmal (cough) phase, and recovery phase. The catarrhal stage of pertussis begins with symptoms of the common cold (rhinorrhea, conjunctivitis, coryza, and low-grade fever). Infants may present with apneic spells. This phase generally lasts from several days to 1 or more weeks and is indistinguishable from any other upper respiratory infection. After this, the patient develops a mild cough which escalates to severe, violent coughing, or the paroxysmal stage. The typical "whooping cough" is characterized by several brief expiratory coughs in succession followed by a rapid inspiration of air past a swollen glottis (which produces the classic "whoop"). Many patients will not present with the classic "whoop," particularly infants and adults. Vomiting after a paroxysm of coughing is common. The paroxysmal state may last for 1-4 weeks. Coughing paroxysms may continue for up to 6 months after infection. (In China, pertussis has been called the "cough of 100 days".) Potential complications of the paroxysmal state include severe vomiting with subsequent weight loss, dehydration, and malnutrition. Other complications include those related to high intrathoracic pressures (eg, subconjunctival hemorrhages, pneumothorax, hernias, etc). Secondary bacterial infections, such as aspiration pneumonia during vomiting and coughing, are the leading cause of death. Central nervous system manifestations are relatively common in pertussis. These include seizures and encephalopathy in up to 2% of hospitalized pertussis cases. During the recovery or convalescent phase, the cough and frequency of paroxysms slowly decreases. Apparent "relapses" of cough are not uncommon during the recovery phase but are most likely due to common respiratory viruses rather than relapses of *B. pertussis*.
- **"Atypical" pertussis:** The clinical picture described above may be altered in infants and in older individuals who are partially immunized. The catarrhal phase may be shortened or absent in some cases. Adults often do not have a typical "whoop," and thus, the diagnosis of pertussis is often not even considered. In HIV-infected persons, *B. pertussis* has been reported to cause a chronic, paroxysmal cough with dyspnea but otherwise negative cultures.

Diagnosis
Pertussis is often difficult to diagnose, particularly if the typical whooping cough is absent. Pertussis should be considered in the differential diagnosis of any person with a prolonged cough illness, regardless of the childhood DTP vaccination status. The laboratory diagnosis of *B. pertussis* is important, but many of the available laboratory techniques suffer from poor sensitivity, specificity, or both. Thus, a clinical case definition for pertussis has been used. For reporting purposes, the Centers for Disease Control have defined a clinical case of endemic or sporadic pertussis as any cough illness lasting 14 days or more (without apparent cause) with any of the following: paroxysms of coughing, inspiratory "whoop," or post-tussive vomiting.

In situations where an outbreak of pertussis is occurring, a clinical case has been defined as a cough illness lasting 14 days or more.

Laboratory confirmation of *B. pertussis* should be attempted in all suspected cases. Techniques include:

- Nasopharyngeal culture: This is considered the gold standard for diagnosing pertussis. If possible, a nasopharyngeal wash should be performed to maximize the yield, although a nasopharyngeal swab (calcium alginate swab) is acceptable. Despite careful specimen collection, *B. pertussis* may fail to grow in culture. This is considered a relatively insensitive technique.
- Direct fluorescent antibody (DFA): DFA systems for detection of *B. pertussis* are widely used but are also insensitive and have the additional problem of variable specificity. The CDC has recommended that DFA should not be used as the criterion for laboratory confirmation of pertussis.
- Serologic tests: Antibody tests for *B. pertussis* are only available on a research basis.
- Other techniques: Polymerase chain reaction (PCR) amplification of *B. pertussis* nucleic acid sequences appears promising but has not been standardized and is still considered a research tool.

Individuals with a prolonged cough and a nasopharyngeal culture positive for *B. pertussis* are considered to have a confirmed case of clinical pertussis (although *B. pertussis* can sometimes be cultured from asymptomatic contacts who never develop disease). Those with a positive DFA and cough for more than 14 days without culture confirmation still have a high likelihood of pertussis. Persons with a cough for longer than 14 days but with a negative DFA and negative culture may have pertussis to a variable degree of certainty, since other organisms can occasionally cause an acute respiratory illness followed by prolonged cough. Persons with a positive DFA, negative culture, and a cough less than 14 days have a much lower likelihood of pertussis. Persons with a cough less than 14 days and a negative DFA and culture probably do not have pertussis.

Diagnostic Tests/Procedures
Bordetella pertussis Direct Fluorescent Antibody *on page 282*
Bordetella pertussis Nasopharyngeal Culture *on page 283*
Bordetella pertussis Serology *on page 284*

Treatment Although a variety of antibiotics appear to be effective against *B. pertussis in vitro*, the drug of choice is erythromycin, given at a dose of 50 mg/kg/day, up to about 2 g daily. Erythromycin has been shown to decrease symptoms even if started after the catarrhal phase. Treatment should be at least 14 days, and longer courses may be necessary. Ampicillin has been associated with clinical failures and should not be used. Alternative agents include tetracycline, co-trimoxazole and chloramphenicol, but the data regarding clinical efficacy of these agents is limited. Hospitalization of infants may be warranted to avoid complications. Adjunctive therapies such as corticosteroids and beta-adrenergic agonists are either controversial or unwarranted and should be reserved for severe disease at physician discretion.

Prevention of *B. pertussis* remains the cornerstone for containment of this infection. There are two vaccines available, the whole-cell vaccine and the acellular vaccine. The whole-cell vaccine is used most frequently throughout the world with an efficacy of over 80% in most series. The main drawback of the whole-cell vaccine is its reactogenicity (local pain and swelling, systemic symptoms). The Centers for Disease Control recommends the whole-cell vaccine be administered as part of the diphtheria-tetanus-pertussis combination vaccine at 6-8 weeks, 4 months, 6 months, 15 months, and 4-6 years (before school entry). The acellular pertussis vaccine was developed to minimize the problems of reactogenicity of the whole-cell vaccine. Acellular pertussis vaccine is available in combination with diphtheria and tetanus toxoids (DTaP). DTaP is currently recommended only for use as the fourth and/or fifth doses of the DTP series among children aged 15 months to 6 years. The new acellular pertussis vaccines appear to be immunogenic in adults and less reactogenic (see references).

Drug Therapy
Recommended
Erythromycin *on page 561*
Alternate
Tetracycline *on page 679*
Co-trimoxazole *on page 545*
Chloramphenicol *on page 531*

Selected Readings
Addiss DG, Davis JP, Meade BD, et al, "A Pertussis Outbreak in a Wisconsin Nursing Home," *J Infect Dis*, 1991, 164(4):704-10.
Aoyama T, Takeuchi Y, Goto A, et al, "Pertussis in Adults," *Am J Dis Child*, 1992, 146(2):163-6.
Edwards KM, Decker MD, Graham BS, et al, "Adult Immunization With Acellular Pertussis Vaccine," *JAMA*, 1993, 269(1):53-6.
Farizo KM, Cochi SL, Zell ER, et al, "Epidemiological Features of Pertussis in the United States, 1980-89," *Clin Infect Dis*, 1992, 14(3):708-19.
Herwaldt LA, "Pertussis in Adults. What Physicians Need to Know," *Arch Intern Med*, 1991, 151(8):1510-2.
Hewlett EL, "*Bordetella* Species," *Principles and Practice of Infectious Diseases*, 4th ed, Mandell GL, Bennett JE, and Dolin R, eds, New York, NY: Churchill Livingstone, 1995, 2078-84.
Onorato IM and Wassilak SG, "Laboratory Diagnosis of Pertussis: The State of the Art," *Pediatr Infect Dis J*, 1987, 6(2):145-51.
"Pertussis Surveillance – United States, 1989-1991," *MMWR Morb Mortal Wkly Rep*, 1992, 41(SS-8):11-9.
"Pertussis Outbreaks: Massachusetts and Maryland, 1992," *MMWR Morb Mortal Wkly Rep*, 1993, 42(11):197-200.

Borrelia burgdorferi

Microbiology *Borrelia burgdorferi* is a tick-borne spirochete which causes Lyme disease.

Epidemiology Lyme disease (more properly, Lyme borreliosis) is the most commonly reported vectorborne illness in the United States. The spirochete is transmitted by the bite of the tick *Ixodes dammini*. These ticks are endemic in the northeast coastal regions of the U.S., the midwest, and the west coast. Nine states account for 90% of the cases: Massachusetts, New York, New Jersey, Connecticut, Rhode Island, Pennsylvania, Minnesota, Wisconsin, and California. In very endemic areas, 30% to 75% of *Ixodes dammini* ticks are infected with *B. burgdorferi*. Lyme disease is most common in individuals living near wooded areas with abundant deer, especially transitional zones of woods to brush. Peak seasons for Lyme disease are May to September, in particular June, July, and August.

There are two insect vectors that can transmit *B. burgdorferi*, *Ixodes dammini* and *Ixodes pacificus* (found on the west coast). *Ixodes dammini* is much more efficient in transmitting the disease. The tick has three stages. The larva hatches from eggs during the spring and ingests a blood meal from the white-footed mouse host (*Peromyscus leucopus*) later in the summer. An infected mouse then transmits the infection (*B. burgdorferi*) to the larva. The larva detach from the mouse and develop into nymphs during the following spring. The nymphal ticks feed during the late spring/summer on other white-footed mice and on human hosts. The nymphal ticks mature into adult male and female ticks and feed on white-tailed deer (*Odocoileus virginianus*) in the fall, winter, and early spring. Females lay eggs which will hatch to larva, and the cycle starts again.

Infection can be transmitted during any stage, but the nymphs are the most efficient. Since the nymph is the size of a poppy seed, it is easily missed or just brushed off. When the nymph bites, it secretes a cement-like substance to keep it attached to the host and secretes a coumarin-like substance which maintains the blood capillary feeding lesion. It feeds to engorgement over about 3 days. Approximately 10% of people bitten by infected ticks will acquire Lyme disease.

Clinical Syndromes The clinical manifestations of Lyme disease were originally divided into three stages: stage I, II, III. More recently, manifestations have been divided into early Lyme disease (stage I and II) and late (III).

Stage I: 3-32 days after the tick bite, a rash develops. A papule appears at the site of the bite followed by an annular (ring-like) rash which spreads outwardly. There is often an area of central clearing. This rash is termed erythema chronicum migrans (ECM). The rash usually resolves in time, even if untreated. Patients may complain of additional symptoms such as headache, malaise, and myalgias. In some, the infection progresses.

Stage II: This stage involves the heart and nervous system primarily. Cardiac symptoms begin about 5 weeks after the bite (range 4 days to 7 months). Atrioventricular heart block is the most common finding and is usually self-limited. From 10% to 20% of people will develop neurologic disease weeks to months after the bite. This includes aseptic meningitis, cranial nerve palsy, peripheral radiculopathy, and Bell's palsy. Examination of the cerebrospinal fluid may show a lymphocytic pleocytosis. Intrathecal production of IgG directed against *B. burgdorferi* can be shown in some patients.

Stage III: Arthritis is the hallmark of stage III Lyme disease. The large joints are generally involved (knees, hips, etc). Joint symptoms begin from several days to over 2 years after the erythema chronicum migrans rash.

Diagnosis Lyme disease is a clinical diagnosis, not a laboratory diagnosis. Laboratory tests are not standardized and **never** should be used alone.

Diagnostic Tests/Procedures
Lyme Disease Serology *on page 394*
Lyme Disease Serology by Western Blot *on page 394*

Treatment The treatment for Lyme disease depends in large part on the stage of the disease.
- Erythema chronicum migrans: Doxycycline is the drug of choice, but also effective are amoxicillin, penicillin, and erythromycin.
- Carditis: Ceftriaxone or penicillin
- Neurologic: Ceftriaxone or penicillin
- Arthritis: Ceftriaxone or penicillin

Pediatric Drug Therapy
Recommended
Ceftriaxone Sodium *on page 523*

Alternate
Ampicillin *on page 495*
Penicillin G, Parenteral *on page 633*

Adult Drug Therapy

Recommended
Ceftriaxone Sodium *on page 523*
Doxycycline *on page 557*

Alternate
Ampicillin *on page 495*
Penicillin G, Parenteral *on page 633*

Selected Readings
"Lyme Disease – United States, 1991-1992," *MMWR Morb Mortal Wkly Rep*, 1993, 42(18):345-8.
Rahn DW, Malawista SE, "Lyme Disease: Recommendation for Diagnosis and Treatment," *Ann Intern Med*, 1991, 114(6):472-81.
Sigal LH, "The Polymerase Chain Reaction Assay for *Borrelia burgdorferi* in the Diagnosis of Lyme Disease," *Ann Intern Med*, 1994, 120(6):520-1.
Spach DH, Liles WC, Campbell GL, et al, "Tick-Borne Diseases in the United States," *N Engl J Med*, 1993, 329(13):936-47.
Steere AC, "Lyme Disease," *N Engl J Med*, 1989, 321(9):586-96.

Branhamella catarrhalis *see Moraxella catarrhalis on page 147*

Brucella Species

Microbiology *Brucella* species are small, aerobic, gram-negative coccobacilli which primarily cause disease in domestic animals. There are four species which cause human disease:
- *B. abortus* (cattle)
- *B. melitensis* (goats and sheep)
- *B. suis* (swine)
- *B. canis* (dogs)

The organism is nonmotile and does not form spores. All species tend to be slow-growing and fastidious. Supplemental carbon dioxide is required for optimal growth of *B. abortus*. The cell walls of *B. abortus*, *B. suis*, and *B. melitensis* contain endotoxin and two major surface antigens (A and M). The endotoxin is structurally and biologically different from endotoxins produced by many other enteric gram-negative bacilli.

Epidemiology Human brucellosis occurs worldwide. Approximately 500,000 cases are reported annually. The incidence has declined following mandatory pasteurization of dairy products and immunization of cattle with live-attenuated *Brucella abortus* vaccine. Endemic areas include the Mediterranean basin, South America, and Mexico. In the United States, more than half the cases of human brucellosis occur in Texas, California, Virginia, and Florida. A small number of cases (1% to 2%) result from exposure to *Brucella* in the microbiology or research laboratory.

Transmission to humans occurs by one of three routes:
- Direct contact of infected tissue, blood, or lymph with broken skin or conjunctivae
- Ingestion of contaminated meat or dairy products
- Inhalation of infected aerosols

Clinical Syndromes *Brucella* species enter the human via breaks in the skin or mucous membranes or via inhalation. Normal human serum has good bactericidal activity against *B. abortus* but not *B. melitensis*. Organisms not killed by polymorphonuclear leukocytes travel to regional lymph nodes, then enter the circulation, and localize in organs of the reticuloendothelial system where they are ingested by macrophages. Some will survive intracellularly and multiply, but when the macrophage is activated, the intracellular organisms are killed and release endotoxin. The host response to endotoxin can result in the signs and symptoms of acute brucellosis.

The clinical manifestations depend on both the immune status of the patient and the species of *Brucella* involved.
- **Asymptomatic infection**
- **Acute brucellosis, or "Malta fever":** Acute symptoms appear 1 week to several months following exposure. Symptoms include fever, sweats, chills, weakness, malaise, headache, and anorexia. In 25% to 50% of cases, there is weight loss, myalgias, arthralgias, and back pain. Epididymis is common in some series. Splenomegaly occurs in 20% to 30% of

(Continued)

Brucella Species *(Continued)*

cases and lymphadenopathy in 10% to 20%.

A number of complications of acute brucellosis have been reported. When infection is present for more than 2 months without therapy, the complication rate can approach 30%.

- **Musculoskeletal:** Sacroiliitis, arthritis, osteomyelitis, paraspinal abscess
- **Neurologic:** Meningoencephalitis, myelitis, others
- **Genitourinary:** Epididymo-orchitis, prostatitis
- **Endocarditis**
- **Granulomatous hepatitis**
- **Caseating or noncaseating granulomatous disease**
- **Splenic abscess**
- **Nodular lung lesions; lung abscess**
- **Erythema nodosum; other skin manifestations**
- **Ocular lesions**
- **Localized disease:** Can occur in any of the sites listed above
- **Subclinical infection**

Diagnosis The clinician should suspect brucellosis in any individual presenting with fever and who has a history of travel to endemic areas; exposure to livestock; a history of consuming unpasteurized milk, cheese, or other dairy products; or suggestive occupational risk factors (veterinarians, laboratory workers, etc). Laboratory confirmation is essential since the signs and symptoms of human brucellosis may be nonspecific. The diagnosis is established by recovery of the organism from blood, fluid, or other tissues (bone, abscesses, etc). In patients with *B. melitensis* infections, cultures of blood will be positive in 70% of cases. Bone marrow biopsy for histopathology and culture may be positive when other specimens are negative. In many laboratories, blood cultures for *Brucella* sp are processed using the Castañeda technique which utilizes biphasic media in a bottle. The microbiology laboratory should always be informed if *Brucella* sp are highly suspected.

Serologic techniques for diagnosing brucellosis include a standard tube agglutination test. A *Brucella* titer of ≥1:160 or a fourfold rise in titer is considered presumptive evidence of recent infection with *Brucella* sp.

Diagnostic Tests/Procedures
Aerobic Culture, Appropriate Site *on page 244*
Blood Culture, *Brucella on page 274*
Gram Stain *on page 352*

Treatment The recommendation from the World Health Organization for the treatment of acute brucellosis is doxycycline 200 mg/day with rifampin 600-900 mg/day for 6 weeks. Longer courses may be required in severe infections or if focal suppurative complications are present. Single agent therapy with tetracycline, streptomycin, rifampin, or trimethoprim are associated with a high relapse rate. For relapsed infection or central nervous system infection, the suggested regimens are third generation cephalosporin and rifampin or tetracycline, streptomycin, and rifampin, in combination. A consultation with an infectious disease specialist is recommended for suspected cases in the United States.

Pediatric Drug Therapy
Recommended
Co-trimoxazole *on page 545*
used in combination with
Gentamicin Sulfate *on page 575*

Adult Drug Therapy
Recommended
Doxycycline *on page 557*
used in combination with
Rifampin *on page 662*

Alternate
Co-trimoxazole *on page 545*
used in combination with
Gentamicin Sulfate *on page 575*

Selected Readings

Ariza J, Gudiol F, Pallares R, et al, "Treatment of Human Brucellosis With Doxycycline Plus Rifampin or Doxycycline Plus Streptomycin," *Ann Intern Med*, 1992, 117(1):25-30.

"Brucellosis Outbreak at a Pork Processing Plant – North Carolina, 1992," *MMWR Morb Mortal Wkly Rep*, 1994, 43(7):113-6.

Kaye D, "Brucellosis," *Harrison's Principles of Internal Medicine*, 13th ed, Isselbacher KJ, Braunwald E, Wilson JD, et al, eds, New York, NY: McGraw-Hill, 1994, 685-7.

ORGANISMS

Shehabi A, Shakir K, el Khateeb M, et al, "Diagnosis and Treatment of 106 Cases of Human Brucellosis," *J Infect*, 1990, 20(1):5-10.

Wise RI, "Brucellosis in the United States. Past, Present, and Future," *JAMA*, 1980, 244(20):2318-22.

Young EJ, "Serologic Diagnosis of Human Brucellosis: Analysis of 214 Cases by Agglutination Tests and Review of the Literature," *Rev Infect Dis*, 1991, 13(3):359-72.

Calymmatobacterium granulomatis

Microbiology *Calymmatobacterium granulomatis* is the causative agent of granuloma inguinale, a sexually transmitted disease. The organism is an encapsulated gram-negative bacillus found within vacuoles of large histiocytic cells. The bacteria multiply within these vacuoles (about 30 organisms per vacuole), mature, and eventually rupture the cell.

Epidemiology Granuloma inguinale, also referred to as Donovanosis, is quite rare in the United States, but in many developing countries, it is one of the most prevalent sexually transmitted diseases. Granuloma inguinale is common in India, the Caribbean, and Africa. In 1984, an outbreak of 20 cases was recognized in Texas (Rosen et al). The epidemiology and pathogenesis of donovanosis in the United States (and endemic countries as well) are poorly characterized. The precise role of sexual transmission is unclear, but repeated anal intercourse appears to be a risk factor for rectal and penile lesions in homosexual couples. Available data suggest that the infection is only mildly contagious and repeated exposures to an infected partner are necessary for transmission.

Clinical Syndromes

- **Granuloma inguinale**: The major disease associated with *Calymmatobacterium granulomatis* is granuloma inguinale, an infection characterized by genital ulceration and regional lymphadenopathy. As such, it must be differentiated from other classic STDs which can cause genital ulceration with regional adenopathy, such as primary syphilis, genital herpes simplex virus, chancroid, and lymphogranuloma venereum.

- **Genital ulcers:** The incubation period for granuloma inguinale varies from 8-80 days. Genital lesions initially appear as subcutaneous nodules (either single or multiple) which later erode. The ulcerations that form above the nodules are painless, clean, granulomatous, and often "beefy-red" with occasional contact bleeding. The lesions are most common on the glans or prepuce of the male and labial area in the female. The ulcers progressively enlarge in a chronic, destructive fashion. The ulcerations of donovanosis may be misidentified as carcinoma of the penis, chancroid, condyloma lata of secondary syphilis (when perianal lesions are present), and others.

- **Inguinal enlargement:** Infection with *Calymmatobacterium granulomatis* does not produce true regional lymphadenopathy. Instead, the granulomatous process in the genitals may extend into the inguinal region causing further fibrosis and granulation tissue, termed "pseudobuboes." These are present in only 10% of patients with donovanosis and are variably painful.

- **Constitutional symptoms:** In most cases of granuloma inguinale, constitutional symptoms are usually absent.

Diagnosis The diagnosis of granuloma inguinale can be confirmed by finding the characteristic "**Donovan bodies**" in a crush preparation. Fresh granulation tissue from a genital ulcer is spread over a clean microscope slide, air-dried, and stained with Wright or Giemsa stain. "Donovan bodies" are multiple, darkly-staining intracytoplasmic bacteria (*Calymmatobacterium granulomatis*) found within the vacuoles of large mononuclear cells. Donovan bodies can also be identified in formal biopsy specimens using standard light microscopy.

Treatment Granuloma inguinale responds well to the following first-line oral antibiotics (used singly): tetracycline 500 mg orally 4 times/day, ampicillin 500 mg 4 times/day, or co-trimoxazole (Bactrim™ DS) twice daily. Antibiotics are continued until the lesions are completely healed, usually 21 days or more; shorter courses are associated with relapses. Alternative therapies include chloramphenicol 500 mg orally 3 times/day or gentamicin 1 mg/kg twice daily. In pregnancy, erythromycin 500 mg orally 4 times/day is recommended. The treatment for HIV-infected individuals with granuloma inguinale is the same.

Drug Therapy

Recommended

Tetracycline *on page 679*
Ampicillin *on page 495*
Co-trimoxazole *on page 545*

ORGANISMS

Alternate
Chloramphenicol *on page 531*
Gentamicin Sulfate *on page 575*
Erythromycin *on page 561*

Selected Readings

Holmes KK, "Donovanosis (Granuloma Inguinale)," *Harrison's Principles of Internal Medicine*, 13th ed, Isselbacher KJ, Braunwald E, Wilson JD, et al, eds, New York, NY: McGraw-Hill, 1994, 694-5.

Krockta WP and Barnes RC, "Sexually Transmitted Diseases. Genital Ulceration With Regional Adenopathy," *Infect Dis Clin North Am*, 1987, 1(1):217-33.

Rosen T, Tschen JA, Ramsdell W, et al, "Granuloma Inguinale," *J Am Acad Dermatol*, 1984, 11(3):433-7.

"1993 Sexually Transmitted Diseases Treatment Guidelines. Centers for Disease Control and Prevention," *MMWR Morb Mortal Wkly Rep*, 1993, 42(RR-14):1-102.

Campylobacter jejuni

Microbiology *Campylobacter jejuni* is a curved, gram-negative bacillus which is the most common cause of bacterial diarrhea in the United States. On Gram stain, *Campylobacter jejuni* appears as a curved, comma-shaped, gram-negative rod which often has a distinctive "seagull wing" appearance.

Campylobacter jejuni is a microaerophilic organism and fails to grow under routine aerobic and anaerobic conditions. The laboratory should be informed that *C. jejuni* is suspected clinically and a special request made for *Campylobacter* culture. A 5% to 10% oxygen, 5% to 10% carbon dioxide, and 80% to 90% nitrogen atmosphere is generally used to facilitate growth.

Epidemiology Infection with this agent occurs worldwide. With over 2 million cases per year in the U.S., *Campylobacter*-induced enteritis is more common than *Salmonella* and *Shigella* combined. The organism is found in the gastrointestinal flora of a number of wild and domestic animals, most notably in chickens. Transmission to humans generally occurs by consumption of the meat or milk of an infected animal, consumption of water contaminated with the feces of infected animals (eg, mountain streams), or fecal-oral transmission from an infected human or household pet. Undercooked chicken is notorious for transmission of *C. jejuni*, accounting for more than 50% of the cases of campylobacteriosis. Outbreaks have been linked to unpasteurized goat's cheese, clams, and untreated stream water in Wyoming. Infection occurs year round but is most common in the summer months.

Clinical Syndromes

- **Acute enteritis:** The organism can cause destructive, ulcerative changes in the mucosal surfaces of the small intestine (especially jejunum and distal ileum) and colon. Invasion of the organism causes inflammation of the lamina propria, bowel wall edema, and crypt abscesses. Patients initially present with nonspecific symptoms such as fever, headache, and myalgias. One to 2 days later, there is crampy abdominal pain and diarrhea. The quality and severity of the diarrhea is variable (although usually mild), and stools may be frequent and watery or visibly bloody. Most cases resolve spontaneously without antimicrobial therapy within 1 week. Less commonly, a fulminant acute colitis may occur. Again, a nonspecific prodrome of fever and malaise precedes any gastrointestinal complaints. However, the diarrhea which follows is voluminous and bloody with large amounts of mucous. Tenesmus is common and further suggests involvement of the colon. Fevers can reach 40°C and occasionally the patient can appear in extremis. This syndrome may be confused with bacillary dysentery from *Shigella* species, severe salmonellosis, or even the initial presentation of inflammatory bowel disease (particularly if it is in a young adult). Toxic megacolon may complicate the hospital course.

- **Appendicitis-like syndrome:** Occasionally, *C. jejuni* can cause right lower quadrant pain mimicking appendicitis, without diarrhea. This "pseudoappendicitis" has been seen in association with other enteric pathogens including *Yersinia enterocolitica*.

- **Bacteremia:** This is an unusual finding in *C. jejuni* infection (even when the patient is febrile), unlike *Campylobacter fetus* which is commonly recovered from the blood. Blood cultures may turn positive several days after a mild diarrheal illness has already resolved; in such cases, antibiotic therapy is usually unnecessary. In other cases, bacteremia may be sustained, particularly in immunocompromised hosts, and this may suggest a deep focus of infection. Infectious disease consultation is appropriate in such cases since prolonged antimicrobial therapy may be necessary.

- **Septic abortion:** *C. jejuni* infection in the pregnant female may lead to this complication. However, *Campylobacter* bacteremia during pregnancy does not automatically justify a therapeutic abortion since the outcome is not uniformly poor.

- **Reactive arthritis:** Following *Campylobacter* enteritis, a reactive arthritis may be seen, particularly in patients who are HLA-B27 positive.
- **Miscellaneous:** Guillain-Barré syndrome, hepatitis, and the hemolytic-uremic syndrome have been associated with *C. jejuni.*

Diagnosis *Campylobacter jejuni* should be suspected in any case of acute gastroenteritis or fulminant colitis. The findings of fecal leukocytes and occult blood in the stool is suggestive of campylobacteriosis and other gastrointestinal infections such as those caused by *Salmonella* sp, *Shigella* sp, enteroinvasive *E. coli,* enterohemorrhagic *E. coli* (0157:H7), Crohn's disease or ulcerative colitis, and others. The diagnosis is confirmed by a positive stool culture for *C. jejuni* or positive blood cultures for the organism.

Diagnostic Tests/Procedures
Blood Culture, Aerobic and Anaerobic *on page 271*
Stool Culture *on page 448*

Treatment The organism is sensitive *in vitro* to many common antimicrobial agents including erythromycin, ciprofloxacin, tetracyclines, aminoglycosides, and others. Ampicillin or penicillin should usually be avoided, and the susceptibility to co-trimoxazole is variable. Most patients with *Campylobacter* enteritis do not require antibiotics; they recover quickly without sequelae. Antimicrobial therapy should be targeted towards the more acutely ill patient. Limited clinical trials suggest that the following groups may benefit from the prompt use of antibiotics: children with severe dysentery, adults with severe bloody diarrhea and fever, individuals with worsening symptoms when seeking medical attention, and prolonged diarrhea (more than 1 week). Treatment with antibiotics does not prolong the fecal carriage of *C. jejuni* (as opposed to *Salmonella*). The drug of choice is erythromycin. For the toxic patient, combination therapy may be useful, but consultation should be made with an Infectious Disease specialist.

Drug Therapy
Recommended
Erythromycin *on page 561*
Doxycycline *on page 557*
Alternate
Fluoroquinolones *on page 571*

Selected Readings
Blaser MJ, Wells JG, Feldman RA, et al, "*Campylobacter* enteritis in the United States. A Multicenter Study," *Ann Intern Med*, 1983, 98(3):360-5.
Johnson RJ, Nolan C, Wang SP, et al, "Persistent *Campylobacter jejuni* Infection in an Immunocompromised Patient," *Ann Intern Med*, 1984, 100(6):832-4.
Peterson MC, Farr RW, and Castiglia M, "Prosthetic Hip Infection and Bacteremia Due to *Campylobacter jejuni* in a Patient With AIDS," *Clin Infect Dis*, 1993, 16(3):439-40.
Sorvillo FJ, Lieb LE, and Waterman SH, "Incidence of Campylobacteriosis Among Patients With AIDS in Los Angeles County," *J Acquir Immune Defic Syndr*, 1991, 4(6):598-602.

Campylobacter pylori see Helicobacter pylori on page 121

Candida Species

Microbiology *Candida* species are normal host saprophyte yeasts found commonly in the gastrointestinal tract, genitourinary tract, and oropharynx. On direct mounts of infected material, they appear as small, oval, thin-walled, budding cells 2-5 μm in diameter with or without the presence of pseudohyphae. They stain gram-positive.

C. albicans is identified by the ability to produce germ tubes and/or chlamydospores in cornmeal agar. All *Candida* species may be distinguished by sugar fermentation and assimilation tests.

Epidemiology *Candida* species are found worldwide. Seventy percent of nosocomial candidal infections are due to *Candida albicans*. The other 30% are due to *C. glabrata, C. guilliermondii, C. krusei, C. pseudotropicalis, C. stellatoidea,* and *C. tropicalis.* According to the National Nosocomial Infections Surveillance System, *Candida* is now the fifth most common blood pathogen isolated from hospitalized patients and the fourth most common in ICU patients.

Risk factors for candidiasis include age extremes, central venous catheters, TPN, burns, exogenous hormone therapy, prosthetic devices, malnourishment, metabolic disease, concurrent infections with other pathogens, antibiotic therapy, uncontrolled diabetes mellitus, GI surgery, AIDS, mechanical disruption of epithelial surfaces, and physiological impairment of epithelial barrier function.

(Continued)

Candida Species *(Continued)*

Clinical Syndromes

- **Cutaneous:** Intertriginous infection occurs most commonly in diabetes and obesity. Patients present with pain, burning and/or itching. Skin appears uniformly erythematous and inflamed with small papules and pustules. May have satellites distal to the border of the lesion. Follicular candidiasis usually occurs in areas that are occluded (ie, under bandages). Paronychial infection is characterized by swelling, tenderness, and redness around the nail.

- **Oral candidiasis:** Early premonitory sign of HIV. Presents as pseudomembranous, hyperplastic, atrophic, or angular cheilitis. Most commonly appears as erythematous patches with white discharge on the buccal mucosa with complaints of burning. The most efficient and cost-effective method of diagnosis is direct microscopic detection of *Candida* in a scraped sample of the oral lesion.

- **Candiduria:** Significance and natural history of progression are not known. Colony count not predictive of severity of infection or location. Treatment based on clinical judgment of severity of illness and risk factors. Symptoms include nocturia, frequency, and dysuria. Associated with urethritis, cystitis, and primary renal candidiasis.

- **Disseminated:** Requires pathological identification of organism (yeast) in tissues and growth of the yeast in culture. Thirty percent of patients with fungemia have endophthalmitis. Rarely occurs early postoperatively. It is indistinguishable from bacterial sepsis and can occur simultaneously with bacterial pathogens. Only 25% of the patients with extensive invasive organ infection will have positive blood cultures. Mortality exceeds 80%. Ten percent to 13% will have cutaneous manifestations. Other foci include septic arthritis, osteomyelitis, pericarditis (especially status post open heart surgery), suppurative phlebitis, and abscesses. Dissemination is likely if three or more colonized sites are present.

- **Vulvovaginitis:** Second most common cause of vaginal infections. Seventy-five percent childbearing age women will acquire this infection, and 40% will have a second occurrence. Less than 5% experience recurrent disease defined as more than four infections in a 12-month period. Eighty-five percent are due to *C. albicans*. Associated with pregnancy, high estrogen oral contraceptives, uncontrolled diabetes mellitus, tight-fitting clothes, antibiotic therapy, dietary factors, intestinal colonization, AIDS, and sexually transmitted disease. Human to human transmission is questionable, although male sexual partners may experience a transient rash, erythema, pruritus or burning sensation of the penis minutes to hours after unprotected sexual intercourse. May cause balanitis. Present with marked itching, watery to cottage cheese thick discharge, vaginal erythema with adherent white discharge, dyspareunia, external dysuria, erythema, and swelling of labia and vulva with discrete pustulopapular peripheral lesions. Cervix appears normal. Symptoms exacerbate the week preceding menses with some relief once menstrual flow begins.

Diagnosis Diagnosis is dependent on visualization of budding yeast with or without pseudohypha and the presence of clinical symptoms. If wet mounts, KOH, or histological stains are negative, need growth of yeast in culture. Endophthalmitis diagnosed by vitrectomy or anterior chamber aspiration (presumptive diagnosis by indirect fundoscopic exam). Serological tests such as nonspecific antigen tests vary in sensitivity and specificity. Serological detection of mannan, beta-1,3-glucan, and enolase are still investigational.

Diagnostic Tests/Procedures

Fungus Culture, Appropriate Site *on page 340*
Gram Stain *on page 352*
KOH Preparation *on page 379*

Treatment

Cutaneous: Requires drying. Nystatin powder or imidazole (butoconazole, clotrimazole, miconazole, tioconazole) powder. Topical steroids may be used to reduce inflammation for the first 5-7 days of therapy. Paronychia infections may require, topical imidazole up to 3 months.

Oral candidiasis: Nystatin 100,000 units 3-5 times/day for 14 days versus azoles topically or orally.

Candiduria: Remove predisposing factors, (ie, Foley catheter). Recommend amphotericin B irrigation 50 mg in 1 L sterile water continuous for 5 days. Alternate therapy includes flucytosine or azoles (fluconazole 50-100 mg/day for 7 days).

Disseminated: Drainage or debridement of accessible sites. Recommended therapy is amphotericin B 0.5 mg/kg daily for 14 days. Fluconazole at doses 200-400 mg/day has been shown to be effective but not against *C. krusei* or *C. glabrata*. Endophthalmitis may require subtenonian or intracameral injection of amphotericin B.

Vulvovaginitis: Imidazole derivatives (butoconazole, clotrimazole, miconazole, tioconazole) and triazole derivative (terconazole) (85% to 90%) are better than polyene preparations (nystatin) (75%). Extensive vulvar inflammation usually requires topical cream. For resistant or recurrent infections, oral agents are preferred (ketoconazole 400 mg orally 5-14 days, fluconazole 100 mg orally one dose, or itraconazole 200 mg orally 3 days). Both ketoconazole and fluconazole are effective prophylactic agents. Single dose fluconazole 150 mg has also been approved for use.

Drug Therapy
Recommended
Amphotericin B *on page 493*
Fluconazole *on page 569*
Ketoconazole *on page 598*
Antifungal, Topical *on page 498*
Alternate
Itraconazole *on page 594*

Selected Readings
Burchard, KW, "Fungal Sepsis," *Infect Dis Clin North Am*, 1992, 6(3):677-92.
Gubbins PO, Piscitelli SC, and Danziger LH, "Candidal Urinary Tract Infections: A Comprehensive Review of Their Diagnosis and Management," *Pharmacotherapy*, 1993, 13(2):110-27.
Pariser DM, "Cutaneous Candidiasis. A Practical Guide for Primary Care Physicians," *Postgrad Med*, 1990, 87(6):101-3, 106-8.
Peterson DE, "Oral Candidiasis," *Clin Geriatr Med*, 1992, 8(3):513-27.
Sobel JD, "Candidal Vulvovaginitis," *Clin Obstet Gynecol*, 1993, 36(1):153-65.

Cestodes

Synonyms Tapeworms

Microbiology Cestodes (tapeworms; segmented worms) are intestinal and tissue parasites of mammals and some fish and are found worldwide. Cestodes have complex life cycles which involve intermediate hosts, in which the worms develop into only a larvae, and definitive hosts, in which worms have sexual reproduction and develop into adults. Humans can serve as both kinds of hosts. Cestodes can be divided into two groups according to the common sites they infect in humans, intestinal and tissue cestodes (see table). Cestodes cause illness in humans in two stages of their life cycles, larvae and adults. If larvae are ingested, the larvae mature into adults which attach by their heads to the intestinal mucosa, grow, lay eggs, and usually produce only minimal damage and discomfort to the host. If eggs are ingested, stomach acid releases larvae from eggs, larvae migrate to specific organs, and encyst. Cysts can grow and damage surrounding tissue. The form of the cyst (cysticercus, coenurus, hydatid cyst, etc) depends on the type of cestode.

Epidemiology Cestodes are parasites of humans, wild animals, domestic animals, and fish. Cestodes and cestode diseases have been recognized since the time of Hippocrates and continue to occur worldwide. Infections occur almost invariably because of poor sanitation habits, carelessness, ingestion of poorly cooked meat, or letting infected animals lick oral membranes (eg, child being licked by dog or cat which has crushed infected fleas in its mouth).

Clinical Syndromes The presentation of someone infected with cestodes is astonishingly varied and includes but is not limited to the following: unusual "things" in stools, "uncomfortable" intestinal symptoms, change in mental status, abdominal cramps, "hunger pains", etc. In addition CNS symptoms (headache, hemiparesis, altered vision, seizures, etc) can suggest cystic disease.

Diagnosis Diagnosis is most commonly made by ova and parasite examination (for eggs and proglottids) of stool. Cystic disease is visualized best by CT or MRI of suspected infected organs (often, brain and liver). Sensitive and specific serological tests (enzyme immunoassay and Western blot) are available for detecting antibody to *Echinococcus*.

Diagnostic Tests/Procedures
Brain Biopsy *on page 285*
Computed Transaxial Tomography, Appropriate Site *on page 307*
Magnetic Resonance Scan, Brain *on page 397*
Ova and Parasites, Stool *on page 416*

Cestodes

Cestode	Ingested Infectious Form and Source
Intestinal	
Diphyllobothrium latum	Larvae in freshwater fish
Taenia solium	Larvae in undercooked pork or eggs in soil or feces
Taenia saginata	Larvae in undercooked beef or eggs in soil or feces
Hymenolepis nana	Larvae in arthropods or eggs in human feces
Hymenolepis diminuta	Larvae in arthropods or eggs in human feces
Dipylidium caninum	Larvae in dog fleas
Tissue	
Echinococcus granulosus	Eggs in dog feces
Echinococcus multilocularis	Eggs in fox and cat feces
Spirometra mansonoides	Larvae in freshwater fish
Diphyllobothrium latum	Larvae in freshwater fish
Multiceps sp	Eggs in dog fleas

Drug Therapy
Recommended
  Praziquantel *on page 650*
Alternate
  Niclosamide *on page 622*
Selected Readings
  Garcia LS and Bruckner DA, *Diagnostic Medical Parasitology*, Washington DC: American Society for Microbiology, 1993, 266-301.
  King CH, "Cestodes (Tapeworms)," *Principles and Practice of Infectious Diseases*, 4th ed, Mandell GL, Bennett JE, and Dolin R, eds, New York, NY: Churchill Livingstone, 1995, 2544-53.
  Maddison SE, "Serodiagnosis of Parasitic Diseases," *Clin Microbiol Rev*, 1991, 4(4):457-69.

Chlamydia pneumoniae

Synonyms *Chlamydia* TWAR; TWAR

Microbiology *Chlamydia pneumoniae*, like all *Chlamydia*, is an obligate intracellular bacterium, which stains gram-negative. This newly described agent was originally named *Chlamydia* TWAR, named after the first two clinical isolates (TW-183 from the eye of a child in a trachoma vaccine study, and AR-39 from a throat swab of a student with pharyngitis). Both names are used interchangeably. *Chlamydia pneumoniae* is one of three distinct species within the genus *Chlamydia*. The two other species of *Chlamydia* are *C. psittaci* (the cause of psittacosis) and *C. trachomatis* (a cause of nongonococcal urethritis and the eye infection called trachoma). *C. pneumoniae* shares about 5% DNA sequence homology with *C. trachomatis* and about 10% with *C. psittaci*. *Chlamydia* species are unique in having two separate forms with separate functions: the elementary body (EB), which is well-suited for extracellular life but lacks the ability to replicate and the reticulate body (RB), which is adapted to intracellular life and can divide by binary fission.

The life cycle of *Chlamydia pneumoniae* is as follows:
1. Elementary bodies attach to the host cell,
2. EBs enter the cell by inducing their own phagocytosis,
3. EBs transform into larger reticulate bodies,
4. The RBs grow and replicate by binary fission within vacuoles; these vacuoles become filled with EBs and appear as inclusion bodies in the host cytoplasm,
5. Vacuoles rupture and release infectious organisms, and the cycle begins again.

Epidemiology There is no known animal reservoir for *C. pneumoniae*, unlike *C. psittaci* which is highly associated with birds. Transmission is person-to-person. Seroprevalence studies have shown that infection is uncommon in early childhood and increases during the teenage years (prevalence 25% to 50%). Many adults are seropositive, and some believe that nearly all adults are infected at least once.

Clinical Syndromes

- **Atypical pneumonia:** *C. pneumoniae* has been recognized as an important cause of community-acquired pneumonia. Approximately 10% of both outpatient and inpatient pneumonias are caused by this agent. Patients present with subacute malaise, cough, and low-grade fever. Hoarseness and pharyngitis are prominent. Chest x-ray show a single subsegmental infiltrate in most cases. The disease is usually mild to moderate in severity, but symptoms may be prolonged.

- **Bronchitis:** *C. pneumoniae* is also a frequent cause of bronchitis, accounting for about 45% of bronchitis cases in young adults. Typically, patients present with pharyngitis followed by dry cough. Chest x-rays are clear.

- **Pharyngitis:** Cases may be quite severe, with prolonged hoarseness. Some cases progress to lower respiratory tract infections.

- **Sinusitis:** The spectrum of *C. pneumoniae* sinusitis is becoming better recognized. In young adults, about 5% of cases of primary sinusitis are due to *C. pneumoniae*.

- **Other:** Fever of unknown origin, influenza-like illness

Diagnosis *Chlamydia pneumoniae* should be suspected in any case of atypical pneumonia, particularly if there is pharyngitis and hoarseness. Other diagnostic considerations for atypical pneumonia should include *Mycoplasma pneumoniae*, *Legionella* infections, viral lower respiratory infections, and others. The diagnosis can be confirmed primarily with serologic studies. The antigens which are used for antibody tests include lipopolysaccharide antigens and major outer membrane protein antigens. Lipopolysaccharide antigen is common to all members of the *Chlamydia* genus. This antigen is measured using complement fixation. Thus, positive studies are not specific for *C. pneumoniae* and can be positive during *C. trachomatis* and *C. psittaci* infections. Major outer membrane proteins (MOMPs) are specific for the different species of *Chlamydia*. These proteins are the basis for microimmunofluorescence (MIF) studies.

There are two patterns of antibody response with Chlamydial infections. Primary infection: Early on, complement fixation antibody is positive; 10 days to 1 month, MIF IgM is positive; 6 weeks, IgG is positive. Secondary infection: Complement fixation antibody is negative; IgM is positive in low titer; IgG response is more prompt. *C. pneumoniae* can also be isolated in cell culture systems but is difficult to do. The organism grows in HeLa cell culture, and identification has been enhanced by development of monoclonal antibodies specific for *C. pneumoniae*.

Diagnostic Tests/Procedures

Chlamydia Culture *on page 294*
Chlamydia pneumoniae Serology *on page 295*
Chlamydia Species Serology *on page 296*

Treatment Large controlled studies comparing different antimicrobial agents have not been performed. Available data suggest that tetracycline and doxycycline are clinically effective. Failure with erythromycin has been reported. Therapy is usually continued for 10-14 days.

Pediatric Drug Therapy
Recommended
Erythromycin *on page 561*

Adult Drug Therapy
Recommended
Doxycycline *on page 557*
Tetracycline *on page 679*
Alternate
Erythromycin *on page 561*

Selected Readings
Grayston JT, "*Chlamydia pneumoniae*, Strain TWAR," *Chest*, 1989, 95(3):664-9.
Grayston JT, Campbell LA, Kuo CC, et al, "A New Respiratory Tract Pathogen: *Chlamydia pneumoniae*, Strain TWAR," *J Infect Dis*, 1990, 161(4):618-25.
Saikku P, Leinonen M, Tenkanen L, et al, "Chronic *Chlamydia pneumoniae* Infection as a Risk Factor for Coronary Heart Disease in the Helsinki Heart Study," *Ann Intern Med*, 1992, 116(4):273-8.

Chlamydia psittaci

Microbiology *Chlamydia psittaci* is an obligate intracellular bacterium and is the causative agent of psittacosis, or parrot fever. In the past, *Chlamydia* was classified as a virus, in part because of its nature as a cellular parasite. However, the organism also has many bacteria-like characteristics and is now regard-

(Continued)

Chlamydia psittaci (Continued)

ed as a specialized bacterium. *Chlamydia psittaci* is one of three distinct species within the genus *Chlamydia*. *Chlamydia pneumoniae* (also called *Chlamydia* TWAR) and *Chlamydia trachomatis*, the cause of trachoma (an eye infection) and a cause of urethritis, are the other two. All *Chlamydia* species are obligate parasites of eukaryotic cells and are unable to replicate extracellularly. *Chlamydia* species are unique in having two separate forms with separate functions; the elementary body (EB), which is well-suited for extracellular life but lacks the ability to replicate, and the reticulate body (RB), which is adapted to intracellular life and can divide by binary fission.

Epidemiology Infections from *C. psittaci* occur sporadically. Approximately 50 cases are reported annually in the United States, with 50% occurring in individuals who own pet birds. High risk groups include pigeon collectors, employees of pet shops, and veterinarians. Outbreaks of psittacosis have been reported in turkey processing plants. Psittacosis has been traditionally associated with psittacine birds such as parrots, and this group remains an important reservoir for infection. However, it is clear that many other bird species can act as reservoirs, such as pigeons, turkeys, canaries, cockatiels, ducks, and many others. *C. psittaci* can be harbored in several sites within an infected bird including the bloodstream, feathers, liver, spleen, and feces. The organisms remain viable for prolonged periods of time within bird excreta. Some infected birds appear only mildly ill (anorexia, diarrhea), and the sympathetic pet owner may deliberately increase the amount of physical contact and time spent with the bird. Transmission can take place by several routes such as inhalation of dried, infected bird feces (this appears to be the most common route of human infection), touching contaminated bird feathers, physical intimacy with a highly infected bird, and person-to-person spread (very rare).

Prolonged, intimate contact with an infected bird is not necessary for transmission. Cases have been reported following brief avian contact. Birds can also be infected but show no signs of clinical disease; viable organisms continue to be shed in the feces for weeks.

Clinical Syndromes

- **Psittacosis (parrot fever):** Infection occurs in two stages. In the first stage, the organisms enter the host via the respiratory tract and travel to the liver and spleen. The organisms replicate in these sites. In the second stage, the organisms disseminate via the blood stream to various sites, especially the lungs. Patients present with the sudden onset of high fevers and a severe headache. The presence of a severe headache, although nonspecific, is important in suggesting psittacosis and is highly characteristic of this infection. A variable number of days into the illness, patients frequently develop a nonproductive cough which can be paroxysmal and severe. Other symptoms include chills, muscle aches, gastrointestinal upset, and anorexia. On physical examination, the patient presentation can range from comfortable to acutely ill. As with other infections from intracellular pathogens, there may be a pulse-temperature dissociation (ie, the pulse is slow relative to the degree of fever). Lung examination usually shows localized inspiratory rales. Signs of lung consolidation can occur with severe disease. An important physical finding is the presence of hepatomegaly and/or splenomegaly which frequently develop in psittacosis. Routine laboratory studies are usually not helpful and Gram stain of sputum reveals no predominant microorganisms and few polymorphonuclear leukocytes. A variety of chest x-ray findings have been reported including a patchy interstitial lower lobe infiltrate (most common), a miliary pattern resembling tuberculosis, and occasionally a densely consolidated lobar pneumonia.
- **Endocarditis:** *C. psittaci* is a rare but reported cause of endocarditis. The diagnosis may be entertained in difficult cases of "culture negative endocarditis" where multiple blood cultures properly collected are negative for pathogens. An infectious disease specialist may be useful in approaching this problem.

Diagnosis *Chlamydia pneumoniae* should be suspected in any case of atypical pneumonia, particularly if there is pharyngitis and hoarseness. The other diagnostic considerations for atypical pneumonia should include *Mycoplasma pneumoniae*, *Legionella* infections, viral lower respiratory infections, and others. The diagnosis can be confirmed primarily with serologic studies. The two major antigens which are used for antibody tests are lipopolysaccharide antigens and major outer membrane protein antigen. Lipopolysaccharide antigen, which is common to all members of the *Chlamydia* genus. This antigen is measured using complement fixation. Thus, positive studies are not specific for *C. pneumoniae* and can be positive during *C. trachomatis* and *C. psittaci*. Major outer membrane proteins (MOMPs), which are specific for the different species of *Chlamydia*. These proteins are the basis for microimmunofluorescence (MIF) studies.

There are two patterns of antibody response with chlamydial infections. Primary infection: Early, complement fixation antibody is positive; 10 days to 1 month, MIF IgM is positive; 6 weeks, IgG is positive. Secondary infection: Complement fixation antibody is negative; IgM is positive in low titer; IgG response is more prompt. *C. pneumoniae* also can be isolated in cell culture systems, but can be difficult. The organism grows in HeLa cell culture and identification has been enhanced by development of monoclonal antibodies specific for *C. pneumoniae*.

Diagnostic Tests/Procedures
Chlamydia psittaci Serology *on page 296*

Treatment Large controlled studies comparing different antimicrobial agents have not been performed. Available data suggest that tetracycline and erythromycin are clinically effective. Failure with erythromycin have been reported. Therapy is usually continued for 10-14 days.

Pediatric Drug Therapy
Recommended
Erythromycin *on page 561*

Adult Drug Therapy
Recommended
Doxycycline *on page 557*
Alternate
Erythromycin *on page 561*

Selected Readings
Barnes RC, "Laboratory Diagnosis of Human Chlamydial Infections," *Clin Microbiol Rev*, 1989, 2(2):119-36.
Kuritsky JN, Schmid GP, Potter ME, et al, "Psittacosis. A Diagnostic Challenge," *J Occup Med*, 1984, 26(10):731-3.
Potter ME, Kaufmann AK, and Plikaytis BD, "Psittacosis in the United States 1979," *MMWR Surveill Summ*, 1983, 32(1):27SS-31SS.
Schlossberg D, "*Chlamydia psittaci* (Psittacosis)," *Principles and Practice of Infectious Diseases*, 4th ed, Mandell GL, Bennett JE, and Dolin R, eds, New York, NY: Churchill Livingstone, 1995, 1693-6.
Yung AP and Grayson ML, "Psittacosis – A Review of 135 Cases," *Med J Aust*, 1988, 148(5):228-33.

Chlamydia trachomatis

Microbiology *Chlamydia trachomatis* is a bacterium-like obligate intracellular organism. There are at least 15 recognized serotypes (immunotypes, serovars, biovars) of *C. trachomatis* which can be distinguished by immunofluorescent techniques. Certain serotypes are highly associated with disease syndromes. For example, *C. trachomatis* types L1, L2, and L3 are found only in patients with the disease lymphogranuloma venereum; whereas types A, B, and C are associated with trachoma, an infection of the eye.

C. trachomatis is one of three distinct species within the genus *Chlamydia*. The two other species are *Chlamydia psittaci* (the cause of psittacosis) and *Chlamydia pneumoniae* (a cause of community-acquired tracheobronchitis and pneumonia). *Chlamydia* species are unique in having two separate forms with separate functions: the **elementary body (EB)**, which is well-suited for extracellular life but lacks the ability to replicate and the **reticulate body (RB)**, which is adapted to intracellular life and can divide by binary fission.

The life cycle of *Chlamydia trachomatis* is as follows:
1. Elementary bodies attach to the host cell,
2. EBs enter the cell by inducing their own phagocytosis,
3. EBs transform into larger reticulate bodies,
4. The RBs grow and replicate by binary fission within vacuoles; these vacuoles become filled with EBs and appear as inclusion bodies in the host cytoplasm,
5. Vacuoles rupture and release infectious organisms, and the cycle begins again.

C. trachomatis is difficult to identify on a Gram stain. The Giemsa stain can be used for staining elementary bodies, reticulate bodies, and intracellular inclusion bodies but should not be trusted for definitive diagnosis.

(Continued)

Chlamydia trachomatis *(Continued)*

Epidemiology Is specific for each disease state and clinical syndrome for which it is responsible. This information is included below.

Clinical Syndromes

Infections in Adults:

- **Nongonococcal urethritis (NGU) in men:** *Chlamydia trachomatis* accounts for about 50% of the cases of NGU. The organism is usually sexually acquired and is harbored in the urethra. About 25% of infected men are asymptomatic but are still able to transmit the organism. When symptoms such as dysuria and/or penile discharge occur, they tend to be mild. This is in contrast to gonococcal urethritis, which tends to be more severe. The characteristic watery or mucoid urethral discharge should be examined under Gram stain to rule out *Neisseria gonorrhoeae*. Serious complications from chlamydial NGU are rare in males.

- **Mucopurulent cervicitis:** This is the female counterpart of NGU in the male. *Chlamydia trachomatis* is an important cause of mucopurulent cervicitis, usually acquired through sexual intercourse. The differential diagnosis of acute cervicitis includes *C. trachomatis*, *Neisseria gonorrhoeae*, herpes simplex virus, and others, making accurate diagnosis important. Many patients with chlamydial infections of the cervix remain asymptomatic. The diagnosis is further suggested by a positive "swab test" (ie, endocervical mucous appearing yellow-green when collected on a white cotton-tipped swab). Gram staining of endocervical secretions is essential to confirm the presence of inflammatory cells (>10 polymorphonuclear cells per high power field correlates well with infectious cervicitis) and to exclude *Neisseria gonorrhoeae*. Complications of chlamydial cervicitis include pelvic inflammatory disease.

- **Pelvic inflammatory disease (PID):** This is probably the most important manifestation of *C. trachomatis* infection with respect to morbidity, permanent sequelae, and cost. In some women, chlamydial infection ascends from the cervix to the upper reproductive tract. The incidence and predisposing factors for this are unclear. Symptoms may be mild, with only nonspecific abdominal discomfort, but at laparoscopy, inflammation can be severe. Salpingitis, endometritis, and peritonitis can occur. Perihepatitis due to *C. trachomatis* has been described (the **Fitz-Hugh Curtis syndrome**).

  Complications of PID include involuntary infertility, chronic and recurrent pelvicoabdominal pain, and ectopic pregnancy. PID is also commonly caused by *Neisseria gonorrhoeae*. The number of cases due to either *Neisseria* or *Chlamydia* varies widely depending on the population studied.

- **Lymphogranuloma venereum (LGV):** Several serotypes of *C. trachomatis* cause LGV, a rare sexually transmitted disease in the United States (170 cases reported in the U.S. in 1984). LGV is an important cause of the syndrome of genital lesions with regional adenopathy. The incubation period for LGV ranges from 3-21 days. The LGV genital lesion is not striking and may be missed by the patient or the physician. The lesion is usually single and painless; it may be a papule, vesicle, or an ulcer. It resolves within several days. The key to the diagnosis of LGV is the nature of the regional adenopathy, not the genital lesion. The inguinal nodes in LGV develop 2-6 weeks after the primary lesion. The nodes are matted, fluctuant, and large. They tend to be unilateral (66% of the cases) and painful. Fistulas have been described, especially after diagnostic needle aspiration. Constitutional symptoms are very prominent, with complaints of fever, headache, myalgias, and malaise.

- **Acute urethral syndrome:** *C. trachomatis* may play an important role in a subgroup of young women who present with recurrent dysuria and pyuria but who have repeatedly sterile urine cultures.

- **Ocular infections:** Worldwide, *C. trachomatis* is one of the leading causes of blindness. Over 400 million people suffer from trachoma, a chronic keratoconjunctivitis caused by *C. trachomatis*. Trachoma is an ancient disease described thousands of years ago. Initial infection occurs in childhood: a gradual onset of epithelial keratitis, infiltrates in the subepithelium, and invasion of blood vessels into the cornea (pannus formation). Bacterial coinfection and scarring of the conjunctiva are common. Trachoma is endemic in Africa, Asia, and the Mediterranean basin. Sporadic cases still occur in the U.S.

  C. trachomatis can also cause inclusion conjunctivitis, an ocular infection different from trachoma (but possibly related). This is most commonly seen in sexually active young adults. The pathogenesis of this ocular infection is either self-inoculation with infected genital secretions or exposure of the eye to infected secretions during orogenital contact.

- **Proctocolitis:** An acute proctocolitis can be caused by *C. trachomatis*, particularly in homosexual males who practice receptive anal intercourse. Symptoms include tenesmus, watery rectal discharge, and rectal pain, but many patients remain asymptomatic.
- **Epididymitis:** *C. trachomatis* accounts for nearly 50% of cases of epididymitis in adolescents and young adults. *Neisseria gonorrhoeae* usually makes up the remainder of cases in this age group.
- **Reiter's syndrome (conjunctivitis, reactive arthritis, and urethritis):** The majority of cases of Reiter's syndrome appear to be related to *C. trachomatis*, although a "postdiarrheal" Reiter's syndrome is well recognized. *C. trachomatis* can be cultured from the urethra in majority of cases of Reiter's syndrome. Untreated chlamydial urethritis appears to be a risk factor. Although *C. trachomatis* has not been isolated from synovial fluid from patients with Reiter's syndrome, elementary bodies suggestive of *Chlamydia* have been found in joint fluid.

Infections in Infants: Newborns acquire *C. trachomatis* infection usually during passage through an infected birth canal. About 66% of those exposed during vaginal delivery ultimately become infected.

- **Pneumonia in infants:** *C. trachomatis* is one of the leading causes of pneumonia in infants 1-6 months of age. About 16% of neonates exposed to *C. trachomatis* during delivery will develop pneumonia. Infants present subacutely with rhinitis and a characteristic "staccato cough" followed by tachypnea and inspiratory rales. Fever is absent. Many have had a preceding conjunctivitis or will develop it during the course of the pneumonia. Chest radiographs show a diffuse interstitial pneumonitis. There is an increased incidence of pulmonary function test abnormalities later in childhood.
- **Conjunctivitis in infants:** Approximately 25% of newborns exposed to *C. trachomatis* during delivery will develop *Chlamydia* conjunctivitis. *C. trachomatis* remains the most common cause of neonatal conjunctivitis, despite prophylaxis with ophthalmic silver nitrate. Newborns present with a mucopurulent ocular discharge and inflamed conjunctivae 2 days to 3 weeks after birth. Most cases resolve spontaneously within several months without long-term sequelae, but some may develop a chronic ocular infection resembling a mild case of trachoma.

Diagnosis Recent recommendations by the Centers for Disease Control (1993) have emphasized the importance of more aggressive testing for the confirmation of *Chlamydia*. A variety of newer, more accurate tests are available, and the CDC now recommends laboratory testing of clinically suspected cases, sex partners of known or suspected cases, and certain asymptomatic individuals in high risk groups (sexually active women younger than 20 year of age, women 20-24 years of age who do not use barrier contraceptives and who have a new sex partner in the previous 3 months, and others).

Diagnostic tests can be classified as follows:
1. Cell culture
2. Nonculture tests:
   - Direct fluorescent antibody (DFA) tests
   - Enzyme immunoassays (EIA) tests
   - Nucleic hybridization (DNA probe) tests

For further information regarding the different tests, see the Laboratory Diagnosis section and the referenced article by the Centers for Disease Control.

For the diagnosis of lymphogranuloma venereum (LGV), serologic titers for LGV may be useful. The complement fixation (CF) test is positive in most cases of active LGV at titers ≥1:64. Such titers become positive between 1 and 3 weeks postinfection. Occasionally, high CF titers have been found in individuals with other chlamydial infections and in asymptomatic patients. Titers <1:64 are suggestive but not diagnostic of LGV. It is difficult to demonstrate a classical fourfold rise in specific antibody titer in LGV due to the late presentation of many patients. Microimmunofluorescent tests are more sensitive than CF for the detection of LGV-producing *C. trachomatis* strains. However, the microimmunofluorescent antibody test is available only in a select number of research laboratories. Finally, *Chlamydia* species can be isolated in cell culture systems in some laboratories. The rate of recovery of LGV *Chlamydia* from buboes or genital lesions is about 30% or less.

(Continued)

Chlamydia trachomatis (Continued)

Diagnostic Tests/Procedures
Chlamydia Culture *on page 294*
Chlamydia trachomatis by DNA Probe *on page 297*
Chlamydia trachomatis DFA Test *on page 298*
Ocular Cytology *on page 416*

Treatment Current treatment recommendations: Oral: Doxycycline 100 mg twice daily for 21 days. Alternatives: Tetracycline 500 mg 4 times/day for 21 days or erythromycin 500 mg 4 times/day for 21 days. In pregnancy, use erythromycin 500 mg 4 times/day. Treatment is the same in HIV-infected individuals.

Pediatric Drug Therapy
Recommended
Erythromycin *on page 561*

Adult Drug Therapy
Recommended
Doxycycline *on page 557*
Tetracycline *on page 679*

Alternate
Erythromycin *on page 561*

Selected Readings
Batteiger BE and Jones RB, "Chlamydial Infections," *Infect Dis Clin North Am*, 1987, 1(1):55-81.

Smith TF, Brown SD, and Weed LA, "Diagnosis of *Chlamydia trachomatis* Infections by Cell Cultures and Serology," *Lab Med*, 1982, 13:92-100.

"Recommendations for the Prevention and Management of *Chlamydia trachomatis* Infections, 1993. Centers for Disease Control and Prevention," *MMWR Morb Mortal Wkly Rep*, 1993, 42(RR-12):1-39.

U.S. Department of Health and Human Services, "1993 Sexually Transmitted Diseases Treatment Guidelines," *MMWR Morb Mortal Wkly Rep*, 1993, 42(RR-14).

Chlamydia **TWAR** *see Chlamydia pneumoniae on page 76*

Citrobacter Species

Microbiology *Citrobacter* species are gram-negative rods which are important causes of nosocomial infection and are only rarely associated with community-acquired infections in normal hosts. *Citrobacter* species are moderate-sized, aerobic, gram-negative bacilli which belong to the large family Enterobacteriaceae. The organism cannot be identified on the basis of its morphologic appearance on Gram stain alone, and is morphologically indistinguishable from other Enterobacteriaceae. *Citrobacter* species are closely related to such gram-negative bacilli as *Klebsiella*, *Serratia*, *Salmonella*, and *E. coli* (about 40% DNA sequence homology with *Citrobacter*). Currently recognized *Citrobacter* species are *C. diversus*, *C. freundii*, and *C. amalonaticus*, all of which are potential human pathogens. Laboratory identification is generally straightforward. Special requests for isolation of *Citrobacter* are not necessary.

Citrobacter shares several potential virulence factors with other Enterobacteriaceae, including endotoxin, the lipopolysaccharide (LPS) associated with the outer membrane of the bacteria. When cell lysis occurs (as with antibiotic therapy), the LPS is released into the host and can lead to such inflammatory responses as fever, leukopenia or leukocytosis, hypotension, and disseminated intravascular coagulation. Thus, LPS is regarded as an important mediator of the sepsis syndrome.

Epidemiology Because *Citrobacter* commonly inhabits the human gastrointestinal tract, it is considered one of the "enteric bacteria." In hospitalized patients, *Citrobacter* can asymptomatically colonize the urine, respiratory tract, abdominal wounds, decubitus ulcers, and others. Community-acquired infection is rare.

Clinical Syndromes
- **Lower respiratory tract infection:** Nosocomial *Citrobacter* infections are often seen in debilitated and ventilator-dependent patients. It should be noted that *Citrobacter* and other gram-negative bacilli can asymptomatically colonize the upper respiratory tract of hospitalized patients. Thus, the recovery of *Citrobacter* in a sputum or tracheal aspirate culture does not necessarily indicate a significant infectious disease. The diagnosis of a pneumonia still rests on standard criteria such as the presence of purulence (many leukocytes) on the Gram stain of sputum, the presence of a pulmonary infiltrate, and signs of systemic inflammation in the patient. A

positive sputum culture alone is not sufficient justification for initiating anti-microbial therapy.

- **Urinary tract infection:** Seen in hospitalized patients, often in those with indwelling Foley catheters. However, *Citrobacter* may harmlessly colonize the urine of patients with chronic bladder catheters without causing disease. The decision to initiate antibiotics in such patients should be based on the clinical situation (the presence of pyuria on urinalysis, suprapubic pain, fever, etc). Even the finding of large numbers of *Citrobacter* in a urine culture ($>10^5$ colony forming units/mL) by itself does not automatically indicate antibiotic therapy.
- **Hospital-associated bacteremias:** *Citrobacter* may be recovered from blood cultures in association with a known focus of infection (eg, pneumonia or catheter infection) or may be a "primary bacteremia" with no clear source. *Citrobacter* may also be cultured as part of a polymicrobial bacteremia, usually from an intravascular catheter or intra-abdominal sepsis. Endocarditis has rarely been reported.
- **Neonatal central nervous system infections:** *Citrobacter diversus* is a recognized cause of meningitis and brain abscesses in this age group.

Diagnosis The clinical presentations of the various nosocomial infections caused by *Citrobacter* are not distinctive, and laboratory isolation is necessary.

Diagnostic Tests/Procedures

Aerobic Culture, Appropriate Site *on page 244*
Gram Stain *on page 352*

Treatment *Citrobacter* species present a challenging therapeutic problem, especially with nosocomial infection. High level drug resistance has been described in some isolates. Preliminary data suggest that the popular third generation cephalosporins may act to select mutants of *Citrobacter* that are resistant to a wide variety of antibiotics, including both cephalosporins and extended spectrum penicillins. These "stably derepressed mutants" are becoming more common in intensive care units and pose a significant and growing problem. Infectious disease consultation may be useful in such cases.

Drug Therapy
Recommended

Cephalosporins, 3rd Generation *on page 528*
Penicillins, Extended Spectrum *on page 637*

Alternate

Imipenem/Cilastatin *on page 586*

Selected Readings

Drelichman V and Band JD, "Bacteremia Due to *Citrobacter diversus* and *Citrobacter freundii*: Incidence, Risk Factors, and Clinical Outcome," *Arch Intern Med*, 1985, 145(10):1808-10.

Lipsky BA, Hook EW 3d, Smith AA, et al, "*Citrobacter* Infections in Humans: Experience at the Seattle Veterans Administration Medical Center and a Review of the Literature," *Rev Infect Dis*, 1980, 2(5):746-60.

Samonis G, Ho DH, Gooch GF, et al, "*In Vitro* Susceptibility of *Citrobacter* Species to Various Antimicrobial Agents," *Antimicrob Agents Chemother*, 1987, 31(5):829-30.

Williams WW, Mariano J, Spurrier M, et al, "Nosocomial Meningitis Due to *Citrobacter diversus* in Neonates: New Aspects of the Epidemiology," *J Infect Dis*, 1984, 150(2):229-55.

Clostridium botulinum

Related Information

Timing of Food Poisoning *on page 723*

Microbiology The etiologic agent of botulism is *Clostridium botulinum*. The organism is a gram-positive, anaerobic bacillus. The natural reservoir is soil and sediment where the organism survives by forming spores. Most foodborne epidemics are associated with home canned foods. Restaurants and commercially canned products are also the source of outbreaks.

As the bacteria grow and undergo autolysis, a powerful polypeptide neurotoxin is released. The toxin is heat labile and thus, is destroyed by appropriate heating in commercial canning processes. An acidic pH inhibits spore germination. This is the basis for adding ascorbic acid to home-canned products. Ingestion of even a small amount of contaminated food may cause severe clinical symptoms.

Epidemiology *Clostridium botulinum* is found in soil worldwide. Incidence of reported botulism is increasing. Most cases are individual or occur as a small cluster. If the outbreak is the result of contaminated commercially distributed food, the cases may occur in a widespread area. Early consultation with the

(Continued)

Clostridium botulinum (Continued)

State Health Department in conjunction with the Center for Disease Control is imperative for case management and epidemic control. Botulism is almost always caused by *C. botulinum* types A, B, and E in the western U.S., eastern U.S., and Alaska, respectively.

Clinical Syndromes

- **Infant botulism:** The most commonly reported form of botulism in the United States is infant botulism. *C. botulinum* toxin is released from organisms colonizing the intestinal tract. The toxin binds to synaptic membranes of cholinergic nerves and prevents the release of acetylcholine. Transmission of nerve fiber impulses to muscle is interrupted with resultant autonomic nerve dysfunction which progresses to motor weakness (flaccid paralysis).

  Subsequently, cranial and peripheral nerve weakness, constipation, and autonomic instability is the result of toxin effect on the ganglionic and postganglionic parasympathetic synapses. Typically, infants 1 week to 1 year of age present with progressive descending weakness following a period of constipation. Weak suck and poor feeding are frequent complaints.

- **Foodborne botulism:** Symptoms of botulism begin as descending paralysis or weakness within a few hours to 1-2 days following ingestion of contaminated food. Symptoms may commence as late as 1 week. Dizziness, lassitude, and weakness are common. Nausea and vomiting are less common. Blockage of autonomic nerve impulse transmission causes dry tongue, mouth, and pharynx which is unrelieved by fluids. Urinary retention, ileus, and constipation frequently follow. Paralysis descends from cranial nerves to extremities and the respiratory muscles. Speech and vision are often impaired. Key clinical observations include the fact that the patients are oriented, alert, or easily roused and afebrile. They may demonstrate postural hypotension and dilated unreactive pupils.

- **Wound botulism:** Botulism may result from germination of spores contaminating traumatic wounds. Wounds caused by intravenous drug and nasal cocaine abuse have also been reported as sources. The clinical syndrome resembles that of foodborne botulism. Toxin can be recovered from the serum and wound drainage of affected patients. *C. botulinum* may be recovered from debrided tissue and drainage.

Diagnosis Outbreaks of botulism may be documented by identifying toxin in the stool or serum of symptomatic patients or from suspected food. Isolation of *C. botulinum* from stool or demonstration of the toxin by the mouse neutralization test establishes the diagnosis. Toxin is difficult to recover from serum; therefore, toxin recovery from stool may be more productive, but acquiring a stool specimen may be difficult because of the constipation. A low volume, normal saline, colonic irrigation may yield a useful specimen. Electromyography and repetitive nerve stimulation may yield corroborative evidence. The electromyographer should be alerted to the suspicion of botulism so that the study can be directed toward the diagnosis. A cerebrospinal fluid analysis to exclude meningitis, poliomyelitis, and Fisher Guillain-Barré syndrome is a useful part of the work-up.

Diagnostic Tests/Procedures

Botulism, Diagnostic Procedure *on page 285*
Cerebrospinal Fluid Analysis *on page 288*

Treatment

Infant botulism: The primary modes of treatment for infant botulism are supportive involving rehydration, nutritional supplementation, and respiratory support. Nasogastric tube feedings have been used relatively early in the course; however, the patients should be monitored for ileus. Oral feeding should not be reinstituted until ileus is gone, a gag reflex is present, and swallowing is normal. Intubation is required in the majority of cases for airway protection and, in about 25%, for ventilation. These patients have a significant risk of atelectasis and aspiration. Antitoxin is usually not used because the level of circulating toxin available to be bound is very low. In addition, there are significant complications of antitoxin therapy which include serum sickness, anaphylaxis, and life-long sensitivity to horse serum. Aminoglycoside antimicrobial therapy is contraindicated because aminoglycosides can cause neuromuscular blockade. Since sepsis is a key differential diagnosis, alternatives to aminoglycosides such as third generation cephalosporins should be considered in cases where botulism is in the differential. Therapy directed at eradication of *C. botulinum* toxin from the bowel has not been shown to produce objective clinical benefit.

Hospitalizations have a mean of about 50 days with complications including atelectasis, inappropriate antidiuretic hormone, autonomic instability, urinary tract infection, pneumonia sepsis, seizures, and subglottic stenosis as a complication of intubation. Despite the complications, mortality is very low (<3%), and prognosis for complete recovery is good.

Foodborne botulism: In cases of foodborne botulism, administration of equine antitoxin should be considered. In conjunction with the State Department of Health, consultation with the Foodborne Diseases branch of the Center for Disease Control is available, (404) 639-2206. The electromyogram, cerebrospinal fluid analysis, summary of the clinical syndrome, and chronology of the patient's illness should be available to facilitate the consultation. The main tenant of therapy for botulism is respiratory support.

Wound botulism: Treatment is similar to the therapy for foodborne botulism. Incision and debridement of the wound should also be considered.

Drug Therapy
Recommended
Botulinum Toxoid, Pentavalent Vaccine (Against Types A, B, C, D, and E Strains of *C. botulinum*) *on page 506*

Selected Readings
Hurst DL and Marsh WW, "Early Severe Infantile Botulism," *J Pediatr*, 1993, 122(6):909-11.
McDonald TD and Lange DJ, "Botulism: Diagnosis and Treatment," *Hosp Med*, March, 1992, 42-57.
Schmidt RD and Schmidt TW, "Infant Botulism: A Case Series and Review of the Literature," *J Emerg Med*, 1992, 10(6):713-8.
Wigginton JM and Thill P, "Infant Botulism. A Review of the Literature," *Clin Pediatr (Phila)*, 1993, 32(11):669-74.

Clostridium difficile

Microbiology *Clostridium difficile* is a spore-forming, gram-positive, anaerobic rod which is the most frequent cause of antibiotic-associated colitis. This organism can be cultured from the stool of about 3% of normal adults. The percentage of hospitalized patients who are colonized with this agent is higher. The bacterium is capable of producing several toxins within the intestinal lumen, the best characterized being toxins A and B.

Epidemiology *C. difficile* colitis is most frequent in elderly persons and in hospitalized patients. The organism causes disease when antibiotics cause an alteration in the normal intestinal flora allowing the bacterium to colonize and ultimately produce toxins. *C. difficile* has been isolated from several sources besides stool, including the hands of health care workers, fomites, endoscopy equipment, and other instruments.

Clinical Syndromes *C. difficile* colitis: The range of severity of symptoms is broad, ranging from mild diarrhea to a more profuse, watery, and mucoid diarrhea. In general, symptoms begin several days after receiving antibiotics. In most cases, the stool is guaiac-negative, although bloody stools can occur. A more severe, sepsis-like presentation has been well-described, in which patients present with high fevers, marked abdominal pain, hypotension, hypoalbuminemia, and evidence of serositis. In some cases, patients may present with a syndrome resembling a toxic megacolon and have little or no diarrhea.

Diagnosis Some cases of antibiotic-associated colitis caused by *C. difficile* are associated with the formation of pseudomembranes in the colon. These are recognized by sigmoidoscopy with or without biopsy. More commonly the condition is confirmed by obtaining stool samples for the toxin produced by *C. difficile*, rather than culture of the stool for this organism.

Diagnostic Tests/Procedures
Clostridium difficile Toxin Assay *on page 300*
Fecal Leukocyte Stain *on page 334*

Treatment The mainstay of treatment for *C. difficile* colitis is discontinuation of all offending antibiotics, whenever feasible. Oral vancomycin is very effective in this condition, but its high cost is almost prohibitive. Metronidazole is also effective in antibiotic-associated colitis and is considerably less expensive.

Drug Therapy
Recommended
Metronidazole *on page 610*
Alternate
Vancomycin Hydrochloride *on page 691*

Selected Readings
Bartlett JG, "Antibiotic-Associated Diarrhea," *Clin Infect Dis*, 1992, 15(4):573-81.
Bartlett JG, "*Clostridium difficile*: Clinical Considerations," *Rev Infect Dis*, 1990, 12(Suppl 2):S243-51.

(Continued)

ORGANISMS

Clostridium difficile (Continued)

Kelly CP, Pothoulakis C, and LaMont JT, "*Clostridium difficile* Colitis," *N Engl J Med*, 1994, 330(4):257-62.

McFarland LV, Mulligan ME, and Kwok RY, "Nosocomial Acquisition of *Clostridium difficile* Infection," *N Engl J Med*, 1989, 320(4):204-10.

Clostridium perfringens
Related Information

Timing of Food Poisoning *on page 723*

Microbiology *Clostridium perfringens* is an anaerobic gram-positive rod; occasionally it can appear gram-negative or gram-variable. It is a spore-forming organism, but the spores are not usually seen on Gram stain. It has been termed "aerotolerant" because of its ability to survive when exposed to oxygen for limited periods of time.

The organism produces 12 toxins active in tissues and several enterotoxins which cause severe diarrhea. Four toxins can be lethal. The toxins separate the species into five types, A-E.

- Alpha toxin: A lecithinase which damages cell membranes. It is produced by *C. perfringens* type A. It is the major factor causing tissue damage in *C. perfringens*-induced gas gangrene (myonecrosis). The toxin is a phospholipase which hydrolyzes phosphatidylcholine and sphingomyelin and leads to increased vascular permeability, myocardial depression, hypotension, bradycardia, and shock.
- Enterotoxin: Produced mainly by *C. perfringens* type A but also by types C and D. This toxin is responsible for the diarrheal syndromes classically ascribed to this organism. The enterotoxin binds to intestinal epithelial cells after the human ingests food contaminated with *C. perfringens*. The small bowel (ileum) is primarily involved. The toxin inhibits glucose transport and causes protein loss.
- Beta toxin: Produced by *C. perfringens* type B and C. This toxin causes enteritis necroticans or pigbel. This disease is seen in New Guinea where some natives ingest massive amounts of pork at feasts after first gorging on sweet potatoes. The sweet potatoes have protease inhibitors which prevent the person from degrading the beta toxin which is ingested in the contaminated pork.

Epidemiology *C. perfringens* is ubiquitous in the environment, being found in soil and decaying vegetation. The organism has been isolated from nearly every soil sample ever examined except in the sand of the Sahara desert. In the human, *C. perfringens* is common in the human gastrointestinal tract. In one study, it was found in 28 of 40 adults. It can also be commonly recovered from many mammals including cats, dogs, whales, and others.

Clinical Syndromes The organism can be pathogenic, commensal, or symbiotic. Important diseases caused by *C. perfringens* include the following:

- **Food poisoning:** *C. perfringens* is one of the most common causes of food poisoning in the United States. Foods commonly contaminated with *C. perfringens* are meat, poultry, and meat products such as gravies, hash, and stew. Human disease is caused by ingestion of heat-labile toxin. The highest risk comes from meats which are partially cooked, cooled, then reheated. Spores present in the food germinate during the reheating process. Symptoms include watery diarrhea and abdominal cramps, which occur about 12 hours after the meal. Fever is generally not part of this illness. Vomiting is unusual. Duration of symptoms is about 24 hours. The diagnosis is made by culturing the stools and, for epidemiological purposes, the food.
- **Pigbel:** See description under Microbiology above. This follows massive ingestion of contaminated pork and sweet potatoes. Incubation period is 24 hours. There is intense abdominal pain, bloody diarrhea, vomiting, shock, and intestinal perforation in some cases. A vaccine is available for travelers.
- **Gynecologic infections:** *C. perfringens* has been isolated in association with septic abortions, tubo-ovarian abscesses, and uterine gas gangrene. Interestingly, *C. perfringens* has been isolated from the blood of healthy females in the immediate postnatal period; the organism appeared to be a commensal in the blood since the patients remained well without antibiotic therapy. This underscores the often enigmatic nature of *C. perfringens*.
- **Skin and soft tissue infection colonization:** Many wounds can be contaminated with *C. perfringens*, particularly when there is an open wound exposed to soil. The organism may or may not be causing disease, and its

relevance should be based on clinical findings; a superficial wound growing *C. perfringens* can often be treated using local care alone.

- **Anaerobic cellulitis:** *C. perfringens* alone or in a mixed infection causes a local tissue invasion with some necrosis. Patients are afebrile, and there is little pain or swelling. Gas may be quite noticeable in the infected tissues. Anaerobic cellulitis is seen in patients with infected diabetic foot ulcers and patients with perirectal abscesses. Localized infection can spread if not appropriately treated.

- **Fasciitis:** Patients with *C. perfringens* fasciitis present with rapidly progressive infection through soft tissue planes. **This is a medical emergency.** Anaerobic organisms cause pain, swelling, and gas formation; and patients frequently present in a florid sepsis syndrome. The classic setting for this is the patient with known colonic cancer with presumed abdominal fascial metastases; this is the nidus for colonic contamination, followed by rapid movement along the fascial planes. Although the muscle is not involved, the mortality of anaerobic cellulitis remains very high even with early surgical intervention.

- **Clostridial myonecrosis:** This entity has been described after traumatic wounds, especially during war time when wounds are grossly contaminated with soil. In World War II, 30% of battlefield wounds were associated with this, but in Vietnam only 0.02%. Clostridial myonecrosis can also be seen with crush injury, colon resections, septic abortions, and other conditions. Clinically, there is systemic toxicity, with tissue hypoxia and vascular insufficiency. The involved muscles appear black and gangrenous. Often there is abundant gas felt as crepitance in the wound. Treatment is surgical removal of devitalized tissue and, often, amputation.

Diagnosis The diagnosis of infection by *C. perfringens* begins with a high index of suspicion when a patient presents with one of the clinical syndromes described above. One important caveat is that the laboratory isolation of *C. perfringens* from a necrotic wound does not necessarily imply disease from this organism; many wounds can be colonized. In the right clinical setting, however, a positive *C. perfringens* culture and a compatible clinical presentation are highly suggestive of disease caused by this agent. Gram stain preparations of wound material, uterine tissue, cervical discharge, muscle tissues, and other relevant materials should be made; a predominance of gram-positive rods should bring anaerobic infection, including *C. perfringens*, to mind.

In patients with clostridial septicemia, accompanying abnormalities may be a clue to clostridial disease before culture confirmation is made. Patients may have disseminated intravascular coagulation with a brisk hemolysis, hemoglobinuria, and proteinuria. X-rays of diseased areas may reveal the presence of gas in muscle or soft tissue; this is suggestive of clostridial infection, although other anaerobes (and aerobes) can cause gas formation. If clostridial myonecrosis is suspected, a muscle biopsy usually performed at the time of tissue debridement, can be diagnostic.

Diagnostic Tests/Procedures

Anaerobic Culture *on page 250*
Gram Stain *on page 352*
Skin Biopsy *on page 443*

Treatment In general, the treatment of clostridial infection is high-dose penicillin G, to which the organism has remained susceptible. For skin and soft tissue infections, the extent of infection determines the need for surgical debridement. When wounds are simply colonized with clostridia, neither antibiotics nor surgery are indicated. Localized soft tissue infections can often be managed by surgical debridement alone, without antibiotics. When systemic symptoms are present and there is extension of infection into deeper tissues, antibiotics and surgical intervention are required. In fulminant cases of gas gangrene with myonecrosis, immediate surgical intervention (debridement, amputation) is the primary treatment of choice, and antibiotics have little effect.

Drug Therapy
Recommended

Penicillin G, Parenteral *on page 633*
Metronidazole *on page 610*

Alternate

Imipenem/Cilastatin *on page 586*
Clindamycin *on page 540*

Selected Readings

"*Clostridium perfringens* Gastroenteritis Associated With Corned Beef Served at St Pat-

(Continued)

Clostridium perfringens (Continued)

rick's Day Meals – Ohio and Virginia, 1993," *MMWR Morb Mortal Wkly Rep*, 1994, 43(8):137, 143-4.

Lorber B, "Gas Gangrene and Other *Clostridium*-Associated Diseases," *Principles and Practice of Infectious Diseases*, 4th ed, Mandell GL, Bennett JE, and Dolin R, eds, New York, NY: Churchill Livingstone, 1995, 2182-95.

Shandera WX, Tacket CO, and Blake PA, "Food Poisoning Due to *Clostridium perfringens* in the United States," *J Infect Dis*, 1983, 147(1):167-70.

Clostridium tetani

Microbiology *Clostridium tetani* is a strictly anaerobic, gram-positive, motile, spore-forming rod. Bacteria in very young or very old cultures can be gram-negative. Under adverse conditions, vegetative cells form polar ("drumstick" or "tennis racquet" appearance) spores which are extremely resistant to drying, boiling for 1 hour, and chemical disinfectants; the spores are killed by autoclaving. *C. tetani* is the etiological agent of tetanus, a strikingly dramatic infectious disease which has been recognized for many centuries. *C. tetani* was first isolated in pure culture in 1889 by Kirtasato, and the tetanus toxoid was first prepared the following year.

Epidemiology *Clostridium tetani* and its spores are found in the soil (especially manured soil) worldwide; the spores can survive in soil for many years. Sometimes *C. tetani* is also found in the lower intestinal tracts of humans and animals. In the United States since the mid 1970s, the number of cases of tetanus per year has remained at about 0.5 per 100,000 persons. Tetanus is most prevalent in the older age group (>60 years of age) and, in all populations, is directly related to an absence of immunization or to inadequate immunization. Tetanus is not uncommon (1 million cases per year) in developing countries, where mortality rates are high, probably because of a lack of intensive and proper supportive care. In developing countries, most cases occur in mothers with incompletely removed and subsequently infected placentas and in their newborns with unclean and infected umbilical cord stumps.

The portal of entry of *C. tetani* is usually a traumatized site (eg, piercing wound, burn, parenteral drug abuse, implantation of infected soil, war, and traumatic motor vehicle accident). Predisposing wounds often are quite small (eg, prick of a rose thorn or small splinter) and not recognized. Resulting traumatized or deep necrotic tissue environment is conducive to germination of implanted spores and the subsequent production of tetanospasmin, the potent neurotoxin of *C. tetani*. The vegetative cells produce the neurotoxin at the site of trauma and do not invade. Tetanospasmin circulates through the blood and lymphatic systems, attaches strongly to ganglioside receptors of presynaptic inhibitory neuron synapses, and inhibits the release of glycine, an inhibitory transmitter. The result of this binding and inhibition is simultaneous contraction of opposing flexor and extensor muscle groups and subsequent, often extremely violent, local and generalized muscle spasms.

Clinical Syndromes Tetanus: The incubation period for tetanus can be from a few days to several months. Shorter incubation periods are associated with more severe disease. The initial presentation of tetanus usually is characterized by general weakness, cramping, stiffness, and/or difficulty swallowing or chewing. "Lockjaw" can be an early sign. During the first week, spasms occur more frequently and become more generalized. Later, spasms can become intensely painful and more severe to the point of affecting breathing, speech, swallowing, and cardiac function. Cardiac, respiratory, and renal failure are the major causes of death. Mortality rates for mild, moderate, severe, and neonatal tetanus have been reported to be 0%, 9%, 44%, and 75%, respectively.

Diagnosis The diagnosis of tetanus is made by clinical judgment and patient history. Culture of specimens is not productive and not clinically useful. A history of appropriate immunization against tetanus almost always eliminates the possibility of tetanus. A differential diagnosis can include rabies, meningitis, peritonitis, antipsychotic drugs, poisoning, and epilepsy.

Treatment Supportive therapy with emphasis on appropriate ventilation should be the major consideration in the treatment of patients with tetanus. The neuromuscular symptoms and spasms from tetanus may be managed with benzodiazepines. Additional sedation may also be necessary. Tetanus immune globulin (TIG) should be administered immediately in a dose of 500-3000 units. Intrathecal TIG (250 units) may be administered, but its use is still investigational. Equine antiserum has also been used but is associated with significantly more adverse reactions than TIG.

Patients should also be treated with antimicrobial therapy. Although intravenous penicillin is often used, metronidazole is at least as effective. Theoretically, TIG should be administered prior to antibiotic therapy to abate any increase in toxin release caused by antibiotic administration. Local wound care is also important.

Other clinical manifestations that may require therapeutic intervention include autonomic instability, increased risk of pulmonary embolus, increased risk of stress ulceration, decubitus ulcers, fluid and electrolyte imbalance, and nutritional imbalance.

Tetanus can be prevented by appropriate immunization. Immunization guidelines can be found in the appendix.

Drug Therapy
Recommended

Tetanus Immune Globulin, Human *on page 677*
used in combination with
Metronidazole *on page 610*
or
Tetanus Immune Globulin, Human *on page 677*
used in combination with
Penicillin G, Parenteral *on page 633*

Selected Readings

Bleck TP, "*Clostridium tetani,*" *Principles and Practice of Infectious Diseases*, 4th ed, Mandell GL, Bennett JE, and Dolin R, eds, New York, NY: Churchill Livingstone, 1995, 2173-8.

Centers for Disease Control, "Tetanus Fatality – Ohio, 1991," *MMWR Morb Mortal Wkly Rep*, 1993, 42(8):148-9.

CMV *see* Cytomegalovirus *on page 97*

Coccidioides immitis

Microbiology *Coccidioides immitis* is a dimorphic fungus. In the mycelial form on culture, the mold grows relatively fast producing a flat, moist, gray colony in 3-5 days and then developing fluffy white aerial mycelium. Wet mount reveals branching septate hyphae and chains of thick-walled, barrel-shaped arthrospores (up to 10 μm) separated by "ghost" spaces (remnants of empty cells). **Arthrospores are highly infectious to laboratory workers.** The yeast form can be seen on direct examination of infected material as round, thick-walled spherules 20-80 μm with many small endospores.

Epidemiology *Coccidioides immitis* is a normal inhabitant of the sandy, salty, dry soil of the lower Sonora Desert. It is found only in the western hemisphere and has been isolated in specific areas of Argentina and Central America, as well as the southwestern United States. The warm, dry environment facilitates the growth of arthroconidia that break from the parent mycelium and become airborne. The infectious arthroconidia are inhaled and within the pulmonary acinus convert to spherules and reproduce by endosporulation.

Coccidioides infects more than 50,000 people each year and is increasing in incidence. In 1991, there was a threefold increase followed by a tenfold increase in 1992 in California as compared to the previous 5 years. Most cases occur in late childhood and early middle age. Epidemics are typically associated with dust storms, construction, archaeological digs, and exploration for oil. Infections in persons residing outside endemic areas arise from travel exposure, laboratory exposure, or inhalation of contaminated fomites.

Impaired T-cell immunity is associated with severe pulmonary and disseminated disease. Approximately 33% of AIDS patients have no focal lesion or only focal pulmonary lesions despite evidence of systemic disease. *Coccidioides* is an AIDS defining illness.

Risk factors for dissemination include infants and elderly, male sex, race (Filipinos > Blacks > Native Americans > Hispanic > Oriental), negative skin test, serum complement fixation > 1:64, immunosuppression, second half of pregnancy, and postpartum.

Clinical Syndromes

- **Asymptomatic:** Subclinical infection. Positive skin test without clinical evidence of disease. Occurs in approximately 60% of cases.
- **Primary pulmonary:** Acute respiratory illness characterized by fever, cough, headache; often associated with malaise, myalgias, and fatigue. Self-limited. Approximately 25% develop more severe disease associated with pleuritic chest pain, yet very few will progress. May have erythema nodosum or erythema multiforme. May develop arthritis, most commonly in

(Continued)
89

Coccidioides immitis (Continued)

the knee, which is an immune complex reaction and not dissemination (referred to as Desert Rheumatism).

- **Pulmonary sequelae:** Characterized by pulmonary infiltrates that are frequently subpleural with overlying pleural effusions (12%), which is usually self-limited. Hilar adenopathy is common, but paratracheal or superior-mediastinal adenopathy suggests dissemination as does diffuse miliary infiltrates. Five percent develop persistent cavities or thin-walled coccidioidal abscesses or nodules (coccidioidoma). One-third of the cavities will close within 2 years while the rest may rupture, bleed, or develop secondary infections which may require surgical excision.
- **Chronic persistent fibrocavitary disease:** Associated with pre- existing bronchopulmonary disease.
- **Disseminated disease:** In approximately 1% of infected individuals. Spreads beyond pulmonary parenchyma or hilar nodes. Found in every organ except GI. Most common site of spread is the skin (granulomas) followed by subcutaneous abscesses, synovitis, and osteomyelitis. Majority of deaths secondary to meningitis which occurs 2-3 weeks to years after initial infection. Hydrocephalus is frequent and is a severe complication. Direct cranial nerve involvement is secondary to a vasculitis that may present as a stroke-like syndrome or transverse myelitis.

Diagnosis Skin tests and serological markers are useful epidemiologic, as well as prognostic tools. Greater than 50% of the population in endemic areas are skin test positive. The presence of substantial or prolonged infection in the presence of negative skin test is a poor prognostic marker. Similarly, high complement fixation titers (>1:64) are associated with extrapulmonic spread and poor prognosis. Serial rising titers are significant.

Diagnosis is made by biopsy material revealing granulomatous response with characteristic spherules with evidence of endosporulation or isolation in culture.

Diagnostic Tests/Procedures
Fungal Serology *on page 337*
Fungus Culture, Appropriate Site *on page 340*
KOH Preparation *on page 379*

Treatment Severe infection requires 1-3 g amphotericin B. Mild to moderate pulmonary disease may be treated with ketoconazole, 400 mg, or fluconazole, 400 mg. There is approximately a one-third relapse when treated with azoles. Primary disease requires no treatment. Meningitis must be treated with intrathecal amphotericin B. Fluconazole is still under investigation.

Drug Therapy
Recommended
Amphotericin B *on page 493*
Alternate
Ketoconazole *on page 598*

Selected Readings
Centers for Disease Control, "Coccidioidomycosis – California, 1991-1993," *MMWR Morb Mortal Wkly Rep*, 1994, 43(23):421-3.
Centers for Disease Control and Prevention, "Coccidioidomycosis - United States, 1991-1992," *JAMA*, 1993, 269(9):1098-9.
Einstein HE and Johnson RH, "Coccidioidomycoses: New Aspects of Epidemiology and Therapy," *Clin Infect Dis*, 1993, 16(3):349-54.
Saubolle MA and Sutton J, "Coccidioidomycosis: Centennial Year on the North American Continent," *Clin Microbiol Newslet*, 1994, 16(18):137-44.

Corynebacterium Group JK *see Corynebacterium jeikeium*
on this page

Corynebacterium jeikeium

Synonyms *Corynebacterium* Group JK

Microbiology *Corynebacterium jeikeium* was only recently described as a human pathogen in 1976. Like other *Corynebacterium* species, it is a gram-positive, aerobic bacterium but tends to have a more coccobacillary (rather than bacillary) appearance and must be distinguished from streptococci. It is considered one of the "diphtheroids," a term which encompasses several similarly-appearing gram-positive bacilli or coccobacilli which morphologically resemble *Corynebacterium diphtheriae*.

Epidemiology *Corynebacterium jeikeium* can colonize the skin of many hospitalized patients. *Corynebacterium jeikeium* has been cultured from the skin of

50% of hospitalized oncology patients. Sites of colonization include the rectum, axilla, and inguinal areas. Oncology patients who have received broad-spectrum antibiotics are at risk for colonization. Healthy individuals living in the community are less likely to be colonized with this organism.

Clinical Syndromes
- **Septicemia:** *Corynebacterium jeikeium* has been increasingly recognized as a cause of blood stream infections, particularly in those with underlying malignancies. There are also reports of bacteremias in cardiac surgery patients. In many cases, the portal of entry appears to be a skin defect, and often a blood stream infection is associated with an indwelling vascular catheter. Risk factors also include neutropenia, lengthy hospitalization, and multiple prior antibiotics.
- **Endocarditis:** Several cases of early prosthetic valve endocarditis from *Corynebacterium jeikeium* have been described.
- **Other infections:** Infected peritoneal dialysis catheters, prosthetic central nervous system shunt infections, prosthetic orthopedic implant infections, pneumonitis, and others.

Diagnosis *Corynebacterium jeikeium* diagnosis is made by identification of the organism by Gram stain and culture in a patient with a relevant clinical syndrome. No special media or conditions are necessary for growth. Any *Corynebacterium* isolated from the blood or catheter of an immunocompromised patient should be examined to determine if the isolate is *Corynebacterium jeikeium*.

Diagnostic Tests/Procedures
Aerobic Culture, Appropriate Site *on page 244*
Anaerobic Culture *on page 250*
Gram Stain *on page 352*

Treatment *Corynebacterium jeikeium* is unique in that it is highly resistant to antimicrobial therapy. The clinically-isolated strains of JK tend to be resistant to cephalosporins and penicillins; some data suggest that antibiotic-susceptible strains of *C. jeikeium* are replaced by resistant strains during prolonged hospitalization. The antibiotic of choice is vancomycin.

Drug Therapy
Recommended
Vancomycin Hydrochloride *on page 691*
Alternate
Penicillin G, Parenteral *on page 633*
  used in combination with
Gentamicin Sulfate *on page 575*

Selected Readings
Holmes RK, "Diphtheria, Other Corynebacterial Infections, and Anthrax," *Harrison's Principles of Internal Medicine*, 13th ed, Isselbacher KJ, Braunwald E, Wilson JD, et al, eds, New York, NY: McGraw-Hill, 1994, 623-30.

Rozdzinski E, Kern W, Schmeister T, et al, "*Corynebacterium jeikeium* Bacteremia at a Tertiary Care Center," *Infection*, 1991, 19(4):201-4.

Spach DH, Opp DR, and Gabre-Kidan T, "Bacteremia Due to *Corynebacterium jeikeium* in a Patient With AIDS," *Rev Infect Dis*, 1991, 13(2):342-3.

Corynebacterium Species, Other than *C. jeikeium*

Microbiology *Corynebacterium* species are gram-positive bacteria which are part of the normal flora of humans. They are important members of a larger group of loosely related organisms referred to as "coryneform bacteria" or "diphtheroids" because they morphologically resemble the organism *Corynebacterium diphtheriae*. All members of the diphtheroid group (including *Corynebacterium* species) are aerobic, gram-positive bacilli or coccobacilli that often appear pleomorphic in clinical samples. Medically important coryneform bacteria include *Corynebacterium jeikeium* (see entry *Corynebacterium jeikeium*), *Corynebacterium* CDC group D-2, *Corynebacterium ulcerans*, *Arcanobacterium haemolyticum* (formerly *Corynebacterium haemolyticum*), and *Corynebacterium minutissimum*. A number of additional *Corynebacterium* species are potential pathogens.

Epidemiology Many *Corynebacterium* species are part of the normal flora of humans and are thus common isolates in a clinical microbiology laboratory. Various sites that are commonly colonized by *Corynebacterium* species include the skin of healthy persons (eg, *C. pseudodiphtheriticum*, *C. xerosis*), the skin of hospitalized patients (eg, *Corynebacterium* CDC group D-2), and the nasopharynx (several species). It may be difficult to determine the significance of a single isolate of *Corynebacterium* from a clinical specimen since it may represent colonization, skin contamination, or true disease.

(Continued)

Corynebacterium Species, Other than *C. jeikeium*
(Continued)

Clinical Syndromes As noted above, the isolation of *Corynebacterium* species from a clinical specimen (eg, wound culture, vascular catheter culture, blood culture) requires careful interpretation by the physician. Serious disease has been associated with some *Corynebacterium* species, and the finding of a positive culture does not necessarily imply skin contamination or colonization. *Corynebacterium* species are considered organisms of low pathogenicity, and patients may present with a mild or chronic illness. Some species have been associated with specific illnesses as follows:

- **Urinary tract infections:** *Corynebacterium* CDC group D-2 has recently been recognized as a potential cause of urinary tract infections. This organism is similar to *Proteus mirabilis* in its ability to use the enzyme urease to hydrolyze urea; this leads to alkalinization of the urine and formation of struvite kidney stones which can become chronically infected. Complications include chronic cystitis secondary to infected stones and pyelonephritis. Again, the finding of a positive urine culture for "diphtheroids" or corynebacteria should be interpreted cautiously since this could also represent contamination of the urine sample from normal flora in the urethral region.

- **Erythrasma:** This common infection of the skin has been associated with *Corynebacterium minutissimum*, although the precise etiology of erythrasma is still unknown. Patients with erythrasma present with a patchy, erythematous rash often in the groin region. Under the fluorescent light of a Wood's lamp, the rash of erythrasma characteristically appears coral red. Cultures for *C. minutissimum* from patients with suspected erythrasma are not usually necessary since the diagnosis can usually be made clinically.

- **Pharyngitis:** *Arcanobacterium haemolyticum* (formerly *Corynebacterium haemolyticum*) can cause a pharyngitis associated with a scarlatiniform skin rash, particularly in young adults. The organism *C. ulcerans* (part of the flora of cows and horses) has occasionally been associated with a diphtheria-like pharyngitis in humans.

- **Pneumonia:** *Corynebacterium* species only rarely have been associated with pneumonia. There are case reports describing pneumonia in AIDS patients from *C. pseudodiphtheriticum*.

- **Bacteremia:** Since many *Corynebacterium* species are part of the normal skin flora, they may contaminate blood cultures (reported as "diphtheroids" in many laboratories). However, these organisms have been reported to cause both true bacteremia and endocarditis.

Diagnosis Most of the clinical manifestations of *Corynebacterium* species (with the exception of erythrasma) are nonspecific and isolation of the organism in the laboratory is necessary. The organisms, in general, grow readily on standard media. At times, *Corynebacterium* CDC group D-2 may be more difficult to grow from urine cultures, and the laboratory should be notified that this organism is suspected (alkaline urine, gram-positive bacilli on Gram stain, presence of stones, etc).

Diagnostic Tests/Procedures
Aerobic Culture, Appropriate Site *on page 244*
Anaerobic Culture *on page 250*
Gram Stain *on page 352*

Treatment Treatment of *Corynebacterium* depends on the severity of the infection and to some extent on the species involved. *Corynebacterium* CDC Group D-2 tends to be somewhat more antibiotic resistant than other species, and some isolates are resistant to the quinolones, which are commonly used for urinary tract infections. *Corynebacterium* species are generally susceptible to erythromycin, vancomycin, and to most beta-lactam antibiotics. If serious infections are documented, full susceptibility testing of the organism should be performed. Note that *Corynebacterium jeikeium* (see entry) is often resistant to multiple antibiotics.

Drug Therapy
Recommended
Erythromycin *on page 561*
Alternate
Penicillin G, Parenteral *on page 633*

Selected Readings
Cohen Y, Force G, Gros I, et al, "*Corynebacterium pseudodiphtheriticum* Pulmonary Infection in AIDS Patients," *Lancet*, 1992, 340(8811):114-5.

Coyle MB and Lipsky BA, "Coryneform Bacteria in Infectious Diseases: Clinical and Laboratory Aspects," *Clin Microbiol Rev*, 1990, 3(3):227-46.

Holmes RK, "Diphtheria, Other Corynebacterial Infections, and Anthrax," *Harrison's Principles of Internal Medicine*, 13th ed, Isselbacher KJ, Braunwald E, Wilson JD, et al, eds, New York, NY: McGraw-Hill, 1994, 623-30.

Soriano F, Aguado JM, Ponte C, et al, "Urinary Tract Infection Caused by *Corynebacterium* Group D2: Report of 82 Cases and Review," *Rev Infect Dis*, 1990, 12(6):1019-34.

Coxiella burnetii

Microbiology *Coxiella burnetii* is an obligately intracellular, gram-negative coccobacillus and a member of the group of organisms known as rickettsiae (*Rickettsia, Ehrlichia, Rochalimaea*, and *Coxiella*). *C. burnetii* survives extracellularly probably in spore form and can survive weeks to years in adverse environmental conditions. *C. burnetii* exists in two antigenic forms or "phases". Phase I organisms are avirulent, exist in nature and in laboratory animals, and react serologically with convalescent sera. Phase II organisms are virulent and react with acute sera. If phase I organisms are passed through chicken eggs, the phase I organisms become phase II organisms. **C. burnetii is extremely infectious to humans; a single organism can cause infection.**

Epidemiology Q fever was first described in Australia in 1937 (Q: "query"), occurs worldwide, and is not uncommon. Cattle, goats, sheep, and ticks are natural reservoirs. Persons at high risk for Q fever are persons associated with slaughter houses, persons who work with the aforementioned animals, persons who work with hides and wool, farmers, veterinarians, and researchers. The most common causes of infection are inhalation of organisms, handling of infected birth products (especially cat and cattle placentas), skinning infected animals, and transport of infected animals. *C. burnetii* is not transmitted person-to-person and only rarely by blood products.

Clinical Syndromes The most common form of Q fever is a self-limited febrile illness. Humans are the only known animals which regularly develop infection with *C. burnetii*. Incubation period is 2-4 weeks. Pneumonia, hepatitis, and endocarditis are the most common manifestations. Q fever usually presents as an atypical pneumonia; Q fever can also present as a rapidly progressive disease or as a secondary finding in someone with fever of unknown origin. The hepatitis form can present as infectious hepatitis. Endocarditis is the primary manifestation of chronic Q fever.

Diagnosis Typical signs and symptoms include headache, usually high fever, chills, fatigue, and myalgia. Other symptoms depend on which organ is affected. A rash can occur in the chronic endocarditis form of Q fever; a rash occurs only rarely in acute Q fever. Isolation of *C. burnetii* is an extremely dangerous laboratory procedure and is not practical. The most practical and clinically relevant method is serology. Complement fixation (CF) and immunofluorescence (IF) are the two most commonly used serological methods. CF is widely available and can demonstrate a fourfold rise in titer; however, CF does not separate IgG from IgM. Immunofluorescence uses separate phase I and II antigens and is more clinically useful. Phase II and I antibody titers are usually high in acute and convalescent disease, respectively. IgM antibody can persist for more than a year in some cases, but this is not a common finding. Some laboratories offer enzyme immunoassay (EIA) serology. EIA probably is the most sensitive of the three tests.

Diagnostic Tests/Procedures
Q Fever Serology *on page 433*

Pediatric Drug Therapy
Recommended
  Chloramphenicol *on page 531*

Adult Drug Therapy
Recommended
  Doxycycline *on page 557*
  Tetracycline *on page 679*
Alternate
  Chloramphenicol *on page 531*

Selected Readings

Feld RD, "Q Fever," *Diag Clin Test*, 1990, 28:30-2.

Marrie TJ, "*Coxiella burnetii* (Q Fever)," *Principles and Practice of Infectious Diseases*, 4th ed, Mandell GL, Bennett JE, and Dolin R, eds, New York, NY: Churchill Livingstone, 1995, 1727-35.

Reimer L, "Q Fever," *Clin Microbiol Rev*, 1993, 6(3):193-8.

ORGANISMS

Coxsackieviruses

Microbiology The name "Coxsackievirus" is derived from the town where this agent was first isolated: Coxsackie, New York. These viruses are composed of single-stranded RNA and have a positive-sense linear genome. They belong to the genus Enterovirus and the family Picornaviridae. The name "Picornaviridae" summarizes the nature of the family: pico (small), -rna (ribonucleic acid), -viruses. Coxsackieviruses are related to poliovirus, echovirus, and rhinovirus. There are two major types of Coxsackieviruses, types A and B. These are further subdivided into numbered serotypes.

Epidemiology Coxsackieviruses can infect all age groups. The virus is found worldwide and predominantly during the summer months. Transmission is mainly by the fecal-oral route, but droplet infection by the respiratory route is also possible. Infection rates are higher in communities with poor sanitation and crowding.

Clinical Syndromes

Diseases caused by Coxsackieviruses, group A:
- **Herpangina:** Patients present with sore throat, fever, and sometimes nausea and vomiting. On examination, there are vesicles present on the soft palate, a location unusual for other agents. Lesions are also seen on the uvula, and less commonly on the hard palate. Cultures of active ulcerating vesicles will yield the organism. Symptoms resolve spontaneously over several days.
- **Hand-foot-and-mouth syndrome**
- **Epidemic conjunctivitis**
- **Pharyngitis**

Diseases caused mainly by Coxsackieviruses, group B:
- **Epidemic pleurodynia:** Group B Coxsackieviruses cause this syndrome of fever, sharp pleuritic pain in the rib cage or upper abdomen. Patients describe this as a "stitch" in the side and is caused by disease of the muscle (not pleura or ribs). The pain is spasmodic in nearly all cases. The diagnosis can be confirmed by obtaining cultures of the throat and/or stool for this virus, or by demonstrating a rise in antibody titer.
- **Myocarditis, pericarditis**
- **Overwhelming infection of the newborn**

Diseases caused by either group A or B Coxsackieviruses:
- **Acute aseptic meningitis**
- **undifferentiated febrile illness**
- **fever with upper respiratory infection**
- **encephalitis**
- **asymptomatic infection**

In addition, the Coxsackieviruses have been linked with such diverse diseases as the Guillain-Barré syndrome, hemolytic uremic syndrome, diarrheal illnesses, myositis, Reye's syndrome, and a syndrome similar to infectious mononucleosis.

Diagnosis Coxsackievirus infection is suspected when an individual presents with one of the syndromes mentioned above. The differential diagnosis of these syndromes is wide, and laboratory confirmation is often necessary. Appropriate specimens of cerebrospinal fluid, rectal swabs, conjunctival swabs, or throat swabs should be promptly submitted to the microbiology laboratory. A special request for a Coxsackievirus (or enterovirus) culture should be made.

Diagnostic Tests/Procedures
Coxsackie A Virus Serology *on page 310*
Coxsackie B Virus Serology *on page 310*
Enterovirus Culture *on page 331*

Drug Therapy Comment
No antiviral agents have been proven effective.

Selected Readings
Kaplan MH, Klein SW, McPhee J, et al, "Group B Coxsackievirus Infections in Infants Younger Than Three Months of Age: A Serious Childhood Illness," *Rev Infect Dis*, 1983, 5(6):1019-32.
Modlin JF, "Coxsackieviruses, Echoviruses, and Newer Enteroviruses," *Principles and Practice of Infectious Diseases*, 4th ed, Mandell GL, Bennett JE, and Dolin R, eds, New York, NY: Churchill Livingstone, 1995, 1620-36.

Cryptococcus neoformans

Microbiology *Cryptococcus neoformans* is an encapsulated round to oval yeast 4-6 μm with a surrounding polysaccharide capsule ranging in size from

1 to over 30 μm. In its natural environment, it is smaller and poorly encapsulated.

In its perfect state (*Filobasidiella neoformans*), mycelia are produced bearing basidiospores 1-3 μm. This state has never been isolated in nature nor patients, although it has been postulated that it may be in this state that route of transmission occurs via inhalation of the basidiospores or unencapsulated forms leading to colonization of the airways and subsequently respiration infection.

It is distinguished from other yeasts by its ability to assimilate urea and possesses membrane bound phenoloxidase enzymes that convert phenolic compounds to melanin as demonstrated on certain agars (ie, birdseed agars).

Epidemiology There are four serotypes designated A, B, C, and D. Serotypes A and D (*C. neoformans* var *neoformans*) is the most common cause of infection and usually occurs in immunocompromised hosts. Serotypes B and C (*C. neoformans* var *gattii*) is typically seen in normal hosts and has a predilection for CNS invasion.

Cryptococcus is found worldwide. *C. neoformans* var *gattii* is endemic in the tropical and subtropical regions (Southern California, Australia, Southeast Asia, Brazil, Central America), particularly in the soils under eucalyptus trees. *Cryptococcus* grows readily from soil contaminated with avian excreta, particularly pigeon droppings but also has been isolated from non-avian sources such as fruits, vegetables, and dairy products. There have been no outbreaks attributable to environmental sources.

The incidence of cryptococcosis is steadily increasing secondary to AIDS and is the fourth most common opportunistic infection in AIDS patients. Five percent to 10% AIDS patients develop cryptococcosis with two-thirds developing meningoencephalitis. Prior to AIDS, 50% of patients had no known underlying immune defect. Risk factors prior to AIDS include diabetes, rheumatoid arthritis, cirrhosis, leukopenia, and malignancy. It was rarely seen in children, and the incidence in men was three times that of women.

Mortality risk factors include positive India ink, increased opening CSF pressure, decreased CSF glucose, CSF leukocyte count <20 cells/μL, extraneural site, absent *Cryptococcus* antibody, *Cryptococcus* antigen >1:32, and steroids or lymphoreticular malignancy. Good prognostic indications include headache as a symptom, normal mental status, and CSF leukocytes >20 cells/μL. Most important prognostic factor is patient's underlying disease process. Morbidity, mortality, and relapse are all increased in immunocompromised hosts.

Clinical Syndromes

- **Asymptomatic:** Solitary or multiple nodules found on plain chest x-ray.
- **Pulmonary cryptococcosis:** Most common infection. Present with cough, fever, and lobar infiltrates or mass. May see diffuse interstitial pattern or pleural effusion. If positive serum *Cryptococcus* antigen, look for disseminated disease.
- **CNS:** Second most common site of infection. Presents as either acute (headache, fever, nuchal rigidity) or chronic (headache, altered mental status) meningitis. May see cryptococcomas on CT or MRI. Usually secondary to lung but may represent reactivation similar to *Histoplasma* and tuberculosis.
- **Cutaneous:** Wide variation, may appear as papules, tumors, vesicles, plaques, abscesses, cellulitis, purpura, draining sinus, ulcers, bullae, or subcutaneous swelling. Usually a sign of dissemination.
- **Other:** Rarely invades eyes, bones, joints, liver, kidneys, or adrenal.

Diagnosis *Cryptococcus* skin test is not standardized as it is not completely characterized; therefore, its sensitivity and specificity is unknown and not used as a diagnostic aid. Diagnosis is confirmed by isolation from sterile body fluids including blood or histopathology revealing encapsulated yeast cells by alcian blue or mucicarmine. The India ink stain is positive in only approximately 50% of the time in normal hosts and >80% of the time in AIDS patients.

Cryptococcal antigen has >95% sensitivity and specificity but does cross react with *Trichosporon beigelii*. It is difficult to interpret a persistently high titer but has been associated with poor prognosis. Cryptococcal antigen in the CSF is produced locally in the subarachnoid space by the invading yeast and not by passive or active diffusion from the serum into the CNS. CSF findings include a pleocytosis lasting 6-12 months, low glucose concentrations, and high protein concentrations.

(Continued)

Cryptococcus neoformans (Continued)

Diagnostic Tests/Procedures
Cryptococcal Antigen Serology, Serum or Cerebrospinal Fluid *on page 312*
Cryptococcus Serology *on page 313*
Fungus Culture, Appropriate Site *on page 340*
India Ink Preparation *on page 373*
KOH Preparation *on page 379*

Treatment Amphotericin B remains the treatment of choice. Ketoconazole may be used for skin and pulmonary infections 1-3 months but has very poor penetration into the CNS so should not be used in serious or disseminated disease. Amphotericin B (dose 0.4-1.0 mg/kg per day with total dose 1.5 g) may be used in conjunction with flucytosine (100-150 mg/kg per day) for 6 weeks. May need to use amphotericin B intraventricular. Either amphotericin B or fluconazole can be used for chronic suppressive therapy. Itraconazole is still under investigation. The relapse role for non-AIDS is 15% to 25% compared to >50% in the AIDS population. Repeat lumbar punctures should be performed after 2 weeks of therapy and again at 1, 3, 6, and 12 months post therapy.

Drug Therapy
Recommended
Amphotericin B *on page 493*
or
Amphotericin B *on page 493*
used in combination with
Flucytosine *on page 570*

Alternate
Fluconazole *on page 569*

Selected Readings
Levitz SM, "The Ecology of *Cryptococcus neoformans* and the Epidemiology of Cryptococcosis," *Rev Infect Dis*, 1991, 13(6):1163-9.
Perfect JR, "Cryptococcosis," *Infect Dis Clin North Am*, 1989, 3(1):77-102.

Cryptosporidium

Microbiology Although *Cryptosporidium* was identified as early as 1907, it was not recognized as a human pathogen until 1976. *Cryptosporidium* is classified as a protozoan and is structurally related to *Toxoplasma* and *Plasmodium* species. Several species of *Cryptosporidium* have been found; the species most associated with human disease is *C. parvum*. The organism is approximately 2.5 μm in diameter and is about the same size and shape as many yeasts. *Cryptosporidium* can be identified by use of an acid-fast stain or an immunofluorescence test of a fresh stool specimen.

The parasite has four spores (sporozoites) within an oocyst. Its life cycle occurs within a single host. Human infection begins when the mature oocyst form of *Cryptosporidium* is ingested or perhaps inhaled. The four sporozoites excyst and divide asexually into meronts which release merozoites which can either reinvade the human or develop sexually into meronts. The sexual cycle ends in the formation of oocysts. The oocysts then can exit the body of the host through the feces to begin the infectious cycle in a new human or in the same host (autoinfection).

Epidemiology Cryptosporidial infections occur worldwide. In the United States, the organism is most prevalent in persons with AIDS, with infection rates ranging from 3% to 20%. In such countries as Africa and Haiti, *Cryptosporidium* can infect over 50% of the AIDS population. The organism is also a cause of sporadic diarrheal illness in normal individuals. Outbreaks of cryptosporidiosis have been well-described in the U.S. and include a recent outbreak in Wisconsin related to a contaminated metropolitan water supply.

The modes of transmission are as follows:
- Person-to-person: Accounts for spread of infection within day care centers, households, and hospitals. Transmission is usually by a fecal-oral route.
- Environmental contamination: The oocyst can be found in rivers and other natural water supplies, and thus, the traveler and camper is at risk. *Cryptosporidium* resists standard chlorination procedures in many areas and thus, can initiate major outbreaks of diarrheal illness when water supplies are contaminated.
- Animal-to-human
- Foodborne illness

Clinical Syndromes

- **Acute diarrhea in the normal host:** The most common manifestation of human cryptosporidiosis is a syndrome characterized by profuse, watery diarrhea, malaise, and abdominal cramping or pain. Fevers to the 39°C to 40°C range have occurred even in immunologically competent individuals. The incubation period is estimated to be 2-14 days following exposure to the parasite. The diarrhea often has an acute onset and symptoms can last 2 weeks or more.
- **Acute diarrhea in the immunocompromised host:** Cryptosporidiosis can be more subacute in onset. However, it is still characterized by voluminous diarrhea and weight loss over a several-week period can occur.
- **Cryptosporidial cholecystitis:** This has been described in immunocompromised patients. Symptoms include right upper quadrant abdominal pain, nausea, vomiting, and fever. There can be a concomitant diarrheal illness.

Diagnosis The symptoms of human cryptosporidiosis are nonspecific and cannot be distinguished from other causes of acute diarrheal illnesses. A high level of suspicion must be maintained because the organism cannot be readily identified using standard fecal smears.

Standard laboratory studies are not helpful in establishing the diagnosis. The leukocyte count may be normal, and there is usually not a peripheral blood eosinophilia to suggest a parasitic disease. Abnormalities in radiographic studies such as barium enemas and small bowel series have been described but again are not diagnostic of the organism. The only reliable means of identifying *Cryptosporidium* is to perform a direct exam (acid-fast stain) of a stool sample. This allows rapid identification of the organism. Because excretion of the parasite in the feces may be intermittent, it is recommended that two or more separate samples be submitted to the laboratory. Other techniques for identification of *Cryptosporidium* have been developed, including a direct immunofluorescence assay (DFA) and an enzyme immunoassay (EIA).

Diagnostic Tests/Procedures
Acid-Fast Stain *on page 239*
Cryptosporidium Diagnostic Procedures, Stool *on page 314*

Treatment At present, there is no widely accepted antimicrobial agent which is effective against *Cryptosporidium*. Some initial reports suggest the extended spectrum macrolides such as clarithromycin may have some use, but further studies are needed.

Drug Therapy Comment
Supportive care as treatment of choice.

Selected Readings
Adams RB, Guerrant RL, Zu S, et al, "*Cryptosporidium parvum* Infection of Intestinal Epithelium: Morphologic and Functional Studies in an *In vitro* Model," *J Infect Dis*, 1994, 169(1):170-7.

Bissuel F, Cotte L, Rabodonirina M, et al, "Paromomycin: An Effective Treatment for Crytosporidial Diarrhea in Patients With AIDS," *Clin Infect Dis*, 1994, 18(3):447-9.

Current WL, Reese NC, Ernst JV, et al, "Human Cryptosporidiosis in Immunocompetent and Immunodeficient Persons: Studies of an Outbreak and Experimental Transmission," *N Engl J Med*, 1983, 308(21):1252-7.

Danziger LH, Kanyok TP, and Novak RM, "Treatment of Cryptosporidial Diarrhea in an AIDS Patient With Paromomycin," *Ann Pharmacother*, 1993, 27(12):1460-2.

Hayes EB, Matte TD, O'Brien TR, et al, "Large Community Outbreak of Cryptosporidiosis Due to Contamination of a Filtered Public Water Supply," *N Engl J Med*, 1989, 320(21):1372-6.

Jokipii L and Jokipii AM, "Timing of Symptoms and Oocyst Excretion in Human Cryptosporidiosis," *N Engl J Med*, 1986, 315(26):1643-7.

Kotler DP, Francisco A, Clayton F, et al, "Small Intestinal Injury and Parasitic Diseases in AIDS," *Ann Intern Med*, 1990, 113(6):444-9.

Newman RD, Zu SX, Wuhlib T, et al, "Household Epidemiology of *Cryptosporidium parvum* Infection in an Urban Community in Northeast Brazil," *Ann Intern Med*, 1994, 120(6):500-5.

Cytomegalovirus

Synonyms CMV

Microbiology As a member of the herpesvirus family, CMV is a DNA virus which replicates in the cell nucleus. Human CMV's are antigenically heterogeneous with differences expressed through endonuclease mapping. No serological distinctions are made. Although difficult to grow in experimental animals, it can be cultured (1-4 weeks) in human fibroblasts. Monoclonal antibody techniques can shorten the identification time to 48 hours.

(Continued)

Cytomegalovirus *(Continued)*

Epidemiology CMV infections occur worldwide. About 50% of the general population is seropositive by the third decade of life. The incidence of CMV infection is more common in underdeveloped countries, lower socioeconomic groups, and in individuals who are sexually promiscuous. Virus can be isolated from several body fluids including saliva, feces, urine, and milk. Transmission requires repeated, prolonged contact. Spread is common in day care centers. In young adults, CMV is often a sexually transmitted disease, with asymptomatic carriage in the semen and cervical secretions. CMV may also be acquired from blood transfusions or organ transplantation.

Clinical Syndromes

- **Congenital CMV infection:** The fetus may become infected with CMV in two ways, primary CMV infection of the mother during pregnancy or reactivation of latent CMV in the mother during pregnancy. Primary maternal infection is much more likely to cause significant fetal infection. The manifestations of disease in the fetus are quite variable. Severe CMV disease is seen in only a small percentage of infected fetuses (5%). At birth, infants have hepatosplenomegaly, jaundice, microcephaly, and other abnormalities. Prognosis depends on the severity of the disease. The majority of congenitally-infected neonates appear healthy at birth. Up to 25% of these asymptomatically infected infants will show developmental disorders later in childhood, such as deafness and mental retardation. Severe CMV infections are associated with a mortality approaching 30%.

- **Perinatal infection:** These infants are not infected in utero but instead acquire CMV during delivery. Seropositive mothers may shed virus into the birth canal due to CMV reactivation. Many infants infected in this manner remain healthy. In a small number of cases, neonates may develop pneumonia, lymphadenopathy, and rash. Infants excrete CMV for months. Neonatal infection can also be transmitted by breast milk.

- **CMV mononucleosis syndrome:** In normal adults, primary infection with CMV is usually asymptomatic. The most common form of clinically apparent disease in previously healthy adults is a febrile illness resembling Epstein-Barr virus mononucleosis. Typically, the patient presents with fever, chills, myalgias, and headache. Examination reveals an enlarged spleen and liver, but unlike EBV infection, adenopathy and pharyngitis are minimal. Most patients recover without incident but occasionally symptoms may persist for weeks. Laboratory studies show elevated liver function tests and circulating atypical lymphocytes on blood smear. Heterophil antibody tests are negative. CMV can be recovered in urine and saliva for an extended period of time. The physician must rely on serologic tests and appropriate viral cultures to distinguish CMV mononucleosis from similar syndromes caused by either EBV or *Toxoplasma gondii.*

- **CMV in the transplant recipient:** One of the most feared complications of transplantation is CMV infection, particularly pneumonia. The peak time for CMV disease occurs several weeks post-transplantation, the so-called "40-day fever". CMV pneumonitis carries a high morbidity. Patients present with dyspnea, fever, cough, and interstitial infiltrates on chest x-ray. Bronchoscopy is usually necessary for both culture and lung biopsy. The diagnosis of CMV pneumonia has been somewhat controversial; it is apparent that a bronchial lavage culture positive for CMV is not necessarily diagnostic of pneumonia. Many clinicians prefer to see the characteristic CMV "owl's eye" inclusion bodies on lung biopsy before diagnosing true pneumonia. Treatment of CMV pneumonia is with ganciclovir intravenously, but failures still occur. Some researchers advocate the use of CMV hyperimmune globulin (concentrated CMV immunoglobulins) in conjunction with ganciclovir, but results of such use have been mixed.

  In an effort to decrease serious CMV infections, transplant centers have adopted a variety of strategies. One approach is to use ganciclovir prophylactically, that is, to give the drug prophylactically as a means of preventing CMV disease. This prophylactic treatment is based on the observation that patients who develop CMV pneumonia often do not have positive buffy coats for CMV (or other culture sites) consistently. Recent clinical trials have supported the prophylactic use of ganciclovir for bone marrow transplants at risk for CMV infection; ganciclovir is begun soon after transplantation and continued for 100 days. Another approach is to develop a reliable laboratory marker to detect CMV disease early. The CMV antigenemia assay appears to be promising. Detection of the pp65 matrix antigen in peripheral polymorphonuclear leukocytes may be a good predictor of impending clinical disease. Potentially, this would allow the "pre-emptive" use of ganciclovir, but clinical trials are needed to confirm this.

- **CMV in AIDS:** Several different organs may be infected with CMV in individuals with AIDS. CMV retinitis occurs in >10% of patients with AIDS. Patients typically complain of altered vision or "floaters" in one or both eyes. Examination reveals characteristic retinal lesions with exudates and hemorrhages ("cottage cheese and catsup"). Patients require lifetime antiviral therapy. Foscarnet or ganciclovir are usually given via a permanent indwelling catheter. Progression is inevitable, although the retinitis can be suppressed for extended periods of time. Other CMV infections are common in AIDS including CMV colitis, adrenalitis, and esophagitis. The incidence of CMV pneumonia in AIDS is unclear but is probably much less common than with the transplant population. Rare manifestations include CMV radiculopathy, encephalopathy, and myelopathy.

Diagnosis CMV-associated disease diagnosis is often very difficult because CMV can often be found in normal patients without the presence of any disease syndrome. Diagnosis depends on clinical symptoms consistent with CMV disease along with the appropriate cultures and serologies for CMV. Positive serologies should be confirmed by culture of the organism with the presence of CMV inclusion bodies from biopsy material of appropriate sites. A significant rise in serology titers also may be useful, but culture confirmation is always preferred. The presence of virus in the blood by buffy coat is also helpful. Presence of a positive culture from lung or gut for example, may not be sufficient to make the diagnosis of pulmonary or colonic CMV disease without confirmation by the presence of CMV inclusions.

Diagnostic Tests/Procedures
Cytomegalovirus Culture *on page 319*
Cytomegalovirus Culture, Blood *on page 320*
Cytomegalovirus Isolation, Rapid *on page 320*
Cytomegalovirus Serology *on page 321*
Immunofluorescent Studies, Biopsy *on page 372*

Treatment Ganciclovir is presently the treatment of choice for all CMV diseases including "CMV syndrome", retinitis, colitis, pneumonitis, and hepatitis. In patients with immunosuppressive agents, decreasing the amount of immunosuppressant may also be helpful. An alternative agent in failures or those patients who are intolerant to ganciclovir is foscarnet. Foscarnet is at least as active as ganciclovir against CMV but is more toxic. The addition of cytomegalovirus immune globulin (CMVIG) has not been proven to be any more effective than either of the antiviral agents alone. In bone marrow transplant patients with severe CMV infections, the addition of intravenous immune globulin (IVIG) to ganciclovir may be useful for CMV prophylaxis in transplant recipients, a variety of agents have been utilized including acyclovir, ganciclovir, IVIG, and CMVIG. CMVIG is effective in preventing primary disease in kidney transplant patients at highest risk for disease (patients who are CMV serology negative, receiving a serologically positive organ) but has not been proven to be effective in these high risk patients undergoing other organ transplants. Ganciclovir and CMVIG are each effective in preventing secondary CMV disease in transplant recipients who are already CMV serology positive. Acyclovir, which is not effective in treating CMV disease, has also been shown to be an effective prophylactic agent, but controversy remains.

Drug Therapy
Recommended
Ganciclovir *on page 574*
Alternate
Foscarnet *on page 571*

Selected Readings
Balfour HH Jr, "A Randomized, Placebo-Controlled Trial of Oral Acyclovir for the Prevention of Cytomegalovirus Disease in Recipients of Renal Allografts," *N Engl J Med*, 1989, 320(21):1381-7.

Chou S, "Newer Methods for Diagnosis of Cytomegalovirus Infection," *Rev Infect Dis*, 1990, 12(Suppl 7):S727-36.

Hirsch MS, "Cytomegalovirus Infection," *Harrison's Principles of Internal Medicine*, 13th ed, Isselbacher KJ, Braunwald E, Wilson JD, et al, eds, New York, NY: McGraw-Hill, 1994, 794-7.

Schmidt GM, Horak DA, Niland JC, "A Randomized, Controlled Trial of Prophylactic Ganciclovir for Cytomegalovirus Pulmonary Infection in Recipients of Allogeneic Bone Marrow Transplants," *N Engl J Med*, 1991, 324(15):1005-11.

ORGANISMS

Dermatophytes

Microbiology Dermatophytes are fungi that invade the keratinized areas of the body (hair, nails, and skin) and are members of the genera *Epidermophyton*, *Microsporon*, or *Trichophyton*. Dermatophytes may be classified by the organism's name, their ecology (anthropophilic, geophilic, or zoophilic), or anatomical location of invasion.

They are differentiated by their colonial morphology, microscopic appearance of conidia, hair perforation or fluorescence, and biochemical/nutritional requirements.

Epidemiology Dermatophytes are the most common fungal infections in humans. They are found worldwide with some species limited geographically. They colonize nonviable structures. Invasion occurs when the role of penetration of the dermatophyte into the keratin exceeds the role of keratin growth and shedding. Local trauma-altered primary host defenses and impaired cell-mediated immunity contribute to infection. *E. floccosum* is the only species of *Epidermophyton* that infects man. It only invades the skin and nails and not hair. *Microsporon* and *Trichophyton* have many species that infect humans. *M. gypseum* is the most important geophilic dermatophyte and typically causes infections secondary to occupational exposure from direct contact with the soil. *M. canis* may be transmitted from animals to their owners and handlers. *T. tonsurans* is the most common cause of tinea capitis worldwide.

Clinical Syndromes

- **Tinea barbae:** Occurs on the bearded areas of face and neck. Most frequently seen in farm workers. May occur as circinate spreading type, vesiculopustular border with central scaling or superficial type characterized by perifollicular involvement with fever, malaise, and regional adenopathy. Most common organism is *T. mentagrophytes*.
- **Tinea capitis:** More common in pediatrics. Present with erythema, marked scaling, and hair loss. Severe form associated with large, boggy pustules, fever, leukocytosis, and regional lymphadenopathy. Associated with erythema nodosum. Transmitted person to person. *T. mentagrophytes* is the most common organism, previously *M. audouinii*.
- **Tinea corporis:** Infection of the skin except groin, palms, scalp, or soles. Affects all ages and sexes. More frequent in hot, humid, tropical areas. Transmitted from other humans, animals, fomites, and, rarely, soil. Presents as erythematous papules with a red, pruritic, raised scaling border with central cleaning.
- **Tinea cruris:** Pruritic, erythematous eruption with circumscribed inflammatory margins that begins on inner thigh and spreads to groin, perineum, and perianal regions. Risk factors include obesity, diabetes, intertrigo, humidity, and tight fitting clothes. Arthroconidia may survive for years, necessitating sterilization of clothes and linens.
- **Tinea pedis:** May occur as intertriginous involvement of toe webs or chronic hyperkeratotic form with minimal inflammation of soles and sides of feet or acutely as erythematous, clear vesicles which may become secondarily infected. Twenty-five percent to 75% of the normal population are culture positive and asymptomatic. Incidence increases with age. Most common organism is *T. rubrum*.
- **Tinea unguium:** Invasion of the nail; must be differentiated from onychomycosis which is a general term for any nail infection.
- **Deep local invasion:** Dissemination; uncommon; seen in immunosuppressed population.

Diagnosis Diagnosis is made by KOH examination of infected material or identification of characteristic macroconidia in culture. Up to 50% of KOH-positive samples may be culture-negative. Some of the organisms may be fluorescent under a Wood's lamp (ie, *M. canis* yellow and green, *T. schoenleinii* dull bluish white). Erythrasma caused by *Corynebacterium minutissimum* will be coral red under Wood's lamp. Other diagnostic tests employed are the hair perforation test and DTM (dermatophyte test media).

Diagnostic Tests/Procedures

Fungus Culture, Skin *on page 343*
KOH Preparation *on page 379*

Treatment The most important aspect of therapy is educating patients for the need to continue therapy for a period of time after the infection appears resolved. Therapy is directed at anatomical location.

- **Tinea barbae:** Griseofulvin for 4-6 weeks
- **Tinea capitis:** Griseofulvin for 1-2 weeks after lesion cleared for a total of 4-8 weeks. Alternative therapy is ketoconazole.

- **Tinea corporis:** Imidazole creams or topical keratolytics. In severe infection, griseofulvin or ketoconazole.
- **Tinea cruris:** Topical imidazole 3-4 weeks.
- **Tinea pedis:** Topical imidazole 3-4 weeks. Chronic form requires griseofulvin, however, *T. rubrum* may develop resistance.
- **Tinea unguium:** Requires griseofulvin for 12 months. May cause hepatotoxicity. Alternate therapy is ketoconazole.
- **Deep or disseminated:** Amphotericin B

Drug Therapy

Recommended

Superficial infection:

Antifungal, Topical *on page 498*

Deep infection:

Griseofulvin *on page 578*

Disseminated infection:

Amphotericin B *on page 493*

Selected Readings

Elewski BE and Hazen PG, "The Superficial Mycoses and the Dermatophytes," *J Am Acad Dermatol*, 1989, 21(4 Pt 1):655-73.

Salata RA, "Ringworm and Other Superficial Mycoses," *Tropical and Geographical Medicine Companion Handbook*, 2nd ed, Mahmoud AAF, ed, New York, NY: McGraw-Hill 1993, 371-7.

Eaton's Agent *see Mycoplasma pneumoniae on page 159*

EBV *see Epstein-Barr Virus on page 110*

E. coli 0157:H7 *see Escherichia coli, Enterohemorrhagic on page 112*

EHEC *see Escherichia coli, Enterohemorrhagic on page 112*

Ehrlichia Species

Microbiology *Ehrlichia* sp are small gram-negative bacilli (0.5 μm) related to the *Rickettsia* species in terms of DNA content, geographic distribution, and clinical disease. The organisms are obligate intracellular aerobes which grow in vacuoles within the host cell. Clusters of these organisms growing within membrane-bound vacuoles have been visualized by light and electron microscopy and given the name morulae. The genus *Ehrlichia* contains several species which are primarily pathogenic for animals (eg, dogs, horses, jackals, and others). **The etiologic agent of human ehrlichiosis has yet to be identified.** The organism causing human disease has not been cultured or sequenced. It is tentatively called "an *Ehrlichia canis*-like agent" because of its serologic cross-reactivity with *E. canis*. Some experts speculate that human ehrlichiosis is probably caused by *E. canis* or a closely related *Ehrlichia* species such as *E. schaffeensis* or *E, phagocytophila*.

Evidence suggests human ehrlichiosis is a tickborne illness. The tick involved in transmission has not been identified, although *Rhipicephalus sanguineus* and *Amblyomma americanum* are distinctly possible vectors. This tick transmits *E. canis*. The infectious cycle for *E. canis* is a possible model for human ehrlichiosis. *E. canis* infection begins when the tick feeds on a dog already infected with *E. canis*. The organisms are harbored in the tick and later transmitted to uninfected dogs during a subsequent blood meal. It is speculated that infection may spread to humans in a similar fashion. The incubation period between the tick bite and initial clinical symptoms is estimated to be 9 days.

Epidemiology Over 100 cases of human ehrlichiosis have been reported but the true number of cases is probably much higher. The peak incidence is from May to July. Infection is four times more common in males. Geographic areas at highest risk are in the southern and south-central regions, as follows: South: South Carolina, North Carolina, Florida, Alabama, Kentucky, Tennessee, Georgia, Virginia, Maryland; South-Central/Central: Arkansas, Oklahoma, Missouri, Texas, Louisiana; others: New Jersey, Wyoming, Vermont, Washington.

As noted, transmission is likely by a tick that has not yet been identified. Person-to-person transmission has not been seen.

Clinical Syndromes

- **Human ehrlichiosis:** Patients present initially with fever, chills, headache, and myalgias. Later, there may be anorexia, vomiting and weight loss. Some patients also present with respiratory symptoms such as cough and dyspnea. A rash may be present but in less than half the reported cases.

(Continued)

Ehrlichia Species *(Continued)*

The rash is usually maculopapular and less commonly petechial. Otherwise, examination findings may be normal. Laboratory studies often show leukopenia and thrombocytopenia, important clues to the diagnosis. Elevated liver function tests are also common during the acute phase of the illness. The chest x-ray may show transient infiltrates. Anemia is seen after about 1 week of illness. The clinical course of human ehrlichiosis is variable, and can range from a mild febrile illness to multiorgan system failure with protracted fever. It is clear that ehrlichiosis can be a systemic disease with a number of visceral organs infiltrated with mononuclear cells. Serious complications have been reported in 40% of hospitalized patients. These include hypotension, neurologic (ie, encephalitis, cerebrospinal fluid pleocytosis), coagulopathies, acute renal failure, hepatocellular necrosis, and death.

Diagnosis Human ehrlichiosis should be suspected in any patient with an unexplained febrile illness who resides in or has traveled to an area endemic for this disease. A history of a tick bite is useful but not necessary. The disease may be difficult to distinguish from Rocky Mountain spotted fever (RMSF) which has a similar geographic distribution. Several characteristics may be used to separate the two diseases: skin rash is less common in ehrlichiosis; when a skin rash is present in ehrlichiosis, it is less often petechial, as is the case with RMSF; leukopenia is more common in ehrlichiosis.

Laboratory confirmation rests primarily on serologic studies. Indirect immunofluorescence assays (IFA) for *Ehrlichia canis* have been used to diagnose human infections. A fourfold rise in titer between acute and convalescent samples is diagnostic. However, false-positive results may occur. Although the direct visualization of ehrlical morulae in host white blood cells has been reported in some cases, this appears to be a rare finding and is insensitive. As mentioned, the agent of human ehrlichiosis has not been cultured as yet, and cannot be used for diagnosis. The differential diagnosis of human ehrlichiosis includes RMSF, viral syndromes. and bacterial septicemia. Because of the variable clinical presentation, consultation with an Infectious Diseases specialist may be useful if this infection is suspected.

Diagnostic Tests/Procedures
Ehrlichia Serology on page 325

Treatment Tetracycline and doxycycline appear to be useful. Intravenous chloramphenicol also has been used successfully.

Pediatric Drug Therapy
Recommended
Chloramphenicol on page 531

Adult Drug Therapy
Recommended
Tetracycline on page 679
Doxycycline on page 557

Selected Readings
Eng TR, Harkess JR, Fishbein DB, et al, "Epidemiologic, Clinical, and Laboratory Findings of Human Ehrlichiosis in the United States, 1988," *JAMA*, 1990, 264(17):2251-8.

Everett ED, Evans KA, Henry RB, "Human Ehrlichiosis in Adults After Tick Exposure. Diagnosis Using Polymerase Chain Reaction," *Ann Intern Med*, 1994, 120(9):730-5.

Fichtenbaum CJ, Peterson LR, and Weil GJ, "Ehrlichiosis Presenting as a Life-Threatening Illness With Features of the Toxic Shock Syndrome," *Am J Med*, 1993, 95(4):351-7.

Fishbein DB, Dawson JE, and Robinson LE, "Human Ehrlichiosis in the United States, 1985 to 1990," *Ann Intern Med*, 1994, 120(9):736-43.

"Human Ehrlichiosis – United States," *MMWR Morb Mortal Wkly Rep*, 1988, 37(17):270, 275-7.

Maeda K, Markowitz N, Hawley RC, et al, "Human Infection With *Ehrlichia canis*, a Leukocytic Rickettsia," *N Engl J Med*, 1987, 316(14):853-6.

McDade JE, "Ehrlichiosis – A Disease of Animals and Humans," *J Infect Dis*, 1990, 161(4):609-17.

Rikihisa Y, "The Tribe Ehrlichieae and Ehrlichial Diseases," *Clin Microbiol Rev*, 1991, 4(3):286-308.

Entamoeba histolytica

Microbiology *Entamoeba histolytica* is an enteric protozoan that exists in two forms, cyst and trophozoite. The cyst ranges in size from 5-20 μm and contains one to four nuclei. The trophozoite is an ameba, ranges in size from 12-60 μm, and contains a single nucleus with a centrally located nucleolus with a uniformly distributed peripheral chromatin. Although all strains of *E. histolytica* are morphologically identical, there is epidemiological and biological evidence that

ORGANISMS

there are pathogenic and nonpathogenic strains. Isoenzyme analysis reveal that there are four distinct zymodemes which appear to correlate with the virulence of the ameba.

Epidemiology It is estimated that 10% of the world is infected with *E. histolytica*, with 50,000-100,000 *E. histolytica*-associated deaths per year, making amebiasis the third leading parasitic cause of death in the world. It is endemic in Mexico, India, West and South Africa, and portions of Central and South America. It appears to be most virulent in the tropics. The vast majority (90%) of patients remain asymptomatic. High risk factors for invasive diseases in the United States include recent immigration, institutionalization, and homosexuality, although 30% to 40% of male homosexuals harbor a nonpathogenic strain. It is imperative to exclude other etiologies of diarrhea in patients with AIDS given the large number of asymptomatic carriers. Infection with *E. histolytica* begins with ingestion of the cyst via contaminated food or water or fecal-oral route. The ingested mature cyst excysts in the lower ileum and multiplies by binary fission producing eight trophozoites. The trophozoites may remain in the lumen of the colon and multiply or invade the wall of the colon and spread hematogenously. Trophozoites encyst in the colon, and both mature and immature cysts are excreted in the feces.

Clinical Syndromes
Intestinal:
- **Asymptomatic colonization:** Affects 90% of those infected. Also referred to as cyst passage.
- **Acute amebic colitis:** Present with lower abdominal pain and explosive bloody diarrhea. Approximately 30% to 40% will have fever. Onset over 7-10 days with a 1- to 4-week duration. More severe in children, pregnant women, and immunosuppressed individuals, especially those on steroids. Toxic megacolon associated with steroid use. Almost all patients will have heme-positive stools but few or no leukocytes presumably due to ability of ameba to lyse leukocytes hence the name "histolytica". Chronic colitis must be differentiated from inflammatory bowel disease.
- **Fulminant colitis:** More common in children. Diffuse abdominal pain and profuse bloody diarrhea. Seventy-five percent of children may develop colonic perforation.
- **Ameboma:** Develops in 1% of patients with colitis. Localized chronic amebic infection usually in cecum or ascending colon. Presents as a tender mass.

Extraintestinal:
- **Hepatic abscess:** Acute hepatic abscess presents with dull, pleuritic, right upper quadrant pain and fever. Subacute less likely to have fever. Ten percent to 15% may present with fever and no pain. Fifty percent acute presentations will have multiple hepatic lesions, whereas 80% subacute will have a single lesion located in the right lobe liver. Fifty percent will have no history of antecedent dysentery. Laboratory reveals leukocytosis without eosinophilia, alkaline phosphatase elevated >75%, transaminase elevated >50%.

  Other rare complications of hepatic abscess include genitourinary, skin, adrenal, and kidney invasion.
- **Pleuropulmonary:** Most common complication of hepatic abscess, occurring 20% to 35%. Typically associated with lesion from left lobe liver. Present with pleuritic pain, cough. May have serous effusions, consolidation, empyema, or hepatobronchial fistula.
- **Peritoneal:** Second most common complication of hepatic abscess is intraperitoneal rupture in 2% to 7.5%. Indolent leaks much more common than rupture or abscess.
- **Pericardial:** Most serious complication of hepatic abscess. Perforation of abscess into the pericardium usually results in tamponade and/or shock. Greater than 60% have abscesses in left lobe liver. Mortality is 40%.
- **CNS:** Brain abscesses occur where intestinal amebiasis is endemic. Aggressive, multifocal disease known as secondary cerebral amebiasis (SCA). Must be differentiated from *Naegleria* and *Acanthamoeba* as treatment differs. Rapidly progressive disease with spreading abscesses with internal necrosis of gray-white junction of cerebral cortex. SCA occurs in 0.6% to 0.8% patients with hepatic abscess. Extremely rare without hepatic invasion. Presentation depends on size, location, and number of lesions. May present as chronic infection with fever, weight loss, hepatomegaly, abdominal pain, dyspnea, and pleuritic pain. Diarrhea may be absent. Less than one-third will have positive ova and parasite fecal exam. Incubation

(Continued)
103

Entamoeba histolytica (Continued)

period is typically 2-5 months. Male to female ratio is 5:1. CSF examination reveals mononuclear cells with normal and low glucose. CT scan reveals ring enhancing lesions.

Diagnosis Eighty percent to 90% of patients with acute dysentery will have cysts or trophozoites on fecal examination after examining three samples. Trophozoites rapidly die after passage; therefore, feces must be examined within 20 minutes of collection. Serology titers are positive in 60% to 90% of the cases after 7 days, however 6% to 20% of patients in endemic areas will have positive serologies which may persist for years after acute infection. Sigmoidoscopy or colonoscopy with biopsy is recommended for patients with chronic colitis to differentiate between inflammatory bowel versus amebiasis. Extraintestinal disease should be diagnosed by aspiration of abscess or biopsies. Liver abscesses aspirate is classically chocolate colored or has an anchovy paste appearance. More than 90% will have positive serology. Absence of serology titer is strong evidence against amebiasis.

Diagnostic Tests/Procedures
Entamoeba histolytica Serology *on page 330*
Ova and Parasites, Stool *on page 416*
Ova and Parasites, Urine or Aspirates *on page 419*

Treatment

Dysentery: Metronidazole 750 mg three times/day for 10 days plus luminal amebicide either iodoquinol, diloxanide furoate (from CDC) or paromomycin. Fluid electrolyte support. May need surgical decompression if megacolon.

Hepatic: Metronidazole plus iodoquinol 650 mg three times/day for 10 days. May need percutaneous draining.

CNS: Metronidazole plus surgical drainage. If no surgical drainage, metronidazole 500 mg four times/day for 4 weeks, chloroquine 300 mg once daily for 4 weeks, tetracycline 500 mg four times/day for 4 weeks followed by dehydroemetine 80 mg once daily for 10 days.

Prevention: Boiling is only means of eradicating *E. histolytica* cysts in water. Vegetables must be cleansed in strong detergent soap and soaked in acetic acid or vinegar for 10-15 minutes. Travelers to endemic areas should be advised to avoid uncooked vegetables, salads, fruits that cannot be peeled, and ice cubes.

Drug Therapy
Recommended
Asymptomatic (cyst passers):
Diloxanide Furoate *on page 553*
Invasive infection:
Metronidazole *on page 610*
followed by
Diloxanide Furoate *on page 553*

Alternate
Invasive infection:
Metronidazole *on page 610*
followed by
Paromomycin Sulfate *on page 630*

Selected Readings
Aucott JN and Ravdin JI, "Amebiasis and "Nonpathogenic" Intestinal Protozoa," *Infect Dis Clin North Am*, 1993, 7(3):467-85.
Campbell S, "Amebic Brain Abscess and Meningoencephalitis," *Semin Neurol*, 1993, 13(2):153-60.
Reed SL, "Amebiasis: An Update," *Clin Infect Dis*, 1992, 14(2):385-93.

Enterobacter Species

Microbiology *Enterobacter* species are gram-negative rods which are increasingly important causes of nosocomial infection, particularly because of the emergence of highly antibiotic-resistant isolates. *Enterobacter* species (formerly called *Aerobacter* species) are aerobic gram-negative bacilli which normally colonize the intestinal tract. The genus name "*Enterobacter*" should not be confused with the broader family name "Enterobacteriaceae;" the latter designation refers to many gram-negative bacteria including *Enterobacter* species, *E. coli*, *Klebsiella*, *Serratia*, and others. Based on studies of DNA relatedness, *Enterobacter* is most closely related to *Klebsiella*, with >50% DNA sequence homology. The organism cannot be distinguished from other related

GNBs on the basis of Gram stain alone, and culture identification is necessary. The major species of *Enterobacter* which are pathogenic for humans include *E. cloacae* (accounting for most infections), *E. aerogenes*, and *E. agglomerans*.

Enterobacter produces endotoxin, the lipopolysaccharide (LPS) component which is associated with the outer membrane of the bacteria. When cell lysis occurs (as with antibiotic therapy) the LPS is released into the host and can lead to such inflammatory responses as fever, leukopenia or leukocytosis, hypotension, and disseminated intravascular coagulation. Thus, LPS is regarded as an important mediator of the sepsis syndrome.

Epidemiology Because *Enterobacter* commonly inhabits the human gastrointestinal tract, it is considered one of the "enteric bacteria." In hospitalized patients, it often asymptomatically colonize the urine, respiratory tract, abdominal wounds, decubitus ulcers, and other sites. Community-acquired infection is rare, and *Enterobacter* is generally considered an opportunist of the hospitalized, debilitated individual.

Clinical Syndromes

- **Lower respiratory tract infection:** Nosocomial *Enterobacter* infections are seen in patients with extended hospitalizations, particularly those who are ventilator-dependent. Patients who have been on prolonged broad spectrum antibiotics seem at particular risk for *Enterobacter* infection. Lengthy courses of broad spectrum antibiotics do not "protect" the patient from opportunistic *Enterobacter* infections. It should be noted that *Enterobacter* and other gram-negative bacilli can asymptomatically colonize the upper respiratory tract of hospitalized patients. Thus, the recovery of a sputum or tracheal aspirate culture for *Enterobacter* does not necessarily indicate a significant infectious disease. The diagnosis of a pneumonia still rests on standard criteria such as the presence of purulence (many leukocytes) on the Gram stain of sputum, the presence of a pulmonary infiltrate, and signs of systemic inflammation in the patient. A positive sputum culture alone is not sufficient justification for initiating antibiotic therapy.

- **Burn wound infections:** Outbreaks of serious *Enterobacter* infections (primarily septicemias) have been reported in burn units.

- **Urinary tract infection:** Seen in hospitalized patients, often those with indwelling Foley catheters. However, *Enterobacter* may harmlessly colonize the urine of patients with chronic bladder catheters without causing disease. The decision to initiate antibiotics in such patients should be based on the clinical situation (the presence of pyuria on urinalysis, suprapubic pain, fever, etc). Even the finding of large numbers of *Enterobacter* in a urine culture ($> 10^5$ colony forming units/mL) by itself does not automatically indicate antimicrobial therapy.

- **Hospital-associated bacteremias:** In 1975, *Enterobacter* strains were associated with a national epidemic of contaminated intravenous products. The organisms were found to grow in commercially available fluids used for intravenous infusions and were the cause of rapid-onset septicemia. There have been no nationwide *Enterobacter* outbreaks since then, but the organism is still recovered periodically from blood cultures.

Diagnosis The clinical presentations of the various nosocomial infections caused by *Enterobacter* are not distinctive, and laboratory isolation is necessary.

Diagnostic Tests/Procedures

Aerobic Culture, Appropriate Site *on page 244*
Gram Stain *on page 352*

Treatment *Enterobacter* species present a challenging therapeutic problem, especially when isolates exhibit high level antibiotic resistance. Preliminary data suggest that the popular third generation cephalosporins may act to select naturally-occurring mutants of *Enterobacter* that are resistant to a wide variety of antibiotics. In the typical case, the cephalosporin is able to eradicate the vast majority of sensitive *Enterobacter* species. However, when the bacterial load is high (as in an abscess), these mutants may be present in small numbers along with the normally susceptible bacteria and continue to divide in the face of selective antibiotic pressure. In time, this resistant strain will dominate and often demonstrates complete resistance to all cephalosporins and all penicillins, even if penicillins were not given. This disturbing trend is particularly common in intensive care units, where prolonged courses of antibiotics are given empirically for fever without a clear focus of infection. Such "type I chromosomal mutants" may still remain susceptible to imipenem; infectious disease consultation may be helpful since imipenem-resistance can develop rapidly as well.

ORGANISMS

Drug Therapy
Recommended
Penicillins, Extended Spectrum *on page 637*
Cephalosporins, 3rd Generation *on page 528*
Alternate
Imipenem/Cilastatin *on page 586*
Selected Readings
Chow JW, Fine MJ, Shlaes DM, et al, "*Enterobacter* Bacteremia: Clinical Features and Emergence of Antibiotic Resistance During Therapy," *Ann Intern Med*, 1991, 115(8):585-90.
Quinn JP, DiVincenzo CA, and Foster J, "Emergence of Resistance To Ceftazidime During Therapy For *Enterobacter cloacae* Infections," *J Infect Dis*, 1987, 155(5):942-7.
Wolff MA, Young CL, and Ramphal R, "Antibiotic Therapy For *Enterobacter* Meningitis: A Retrospective Review of 13 Episodes and Review of the Literature," *Clin Infect Dis*, 1993, 16(6):772-7.

Enterobius vermicularis
Synonyms Pinworm

Microbiology *Enterobius vermicularis*, or pinworm, causes a form of perianal pruritus called enterobiasis, often seen in children. *Enterobius vermicularis* is a nematode, or roundworm, and is thus related to such parasites as *Ascaris lumbricoides*, *Ancylostoma duodenale* (hookworm), and *Strongyloides stercoralis*. *E. vermicularis* is a small, white worm with a cylindric unsegmented body. It is visible to the naked eye. The infectious cycle begins when the human host ingests the embryonated egg, which is infective within hours. The eggs hatch in the small intestine, and the emerging larval forms migrate to the large intestine. There, the larvae penetrate and develop within the mucosa and mature into male and female adult forms over a 2-to 6-week period. Fertilization takes place and the gravid female migrates to the perianal region of the host at night and lays its eggs in the perianal folds. The eggs mature rapidly and are infectious within hours.

Epidemiology Pinworm infection is most common in school children, although infection may occur at all ages. Infection is favored by close living conditions and is typically seen in institutions, schools, and day care centers. Cases frequently are clustered in families. All socioeconomic groups are at risk. Over 500 million cases occur worldwide, with about 40 million individual infections in the United States. Humans are the only known reservoir. Transmission occurs primarily via direct person-to-person spread. Eggs of the parasite frequently are carried beneath the fingernails of children who have been scratching the irritated perianal area. *E. vermicularis* eggs are relatively hardy and remain viable in dust, clothing, day care toys, furniture, and other fomites; infection can occur from inhalation of the eggs contained in infested dust.

Clinical Syndromes
- **Asymptomatic carriage:** Many infected individuals experience no symptoms from *E. vermicularis* but are still capable of spreading the worm.
- **Perianal pruritus:** This is the most common manifestation of pinworm infestation. Often there is severe local pruritus, interfering with sleep. Excessive scratching of the perianal region may lead to bacterial infection in severe cases.
- **Miscellaneous:** Unusual complications include appendicitis, salpingitis, granuloma formation, penetration through the intestinal wall, and bowel lesions.

Diagnosis Pinworm infestation is usually suspected in the individual who presents with refractory itching in the perianal area, particularly in children. The "Scotch tape test" is an accurate and inexpensive means of confirming the diagnosis. Clear adhesive tape is pressed to the perianal region early in the morning, prior to bathing or bowel movement . The eggs deposited overnight by the migrating adult readily adhere to the cellophane tape. This tape may be brought in later for examination by the physician. The thin-walled eggs are easily seen at low power under the microscope. Several examinations over consecutive days may be necessary since a single test may be falsely negative in 50% of cases. Commercial kits may be used in place of the less formal Scotch tape method; these kits utilize an adhesive paddle and follow the same general principles. Stool examinations are rarely diagnostic for pinworm. Peripheral eosinophilia is not characteristically seen.

Diagnostic Tests/Procedures
Pinworm Preparation *on page 430*

Treatment The drug of choice is mebendazole (Vermox®), which leads to a cure in >90% of the cases. Retreatment may be necessary in some cases, especially if reinfection occurs. Family members should be tested, even if asymptomatic, and treated as necessary.

Drug Therapy
Recommended
Mebendazole *on page 604*
Pyrantel Pamoate *on page 651*
Selected Readings
Mahmoud AA, "Intestinal Nematodes (Roundworms)," *Principles and Practice of Infectious Diseases*, 4th ed, Mandell GL, Bennett JE, and Dolin R, eds, New York, NY: Churchill Livingstone, 1995, 2526-31.
Wagner ED and Eby WC, "Pinworm Prevalence in California Elementary School Children, and Diagnostic Methods," *Am J Trop Med Hyg*, 1983, 32(5):998-1001.

Enterococcus Species

Microbiology Historically, the term *Enterococcus* was used to describe hardy, nonfastidious streptococci that were able to be cultured under a variety of conditions. The enterococci, *Streptococcus bovis* and *Streptococcus equinus* were classified as group D streptococci. Subsequently in 1984, the genus streptococci was divided into three genera, *Streptococcus*, *Lactococcus*, and *Enterococcus*. Enterococci, on Gram stain, are gram-positive, oval cocci that occur in pairs or short chains. In culture, they can grow in 6.5% NaCl broth at 10°C to 45°C, can hydrolyze esculin in 4% bile, and hydrolyze L-pyrholidonyl β-napththylamide.

Epidemiology In the human host, the main reservoir for *Enterococcus* species is the intestinal tract. They are also commonly found in the oral cavity, urethra, and vagina. Infections may arise from endogenous flora and may be spread as nosocomial infections by hand and environmental contamination. *E. faecalis* and *E. faecium* are the species recovered in 80% to 90% of enterococcal infections. Isolates of enterococci from blood are generally considered pathogenic because 85% of these patients have clinical infections. Broad spectrum antibiotic therapy may suppress normal flora and allow enterococcal overgrowth of the intestinal flora. Wound colonization is common and superinfection in compromised hosts and those on antimicrobial therapy also occurs frequently. The organism is considered to have low intrinsic virulence and is considered to be primarily an opportunistic pathogen.

Clinical Syndromes The enterococci are recognized as causes of urinary tract infections, bacteremia, endocarditis, intra-abdominal infections, and osteomyelitis primarily in diabetic patients. Pneumonia and meningitis due to *Enterococcus* are rare in adult patients. Fifteen percent to 20% of bacterial endocarditis is caused by enterococci. *Streptococcus viridans* and *Staphylococcus* are the only organisms more frequently isolated. Enterococcal endocarditis occurs in the elderly more in association with urinary tract manipulation (ie, cystoscopy and catheterization); in young women associated with childbirth, Cesarean sections, intrauterine devices (IUDs), curettage (D & Cs), and abortions. Intravenous drug abusers have a high incidence of enterococcal endocarditis which most frequently affects the mitral and/or aortic valves. Bacteremia is frequently detected in patients with serious underlying medical conditions including recent surgery, trauma, or burns. Enterococcal bacteremia is frequently nosocomial and often represents superinfection. Polymicrobic infections are frequently more fulminant with a higher incidence of shock, thrombocytopenia, and disseminated intravascular coagulation (DIC) than infections where enterococci are the sole pathogens. Gram-negative bacilli are the most frequently encountered copathogens. Prior antimicrobial therapy and long hospital stays are risk factors. The urinary tract is a frequent source of enterococcal bacteremia; however, because these cases are almost always associated with host factors enterococcal urinary tract infections (UTIs) are rarely encountered in office patients who are healthy otherwise. In intra-abdominal infections, enterococci are frequently present in part of a mixed infection where they may act synergistically with other bacteria. Neonatal meningitis may occur as nosocomial epidemics associated with prematurely low birth weight, previous antimicrobial therapy, arterial or venous catheterization, and nasogastric intubation.

Diagnostic Tests/Procedures
Aerobic Culture, Appropriate Site *on page 244*
Antimicrobial Susceptibility Testing, Aerobic and Facultatively Anaerobic Organisms *on page 259*
Blood Culture, Aerobic and Anaerobic *on page 271*
Gram Stain *on page 352*

Duration of Therapy Enterococcal endocarditis is commonly treated with combination therapy for 4-6 weeks. Therapy for other enterococcal infections range from 7-14 days.

Treatment Appropriate treatment for enterococcal infections other than those of the urinary bladder includes a bactericidal combination of penicillin or gly-

(Continued)

Enterococcus Species *(Continued)*

copeptide (vancomycin) and an aminoglycoside. In uncomplicated cystitis, the achievable antimicrobial concentrations in urine generally greatly exceed the minimal inhibitory concentration thus monotherapy with a β-lactam (ampicillin) or glycopeptide (vancomycin) can be utilized. The American Heart Association (AHA) currently recommends treating enterococcal endocarditis with penicillin G 20 million units or ampicillin 12 g administered as a continuous infusion or in six equally divided doses in combination with gentamicin 1-2 mg every 8 hours to achieve a postdose peak of 3-5 mg/L. Streptomycin dosages are 7.5 mg/kg, not to exceed 500 mg, every 12 hours to achieve a postdose peak of 15-30 mg/L. Vancomycin dosages are 15 mg/kg every 12 hours to achieve a post-dose concentration of 30-45 μg/L and a predose concentration <10 μg/L. If a vancomycin-resistant organism is encountered in a penicillin-sensitive patient, desensitization should be considered.

Typically enterococci have low level resistance to aminoglycosides. High level aminoglycoside resistance mediated by plasmids and transposons has become an increasing problem. *E. faecalis* frequently exhibits high level resistance to all currently available aminoglycosides. In serious infections, high level synergy testing is recommended for gentamicin and streptomycin. Because of β-lactamase production by some strains, β-lactamase testing (nitrocefin) also is performed by some laboratories. Vancomycin resistance is emerging; therefore, susceptibility testing for vancomycin is also indicated.

The resistance determinants of the enterococci reside on highly mobile genetic elements (plasmids and transposons) which have the potential to spread within the genus as well as to other gram-positive cocci. Thus the recognition, appropriate therapy, and awareness of the potential for nosocomial spread are of particular importance.

Co-trimoxazole frequently may appear to have a low minimal inhibitory concentration (MIC) against enterococci. This is due to low folate concentrations in the test medium. *In vivo*, folate from the host can be used by the enterococci to overcome the metabolic block of the co-trimoxazole thus co-trimoxazole should not be used in the therapy of enterococcal infections.

Cephalosporin *in vitro* susceptibility tests frequently suggest susceptibility; however, **cephalosporins are not effective** *in vivo*.

Drug Therapy
Recommended
Penicillin G, Parenteral *on page 633*
  used in combination with
Gentamicin Sulfate *on page 575*
  or
Ampicillin *on page 495*
  used in combination with
Gentamicin Sulfate *on page 575*

Alternate
Vancomycin Hydrochloride *on page 691*
  used in combination with
Gentamicin Sulfate *on page 575*
  or
Penicillin G, Parenteral *on page 633*
  used in combination with
Streptomycin Sulfate *on page 669*
  or
Ampicillin *on page 495*
  used in combination with
Streptomycin Sulfate *on page 669*

Selected Readings

Herman DJ and Gerding DN, "Antimicrobial Resistance Among Enterococci," *Antimicrob Agents Chemother*, 1991, 35(1):1-4.

Maki DG and Agger WA, "Enterococcal Bacteremia: Clinical Features, the Risk of Endocarditis and Management," *Medicine (Baltimore)*, 1988, 67(4):248-69.

Megran DW, "Enterococcal Endocarditis," *Clin Infect Dis*, 1992, 15(1):63-71.

Moellering RC Jr, "Emergence of Enterococcus as a Significant Pathogen," *Clin Infect Dis*, 1992, 14(6):1173-6.

Tailor SA, Bailey EM, and Rybak MJ, "Enterococcus, An Emerging Pathogen," *Ann Pharmacother*, 1993, 27(10):1231-42.

Watanakunakorn C and Patel R, "Comparison of Patients With Enterococcal Bacteremia Due to Strains With and Without High-Level Resistance to Gentamicin," *Clin Infect Dis*, 1993, 17(1):74-8.

Enterovirus

Microbiology Enteroviruses are small, single-stranded RNA viruses belonging to the family Picornaviridae. The term "enterovirus" may be a source of confusion since it may refer to either the genus Enterovirus (which includes echovirus, coxsackieviruses A and B, poliovirus, and enterovirus) or the species enterovirus. The following discussion applies to the species enterovirus, which is further classified into enterovirus serotypes 68-71. These agents are sometimes referred to as the "newer enteroviruses" because of their recent recognition as agents of disease. The enteroviruses lack a lipid envelope. Important biophysical properties include the ability to survive in conditions of low pH and relatively high temperatures, and resistance to chlorine and alcohol decontamination. Enteroviruses grow best at body temperature. They replicate well in the upper respiratory and gastrointestinal tracts and can survive the acid environment of the stomach.

Epidemiology The newer enteroviruses are widely distributed throughout the world. Enteroviruses 70 and 71 are the two serotypes best characterized from an epidemiological and clinical standpoint. Enterovirus serotype 70 was first reported as a pathogen in 1969 during an outbreak of hemorrhagic conjunctivitis in Indonesia. This previously unrecognized virus has since spread thoughout the globe and has been linked to millions of cases of hemorrhagic conjunctivitis. Pandemics are reported almost yearly. The majority of cases occur in the Far East, India, and Africa, generally in crowded urban areas with tropical climates. In the western hemisphere, most cases have been reported from Central America and the Caribbean, although an outbreak was reported from Florida in 1981 in an indigent population.

Enterovirus 71 was first isolated in 1969 from the stools of an infant in California with encephalitis. Over the next 10 years, a total of 8 epidemics were reported globally. The largest outbreak occurred in 1973 in Japan with over 3000 cases with hand-foot-and-mouth disease and aseptic meningitis. In 1975, an epidemic in Bulgaria involving 700 persons received worldwide attention. Over 20% of cases, mostly children, developed a polio-like paralysis with a significant number of fatalities; this was the first time a virus other than poliovirus was found to cause an epidemic paralytic disease. Small clusters of cases have been reported in the United States including a 1972 New York State outbreak characterized by meningitis and encephalitis in 11 cases and a similar small outbreak in 1977 in Rochester, New York, with two patients developing a self-resolving paralysis. An additional 5 children developed a polio-like paralysis in the summer of 1987 in Philadelphia, which remains the largest series of Enterovirus 71-associated paralysis reported in the United States.

Infections caused by the genus Enterovirus most commonly involve infants and younger children. Although specific data regarding Enterovirus 71 is somewhat limited, infants and younger children are at highest risk for infection with this serotype, based on data derived from the major epidemics of Enterovirus 71. In addition, most of the serious complications of Enterovirus 71, such as muscle paralysis and encephalitis, were reported in young children. Infections caused by Enterovirus 70 seem to involve all age groups equally.

Less is known about the transmission of the newer enteroviruses than related Enteroviruses such as poliovirus or Coxsackievirus. In general, the fecal-oral route is felt to be the major route of spread for the genus Enterovirus. Live virus may be shed from the oropharynx for weeks after acute infection, and there may be persistent shedding of virus in the stools for months. Direct person-to-person spread via the fecal-oral route is likely in this setting. Enterovirus 70 is an exception to this rule in that spread most likely occurs directly from hand-to-eye or indirectly from fomites to the eye.

Clinical Syndromes Infections caused by the newer enteroviruses have a diverse clinical spectrum but tend to be neurovirulent. There is also some overlap in the types of illnesses caused by the newer enteroviruses, poliovirus, Coxsackievirus A and B, and Echovirus.

- **Asymptomatic infection:** Many of the infections caused by viruses of the genus Enterovirus are asymptomatic, with an estimated 90% or more of enteroviral infections resulting in a nonspecific febrile illness. This likely holds true for the newer enteroviruses.
- **Poliomyelitis-like paralysis:** As noted above, Enterovirus 71 is a potential cause of an epidemic, lower motor neuron paralysis similar to polio. Anterior horn cells in the spinal cord are involved, as in poliomyelitis. The disease is acute in onset and usually involves children. Patients present with asymmetric flaccid paralysis of the extremities with absent reflexes in the in-

(Continued)

109

Enterovirus *(Continued)*

volved extremity. The sensory system is typically intact. This clinical syndrome is still rare in the United States but should be considered in the differential diagnosis of a child presenting with an unexplained paralytic disease.

- **Acute hemorrhagic conjunctivitis:** This disease, caused by Enterovirus serotype 70, tends to occur in an epidemic fashion and is highly contagious. Patients present with acute onset of a hemorrhagic conjunctivitis, with pain in the eye, photophobia, and periorbital swelling. Some may have constitutional symptoms such as fever and malaise. Nearly all will have subconjunctival bleeding, and this is distinctive. Complications include keratitis and occasionally neurologic complications such as motor paralysis have been reported following the conjunctivitis. Since only a limited number of cases have been reported from the western hemisphere, this diagnosis is unlikely in the United States but should be considered in immigrants or travelers.

  - **Aseptic meningitis:** Like other enteroviruses, Enterovirus 71 has been associated with the syndrome of aseptic meningitis. Patients present with headache, neck stiffness, and a lymphocytic pleocytosis in the spinal fluid. Enterovirus 71 is a relatively uncommon cause of this syndrome, with many studies demonstrating Coxsackievirus as the major etiologic agent.

  - **Hand-foot-and-mouth syndrome:** Like Coxsackievirus A16, Enterovirus 71 can cause this syndrome of vesicular lesions in the palms of the hands (exanthem) and the mucous membranes of the mouth (enanthem). This is a self-limited disease.

Diagnosis The clinical suspicion of enteroviral infection needs to be confirmed by viral culture. It is less important to differentiate the newer enteroviruses from Coxsackievirus or echovirus, than it is to differentiate it from bacterial causes of infection. The virus can be isolated in cell culture, particularly from rectal swabs or from throat secretions. In addition, it can be grown in cell culture from clinical specimens such as cerebrospinal fluid, skin lesions, or pericardial fluid.

Serologic studies are available to look for specific antibody responses to enterovirus. IgG antibody and IgM antibody against enteroviruses are available, and the finding of a fourfold increase in IgG or the presence of IgM antibody is helpful in establishing the diagnosis. However, it should be noted that recovery of enterovirus from a throat swab or a rectal swab does not necessarily establish enterovirus as the cause of an illness, since asymptomatic viral shedding may persist for periods of time. However, recovery of enterovirus from a site such as spinal fluid or a swab of a conjunctival lesion is confirmatory.

Diagnostic Tests/Procedures
Enterovirus Culture *on page 331*

Drug Therapy Comment Currently, there are no antiviral agents available which are active *in vivo* against enterovirus.

Epstein-Barr Virus
Synonyms EBV

Microbiology EBV is a DNA virus and a member of the herpesvirus family. Two strains of EBV, differing in their B lymphocyte transformation and in viral gene sequence expression, infect humans. The structure of the viral DNA of EBV is unique as compared to other herpesvirus. The virus selectively infects human B lymphocytes and produces "immortalized" cell lives and usually causes latent infection.

Epidemiology Infection with EBV is common, with about 95% of the population demonstrating specific antibodies to this virus. In the U.S., the first peak of EBV infection occurs in children, with nearly 50% of 5 year olds seroconverting. There is a second peak of infection in the 20-30 year old age group.

EBV is transmitted by exchange of saliva containing live virus. EBV often persists in the throat of acutely infected individuals for months. Periodic asymptomatic shedding of virus is common. EBV may be cultured from the throat of 10% to 20% of healthy adults. Many with acute EBV are not aware of a sick contact who may have transmitted the disease. Prolonged intimate contact is necessary for spread. In general, the data suggest that EBV is widespread but is a virus of relatively low pathogenicity. Following the initial exposure to the virus, there is a 1-2 month incubation period prior to clinical disease. During this time, the virus disseminates through the reticuloendothelial system (liver, spleen, lymph nodes).

Clinical Syndromes

- **Infectious mononucleosis:** In the United States, "mono" occurs most commonly in individuals between 15-25 years of age. Characteristically, the patient presents with the "classic triad" of fever, sore throat, and lymphadenopathy. Rash is seen in only 5% of cases, but the rash is seen in nearly 100% of patients who mistakenly receive ampicillin for their symptoms. The tonsils are enlarged and the pharynx is inflamed, often with petechiae. Splenomegaly is an important physical finding in this setting and is present in nearly 50% of cases. Liver enlargement may also occur and liver function tests are frequently elevated. In many cases, the clinician must rely heavily on laboratory confirmation of suspected infectious mononucleosis, since both toxoplasmosis and cytomegalovirus can cause a similar syndrome. A compatible clinical syndrome, a positive heterophil test, and atypical lymphocytosis on blood smear are usually enough to establish the diagnosis of EBV mononucleosis. However, many cases may lack one or more of these findings; children are particularly prone to have heterophil-negative EBV mononucleosis. More detailed serologic testing is often necessary to confirm the diagnosis. Most patients recover completely from infectious mononucleosis over 2-3 weeks. However, a variety of complications have been reported: splenic rupture, hemolytic anemia, airway obstruction, profound thrombocytopenia, encephalitis, and the Guillain-Barré syndrome. Rare patients demonstrate objective evidence of ongoing EBV infection, with leukopenia, pulmonary infiltrates, and progressive neurologic disorders; this is in distinction to the "chronic EBV syndrome" described below. Although acyclovir inhibits EBV *in vitro* and probably *in vivo* as well, it appears to have minimal benefit in acute EBV mononucleosis. In large part, this is likely due to the observation that the clinical events in EBV mononucleosis result from the host's immune response rather than from direct viral invasion. Case reports have described the benefit of acyclovir in life-threatening EBV, but data are limited. The use of corticosteroids is controversial. Some have advocated corticosteroids only in complicated EBV infection (airway obstruction, thrombocytopenia, etc), but the benefits are unclear.
- **Possible relationship with the chronic fatigue syndrome (CFS):** Persistent EBV infection has been theorized to cause the CFS. This controversial syndrome is characterized by overwhelming fatigue, muscle aches, poor concentration, low grade fevers, and minor lymphadenopathy. Initially, this symptom complex was termed the "chronic mononucleosis syndrome" due to its similarities with the prodromal symptoms of infectious mononucleosis. EBV was further implicated as an etiologic cause of "chronic mono" because many such individuals demonstrated high titers of EBV-specific antibody. Carefully controlled studies later showed that EBV titers were equivalent in patients with CFS and matched normal controls. In addition, clinical trials using acyclovir in CFS demonstrated no benefit. Currently, there is little objective evidence to link CFS and EBV.
- **EBV and malignancies:** EBV has been implicated as a cofactor in the development of Burkitt's lymphoma, a malignancy common in Africa. A direct causal relationship is suspected but has yet to be proven. EBV DNA sequences and virions have been identified in biopsy samples of Burkitt's lymphoma. EBV has also been strongly associated with nasopharyngeal carcinoma, a neoplasm most common in the Orient. Again, EBV nucleic acid has been found within malignant tissues.
- **EBV in transplant recipients:** In patients who have undergone solid organ or bone marrow transplantation, EBV has been reported to cause an unusual lymphoma-like syndrome called the "post-transplantation lymphoproliferative disorder." Patients receiving cyclosporin A, a medication used to prevent organ rejection, appear to be at increased risk. Biopsies of involved organs reveal a B-cell lymphoproliferative malignancy with identifiable EBV nucleic acid sequences. The spectrum of this disorder is still under study. In general, and unlike cytomegalovirus or herpes simplex virus, EBV is an unusual opportunistic pathogen in the transplant population.
- **EBV infection in patients with AIDS:** An EBV-related lymphoproliferative syndrome has also been reported in patients with advanced HIV infection. Another disease associated with EBV infection is oral hairy leukoplakia. This disease is a commonly seen lesion of the tongue and is frequently noted in advanced AIDS. EBV has been implicated as a possible etiologic cause (or cofactor) in this disorder.

(Continued)

Epstein-Barr Virus *(Continued)*

Diagnostic Tests/Procedures
Epstein-Barr Virus Culture *on page 332*
Epstein-Barr Virus Serology *on page 332*
Immunofluorescent Studies, Biopsy *on page 372*
Infectious Mononucleosis Serology *on page 374*

Drug Therapy Comment
No antiviral agents have been proven to be effective in the treatment of Epstein-Barr virus infections. Supportive care is the treatment of choice.

Selected Readings
Schooley RT, "Epstein-Barr Virus Infections, Including Infectious Mononucleosis," *Harrison's Principles of Internal Medicine*, 13th ed, Isselbacher KJ, Braunwald E, Wilson JD, et al, eds, New York, NY: McGraw-Hill, 1994, 790-3.

Straus SE, Cohen JI, Tosato G, et al, "Epstein-Barr Virus Infections: Biology, Pathogenesis, and Management," *Ann Intern Med*, 1993, 118(1):45-58.

Escherichia coli, Enterohemorrhagic

Synonyms
E. coli 0157:H7; EHEC

Microbiology
Enterohemorrhagic *E. coli* causes a distinct form of hemorrhagic colitis in humans. Like other *E. coli* strains, enterohemorrhagic *E. coli* is a facultative, gram-negative bacillus. The most common serotype is 0157:H7. Essentially all published information regarding enterohemorrhagic *E. coli* refers only to this serotype.

Epidemiology
In 1982, the first large-scale outbreak of *E. coli* 0157:H7 colitis was described. Multiple cases of severe bloody diarrhea were found to be epidemiologically linked to ingestion of contaminated hamburger meat. Since then, the organism has been recognized as an important cause of bloody diarrhea and the hemolytic uremic syndrome. Over 12 major outbreaks have been reported, along with numerous sporadic cases. The majority of cases have been traced to contaminated ground beef, although other potential sources have been cited, including unpasteurized milk, apple cider, municipal water, and roast beef. The organism inhabits the gastrointestinal tract of some healthy cattle and is thought to contaminate meat during slaughter and the processing of ground beef ("internal contamination"). If the ground beef is undercooked, the organism remains viable; undercooking of hamburger patties has proven important in several outbreaks.

In 1993, a well-publicized multistate outbreak of *E. coli* 0157:H7 took place in the western United States (Washington, California, Idaho, and Nevada). Over 500 infections and four deaths were documented. The vast majority of cases were ultimately linked to contaminated hamburger meat from a particular restaurant chain. Further investigation by the Centers for Disease Control identified several slaughter plants in the United States and one in Canada as the probable source. Thousands of contaminated patties not yet consumed were discovered. In March, 1994, the USDA Food Safety and Inspection Service recommended that all raw meat should be cooked thoroughly, with an increase in the internal temperature for cooked hamburgers to 155°F.

A 2-year nationwide surveillance study by the Centers for Disease Control has found *E. coli* 0157:H7 to be the most commonly identified pathogen associated with bloody diarrhea. In many parts of the U.S., *E. coli* 0157:H7 is the second most common cause of bacterial diarrhea.

Acquisition of disease is usually by ingestion of contaminated food, but person-to-person transmission has been documented, especially in day care centers. Children and elderly individuals are at highest risk for severe infections. Simple and careful hand washing essentially eliminates the probability of person-to-person transmission.

Clinical Syndromes
- **Hemorrhagic colitis:** *E. coli* 0157:H7 causes a bloody diarrhea associated with abdominal cramps. Pathologically, there is no invasion or inflammation of the intestinal mucosa, and thus fever is often absent. The diarrhea is caused by shiga-like toxins. In most cases, the illness resolves within 7 days, but death can occur in the elderly.
- **Hemolytic uremic syndrome:** Approximately 5% to 10% of patients with *E. coli* 0157:H7 diarrhea develop a syndrome characterized by acute renal failure, thrombocytopenia, and evidence of hemolysis on a peripheral blood smear. Children are at high risk for this syndrome. The patient may be toxic-appearing, and the presentation may be confused with a variety of

diseases including sepsis with disseminated intravascular coagulation, vasculitis, thrombotic thrombocytopenia purpura, and others. The estimated mortality is 3% to 5%.

Diagnosis Enterohemorrhagic *E. coli* should be strongly considered in any patient presenting with bloody diarrhea, whether or not hemolytic uremic syndrome is present. It is likely that many sporadic cases of *E. coli* 0157:H7 diarrhea occur in the community and go unrecognized for two reasons: many clinicians do not order stool cultures for stable patients with diarrhea; many microbiology laboratories do not routinely culture stools for *E. coli* 0157:H7 unless there is a specific order from the physician.

Diagnosis is confirmed by isolation of *E. coli* 0157:H7 from stool specimens and subsequent serological confirmation. This requires special media in the microbiology laboratory (sorbitol-MacConkey medium). Other methods for the rapid detection of this organism are currently under study.

Diagnostic Tests/Procedures
Stool Culture, Diarrheagenic *E. coli* on page 449

Drug Therapy Comment
No antibiotics proven effective.

Selected Readings
"*Escherichia coli* 0157:H7 Outbreak Linked to Home-Cooked Hamburger – California, July 1993," *MMWR Morb Mortal Wkly Rep*, 1994, 43(12):213-6.

Griffin PM, Ostroff SM, Tauxe RV, et al, "Illnesses Associated With *Escherichia coli* 0157:H7 Infections: A Broad Clinical Spectrum," *Ann Intern Med*, 1988, 109(9):705-12.

Riley LW, Remis RS, Helgerson SD, et al, "Hemorrhagic Colitis Associated With a Rare *Escherichia coli* Serotype," *N Engl J Med*, 1983, 308(12):681-5.

"Update: Multistate Outbreak of *Escherichia coli* 0157:H7 Infections From Hamburgers – Western United States, 1992-1993," *MMWR Morb Mortal Wkly Rep*, 1993, 42(14):258-63.

Escherichia coli, Nonenterohemorrhagic

Microbiology *Escherichia coli* is a lactose-positive, gram-negative, facultative bacillus with variable motility. A member of the Enterobacteriaceae family, *E. coli* is probably the most widely studied free-living organism. Most *E. coli* are nonpigmented, produce lysine decarboxylase, utilize acetate as a carbon source, and hydrolyze tryptophan to indole. Serologic typing is based on three surface antigens (O, H, K). The lipopolysaccharide of the cell wall is known as endotoxin and is a factor in sepsis and septic shock in infected individuals.

Epidemiology *E. coli*, as well as other Enterobacteriaceae, are normal colonizers of the human and animal gastrointestinal tract. It is often considered an opportunistic pathogen in hospitalized or debilitated patients but is the most common cause of urinary tract infections among "normal" hosts.

Clinical Syndromes
- **Urinary tract infections:** In the United States, *E. coli* is the most common cause of urinary tract infections both in normal hosts and immunocompromised or hospitalized patients. Although most common in sexually active young women, *E. coli* urinary tract infections occur in patients who are at increased risk of urinary tract infections in general (catheterized, obstructed, diabetic, prostatitis, etc).
- **Lower respiratory infections:** *E. coli* causes a significant number of nosocomial pneumonias in the United States and is an uncommon cause of community-acquired pneumonia or bronchitis. *E. coli* may also colonize the respiratory tract of hospitalized patients without causing disease, and its treatment in the absence of clinically relevant findings is usually unwarranted.
- **Neonatal meningitis:** Although uncommon in older populations, *E. coli* is a rare but important cause of meningitis and subsequent mortality in neonates.
- **Peritonitis:** *E. coli* is a major pathogen in polymicrobial intra-abdominal infections.
- **Sepsis and other infections:** *E. coli* is one of the leading causes of bacteremia, sepsis, and septic shock. It can also cause a variety of other infections including wound infections, cellulitis, and diarrhea.

Diagnosis *E. coli* infection diagnosis can be made by identification through Gram stain and culture in patients with relevant clinical syndromes. No special media or conditions are necessary to grow this organism. *E. coli* should always be one of several suspected organisms in patients with peritonitis.

Diagnostic Tests/Procedures
Aerobic Culture, Appropriate Site on page 244
Gram Stain on page 352

(Continued)

113

Escherichia coli, Nonenterohemorrhagic *(Continued)*

Treatment Although the majority of *E. coli* are still sensitive to ampicillin, amoxicillin, and first generation cephalosporins, increasing resistance is being noted, especially in nosocomial isolates. Most mild to moderate urinary tract infections can be treated with amoxicillin or co-trimoxazole until susceptibility confirmation. In more serious or nosocomial infections, more broad spectrum antibiotics, such as third generation cephalosporins, should be initiated until susceptibility data is available. In patients who are septic, supportive care will also be necessary along with appropriate antibiotics.

Drug Therapy

Recommended

Severe infection:

Cephalosporins, 3rd Generation *on page 528*

Mild to moderate infection:

Ampicillin *on page 495*

Co-trimoxazole *on page 545*

Alternate

Cephalosporins, 1st Generation *on page 527*

Cephalosporins, 2nd Generation *on page 527*

Selected Readings

Eisenstein BI, "*Enterobacteriaceae,*" *Principles and Practice of Infectious Diseases,* 4th ed, Mandell GL, Bennett JE, and Dolin R, eds, New York, NY: Churchill Livingstone, 1995, 1964-80.

Zwadyk P, "*Enterobacteriaceae:* General Characteristics," *Zinsser Microbiology,* 20th ed, Joklik WK, Willett HP, Amos DB, et al, eds, Norwalk, CT: Appleton & Lange, 1992, 538-43.

Zwadyk P, "Opportunistic Enterobacteriaceae," *Zinsser Microbiology,* 20th ed, Joklik WK, Willett HP, Amos DB, et al, eds, Norwalk, CT: Appleton & Lange, 1992, 544-55.

GABHS *see Streptococcus pyogenes on page 207*

Gardnerella vaginalis

Microbiology *Gardnerella vaginalis* is a small gram-negative rod which is part of the normal vaginal flora in many healthy women. It has been implicated as the cause of bacterial vaginosis, a common superficial infection of the vaginal mucosa. The organism is a nonmotile, pleomorphic, gram-negative (or gram-variable) rod. It lacks a capsule and does not form spores. Although *Gardnerella vaginalis* stains gram negative in clinical specimens, the cell wall is morphologically more characteristic of gram-positive bacteria. Most isolates are facultatively anaerobic, and the organism can be isolated in the laboratory without anaerobic culture techniques. The organism tends to be fastidious in its growth and nutritional requirements. Specific enrichment media may be used in the laboratory to optimize its recovery in culture; these media are combinations of Columbia agar base and human blood.

Epidemiology *Gardnerella vaginalis* can be recovered from the vagina in up to 60% of asymptomatic females. In the condition called bacterial vaginosis, it can be cultured in 95% to 100% of women. Its role as the causative agent of bacterial vaginosis is controversial, since it is so frequently found in healthy individuals. Other organisms comprising the normal vaginal flora can also significantly increase in women with bacterial vaginosis, including the obligate anaerobes *Peptococcus, Eubacterium,* and *Mobiluncus.* Some believe these other bacteria work in combination with *Gardnerella* to alter the physiologic environment within the vagina which ultimately leads to bacterial vaginosis. This is not a sexually transmitted disease. Although *Gardnerella* may at times be cultured from the urethra of the male sexual partner of a woman with bacterial vaginosis, there is no clinical counterpart of this condition in men.

Clinical Syndromes

• **Bacterial vaginosis:** As noted above, the precise role of *Gardnerella vaginalis* in the pathogenesis of this condition is not known. In bacterial vaginosis, there is characteristically a new vaginal discharge with a "fishy odor." The woman may be otherwise asymptomatic or may have mild vaginal irritation. Vaginal pruritus or severe burning are not seen. Bacterial vaginosis may be diagnosed clinically if the following are present: 1. a thin, homogeneous vaginal discharge is present on pelvic examination; 2. the pH of the vaginal mucosa/discharge is >4.5 (normal is <4); 3. the vaginal discharge has a "fishy odor" when a drop of 10% KOH is added to the discharge on a microscope slide ("whiff test"); 4. "clue cells" are seen on a wet mount of the vaginal discharge. These distinctive cells are actually the normal large vaginal epithelial cells which have been covered by sheets of gram-negative *Gardnerella* organisms. Generally, the presence of three of these four criteria is sufficient to establish bacterial vaginosis and to separate this condition from the two other common causes of vaginitis, namely *Candida albicans* and *Trichomonas vaginalis*.

- **Urinary tract infections:** *Gardnerella* is a rare (<1%) cause of either lower or upper urinary tract infections. Since the organism so often colonizes the normal vaginal flora, it is often difficult to determine if a positive urine culture for *Gardnerella* represents vaginal contamination. However, case reports have argued that it may be truly pathogenic in the urinary tract in a small number of patients, particularly young women and men with underlying renal disease.

- **Bacteremia:** Isolation of *Gardnerella* in blood cultures has been reported following various obstetric and gynecologic manipulations, including septic abortion and postpartum endometritis. It has also been reported in men following transurethral resection of the prostate (TURP).

- **Miscellaneous infections:** Less commonly, *Gardnerella* has also been associated with salpingitis, vaginal abscesses, and infection following cesarian section. Preliminary studies have implicated bacterial vaginosis as a potential cause of premature delivery and premature rupture of membranes in pregnant women. It is hypothesized that *Gardnerella* has phospholipase A_2 activity which may initiate labor. This relationship is still under study.

Diagnosis The diagnosis of bacterial vaginosis is made clinically, based on the criteria outlined above. Routine laboratory studies such as the complete blood count or electrolyte panel are not necessary. The Gram stain of vaginal discharge is helpful in identifying clue cells, which are pathognomonic for bacterial vaginosis. A striking decrease in the number of lactobacilli (gram-positive rods) normally dominant in the vaginal flora is also characteristic of bacterial vaginosis. A direct wet mount of vaginal secretions is useful in identifying clue cells and ruling out the presence of trichomonads (as seen in vaginal trichomoniasis) or yeast cells (as seen in candidal vaginitis). Although often obtained, cultures of the vagina for *Gardnerella* do little to establish the presence of bacterial vaginosis and are not indicated in the majority of cases. Vaginal Gram stains have been shown to be as sensitive as vaginal cultures (including semiquantitative culture techniques), with greater specificity and positive predictive value. Cultures for *Gardnerella vaginalis* from extravaginal sites (such as blood) are appropriate in the proper clinical setting. *Gardnerella* can be grown in blood culture media which is free of sodium polyanetholsulfonate (SPS).

Diagnostic Tests/Procedures
Gram Stain *on page 352*
KOH Preparation *on page 379*
Trichomonas Preparation *on page 462*

Treatment Unlike other gram-negative bacilli, *Gardnerella vaginalis* is susceptible to penicillin, ampicillin, vancomycin, and clindamycin. Most strains are resistant to nalidixic acid, sulfadiazine, and neomycin. The organism is resistant to metronidazole *in vitro*, but is effective *in vivo*, probably due to an active metabolite of metronidazole. Treatment guidelines are as follows:

1. For nonpregnant women with bacterial vaginosis, metronidazole (Flagyl®) is the drug of choice, 500 mg orally 2 times a day for 7 days. As an alternative, clindamycin may be used, 300 mg orally 2 times a day for 7 days. Since bacterial vaginosis is not a sexually transmitted disease, there is no need to routinely treat the male sexual partner.

2. For the pregnant female, treatment is at the physician's discretion. Limited data has linked bacterial vaginosis with premature delivery, but the benefits of antibiotic therapy, if any, are presently unknown. Metronidazole is contraindicated in the first trimester of pregnancy. The Centers for Disease Control have recommended clindamycin in this situation, should treatment be initiated.

3. For bacteremia with *Gardnerella*, a variety of antibiotics may be used including ampicillin.

Drug Therapy
Recommended
Metronidazole *on page 610*
Alternate
Ampicillin *on page 495*

Selected Readings
Josephson S, Thomason J, Sturino K, et al, "*Gardnerella vaginalis* in the Urinary Tract: Incidence and Significance in a Hospital Population," *Obstet Gynecol*, 1988, 71(2):245-50.

(Continued)

Gardnerella vaginalis (Continued)

Spiegel CA, "*Gardnerella vaginalis* and *Mobiluncus* Species," *Principles and Practice of Infectious Diseases*, 4th ed, Mandell GL, Bennett JE, and Dolin R, eds, New York, NY: Churchill Livingstone, 1995, 2050-3.

"1993 Sexually Transmitted Diseases Treatment Guidelines. Centers for Disease Control and Prevention," *MMWR Morb Mortal Wkly Rep*, 1993, 42(RR-14):1-102.

Gemella morbillorum see *Streptococcus*, Viridans Group
on page 213

Giardia lamblia

Microbiology *Giardia lamblia* is an important intestinal parasite classified as a protozoan flagellate. It is related to other clinically relevant protozoans such as *Trichomonas vaginalis* and *Dientamoeba fragilis*. The organism exists as either a trophozoite or a cyst, and both can be detected in stool samples. Microscopically, *G. lamblia* trophozoites are characterized by long flagella at one end (which provide motility in fluid environments), a ventral adhesive disk (which attaches to the intestinal villi of humans), and two parabasal bodies located near the nucleus. These paired bodies give a characteristic and easily identifiable appearance of "two eyes" looking at the examiner. The cyst form of *Giardia* is somewhat smaller than the trophozoite and is considered the infective form of *Giardia*.

The infectious cycle for humans begins with ingestion of *Giardia lamblia* cysts (eg, from contaminated water or food). As few as 10 organisms can initiate human disease. In the stomach, excystation is promoted by gastric acid, and trophozoites are released in the duodenum and multiply by longitudinal binary fission. The trophozoites attach to the intestinal villi by means of the ventral sucking disk. Histologically, there is a mild to moderate inflammation of the small bowel mucosa. Both the cyst and trophozoite are passed into the human feces.

Epidemiology Infection with *Giardia* occurs worldwide. In particular, it can be found in wilderness streams, lakes, and mountainous areas. Beavers, muskrats, and other wild animals serve as another reservoir for this organism. Common means of acquisition include:

- Ingestion of contaminated water. Outbreaks from contaminated water in mountain resorts have been described. *Giardia lamblia* cysts are not killed by the chlorine concentrations used in many water treatment facilities. It is important to obtain a travel history (including recent camping) in patients with acute giardiasis.
- Ingestion of contaminated food.
- Oral-anal sexual contact. This is an important means of person-to-person spread, particularly amongst male homosexuals.
- Fecal-oral spread, especially in children attending day care centers.

Clinical Syndromes

- **Asymptomatic carriage:** In almost 50% of cases, infection with *Giardia lamblia* occurs in the absence of symptoms. This state of carriage can persist indefinitely in some individuals.
- **Gastrointestinal disease:** The spectrum of symptomatic giardiasis is variable and ranges from a mild nonspecific diarrheal illness to a more severe illness characterized by abdominal pain, bloating, and profuse diarrhea. A chronic malabsorption syndrome has been described. The diarrhea tends to be watery and associated with abdominal cramping; stools are almost always guaiac-negative since *Giardia* does not invade the mucosal tissues. Patients at particular risk for severe or relapsing giardiasis are individuals with an underlying IgA deficiency or diverticulosis.

Diagnosis Diagnosis can be made by wet mount of liquid stool for cysts or trophozoites, or exam of fresh semiformed stool for cysts, preserved stool (formalin or PVA) can be stained with trichrome or iron hematoxylin. If stool is negative, duodenal biopsy aspiration or sting test can be performed. The sting test consists of a gelatin capsule or a nylon string that is swallowed. After a testing incubation period (at least 4-6 hours), the sting is removed and examined/stained for the organism.

Diagnostic Tests/Procedures
Giardia Specific Antigen (GSA65) *on page 352*
Ova and Parasites, Stool *on page 416*

Treatment Many cases of giardiasis are self-resolving without specific therapy. However, both symptomatic and asymptomatic *G. lamblia* infections should be treated. The drug of choice is metronidazole, with quinacrine being a good alternative.

Drug Therapy
Recommended
  Metronidazole *on page 610*
Alternate
  Quinacrine Hydrochloride *on page 655*
Selected Readings
  Adam RD, "The Biology of *Giardia* spp," *Microbiol Rev*, 1991, 55(4):706-32.
  Lengerich EJ, Addiss DG, and Juranek DD, "Severe Giardiasis in the United States," *Clin Infect Dis*, 1994, 18(5):761-3.
  Overturf GD, "Editorial Response: Endemic Giardiasis in the United States – Role of the Day Care Center," *Clin Infect Dis*, 1994, 18:764-5.
  Pickering LK and Engelkirk PG, "*Giardia lamblia*," *Pediatr Clin North Am*, 1988, 35(3):565-77.
  Pickering LK, Woodward WE, DuPont HL, et al, "Occurrence of *Giardia lamblia* in Children in Day Care Centers," *J Pediatr*, 1984, 104(4):522-6.
  Steketee RW, Reid S, Cheng T, et al, "Recurrent Outbreaks of Giardiasis in a Child Day Care Center, Wisconsin," *Am J Public Health*, 1989, 79(4):485-90.

Gram-Negative Bacilli
Synonyms GNB
Refer To
  Acinetobacter Species *on page 50*
  Bartonella Species *on page 62*
  Bordetella pertussis on page 65
  Brucella Species *on page 69*
  Campylobacter jejuni on page 72
  Citrobacter Species *on page 82*
  Enterobacter Species *on page 104*
  Escherichia coli, Enterohemorrhagic *on page 112*
  Escherichia coli, Nonenterohemorrhagic *on page 113*
  Gardnerella vaginalis on page 114
  HACEK Group *on this page*
  Haemophilus ducreyi on next page
  Haemophilus influenzae on page 119
  Helicobacter pylori on page 121
  Klebsiella Species *on page 137*
  Legionella pneumophila on page 139
  Pasteurella multocida on page 170
  Proteus Species *on page 176*
  Pseudomonas aeruginosa on page 177
  Salmonella Species *on page 185*
  Serratia Species *on page 190*
  Shigella Species *on page 191*
  Vibrio cholerae on page 230
  Xanthomonas maltophilia on page 231
  Yersinia enterocolitica on page 232
  Yersinia pestis on page 233

Group A β-Hemolytic *Streptococcus* *see Streptococcus pyogenes on page 207*

Group A *Streptococcus* *see Streptococcus pyogenes on page 207*

Group B *Streptococcus* *see Streptococcus agalactiae on page 203*

Group D Streptococci *see Streptococcus bovis on page 205*

HACEK Group
Microbiology HACEK is a pneumonic which includes *Haemophilus aphrophilus*, *Actinobacillus actinomycetemcomitans*, *Cardiobacterium hominis*, *Eikenella corrodens*, and *Kingella* species. These organisms are pleomorphic, coccobacilli and bacilli and occur as chains or filamentous forms. These organisms are all fastidious, gram-negative bacteria which require specific types of growth conditions. These conditions include enhanced CO_2, specific growth factors (*Haemophilus*), growth only on chocolate and/or blood agar, and often increased time for incubation. Organisms in this group may be differentiated by reaction to oxidase and catalase, cell shape, indole positivity, nitrate to nitrite, and fermentation of carbohydrates. In a microbiology laboratory, these five bacteria are identified and reported separately.
(Continued)

ORGANISMS

HACEK Group *(Continued)*

Epidemiology Members of the HACEK group are normal flora of the mouth and respiratory tract and are opportunistic organisms that cause infections in patients with oral cavity disease or trauma and in immunocompromised hosts. *Eikenella* infections are often associated with other mouth flora organisms.

Clinical Syndromes Although many of the HACEK organisms have been know to cause disease in several organ systems and clinical settings, endocarditis is by far the most common. Endocarditis is usually subacute with a very insidious onset, often in patients with previously damaged or prosthetic valves. Although medical treatment is often successful, reporting bias must be considered.

Diagnosis The diagnosis of a HACEK group infection can only be made by identification of the specific pathogen through culture in a patient with a relevant clinical syndrome. Patients with seemingly culture-negative endocarditis should have their cultures held, as prolonged incubation time may be needed. Also, special media and conditions may be necessary as described above.

Diagnostic Tests/Procedures
Blood Culture, Aerobic and Anaerobic *on page 271*
Gram Stain *on page 352*

Treatment Empiric therapy with ampicillin plus gentamicin sulfate or a third generation cephalosporin should be considered if a HACEK organism is suspected. There are strains of these organism which have been shown to produce beta-lactamases that inactivate ampicillin. The final therapeutic decision should be based on clinical condition of the patient (especially while cultures are pending or negative) and sensitivity testing.

Drug Therapy
Recommended
Cephalosporins, 3rd Generation *on page 528*
or
Ampicillin *on page 495*
used in combination with
Gentamicin Sulfate *on page 575*

Selected Readings
Baron EJ and Finegold SM, eds, "Gram-Negative Facultatively Anaerobic Bacilli and Aerobic Coccobacilli," *Bailey & Scott's Diagnostic Microbiology*, St Louis, MO: CV Mosby Co, 1990, 408-30.
Ellner JJ, Rosenthal MS, Lerner PI, et al, "Infective Endocarditis Caused by Slow-Growing, Fastidious, Gram-Negative Bacteria," *Medicine (Baltimore)*, 1979, 58(2):145-58.
Meyer DJ and Gerding DN, "Favorable Prognosis of Patients With Prosthetic Valve Endocarditis Caused by Gram-Negative Bacilli of the HACEK Group," *Am J Med*, 1988, 85(1):104-7.
Murray PR, Drew WL, Kobayashi GS, et al, eds, "Miscellaneous Gram-Negative Bacilli," *Medical Microbiology*, St Louis, MO: CV Mosby Company, 1990, 175-9.

Haemophilus ducreyi

Microbiology *Haemophilus ducreyi* is a gram-negative coccobacillus which causes a sexually transmitted disease called chancroid. It is indistinguishable on Gram stain from other *Haemophilus* species (such as *H. influenzae*).

Epidemiology In 1838, chancroid (soft chancre) was first differentiated from syphilis (or hard chancre) by the French microbiologist Ricord. Although chancroid has remained an uncommon sexually transmitted disease in the U.S., its worldwide incidence may exceed that of syphilis. In 1986, there were 3418 cases reported, the largest number since the 1950s.

From 1981 to 1987, nine major outbreaks of chancroid were reported in the U.S. Chancroid was seen mainly in hispanic and black heterosexual men who patronized prostitutes. In Florida, chancroid was seen in highly sexually active men without clear prostitute exposure. In Boston, the outbreak may have been related to individuals who had been originally infected in endemic foreign countries, such as Haiti and the Dominican Republic.

Clinical Syndromes *H. ducreyi* is an important cause of the syndrome of **genital ulceration with regional adenopathy**. Other sexually transmitted diseases that can cause this syndrome include primary syphilis, genital herpes simplex virus, lymphogranuloma venereum, and others. The incubation period for *H. ducreyi* is 1-21 days with an average of 7 days. Chancroid ulcers are painful, deep, shaggy and friable. The borders of the ulcer are undermined. In men, ulcers are more commonly single, but in women, the ulcers are multiple. Regional adenopathy occurs simultaneously with the ulcer and is seen in 50% to 65% of cases. The nodes are quite tender and tend to be unilateral. In addition, they tend to be fluctuant and can easily fistulize. Constitutional symptoms are uncommon.

Diagnosis Isolation of *Haemophilus ducreyi* from an active genital ulcer is the only accurate means of confirming a case of chancroid. However, special media and culture techniques are required to culture this fastidious organism, and the microbiology laboratory must be alerted to the possibility of *H. ducreyi*. Cotton or calcium alginate swabs should be rolled over a purulent ulcer base. The Gram's stain of an ulcer specimen may be misleading because of the presence of polymicrobial flora colonizing genital ulcers. Isolation of *H. ducreyi* from active genital ulcers is variable (50% to 80% depending on the culture medium). *H. ducreyi* is almost never isolated from aspiration of inguinal buboes.

Unfortunately, it is difficult to diagnose chancroid on the basis of clinical suspicion alone. Chancroid is presumptively diagnosed in patients presenting with genital ulcers with a negative RPR/VDRL, darkfield-negative for *T. pallidum*, and negative for HSV (by clinical appearance). However, as pointed out by Salzman et al, many such presumptive cases are ultimately found not to be chancroid.

Treatment Chancroid is an unusual disease in the U.S., and consultation with an Infectious Disease Specialist is appropriate. Suggested therapy is erythromycin 500 mg orally 4 times/day for 7 days or ceftriaxone 250 mg I.M. times 1. Alternatives include co-trimoxazole (Bactrim™ DS) orally twice daily for 7 days, or Augmentin® 500 mg orally 3 times/day for 7 days, or ciprofloxacin hydrochloride 500 mg orally twice daily for 3 days. The choice of antibiotics is the same in pregnancy.

Drug Therapy
Recommended
Erythromycin *on page 561*
Ceftriaxone Sodium *on page 523*
Alternate
Co-trimoxazole *on page 545*
Amoxicillin and Clavulanic Acid *on page 490*
Ciprofloxacin Hydrochloride *on page 537*

Selected Readings
Hammond GW, Slutchuk M, Scatliff J, et al, "Epidemiologic, Clinical, Laboratory, and Therapeutic Features of an Urban Outbreak of Chancroid in North America," *Rev Infect Dis*, 1980, 2(6):867-79.
Ronald AR and Plummer FA, "Chancroid and *Haemophilus ducreyi*," *Ann Intern Med*, 1985, 102(5):705-7.
Schmid GP, Sanders LL Jr, Blount JH, et al, "Chancroid in the United States. Reestablishment of an Old Disease," *JAMA*, 1987, 258(22):3265-8.
"1993 Sexually Transmitted Diseases Treatment Guidelines. Centers for Disease Control and Prevention," *MMWR Morb Mortal Wkly Rep*, 1993, 42(RR-14):1-102.

Haemophilus influenzae
Related Information
Immunization Guidelines *on page 710-717*
Vaccines *on page 706-709*

Microbiology *Haemophilus influenzae* are typically gram-negative, aerobic (facultatively anaerobic), coccobacilli; however, they are often pleomorphic, gram-variable, and filamentous. There are six types (a–f) based on polysaccharide capsular properties; type b is the most invasive. There are also nonencapsulated, nontypable *Haemophilus influenzae*. There are eight different biotypes (with different biochemical properties) of which biotype 1 is most prevalent as a pathogen.

Haemophilus influenzae grows on chocolate agar which has X and V factors necessary for growth. It can also grow on Levinthal and Fildes enriched agar which are useful in determining encapsulation properties.

Epidemiology The epidemiology of *Haemophilus influenzae* is changing in the 1990s because of successful early childhood immunization, which is dramatically decreasing the incidence of invasive disease caused by *Haemophilus influenzae* b. *Haemophilus influenzae* is often found in the nasopharynx of normal asymptomatic individuals. Most *Haemophilus influenzae* isolates in the United States are nonencapsulated and rarely are pathogenic. Historically, the frequency of invasive disease was based on age with meningitis most common in children 2 month to 2 years of age, epiglottitis in the 3-5 years of age range, and other infections having an increasing incidence in older adults. The total increase incidence over the past two decades may have been due in part to improved laboratory identification of organisms.

(Continued)

Haemophilus influenzae (Continued)

Clinical Syndromes Early *Haemophilus influenzae* b vaccination has decreased the incidence of serious *Haemophilus influenzae* b disease dramatically over the past few years. *Haemophilus influenzae* can cause a variety of clinical syndromes including meningitis, epiglottitis, cellulitis, otitis, respiratory tract infection, and other infections.

- **Meningitis:** Although not a high mortality when diagnosed early, *Haemophilus influenzae* meningitis often causes permanent neurologic sequelae even when "successfully" treated. Meningitis characteristically occurred in infants up to 2 years of age.
- **Epiglottitis (ages 3-5 years):** Is a medical emergency which often requires ventilatory support if not managed promptly.
- ***Haemophilus influenzae* otitis:** Common in children of various ages.
- **Respiratory tract infections:** More common in adults, especially those with chronic obstructive pulmonary disease and smokers.

Diagnosis Diagnosis can be made by Gram stain and culture of specimens from appropriate sites. Gram stain will reveal gram-negative coccobacilli but is neither sensitive nor specific enough to be diagnostic. *Haemophilus influenzae* grows well on chocolate agar supplemented by growth factors V and X. These factors differentiate it from other *Haemophilus* species. Satellite colonies may appear around *S. aureus* species. Antigen detection for the polyribophosphate capsule is available but is no more sensitive than Gram stain or culture. Subgrouping may be performed for epidemiologic purposes.

Diagnostic Tests/Procedures
Aerobic Culture, Appropriate Site *on page 244*
Gram Stain *on page 352*

Treatment Meningitis and epiglottitis should be treated with a third generation cephalosporin when *Haemophilus influenzae* is suspected, as these are medical emergencies. Up to 30% of *Haemophilus influenzae* b strains are resistant to ampicillin. Less serious infections may be treated with ampicillin or amoxicillin (when susceptible), co-trimoxazole, or a second generation cephalosporin. Most strains are also susceptible to chloramphenicol and quinolones (not first line agents). *Haemophilus influenzae* b vaccine is now a part of routine vaccinations administered in the first few months of life.

Prophylaxis may be desirable in *H. influenzae* outbreaks or in close contacts with invasive disease. Rifampin is the recommended agent for prophylaxis in a 4-day regimen of 600 mg daily for adults and 20 mg/kg daily for infants and children.

Drug Therapy
Recommended
Severe infection:
Cephalosporins, 3rd Generation *on page 528*
Mild infection:
Co-trimoxazole *on page 545*
Alternate
Severe infection:
Cephalosporins, 2nd Generation *on page 527*
Chloramphenicol *on page 531*
Mild infection:
Ampicillin *on page 495*
Amoxicillin and Clavulanic Acid *on page 490*
Cefaclor *on page 508*
Amoxicillin Trihydrate *on page 491*

Selected Readings
Adams WG, Deaver KA, Cochi SL, et al, "Decline of Childhood *Haemophilus influenzae* Type b (Hib) Disease in the Hib Vaccine Era," *JAMA*, 1993, 269(2):221-6.
Baron EJ and Finegold SM, eds, "Gram-Negative Facultatively Anaerobic Bacilli and Aerobic Coccobacilli," *Bailey & Scott's Diagnostic Microbiology*, St Louis, MO: CV Mosby Co, 1990, 408-30.
Murray PR, Drew WL, Kobayashi GS, et al, eds. "Pasteurellaceae," *Medical Microbiology*, St Louis, MO: CV Mosby Co, 1990, 139-47.
Quagliarello V and Scheld WM, "Bacterial Meningitis: Pathogenesis, Pathophysiology, and Progress," *N Engl J Med*, 1992, 327(12):864-72.
Willett HP, "*Haemophilus*," *Zinsser Microbiology*, 20th ed, Joklik WK, Willett HP, Amos DB, et al, eds, Norwalk, CT: Appleton & Lange, 1992, 461-73.

HBV *see* Hepatitis B Virus *on page 122*
HDV *see* Hepatitis D Virus *on page 126*

ORGANISMS

Helicobacter pylori

Synonyms *Campylobacter pylori*

Microbiology Controversy surrounds *Helicobacter pylori*, a gram-negative bacillus recently implicated as a cause of duodenal and gastric ulcers and a potential cause of the non-ulcer dyspepsia syndrome. Originally named *Campylobacter pyloridis*, then *Campylobacter pylori*, this organism was renamed *Helicobacter pylori* in 1989. It is a spiral-shaped gram-negative bacillus which is susceptible *in vitro* to a variety of antimicrobial agents including tetracycline, metronidazole, amoxicillin, and clarithromycin. Resistance to these antibiotics has been described in some isolates, including metronidazole-resistant strains which have been associated with treatment failures. The organism is unique in its ability to survive the acidic pH of gastric fluids, which is otherwise sterile in healthy individuals. *H. pylori* is most commonly recognized in histologic analysis of gastric biopsies. Cultures for the organism are available in many laboratories but have variable sensitivity.

Epidemiology *H. pylori* has been associated with infection in adults over the age of 20 years, with an increased incidence with aging. The natural reservoir appears to be in humans, although the precise source is unknown. Transmission has been theorized to be fecal-oral. In some studies, *H. pylori* has been recovered from nearly 100% of patients with duodenal ulcers and has thus stimulated much research concerning its role as a possible etiologic agent of peptic ulcer disease.

Clinical Syndromes

- **Duodenal ulcers:** *H. pylori* has been implicated as a cause of duodenal ulcers in patients who are not receiving nonsteroidal anti-inflammatory agents. This is based on a number of lines of evidence. The prevalence of *H. pylori* in duodenal ulcer cases is nearly 100%. Eradication of *H. pylori* decreases the relapse rate of duodenal ulcers when compared with patients with duodenal ulcers who have persistent infection with *H. pylori*. Other experts have strongly disagreed with these findings and conclusions and suggest that *H. pylori* is only a cofactor in causation of duodenal ulcers.
- **Gastric ulcers:** Again, epidemiologic evidence suggests a relationship between *H. pylori* and gastric ulcers. Studies have suggested a weaker relationship with gastric ulcers than with duodenal ulcers, with 60% of gastric ulcer cases positive for *H. pylori*. (Some studies has shown a higher rate of recovery, approaching 100%). Relapse rates in patients who have been successfully treated for *H. pylori* have been close to 0% at 1 year, as compared with 60% in controls.
- **Non-ulcer dyspepsia:** In this difficult to define entity, individuals complain of chronic symptoms of abdominal pain similar to peptic ulcer disease but have no objective disease on upper endoscopy. *H. pylori* has also been associated with this condition. The results of studies eradicating *H. pylori* in non-ulcer dyspepsia have been inconclusive to date. The data suggest a subgroup of patients may in fact benefit from eradication of the organism, but the difficulty has been identifying such individuals prior to therapy.
- **Gastric carcinoma:** Limited evidence has linked chronic *H. pylori* infection with some individuals with gastric cancer.

Diagnostic Tests/Procedures

Helicobacter pylori Culture and Urease Test *on page 356*
Helicobacter pylori Culture, Gastric Biopsy *on page 357*

Treatment The decision to treat an individual for *H. pylori* infection should be made after review of the conflicting opinions and the published data. Recent reviews on both sides of the issue are referenced below. An increasing body of literature is supporting the practice of treating individuals with histologically proven *H. pylori* infection. Patients who appear to benefit the most from therapy are those with recurrent duodenal ulcers (endoscopically proven), duodenal ulcers resistant to conventional therapy, or perforated duodenal ulcers. The data do not suggest that all patients with peptic ulcer disease will benefit from antibiotics. Only patients who have chronic *H. pylori* infection associated with peptic ulcer disease benefit from therapy; those with other mechanisms to produce ulcers (such as nonsteroidal-induced ulcers or Zollinger-Ellison syndrome) are not likely to benefit. One currently accepted treatment is a three drug regimen for 10-14 days, such as tetracycline, bismuth subsalicylate (Pepto-Bismol®), and metronidazole. Other successful regimens have substituted amoxicillin for tetracycline. There is a significant incidence of minor side effects such as nausea, vomiting, and diarrhea with these oral regimens. Patient compliance may be low, and close monitoring and encouragement is necessary. Some regimens have combined an H_2-antagonist or omeprazole with a combination antibiotic regimen with good results.

Drug Therapy
Recommended
    Amoxicillin Trihydrate *on page 491*

    Tetracycline *on page 679*

    Metronidazole *on page 610*

Alternate
    Bismuth *on page 505*

Selected Readings
Dooley CP, Cohen H, Fitzgibbons PL, et al, "Prevalence of *Helicobacter pylori* Infection and Histological Gastritis in Asymptomatic Persons," *N Engl J Med*, 1989, 321(23):1562-6.

Graham DY, Lew GM, Klein PD, et al, "Effect of Treatment of *Helicobacter pylori* Infection on the Long-Term Recurrence of Gastric or Duodenal Ulcer. A Randomized Controlled Study," *Ann Intern Med*, 1992, 116(9):705-8.

Kendall BJ and Marshall BJ, "The Coming of Age of *Helicobacter pylori*," *Contemp Int Med*, 1993, 5(3):48-66.

Hepatitis A Virus

Related Information
Immunization Guidelines *on page 710-717*

Occupational Exposure to Bloodborne Pathogens (Universal Precautions) *on page 751-756*

Microbiology Hepatitis A virus (HAV; enterovirus 72) is a member of the picovirus family (poliovirus, Coxsackievirus, echovirus). Mature HAV virions are nonenveloped, have icosahedral capsids, and contain single-stranded RNA.

Epidemiology HAV caused "infectious" hepatitis which was observed and recorded by Hippocrates. Epidemics of infectious hepatitis have been recorded throughout modern history, especially during World Wars I and II. Today, infectious hepatitis occurs worldwide and is very common in areas with poor sanitation and in institutional settings such as facilities for the developmentally disabled, the military, prisons, and day care centers. In developing countries, almost all persons become infected with HAV (or at least become HAV antibody-positive) during childhood. In developed countries, the number of HAV antibody-positive persons is age-dependent and increases sharply with adulthood. The natural reservoir for HAV is humans. HAV is spread by the oral-fecal route. Transmission of HAV by blood and blood products occurs, but it is a rare event. Chronic excretion of HAV has not been documented.

Clinical Syndromes HAV causes acute infectious hepatitis which is usually mild in children and young patients, more severe in adults, and almost impossible to distinguish from acute hepatitis caused by other viruses. The incubation period for infectious hepatitis is about 30 days (range, 10-50 days). Typically, infectious hepatitis is characterized by a 1- to 7-day prodrome phase (fever, headache, fatigue, vomiting, abdominal pain, elevated serum ALT and AST levels [especially ALT]). (In all types of hepatitis, ALT levels are higher than AST levels.) Subsequently, more specific characteristics develop (dark urine, light-colored stool, jaundice, ±right upper quadrant pain, ±enlarged liver and spleen). Infectious hepatitis usually is acute and self-limiting. Infectious hepatitis is not chronic.

Diagnosis Infectious hepatitis is diagnosed clinically and serologically. The most useful methods for the laboratory diagnosis of infectious hepatitis are enzyme immunoassays for HAV-specific antibody (total and IgM). Almost all patients have anti-HAV IgM by the time symptoms are observed; IgM levels usually are not detectable 3-6 months after infection.

Diagnostic Tests/Procedures
Hepatitis A Profile *on page 358*

Drug Therapy Comment
No antiviral agents active against hepatitis A, but for pre-exposure and postexposure, prophylaxis intravenous immunoglobulins may be appropriate.

Drug Therapy
Recommended
    Immune Globulin *on page 588*

Selected Readings
Battegay M, Gust ID, and Feinstone SM, "Hepatitis A Virus," *Principles and Practice of Infectious Diseases*, 4th ed, Mandell GL, Bennett JE, and Dolin R, eds, New York, NY: Churchill Livingstone, 1995, 1636-56.

Hojvat SA, "Diagnostic Tests for Viral Hepatitis," *Clin Microbiol Newslett*, 1989, 11:33-9.

Hepatitis B Virus

Related Information
Immunization Guidelines *on page 710-717*

Occupational Exposure to Bloodborne Pathogens (Universal Precautions) *on page 751-756*
Postexposure Prophylaxis for Hepatitis B *on page 719-720*
Vaccines *on page 706-709*

Synonyms HBV

Microbiology Hepatitis B virus (HBV) is the etiological agent of serum hepatitis. HBV (archaic term, Dane particle) is a nonenveloped, partially double-stranded DNA virus which is trophic for liver cells. HBV is composed of a surface protein coat, a nucleocapsid, and internal proteins and nucleic acid. HBV usually is referred to as being composed of three antigens, surface (HB_sAg), core (HB_cAg), and e (HB_eAg). The surface of HBV is a complex antigen with many determinants/epitopes. The amount of HB_sAg produced during an infection usually is excessive, extremely large, and out of proportion to the amount needed to assemble mature, complete circulating HBV virions produced during infection. The HB_cAg (nucleocapsid) is found in the blood only as an internal part of the complete HBV virion; HB_cAg has not been detected free in blood. The HB_eAg is always associated with complete infectious HBV particles and, therefore, with infectivity.

Epidemiology Serum hepatitis is a common and serious endemic disease throughout the world. The prevalence of serum hepatitis depends on age and socioeconomic situation. At least 280 million cases and 1 million persons are chronic carriers of HBV worldwide and in the United States, respectively. The carrier rate in some parts of Asia is 15%. The natural reservoirs of HBV are humans and probably a few other primates, such as chimps and monkeys. HBV is transmitted parenterally by needles and intravenous equipment, sexually, in unscreened blood products, and perinatally. HBV is not transmitted by the fecal-oral route. One of the sequelae of HBV infection, hepatocellular carcinoma, is a major public health problem worldwide. HBV probably is the cause of 80% of all cases of hepatocellular carcinoma worldwide. HBV has been found in almost all body secretions, but only blood, serum, semen, and vaginal fluids have been shown to be infectious. Perinatal transmission in developing countries is believed to be the main reason HBV is so prevalent worldwide. Perinatal infection has a high incidence resulting in chronic hepatitis, cirrhosis, and hepatocellular carcinoma.

Clinical Syndromes Most primary HBV infections are subclinical, self-limiting, and resolve within 3-6 months. HBV can produce mild to fulminant acute hepatitis, chronic persistent hepatitis, chronic active hepatitis, and hepatocellular carcinoma. The incubation period for serum hepatitis is 4-28 weeks. Signs and symptoms of acute serum hepatitis are quite variable and often include insidious onset of serum sickness-like illness, rash, and fever for several days to weeks. Subsequently, liver disease and joint involvement become clinically apparent. The presence of jaundice and abdominal pain are variable. This clinical condition usually is not distinguishable from that of acute disease caused by hepatitis A virus. Several variant forms of serum hepatitis have been described.

Diagnosis Diagnosis usually is made clinically, and determination of the specific etiological agent is made by serological and specific viral tests. Serological tests for several HBV antigens (surface and core) and antibodies to those antigens (anti-surface, anti-core, and anti-e) are widely available and clinically useful. Results of these tests are interpreted by consulting widely available charts which correlate various results (antigen and antibody patterns) with stages of infection. See the following tables and Hepatitis B Profile test entry for interpretation of the results of serology testing.

Diagnostic Tests/Procedures
Hepatitis B Profile *on page 358*

Drug Therapy Comment
Alpha interferon for chronic active hepatitis only. No drug therapy for acute hepatitis B.

Drug Therapy
Recommended
Interferon Alfa-2b *on page 590*

Selected Readings
Hojvat SA, "Diagnostic Tests for Viral Hepatitis," *Clin Microbiol Newslett*, 1989, 11:33-9.
Robinson WS, "Hepatitis B Virus and Hepatitis D Virus," *Principles and Practice of Infectious Diseases*, 4th ed, Mandell GL, Bennett JE, and Dolin R, eds, New York, NY: Churchill Livingstone, 1995, 1406-39.

Hepatitis B Serological Profiles

Core Window Identification

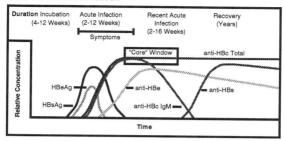

Hepatitis B Chronic Carrier No Seroconversion

Hepatitis B Chronic Carrier Late Seroconversion

Reprinted from Abbott Diagnostics

Hepatitis C Virus

Related Information

Immunization Guidelines *on page 710-717*

Occupational Exposure to Bloodborne Pathogens (Universal Precautions) *on page 751-756*

Microbiology Since its initial identification in 1988, there has been a tremendous amount of information regarding hepatitis C virus (HCV), an RNA virus related to the flaviviruses. Although the virus has yet to be grown in cell culture, the genome is well characterized and has been sequenced and cloned.

Epidemiology HCV is one of the most common causes of liver disease in the United States, behind alcoholic liver disease. Routes of transmission include:

Blood transfusions. HCV is the most common cause of transfusion-related hepatitis. Formerly termed non-A, non-B hepatitis, it is now clear that HCV is responsible for the majority of these cases. However, blood transfusion is not the most common route of transmission of HCV; in 1990, transfusions accounted for only 6% of new HCV cases. Aggressive screening of blood donors has helped decrease the incidence of HCV infection.

Intravenous drug use, which is the most commonly identified means of transmission. Up to 85% of I.V. drug users have serologic evidence of HCV infection. In 1990, about 40% of HCV cases appeared to be related to I.V. drug use.

Sexual transmission. Current data suggests that sexual transmission of HCV is inefficient. Some studies have shown no increased risk of HCV transmission between sex partners in a stable and monogamous relationship. Hepatitis B virus and HIV are much more easily acquired sexually.

Sporadic hepatitis. A number of individuals with serologic evidence of HCV infection have no obvious risk factor for acquisition. The extent of these "sporadic" cases has been debated with some estimates around 20% of all acute cases.

Miscellaneous. Other higher risk groups include health care workers, hemodialysis patients, individuals requiring multiple transfusions (hemophiliacs), and others.

Clinical Syndromes

- **Asymptomatic infection:** The majority of cases (~75%) of HCV infection are asymptomatic. Some individuals are identified by serologic testing (eg, blood donor screening programs), but many remain undetected. This is particularly problematic for several reasons. The virus can be unknowingly transmitted to others, liver damage occurs despite the absence of symptoms, and >50% will develop a chronic hepatopathy.

- **Acute HCV infection:** Following an initial incubation period (2 weeks to 6 months), the patient enters a "preicteric" phase. Symptoms tend to be non-specific, with malaise and anorexia. In some cases, there is also right upper quadrant pain, nausea, and vomiting. This is followed by the "icteric" phase, where the patient presents with jaundice and dark urine. Systemic symptoms usually improve during the icteric phase. Several points should be noted: Infection with HCV cannot be accurately distinguished from other causes of viral hepatitis (including hepatitis B) on the basis of clinical presentation alone; the course of acute HCV tends to be more indolent than hepatitis B; clinical symptoms may be quite variable; a high clinical suspicion should be maintained since serologic tests for HCV may be negative early on. Fulminant hepatic failure secondary to acute HCV infection is a rare but important complication.

  Although a serum sickness-like illness with fever, arthritis, and skin rash has been well recognized in acute hepatitis B infection, only rarely has this been reported with hepatitis C infection. Other extrahepatic complications of acute HCV include aplastic anemia and pancreatitis.

- **Chronic HCV infection:** Over 50% of individuals infected with HCV develop chronic liver disease (hepatitis B, 5% to 10%). Symptoms are usually mild and nonspecific, with the main complaint being fatigue. The diagnosis is often difficult since liver function tests may be normal or only minimally elevated much of the time. Liver abnormalities include chronic persistent hepatitis, chronic active hepatitis, and cirrhosis.

  Chronic HCV infection has been associated with several syndromes, including membranoproliferative glomerulonephritis, type II cryoglobulinemia, hepatocellular carcinoma; growing evidence supports an epidemiologic link between chronic HCV and hepatocellular carcinoma, independent of hepatitis B infection or alcoholic liver disease.

Diagnosis

As noted above, the diagnosis of HCV infection is quite difficult on clinical grounds alone and routine liver function tests may intermittently be normal. Thus, laboratory confirmation is essential.

Serologic tests: These assays are designed to detect host antibodies to HCV. Several caveats: antibodies to HCV remain undetectable until weeks or months after the initial infection; serologic studies may be needed at 6 months (90% of seroconverters identified) and possibly 12 months; in a few individuals, antibodies to HCV fail to develop for unclear reasons at any time postinfection. Available tests include:

- Enzyme-linked immunosorbent assay (ELISA) for detection of antibody against the C100-3 protein. One of the earlier tests made available, it has been found to have a high false-positive rate.
- ELISA for antibody to core protein C22. This "second generation" test is currently a popular screening test in many laboratories. False-negative reactions are still possible.

(Continued)

Hepatitis C Virus *(Continued)*

- Radioimmunoblot assay (RIBA) is used as a supplemental or confirmatory test for patients who are anti-HCV positive by ELISA. Currently the RIBA is designed to detect distinct antibodies to four different HCV proteins, including protein C1OO-3.

Molecular detection methods: These tests are still experimental but hold promise.
- Polymerase chain reaction for amplification and detection of small quantities of HCV RNA (target amplification) directly from blood specimens.
- Branched chain detection for detection of HCV RNA from blood without target amplification (signal amplification).

Treatment Acute HCV infection: No specific therapy is recommended at this time. The role of interferon therapy is still under study.

Chronic HCV infection: Large, multicenter clinical trials have shown that interferon alpha is beneficial in patients with HCV-related chronic active hepatitis, chronic persistent hepatitis, and well-compensated cirrhosis. About 25% showed a long-term response.

Drug Therapy
Recommended
Interferon Alfa-2b *on page 590*

Selected Readings
Carey WD and Patel G, "Viral Hepatitis in the 1990s, Part III: Hepatitis C, Hepatitis E, and Other Viruses," *Cleve Clin J Med*, 1992, 59(6):595-601.

Johnson RJ, Gretch DR, and Yamabe H, "Membranoproliferative Glomerulonephritis Associated With Hepatitis C Virus Infection," *N Engl J Med*, 1993, 328(7):465-70.

Lemon SM and Brown EA, "Hepatitis C Virus," *Principles and Practice of Infectious Diseases*, Mandell GL, Bennett JE, and Dolin R, eds, New York, NY: Churchill Livingstone, 1995, 1474-86.

Hepatitis D Virus
Related Information
Occupational Exposure to Bloodborne Pathogens (Universal Precautions) *on page 751-756*

Synonyms HDV

Microbiology Hepatitis D virus (HDV) is the etiological agent of delta hepatitis. HDV was first recognized in an Amazon tribe in 1969 and was first described in 1977. HDV is a small (35-40 nm) virus composed of only a circular single-strand RNA genome and a two-protein complex (the delta antigen) which surrounds and is intimately associated with the RNA. The RNA genome is the smallest of any animal virus. HDV can replicate on its own but requires the presence of HBV for transmission. Therefore, HDV is a defective/incomplete virus and invariably is found only in persons with acute or chronic HBV infection. During coinfection and when HBV and HDV are within the same cell, the HDV acquires a protein coat (envelope) composed of HBV surface antigen. This coat allows HDV to infect other cells. HDV will not be found in a HBV surface antigen-negative person.

Epidemiology HDV is present in extremely high numbers in circulating blood and usually is transmitted parenterally in ways similar to those of HBV (eg, by blood, blood products, and contaminated needles). In general, delta hepatitis is most prevalent in populations at high risk for hepatitis B (eg, multiply infused patients, intravenous drug users, hemophiliacs, inhabitants of underdeveloped countries, etc). Sexual transmission of HDV has been reported. Hepatitis D is a worldwide problem because the many millions of worldwide carriers of HBV surface antigen are potentially susceptible to HDV. Worldwide, HDV is present in about 5% of HBV carriers. Many epidemics of hepatitis D outside of the United States have been described, particularly in Africa and South America. In the United States, hepatitis B is a reportable disease, but hepatitis D is not reportable. This is probably because hepatitis D is not easy to diagnose, it is not common in the United States, and it is not yet a public health problem. HDV causes less than 1% of all viral hepatitis diseases.

Clinical Syndromes Acute viral hepatitis is a distinct clinical entity and usually is not too difficult to diagnose. In general, the diseases produced by hepatitis A, B, C, D, and E viruses are clinically indistinguishable. The clinical presentations of the diseases vary drastically from asymptomatic infections to icteric hepatitis to fulminant and fatal hepatitis.

Acute delta hepatitis occurs either as a coinfection at the same time as acute hepatitis B or as a superinfection during chronic hepatitis B. In both cases, the resulting disease is more severe than hepatitis B alone. A third type of hepatitis D has been suggested, a latent HDV infection which is active only after a subsequent HBV infection. Hepatitis D coinfection usually is clinically indistinguishable from acute hepatitis B, except the course is more severe. Less than 5% of patients with acute HDV coinfection develop chronic hepatitis D; however, most patients with hepatitis D acquired as a superinfection develop chronic hepatitis D. Patients who experience a superinfection can deteriorate rapidly and experience abrupt liver failure. Both acute and chronic hepatitis D are usually severe. Mortality rates for acute hepatitis D are 2% to 20%. Sixty percent to 70% of patients with chronic hepatitis D develop cirrhosis; most of these patients die of liver disease.

Diagnosis Viral hepatitis usually is diagnosed clinically, and determination of the specific etiological agent is made by serological and specific viral tests. Serological tests for anti-HDV IgG and IgM antibodies are widely available and clinically useful. Results of these tests are interpreted by consulting widely available charts which correlate various results (antigen and antibody patterns) with stages of infection. Tests for HDV antigen are available but are technically demanding and are not particularly diagnostically useful. Hepatitis A, B, C, D, and E viruses produce somewhat characteristic, but essentially indistinguishable, lesions in the liver. Polymerase chain reaction and associated nucleic acid probe tests for HDV RNA and HDV antigen have been reported.

Diagnostic Tests/Procedures

Hepatitis D Serology *on page 361*

Drug Therapy Comment Currently, no antiviral therapy effective against hepatitis D.

Selected Readings

Gupta S, Govindarajan S, Cassidy WM, et al, "Acute Delta Hepatitis: Serological Diagnosis With Particular Reference to Hepatitis Delta Virus RNA," *Am J Gastroenterol*, 1991, 86(9):1227-31.

Hojvat SA, "Diagnostic Tests for Viral Hepatitis," *Clin Microbiol Newslett*, 1989, 11:33-9.

Holt DA, Baran DA, Oehler RL, et al, "Delta Hepatitis: A Diagnostic Algorithm," *Infect Med*, 1993, 10:23-9.

Hsu HH, Feinstone SM, and Hoofnagle JH, "Acute Viral Hepatitis," *Principles and Practice of Infectious Diseases*, 4th ed, Mandell GL, Bennett JE, and Dolin R, eds, New York, NY: Churchill Livingstone, 1995, 1136-53.

Hepatitis E Virus

Related Information

Occupational Exposure to Bloodborne Pathogens (Universal Precautions) *on page 751-756*

Synonyms HEV

Microbiology Hepatitis E virus (HEV) is an unenveloped single-strand RNA virus, is structurally similar to calicivirus, and is found in the stool of hepatitis E patients during incubation and early acute phase of the disease. HEV is the etiological agent of "epidemic" or "enterically transmitted" non-A, non-B hepatitis and is associated with epidemics and contaminated water. ("Classic" non-A, non-B hepatitis is caused by hepatitis C virus and is associated with parenteral exposure.)

Epidemiology HEV causes less than 1% of all viral hepatitis diseases. Hepatitis E is transmitted by the fecal-oral route, is found in stool, and has been reported to be the cause of several large outbreaks of hepatitis in India, China, Peru, Russia, Africa, and Mexico. None of these epidemics were associated with either HAV or HBV; most of these outbreaks were associated with fecally contaminated water supplies and poor sanitation. Hepatitis E is very rare in the United States. HEV has not caused outbreaks in the United States and western Europe. Hepatitis E occurs only rarely in the United States, where persons with hepatitis E are almost always immigrants from endemic areas. Mortality rates of pregnant females who acquire hepatitis E are very high (15% to 30%), and fetal wastage is common.

Clinical Syndromes Clinically, hepatitis E is similar to hepatitis A except for the following: early presentations tend to include puritis and joint pain; cholestasis is common; concentrations of serum aminotransferase and alkaline phosphatase tend to be lower and higher, respectively.

Diagnosis Hepatitis E is diagnosed clinically. Antibody to HEV develops early in the disease. Laboratory tests to detect antibody to HEV (immune electron microscopy and inhibition of immunofluorescence) are available in only a few (usually research) laboratories.

(Continued)

Hepatitis E Virus *(Continued)*

Drug Therapy Comment Currently, no antiviral therapy effective against hepatitis E.

Selected Readings

Center for Disease Control, "Hepatitis E Among U.S Travelers, 1989-1992," *MMWR Morb Mortal Wkly Rep*, 1993, 42(1):1-3.

Hsu HH, Feinstone SM, and Hoofnagle JH, "Acute Viral Hepatitis," *Principles and Practice of Infectious Diseases*, 4th ed, Mandell GL, Bennett JE, and Dolin R, eds, New York, NY: Churchill Livingstone, 1995, 1136-53.

Yarbough PO, "Hepatitis E: Diagnosis of Infection," *Clin Microbiol Newslett*, 1993, 15(15):113-5.

Herpes Simplex Virus

Synonyms HSV

Microbiology Herpes simplex is a member of the DNA virus family herpesvirus. Herpes simplex 1 and 2 can be differentiated by neutralization titrations but often cross react. Differentiating the simplex virus from other members of the family is performed by antigenic analysis, and DNA, polypeptide, and molecular analysis.

Epidemiology Herpes simplex virus (HSV) infections occur worldwide. HSV 1 infection is common in childhood. By the fourth decade, approximately 90% of individuals will be seropositive for HSV 1. In lower socioeconomic groups, the incidence is even higher. HSV 2 is less common than HSV 1, and primary infections tend to occur in an older age group. The seroprevalence of HSV 2 in the U.S. is 10% to 40%. Clearly, HSV 2 is an important sexually transmitted disease (STD), and seroprevalence correlates well with increasing sexual activity. Up to 50% of young adults attending an STD clinic may demonstrate seropositivity for HSV 2. The general rule that HSV 1 causes "above the waist" infections and HSV 2 causes "below the waist" infections still holds true in many cases, but cross infections are increasingly common.

The incubation period following exposure to the virus is about 1 week (range 1-26 days). HSV transmission is most efficient in individuals with active ulcerations of the mucous membranes or genitalia but can still occur when virus is shed asymptomatically. HSV 1 can be cultured from the oropharynx of 2% to 9% of healthy adults and 5% to 8% of healthy children, indicating that asymptomatic shedding of the virus is common. Similarly, HSV 2 can be recovered from the genital tracts of asymptomatic, sexually active patients.

Clinical Syndromes

- **Genital herpes:** Herpes genitalis is still more commonly caused by HSV 2 (70% to 90% of cases), although there are a sizeable number of cases caused by HSV 1 (10% to 30%). Young adults and adolescents are most commonly infected. In males, vesicular lesions occur on the penile shaft or glans. In the female, similar lesions are seen in a variety of areas, including the cervix, perineum, vulva, and vagina. Symptoms are most severe during the primary infections, and patients may display fever and inguinal lymph node enlargement. The vesicles are typically tender and have an erythematous base. Lesions may persist for weeks with severe primary infections but eventually crust over. Recurrent genital lesions occur in both sexes. The systemic symptoms and severity of the lesions are diminished in comparison with primary infection. Patients will often complain of a prodrome of burning prior to an outbreak. Lesions typical for HSV develop during recurrences and heal over 7-10 days. Some patients experience frequent recurrences. Data suggests that chronic suppression with acyclovir may be useful in decreasing the number of outbreaks per year.

- **Oral HSV infections:** Primary herpes gingivostomatitis is seen mainly in children and is caused by HSV 1 in 90% of cases. Less commonly, primary infection occurs in the young adult; in such cases infection may be from either HSV 1 or 2. The incubation period following exposure is 2-12 days. Vesicles develop in the oral cavity, including the pharynx, palate, buccal mucosa, and/or tongue. The vesicles rapidly break down into small ulcers and are covered with an exudate. Lesions may extend to involve the lips and cheek. Severe primary lesions can be accompanied by high fevers, malaise, cervical lymphadenopathy, and dehydration. However, it is known that primary oral HSV infections are most commonly asymptomatic or mild. The lesions generally resolve without therapy in 2 weeks. HSV pharyngitis is probably under-recognized in the college-aged population, where it may be misdiagnosed as "strep throat." Recurrent HSV labialis (lip lesions) is problematic in some adults. Recent data suggest that chronic daily acyclovir may have some minor benefit in this group. In patients who are immunosuppressed, recurrences of HSV labialis can be quite severe.

- **Herpetic keratitis:** HSV 1 is one of the most common causes of corneal blindness. Patients typically present with unilateral eye pain, lacrimation, conjunctivitis, and blurred vision. It is important to identify HSV because topical corticosteroids can worsen the condition. Recurrences are common. Permanent visual damage may occur if there is significant corneal scarring. Other eye diseases associated with HSV infection include chorioretinitis (seen in HIV-infected individuals as a result of disseminated HSV) and the acute retinal necrosis syndrome (a rare cause of visual loss seen in healthy adults).

- **Herpetic whitlow:** This is the term used for HSV infection of the finger. It may result from occupational exposure, as in a respiratory technologist whose finger is inoculated with virus from a patient excreting the virus orally. Characteristically, there are vesicular lesions on the finger, with redness and edema. Recurrences are common. The lesions may be mistaken for bacterial pustules, especially when the patient presents with fever and regional lymphadenopathy. Many physicians mistake these lesions as being filled with pus and, subsequently, lance the lesions. The lesion can then develop a secondary bacterial infection.

- **HSV infections of the central nervous system:** HSV 1 is the most common cause of sporadic encephalitis in the United States. Encephalitis may result from primary HSV 1 infection, reactivation, or reinfection. It is theorized that the virus travels along the olfactory nerve of a susceptible host and reaches the temporal lobe of the brain. Patients present with the subacute onset of confusion. Other features include fever, headache, focal seizures, and olfactory hallucinations. It is difficult to distinguish encephalitis caused by HSV from other etiologies of encephalitis (such as arboviruses, tuberculosis, fungal infections, etc). Cerebrospinal fluid findings are usually nondiagnostic, and HSV 1 is only rarely isolated from spinal fluid culture. Electroencephalography (EEG) is helpful in localizing the area of inflammation to the temporal lobe. CT scan or MRI scan of the brain can reveal necrosis of the temporal lobe in some cases, a finding highly suggestive of HSV encephalitis. The definitive diagnostic test is the brain biopsy, with viral culture and histopathology. However, surgeons are becoming less willing to perform this invasive procedure and may suggest an empiric course of intravenous acyclovir instead.

- **HSV and AIDS:** Severe and recurrent HSV infections are frequently seen in AIDS. Progressive perianal ulcerations with proctitis may be due to either HSV 1 or 2. This infection may be quite debilitating, with anorectal pain, bloody stools, tenesmus, and fever. Such patients usually respond to I.V. or oral acyclovir. Since recurrences are the rule, these patients are often placed on chronic acyclovir suppression. This has led to the emergence of acyclovir-resistant HSV mutants and progressive rectal infection. HSV esophagitis may result from direct extension of oral HSV lesions into the esophagus or from reactivation of HSV in the vagus nerve which innervates the esophagus. The clinical presentation is indistinguishable from *Candida* esophagitis, another common condition in AIDS. Unfortunately, HSV esophageal lesions have a nonspecific appearance both on barium swallow and upper endoscopy, and tissue biopsy is required to rule out *Candida* (or cytomegalovirus) esophagitis.

- **HSV pneumonia:** This unusual manifestation of HSV is seen in the immunosuppressed. Cases have also been reported in burn unit patients. The pathogenesis is direct extension of herpetic tracheobronchitis into the lungs. A necrotizing pneumonia results, and bronchoscopy is usually required to confirm the diagnosis.

- **Neonatal infection:** HSV infection in newborns (less than 6 weeks of age) is frequently devastating. Visceral dissemination of the virus and central nervous system infection are common. Untreated, the mortality exceeds 65%. Many who survive exhibit developmental disabilities. Infection occurs most commonly during delivery as the neonate passes through an infected birth canal. *In utero* infection, while reported, is much less common.

Diagnosis Diagnosis can be made by culture, stain and/or serology depending on the clinical setting. Culture is performed on cell culture, with cytopathic effects appearing as early as 24-48 hours after inoculation. Monoclonal antibodies are also used to identify and type HSV isolates. Direct examination of a lesion can be done, staining a scraping with Giemsa stain (Tzanck smear). A variety of serology tests are also available with a fourfold rise in convalescence titers necessary in primary disease.

(Continued)

Herpes Simplex Virus (Continued)

Diagnostic Tests/Procedures
Herpes Cytology on page 362
Herpes Simplex Antibody on page 363
Herpes Simplex Virus Culture on page 364
Herpes Simplex Virus, Direct Immunofluorescence on page 365
Herpes Simplex Virus Isolation, Rapid on page 366

Treatment Acyclovir is the drug of choice for most herpes infections. For primary genital lesions, a 7-10 day course of oral acyclovir may decrease pain and viral shedding by several days. Topical acyclovir is less effective. Acyclovir is of limited utility in recurrences of genital herpes lesions, although long-term low dose oral acyclovir may be of benefit in preventing chronic recurrences (>6 per year). Herpes keratitis is often best treated with topical ophthalmic idoxuridine or trifluridine. Disseminated herpes simplex or HSV encephalitis should be treated aggressively with high-dose I.V. acyclovir. In patients who are failing therapy or who are intolerant to acyclovir, ganciclovir or foscarnet may be utilized. In immunocompromised patients, such as transplant or chemotherapy patients, HSV infection can be prevented with prophylactic administration of acyclovir or ganciclovir.

Drug Therapy
Recommended
Acyclovir on page 484
Alternate
Foscarnet on page 571
Ganciclovir on page 574

Selected Readings
Corey L, Spear PG, "Infections with Herpes Simplex Viruses," N Engl J Med, 1986, 314(11):686-91 and 314(12):749-57.

Erlich KS, Mills J, Chatis P, et al, "Acyclovir-Resistant Herpes Simplex Virus Infections in Patients With the Acquired Immunodeficiency Syndrome," N Engl J Med, 1989, 320(5):293-6.

Stone KM and Whittington WL, "Treatment of Genital Herpes," Rev Infect Dis, 1990, 12(Suppl 6):S610-9.

HEV see Hepatitis E Virus on page 127

HHV-6 see Human Herpesvirus-6 on next page

Histoplasma capsulatum

Microbiology Histoplasma capsulatum is a dimorphic fungus of low pathogenicity. It differs from other pathogenic fungi in that it is primarily a parasite of the reticuloendothelial system and rarely is found extracellular.

In the mold form, it has microconidia (2-6 μm) on short lateral branches or sessile on the sides of hyphae and large round to pyriform tuberculate macroconidia (8-14 μm) . This mold form is found in the soil and grows best in humid, shady environments at modest temperatures. Bird droppings and bat guano facilitate its growth. The spores become airborne and are inhaled.

The yeast form may be seen in human infections by direct examination. The cells are ovoid, 1-2 μm by 3-3.5 μm, and proliferate in macrophages (and occasionally neutrophils) which can be seen intracellular throughout the reticuloendothelial system including lymph nodes, bone marrow, spleen, liver, and adrenal glands.

Epidemiology Histoplasmosis is the most frequently diagnosed systemic fungal disease with approximately 500,000 cases per year in the United States. Endemic areas include the Mississippi and Ohio River Valleys, as well as some parts of Central America. Environmental sources include caves, chicken coops, bamboo canebrakes, bird roosts, school yards, prison grounds, decayed wood piles, dead trees, chimneys, and old buildings. Epidemics typically occur where contaminated soil is disturbed causing the spores to become airborne.

Clinical Syndromes
- **Asymptomatic:** Approximately 99% of all cases of histoplasmosis are asymptomatic and is an incidental finding on autopsy or seen as calcification on plain films of the lungs or spleen or noted as lymphadenopathy.
- **Acute histoplasmosis:** Typically presents as a flu-like syndrome with fever (95%), anorexia (85%), nonproductive cough (75%), and chest pain (75%). Retrosternal pain is a prominent feature and may be related to mediastinal

adenopathy. Skin and joint involvement is more common in women. Physical exam is typically normal except for pulmonary crackles and adenopathy. Chest x-ray may reveal hilar and mediastinal adenopathy with or without patchy or diffuse infiltrates. Rarely, patients present with pericarditis with or without tamponade. This syndrome is typically self-limited, lasting approximately 2 weeks.

- **Histoplasmomas:** Granulomatous nodules form on the lungs, usually in the lower lobes and less than 3 cm. Usually associated with hilar lymph node calcification, and 75% are found to be solitary lesions.
- **Acute pulmonary histoplasmosis:** Self-limited interstitial pneumonitis.
- **Chronic histoplasmosis:** Chronic pulmonary disorder that typically occurs in older patients with emphysema. Mimics tuberculosis. Referred to as the "marching cavity" because, in more than 50% of the cases, the walls of the lung cavity gradually enlarge.
- **Mediastinal histoplasmosis:** Approximately 25% of patients who develop this syndrome present with SVC syndrome, pulmonary vessel or esophageal or large airway obstruction, which may require surgical intervention. Rarely, associated with fibrosing mediastinitis.
- **Disseminated:** Defined as extrapulmonic spread with progressive clinical illness (ie, intestinal or oral ulcers, endocarditis, adrenal involvement). Typically, reactivated secondary to impaired cellular immunity. Classified as an AIDS-defining illness.

Diagnosis Skin tests are usually not helpful. Over 50% of the population in endemic areas may have positive skin tests. Approximately 50% of patients that do have disseminated diseases may have negative skin tests secondary to impaired immunity. False-positive skin tests may occur secondary to other systemic fungal diseases. Similar results are found with the complement fixation tests, however, a fourfold rise in titer is significant. Direct examination and isolation in culture is the preferred diagnostic procedure.

Diagnostic Tests/Procedures
Fungal Serology *on page 337*
Fungus Culture, Appropriate Site *on page 340*
Histoplasmosis Serology *on page 367*
KOH Preparation *on page 379*

Treatment No antifungal treatment is necessary for mild or asymptomatic histoplasmosis. Acute, nondisseminated disease is self-limited and requires only symptomatic care unless it persists for more than 3 weeks, at which time ketoconazole may be initiated. Heavy exposure, acute diffuse pulmonary involvement with respiratory insufficiency, and disseminated disease requires treatment with amphotericin B.

Patients with erythema nodosum or erythema multiform and arthralgias/arthritis may be treated with NSAIDs or corticosteroids. Eighty percent of patients with chronic pulmonary histoplasmosis respond to ketoconazole but have a higher relapse than those treated with amphotericin B.

Drug Therapy
Recommended
Severe infection:
Amphotericin B *on page 493*
Chronic infection:
Ketoconazole *on page 598*
Alternate
Itraconazole *on page 594*

Selected Readings
Hammarsten JE and Hammarsten JF, "Histoplasmosis Recognition and Treatment," *Hosp Pract (Off Ed)*, June, 1990, 95-9, 103, 106.
Lloyd JE, DesPrez RM, Goodwin RA, "Histoplasmosis," *Tropical and Geographical Medicine*, 2nd ed, Warren KS, Mahmoud AAF, eds, New York, NY: McGraw-Hill Inc, 1990, 965-72.

HIV *see* Human Immunodeficiency Virus *on page 133*

HIV Clinical Practice Guidelines *see page 765*

Hookworm *see* Ancylostoma duodenale *on page 54*

HSV *see* Herpes Simplex Virus *on page 128*

HTLV III *see* Human Immunodeficiency Virus *on page 133*

Human Herpesvirus-6

Synonyms HHV-6

Microbiology In 1986, a novel cytopathic virus was isolated from peripheral blood cells from patients with lymphoproliferative disease. The virus was origi-

(Continued)

Human Herpesvirus-6 *(Continued)*

nally named human β-lymphotropic virus because of its ability to infect B cells *in vitro* but later was found to be tropic for primarily T lymphocytes. It has since been classified as one of the human herpesviruses. It is a double-stranded DNA virus with an icosahedral capsid and outer envelope. HHV-6 is indistinguishable from other herpesviruses by electron microscopy, with the same morphology and size. In addition to its T-lymphocyte tropism, HHV-6 can infect B cells, monocytes, macrophages, and other cell lines. CD4$^+$ T cells, in particular, are targets for viral infection. The genome has been analyzed and sequenced for research purposes. A close homology between HHV-6 DNA and cytomegalovirus DNA has been found. The degree of relatedness of these two viruses remains to be seen since the gene products of HHV-6 are still being studied. There appear to be two general types of HHV-6, types A and B. The clinical significance of these two types is unknown, although most clinical isolates are type B.

Epidemiology Knowledge of the epidemiology of HHV-6 is still evolving. Much of the epidemiologic data for this virus will rest on the use of specific serologic tests. Unfortunately, serologic techniques are still being developed and have yet to be standardized. Earlier use of an immunofluorescence assay for antibody detection has been criticized on technical grounds and is probably too insensitive. To date there is no accepted gold standard for serologic tests and "borderline" positive specimens are difficult to interpret.

Available data indicate that HHV-6 infection occurs at an early age, between 6 months and 3 years most commonly. The seroprevalence is about 80% in the general population. It is likely to be as common as other herpesvirus infections. Newborns have a high level of antibody, probably from passive transfer from the mother. The titer of antibody rapidly decreases in the neonate as maternal antibody is lost; this is followed later by a second peak of antibody signifying primary infection in childhood.

Preliminary data suggest that asymptomatic HHV-6 shedding occurs in seropositive individuals. The virus has been isolated from the saliva of healthy children and adults who have had prior HHV-6 infection. Asymptomatic salivary excretion in the general population has been hypothesized as the main reservoir of the virus in the community and potentially could explain the large number of children who become infected. Initial studies reported very high salivary excretion rates, but later studies failed to confirm these results. Some experts have been critical of the methodologies employed in the earlier studies, suggesting that some of the viral isolates could have been HHV-7 rather than HHV-6. At the present time, it is clear that salivary excretion does take place, but the precise incidence is still debatable.

The mechanism(s) of HHV-6 transmission have not been definitively established. It is also unclear whether the virus can be transmitted by transfusion of blood products or by transplantation of organs.

Clinical Syndromes

- **Exanthem subitum (roseola):** Also known as roseola infantum, exanthem subitum is a benign disease of childhood that is caused by HHV-6. The disease is most common in children aged 6 months to 3 years old. In typical cases, there is an abrupt onset of high fever (often 40°C), and in a variable number of cases there may be additional symptoms such as sore throat, otitis, or cervical adenopathy. After 3-5 days, the fever resolves completely. This is followed 24-48 hours later by a maculopapular rash involving the trunk and neck. Although the rash itself is nonspecific in appearance, the timing of the rash is distinctive for roseola. The rash also resolves spontaneously after several days. Roseola is nearly always a benign disease. More serious complications of acute HHV-6 infection have been described (meningoencephalitis, hepatitis). During the febrile phase of exanthem subitum, HHV-6 can be cultured from peripheral blood mononuclear cells. Seroconversion can also be documented.

- **Undifferentiated febrile illness:** Primary HHV-6 infection appears to be a common, identifiable cause of high fevers in children. In a recent study, 14% of children who presented to an emergency room for evaluation of fever were found to have HHV-6 viremia. Of note, the rash of classic roseola was absent in many children, and the most common presentation was irritability, inflamed tympanic membranes, and temperatures higher than 40°C. Although the full range of HHV-6 infection has yet to be determined, it is likely that many primary infections are either nonspecific, febrile syndromes or entirely asymptomatic.

- **HHV-6 in adults:** Primary infection with HHV-6 is probably uncommon in adults. The clinical course of such infections have been described in small numbers of adults with documented seroconversion. Symptoms included fever, headache, and fever lasting over 1 week. Cervical lymphadenopathy was noted in several cases and was persistent for months. Laboratory abnormalities included a minor elevation in liver function tests, leukopenia, and atypical lymphocytosis. Latent HHV-6 infection appears to take place following primary infection, as with other herpesviruses. Reactivation has also been reported in adults. Little is known about the incidence or mechanisms underlying either latency or reactivation.

- **HHV-6 in immunocompromised hosts:** The role of HHV-6 in transplant recipients is still largely unknown. The following observations have been made: 1. Many individuals are seropositive for HHV-6 prior to transplantation. 2. An increase in specific antibody against HHV-6 is commonly seen after transplantation. Viremia with HHV-6 also appears to be common at 2-3 weeks post-transplantation, earlier than the peak for cytomegalovirus. The importance of these findings has yet to be determined. 3. Primary infection with cytomegalovirus in the transplant patient is often associated with a significant rise in HHV-6 antibodies. The significance of this simultaneous seroconversion is unclear. 4. Some kidney biopsy specimens which have demonstrated acute rejection have stained positive for HHV-6. The relationship between HHV-6 and acute rejection is unknown.

HHV-6 has also been implicated by some as a possible cofactor in HIV infection. This is based on several observations, including the mutual tropism for the host's CD4$^+$ T lymphocytes. Whether HHV-6 alters the natural course of HIV infection is still under study.

Diagnosis Viral isolation can be performed in specialized laboratories. HHV-6 can be cultured in peripheral blood mononuclear cells (with or without the addition of donor cells). Standard tissue culture used for isolation of other viruses is suboptimal for HHV-6. Even under optimal conditions, the cytopathic effect of HHV-6 in peripheral blood mononuclear cells can be subtle; multiple passages of the virus in culture may be necessary. Detection methods are then necessary to confirm the presence of this virus.

HHV-6 has also been isolated from clinical samples of saliva and blood. Antigen detection methods, while still being perfected, have been used to identify the virus directly from biopsy samples. Polymerase chain reaction has been used successfully in limited reports. A serologic test has recently become available.

Diagnostic Tests/Procedures
Human Herpesvirus 6, IgG and IgM Antibodies, Quantitative
on page 369

Treatment Most infections caused by HHV-6 are mild and self-limiting. Susceptibility to antiviral agents are probably similar to CMV, where acyclovir only inhibits the organism at high concentrations. Ganciclovir has been shown to inhibit HHV-6 at achievable concentrations, although this data is inconsistent.

Drug Therapy Comment No drug therapy is recommended.

Selected Readings
Carrigan DR, Drobyski WR, Russler SK, et al, "Interstitial Pneumonitis Associated With Human Herpesvirus-6 Infection After Marrow Transplantation," *Lancet*, 1991, 338(8760):147-9.

Chou S, "Human Herpesvirus 6 Infection and Associated Disease," *J Lab Clin Med*, 1993, 121(3):388-93.

Pruksananonda P, Hall CB, Insel RA, et al, "Primary Human Herpesvirus-6 Infection in Young Children," *N Engl J Med*, 1992, 326(22):1445-50.

Yamanishi K, "Pathogenesis of Human Herpesvirus 6 (HHV-6)," *Infect Agents Dis*, 1992, 1(3):149-55.

Human Immunodeficiency Virus

Related Information
HIV Clinical Practice Guidelines *on page 765-774*
Occupational Exposure to Bloodborne Pathogens (Universal Precautions)
on page 751-756

Synonyms AIDS Virus; HIV; HTLV III; Human T-Cell Lymphotrophic Virus

Microbiology HIV is one of the four known pathogenic human retroviruses and a member of the Lentiviruses. There are two recognized subtypes of HIV; HIV-1 causes AIDS worldwide, and HIV-2 produces an AIDS-like illness that appears to be less pathogenic than HIV-1. HIV is an enveloped virus about 100 μm in diameter that forms by budding from cell membranes. HIV is diploid, meaning that an electron-dense central core surrounds two identical copies of

(Continued)

a single-stranded viral RNA genome. Reverse transcriptase catalyzes the transcription of the RNA genome into a double-stranded DNA (known as the "provirus") that migrates from the cytoplasm to the nucleus, integrates into the host cell DNA, and remains integrated for the lifetime of the cell. HIV contains three essential genes for viral replication, "gag", "pol", and "env". "Gag" (glycosaminoglycan) refers to genes which code for group antigens associated with viral core proteins which include p24. "Pol" (polymerase) encodes reverse transcriptase. "Env" (envelope) encodes the envelope surface glycoproteins gp 120 and gp 41.

Epidemiology HIV is now the leading cause of death of men aged 25-40, the sixth leading cause of death of adolescent males aged 15-24, and the fourth leading cause of death in women aged 25-44. It is estimated that over 1 million U.S. residents are HIV infected; roughly 1 out of 250. By the year 2000, it is estimated by the World Health Organization that there will be 40 million HIV-infected individuals worldwide.

Male homosexuality continues to be the most common mode of transmission. HIV secondary to I.V. drug use and heterosexual transmission continues to rise. Approximately 14% of reported cases of AIDS in 1994 are women as compared to 5% in 1991. Nationally for both men and women, 7% of cases are secondary to heterosexual contact, however in Florida, New York, and California that number approaches 30%. Minorities account for a disproportionate amount of AIDS as expected by population statistics.

Clinical Syndromes During initial HIV infection, CD4 counts transiently decrease and HIV antigen (viremia) rises; antibody is detectable usually by 3 months. At 2-6 weeks after infection, patients may develop viral-like illness consisting of fever, sweats, fatigue, malaise, lymphadenopathy, sore throat, and sometimes splenomegaly. Patients may remain asymptomatic for months to years depending on the progression of their disease. In 1993, the Centers for Disease Control revised the previous classification of HIV (see table).

1993 Revised CDC HIV Classification System and Expanded AIDS Surveillance Definition for Adolescents and Adults
(*MMWR* 41:RR-17, Dec 18, 1992)

The revised system emphasizes the importance of CD4 lymphocyte testing in clinical management of HIV infected persons. The system is based on three ranges of CD4 counts and four clinical categories giving a matrix of nine exclusive categories. The system replaces the 1986 classification.

Criteria for HIV Infection

Persons 13 years of age or older with repeatedly (2 or more) reactive screening tests (ELISA) plus specific antibodies identified by a supplemental test, eg, Western blot ["reactive" pattern = positive for any two of p24, gp41, or gp120/160 (*MMWR*, 1991, 40:681)]. Other specific methods of diagnosis of HIV-1 include virus isolation, antigen detection, and detection of HIV genetic material by PCR.

Classification System

CD4 Cell[†] Category	Clinical Category*		
	A	B	C
$\geq$500/mm^3	A1	B1	*C1*
200-499/mm^3	A2	B2	*C2*
<200/mm^3	*A3*	*B3*	*C3*

*See following clinical definitions. Italics indicate expansion of AIDS surveillance definition. Category C currently "reportable." Categories A3 and B3 are "reportable" as AIDS effective January 1, 1993.

†There is a diurnal variation in CD4 counts averaging 60/mm^3 higher in the afternoon in HIV-positive individuals and 500/mm^3 in HIV-negative persons. Blood for sequential CD4 counts should be drawn at about the same time of day each time (*J AIDS*, 1990, 3:144). The equivalence between CD4 counts and CD4 % of total lymphocytes: $\geq$500 = $\geq$29%, 200-499 = 14%-28%, <200 = <14%.

Clinical Category A

Asymptomatic HIV infection
Persistent generalized lymphadenopathy (PGL)‡
Acute (primary) HIV illness

‡Nodes in 2 more extrainguinal sites, at least 1 cm in diameter for ≥3 months.

Clinical Category B

Symptomatic, not A or C conditions
Examples include but not limited to:
    Bacillary angiomatosis
    Candidiasis, vulvovaginal: persistent >1 month, poorly responsive
      to therapy
    Candidiasis, oropharyngeal
    Cervical dysplasia, severe, or carcinoma *in situ*
    Constitutional symptoms, eg, fever (>38.5°C) or diarrhea >1
      month

The above must be attributed to HIV infection or have a clinical course
or management complicated by HIV.

Clinical Category C§

Candidiasis: esophageal, trachea, bronchi
Coccidioidomycosis, extrapulmonary
Cryptococcosis, extrapulmonary
Cervical cancer, invasive§
Cryptosporidiosis, chronic intestinal (>1 month)
CMV retinitis, or other than liver, spleen, nodes
HIV encephalopathy
Herpes simplex with mucocutaneous ulcer >1 month, bronchitis,
    pneumonia
Histoplasmosis: disseminated, extrapulmonary
Isosporiasis, chronic (>1 month)
Kaposi's sarcoma
Lymphoma: Burkitt's, immunoblastic, primary in brain
M. avium or *M. kansasii*, extrapulmonary
M. tuberculosis,§ pulmonary or extrapulmonary
Mycobacterium, other species disseminated or extrapulmonary
Pneumocystis carinii pneumonia
Pneumonia,§ recurrent (≥2 episodes in 1 year)
Progressive multifocal leukoencephalopathy
Salmonella bacteremia, recurrent
Toxoplasmosis, cerebral
Wasting syndrome due to HIV

§These are the 1987 CDC case definitions (*MMWR*, 1987, 36:15). The 1993 CDC
Expanded Surveillance Case Definition includes all conditions contained in the
1987 definition (above) plus persons with documented HIV infection and any of
the following: (1) CD4 T-lymphocyte count <200/mm^3 (or CD4 <14%), (2)
pulmonary tuberculosis,§ (3) recurrent pneumonia§ (≥2 episodes within 1 year)
or, (4) invasive cervical carcinoma.§

Diagnosis Is made serologically. Detection of HIV antibody by ELISA must be
confirmed by Western blot. Alternate diagnosis may be made by viral culture,
antigen detection, or HIV by polymerase chain reaction (PCR). Maternal antibodies may persist in infants until 18 months of age; therefore, CD4 counts,
viral culture, and/or PCR followed by antibody detection after 18 months must
be performed in order to diagnose HIV in infants.

Human Immunodeficiency Virus (Continued)

Diagnostic Tests/Procedures
HIV-1 Serology on page 368
Human Immunodeficiency Virus Culture on page 370
Human Immunodeficiency Virus DNA Amplification on page 370
p24 Antigen on page 420
T4/T8 Ratio on page 453

Treatment Previous recommendations were that antiretrovirals (AZT, DDI, DDC) were initiated once CD4 counts were <500/mm^3. After publication of the European Concorde study, many clinicians began to question the efficacy of starting antiretroviral therapy early in asymptomatic patients. In summary, the Concorde study suggested benefit in a subset of patients by noting a delay of progression to opportunistic infections but failed to show prolongation of survival. Due to concerns of drug resistance and potential side effects, it is a clinical judgment decision as when to initiate antiretrovirals. Most investigators recommend starting therapy when there is a decline of >80 CD4 cells per year or a change in the patient's clinical status. Again, debate exists as to when to start combination therapy or switch antiretrovirals. Zidovudine has been found to reduce perinatal transmission from 25% to 8% when taken during pregnancy. See specific organisms for treatment of AIDS-related infections.

Drug Therapy
Recommended
Zidovudine on page 696
Alternate
Didanosine on page 552
Zalcitabine on page 695

Selected Readings
American College of Physicians and Infectious Diseases Society of America, "Human Immunodeficiency Virus," Clin Infect Dis, 1994, 18(6):963-73.

Cotton P, "Use of Antiretroviral Drugs in HIV Disease Declines Following Preliminary Results From Concorde Trial," JAMA, 1994, 271(7):488-9.

U.S. Department of Health and Human Resources, Evaluation and Management of Early HIV Infection, Agency for Health Care Policy and Research Pub No. 94-0572, January 1994 (to obtain copy call 1-800-342-AIDS).

Human T-Cell Lymphotrophic Virus see Human Immunodeficiency Virus on page 133

Immunization Guidelines see page 710

Influenza Vaccine see page 718

Influenza Virus
Related Information
Immunization Guidelines on page 710-717
Influenza Vaccine on page 718
Vaccines on page 706-709

Microbiology Influenza virus is the etiological agent of influenza, is an enveloped, double-stranded (multi-segmented) RNA virus, and is the only member of the Orthomyxovirus family. Influenza virus is broadly classified into three groups (A, B, and C) which are based primarily on antigenic (serological) differences in internal proteins. The envelope of influenza virus contains transmembrane proteins H (three types) and N (two types) which are associated with hemagglutination and neuraminidase activities, respectively. Gradual and continual antigenic changes in the H and N proteins (usually the H) are called "antigenic drift" and are responsible for bypassing human immunity from year to year. Sudden and major antigenic changes in the H and N proteins are called "antigenic shift" and are responsible for worldwide epidemics (pandemics) of influenza every 10 to 20 years or so. Strains of influenza are designated by the type of internal protein, host species (human if not designated), strain number, year of isolation, and H/N types (eg, A/California/10/78/H1N2). The natural reservoirs of influenza virus are as follows: type A, humans and many types of animals; type B, humans; type C, swine. Type A is by far the most prominent and important because of its association with pandemics of influenza.

Epidemiology Influenza virus causes influenza and is an important cause of worldwide respiratory disease. Recurrent episodes of influenza (due to antigenic drift and usually in isolated countries or regions of the world) have been observed every 1 to 3 years for the last 400 years. Worldwide pandemics of influenza occur every 10 to 20 years and have been responsible for an estimated

21 million deaths. Influenza virus is spread person to person by inhalation of the virus in aerosolized droplets and possibly by contaminated fomites.

Clinical Syndromes Signs and symptoms of influenza vary greatly and can range from a mild upper respiratory tract illness to rapidly fatal pneumonia. There are three basic clinical presentations of influenza virus infection:

- **Uncomplicated rhinotracheitis:** Abrupt onset of headache, myalgia, malaise, runny nose, chills, and cough. The course of this disease is usually 7-10 days.
- **Rhinotracheitis and subsequent bacterial pneumonia:** Typical rhinotracheitis, a brief period of feeling well, and subsequent secondary bacterial pneumonia typically caused by *Streptococcus pneumoniae*, *Staphylococcus*, or *Haemophilus influenzae*.
- **Frank viral pneumonia:** Can be fulminating and can lead to hypoxia and death in only a few days.

Diagnosis Influenza usually is diagnosed clinically, but laboratory diagnosis and confirmation is highly recommended because symptoms of influenza often are not readily distinguishable from those caused by other respiratory pathogens. Influenza virus is rather easily grown in cell culture, and positive cultures can be observed within 4 days. Some laboratories offer direct detection of influenza-infected cells obtained from nasopharyngeal aspirates or swabs, or from sputum. Serological tests for antibodies for influenza virus are easy to perform and are cost-efficient. Influenza-specific antibodies often can be detected as soon as 4-7 days after the onset of symptoms and can reach peak titers at 14-21 days after symptoms. However, serological tests are retrospective, and acute and convalescent sera must be examined for a fourfold rise in titer.

Diagnostic Tests/Procedures

Influenza A and B Serology *on page 375*
Influenza Virus Culture *on page 375*
Viral Culture, Throat *on page 479*
Virus, Direct Detection by Fluorescent Antibody *on page 480*

Drug Therapy Comment

Use amantadine hydrochloride for influenza A infections only. No antiviral therapy for influenza B infections.

Drug Therapy
Recommended

Amantadine Hydrochloride *on page 486*

Selected Readings

Betts RF, "Influenza Virus," *Principles and Practice of Infectious Diseases*, 4th ed, Mandell GL, Bennett JE, and Dolin R, eds, New York, NY: Churchill Livingstone, 1995, 1546-67.

Greenberg SB, "Viral Pneumonia," *Infect Dis Clin North Am*, 1991, 5(3):603-621.

Shaw MW, Arden NH, and Maassab HF, "New Aspects of Influenza Viruses," *Clin Microbiol Rev*, 1992, 5(1):74-92.

"Update: Influenza Activity – United States, 1993-94 Season," *MMWR Morb Mortal Wkly Rep*, 1994, 43(1):1-3.

Klebsiella Species

Microbiology *Klebsiella* species are aerobic gram-negative bacilli belonging to the tribe Klebsielleae and the family Enterobacteriaceae. The main species causing human disease are *K. pneumoniae* and *K. oxytoca*. A distinctive characteristic of most isolates of *Klebsiella* is the polysaccharide capsule which imparts a mucoid appearance of the organisms when growing on solid media. The prominent capsule also makes the organism appear large on Gram stain. The presence of the capsule is a virulence factor. As with other gram-negative bacilli of this family, *Klebsiella* produces endotoxin, a mediator of the sepsis syndrome.

Epidemiology *Klebsiella* sp are primarily nosocomial pathogens. However, the organism is associated with one important community-acquired infection, primary lobar pneumonia.

Clinical Syndromes

- **Primary lobar pneumonia:** This infection is community-acquired and is seen in alcoholics and other patients with chronic debilitating underlying illnesses (such as chronic obstructive pulmonary disease). It is rarely seen in the otherwise healthy individual and is considered a type of opportunistic infection. Characteristically, a patient with underlying alcoholism presents with the acute onset of fever, purulent sputum with a "currant jelly" appearance (reflecting lung necrosis and blood), and dyspnea. The classic x-ray finding is the "bowed fissure;" the lobe is swollen and the fissure appears to be sagging and widened. Complications include lung abscess, empy-

(Continued)

Klebsiella Species *(Continued)*

ema, cavity formation, and progressive infiltrates. This form of pneumonitis is severe with extensive necrosis. Many patients expire, in part due to their comorbidity conditions.

- **Bronchitis and bronchopneumonia:** Not all forms of *Klebsiella* lung infection lead to the severe form of necrotizing pneumonia described above. Community-acquired *Klebsiella* bronchitis and bronchopneumonia do occur but are much less frequently seen than hospital-acquired respiratory infections.
- **Nosocomial pneumonia:** Hospital-acquired *Klebsiella* lower respiratory infections are seen in debilitated, ventilator-dependent patients. *Klebsiella* and other gram-negative bacilli can asymptomatically colonize the upper respiratory tract of hospitalized patients. Thus, the recovery of *Klebsiella* from a sputum or tracheal aspirate culture does not necessarily indicate a significant infection. The diagnosis of a nosocomial pneumonia still rests on standard criteria such as the presence of purulence (many leukocytes) on the Gram stain of sputum, the presence of a pulmonary infiltrate, and signs of systemic inflammation in the patient. **A positive sputum culture alone is not sufficient justification for initiating antibiotic therapy**.
- **Nosocomial urinary tract infections:** Hospitalized patients with indwelling Foley catheters are at risk for cystitis or pyelonephritis from *Klebsiella*. *Klebsiella* may be recovered more frequently from the urine than from any other site, including the respiratory tract. However, the organism may also harmlessly colonize the urine of patients with chronic bladder catheters without causing disease. The decision to initiate antibiotics in such patients should be based on the clinical situation (the presence of pyuria on urinalysis, suprapubic pain, fever, etc). Even the finding of large quantity of *Klebsiella* in a urine culture ($>10^5$ colony forming units/mL) by itself does not automatically indicate antibiotic therapy.
- **Hospital-associated bacteremias:** *Klebsiella* is a common cause of primary bacteremia. In some series, it approaches *E. coli* as one of the most frequently recovered gram-negative bacillus from the bloodstream.
- **Surgical wound infections.**
- **Biliary tract infections, especially following instrumentation.**

Diagnosis The diagnosis of lobar pneumonia secondary to *Klebsiella* should be considered in any debilitated patient who presents with a necrotizing pneumonia. The history of "currant jelly" sputum and the finding of a "bowed fissure" on chest x-ray are highly suggestive but are not always present. The differential diagnosis of such cases should include anaerobic lung abscess, tuberculosis, *Pseudomonas* and other gram-negative bacilli, and mixed aspiration pneumonitis, among others. The presentation of nosocomial *Klebsiella* infections are more nonspecific and can be due to a variety of pathogenic gram-negative bacilli. Culture and Gram stain of appropriate clinical specimens (sputum, urine, blood, catheter tips, etc) is necessary to make the diagnosis.

Diagnostic Tests/Procedures
Aerobic Culture, Appropriate Site *on page 244*
Gram Stain *on page 352*

Treatment Like many other nosocomial pathogens, *Klebsiella* sp may be difficult to treat because of antimicrobial resistance. Although the organisms have been traditionally susceptible to cephalosporins, including the first generation agents, increasing problems with resistance are emerging. Isolates of *Klebsiella* which are resistant to cephalosporins and aminoglycosides have emerged because of widespread use of these antimicrobial agents. Resistance is spread bacterium to bacterium by plasmid-mediated resistance mechanisms. In all cases, the final selection of antibiotics must be based on the susceptibility pattern of the particular isolate because the organism is no longer predictably sensitive to all agents.

Drug Therapy
Recommended
Cephalosporins, 1st Generation *on page 527*
Cephalosporins, 2nd Generation *on page 527*
Cephalosporins, 3rd Generation *on page 528*
Alternate
Penicillins, Extended Spectrum *on page 637*
Imipenem/Cilastatin *on page 586*
Aztreonam *on page 501*

Selected Readings
Carpenter JL, "*Klebsiella* Pulmonary Infections: Occurrence at One Medical Center and Review," *Rev Infect Dis*, 1990, 12(4):672-80.

ORGANISMS

Garcia de la Torre M, Romero-Vivas J, Martinez-Beltran J, et al, "*Klebsiella* Bacteremia: An Analysis of 100 Episodes," *Rev Infect Dis*, 1985, 7(2):143-50.

Meyer KS, Urban C, Eagan JA, et al, "Nosocomial Outbreak of *Klebsiella* Infection Resistant to Late-Generation Cephalosporins," *Ann Intern Med*, 1993, 119(5):353-8.

Legionella pneumophila

Microbiology *Legionella pneumophila* is an aerobic, gram-negative rod first isolated in 1947 which causes a pneumonia called Legionnaires' disease (or legionellosis), as well as a distinct febrile illness called Pontiac fever. There are over 30 *Legionella* species, with *L. pneumophila* accounting for about 90% of human infections. The organism is very difficult to visualize on Gram stain of clinical specimens. Other stains are more effective in identifying the organism, such as the silver stain (Dieterle or Warthin-Starry stains), Gimenez stain, and others. The organism also requires special medium for growth and cannot be cultured using standard bacteriologic media. Charcoal yeast extract is the medium most commonly used for culture isolation.

Epidemiology The importance of this organism was recently recognized in 1976 following an outbreak of pneumonia involving an American Legion convention in Philadelphia, Pennsylvania. The cause of this well-publicized outbreak which involved over 200 individuals was initially unknown. Only later was the bacterium *Legionella pneumophila* isolated from lung autopsy specimens by the Centers for Disease Control. Another epidemic of Legionnaires' disease had been described in 1965, where the diagnosis was established using serologic studies rather than identification of the organism. Since then, prospective studies have shown *L. pneumophila* to be one of the three most common causes of community-acquired pneumonia. The prevalence of *L. pneumophila* varies geographically. In some areas of the United States, it is the most common cause of community-acquired pneumonia.

The bacterium typically inhabits lakes, ponds, polluted waters, and hot water systems in buildings and homes. Evidence suggests that human disease is likely caused by aspiration of contaminated water. Airborne transmission by aerosolization has been theorized as well but cannot explain many cases.

Clinical Syndromes

- **Community-acquired pneumonia:** The incidence of *L. pneumophila* as a cause of community-acquired pneumonia has ranged from 1% to 15%. There is a well-recognized, broad spectrum of clinical symptoms. Patients may present with a minor cough or with a progressive five-lobe pneumonia with shock. Fever is almost always present, and often over 40°C. Typically, the cough is nonproductive although pleuritic chest pain may occur. Other accompanying features are shaking chills, relative bradycardia, diarrhea and other gastrointestinal symptoms (up to 50% of cases), and hyponatremia. No single symptom or constellation of symptoms is diagnostic of legionellosis. In one study, the extrapulmonary symptoms such as diarrhea and neurologic findings were not found more frequently with Legionnaires' disease in comparison with other forms of pneumonia. The chest radiograph classically shows unilateral patchy infiltrates early on, which progress over several days to consolidation. However, a very wide variety of x-ray abnormalities has been described with this infection. Pleural effusions are common.
- **Nosocomial pneumonia:** *L. pneumophila* is a sporadic cause of hospital-acquired pneumonias.
- **Pontiac fever:** This is a febrile illness caused by *L. pneumophila* which tends to be self-resolving without antibiotics. Patients present with fever, myalgias, headache and malaise, mimicking the flu, however, pneumonia is not present.
- **Miscellaneous:** *L. pneumophila* has been described rarely as a cause of endocarditis, sinusitis, pericarditis, peritonitis, pancreatitis, encephalopathy, and wound infections.

Diagnosis A high level of suspicion must be maintained by the clinician since the presentation of Legionnaires' disease is varied and notoriously nonspecific. Laboratory testing is essential in making the diagnosis since the organism cannot be reliably recovered in routine cultures of sputum, blood, or bronchoscopy specimens. The clinician must specify both special stains and cultures for *L. pneumophila*.

Diagnostic Tests/Procedures

Legionella Antigen, Urine *on page 380*
Legionella DNA Probe *on page 381*
Legionella pneumophila Culture *on page 381*
(Continued)

Legionella pneumophila (Continued)

Legionella pneumophila Smear *on page 383*
Legionella Serology *on page 384*

Treatment The antibiotic of choice is erythromycin, which has been shown to improve survival in several studies. The preferred regimen is erythromycin 2-4 g/day intravenously. Some authors recommend a combination of erythromycin and rifampin for known cases of Legionnaires' disease, based mainly on *in vitro* susceptibility data.

Drug Therapy
Recommended

Erythromycin *on page 561*
or
Erythromycin *on page 561*
used in combination with
Rifampin *on page 662*

Alternate

Clarithromycin *on page 539*
Azithromycin Dihydrate *on page 500*
Ciprofloxacin Hydrochloride *on page 537*

Selected Readings

Bernstein MS, Locksley RM, "*Legionella* Infections," *Harrison's Principles of Internal Medicine*, 13th ed, Isselbacher KJ, Braunwald E, Wilson JD, et al, eds, New York, NY: McGraw-Hill, 1994, 654-8.

Blatt SP, Dolan MJ, Hendrix CW, et al, "Legionnaires' Disease in Human Immunodeficiency Virus-Infected Patients: Eight Cases and Review," *Clin Infect Dis*, 1994, 18(2):227-32.

Edelstein PH, "Legionnaires' Disease," *Clin Infect Dis*, 1993, 16(6):741-7.

Lowry PW, Blankenship RJ, Gridley W, et al, "A Cluster of *Legionella* Sternal-Wound Infections Due to Postoperative Topical Exposure to Contaminated Tap Water," *N Engl J Med*, 1991, 324(2):109-13.

Nguyen MH, Stout JE, and Yu VL, "Legionellosis," *Infect Dis Clin North Am*, 1991, 5(3):561-84.

Leptospira interrogans

Microbiology *Leptospira interrogans* is an aerobic spirochete which causes the febrile human disease leptospirosis. *L. interrogans* is the main pathogenic species of the genus *Leptospira*, which is divided into 170 serotypes. A second species, *L. biflexa*, is saprophytic. The organism is a finely coiled, motile, helical rod 0.1 μm in width and 6-20 μm in length. One or both ends of the rod are usually hooked, giving the appearance of a question mark (thus the name *L. interrogans*).

Epidemiology Leptospirosis is an unusual disease in the U.S., with 50-100 cases reported annually. It is primarily a disease of wild and domestic mammals. Humans are infected only occasionally through direct animal contact or through indirect contact with soil or water that is contaminated with infected urine. Groups at risk include farmers, veterinarians, abattoir workers, campers, and swimmers. Worldwide, rats are the most common source of human infection with a 90% carriage rate. In the U.S., the most important sources of infection are dogs, livestock, rodents, wild mammals, and cats. Person-to-person transmission is extremely rare. Most cases of leptospirosis occur in young adult men, and the peak incidence is in the summer and early fall.

Clinical Syndromes The organisms are capable of penetrating intact mucous membranes or abraded skin of the host. The leptospires enter the blood stream and are rapidly disseminated even to "sequestered sites" such as the cerebrospinal fluid and the eye. The primary pathologic lesion is damage to the endothelium of small blood vessels.

- **Subclinical leptospirosis:** Some individuals may have minimal symptoms after infection with *L. interrogans*. This occurs most commonly in those who are frequently exposed to infected animals. Leptospires can establish a symbiotic relationship with many animal hosts, persisting for long periods in the renal tubules without producing disease or pathologic changes in the kidney.

- **Anicteric leptospirosis:** Among patients ill with leptospirosis, 90% have a mild anicteric disease. The incubation period is 7-12 days usually. Individuals with anicteric leptospirosis have an abrupt onset of remitting fever, headache, abdominal pain, nausea and vomiting, severe myalgias, and malaise. Prostration may persist for 4-7 days. The illness may be biphasic. Following this initial flu-like illness, the patient is then afebrile for several days. The second phase, called the "immune phase" occurs in some, but not all, patients and is characterized by low grade fever, throbbing headaches, and sometimes delirium without encephalitis. Up to 90% will have evidence of meningitis, with a cerebrospinal fluid pleocytosis. Although the CSF pressure is normal, characteristically the spinal tap will improve the headaches. Other symptoms include ocular manifestations, in particular suffusion of the bulbar conjunctiva, photophobia, ocular pain, and conjunctival hemorrhage; abdominal pain, with nausea and vomiting; myalgias; splenomegaly (15% to 25% of cases); lymphadenopathy; rash, with raised 1-5 cm erythematous lesions in the pretibial area (so-called Fort Bragg fever caused by *L. autumnalis*).

- **Icteric leptospirosis:** Also known as Weil syndrome, this severe form of leptospirosis is characterized by hepatic dysfunction, jaundice, impaired renal function, hemorrhage, vascular collapse, and severe mental status changes. Mortality is 5% to 10%. Jaundice is due to hepatocellular damage without necrosis. Marked elevation of the serum creatine phosphokinase, with only modest elevations of transaminases is seen. Severely jaundiced patients are the ones most likely to exhibit renal failure and subsequent loss of intravascular volume. Renal failure is primarily the result of tubular damage, with the leptospires visible in the tubular lumen. Immune complex glomerulonephritis may be seen. Urinalysis shows proteinuria, hematuria, and casts. Hemorrhagic myocarditis often contributes to fatal cases.

Diagnosis Definitive diagnosis can only be made by isolation of the organism as seroconversion (greater than 4 times rise in serologic titer) in patients with relevant clinical syndromes. There are a variety of serological tests available including a macroscopic slide agglutination test (killed antigen), microscopic agglutination test (live antigen), indirect hemagglutination test, an ELISA and a Dot-ELISA test.

Culture of organism requires special media (Tween® 80-albumin medium is preferred) and takes 5-6 weeks at 28°C to 30°C to grow (in the dark). A rapid method using the Bactec® 460 system may detect organisms from blood with 2-5 days. Organisms will be present in the blood only during the first 10 days of an acute illness and are present in urine during week two. These organisms can be seen by the experienced microbiologist upon darkfield examination.

Diagnostic Tests/Procedures

Darkfield Examination, Leptospirosis *on page 322*

Leptospira Culture *on page 384*

Leptospira Serology *on page 385*

Treatment Early studies suggested that penicillin or tetracycline might shorten the duration of fever and reduce the incidence of renal, hepatic, meningeal, and hemorrhagic complications, but only if therapy was started by the fourth day of illness. Recently it was found that therapy may be effective in severe disease even when treatment was delayed. Administration of a single dose of doxycycline, 200 mg once a week, prevented infection in soldiers in Panama.

Treatment recommendations are for penicillin G, 1.5 million units every 6 hours or ampicillin, 1000 mg I.V. every 6 hours in severe disease. In less severe disease, oral therapy with doxycycline, 100 mg orally twice daily or ampicillin, 500-750 mg orally every 6 hours for 5-7 days.

In the U.S., there is no licensed human vaccine, but in other countries, human vaccine against leptospirosis has been reported to be useful.

Pediatric Drug Therapy

Recommended

Penicillin G, Parenteral *on page 633*

Adult Drug Therapy

Recommended

Penicillin G, Parenteral *on page 633*

Alternate

Tetracycline *on page 679*

Doxycycline *on page 557*

Selected Readings

Emmanouilides CE, Orly FK, and Garibaldi R, "Leptospirosis Complicated by a Jarisch-Herxheimer Reaction and Adult Respiratory Distress Syndrome," *Clin Infect Dis*, 1994, 18:1004-6.

Farrar WE, "*Leptospira* Species (Leptospirosis)," *Principles and Practice of Infectious Diseases*, 4th ed, Mandell GL, Bennett JE, and Dolin R, eds, New York, NY: Churchill Livingstone, 1995, 2137-41.

Kennedy ND, Pusey CD, Rainford DJ, et al, "*Leptospirosis* and Acute Renal Failure – Clinical Experiences and a Review of the Literature," *Postgrad Med J*, 1979, 55(641):176-9.

(Continued)

Leptospira interrogans (Continued)

O'Neil KM, Rickman LS, and Lazarus AA, "Pulmonary Manifestations of Leptospirosis," *Rev Infect Dis*, 1991, 13(4):705-9.

Takafuji ET, Kirkpatrick JW, Miller RN, et al, "An Efficacy Trial of Doxycycline Chemoprophylaxis Against Leptospirosis," *N Engl J Med*, 1984, 310(8):497-500.

Lice

Synonyms *Pediculus humanus*; *Philhirus pubis*

Microbiology Human lice are ectoparasites and thus tend to live on or in the skin of the host. They belong to the insect class *Hexapoda*. There are three species important in human infection. *Pediculus humanus* var. *corporis* is the human body louse, *Pediculus humanus* var. *capitis* is the human head louse, and *Phthirus pubis* is the crab louse. The body and head louse have similar appearances and are about 4 mm long. The pubic louse is much wider and has a crab-like appearance from which its name is derived. The eggs adhere to human hair and to clothing and are termed nits.

Epidemiology Humans are the reservoir for lice. Infestations have been described worldwide especially in areas of overcrowding. The incubation period is about 1-4 weeks following exposure. Individuals are communicable until all the lice and eggs have been treated and destroyed. Pediculosis capitis is a particular problem with school-aged children, where the practice of sharing combs or brushes facilitates epidemic transmission. All socioeconomic backgrounds are at risk for head lice. In contrast, pediculosis corporis is seen mainly in areas of poor sanitation. The body louse resides almost exclusively in soiled clothing, rather than the skin, and only leaves the clothing for a blood meal from the host. Pediculosis corporis also transmits the rickettsial infection epidemic typhus, as well a several others. *Phthirus pubis* is usually sexually transmitted, although spread via infested bedding or clothing can occur.

Clinical Syndromes

- **Pediculosis corporis:** Typically, the patient complains of severe pruritus, and small, erythematous papules are found on the body. Often extensive self-induced excoriations across the trunk are noted. If left untreated for long periods, hyperpigmentation and scarring may occur, called "vagabond's disease."

- **Pediculosis capitis:** The most common presentation is intractable scalp pruritus. On examination there may be evidence of secondary bacterial infection of the scalp from excoriations. At times, an "id reaction" occurs, characterized by a dramatic skin eruption over the arms and trunk, felt to be a hypersensitivity reaction.

- **Pediculosis pubis:** Most patients present with pruritus in the region of the pubic hairs, but other areas may be involved including the eyelashes and hairs in the axilla. Secondary bacterial infections are less common.

Diagnosis The diagnosis of pediculosis is often suspected when an individual presents with severe pruritus. On some occasions, the patient may have identified lice themselves or have had a recent contact history. The diagnosis is confirmed by finding lice (1-4 mm long, depending on species) and/or the "nits" (usually 1 mm or less, attached to hairs).

Diagnostic Tests/Procedures

Arthropod Identification *on page 268*

Treatment General principles of treating pediculosis include discarding or carefully laundering clothing, discarding infested combs or hats, and laundering bedsheets. In general, clothes and bedsheets can be effectively decontaminated by dry cleaning or by machine washing and drying in a hot cycle. Secondary bacterial infections of the skin are common and generally respond to antibiotics effective against *Staphylococcus aureus* (dicloxacillin, erythromycin, and others). Pruritus is typically quite severe and may be alleviated by hydroxyzine (Atarax®), diphenhydramine (Benadryl®), and/or topical steroid creams. Treatment guidelines are as follows:

1. Pediculosis corporis: Since the louse resides mainly in the creases of clothes and not on the host, the infection can often be eradicated by delousing contaminated items and maintaining careful hygiene.

2. Pediculosis capitis: Several agents are effective: 1% lindane (Kwell®) shampoo to the scalp, pyrethrin liquid (RID), or permethrin creme rinse (Nix™) These insecticides are probably equal in efficacy. Only lindane requires a prescription. Caution: Lindane has been associated with seizures and other nervous system toxicities. However, the risk of serious adverse effects during treatment for pediculosis is small due to its minimal systemic absorption. Nevertheless, lindane should be avoided in pregnancy and in lactating women.

3. Pediculosis pubis. The treatment recommendations are the same as for pediculosis capitis. In addition, sexual partners should be identified and treated in the same manner. Pediculosis involving the eyelashes should **not** be
treated with insecticides. Instead, occlusive ophthalmic ointment should
be applied to the eyelashes twice daily for at least 8 days in an attempt to
smother the parasites.

Patients should be seen in follow-up if symptoms persist 1 week after treatment. A second application may be necessary. Some clinicians routinely instruct patients to reapply the insecticide at the 1 week point.

Drug Therapy
Recommended
Lindane *on page 599*
Pyrethrins *on page 653*
Permethrin *on page 640*
Malathion *on page 602*

Listeria monocytogenes

Microbiology *Listeria monocytogenes* is a gram-positive bacillus which causes
sporadic cases of meningoencephalitis, neonatal infection, septicemia, and
several less common syndromes. It is a leading cause of meningitis in immunocompromised individuals, especially renal transplant patients.

The organism is an aerobic, gram-positive rod which does not produce spores.
At times it may assume a more coccoid appearance on Gram stain of clinical
samples (eg, cerebrospinal fluid) and may thus be mistaken for gram-positive
cocci such as *Streptococcus pneumoniae*. *Listeria* can also be confused morphologically with the more commonly seen *Corynebacterium* species, which
are also gram-positive bacilli (but are often contaminants). *Listeria* is primarily
an intracellular pathogen, and tends to reside within mononuclear phagocytes
of the host. This feature is thought to contribute to its pathogenicity, since the
organism can spread from cell to cell in a somewhat protected fashion.

When *Listeria monocytogenes* meningitis is suspected, the clinician should try
to submit at least 10 mL of cerebrospinal fluid for bacterial culture, since only
a few *Listeria* organisms may be present. The organism generally grows well
on most routine media used in the laboratory, and special requests for selective or enrichment cultures for *Listeria* are usually not necessary. It is important
that the clinician does not automatically dismiss a report of a "gram-positive
rod" isolated from multiple blood or a sterile body site as a contaminant, particularly in an immunocompromised host in whom *Listeria* infection is possible.

Epidemiology The epidemiology of listeriosis can be important in certain cases,
since clinical presentations may be nonspecific. The precise prevalence of
human infection is unclear, but the attack rate appears to be increasing (perhaps due to better reporting or laboratory recognition). Asymptomatic carriage
of *Listeria* in stools is relatively frequent; some studies suggest a fecal excretion rate of 1% or more in healthy humans. Humans may be exposed to *Listeria*
by one of several routes: consumption of contaminated food, direct exposure
to infected animals, or exposure to environmental reservoirs (soil, water, etc).

Cases of listeriosis tend to be sporadic and difficult to predict. Most infections
occur in the summer months and are more common in urban than rural settings, despite its reputation as a zoonotic infection. Often, the source of the
Listeria remains unknown. Increasing attention has been given to foodborne
transmission, particularly in the setting of a traceable outbreak. Mexican-style
cheese, coleslaw, undercooked chicken, hot dogs, dairy products, and other
foods have caused outbreaks. The ability of the organism to survive (and even
multiply) during refrigeration probably contributes to food-related transmission.

Infection with *Listeria* usually occurs in definable groups in the community. Cell
mediated immunity is critically important in defense against *Listeria*, whereas
neutropenia is not clearly a risk factor. Those at highest risk include patients
with solid organ transplants, malignancies (particularly lymphoma), and patients receiving corticosteroids. Pregnant females, neonates, and alcoholics
are additional groups at risk for infection. Interestingly, listeriosis does not appear to be a common pathogen in patients with AIDS, despite the deficiencies
in T-cell function. Although uncommon, serious infections with *Listeria* have
been described in otherwise healthy individuals.

Clinical Syndromes
• **Adult meningoencephalitis:** *Listeria* is the most common cause of com-

(Continued)
143

Listeria monocytogenes (Continued)

munity-acquired meningitis in immunosuppressed individuals. *Listeria* meningitis can be quite variable in its presentation and can range from a subacute course to a rapid and fulminant one. In some cases the diagnosis may be quite difficult when high fevers and nuchal rigidity are absent. There are no pathognomonic features of *Listeria* meningitis which allow diagnosis on clinical grounds alone. CSF chemical analysis is variable and frequently nondiagnostic. The degree of CSF pleocytosis can range from several cells to > 12,000 cells/mm^3. Differential cell counts vary from nearly 100% polymorphonuclear cells to 100% mononuclear cells. Often a modest elevation of CSF protein is seen, along with a minor decrease in CSF glucose. The differential diagnosis of a subacute meningitis in an immunosuppressed host must also include *Cryptococcus neoformans*. The finding of focal brain lesions by CT scan or MRI broadens the differential to include toxoplasmosis, *Nocardia asteroides*, bacterial brain abscess, fungal meningitis, and others. Meningoencephalitis has also been sporadically reported in otherwise healthy individuals and should be considered in the differential diagnosis of any community-acquired meningitis.

- **Meningoencephalitis of the neonate:** This is a "late-onset" neonatal disease, occurring several days to weeks postpartum. As with adult cases, isolated neonatal meningitis from *Listeria* can be variable in its presentation. Fever may be low grade or absent, and irritability and failure to thrive may be the only clues. CSF findings in the neonate are similar to those in the adult. It is important to review the Gram stain of CSF carefully to avoid confusing *Listeria* with Group B streptococci, a common cause of neonatal meningitis.

- **Cerebritis:** This form of nonmeningeal central nervous system infection is gaining increased recognition. Patients may complain of fever, cephalgia, and hemiparesis. This form of listeriosis may be mistaken for a stroke, vasculitis, brain tumor, or abscess. CT and MRI scans suggest focal inflammation without a discrete abscess or ring enhancement. Cerebrospinal fluid is usually normal and CSF cultures are negative for *Listeria*. The diagnosis is usually made when *Listeria* is isolated from blood cultures.

- **Listeriosis in pregnancy:** Unfortunately, this is often difficult to diagnose, since the woman may be asymptomatic or complain of only a mild fever and malaise. Other symptoms variably present include diarrhea and flank pain. The differential diagnosis is usually broad and listeriosis may be mistaken for pyelonephritis, lower urinary tract infection, and viral syndromes (eg, influenza). Blood cultures may be positive and should be performed. Complications include premature delivery, septic abortion, and *in utero* fetal infection.

- **Granulomatosis infantiseptica:** This unique, transplacentally acquired infection is severe and often lethal. It is an "early onset" neonatal infection apparent within hours of birth. Typically, the infants are seriously ill. There are widespread abscesses involving visceral organs such as the liver, spleen, lungs, intestinal tract, and brain. The lesions are usually abscesses with polymorphonuclear leukocytes, but granulomas have also been seen (referred to as "miliary granulomatosis"). Dark papular skin lesions may be present on the trunk and lower extremities, suggesting the diagnosis. Gram stain and culture of meconium, amniotic fluid, conjunctival exudates, CSF, throat, blood, or skin lesions frequently are positive for *L. monocytogenes*. Antibiotic therapy should be started immediately if this diagnosis is suspected, since death may occur if treatment is withheld until cultures are finalized.

- **Septicemia:** *Listeria* can be isolated from the blood in adults and neonates who present from the community with nonspecific fever and chills. Bacteremias are more likely in profoundly immunosuppressed hosts but have been seen in alcoholics, diabetics, pregnancy, and normal healthy individuals. The clinical presentation can be indistinguishable from gram-negative sepsis, with high fevers and hypotension (so-called "typhoidal listeremia"). On rare occasion, the diagnosis is suggested by the finding of a monocytosis on the peripheral blood smear, but blood cultures remain the highest yield.

- **Miscellaneous:** Endocarditis, ocular infections, lymphadenitis, osteomyelitis, brain abscess, peritonitis, and other focal infections have been rarely reported.

Diagnosis Except for granulomatosis infantiseptica, the clinical presentations of listeriosis are not unique and microbiological confirmation is necessary. Depending on the clinical site of infection, specimens of blood and body fluids should be sent, as described above. Agglutination studies for antibodies directed against *L. monocytogenes* have little value.

Diagnostic Tests/Procedures
Aerobic Culture, Cerebrospinal Fluid *on page 245*
Blood Culture, Aerobic and Anaerobic *on page 271*
Cerebrospinal Fluid Analysis *on page 288*
Gram Stain *on page 352*
Lumbar Puncture *on page 390*

Treatment No randomized comparison trials have been performed to determine the drug(s) of choice for listeriosis. *In vitro* data show the organism is susceptible to many antibiotics. The most clinical experience has been limited to penicillin and ampicillin, and they are probably equivalent. Occasionally, penicillin-resistant strains of *Listeria* have been reported, and thus results of susceptibility testing should be followed up on. There is some *in vitro* evidence to suggest the combination of penicillin (or ampicillin) with an aminoglycoside may be synergistic against *Listeria*, and this combination has been used in serious, life-threatening infections. Cephalosporins do not reliably cover this organism and should not be used for cases of *Listeria* meningitis. Consultation with an infectious disease specialist is appropriate in complicated cases or in the patient with a penicillin allergy.

Drug Therapy
Recommended
Ampicillin *on page 495*
  or
Ampicillin *on page 495*
  used in combination with
Gentamicin Sulfate *on page 575*
  or
Penicillin G, Parenteral *on page 633*
  or
Penicillin G, Parenteral *on page 633*
  used in combination with
Gentamicin Sulfate *on page 575*

Alternate
Co-trimoxazole *on page 545*

Selected Readings
Armstrong D, "*Listeria monocytogenes*," *Principles and Practice of Infectious Diseases*, 4th ed, Mandell GL, Bennett JE, and Dolin R, eds, New York, NY: Churchill Livingstone, 1995, 1880-5.

Gellin BG and Broome CV, "Listeriosis," *JAMA*, 1989, 261(9):1313-20.

Nieman RE and Lorber B, "Listeriosis in Adults: A Changing Pattern. Report of Eight Cases and Review of the Literature, 1968-1978," *Rev Infect Dis*, 1980, 2(2):207-27.

MAC *see Mycobacterium avium-intracellulare on page 152*

MAI *see Mycobacterium avium-intracellulare on page 152*

Maltophilia *see Xanthomonas maltophilia on page 231*

Measles Virus
Related Information
Immunization Guidelines *on page 710-717*
Vaccines *on page 706-709*

Synonyms Rubeola Virus

Microbiology Measles virus is a member of the Paramyxoviridae family (measles virus, mumps virus, parainfluenza virus, canine distemper virus, respiratory syncytial virus, and others). Measles virus is enveloped and contains single-stranded RNA. Measles virus has specific envelope proteins H and F which are responsible for adsorption/hemagglutination and cell penetration/fusion, respectively. Measles virus is extremely labile and is sensitive to light, drying, and naturally occurring enzymes and acids. Measles virus remains extremely infective for several hours as long as it remains moist and in aerosolized droplets. The fact that measles virus is easily spread by inhalation of such droplets and by direct contact with nasal secretions explains why measles virus causes one of the most contagious of all infectious diseases, measles. Measles virus exists in two forms, wild type and vaccine form. The wild type is extremely genetically stable; the same genotype and phenotype exists worldwide.

Epidemiology Measles (archaic term, rubeola) has been observed and recorded for over 2000 years and occurs today in every country. In developing
(Continued)

Measles Virus (Continued)

countries, measles affects almost all children younger than 5 years of age and causes 1-2 million deaths per year in children. In the United States, in 1990, there were ca. 27,000 reported cases of measles. More than 80% of the persons who represented these cases had previously received measles vaccine, and ca. 50% of these cases were represented by poor, inner-city pre-school children. Humans are the natural reservoir and, for all practical purposes, the only hosts of measles virus.

Clinical Syndromes Measles is an infection of the respiratory tract and central nervous system and can present in at least three syndromes.

- **Conventional measles:** Incubation period, 10-14 days; prodrome of "flu"-like symptoms, conjunctivitis, and other upper respiratory tract symptoms; Koplik spots; typically a 5-day rash which spreads from head to trunk to extremities to palms and soles. Most patients are not contagious after the rash reaches its peak.

- **Mild measles:** Usually observed in infants younger than 1 year of age; similar to conventional measles but is milder and usually is not characterized by all of the typical signs and symptoms of conventional measles.

- **Atypical measles:** More severe and lasts longer than conventional measles; rash usually begins peripherally and progresses toward the trunk; can be confused with chickenpox or Rocky Mountain spotted fever; antibody titers to measles virus often are extremely high.

Diagnosis Measles is usually diagnosed clinically. Measles virus can be isolated in cell culture, but this method is somewhat difficult and usually not practical. The specimens of choice are throat and nasopharyngeal washings. Serology is the diagnostic method of choice. As with most viral serology, diagnosis is made by demonstration of a fourfold rise in measles virus-specific antibody; however, the most widely used tests are immunofluorescence antibody and enzyme immunoassays for measles-specific IgM. A minimal protective IgG antibody level has not been determined. Some laboratories offer direct detection of measles virus-infected cells from nasopharyngeal washings and nasal swabs.

Diagnostic Tests/Procedures
Measles Antibody *on page 399*
Virus, Direct Detection by Fluorescent Antibody *on page 480*

Drug Therapy Comment
No antiviral agents active against measles, but for immune suppressed patients, intravenous immunoglobulins may be indicated.

Drug Therapy
Recommended
Immune Globulin *on page 588*

Selected Readings
Gershon AA, "Measles Virus (Rubeola)," *Principles and Practice of Infectious Diseases*, 4th ed, Mandell GL, Bennett JE, and Dolin R, eds, New York, NY: Churchill Livingstone, 1995, 1519-26.

"Measles – United States, First 26 Weeks, 1993," *MMWR Morb Mortal Wkly Rep*, 1993, 42(42):813-6.

Schlenker T, "Measles Resurgent," *Clin Microbiol Newslett*, 1991, 13:156-7.

Siegel CS, "Measles – A Review of the Virological and Serological Methods for Early Detection," *Clin Microbiol Newslett*, 1991, 13:177-9.

Microaerophilic Streptococci *see Streptococcus*-Related Gram-Positive Cocci *on page 212*

Microsporidia

Microbiology Microsporidia are single-cell obligate intracellular parasites which can form spores under extracellular (adverse) environmental conditions. Microsporidia spores are oval to spherical and are 1-20 μm long, depending on the species; however, the spores typically are only 1-5 μm long when found in humans and other mammals. In stained stool preparations, the spores appear as large, fat, gram-negative rods and often have a central and darkly stained band or dot. There are many genera of microsporidia; however, only five genera have been associated with human disease, *Enterocytozoon*, *Encephalitozoon*, *Nosema*, *Pleistophora*, and *Septata*.

Epidemiology Microsporidia are found in many animal species, particularly invertebrates. Microsporidia have been isolated from many human specimens, including stool (by far the most common clinical source), intestine (only the jejunum and duodenum), urine, CSF, liver, skin, sinus/nasal mucosa, cornea, conjunctiva, kidney, and lungs. Microsporidia in the intestines are usually found as complete organisms in the enterocytes and as spores in the stool. Microsporidia, particularly *Enterocytozoon* and *Septata*, probably are pathogens in AIDS patients and probably are responsible for 10% to 20% of the cases of chronic diarrhea in AIDS patients. Less than 20 of the approximately 400 reported cases of microsporidia-associated diarrhea were reported from non-AIDS cases; the remainder were AIDS cases. Most cases have been associated with male homosexuals with AIDS and extremely low CD4 cell counts.

Clinical Syndromes Microsporidia-associated diarrhea: The most common clinical presentation of microsporidia-associated diarrhea in AIDS patients is gradual onset (eventually chronic) of diarrhea (no blood or mucus), weight loss, nausea, abdominal cramps, and anorexia.

Diagnosis Diagnosis is made by clinical impression and a few laboratory tests. D-xylose and fat malabsorption frequently are present. Histological examination of jejunal and duodenal biopsies can be helpful if pathologists are notified of a suspected case, use appropriate stains, and are familiar with the characteristic morphology of the organism and histological alterations elicited by the organism. The staining characteristics of microsporidia in sections of tissue are variable and unpredictable, and microsporidia often are difficult to recognize in paraffin sections; they are more easily recognized in plastic sections. Microsporidia are easily and reproducibly stained and recognized outside of tissue, specifically in tissue imprint preparations and direct stool smears. Such preparations are best stained by a modified trichrome stain such as that described by Weber (see references).

Diagnostic Tests/Procedures
Microsporidia Diagnostic Procedures *on page 400*
Note: Contact laboratory for availability of tests and special instructions.

Treatment Microsporidia-induced diarrhea should be managed with supportive fluid and electrolyte replacement. Although a variety of antiprotazoals have been utilized in the treatment of this infection, success has been limited. Albendazole, an investigational drug, may have the most clinical success. Metronidazole may also be a useful therapy especially in non-HIV infected patients.

Drug Therapy Comment Not available on the market in the United States is the drug of choice, albendazole. Call SmithKline Beecham for compassionate use.

Drug Therapy
Recommended
Metronidazole *on page 610*

Selected Readings
Lecuit M, Oksenhendler E, and Sarfati C, "Use of Albendazole for Disseminated Microsporidian Infections in a Patient With AIDS," *Clin Infect Dis*, 1994, 19:332-3.
Shadduck JA and Greeley E, "Microsporidia and Human Infections," *Clin Microbiol Rev*, 1989, 2(2):158-65.
Sun T, "Microsporidiosis in the Acquired Immunodeficiency Syndrome," *Infect Dis Newslett*, 1993, 12:20-2.
Weber R and Bryan RT, "Microsporidial Infections in Immunodeficient and Immunocompetent Patients," *Clin Infect Dis*, 1994, 19:517-21.
Weber R, Bryan RT, Owen RL, et al, "Improved Light-Microscopical Detection of Microsporidia Spores in Stool and Duodenal Aspirates. The Enteric Opportunistic Infections Working Group," *N Engl J Med*, 1992, 326(3):161-6.
Weber R, Bryan RT, Schwartz DA, et al, "Human Microsporidial Infections," *Clin Microbiol Rev*, 1994, 7(4):426-61.

Moraxella catarrhalis

Synonyms *Branhamella catarrhalis*

Microbiology *Moraxella catarrhalis* (*Branhamella*) is an aerobic, gram-negative diplococcus which resembles *Neisseria* species in its Gram stain appearance. Although generally considered an organism of low pathogenicity, *M. catarrhalis* has gained increasing attention as a potential pathogen of the upper and lower respiratory tract, particularly in individuals with chronic bronchitis.

In the medical literature this organism has been variously named *Neisseria catarrhalis*, *Branhamella catarrhalis*, and most recently *Moraxella catarrhalis*. *M. catarrhalis* belongs to the family Neisseriaceae. *M. catarrhalis* is a kidney bean shaped coccus 0.6-1.0 μm in diameter, often appearing in pairs or tetrads. During active infection, the organisms can sometimes be seen within the cytoplasm of polymorphonuclear cells, where it is referred to as gram-negative intracellular diplococci. In the laboratory, the organism is readily grown on routine media such as blood agar and can often grow on ordinary media without blood.

(Continued)

Moraxella catarrhalis (Continued)

Epidemiology *Moraxella catarrhalis* is considered part of the normal flora of the human respiratory tract, particularly in the nasal cavity where it is considered the main natural reservoir for this organism. Thus its isolation in culture does not necessarily imply clinical disease. Less commonly, it has been isolated from the oropharynx of otherwise healthy children and adults, although the prevalence figures vary among different published studies. Higher carriage rates are seen in patients with chronic bronchitis, and there is an established increase in colonization during the winter months.

Clinical Syndromes

- **Exacerbations of chronic obstructive pulmonary disease:** *M. catarrhalis* has been recognized as a potential cause of purulent exacerbations of chronic bronchitis, although still less common than *Streptoccocus pneumoniae* and *Haemophilus influenzae*.
- **Respiratory tract infections in infants and children, particularly in asthmatics.**
- **Acute otitis media.** This organism is the third leading cause of acute otitis media in children, accounting for about 15% of cases, with the highest incidence in the winter months. *M. catarrhalis* can be recovered from specimens of middle ear fluid via tympanocentesis, if clinically indicated.
- **Sinusitis:** *M. catarrhalis* can be a cause of acute sinusitis in both children and adults. It is usually found with other organisms and can be recovered from properly performed sinus aspirates.
- **Acute urethritis:** This organism is occasionally a saprophyte of the genital tract and has been reported to be a rare cause of the urethral syndrome.
- **Other invasive diseases:** Cases of meningitis, endocarditis, septicemia, and peritonitis have been reported, usually in immunosuppressed patients.

Diagnosis The laboratory is easily able to separate it from related *Neisseria* species biochemically. Rapid tests used to speciate *Neisseria* do not react with *Moraxella*. *Moraxella* is frequently recovered from sputum cultures along with a variety of other organisms. Every attempt should be made to obtain a high quality sputum specimen in order to minimize contamination of samples with commensal mouth organisms, which may include *Moraxella*. The finding of many gram-negative diplococci within polymorphonuclear leukocytes on a Gram stain of expectorated sputum is suggestive of true infection, rather than colonization.

Serologic studies looking for a fourfold rise in antibody titer against *M. catarrhalis* play a limited role for most patients and remain primarily epidemiologic or investigational tools.

Diagnostic Tests/Procedures

Aerobic Culture, Sputum *on page 246*
Blood Culture, Aerobic and Anaerobic *on page 271*
Gram Stain *on page 352*

Treatment In past years, *Moraxella catarrhalis* was exquisitely sensitive to penicillin. However, in the early 1980s, an increasing number of community isolates were found to produce the enzyme beta-lactamase, which could be either plasmid or chromosomally mediated. It is now estimated that 75% to 85% of strains of *M. catarrhalis* produce beta-lactamase. Such strains generally remain susceptible to oral erythromycin and tetracycline, with only 1% to 2% *in vitro* resistance. Co-trimoxazole is active against most strains of *M. catarrhalis*, which is particularly helpful when empirically treating a patient with an exacerbation of chronic bronchitis. Ampicillin alone is ineffective in treating beta-lactamase producing *M. catarrhalis* and should not be used even if such an organism appears sensitive to ampicillin *in vitro*. The combination of ampicillin with a beta-lactamase inhibitor such as sulbactam or clavulanate (Augmentin®) is effective against most beta-lactamase positive strains. Finally, the cephalosporins in general appear more stable than penicillins in the presence of *M. catarrhalis* beta-lactamase; however, the results of *in vitro* susceptibility testing remain important in management.

Drug Therapy

Recommended

Co-trimoxazole *on page 545*

Alternate

Amoxicillin and Clavulanic Acid *on page 490*
Cephalosporins, 2nd Generation *on page 527*
Cephalosporins, 3rd Generation *on page 528*

Selected Readings

Catlin BW, "*Branhamella catarrhalis*: An Organism Gaining Respect as a Pathogen," *Clin Microbiol Rev*, 1990, 3(4):293-320.

Hager H, Verghese A, Alvarez S, et al, "*Branhamella catarrhalis* Respiratory Infections," *Rev Infect Dis*, 1987, 9(6):1140-9.

Verghese A, Berk SL, "*Branhamella catarrhalis*: A Microbiologic and Clinical Update," *Am J Med*, 1990, 88(Suppl 5A):1S-56S.

Verghese A, Berk SL, "*Moraxella (Branhamella) catarrhalis*," *Infect Dis Clin North Am*, 1991, 5(3):523-38.

MRSA *see Staphylococcus aureus*, Methicillin-Resistant
   on page 195

MRSE *see Staphylococcus epidermidis*, Methicillin-Resistant
   on page 200

MSSA *see Staphylococcus aureus*, Methicillin-Susceptible
   on page 198

MSSE *see Staphylococcus epidermidis*, Methicillin-Susceptible
   on page 201

Mucor Species

Microbiology Mucormycosis refers to opportunistic fungal infections caused by the mold order Mucorales, class Zygomycetes. Contrary to the name, *Mucor* species are rarely implicated in human disease. The most frequent fungi isolated are *Rhizopus*, *Rhizomucor* and *Absidia*. Mucorales are ubiquitous organisms found worldwide in soil, dust, spoiled fruit, and bread products. They initiate and facilitate decay of organic material.

KOH preparation of infected material reveals sparsely septate mycelia 6-50 μm wide, up to 200 μm long, and rounded sporangia. Growth in culture is rapid at temperatures 25°C to 55°C (optimum temperature 28°C to 30°C) and usually begins as a cottony white mold turning gray to yellow to brown in 3-5 days. Wet mounts reveal sporangiophores arising off clusters of rhizoids (*Mucor* species lack rhizoids). H & E stains typically reveal an abundance of irregular shaped, broad hyphae with right angle branching in the midst of polymorphonuclear infiltrate and round blood vessel walls with or without invasion into the vessel wall.

Epidemiology Mucormycosis is one of the most acute and fulminant fungal infections. It has a distinct predilection for invasion of blood vessel walls with resultant ischemia and necrosis of the adjacent tissue, commonly referred to as "black pus". There are no associations with age, sex, race, or geography. Most frequently seen in poorly controlled diabetics and hematologic malignancies. Infection is secondary to direct inoculation cutaneously or inhalation of spores into the respiratory tract and taken up by alveolar macrophages.

Clinical Syndromes

• **Rhinocerebral:** Generally seen in diabetics, predilection for acidosis. Present with facial pain, headache, and fever. May see black necrotic eschar on palate or nasal mucosa. May involve orbit leading to orbital cellulitis, proptosis, chemosis, cranial nerve involvement, and eventual CNS involvement. Two-thirds develop orbital cellulitis, and one-third develop internal carotid artery thrombosis or cavernous sinus thrombosis. Overall mortality is 80% to 90%.

• **Pulmonary:** Most commonly seen in hematologic malignancies particularly with neutropenia. Present with fever, dyspnea, and chest pain. Typically, no infiltrates seen on chest radiograph secondary to absence of leukocytes. Chest radiograph may reveal necrosis and hemorrhage.

• **Cutaneous:** Usually secondary to direct inoculation from trauma burns. May be secondary to dissemination.

• **Gastrointestinal:** Present with nonspecific signs and symptoms of intra-abdominal abscess. Associated with severe malnutrition, kwashiorkor. Usually diagnosed at autopsy.

• **CNS:** Direct extension from nose or paranasal sinuses. Direct inoculation via intravenous drug abuse. Disseminated disease associated with deferoxamine therapy.

• **Miscellaneous:** Rarely affects bones, kidneys, or mediastinum. Cardiac invasion associated with myocardial infarction, congestive heart failure, valvular incompetence, and pericarditis.

Diagnosis CT scans are useful in delineating extent of rhinocerebral disease. Definitive diagnosis depends on direct examination of infected material revealing characteristic histopathology as cultures of biopsied material frequently do not grow.

(Continued)

Mucor Species *(Continued)*

Diagnostic Tests/Procedures
Fungus Culture, Biopsy *on page 340*
Fungus Culture, Bronchial Aspirate *on page 342*
KOH Preparation *on page 379*

Treatment Treatment requires extensive surgical debridement, amphotericin B 1-1.5 mg/kg per day and, if possible, correction of the underlying illness. Azoles are still under investigation. Unproven therapies include rifampin, tetracycline, and hyperbaric oxygen.

Drug Therapy
Recommended
Amphotericin B *on page 493*

Selected Readings
Morrison VA and McGlave PB, "Mucormycosis in the BMT Population," *Bone Marrow Transplant*, 1993, 11(5):383-8.
Rinaldi MG, "Zygomycosis," *Infect Dis Clin North Am*, 1989, 3(1):19-41.
Sugar AM, "Mucormycosis," *Clin Infect Dis*, 1992, 14(Suppl 1):S126-9.

Mumps Virus

Related Information
Immunization Guidelines *on page 710-717*
Vaccines *on page 706-709*

Microbiology Mumps virus is the cause of an acute, nonsuppurative infection of the parotid glands (viral parotitis) which is primarily seen in children and adolescents. Mumps infection can also lead to serious systemic diseases including encephalitis and orchitis.

Mumps virus is an RNA virus of intermediate size (120-200 nm diameter), and belongs to the family Paramyxoviridae. It has two antigens (S and V) which can fix complement. Mumps virus can be grown in cell culture in a diagnostic virology laboratory.

Epidemiology Mumps occurs worldwide and throughout the year, with a peak in the spring (April and May). Humans are the only known reservoir. Epidemics are limited to groups where people live in close quarters, such as military barracks, institutions, or prisons. The incidence of mumps in the United States has declined by 95% since the institution of the mumps vaccine in the late 1960s. However, a significant rise in the number of mumps cases was reported in 1986 and 1987.

The virus has a reputation as being "less contagious" than other childhood illnesses such as measles or chicken pox, but this may not accurately reflect the many mumps infections which are asymptomatic or subclinical. Over 90% of adults are seropositive for mumps, indicating widespread exposure. The infection is rare in children less than 2 years of age, and peak incidence is between 5 and 9 years of age. Transmission is by direct person-to-person spread of infected salivary secretions. An individual may be infectious for up to 1 week prior to the onset of clinical parotitis, with a peak infectivity 1-2 days before salivary gland swelling. Thus, control of spread is difficult. Mumps has also been isolated from the urine, and this remains a less important but potential route of spread (viruria may persist for weeks). After exposure, the incubation period is 2-4 weeks.

Immunity is life-long. One episode of mumps (even if subclinical) confers protection in almost all cases, and reinfections with mumps have only rarely been reported.

Clinical Syndromes During the several-week incubation period, the virus replicates in the upper respiratory tract and the cervical lymph nodes. Following this period of asymptomatic localized infection, the virus disseminates hematogenously to other organs, including the parotid glands, testes, central nervous system, ovaries, inner ear, and others. Common clinical manifestations include:

- **Acute salivary adenitis:** The salivary glands are thought to be infected during the phase of viremia, although direct extension from the respiratory tract has also been postulated. Typically, there is an abrupt onset of fever and swelling of the salivary glands. The patient may complain of earache, difficulty chewing, and swallowing. Systemic symptoms (ie, malaise, headache, sore throat, chills) may sometimes precede the acute adenitis, or may follow the onset of parotid swelling. Of the salivary glands, the parotid gland is most commonly involved and is bilateral in two-thirds. The submaxillary and/or the sublingual glands may be infected, alone or in combination with the parotids. In most (but not all) cases, the gland is exquisitely tender to palpation for several days and has a "gelatinous" texture. The ostium of Stensen's duct appears erythematous but frank pus is not expressible, as in bacterial parotitis. Inflammation of the parotid leads to release of salivary amylase, which can be detected in the serum. Most cases resolve in about 1 week without specific intervention.

- **Mumps meningitis:** It is estimated that the mumps virus involves the central nervous system in 50% of cases, although only 10% or less of patients with mumps parotitis develop clinical meningitis. Over 50% of cases of mumps meningitis will have no evidence of parotitis. Patients typically present with an "aseptic meningitis" picture, with headache, photophobia, fever, and stiff neck. Cerebrospinal fluid (CSF) reveals a lymphocytic pleocytosis, sometimes >2000 cells/mm^3, but up to 25% of patients will have a predominance of polymorphonuclear leukocytes, leading to confusion with bacterial meningitis. CSF protein levels are modestly elevated. Hypoglycorrhachia, or a low CSF glucose, is common with mumps meningitis, again potentially causing confusion with bacterial meningitis. Mumps meningitis is self-resolving and benign, and comprises about 1% of aseptic meningitis cases.

- **Mumps encephalitis:** This is a more serious infection than mumps meningitis. Encephalitis may be either "early", occurring at the time of onset of parotitis, or "late", occurring 1-2 weeks later. The "early" cases may be due to direct viral invasion of brain tissue, whereas the "late" cases may be due to an autoimmune, postinfectious demyelinating syndrome (similar to Guillain-Barré). Patients typically present with marked personality changes, decreased sensorium, and high fevers; seizures and aphasia have also been reported. CSF findings are similar to mumps meningitis. Mortality is about 1% to 2%. In the absence of active parotitis, mumps encephalitis is almost impossible to distinguish from herpes simplex encephalitis on clinical grounds. Of all viral encephalitides, mumps is etiologic in only 1% or less due to the success of the mumps vaccine.

- **Epididymoorchitis:** Most cases occur within the first 1-2 weeks following the onset of parotid symptoms, but in some cases, orchitis may occur prior to or without salivary gland involvement. About 25% of mumps cases in postpubertal males are complicated by orchitis. Characteristically, this is part of a biphasic illness, with a dramatic return of systemic symptoms (fever to 40°C, chills, vomiting, headache) accompanied by acute pain and swelling in the testicle. In most cases, there is unilateral testicular pain. Epididymitis is present in the majority of cases. Symptoms usually begin to resolve within 1 week. Sterility is unusual unless there is bilateral testicular involvement complicated by testicular atrophy.

- **Miscellaneous:** Mumps has been reported to cause pancreatitis, oophoritis (5% of postpubertal women), migratory polyarthritis, electrocardiographic abnormalities, myocarditis (rare), and others.

Diagnosis The diagnosis of mumps infection is usually made on clinical grounds, particularly if the characteristic parotid gland inflammation is present. The WBC count is often normal but may show a leukopenia, lymphocytosis, or leukocytosis (with extrasalivary involvement). The serum amylase level stays elevated for several weeks in many cases, even without obvious parotid swelling, and may be useful when mumps encephalitis is suspected.

Laboratory confirmation of the mumps virus is usually not necessary. However, culture or serologic confirmation may be important when mumps encephalitis is a reasonable possibility, extrasalivary mumps is suspected but no parotitis is present, or parotitis is unusually fulminant or prolonged. Laboratory techniques include:

1. Viral culture in cell culture systems. Appropriate specimens include viral swabs of Stensen's duct, saliva, CSF, biopsy material, and sometimes urine. Blood cultures for mumps virus are low yield. The virus grows well in monkey kidney cells and demonstrates a distinctive cytopathic effect.
2. Serologic studies. Detection of mumps specific IgM antibody is presumptive evidence of recent infection. A fourfold rise in specific IgG titer is also diagnostic.

Diagnostic Tests/Procedures
Mumps Serology *on page 402*
Mumps Virus Culture *on page 402*
Virus, Direct Detection by Fluorescent Antibody *on page 480*

Treatment There are no antiviral agents proven effective in mumps infection. Mumps immune globulin has been used prophylactically in susceptible individ-
(Continued)

151

Mumps Virus *(Continued)*

uals during outbreaks but without benefit. A live-attenuated vaccine has been in use in the United States since 1967 and is part of routine pediatric immunizations. The first dose is given around 15 months of age along with the vaccines for measles and rubella, the MMR. The live attenuated vaccine should not be administered to patients with severe immunodeficiencies, including AIDS. An inactivated vaccine is available in such instances.

Drug Therapy Comment
No antiviral agents proven effective.

Selected Readings
Hersh BS, Fine PE, Kent WK, et al, "Mumps Outbreak in a Highly Vaccinated Population," *J Pediatr*, 1991, 119(2):187-93.
Ray CG, "Mumps," *Harrison's Principles of Internal Medicine*, 13th ed, Isselbacher KJ, Braunwald E, Wilson JD, et al, eds, New York, NY: McGraw-Hill, 1994, 830-2.

***Mycobacterium avium* complex** *see Mycobacterium avium-intracellulare on this page*

Mycobacterium avium-intracellulare

Synonyms MAC; MAI; *Mycobacterium avium* complex

Microbiology MAI is an acid-fast bacillus that grows best at 37°C after 10-21 day incubation on selective agar media.

See table in *Mycobacterium tuberculosis* entry for a listing of important and major species of *Mycobacterium* and the pathogenic potential of each species.

Epidemiology Prior to the AIDS epidemic, MAI was extremely rare. Infection is acquired by ubiquitous environmental exposure either ingestion or inhalation as opposed to reactivation as occurs with tuberculosis. It is estimated that 15% to 40% of patients with AIDS have MAI. Five percent of patients at the time of diagnosis of AIDS will have MAI and increases by 20% each year after AIDS diagnosis. MAI infection appears unrelated to age, sex, race, or risk category for HIV. The number of MAI infections continues to steadily increase which may be related to the overall increased survival of patients with AIDS. MAI is associated with CD4 counts below 100/mm^3.

Clinical Syndromes
- **Asymptomatic:** Normal hosts may have colonization in the respiratory or gastrointestinal tracts. Duration of asymptomatic to dissemination in HIV is unknown.
- **Localized:** Focal pneumonia, skin, endophthalmitis, and CNS infections are rare. Localized infection of the GI tract is more common with infection in the duodenum most common. Patients present with nausea, diarrhea, abdominal pain, and, less commonly, biliary obstruction secondary to lymphadenopathy.
- **Disseminated:** Patients present with fever, weight loss, night sweats, anemia, and elevated alkaline phosphatase. Factors associated with MAI include time since diagnosis of AIDS, presence of significant anemia (hemoglobin <8 g/dL), previous opportunistic infection and interruption of antiretroviral therapy. Average lifespan of patient with AIDS and untreated MAI is 4 months. Pathology of infected organs reveal organomegaly, organs which may be yellow secondary to color of organism, histiocytes filled with acid-fast bacilli, and poorly formed granulomas.

Diagnosis Positive blood, bone marrow, lymph node, liver, or stool culture

Diagnostic Tests/Procedures
Acid-Fast Stain *on page 239*
Blood Culture, Mycobacteria *on page 276*
Mycobacteria Culture, Biopsy or Body Fluid *on page 404*
Mycobacteria Culture, Sputum *on page 406*

Treatment Treatment is variable given the susceptibility testing of the organism. Resistance is common. Current recommendations include a two- or three-drug regimen being: 1. clarithromycin or azithromycin, 2. ethambutol, 3. clofazimine, ciprofloxacin, rifampin, amikacin, or rifabutin.

Current prophylaxis recommendation is either rifabutin or clarithromycin. Patients typically need to be treated for 2-8 weeks and then remain on suppressive therapy for life. Anemia usually does not resolve and frequently requires blood transfusion. Attempt to fully eradicate MAI have been unsuccessful.

Drug Therapy
Recommended
Treatment includes 2 to 5 of the following drugs used in combination:

Rifampin *on page 662*
Ethambutol Hydrochloride *on page 565*
Clofazimine *on page 542*
Amikacin Sulfate *on page 487*
Ciprofloxacin Hydrochloride *on page 537*
Clarithromycin *on page 539*
Imipenem/Cilastatin *on page 586*
Rifabutin *on page 661*

Selected Readings

Benson CA and Ellner JJ, "*Mycobacterium avium* Complex Infection and AIDS. Advances in Theory and Practice," *Clin Infect Dis*, 1993, 17(1):7-20.

Masur H, "Management of *Mycobacterium avium* Complex in Patients With HIV Infection," *Clin Infect Dis*, 1994, 18(Suppl 3):S217-43.

Masur H, "Recommendations on Prophylaxis and Therapy for Disseminated *Mycobacterium avium* Complex Disease in Patients Infected With Human Immunodeficiency Virus," *N Engl J Med*, 1993, 329(12):898-904.

Nightingale SD, Cameron DW, Gordin FM, et al, "Two Controlled Trials of Rifabutin Prophylaxis Against *Mycobacterium avium* Complex Infections in AIDS," *N Engl J Med*, 1993, 329(12):828-33.

"Recommendations on Prophylaxis and Therapy for Disseminated *Mycobacterium avium* Complex for Adults and Adolescents Infected With Human Immunodeficiency Virus. U.S. Public Health Service Task Force on Prophylaxis and Therapy for *Mycobacterium avium*, Complex," *MMWR Morb Mortal Wkly Rep*, 1993, 42(RR-9):14-20.

Mycobacterium kansasii

Microbiology *Mycobacterium kansasii* is an acid-fast bacillus that is a "nontuberculous" *Mycobacterium*. It is a photochromogen and appears as a long, thick bacillus on clinical specimens. The organism is not well visualized using the Gram stain and an acid-fast stain is necessary. Similarly, the organism does not grow well on routine bacteriologic media.

See table in *Mycobacterium tuberculosis* entry for a listing of important and major species of *Mycobacterium* and the pathogenic potential of each species.

Epidemiology *M. kansasii* has been reported to cause disease worldwide. The highest incidence of disease in the United States has been reported in the southwest and midwest regions. Infection in children is unusual, with most cases reported in the fifth decade of life. Occupational groups at increased risk for *M. kansasii* infection include miners, welders, and painters, among others. There is also an increased incidence of chronic obstructive pulmonary disease in individuals infected with *M. kansasii*. Healthy individuals can be infected by this organism.

Clinical Syndromes

- **Pulmonary infection:** Infection by *M. kansasii* frequently causes a pneumonitis similar to that caused by *Mycobacterium tuberculosis*. Patients present with subacute onset of cough, low grade fevers, and malaise. Routine blood studies are not helpful. A variety of radiographic abnormalities have been reported including cavitary lung disease, pleural effusions, and a miliary pattern. In many cases it is difficult to distinguish the x-ray from tuberculosis. Some individuals are chronically colonized with this organism, making the clinical interpretation of a positive respiratory culture difficult.

- **Extrapulmonary infection:** *M. kansasii* has been reported to cause cervical lymph node infection, skin lesions (from local inoculation), osteomyelitis, soft tissue infection, renal pelvis obstruction, and dissemination.

Diagnosis Infection with *M. kansasii* mimics tuberculosis both clinically and radiographically. Culture confirmation is essential. Most commonly the diagnosis is established by sending respiratory samples (sputum, bronchoscopy specimens) for acid-fast bacilli (AFB) stain and culture. In cases of extrapulmonary disease, the appropriate body fluid or tissue (urine, lymph node biopsy, etc) should be specified for AFB stain and culture.

Diagnostic Tests/Procedures

Acid-Fast Stain *on page 239*
Mycobacteria Culture, Biopsy or Body Fluid *on page 404*

Treatment In general, *M. kansasii* responds well to antimicrobial therapy. The role on isoniazid has been controversial since this agent has only minimal efficacy against *M. kansasii in vitro*. Current recommendations suggest the combination of isoniazid, rifampin, and ethambutol for initial therapy.

Drug Therapy
Recommended
Isoniazid *on page 592*
Rifampin *on page 662*
Ethambutol Hydrochloride *on page 565*
all 3 used in combination

Selected Readings
Bamberger DM, Driks MR, Gupta MR, et al, "*Mycobacterium kansasii* Among Patients Infected With Human Immunodeficiency Virus in Kansas City," *Clin Infect Dis*, 1994, 18(3):395-400.

Mycobacterium Species, Not MTB or MAI

Microbiology Mycobacteria other than *M. tuberculosis* (MTB) and *M. avium-intracellulare* (MAI) (hereafter called "other" mycobacteria) are acid-fast bacilli which have cell walls with high lipid content and are morphologically similar to MTB and MAI. Other mycobacteria are different from MTB and MAI in biochemical reactions, pigmentation, growth rates, natural reservoirs, pathogenesis, manifestations of disease, and susceptibilities to antimicrobial agents. Like MTB, other mycobacteria tend to cause chronic diseases and lesions. There are many species of other mycobacteria, the most commonly isolated are the following: *M. kansasii, M. marinum, M. gordonae, M. ulcerans, M. fortuitum, M. chelonae* subsp *chelonae, M. chelonae* subsp *abscessus*, and *M. scrofulaceum. M. genavense* and *M. haemophilum* are recently recognized other mycobacteria with which most physicians are not familiar. These other mycobacteria are pathogens to humans (usually immunocompromised hosts), grow in blood culture broth but require special growth media for subculture, and can require 4-9 weeks to grow on solid culture media.

See table in *Mycobacterium tuberculosis* entry for a listing of important and major species of *Mycobacterium* and the pathogenic potential of each species.

Epidemiology Other mycobacteria are ubiquitous in nature. Natural reservoirs include soil, cattle and other domestic livestock, fish, water, milk and other foods, wild animals, and nonhuman primates. The CDC has reported that other mycobacteria accounted for 35% of non-MTB mycobacteria clinical isolates. Humans become infected with other mycobacteria by inhalation of the mycobacteria through the mouth and nose and by direct inoculation into breaks in the skin. Other mycobacteria generally are not transmitted person to person.

Clinical Syndromes Other mycobacteria can cause numerous clinical syndromes, the most common of which are presented in the following table.

Mycobacterium Infection	Relatively Common Cause
Chronic pulmonary	*M. kansasii, M. fortuitum*
Cervical lymphadenitis	*M. kansasii, M. scrofulaceum*
Soft tissue	*M. marinum, M. abscessus*
Disseminated	*M. kansasii*
Surgical wound	*M. fortuitum, M. chelonae* subsp
Skeletal, joint	*M. kansasii, M. fortuitum, M. ulcerans*
Skin, ulcer, abscess	*M. marinum, M. fortuitum, M. abscessus, M. ulcerans, M. chelonae* subsp

Mycobacterium fortuitum and *M. chelonei* are two important Runyon group IV "rapid growers", so-named because of their ability to grow in several days when subcultured (initial isolation of the organism may require 1 or more weeks). Both healthy and immunocompromised persons may develop infection with these agents. Skin and soft tissue infections are relatively common manifestations of these organisms and are usually associated with trauma or the presence of a foreign body; this includes infection of postoperative wounds (eg, sternal wounds after cardiac surgery), infections of orthopedic devices such as arthroplasties, breast implant infections, post-traumatic wound infections, and others. Pulmonary infection from inhalation may occur with microabscess formation in the lungs (granuloma formation is less common). Other manifestations include endocarditis, osteomyelitis, and lymphadenitis, but visceral dissemination outside of the lungs is rare. Although disseminated disease has been reported in immunocompromised individuals, a recent review suggests this is an unusual occurrence.

Mycobacterium marinum is the cause of "fishtank granuloma." Infections are characterized by multiple ulcerative skin lesions on an extremity that spread proximally along the lymphatics. The organism grows well in fresh and salt water and is associated with fishtanks, pools, and aquariums. Human disease occurs usually through direct inoculation through a break in the skin. Patients with this clinical syndrome should be asked about exposure to aquarium water or other aquatic activities. Other mycobacteria besides *M. marinum* can cause a similar syndrome, as can infection with *Sporothrix schenckii.*

Mycobacterium scrofulaceum is an important cause of cervical lymphadenitis in children. The disease remains localized, but cure often requires both antimicrobial therapy and surgery.

Mycobacterium ulcerans is pathogenic mainly in tropical countries such as Africa. It characteristically causes a necrotic ulcer on the extremities.

Diagnosis The aforementioned diseases are diagnosed by culture of tissues (**not** swab specimens). Most other mycobacteria will grow in culture in 2-4 weeks. However, growth rates depend on the species and range from 3-60 days. *M. abscessus* soft tissue infections of an extremity can resemble sporotrichosis.

Diagnostic Tests/Procedures
Acid-Fast Stain *on page 239*
Mycobacteria Culture, Biopsy or Body Fluid *on page 404*

Treatment

M. fortuitum: Typically resistant to all common antitubercular agents. Amikacin and cefoxitin can be administered for 2-6 weeks followed by oral therapy with co-trimoxazole or doxycycline for 2-6 months.

M. scrofulaceum: Treatment of choice is usually surgical excision. If necessary, drug therapy regimen should include isoniazid, rifampin, and streptomycin. This organism is also sensitive *in vitro* to the macrolides and cycloserine.

M. marinum: A 6-week (6-month, if deep infection) course of co-trimoxazole or minocycline or rifampin in combination with ethambutol can be used. Surgical excision may also be required.

M. chelonae: Sensitive to amikacin and the macrolides. A 6-month course of clarithromycin may be the regimen of choice.

M. ulcerans: A useful regimen includes a 6-week course of either rifampin in combination with amikacin or ethambutol in combination with co-trimoxazole.

Treatment regimens remain controversial for some of these mycobacterial agents due to a lack of formal clinical trials. Combination therapy is of use with severe infections, but even less data is available concerning the optimal agents to be used. **Antibiotic susceptibility testing is strongly recommended since the drug-susceptibility patterns are not reliably predictable.** Consultation with an Infectious Disease specialist should also be considered.

Selected Readings
Horowitz EA and Sanders WE Jr, "Other *Mycobacterium* Species," *Principles and Practice of Infectious Diseases*, 4th ed, Mandell GL, Bennett JE, and Dolin R, eds, New York, NY: Churchill Livingstone, 1995, 2264-73.

Wayne LG and Sramek HA, "Agents of Newly Recognized or Infrequently Encountered Mycobacterial Diseases," *Clin Microbiol Rev*, 1992, 5(1):1-25.

Woods GL and Washington JA 2d, "Mycobacteria Other Than *Mycobacterium tuberculosis*: Review of Microbiologic and Clinical Aspects," *Rev Infect Dis*, 1987, 9(2):275-94.

Mycobacterium tuberculosis
Related Information
HIV Clinical Practice Guidelines *on page 765-774*

Synonyms Tubercle Bacillus

Microbiology *Mycobacterium tuberculosis* (MTB) is a fastidious, slowly-growing, aerobic bacterium with a complex cell wall composed of peptidoglycans and many complex, long-chain lipids. The free lipids on the outer layer make *M. tuberculosis* relatively hydrophobic and resistant to many stains used in the laboratory including the Gram stain and Giemsa stain. It is an acid-fast bacillus, meaning once the organism is stained, it cannot be decolorized by acid solutions.

(Continued)

ORGANISMS
Mycobacterium tuberculosis (Continued)

Mycobacteria can be isolated on solid agar media or in broth cultures (which can be read by automated devices). Growth in broth is usually much more rapid than on agar.

See table for listing of important and major species of *Mycobacterium* and the pathogenic potential of each species.

Clinically Relevant Major Species of *Mycobacterium*

Group	Strict Human Pathogens	Occasional/Potential Human Pathogens	Usually Environmental/ Rarely Human Pathogens
M. tuberculosis complex	M. tuberculosis M. leprae M. africanum M. ulcerans	M. bovis	
Photochromogens		M. kansasii M. marinum M. simiae M. asiaticum	
Scotochromogens		M. scrofulaceum M. szulgai M. xenopi	M. gordonae M. flavescens
Nonchromogens	M. genavense	M. avium M. intracellulare M. hemophilum M. malmoense	
Rapid Growers		M. fortuitum M. chelonei	M. smegmatis

Epidemiology Tuberculosis remains one of the most common and deadly diseases throughout the world. It is estimated that one-third of the world's population has been infected with *M. tuberculosis*. There are approximately 30 million active cases of tuberculosis at any time.

In the past 10 years there has been a resurgence of tuberculosis in the United States. In prior years, the number of new cases of tuberculosis had been declining at a rate of about 5% per year, but since the mid 1980s, the case rate began to rise at a rate of about 3% per year; this disturbing reversal has been attributed in large part to the AIDS epidemic. In the United States, over 10 million individuals in the U.S. have been infected with MTB at some point in their lives based on the results of tuberculin skin testing. The majority of active cases of tuberculosis come from this large pool of individuals who have been exposed to MTB in the past and later present with reactivation of latent infection. A smaller number of active cases are attributable to recent exposure of a healthy individual to a person with active tuberculosis.

In the United States, there are many defined groups at high risk for MTB infection:
- individuals with HIV infection
- close contacts (ie, family members and others) of infectious TB cases
- persons with underlying medical conditions which increase the risk of TB (see below)
- persons from foreign countries with a high prevalence of TB
- indigent populations
- alcoholics and persons who use intravenous drugs
- persons residing in nursing homes, prisons, and other long-term care facilities
- health care workers

Certain medical conditions predispose a person to the development of active tuberculosis once a person has been infected with the organism:
- HIV infection
- silicosis
- chest x-ray which shows fibrotic lesions, consistent with prior TB
- diabetes
- steroids or other immunosuppressive medications
- lymphomas and other hematologic diseases

- end-stage renal disease, especially those on chronic dialysis
- intestinal bypass
- postgastrectomy
- chronic malabsorption syndromes
- head and neck malignancies
- weight loss of 10% below ideal body weight, from any cause

MTB is transmitted via the respiratory route when an infected individual comes in close contact with a susceptible person. The organism is carried in droplets of respiratory secretions ("airborne droplets") during coughing, sneezing, and speaking; the organism can remain airborne and infectious for a period of time. Person-to-person transmission occurs when a susceptible individual inhales the infectious droplet nuclei. Close household contacts of infected individuals puts others at risk for acquiring infection, although typically several months of exposure may be needed. The degree of contagiousness of a given patient depends on a variety of factors including the number of organisms in the sputum, presence or absence of cavitary lung disease, amount of coughing, length of time on antituberculous therapy, and others.

Clinical Syndromes

- **Primary tuberculosis:** Primary infection, or first exposure to *M. tuberculosis*, often is asymptomatic. Typically, there is a pulmonary infiltrate in the mid or lower lung fields with or without hilar adenopathy. The infiltrates are nonspecific in appearance and are not cavitary. In most cases, the pneumonitis clears without specific therapy and latent infection is established. In some cases, the primary infection progresses and mimics reactivation disease.
- **Latent infection:** Many individuals remain asymptomatic following the primary infection with *M. tuberculosis*. The organism remains latent within macrophages indefinitely. The tuberculin skin test is extremely important in identifying these individuals (see Tuberculin Skin Testing, Intracutaneous). Approximately 1 in 10 persons with infection from *M. tuberculosis* will develop clinical disease at some time in their life unless given preventative therapy.
- **Reactivation tuberculosis:** Patients with reactivation tuberculosis present with weight loss, fever, constitutional symptoms, and a generalized wasting syndrome. Drenching night sweats are common. Often, these individuals are diagnostic dilemmas since pulmonary symptoms may be very mild or absent.
- **Pulmonary tuberculosis:** The majority of cases of active pulmonary tuberculosis are due to reactivation of the latent organism. Reactivation is likely to occur in the upper lobes and the superior segments of the lower lobes due to the oxygen-rich environment. However, disease can involve any area of the lung, especially in diabetics, elderly persons, and persons with AIDS. The absence of apical infiltrates should not be used to exclude tuberculosis; and for practical purposes, TB should be included in the differential diagnosis of any undiagnosed pneumonia. The extent of disease is also variable, ranging from subtle infiltrates in chest x-ray with minimal cough to the classic cavitary tuberculosis with hemoptysis. If untreated, the pulmonary lesions develop areas of caseation or central necrosis with partial liquefaction.
- **Extrapulmonary tuberculosis:** See references. Tuberculous disease outside the lung parenchyma can be even more difficult to diagnose. Extrapulmonary TB can become clinically apparent during the phase of primary infection, particularly in children. More commonly, extrapulmonary TB represents reactivation of latent infection. It is important to note that a pulmonary lesion of any type will be absent in 50% or more cases of extrapulmonary TB; it is even more uncommon to have a chest x-ray showing active pulmonary infiltrates or cavities. Extrapulmonary TB includes:
  - pleural disease with effusion; the most common form of extrapulmonary TB
  - tuberculous meningitis; often a difficult diagnosis to confirm. Classically, patients present with a chronic meningitis, but a more fulminant variety resembling pyogenic meningitis is well recognized. Because there is often a basilar meningitis, patients frequently develop cranial nerve signs; tuberculous meningitis should be strongly considered in any patient with signs or symptoms of meningitis with cranial nerve deficits. The spinal fluid typically has an elevated protein, low glucose, and a lymphocytic pleocytosis (see Lumbar Puncture), but this pattern can be seen in a number of other disease entities. Often repeated lumbar

(Continued)

Mycobacterium tuberculosis (Continued)

puncture with high volumes of spinal fluid submitted for mycobacterial culture are required to confirm the diagnosis. However, if the clinical suspicion for tuberculous meningitis is high (ie, positive tuberculin skin test, lymphocytic pleocytosis, etc), antituberculous therapy should be initiated.

- pericarditis
- peritonitis
- tuberculous adenitis or "scrofula" (chronic tuberculous infection of the cervical lymph nodes)
- osteomyelitis including tuberculosis of the spine (Pott's disease)
- genitourinary tuberculosis
- ocular infections including chorioretinitis
- gastrointestinal tuberculosis
- cutaneous tuberculosis (lupus vulgaris)
- miliary tuberculosis; *M. tuberculosis* can disseminate into the lympho-hematogenous system either during primary tuberculous infection or during reactivation (more common). This can be a difficult diagnosis to establish, and the chest x-ray can be normal early on.

Diagnosis A high index of suspicion must be maintained for tuberculosis. Laboratory confirmation of suspected cases is essential since the manifestations of MTB are protean. The tuberculin skin test is an important first step in identifying infected patients. Laboratory techniques for identifying *M. tuberculosis* include:

- acid-fast smears and cultures of respiratory secretions
- acid-fast smears and cultures of other potentially infected body fluids or tissues (cerebrospinal fluid, gastric fluid, urine, bone marrow biopsies, joint fluids, and many others)
- rapid methods – amplification of nucleic acid of MTB by the polymerase chain reaction (PCR) and subsequent detection by nucleic acid probes

Diagnostic Tests/Procedures

Acid-Fast Stain *on page 239*

Lumbar Puncture *on page 390*

Mycobacteria Culture, Biopsy or Body Fluid *on page 404*

Mycobacteria Culture, Sputum *on page 406*

Tuberculin Skin Testing, Intracutaneous *on page 463*

Treatment The treatment of tuberculosis is based on the following principles.

- *M. tuberculosis* becomes resistant to drugs through random, spontaneous genetic mutations. For isoniazid, the proportion of naturally occurring resistant bacteria has been established as 1 in 10^6, and for rifampin, the ratio is 1 bacterium in 10^8.
- A regimen containing multiple drugs to which the organisms are susceptible should be used; susceptibility testing should be done on all isolates.
- Both isoniazid-resistant MTB and multidrug-resistant MTB are becoming increasing problems (see references).
- When patient compliance is poor, directly observed therapy given 3 times per week in an outpatient setting should be strongly considered.
- Failures of therapy are often due to noncompliance with the regimen. The emergence of multidrug therapy is partly due to noncompliance as well.
- Physicians must take into account the immune status of the patient.

The Centers for Disease Control has recommended the initial treatment of TB should include four drugs. During the first 2 months, the drug regimen should include isoniazid, rifampin, pyrazinamide, and ethambutol or streptomycin. When drug susceptibility results are available, this regimen should be altered appropriately. In some cases, the four-drug regimen is not necessary but should be based on analysis of the local rate of both isoniazid resistance and multidrug resistance. If the rate of isoniazid resistance in the community is less than 4%, a two- or three-drug regimen could be used at physician discretion.

Drug Therapy
Recommended

Isoniazid *on page 592*

Rifampin *on page 662*

Pyrazinamide *on page 652*

Ethambutol Hydrochloride *on page 565*

Streptomycin Sulfate *on page 669*

Note: See Treatment for appropriate regimen.

Alternate

If intolerant of a first-line antitubercular agent or if multidrug resistant and TB is present, one or more of the alternative antitubercular agents should be substituted:

Antituberculars *on page 499*

Selected Readings

Barnes PF and Barrows SA, "Tuberculosis in the 1990s," *Ann Intern Med*, 1993, 119(5):400-10.

Berenguer J, Moreno S, Laguna F, et al, "Tuberculosis Meningitis in Patients Infected With the Human Immunodeficiency Virus," *N Engl J Med*, 1992, 326(10):668-72.

Centers for Disease Control/American Thoracic Society, *Core Curriculum on Tuberculosis*, 2nd ed, Atlanta, GA: U.S. Department of Health and Human Services, Public Health Service, 1991.

Frieden TR, Sterling T, Pablos-Mendez A, et al, "The Emergence of Drug Resistant Tuberculosis in New York City," *N Engl J Med*, 1993, 328(8):521-6.

Goble M, Iseman MD, Madsen LA, et al, "Treatment of 171 Patients With Pulmonary Tuberculosis Resistant to Isoniazid and Rifampin," *N Engl J Med*, 1993, 328(8):527-32.

"Initial Therapy for Tuberculosis in the Era of Multidrug Resistance," *MMWR Morb Mortal Wkly Rep*, 1993, 42(RR-7):1-8.

Snider DE Jr and Roper WL, "A New Tuberculosis," *N Engl J Med*, 1992, 326(10):703-5.

"Treatment of Tuberculosis and Tuberculosis Infection in Adults and Children. American Thoracic Society and the Centers for Disease Control and Prevention," *Am J Respir Crit Care Med*, 1994, 149(5):1359-74.

Mycoplasma pneumoniae

Synonyms Eaton's Agent

Microbiology *Mycoplasma pneumoniae*, also called Eaton's agent, is the smallest and simplest prokaryote capable of self-replication. Originally, this free-living, strictly aerobic organism was thought to be a virus but later determined to be a bacterium. The diameter of *M. pneumoniae* is 0.2-0.8 μm, and the organism is highly pleomorphic. The organism lacks a cell wall and has only a trilaminar membrane (similar to the structure of the trilaminar membrane which surrounds all bacterial and mammalian cells) enclosing the cell cytoplasm. Although *M. pneumoniae* is classified as a gram-negative bacterium, it retains the Gram stain poorly and, thus, cannot be reliably seen on routine Gram stain of clinical specimens such as sputum.

Growth of *M. pneumoniae* in culture requires special laboratory techniques, and a special request for *Mycoplasma* culture must be made. The organism does not grow on routine culture media used for isolating common bacterial respiratory pathogens. *Mycoplasma pneumoniae* requires an exogenous supply of cholesterol and other sterols for membrane synthesis; these nutrients can be supplied by animal sera added to the culture medium, and an exogenous supply of nucleic acids, for synthesis of purines and pyrimidines; this can be supplied by yeast extracts. An artificial, cell-free, selective culture medium is used in many laboratories. This diphasic media is composed of broth (liquid medium) overlying agar. A pH indicator in the agar is used to detect acid produced by *Mycoplasma* as it ferments glucose; a visible color change in the agar is presumptive evidence of *M. pneumoniae*. The colonies of *M. pneumoniae* in culture are 50-100 μm in diameter and have a unique "fried egg" colonial morphology.

Epidemiology *Mycoplasma pneumoniae* infections occur worldwide, with a tendency towards temperate climates. Epidemics of mycoplasmal infections seem to occur every 4-6 years, although outbreaks of epidemic proportions can occur in small communities at any time. Infections with *M. pneumoniae* do not follow a seasonal pattern, unlike many other respiratory pathogens which cause bronchitis and/or pneumonia in the winter and spring months (*Streptococcus pneumoniae*, respiratory syncytial virus, influenza A and B, and others). Thus, during summer months, the proportion of respiratory infections due to *Mycoplasma pneumoniae* increases (up to 50% of pneumonia cases), although the actual number of cases stays constant month to month.

One important characteristic of *Mycoplasma* infection is its tendency to spread within a family in a step-wise fashion. Spread within the family is slow (often over weeks), but many, if not all, members become infected. Often the point source for infection in a family can be identified. Clustered cases also occur in military barracks, institutionalized setting, day care centers, and college dormitories but tend to be slower and less complete than spread within families.

The highest rates of infection are in the young; school-aged children and young adults are statistically at highest risk. Although mycoplasmal infections

(Continued)

Mycoplasma pneumoniae (Continued)

are less common in children younger than 5 years of age, some studies have shown this organism to be a frequent cause of mild, but symptomatic, respiratory infections in this age group. Similarly, the incidence of mycoplasmal infection decreases with advancing age but still remains a sporadic cause of pneumonia in the older adult, which may be overlooked. Transmission of *M. pneumoniae* is via infected respiratory secretions such as nasal discharge. Close contact appears to be necessary for the infection to be spread. The incubation period between exposure to the infection and the first clinical symptoms is about 2-3 weeks.

Clinical Syndromes *Mycoplasma pneumoniae* is pathogenic for the lower respiratory tract and is able to adhere to respiratory epithelium by means of a special protein called P1. This attachment factor is contained in surface projections of the organism which bind to a receptor protein on the surface of the respiratory epithelial cells. Cellular injury takes place probably by several mechanisms including the production of superoxides. In severe cases, there is likely an immunologic component of cellular destruction as well. The organism remains extracellular during infection.

- **Community-acquired pneumonia:** Also known as "walking pneumonia" or "primary atypical pneumonia", this form of *Mycoplasma* infection is seen mainly between 5 and 20 years of age. *Mycoplasma pneumoniae* is the most common cause of pneumonia in this age group. The disease tends to be mild to moderate in severity but is characteristically very slow to resolve. Hospitalization is usually not necessary, and patients remain ambulatory (hence the term "walking pneumonia").

Patients present with prominent constitutional symptoms: persistent headache, malaise, low grade fevers, and muscle aches. Sore throat and ear pain are also present in some cases. The onset of symptoms is gradual and subacute. Respiratory symptoms usually appear after several days of malaise. Patients develop a persistent, nonproductive cough. Purulent sputum, rigors, chest pain, and gross hemoptysis are not prominent features of this infection (although each has been rarely reported). Examination of the lungs may show wheezing, localized rales and/or rhonchi. In some cases, the lungs may be completely clear. Physical findings suggestive of lung consolidation (such as egophony, bronchial breathing, and dullness to percussion) are uncommon and suggestive of other bacterial pathogens. Examination of the head and neck often shows a mild injection of the tympanic membranes, mild pharyngeal erythema, and cervical adenopathy. More severe ear inflammation may be seen in about 15% of cases, with bullous myringitis being classically associated with mycoplasmal pneumonia. However, hemorrhagic bullous myringitis is uncommon, and its absence should not preclude the diagnosis. A nonspecific maculopapular rash is seen in some patients. Chest x-rays typically reveal patchy areas of bronchopneumonia with peribronchial cuffing. Most often the lower lung fields on one side are involved, but multilobar disease can occur. Radiographic findings of lobar consolidation are less common and large pleural effusions are distinctly unusual, both findings suggestive of respiratory pathogens such as *Streptococcus pneumoniae*. The course of atypical pneumonia tends to be protracted, with or without antibiotic treatment. Most patients recover completely, although life-threatening pneumonia with the adult respiratory distress syndrome (ARDS) has been reported.

Complications of *M. pneumoniae* respiratory infection are statistically uncommon. However, unusual and potentially lethal complications have been well-recognized, and the incidence may exceed 10% in hospitalized patients. Respiratory complications include ARDS, pleural effusions, bronchiolitis obliterans, cavitary lung lesions, and bronchiectasis. Nonrespiratory complications include: 1. Mycoplasmal encephalitis, which can be seen when respiratory complaints are minor. Patients present with variable degrees of fever, confusion, and/or personality changes. Mycoplasmal encephalitis is indistinguishable from other forms of infectious encephalitis such as herpes simplex virus encephalitis. This entity should be considered in the differential diagnosis of any patient who presents with encephalitis and a pulmonary infiltrate. Other neurologic complications: transverse myelitis, stroke, postinfectious leukoencephalitis, optic neuritis, polymyositis syndrome, and others. 2. Autoimmune hemolytic anemia, which at times can be quite severe. Such patients have high titers of cold-reacting autoantibodies (cold agglutinins) 3. Erythema multiforme, erythema nodosum. 4. myocarditis, and pericarditis.

- **Tracheobronchitis:** The majority of *M. pneumoniae* infections do not lead to pneumonia. Tracheobronchitis accounts for 70% to 80% of all infections with *M. pneumoniae*, with only about one-third progressing to pneumonia. The clinical presentation of tracheobronchitis is similar to pneumonia, with prominent constitutional symptoms followed by a dry, persistent cough. The chest x-ray in tracheobronchitis remains clear because inflammation is limited primarily to the bronchi. Overall, the disease course is milder than with pneumonia, although the disease course may be equally protracted.

- **Pharyngitis:** *M. pneumoniae* can cause a primary pharyngitis, or mycoplasmal pharyngitis may develop in association with tracheobronchitis or pneumonia. Again, school-aged children and young adults are most commonly involved. Constitutional symptoms are prominent, with fever, headache, and malaise. Patients complain of a severe sore throat and often have difficulty swallowing. On examination, there is tonsillar enlargement, inflammatory exudate, and pharyngeal edema and erythema. Cervical lymphadenopathy is common. The clinical presentation may be confused with streptococcal pharyngitis or primary infectious mononucleosis (from Epstein-Barr virus). Mycoplasmal pharyngitis is probably underdiagnosed.

Diagnosis Diagnosis is made on a clinical basis as described above. A test for cold hemagglutinins can be performed, especially in seriously ill, hospitalized patients. Diagnosis is definitive when the organism is cultured from sputum or throat swab. A rise in antibody titer from acute to convalescent sera is also diagnostic and may occur in up to 80% of patients with pneumonia.

Diagnostic Tests/Procedures
Cold Agglutinin Titer *on page 302*
Mycoplasma Serology *on page 410*
Mycoplasma/Ureaplasma Culture *on page 410*

Duration of Therapy 2-3 weeks

Treatment The treatment of choice for *M. pneumoniae* infections is erythromycin, although, tetracycline has been shown to be equally effective in clinical trials. Most patients can be treated as outpatients. Patients with severe disease should also receive appropriate supportive care.

Pediatric Drug Therapy
Recommended
Erythromycin *on page 561*
Adult Drug Therapy
Recommended
Erythromycin *on page 561*
Alternate
Tetracycline *on page 679*
Doxycycline *on page 557*

Selected Readings
Lind K, "Manifestations and Complications of *Mycoplasma pneumoniae* Disease: A Review," *Yale J Biol Med*, 1983, 56(5-6):461-8.

Mansel JK, Rosenow EC, Smith TF, et al, "*Mycoplasma pneumoniae* Pneumonia," *Chest*, 1989, 95(3):639-46.

Marrie TJ, "*Mycoplasma pneumoniae* Pneumonia Requiring Hospitalization, With Emphasis on Infection in the Elderly," *Arch Intern Med*, 1993, 153(4):488-94.

Murray HW, Masur H, Senterfit LB, et al, "The Protean Manifestations of *Mycoplasma pneumoniae* Infection in Adults," *Am J Med*, 1975, 58(2):229-42.

Necator americanus see Ancylostoma duodenale *on page 54*

Neisseria gonorrhoeae

Microbiology *Neisseria gonorrhoeae* is an oxidase- and catalase-positive, gram-negative diplococcus. *N. meningitidis* produces acid from only glucose which differentiates it from the other *Neisseria* species. Typing for different strains of *N. gonorrhoeae* can be performed but are useful only for epidemiologic studies.

The organism readily grows on Thayer-Martin or chocolate media and grows best in the presence of CO_2. Growth is more fastidious than that of *N. meningitidis*.

Epidemiology Humans are the only natural reservoir for *N. gonorrhoeae*. The estimate that 1 million new cases of gonorrhea have occurred each year since the early 1960s is most likely a severe underestimate. Transmission is primarily by sexual contact, with the major reservoir in asymptomatically infected per-

(Continued)

161

Neisseria gonorrhoeae (Continued)

sons. The organism and disease is most commonly found in individuals 20-24 years of age. Fifty percent of women will become infected after a single exposure to an infected male while only 20% of men become infected after a single exposure to an infected female.

Clinical Syndromes In men, gonorrhea is usually limited to burning on urination and a purulent urethral discharge. Ten percent of men will be asymptomatic with 1% or less developing the complications of prostatitis, urethral stricture, or epididymitis. Approximately 50% of women are asymptomatic; when symptoms occur they include dysuria, frequency, vaginal discharge, fever, and abdominal pain. Up to 15% of women with gonorrhea develop pelvic inflammatory disease (PID), with fallopian scarring or subsequent chronic PID, sterility, or ectopic pregnancies. Rectal and pharyngeal colonization and disease may also occur in women and homosexual men.

Disseminated disease may include sepsis, peritonitis, or meningitis, but most commonly causes septic arthritis in patients otherwise asymptomatic. Disseminated disease may be accompanied by petechial or papular lesions. In children, the most common form of gonococcal disease is gonorrhea ophthalmia from contamination through an infected birth canal. This is easily prevented with 1% silver nitrate aqueous drops.

Diagnosis In men with urethral symptoms, Gram stain of the purulent material is highly sensitive and specific. Gram stain is less diagnostic in asymptomatic men and clinically useless in diagnosing cervicitis in women because intracellular gram-negative diplococci could be any of the many *Haemophilus* species which are normal vaginal flora. A positive Gram stain is usually characterized by the presence of gram-negative cocci within or closely associated with polymorphonuclear leukocytes. The Gram stain of joint fluid can detect organisms in early septic arthritis but is not particularly sensitive for skin lesions or rectal or pharyngeal disease. Specimens from appropriate sites may be inoculated on Thayer-Martin medium when contaminating organisms are present and on chocolate agar if the specimen is from a normally sterile body site. When asymptomatic or cervical disease is expected, the rectum may yield the only positive specimen. Growth is enhanced by CO_2 inoculated media. Blood cultures are positive in early disseminated disease. Infected joint fluid cultures are also usually positive.

Diagnostic Tests/Procedures

Gram Stain *on page 352*

Neisseria gonorrhoeae Culture *on page 412*

Neisseria gonorrhoeae by Nucleic Acid Probe *on page 411*

Treatment For uncomplicated gonococcal infections, one time single doses of one of the following has been recommended by the Centers for Disease Control (CDC) along with treatment for concomitant *C. trachomatis* infection: ceftriaxone sodium 125 mg I.M., cefixime 400 mg oral, ciprofloxacin 500 mg oral, or ofloxacin 400 mg oral. For disseminated disease, the CDC recommends ceftriaxone 1 g I.V. or I.M. every 24 hours until clinical improvement, then switching to an oral regime of cefixime 400 mg twice daily or ciprofloxacin 500 mg twice daily for at least 1 full week. For other systemic manifestations of disease, ceftriaxone is the drug of choice in both children and adults. A 1% silver nitrate solution is used for prophylaxis of gonococcal ophthalmia.

Pediatric Drug Therapy
Recommended

Ceftriaxone Sodium *on page 523*

Adult Drug Therapy
Recommended

Cefixime *on page 512*

Ceftriaxone Sodium *on page 523*

Ciprofloxacin Hydrochloride *on page 537*

Ofloxacin *on page 626*

Alternate

Spectinomycin Hydrochloride *on page 667*
used in combination with

Doxycycline *on page 557*

Selected Readings

Baron EJ and Finegold SM, eds, "Aerobic, Gram-Negative Cocci, (*Neisseria* and *Branhamella*)," *Bailey & Scott's Diagnostic Microbiology*, St Louis, MO: CV Mosby Co, 1990, 353-62.

Murray PR, Drew WL, Kobayashi GS, et al, eds, "Neisseriaceae," *Medical Microbiology*, St Louis, MO: CV Mosby Co, 1990, 85-97.

U.S. Department of Health and Human Services, "1993 Sexually Transmitted Diseases Treatment Guidelines," *MMWR Morb Mortal Wkly Rep*, 1993, 42(RR-14).

Neisseria meningitidis

Microbiology *Neisseria meningitidis* is an oxidase- and catalase-positive, gram-negative diplococcus. *N. meningitidis* produces acid from glucose and maltose but not from sucrose or lactose, which differentiates it from the other *Neisseria* species. At least nine different serogroups of *N. meningitidis* have been identified on the basis of their polysaccharide capsules. More than 20 serotypes have been identified. Serogroups A, B, C, Y, and W135 are most commonly associated with clinical disease states.

The organism grows on Thayer-Martin or chocolate media and grows best in the presence of CO_2.

Epidemiology *N. meningitidis* is exclusively a human pathogen and causes 3000-4000 cases of meningitis yearly in the United States. *N. meningitidis* is transmitted by droplets among persons with prolonged close contact and who are in direct contact with respiratory secretions. Carriage occurs in 10% to 30% of healthy adults, but disease is rare. Most disease occurs in children 6 months to 5 years of age. Outbreaks occur in other close contact populations such as the military.

Serogroups B and C account for over 75% of cases, and groups W135, Y, and A account for the rest. The last urban epidemic occurred in Brazil in 1971 (serogroups C and A), and the last United States epidemic occurred in 1946 (serogroup A).

Clinical Syndromes *N. meningitidis* causes a wide spectrum of clinical illness which range from a mild nonspecific febrile illness to meningitis and sepsis.

- **Meningitis:** Usually abrupt onset with fever, headache, and meningismus, although the syndrome may be less specific in young children. Mortality is 100% if untreated; 15% if treated appropriately. In meningococcemia, signs and symptoms of sepsis may be seen accompanied by characteristic meningococcal emboli (vasculitic purpura). This syndrome is occasionally preceded by petechial skin lesions. Disseminated intravascular coagulopathy and shock may follow, along with adrenal gland destruction (Waterhouse-Friderichsen syndrome).
- Can also be responsible for urethritis, pneumonias, and arthritis.

Diagnosis Diagnosis is made by Gram stain and culture of cerebrospinal fluid, blood, etc. Occasionally, the organism can be observed on Gram stain of the petechial lesions or detected in buffy coat smears. *N. meningitidis* will grow on blood or chocolate agar (best growth with increased CO_2 concentration) or in Thayer-Martin media when multiple organisms are suspected.

Rapid identification can be performed by several laboratory tests, but definitive identification must be made biochemically.

Diagnostic Tests/Procedures

Aerobic Culture, Cerebrospinal Fluid *on page 245*
Bacterial Antigens, Rapid Detection Methods *on page 269*
Gram Stain *on page 352*

Treatment High dose intravenous penicillin remains the drug of choice for the treatment of meningococcal meningitis. Resistance to penicillin is still exceedingly rare. Chloramphenicol or a third generation cephalosporin are excellent alternatives. Supportive measures are also necessary in patients with meningitis or sepsis.

Prophylaxis for persons with significant exposures to the respiratory secretions of patients with the disease remains controversial. A 2-day regiment of rifampin is recommended (600 mg twice daily for adults, 10 mg/kg twice daily in children, and 5 mg/kg in children younger than 1 month of age). Attempts at eradicating *N. meningitidis* from asymptomatic carriers are impractical and unlikely to be effective.

Drug Therapy
Recommended

Penicillin G, Parenteral *on page 633*

Alternate

Cephalosporins, 3rd Generation *on page 528*
Chloramphenicol *on page 531*

Selected Readings

Baron EJ and Finegold SM, eds, "Aerobic Gram-Negative Cocci (*Neisseria* and *Branhamella*)," *Bailey & Scott's Diagnostic Microbiology*, St Louis, MO: CV Mosby Co, 1990, 353-62.

(Continued)

Neisseria meningitidis (Continued)

Murray PR, Drew WL, Kobayashi GS, et al, eds, "Neisseriaceae," *Medical Microbiology*, St Louis, MO: CV Mosby Co, 1990, 85-97.

Quagliarello V and Scheld WM, "Bacterial Meningitis: Pathogenesis, Pathophysiology, and Progress," *N Engl J Med*, 1992, 327(12):864-72.

Nocardia Species

Microbiology *Nocardia* species are variably acid-fast, "higher order," aerobic bacteria. They belong to the family Nocardiaceae. There are several species of *Nocardia* which are pathogenic for humans, the most common being *Nocardia asteroides* followed by *N. brasiliensis*. Other species occasionally cause human disease such as *N. otitidiscaviarum* (formerly *N. caviae*) and the newly recognized *N. transvalensis*.

Nocardia species have a delicate, branching appearance and may appear fragmented in clinical specimens. The organisms are weakly gram-positive and have a characteristic "beaded" appearance; if present, these characteristics allow rapid preliminary identification. The organisms may be more easily visualized on an acid-fast stain rather than Gram stain. Most (but not all) strains of *Nocardia* are acid-fast and retain carbol fuchsin when decolorized with a weaker alcohol than the acid alcohol commonly used for staining mycobacterial species. It is important to realize that the acid-fast staining properties of *Nocardia* species differ from those of other acid-fast organisms such as *Mycobacterium tuberculosis*. Laboratories use a **modified** acid-fast stain (eg, a modified Ziehl-Neelsen stain and others) to optimally detect *Nocardia* in direct specimens. In most institutions, the clinician must specifically request a modified acid-fast stain for *Nocardia* if this organism is suspected. In some institutions, a *Nocardia* stain may be part of a routine protocol for processing certain clinical specimens, such as bronchoalveolar lavage fluid from immunocompromised patients.

Nocardia species grow on a variety of standard media employed in microbiology laboratories, including blood agar and Sabouraud's dextrose agar. Growth also occurs on media used for isolation of mycobacteria such as the Lowenstein-Jensen medium. Usually 4-10 days are required before growth of the organism is apparent. When *Nocardia* species are present along with other aerobic bacteria, isolation of *Nocardia* may be delayed for several weeks. *Nocardia* species are most frequently isolated from respiratory specimens; only rarely can they be isolated from standard blood cultures.

Epidemiology *Nocardia* species are distributed worldwide, and there appears to be no geographic clustering of cases. The organisms are ubiquitous in soil and areas of plant decay. Approximately 500-1000 cases are reported in the United States annually. The most common age range is 20-50 years, with several series demonstrating a male predominance. Nocardial infections occur mainly in individuals with defective T-cell immunity (cell-mediated immunity), such as organ transplant recipients, patients with malignancies (lymphoma), those receiving corticosteroids or cytotoxic agents, and persons with AIDS. A 13% incidence was once described in one cardiac transplant center, but other institutions have consistently reported much lower rates. Persons with neutrophil dysfunction also appear at increased risk, and nocardiosis has been well-described in children with chronic granulomatous disease. A large number of other diseases have been associated with nocardiosis including tuberculosis, alcoholism with cirrhosis, inflammatory bowel disease, various forms of vasculitis, pulmonary alveolar proteinosis, sarcoidosis, bronchiectasis, and immunoglobulin deficiencies. Nontuberculous mycobacteria has also been reported as a predisposing condition for nocardial infection. Clinically, significant nocardiosis also may occur in otherwise healthy persons, although the incidence of this has been highly variable.

Although occasional clusters of *Nocardia* infection have been described, most experts feel that the organism is not transmitted person-to-person.

Outside the United States, *Nocardia* species are commonly associated with mycetoma (see Clinical Syndromes). Individuals with frequent contact with soil and other plant matter are at risk for this form of nocardiosis.

Clinical Syndromes Disease usually results from inhalation of the organism leading to colonization in the lung. The organisms may resist local pulmonary defenses including macrophages and immunoglobulins. Infections with *Nocardia* species classically result in abscess formation, with numerous polymorphonuclear leukocytes and only a thin abscess wall.

- **Colonization in healthy persons:** Occasionally immunocompetent persons with no significant lung disease may have positive sputum cultures for *Nocardia*. Clinical evaluation is important in deciding on the role of antibiotics.

- **Respiratory colonization in individuals with chronic obstructive pulmonary disease (COPD):** Several series have reported positive sputum cultures from asymptomatic COPD patients; in most cases, there is no active pneumonia and repeat sputum cultures were negative. Repeated isolation of *Nocardia* in these individuals is more worrisome for active disease, and consultation with an Infectious Disease specialist should be considered.
- **Pneumonia:** Immunosuppressed individuals may develop an isolated pneumonia most commonly from *N. asteroides*. The presentation may be subacute or acute. Symptoms are similar to other bacterial pneumonias with fever, purulent sputum, cough, and dyspnea. Some may have pleuritic chest pain mimicking pneumococcal pneumonia. Since *Nocardia* tends to cause suppurative disease, lung cavitation and empyema are common. Chest x-rays may show a nodular infiltrate, cavities, or a lobar pattern. Direct extension of purulent nocardial infections may occur into the pericardium and other mediastinal structures. Disease outside the lungs may be present in up to 50% of cases.
- **Brain abscess:** *Nocardia* commonly disseminates to the brain in immunosuppressed persons. Multiple brain lesions can occur, and the presentation may be subacute. Nocardial infection should be considered in a patient presenting with pneumonia and brain abscess. Meningitis from *Nocardia* is uncommon.
- **Disseminated nocardial infection:** Approximately 20% of patients with nocardiosis have no apparent lung involvement and instead present with extrapulmonary nocardiosis. The most common presentation is brain abscess. A number of other sites may be involved such as bone, skin, abdomen, and others.
- **Mycetoma:** This is usually seen in persons from tropical or subtropical regions. The pathogenesis of mycetoma is from direct inoculation of the organism into the skin rather than inhalation. The feet and/or hands are the most frequent sites. Chronic nocardial infection may develop with disfiguring skin and soft tissue changes and multiple sinus tracts.
- **Cellulitis and lymphocutaneous nodules:** These forms of direct inoculation are more common in the United States than mycetoma. The cellulitis caused by *Nocardia* species may be difficult to distinguish from other forms of bacterial cellulitis. *Nocardia brasiliensis* may cause subcutaneous nodules that spread on an arm or leg following lymphatic drainage. This may mimic infections caused by *Sporothrix schenckii*.
- **Keratitis:** Occasionally, *Nocardia asteroides* is directly inoculated into the eye following trauma.

Diagnosis *Nocardia* infection should be in the differential diagnosis of any immunocompromised patient presenting with an unexplained pneumonia. The clinical suspicion should be high if there is evidence of extrapulmonary involvement as well, particularly the presence of a central nervous system lesion. Respiratory specimens should be submitted for nocardial stain and culture. The organism may be recovered from induced sputum, but bronchoscopy may be necessary in many cases. It is difficult to isolate *Nocardia* species from blood cultures or cerebrospinal fluid but is readily identified from brain abscesses (if the patient has not received prior antibiotics). Serologic studies for *Nocardia* are not clinically helpful at present.

Diagnostic Tests/Procedures

Acid-Fast Stain, Modified, *Nocardia* Species *on page 241*
Nocardia Culture, All Sites *on page 415*

Treatment The optimal regimen for treating *Nocardia* is still controversial and under study. Sulfonamides have been the cornerstone of therapy and appear to be effective in many cases as monotherapy, even in immunocompromised persons. Sulfisoxazole at high doses ($\geq$6 g/day) has been effective in several studies, as has sulfadiazine. Blood levels may be obtained in serious cases. Co-trimoxazole has also been used with success (given at doses up to 20 mg/kg/day of the trimethoprim component). Some experts have been concerned that the commercially available preparations of co-trimoxazole, such as Bactrim™, may not have enough trimethoprim synergistic activity against *Nocardia*. Other problems with co-trimoxazole include a somewhat higher incidence of drug toxicity than sulfonamides alone, occasional treatment failures, and relapses. However, co-trimoxazole is considered by some to be the treatment of choice.

(Continued)

165

Nocardia Species *(Continued)*

Minocycline is effective *in vitro* and *in vivo* and can be used if patients develop hypersensitivity to one of the sulfonamides. Other tetracyclines may be less active. A number of other agents have been reported effective in clinical situations including amikacin and imipenem. Many clinicians use combination therapy in life-threatening or refractory cases, although clinical data is very limited. It is still unclear whether combination therapy (eg, sulfisoxazole and amikacin) is superior to a sulfonamide used as monotherapy.

Since *Nocardia* species tend to form abscesses, surgical drainage may be extremely important, particularly with empyema and brain abscess.

Drug Therapy
Recommended
Co-trimoxazole *on page 545*
Sulfisoxazole *on page 675*
Sulfadiazine *on page 671*
Alternate
Minocycline Hydrochloride *on page 614*

Selected Readings
Lerner PI, "*Nocardia* Species," *Principles and Practice of Infectious Diseases*, 4th ed, Mandell GL, Bennett JE, and Dolin R, eds, New York, NY: Churchill Livingstone, 1995, 2273-80.

Occupational Exposure to Bloodborne Pathogens (Universal Precautions) *see page 751*

Paraflu *see* Parainfluenza Virus *on this page*

Parainfluenza Virus
Related Information
Immunization Guidelines *on page 710-717*
Vaccines *on page 706-709*

Synonyms Paraflu

Microbiology Parainfluenza viruses (also known as "paraflu") are RNA viruses which frequently cause lower respiratory infections in children and are the most common cause of croup (laryngotracheobronchitis). Parainfluenza viruses are single-stranded RNA viruses with an envelope derived from the host. It belongs to the family Paramyxoviridae and is thus related to the mumps virus and respiratory syncytial virus. Isolates causing human disease have been divided into four serotypes, parainfluenza 1-4. Two glycoproteins are found in the envelope, with hemagglutinin and neuraminidase activity associated with one of the two glycoproteins.

Epidemiology The virus is distributed worldwide. Parainfluenza type 4 is the least common of the serotypes isolated clinically, but this may be due to difficulties in culturing *in vitro*. Parainfluenza viruses are usually considered pathogenic in the pediatric population with antibodies to types 1-3 detectable in almost all children by 8 years of age. Longitudinal studies have shown an interesting pattern; outbreaks of parainfluenza types 1 and 2 tend to occur every other year (usually odd-numbered years) and during fall months, whereas outbreaks of type 3 occur during consecutive years most commonly during the spring. Parainfluenza viruses are a common cause of lower respiratory infections in children, second only to respiratory syncytial virus. Parainfluenza type 3 virus can infect infants in the first month of life. Types 1 and 2 tend to infect children and are important causes of croup. Transmission of the virus is by either direct person-to-person contact or by large droplets (eg, sneezing). The incubation period following exposure is about 3-6 days.

Clinical Syndromes
- **Upper respiratory tract infection:** This occurs particularly in children and is manifested by fever (in over 50% of cases), coryza, sore throat, and cough.
- **Croup or laryngotracheobronchitis:** Parainfluenza type 1 is the most common cause of this type of lower respiratory infection. Croup is characterized by a distinctive cough like a "barking seal." In severe cases, the airway may be compromised secondary to subglottal edema, with stridor and respiratory failure. Most cases of croup recover uneventfully within several days. The differential diagnosis must include epiglottitis from *Haemophilus influenzae* or influenza A.
- **Bronchiolitis or pneumonia:** These forms of lower respiratory infection are characterized by progressive cough with wheezing, dyspnea, and inter-

costal retractions. The chest radiograph may demonstrate air trapping and interstitial infiltrates.

- **Infection in adults:** Parainfluenza usually causes a mild respiratory infection in adults and is one cause of the common cold. Often adults may experience hoarseness along with the rhinorrhea, sore throat, and cough. Less commonly, tracheobronchitis has been described both in the adult with underlying chronic bronchitis, as well as the otherwise healthy individual. Pneumonia has also been reported in the elderly.

Diagnosis Infection with parainfluenza is suspected when there is a compatible clinical presentation in the appropriate epidemiologic setting, particularly if the "barking seal" cough of croup is recognized. However, the other manifestations of the disease are generally not specific enough to distinguish parainfluenza from other common respiratory viruses, such as respiratory syncytial virus. Microbiologic confirmation is indicated in severe cases (such as bronchiolitis or pneumonia), atypical cases, or if suspected in the adult. In severe cases, it may also be important to rule out respiratory syncytial virus, for which treatment is available. Rapid identification techniques are offered in many virology laboratories, and the identification of the infecting virus may avoid unnecessary antibacterial agents or invasive diagnostic procedures. In mild upper respiratory infections, virologic confirmation is optional.

The best respiratory sample for detecting parainfluenza virus is the nasopharyngeal wash. This is performed at the bedside by gently administering saline into the nares with a standard syringe then aspirating the fluid back into the syringe, capturing saline, mucous, and respiratory epithelial cells. Alternatively, a viral swab may be inserted into the nasopharynx, but fewer respiratory cells are obtained with this technique and the sensitivity is lower. A "respiratory panel" is offered in some microbiology laboratories, whereby a single nasopharyngeal wash (or swab) may be sent for detection of multiple viruses, such as parainfluenza, influenza, respiratory syncytial virus, and others. Laboratory detection methods include:

1. Cell culture, where the clinical specimen is inoculated onto a monolayer of cells. If parainfluenza virus is present, a characteristic change in the appearance of the monolayer is seen, called cytopathic effect (CPE). The turnaround time is variable, and may be over several days, depending on the quality of the specimen and the amount of virus present.
2. Immunofluorescence. This is a rapid technique designed to detect viral presence without culture. Results may be available within hours of sample submission, if necessary.
3. Direct viral antigen detection. This is another early detection method but is still under study.
4. Serologic studies. Specific antibody titers to parainfluenza may be obtained during the acute and convalescent period. Demonstration of a fourfold increase in specific antibody titer is diagnostic of parainfluenza infection. This may be useful if it is important to diagnose a respiratory illness in retrospect (as for an epidemiologic or outbreak study), but contributes little to the immediate management of a new case.

Diagnostic Tests/Procedures

Parainfluenza Virus Antigen, Direct Fluorescent Antibody *on page 423*

Parainfluenza Virus Culture *on page 423*

Parainfluenza Virus Serology *on page 424*

Treatment There are no antiviral agents currently approved for parainfluenza virus, although several are being studied. Bacterial superinfection is always possible and should be considered as a potentially reversible complication in difficult cases. Most cases of croup respond to supportive therapy alone, but severe cases may require intubation.

Drug Therapy Comment

No antiviral agents proven effective.

Selected Readings

Denny FW, Murphy TF, Clyde WA Jr, et al, "Croup: An 11 Year Study in a Pediatric Practice," *Pediatrics* 1983, 71(6):871-6.

Heilman CA, "Respiratory Syncytial and Parainfluenza Viruses," *J Infect Dis*, 1990, 161(3):402-6.

Parvovirus B19

Microbiology Parvovirus B19 is a small DNA virus which has received increasing attention in recent years. It is the cause of the childhood rash erythema infectiosum ("fifth disease" because it's the "fifth" infectious rash of children) and has been recently linked with a symmetrical adult arthritis, transient aplastic

(Continued)

Parvovirus B19 *(Continued)*

anemia, and chronic anemia in AIDS patients.

Parvovirus B19 is a single-stranded, encapsulated DNA virus which belongs to the family Parvoviridae. There are several other parvoviruses in the same genus as B19, including the common canine parvovirus. However, B19 is a strictly human pathogen and does not cause disease in animals. Infection with B19 is not acquired from dogs (a common misconception); animal parvoviruses have not been shown to cause human disease. The virus predominantly infects erythrocyte precursors in the bone marrow and causes cell lysis. Myeloid precursors in the marrow appear to be spared, although the virus has occasionally been found in peripheral leukocytes. Although parvovirus B19 has been cultured *in vitro* in erythropoietin-stimulated marrow cells, such techniques are not available in clinical virology laboratories. Instead, detection of viral presence is mainly achieved through detection of either specific B19 antibody, viral antigens, or nucleic acid (using polymerase chain reaction).

Epidemiology Infection with parvovirus B19 is common in the United States, beginning in early childhood. Over 50% of the adult population has serologic evidence of prior infection. Many cases are asymptomatic or mild. The primary mode of transmission is most likely respiratory. Outbreaks within families or schools can occur because of a high secondary attack rate which sometimes exceeds 50%. Spread of the virus is facilitated by subclinically infected individuals shedding the virus unknowingly in respiratory secretions. In addition, the individual is infective for several weeks before the characteristic parvovirus rash appears. Based on human volunteer studies, the period of incubation is approximately 1 week (4-14 days).

Clinical Syndromes

- **Erythema infectiosum (slapped cheek):** This is a childhood exanthem caused exclusively by parvovirus B19, also referred to as "fifth disease." Typically, a school-aged child develops a nonspecific febrile illness (low grade fever, malaise, and myalgias), which resolves over several days. Days to weeks later, when the child is feeling well, a brightly erythematous rash develops on the face. This is the characteristic "slapped cheek" rash of erythema infectiosum and is considered benign. Mild constitutional symptoms may accompany the rash (malaise, headache, etc), but the child is usually not infectious at this point. Erythema infectiosum has also been described in the adult and is frequently accompanied by joint symptoms.

- **Adult polyarthropathy:** B19 has recently been associated with a sudden onset, symmetrical polyarthritis syndrome. The great majority of cases have been reported in otherwise healthy women. Patients initially experience a nonspecific viral prodrome, probably corresponding to the period of viremia (B19 nucleic acid has been detected in the serum of some individuals). Several days to weeks later, an acute arthropathy develops, symmetrically involving the small joints of the hands, feet, and knees. Other joints may be involved less commonly (spine, costochondral joints). In addition to these arthralgias, there is often evidence of arthritis and synovitis, with joint stiffness, inflammation, and joint effusions. Arthrocentesis typically shows a mild elevation in WBCs around 3000-6000 cells/mm^3, mostly mononuclear. It is not clear whether B19 arthropathy is due to autoimmune mechanisms or direct viral infection. B19 nucleic acid has been found in the synovial fluid of a single patient (suggesting direct infection) but is generally undetectable in the blood during the arthropathy phase (suggesting an autoimmune etiology). Less than 50% of the cases are accompanied by a rash. When present, the rash appears macular in men and "lace-like" in women. The distribution of the rash is variable but tends to include the arms of legs. In some cases, there is marked involvement of the soles of the feet and the palms (somewhat unusual locations for an exanthem). The typical "slapped cheek" rash of erythema infectiosum is uncommon. The majority of cases of B19 arthropathy resolve completely with observation alone. Occasionally, the polyarthropathy may be persistent or recurrent over a period of years, and recent studies have linked it to a chronic fibromyalgia syndrome. Of note, there are many variations in the presentation of this syndrome, including symmetrical arthritis without a flu-like illness or rash.

- **Transient aplastic crisis:** Parvovirus B19 can cause a severe erythropoietic arrest in patients with a previous underlying blood disorder, especially sickle cell disease, hereditary spherocytosis, thalassemia, hemoglobin SC, and other chronic hemolytic states. (Transient aplastic crisis from B19 usually does not cause anemia in healthy individuals since mature, circulating erythrocytes are spared and continue to circulate for 120 days.) Individuals present with profound fatigue and lethargy, with or without a history of a preceding flu-like illness. Rash and arthralgias are usually not present. Blood counts reveal a severely decreased hemoglobin with absent reticulocytes. Urgent transfusion may be necessary. Examination of the bone marrow shows erythroid hypoplasia with other cell lines usually intact. The finding of giant pronormoblasts in the bone marrow is considered pathognomonic for this infection. B19 viremia has been demonstrated during this time, and patients are potentially still infectious. The aplastic crisis usually resolves within 1-2 weeks.

- **Transient pancytopenia:** Other cells besides the erythrocytes can be involved with an acute parvovirus B19 infection. Potentially life-threatening declines in the neutrophil and/or platelet counts have been reported. In addition, a mild and transient pancytopenia was commonly observed in human volunteers experimentally infected with B19 and likely occurs in natural infections.

- **Chronic anemia in the immunocompromised host:** In these patients, B19 is incompletely cleared after the initial infection and leads to a waxing and waning, persistent infection. Chronic bone marrow suppression may be seen, as the virus causes continued lysis of RBC progenitor cells. Patients may be otherwise asymptomatic despite the chronicity of infection. Cases have been reported in acute leukemia, severe combined immunodeficiency syndrome, bone marrow transplant patients, and HIV-1 infections. The host antibody response to chronic B19 infection is highly variable, and viremia has been seen in patients with a negative parvovirus IgG and IgM. Diagnosis may require demonstration of B19 DNA in the serum by polymerase chain reaction. It is important to recognize this form of chronic anemia because it may respond to immunoglobulin therapy. In 1990, persistent B19 infection was found in a group of HIV-infected patients with red cell aplasia. All patients had giant pronormoblasts in the bone marrow.

- **Perinatal infections:** The developing fetus is at particular risk for complications related to perinatal parvovirus infection. This is due to several factors including the immaturity of the fetal immune system, delayed and incomplete transfer of protective maternal antibody across the placenta, and the need for brisk erythrocyte production in the fetus. Maternal infections with B19 during pregnancy may lead to hydrops fetalis or fetal death. The precise risk of intrauterine transmission to the fetus is unknown, as is the risk of fetal death once transmission has taken place. However, the data available suggest that the majority of pregnant women with acute B19 infections deliver healthy infants. However, fetal demise has been reported following asymptomatic maternal B19 infections. The cause of death in the fetus has been attributed to destruction of erythroid precursors in the liver and bone marrow, followed by edema and congestive heart failure; however, virus has also been identified in tissues such as the heart. Perinatal parvovirus B19 infection has not been associated with congenital abnormalities. Thus, maternal infection is not an indication for an abortion. Although the epidemiology of perinatal parvovirus infections is still evolving, this virus is still an uncommon cause of stillbirths or spontaneous abortions in the general U.S. population (by some estimates, approximately 1% of cases of fetal loss). The Centers for Disease Control has addressed the growing public concern regarding B19 and fetal death by estimating the risks of B19 infection in pregnant women following different exposures to the virus (see references). The risk of fetal death in susceptible women exposed to B19 during epidemic outbreaks (school, day care centers) is roughly 1% to 2%.

Diagnosis In the absence of classic erythema infectiosum, parvovirus infection may be difficult to diagnose. The clinician must maintain a high level of suspicion for B19 in patients with unusual skin rashes, arthritis-arthralgia syndromes, aplastic anemia of unknown etiology, and chronic anemia. Laboratory studies are necessary to confirm the diagnosis. These consist of:

1. IgG and IgM antibodies specific for parvovirus B19. The presence of IgM antibody in the patient (or in cord blood of the fetus) confirms acute infection. A significant rise in parvovirus IgG during acute and convalescent periods is also diagnostic. A single positive IgG only suggests past infection, and a paired sample is necessary for proper interpretation. Chronic B19 infection in immunosuppressed patients may or may not demonstrate IgG or IgM antibodies and are not completely reliable.

(Continued)

Parvovirus B19 *(Continued)*

2. Detection of viral antigen is still a research tool and not commercially available as yet.

3. Polymerase chain reaction (PCR), the most sensitive technique, has been employed successfully in many studies, with viral DNA being detected in the serum of individuals with acute viremia as well as a variety of tissues. Contact a large commercial reference laboratory or the Centers for Disease Control and Prevention (Division of Viral Diseases) for inquiries regarding PCR.

4. Electron microscopy for parvovirus-like particles.

5. Histologic specimens, looking for eosinophilic nuclear inclusions (not pathognomonic for B19)

6. Bone marrow aspiration and biopsy. The finding of giant pronormoblasts in Wright-Giemsa stained marrow is characteristic of parvoviral infection.

B19 cannot be detected using the common cell culture systems available in clinical virology laboratories.

Diagnostic Tests/Procedures

Bone Marrow Aspiration and Biopsy *on page 277*

Parvovirus B19 Serology *on page 425*

Treatment Currently, there is no antiviral agent with significant clinical activity against the B19 virus itself. However, in some cases, the chronic anemia of B19 infection in immunosuppressed patients has been shown to respond dramatically to infusions of intravenous immunoglobulin. This important finding has also been shown in a small cohort of HIV-1 infected individuals with B19-induced anemia.

Drug Therapy Comment

No antiviral agents proven effective.

Selected Readings

Anderson LJ, "Human Parvoviruses," *J Infect Dis*, 1990, 161(4):603-8.

Faden H, Gary GW Jr, and Anderson LF, "Chronic Parvovirus Infection in a Presumably Immunologically Healthy Woman," *Clin Infect Dis*, 1992, 15(4):595-7.

Frickhofen N, Abkowitz JL, Safford M, et al, "Persistent B19 Parvovirus Infection in Patients Infected With Human Immunodeficiency Virus Type 1 (HIV-1): A Treatable Cause of Anemia in AIDS," *Ann Intern Med*, 1990, 113(12):926-33.

Kurtzman G, Frickhofen N, Kimball J, et al, "Pure Red-Cell Aplasia of 10 Years' Duration Due to Persistent Parvovirus B19 Infection and Its Cure With Immunoglobulin Therapy," *N Engl J Med*, 1989, 321(8):519-23.

Kurtzman GJ, Cohen B, Meyers P, et al, "Persistent B19 Parvovirus Infection as a Cause of Severe Chronic Anemia in Children With Acute Lymphocytic Leukaemia," *Lancet*, 1988, 2(8621):1159-62.

Woolf AD, Campion GV, Chishick A, et al, "Clinical Manifestations of Human Parvovirus B19 in Adults," *Arch Intern Med*, 1989, 149(5):1153-6.

Pasteurella multocida

Microbiology *Pasteurella multocida* is a gram-negative rod which is primarily a pathogen in wild and domestic animals but is also capable of causing sporadic human diseases such as animal bite infection, osteomyelitis, pneumonia, and sepsis. *P. multocida* is an aerobic, gram-negative coccobacillus which does not form spores. It belongs to the family Pasteurellaceae, and is thus related to *Haemophilus* species. There are six distinct species of *Pasteurella*, but the most common to cause human disease is *Pasteurella multocida*. Special requests for identification for this organism are helpful for the microbiology laboratory but are usually not necessary; the organism grows readily on several standard culture media such as blood agar or chocolate agar.

Epidemiology *P. multocida* is a normal commensal of the oropharynx and the gastrointestinal tract of several kinds of animals. However, it is only rarely recovered from the respiratory tract of humans and has been found to be part of the normal oral flora only in individuals with significant animal contact (eg, veterinarians). The frequency of recovery of this organism from a healthy animal depends on the particular animal species, as follows: cats, 50% to 75%; dogs, 10% to 60%; pigs, 50%, and rats, 15%.

Pasteurella has been reported in all age groups. Human infection usually occurs following an animal bite or scratch. One study found that up to 17% of patients being treated in an emergency room for an animal bite ultimately developed a *Pasteurella* infection. Cat scratches or bites cause the majority of *Pasteurella* infections (about 65% of cases). Dog bites are responsible for about 35% of cases. A smaller number of cases of *Pasteurella* infections are due to animal exposures without a clear history of an animal bite or scratch.

The patient tends to be frequently exposed to animals (such as a veterinarian, livestock handler, pet shop worker), and the infections are generally in the respiratory tract, although cases of intra-abdominal infection have also been described. A small percentage of patients are infected with *P. multocida* without any significant animal exposure.

Clinical Syndromes

- **Animal bite-wound infections:** Patients who have *Pasteurella* inoculated via a bite wound develop rapid onset of pain, erythema, and edema locally. This may occur within hours of the bite or may be delayed by several days. Common sites include the upper extremities (in particular, hands), legs, and the head and neck region. An important complication is the development of regional lymphadenopathy. Occasionally, *Pasteurella* infection may be the cause of lymph node enlargement of unknown etiology; such patients should be questioned about seemingly minor animal scratches as well. Bite-wound infections are often limited to soft tissue cellulitis or focal abscesses. At times, the course may be complicated by tenosynovitis and osteomyelitis, which can be particularly difficult to treat when involving the hand. Note that the specific entity known as "cat scratch disease" is not caused by *Pasteurella multocida*. The exact cause of this lymphadenopathy syndrome is still being debated.
- **Upper and lower respiratory infections:** This unusual presentation of *Pasteurella* infection may be seen in patients who have had a significant exposure to animals but lack a history of an animal bite. *Pasteurella* has been implicated as a rare cause of bronchitis, sinusitis, and pneumonia in both healthy individuals and those with underlying chronic bronchitis.
- **Infection in the immunocompromised host:** Serious and life-threatening *Pasteurella* infections have been reported in patients with underlying malignancies, organ transplantations, and HIV infection.
- **Miscellaneous infections:** Meningitis, arthritis, peritonitis (particularly patients undergoing peritoneal dialysis), corneal ulcers, ophthalmitis, and urinary tract infections are rarely reported.

Diagnosis *P. multocida* infection should be included in the differential diagnosis of any wound infection following an animal bite or deep scratch. The diagnosis strongly suggested if the onset of local inflammation is within 3-24 hours of the bite and if the animal involved was a cat. Longer periods of incubation are more suggestive of streptococcal or staphylococcal infection, although certainly cases of pasteurellosis may have a delayed onset. The diagnosis is more difficult for nonbite *Pasteurella* infections; the clinician must carefully inquire about unusual or prolonged animal exposures in the workplace and at home.

Diagnostic Tests/Procedures

Blood Culture, Aerobic and Anaerobic *on page 271*
Gram Stain *on page 352*
Wound Culture *on page 480*

Treatment The drug of choice for pasteurellosis is penicillin. If the infection is minor and limited to soft tissue, a trial of oral penicillin may be attempted (eg, penicillin V, 500 mg orally every 6 hours). If the infection is more serious, parenteral penicillin should be used. This includes deep wound infections of the extremities, osteomyelitis, septic arthritic, tenosynovitis, and pneumonia. Consultation with an infectious disease specialist may be useful in complicated cases, where therapy may be prolonged and surgical debridement necessary. Other antimicrobial agents are probably effective but the clinical experience is more limited: tetracycline, ampicillin, possibly ciprofloxacin, and the cephalosporins. Infectious disease consultation may be helpful for therapy with alternative agents.

Drug Therapy

Recommended

Penicillin G, Parenteral *on page 633*

Alternate

Amoxicillin and Clavulanic Acid *on page 490*
Ampicillin Sodium and Sulbactam Sodium *on page 497*

Selected Readings

Weber DJ, Wolfson JS, Swartz M, et al, "*Pasteurella multocida* Infections. Report of 34 Cases and Review of the Literature," *Medicine (Baltimore)*, 1984, 63(3):133-154.

Pediculus humanus see Lice *on page 142*

Peptostreptococcus see *Streptococcus*-Related Gram-Positive Cocci *on page 212*

Philhirus pubis *see* Lice *on page 142*

Pinworm *see* Enterobius vermicularis *on page 106*

Plasmodium Species

Microbiology *Plasmodium* sp are obligate intracellular protozoa related to *Babesia* and *Toxoplasma*. *Plasmodium* sp reproduce sexually in mosquitos. Mosquitos transmit the resulting sporozoites into humans where the organisms reproduce asexually. The sporozoites multiply within the liver; resulting merozoites invade erythrocytes where the merozoites multiply or mature into male and female gametocytes which eventually will be taken up by a mosquito during a blood meal.

Plasmodium sp stain well with Giemsa or Wright-Giemsa and are easily observed in stained peripheral blood smears if parasitemia is heavy enough. There are many species of *Plasmodium*; however, only the following four species infect humans: *P. falciparum*, *P. vivax*, *P. ovale*, and *P. malariae*.

Epidemiology *P. falciparum* is found in tropical areas; *P. vivax* is found throughout many tropical and subtropical parts of the world; *P. ovale* is found in central and west Africa and in some Pacific islands; and *P. malariae* is found sporadically throughout the world. *P. falciparum* and *P. vivax* cause ca. 80% and 15%, respectively, of all cases of malaria. Malaria is the most severe infectious disease of tropical and subtropical areas of the world. One-half of the world's population live in areas where malaria is endemic. Each year ca. 270 million persons become infected with *Plasmodium* sp, ca. 110 million persons develop clinical disease, and 7 million Americans visit areas where malaria is endemic.

Clinical Syndromes After experiencing a prodrome phase of constitutional "flu"-like symptoms, most persons with malaria will experience the hallmark of classic malaria, the paroxysm. A paroxysm is a 3- to 6-hour period of high fever, chills, and rigors. Paroxysms correspond to periodic release of *Plasmodium* merozoites from erythrocytes and the beginning of another life cycle of the organism within erythrocytes. Fever patterns are often irregular, but the paroxysm often occurs regularly (eg, every 2 days). Often, patients are asymptomatic between paroxysms. Patients with malaria can experience severe splenomegaly and hepatomegaly. Rupture of the spleen is not uncommon. Anemia is a common complication. Malaria caused by *P. falciparum* is a medically urgent situation and requires immediate diagnosis and medical intervention. Fulminant complications of malaria include renal failure, pulmonary edema, cerebral involvement, and severe reduction of the flow of blood through capillaries.

Diagnosis Smears of peripheral blood must be stained with Giemsa or Wright-Giemsa stains and examined for parasites. Blood should be collected no less than twice per day (preferably, several times a day) until malaria is ruled out or until parasites are observed and identified. The most important and immediate concerns in the management of malaria are to determine if the patient is infected with *Plasmodium* and, if so, to determine if the parasite is *P. falciparum*.

Diagnostic Tests/Procedures
Peripheral Blood Smear, Thick and Thin *on page 429*

Drug Therapy
  Recommended
    Chloroquine-susceptible:
      Chloroquine Phosphate *on page 534*
      Quinidine *on page 656*
    Chloroquine-resistant:
      Mefloquine Hydrochloride *on page 605*
  Alternate
    Chloroquine-resistant:
      Sulfadoxine and Pyrimethamine *on page 673*

Selected Readings
Garcia LS, "Update on Malaria," *Clin Microbiol Newslett*, 1992, 14:65-9.
Krogstad DJ, "*Plasmodium* Species (Malaria)," *Principles and Practice of Infectious Diseases*, 4th ed, Mandell GL, Bennett JE, and Dolin R, eds, New York, NY: Churchill Livingstone, 1995, 2415-27.

Pneumocystis carinii

Microbiology *Pneumocystis carinii* has traditionally been classified as a protozoan, although more recent evidence suggests it is more closely related to fungi. Studies using molecular techniques have shown a close homology between *P. carinii* and fungi such as *Saccharomyces* than other protozoans such as *Plasmodium* (the cause of malaria). The organism is unicellular and has three stages: trophozoite, precyst, and cyst. In clinical specimens, the trophozoites are most predominant. The life cycle of *P. carinii* has yet to be fully defined. The organism cannot be cultured reliably in the laboratory, even in research settings. The organism requires special staining to be visible in clinical specimens. Several stains will selectively stain the organism (methenamine-silver, toluidine blue, Wright-Giemsa, and others).

Epidemiology *P. carinii* is distributed worldwide and in animals. Serologic data suggests that infection with this organism is common. Most children show serologic evidence of infection by 4 years of age. Most of these primary infections with *Pneumocystis* in the normal child are insignificant, with either mild or no clinical disease. Individuals with normal immune systems generally are asymptomatic; reactivation or significant reinfection occurs only when the immune system is compromised. Transmission of *P. carinii* is probably by an airborne route. The precise reservoir for the organism in nature is not clear; it is not known if the organism can exist outside of a living host. In humans and animals, the natural reservoir is the lung.

P. carinii causes an opportunistic infection in immunocompromised hosts. Early on, cases of *Pneumocystis carinii* pneumonia (PCP) were described in premature and debilitated infants, institutionalized children, patients with primary immunodeficiency disorders, and adults receiving immunosuppressive medications such as corticosteroids. A defect in the host cell-mediated immunity appeared to be the major risk factor for PCP. More recently, PCP has been and continues to be a common infection in persons with AIDS and is an important AIDS-defining opportunistic infection.

Persons with AIDS are at particularly high risk for PCP. Before the advent of preventative therapy for PCP, about 60% to 80% of AIDS patients developed PCP. Infection with *P. carinii* rarely occurs when the CD4 count is >200 cells/mm^3, with most cases occurring when the CD4 count is <100 cells/mm^3.

Clinical Syndromes

- ***Pneumocystis carinii* pneumonia (PCP):** Patients classically present with fever, dyspnea on exertion, and dry cough. AIDS patients often have a very indolent presentation with symptoms present for several weeks. Other symptoms include chills, chest pain, and sputum production. On examination, patients with PCP have tachypnea and tachycardia, but the auscultation of the lungs may be completely normal. Useful laboratory tests include the arterial blood gas, which shows hypoxia, increased alveolar–arterial oxygen gradient, and respiratory alkalosis in most, but not all, patients. The diffusing capacity of the lung (DLCO) at rest or with exercise is decreased in many cases. The chest radiograph usually shows bilateral, symmetrical interstitial pulmonary infiltrates. A variety of unusual chest x-ray findings have been reported including nodules and cavities. In some patients, both the lung examination, arterial blood gas, and chest x-ray are normal.
- **Extrapulmonary pneumocystosis:** Although *P. carinii* most commonly involves the lung, cases of *P. carinii* infection outside the lung have been reported, particularly in AIDS patients receiving aerosolized pentamidine for PCP prophylaxis. These include retinal infection, lymph nodes, liver and spleen, thyroid, ear lesions, skin lesions, and mastoiditis.

Diagnosis The manifestations of *P. carinii* infection in the AIDS patient can be very subtle, and a high index of suspicion must be maintained. Similarly, the non-AIDS patient with PCP may present only with fever and malaise without prominent respiratory symptoms. Laboratory confirmation includes:

- induced sputum for *P. carinii* (usually productive only in immunocompromised patients). Stains for *P. carinii* (toluidine blue, methenamine-silver, Giemsa, immunofluorescence, and calcofluor staining procedures) have been found to be sensitive and convenient.
- bronchoscopy with or without transbronchial biopsy (BAL produces a particularly good specimen)
- open lung biopsy (infrequently required)

Diagnostic Tests/Procedures

Pneumocystis carinii Test *on page 431*

Treatment The mainstays of therapy for *P. carinii* remain co-trimoxazole (Bactrim™) or intravenous pentamidine. Comparison studies have shown these agents are equally efficacious but fewer adverse reactions have been noted with Bactrim™. Thus, co-trimoxazole is considered the agent of choice, usually administered intravenously in serious cases. In mild cases, oral Bactrim™ may be utilized initially. There is still a high incidence (50% or greater) of adverse reactions with Bactrim™ in AIDS patients with PCP; the incidence is much lower in non-AIDS patients.

Drug Therapy
Recommended

Co-trimoxazole *on page 545*

Alternate
Pentamidine Isethionate *on page 639*

Selected Readings

Davey RT Jr, Masur H, "Recent Advances in the Diagnosis, Treatment, and Prevention of *Pneumocystis carinii* Pneumonia," *Antimicrob Agents Chemother*, 1990, 34(4):499-504.

National Institutes of Health – University of California Expert Panel for Corticosteroids as Adjunctive Therapy for *Pneumocystis* Pneumonia, "Consensus Statement on the Use of Corticosteroids as Adjunctive Therapy for *Pneumocystis* Pneumonia in the Acquired Immunodeficiency Syndrome," *N Engl J Med*, 1990, 323(21):1500-4.

Phair J, Munoz A Detels R, et al, "The Risk of *Pneumocystis carinii* Pneumonia Among Men Infected With Human Immunodeficiency Virus Type 1," *N Engl J Med*, 1990, 322(3):161-5.

"Recommendations for Prophylaxis Against *Pneumocystis carinii* for Adults and Adolescents Infected With Human Immunodeficiency Virus," *MMWR Morb Mortal Wkly Rep*, 1992, 41(No. RR-4):1-11.

Telzak EE, Cote RJ, Gold JW, et al, "Extrapulmonary *Pneumocystis carinii* Infections," *Rev Infect Dis*, 1990, 12(3):380-6.

Wachter RM, Russi MB, Bloch DA, et al, "*Pneumocystis carinii* Pneumonia and Respiratory Failure in AIDS," *Am Rev Respir Dis*, 1991, 143(2):251-6.

Poliovirus

Related Information
Immunization Guidelines *on page 710-717*
Vaccines *on page 706-709*

Microbiology Polioviruses are single-stranded RNA viruses which cause poliomyelitis, a central nervous system disease of once epidemic proportions. They belong to the family Picornaviridae (pico-, very small; rna-, ribonucleic acid; -viruses) and the genus Enterovirus. Thus, polioviruses are closely related to such agents as Coxsackieviruses, Enteroviruses, and ECHO viruses. Polioviruses have three distinct serotypes (types 1-3). Infection with one serotype (either natural or vaccine-related) confers serotype-specific immunity; reinfection with a different serotype has been reported.

The virus is tropic for neural tissue. Polioviruses have a narrow tissue tropism in comparison with other Enteroviruses. Polioviruses attach to anterior horn cells of spinal cord gray matter, motor neurons, and dorsal root ganglia by means of a specific receptor (cellular adhesion molecules). The neurovirulence of "wild-type" strains (ie, strains present in the general population) varies enormously. The viral strains used in the polio vaccines are of low neurovirulence and can be distinguished from wild-type strains by means of genomic sequencing and other molecular techniques.

Epidemiology Poliovirus infections were epidemic in the United States in the first half of the twentieth century. In the 1950s, epidemics occurred on a regular basis with an attack rate of 17 cases per 100,000. The introduction of the inactivated polio vaccine (IPV) by Albert Sabin in 1955 was one of the great advances in modern medicine. This introduction was followed soon afterwards by the live-attenuated oral polio vaccine (OPV) developed by Jonas Salk. A striking decline in paralytic and nonparalytic polio cases followed. With the extensive use of the OPV in both North and South America, wild-type strains of polio have nearly disappeared in the Western hemisphere, despite the large number of children who are inadequately immunized. The year 1979 marked the last reported case of endemic, wild-type poliomyelitis in the United States. The most recent case of wild-type paralytic poliomyelitis in either North or South America came from Peru in August 1991. Cases of acute flaccid paralysis continue to be screened by aggressive surveillance programs, but additional wild-type cases have not been recognized through 1992 and the first half of 1993.

Although naturally-occurring cases have been eliminated in this country, rare cases of vaccine-related poliomyelitis still occur. Each of the 5-10 annual cases in the United States can be directly linked to the OPV vaccine. Vaccine-related infections have been reported in recipients of the OPV (usually children), as well as close contacts of vaccine recipients (usually adults). Some experts believe that wild-type polioviruses have essentially been replaced with Sabin vaccine strains; these vaccine strains now circulate widely in the population, presumably causing asymptomatic or mild infections. Poliomyelitis still occurs with some frequency in developing countries outside North and South America. About 120,000 cases were recognized in 1992, mainly in sub-Saharan Africa and the Indian subcontinent. Global eradication of this infection is still possible, although there are multiple factors which account for the persistence of disease. Reintroduction of wild-type polioviruses into the United States from foreign visitors or travelers to endemic areas remains a concern, and justifies continued immunization programs.

Although infection can be induced in experimental animals, humans are believed to be the only natural host of the virus. The infectious cycle begins when the host ingests materials which contain contaminated feces (ie, a fecal-oral route of transmission). Active viral replication takes place in the oropharynx (particularly the tonsils) and in the distal portion of the small bowel (Peyer's patches, intestinal mucosa). This replication is followed by a transient phase of "minor viremia" where virus particles spread hematogenously to various organs and lymph nodes. In the majority of cases, the infection is aborted at this stage by the host immune system; only subclinical or asymptomatic infection results ("abortive poliomyelitis"). Less commonly, viral replication is not controlled by immunologic mechanisms, and virus proliferates in the liver, spleen, marrow, and nodes. This is followed by a "major viremia" in which visceral organs are again seeded hematogenously, including the brain and spinal cord. This "major viremia" corresponds with the prodromal symptoms of poliomyelitis (fever, malaise). The incubation period between exposure and the onset of symptoms has been estimated at 5-35 days.

Clinical Syndromes

- **Asymptomatic illness:** As with other enteroviral infections, the vast majority of infections with poliovirus are asymptomatic, and never go on to develop clinical illness.

- **Aseptic meningitis:** Patients present with fever, headache, and nuchal rigidity. Cerebrospinal fluid characteristically reveals a mild lymphocytic (predominantly polymorphonuclear leukocytes early on, the lymphocytic) with elevated protein in the 40-50 mg/dL range. In some cases the virus may be directly cultured from CSF with cytopathic effect in cell culture in 1 week. There is a rapid clinical recovery within 2-10 days. Poliovirus is a relatively rare cause of the syndrome of aseptic meningitis is indistinguishable from the aseptic meningitis caused by other, more common viruses.

- **Abortive poliomyelitis:** This occurs in less than 10% of polio cases. Patients develop a nonspecific viral syndrome with fever, sore throat, malaise, and abdominal discomfort. Symptoms resolve quickly and there is no progression to paralytic polio.

- **Bulbar poliomyelitis:** In this form of polio, patients initially present with dysphagia and a change in speech due to paralysis of the muscles of the pharynx. Most commonly there is involvement of cranial nerves IX and X, although others may be involved.

- **Polioencephalitis:** Infants are most susceptible to this uncommon manifestation of poliovirus infection. There is alteration in the level of consciousness and seizures are common.

- **Paralytic poliomyelitis:** This is the most feared complication of poliovirus infection and occurs in less that 1 in 1000 cases. Risk factors for this syndrome include prior tonsillectomy, trauma, immunodeficiency, pregnancy, and others. Following an incubation period of 1-5 weeks, patients typically enter a period of "minor illness" (corresponding to viremia), consisting of a flu-like illness with fever, nausea, malaise, headache, sore throat, and vomiting. This nonspecific illness lasts several days then resolves completely. The "major illness" occurs about 1 week later. Patients develop a meningitic syndrome with fever and neck stiffness, along with severe muscle pain often involving the limbs and back. This is followed by the onset of muscle paralysis and weakness. The extent of muscle involvement is highly variable. In mild cases, an isolated muscle group may develop weakness. In severe cases, there may be complete quadriplegia with flaccid paralysis and loss of reflexes. The most common presentation is weakness of one leg or one arm. An important clue to the diagnosis of polio is asymmetric flaccid paralysis. The deficit is purely motor in nearly all cases. Loss of sensation is not part of paralytic poliomyelitis and should bring to mind other diagnoses such as Guillain-Barré syndrome. Following this initial attack, there may be a period of recovery of strength, but this is variable. This is followed by a long period of stability and many persons are able to function at a nearly normal level.

- **Post-polio syndrome:** This syndrome has received much attention in both the medical and lay press. There are roughly 300,000 persons who survived the last epidemic of poliomyelitis in the 1950s, and it appears that all are at risk for the post-polio syndrome. About 30 years after the initial bout of paralytic polio, some individuals have developed fatigue, muscle weak-

(Continued)

Poliovirus *(Continued)*

ness, and sometimes pain. Most commonly the same muscle group(s) originally involved years ago are once again involved, but in some cases "new" muscle groups also develop weakness. This phenomenon was initially dismissed as being nonorganic, but recent evidence strongly suggests it is a disorder of the motor unit, with objective evidence of ongoing denervation by electromyogram and muscle biopsy even in asymptomatic patients. Although many persons may potentially develop this syndrome, the degree of muscle weakness is not as severe as the original bout of polio and it tends not to progress.

Diagnosis Polioviruses are readily isolated in tissue culture. The highest yield for the virus is from the pharynx early in the illness. Later, virus remains viable in the stool for up to 1 month. The virus is difficult to isolate from cerebrospinal fluid.

Diagnostic Tests/Procedures

Poliovirus Serology *on page 432*

Viral Culture, Central Nervous System Symptoms *on page 476*

Viral Culture, Stool *on page 478*

Viral Culture, Throat *on page 479*

Drug Therapy Comment

No antiviral agents proven effective.

Selected Readings

Agre JC, Rodriquez AA, and Tafel JA, "Late Effects of Polio: Critical Review of the Literature on Neuromuscular Function," *Arch Phys Med Rehabil*, 1991, 72(11):923-31.

Foege WH, "A World Without Polio," *JAMA*, 1993, 270(15):1859-60.

Modlin JF, "Poliovirus," *Principles and Practice of Infectious Diseases*, 4th ed, Mandell GL, Bennett JE, and Dolin R, eds, New York, NY: Churchill Livingstone, 1995, 1613-20.

Munsat TL, "Poliomyelitis – New Problems With an Old Disease," *N Engl J Med*, 1991, 324(17):1206-7.

Sharief MK, Hentges R, and Ciardi M, "Intrathecal Immune Response in Patients With the Post-Polio Syndrome," *N Engl J Med*, 1991, 325(11)749-55.

Sonies BC and Dalakos MD, "Dysphagia in Patients With the Post-Polio Syndrome," *N Engl J Med* 1991, 324(17):1162-7.

"Update: Polio Eradication – The Americas, 1993," *MMWR Morb Mortal Wkly Rep*, 1993, 42(35):685-6.

Postexposure Prophylaxis for Hepatitis B *see page 719*

Proteus Species

Microbiology *Proteus* species are facultative, gram-negative bacilli which belong to the large family Enterobacteriaceae. These organisms are considered "enteric bacilli" because they commonly inhabit the gastrointestinal tract. The two most clinically important *Proteus* species are *Proteus mirabilis* and *Proteus vulgaris*. Biochemically, nearly all strains of *P. mirabilis* are indole-positive; all other clinically relevant *Proteus* species such as *Proteus vulgaris* are indole-negative. *Proteus* species characteristically "swarm" (spread) over the surface of a moist agar plate. The organisms have several features that promote urinary tract infections including fimbriae which facilitate colonization of the organism in the urinary tract and flagella which facilitate motility in the urinary system. In addition, *Proteus* species have the unique ability to produce urease to hydrolyze urea (found in urine of the human host) to ammonium hydroxide which can lead to renal calculi formation and urinary tract infections.

Epidemiology *Proteus* species are found in soil, water, and fecally contaminated materials. They are found in human feces and are considered part of the normal fecal flora. *Proteus* species are some of the most frequently isolated and clinically significant Enterobacteriaceae. In some studies, *Proteus mirabilis* is the second leading cause of community-acquired urinary tract infections, second only to *E. coli*. Aside from urinary tract infections, *Proteus* species rarely cause serious disease in otherwise healthy individuals. However, they are an important cause of hospital-acquired infections in debilitated patients and account for up to 10% to 15% of nosocomial infections in the United States.

Clinical Syndromes

- **Urinary tract infections:** The ability of *P. mirabilis* to hydrolyze urea to ammonia causes a rise in the urine pH. This alkaline urine leads to precipitation of magnesium, calcium, and ammonium and ultimately forms a type of kidney stone called struvite or triple phosphate stones. These stones act as obstructing foreign bodies and can lead to hydronephrosis, chronic and recurrent *Proteus mirabilis* urinary tract infections, pyelonephritis, and renal abscess. As a rule, it is difficult to treat urinary tract infections in the presence of a renal stone; medical therapy with antibiotics alone is often unsuccessful and patients are at risk for urosepsis if the stone is not removed.

- **Pneumonia:** Like other gram-negative bacilli, *Proteus* species can cause serious nosocomial pneumonia particularly in debilitated, ventilator-dependent individuals.
- **Surgical wound infections:** *Proteus* species can cause serious postoperative wound infections, either alone or as part of a polymicrobial infection, particularly in contaminated abdominal wounds.
- **Chronic destructive ear infections:** These organisms have been recovered in patients with a chronic, destructive otitis media similar to necrotizing otitis caused by *Pseudomonas aeruginosa*. This entity can involve the mastoids and central nervous system.
- **Septicemia:** Debilitated hospitalized patients can develop a life-threatening *Proteus* septicemia, most often from a urinary source. Other common origins include biliary tract sepsis (*Proteus* sp are part of the normal fecal flora), abdominal abscesses, catheter-associated bacteremia, and others.

Diagnosis The diagnosis of *P. mirabilis* infection is made by isolation of the organism from appropriate body fluids (urine, sputum, blood, etc). No special culture isolation methods are necessary; *Proteus* species grow readily in standard blood cultures and on solid media. The finding of chronic urinary tract infection in the setting of struvite stones is highly suggestive of *Proteus mirabilis* infection; particularly if there is a consistently high urinary pH.

Diagnostic Tests/Procedures

Aerobic Culture, Appropriate Site *on page 244*
Gram Stain *on page 352*

Treatment The treatment of *Proteus* infections depends in part on the species involved. *Proteus mirabilis* (indole-negative *Proteus*) was once generally susceptible to most beta-lactams, cephalosporins, and aminoglycosides, but increasing numbers of community-acquired isolates are becoming resistant to these agents. Final antimicrobial selection should be based on antibiotic susceptibility tests. Indole-positive *Proteus* species (including *Proteus vulgaris*) are more commonly hospital-acquired strains and tend to be more antibiotic-resistant than *P. mirabilis*. Multiple beta-lactam resistant *Proteus* strains are becoming more common, as are aminoglycoside-resistant strains; antimicrobial susceptibility testing is crucial in the proper selection of treatment for hospital-acquired *Proteus* infections.

Drug Therapy

Recommended

Cephalosporins, 3rd Generation *on page 528*

Alternate

Imipenem/Cilastatin *on page 586*
Penicillins, Extended Spectrum *on page 637*

Selected Readings

Eisenstein BI, "Diseases Caused by Gram-Negative Enteric Bacilli," *Harrison's Principles of Internal Medicine*, 13th ed, Isselbacher KJ, Braunwald E, Wilson JD, et al, eds, New York, NY: McGraw-Hill Inc, 1994, 664.

Pseudomonas aeruginosa

Microbiology *Pseudomonas aeruginosa* is a lactose-negative, oxidase-positive, nonfermenting, aerobic, gram-negative bacillus with a single flagellum (usually). Strains that produce polysaccharide capsules (glycocalyx) are mucoid in colony appearance, with some strains producing diffusible blue, yellow, or brown pigments (pyocyanin, fluorescein, pyorubin, respectively). *Pseudomonas aeruginosa* can grow on almost all laboratory media at temperatures from 10°C to 40°C. (Optimal growth is at 35°C.)

Epidemiology *Pseudomonas aeruginosa* is ubiquitous; therefore, isolation of the organism on hospital equipment, sinks, etc, is not unexpected and by itself not meaningful. *Pseudomonas aeruginosa* is often considered an opportunistic pathogen because disease occurs most often in patients with neutropenia or neutrophil dysfunction, tissue damage, or other altered host defenses. Presence of *Pseudomonas aeruginosa* in clinical specimens may be contamination or colonization unless accompanied by a correlating clinical scenario.

In the hospital setting, up to 90% of patients staying in intensive care units for more than 7 days may become colonized with *P. aeruginosa*. In some burn centers, up to 30% of infections can be attributed to *P. aeruginosa*. *Pseudo-*

(Continued)

Pseudomonas aeruginosa (Continued)

monas aeruginosa is also responsible for approximately 10% of nosocomial infections.

Clinical Syndromes *Pseudomonas aeruginosa* can infect any tissue or organ system including blood, lung, heart, ear, eye, urinary tract, gastrointestinal tract, or musculoskeletal system. Syndromes caused by *Pseudomonas aeruginosa* are usually indistinguishable from those caused by the Enterobacteriaceae with several exceptions. Patients with bacteremia or pneumonia caused by *Pseudomonas aeruginosa* have a higher mortality rate that when caused by the Enterobacteriaceae. *Pseudomonas aeruginosa* is the second most common organism infecting burn patients. Malignant otitis externa is characteristically caused by *P. aeruginosa*.

Diagnosis The only way a diagnosis of *Pseudomonas aeruginosa* infection can be made is by identification of the organism through culture in a patient with a relevant clinical syndrome. No special media or conditions are necessary to grow this organism.

Diagnostic Tests/Procedures
Aerobic Culture, Appropriate Site *on page 244*
Gram Stain *on page 352*

Treatment Combination of an antipseudomonal penicillin or ceftazidime plus an aminoglycoside is the standard therapy. Combination therapy is necessary for additive or synergistic affects as well as potentially decreasing the emergence of resistant pseudomonal strains. Combination therapy improves outcome in patients with *Pseudomonas aeruginosa* bacteremia. Quinolones and imipenem are active against *Pseudomonas aeruginosa* and should also be used in combination with aminoglycosides in the treatment of serious infection. Quinolones may be used with an antipseudomonal beta-lactam in the treatment of serious *Pseudomonas aeruginosa* infections; in theory, the different mechanisms of action of the two drug classes should be at least additive. Double beta-lactam therapy should be avoided.

Pediatric Drug Therapy
Recommended
Urinary tract infection
Ceftazidime *on page 520*
Penicillins, Extended Spectrum *on page 637*

Adult Drug Therapy
Recommended
Severe infection
Ceftazidime *on page 520*
used in combination with
Aminoglycosides *on page 489*
or
Penicillins, Extended Spectrum *on page 637*
used in combination with
Aminoglycosides *on page 489*
or
Imipenem/Cilastatin *on page 586*
used in combination with
Aminoglycosides *on page 489*
Urinary tract infection
Ciprofloxacin Hydrochloride *on page 537*

Alternate
Urinary tract infection
Ceftazidime *on page 520*
Penicillins, Extended Spectrum *on page 637*

Selected Readings
Bisbe J, Gatell JM, Puig J, et al, "*Pseudomonas aeruginosa* Bacteremia: Univariate and Multivariate Analyses of Factors Influencing the Prognosis in 133 Episodes," *Rev Infect Dis*, 1988, 10(3):629-35.

Griffith SJ, Nathan C, Selander RK, et al, "The Epidemiology of *Pseudomonas aeruginosa* in Oncology Patients in a General Hospital," *J Infect Dis*, 1989, 160(6):1030-6.

Hilf M, Yu VL, Sharp J, et al, "Antibiotic Therapy for *Pseudomonas aeruginosa* Bacteremia: Outcome Correlations in a Prospective Study of 200 Patients," *Am J Med*, 1989, 87(5):540-5.

Mendelson MH, Gartman A, Szabo S, et al, "*Pseudomonas aeruginosa* Bacteremia in Patients With AIDS," *Clin Infect Dis*, 1994, 18(6):886-95.

Murray PR, Drew WL, Kobayashi GS, et al, eds, "Pseudomonadaceae," *Medical Microbiology*, St Louis, MO: CV Mosby Co, 1990, 119-26.

Pollack M, "*Pseudomonas aeruginosa*," *Principles and Practice of Infectious Diseases*, 4th ed, Mandell GL, Bennett JE, and Dolin R, eds, New York, NY: Churchill Livingstone 1995, 1980-2003.

Widmer AF, Wenzel RP, Trilla A, et al, "Outbreak of *Pseudomonas aeruginosa* Infections in a Surgical Intensive Care Unit: Probable Transmission Via Hands of a Health Care Worker," *Clin Infect Dis*, 1993, 16(3):372-6.

Zwadyk P, "*Pseudomonas*," *Zinsser Microbiology*, 20th ed, Joklik WK, Willett HP, Amos DB, et al, eds, Norwalk, CT: Appleton & Lange, 1992, 576-83.

Rabies Virus
Related Information
Animal and Human Bites Guidelines *on page 736-739*
Immunization Guidelines *on page 710-717*
Vaccines *on page 706-709*

Microbiology Rabies virus is a bullet-shaped single-stranded RNA virus which belongs to the family Rhabdoviridae. A number of important viral proteins have been identified such as viral polymerase, nucleocapsid protein, glycoprotein, and others. Some of these proteins have been used to develop specific diagnostic monoclonal antibodies. Rabies virus can be isolated under the proper conditions in tissue culture. During active rabies infection, the virus can be cultured from a variety of human (and animal) tissues including saliva, brain tissue, respiratory secretions, and urine; the virus is most easily recovered from brain tissue.

The virus is highly neurotropic. When a human is inoculated with rabies virus, the viral glycoprotein attaches to the plasma membrane of cells, possibly the nicotinic acetylcholine receptor. The virus then replicates in skeletal muscle, and when the titer is high enough, it invades nearby sensory and motor nerves and enters the nervous system. It travels along the axon at speeds up to 20 mm/day and eventually reaches the spinal cord. From there, dissemination through the central nervous system occurs rapidly and encephalitis ensues. Other peripheral nerves become involved; the organism can be recovered from the saliva due to infection of nerves in the salivary glands.

Epidemiology Rabies remains primarily a disease of animals, not humans. In many areas of Asia, Africa, and Latin America, canine rabies is poorly controlled, and dogs account for up to 90% of animal rabies cases. In contrast, in Europe and the United States, dogs account for a much lower percentage of cases. In the United States, different species of animals are involved in well-defined geographic areas. For example, raccoons are important in two regions, the eastern seaboard states (New York, New Jersey, Delaware, Maryland, Virginia) and some southeastern states (Florida, South Carolina, Georgia, Alabama). Skunks predominate in the north central states and California, gray foxes in Texas and Arizona, and coyotes in southern Texas. A total of ten distinct geographic areas in the United States have been identified; one terrestrial animal predominates and one antigenic variant of the rabies virus predominates. Bats remain an important reservoir of rabies and cause sporadic cases.

Human rabies is distinctly unusual in the United States although it is still problematic in some areas worldwide. In large part, this is due to the control of canine rabies in this country. Between 1980 and 1993, there were 18 reported cases of rabies in the United States with 10 of these acquired outside the country. Of the rabies cases reported since 1960, the great majority involved males younger than 16 years of age or older than 50 years of age. Most cases in the United States are now reported from the following groups:

- U.S. travelers to foreign countries who sustain a dog bite in a rabies-endemic region
- persons bitten by wild animals in the U.S.
- persons with unknown exposure history

A few cases of "nonbite rabies" have been reported. These include:
- laboratory exposure to rabies virus (aerosolized virus)
- rabies contracted from corneal transplant from an infected donor (4 cases)
- inhalation of aerosolized virus in caves with high concentrations of bat secretions (rare)
- contact of virus on mucous membranes, scratches, or eyes (rare)

Clinical Syndromes
Clinical rabies: There is a variable period of incubation before the onset of symptoms (4 days to 19 years), but most cases occur within 1 year of exposure. The initial prodrome of rabies is nonspecific with malaise, fatigue, and fever. In many patients, there may be pain at the initial exposure site. After about 10 days, the patient enters an acute neurologic phase, characterized

(Continued)

ORGANISMS

Rabies Virus *(Continued)*

by bizarre behavior, hyperactivity, and confusion. A small stimulus can elicit short periods of thrashing, biting, and other behaviors. Many patients will display hydrophobia (fear of water); there is often severe laryngospasm and choking when trying to drink water. This will progress to paralysis, which dominates the clinical picture for some days. Patients typically lapse into coma and develop respiratory failure or arrhythmias, leading to death in most cases despite full support in intensive care units. Occasional cases of recovery from rabies have been reported.

Diagnosis Currently, there are no tests available to detect rabies prior to the development of symptoms. The virus is felt to be immunologically "protected" in the muscle cells or nerve cells near the inoculation site, and antibody production occurs late in infection. Rabies encephalitis may be difficult to distinguish from other forms of viral encephalitis. Laboratory tests available include:

- rabies neutralizing antibody
- rabies viral culture of saliva, cerebrospinal fluid, urine, respiratory secretions
- brain biopsy – specimens may be submitted for rabies viral culture; immunofluorescent rabies antibody staining of brain cells; and pathologic examination for Negri bodies, which are cytoplasmic inculsions characteristic of rabies encephalitis seen in 20% to 30% of cases.

Diagnostic Tests/Procedures

Brain Biopsy *on page 285*
Rabies *on page 433*

Treatment There is currently no treatment for rabies once it has become clinically established. Mortality approaches 100%. Thus, the main treatment issues involve rabies prevention, particularly postexposure prophylaxis. The physician deciding whether or not to initiate rabies treatment (rabies vaccine, rabies immunoglobulin) must answer the following questions: Has a significant exposure occurred, and what is the risk that an animal is rabid?

A significant exposure includes the following.

- An animal bite, defined as penetration of the person's skin by teeth with contamination of the wound with saliva
- Contamination of the mucous membranes with saliva or other potentially infectious tissue from an infected animal
- Certain nonbite exposures, including contamination of scratches, scrapes, wounds, or mucous membranes with saliva or other infectious tissues. The risk of rabies after nonbite exposures is extremely rare, although scattered cases have been reported.

Petting a rabid animal or contacting its blood or body fluids is not an exposure. If it appears that a significant exposure has taken place, the physician must determine whether or not the animal was rabid. As outlined by Fishbein and Robinson, this depends on the percentage of animals found to be rabid in the species in the particular geographical area.

Group 1: Rabies is endemic in animal species involved in exposure. This includes:

- bats – anywhere in the United States (3% to 20% positive for rabies)
- terrestrial animals – skunks, raccoons, foxes in areas of United States where rabies is endemic
- dogs in developing countries
- dogs in the United States along the Mexican border.

For Group 1 exposure, treatment should be initiated for both bite and nonbite exposures.

Group 2: Rabies is not endemic in species involved but is endemic in other wild animals in the area. The risk of rabies is about ten times lower in these animals compared with the predominant species. These animals include:

- wild carnivores such as wolves, bobcats, bears, and groundhogs. Up to 20% may have rabies. Bite exposures from these should be treated. Nonbite exposures should either be treated or the local health department consulted.
- rodents (squirrels, hamsters, guinea pigs, gerbils, rats, mice) have a low incidence of rabies, 0.01%. Bite exposures should not be treated (or in exceptional cases, the local health department could be consulted). Nonbite exposures should not be treated.
- dogs and cats – in the United States, the risk of rabies in dogs is less than 1% (except along the Mexican border) in areas where rabies is

common in other land animals. In addition, dogs almost always show signs of clinical rabies shortly after the virus is present in saliva. Bite exposure should not be treated if a healthy dog (or cat) is captured; the animal should be observed for 10 days. If the animal develops signs of rabies, treatment in the human should be commenced immediately. If the animal is a stray, it should be sacrificed immediately and the head removed and shipped to an appropriate laboratory. Treatment is delayed pending laboratory testing. The same approach is recommended for nonbite exposures.

Group 3: Rabies is not endemic in the animal species involved in the exposure and is uncommon in other wild animals in the region. This incudes most domestic cats and dogs and wild land animals in Idaho, Washington, Utah, Nevada, and Colorado, where the proportion of rabid animals is very low. For bite or nonbite exposures from Group 3 animals, either consult the local health department or do not treat.

Postexposure treatment consists of:

1. Vigorous wound cleaning – this has been shown to decrease the risk of rabies.
2. Administration or rabies vaccine, either human diploid-cell rabies vaccine or rabies vaccine adsorbed. For persons not previously vaccinated, rabies vaccine should be given 1 mL I.M. on days 0, 3, 7, 14, and 28. Abbreviated regimens have been described. For persons previously vaccinated, the rabies vaccine should be given 1 mL I.M. on days 0 and 3.
3. Administration of rabies immunoglobulin. For persons not previously vaccinated, this should be given at 20 IU/kg of body weight. If possible, one-half the dose should be injected locally near the original wound and the rest given I.M. (using a new needle). For persons previously vaccinated, rabies immunoglobulin is not recommended.

Selected Readings

Centers for Disease Control, "Human Rabies – Texas and California, 1993," *MMWR Morb Mortal Wkly Rep*, 1994, 43(6):93-6.

Fishbein DB and Bernard KW, "Rabies Virus," *Principles and Practice of Infectious Diseases*, 4th ed, Mandell GL, Bennett JE, and Dolin R, eds, New York, NY: Churchill Livingstone, 1995, 1527-43.

Fishbein DB and Robinson LE, "Rabies," *N Engl J Med*, 1993, 329(22):1632-8.

Respiratory Syncytial Virus

Synonyms RSV

Microbiology Respiratory syncytial virus (RSV) is the most common cause of bronchiolitis and pneumonia in infants and children. It is also emerging as a pathogen of the elderly and the immunosuppressed.

RSV is a single-stranded, enveloped RNA virus belonging to the family Paramyxoviridae, and comprises its own genus, *Pneumovirus*. The viral genome codes for at least 10 separate genes. The virus lacks neuraminidase or hemagglutinating activity, which differentiates it from other paramyxoviruses, such as parainfluenza and mumps virus. There are two major subgroups of RSV, group A or B, based on the presence of different surface glycoprotein antigens. The clinical significance of this strain variation is still unknown. RSV is rarely isolated from asymptomatic children and is thus not part of the normal flora.

As with other pathogenic viruses, RSV requires a tissue culture system in the laboratory to support its growth. Clinical specimens can be successfully inoculated onto a variety of cell lines. Of note, live virus from patient secretions can survive for a period of time on environmental surfaces. On a nonporous surface such as a countertop, the virus is still viable up to 7 hours. On a porous surface such as tissue paper or clothing, survival is decreased to about 1 hour.

Epidemiology Infections with RSV are common worldwide, regardless of climate. There is a definite seasonal occurrence to RSV infections, tending to occur almost exclusively in the winter and spring in temperate climates; in temperate climates there is a sharp peak in colder months. In many communities, RSV outbreaks occur every year without fail and often in a very predictable pattern, and at its peak in a season, RSV dominates influenza and other respiratory viruses. Based on studies to determine the prevalence of specific RSV antibody, it appears that nearly all children have been infected with RSV before entering school. Estimates of the attack rates vary according to age. In children younger than 2 years of age, the attack rate for lower respiratory infections was from 9-23 out of 1000, from 2-3 years old it was 7-15 out of 1000, and in the 4-5 year age group, it was 5-8 out of 1000. However, the attack rate for all forms of infection including mild infections is probably much higher based

(Continued)

Respiratory Syncytial Virus *(Continued)*

on prospective studies, with some studies estimating 6 per 100. The attack rate is extremely high in day care centers, approaching 100%.

Recurrent infections with RSV are the rule. With each episode of clinical illness, progressively milder forms of infection are seen. Specific neutralizing antibodies develop (IgG, IgM, and secretory IgA) but are not protective. The reason for this is unclear and is not explained by differences in RSV serotypes.

Transmission can be by several routes: self-inoculation of the eyes or nares following contact with contaminated secretions; self-inoculation following contact with contaminated fomites; aerosol spread, when infected individuals are coughing or sneezing (large droplet spread only).

Clinical Syndromes

In children, the major manifestations of RSV include:

- **Upper respiratory infection:** This often mimics the common cold, along with significant fever and profuse rhinorrhea. Typically, lower respiratory infections are preceded by several days of upper tract symptoms.
- **Bronchiolitis:** This is one of the most common manifestations of RSV and is particularly prevalent in infants 2-6 months of age. It is characterized by wheezing, cough, and tachypnea (sometimes 80 breaths per minute) reflecting the hallmark inspiratory and expiratory obstruction of the lower respiratory tract in bronchiolitis. Fever of 38°C to 40°C is common. Chest radiographs may reveal infiltrates, but these are felt to be due to atelectasis and not alveolar consolidation. Most recover spontaneously or with supportive care only, although 1% to 2% may require hospitalization. Bronchiolitis is difficult to separate from pneumonia, and some may have both.
- **Pneumonia:** The presentation of RSV pneumonia is similar to bronchiolitis. Lower respiratory infection in young children is estimated to complicate up to 70% of RSV infections. Chest radiograph abnormalities vary from interstitial infiltrates to consolidation (usually upper and/or middle lobes). Hyperinflation is common. The radiographic findings, however, are not distinctive enough to differentiate RSV pneumonia from other infectious causes of pneumonia, including bacterial pathogens. Fatalities are still uncommon with the notable exception of children with underlying congenital heart disease, pulmonary disease, or compromised immune system.
- **Croup:** RSV is an uncommon cause of croup, accounting for about 5% to 10% of croup cases .
- **Otitis media:** This is quite common in infants. Otitis media may be either primary infection (with symptoms localized to the ear only) or may be secondary to RSV infection elsewhere (usually in the lower respiratory tract).
- **Apnea and the sudden infant death syndrome (SIDS):** Infants with lower respiratory tract infections with RSV have frequent apneic episodes but are self-resolving. Although the cause of SIDS is still unknown, RSV and other respiratory viruses have been implicated due to the frequent recovery of these pathogens from the lungs of infants with SIDS.

Infections in adults:

- **Upper respiratory tract infections:** In adults, RSV commonly causes an upper respiratory infection somewhat more severe than the common cold. Nasal congestion and cough are prominent, and symptoms may be prolonged, lasting over 1 week. Otalgia is less common in adults. Episodes are self-resolving, but the severity of the URI may cause some to be bedridden for several days.
- **Lower respiratory tract infection:** Tracheobronchitis and pneumonia are relatively uncommon in the otherwise healthy adult. In the elderly patient or the individual with chronic bronchitis, pneumonia can be quite fulminant and clinically mimics the disease as seen in infants. Outbreaks of RSV in the elderly are associated with a high incidence of pneumonia, perhaps up to 50%.
- **Nosocomial infection:** RSV is an important cause of nosocomial viral respiratory infections, both in adults and children. This is particularly problematic in pediatric wards where children are hospitalized during an outbreak of RSV; the virus spreads efficiently to the adult staff with nearly 50% infected.

Diagnosis RSV infection is suspected when there is a compatible clinical presentation, particularly in the setting of a known community outbreak. In the infant and young child, the diagnosis is often made clinically during an outbreak, with microbiologic confirmation reserved for serious or atypical cases. In the adult, RSV infection mimics other viral and bacterial causes of respiratory illness. Routine laboratory studies such as the complete blood count and electrolyte panel are not helpful in making the diagnosis. Microbiological confirmation of RSV is generally unnecessary for mild upper respiratory infections but may be useful in suspected lower respiratory infections or infections in the immunocompromised host. Potentially this may avoid unnecessary antibiotics or invasive diagnostic testing.

There are several laboratory methods available:
1. Viral culture: RSV grows best in continuous cell lines of human origin, such as HEp-2 cells. The virus causes a characteristic cytopathic effect in the cell lines, syncytial formation, from which its name is derived. Culture results may not be available for several days.
2. Direct fluorescent antibody (DFA) detection: This rapid method can detect the presence of RSV in specimens within hours but requires a specimen with cellular material.
3. Enzyme immunoassays (EIA): Another rapid test with results available on the same day.
4. Serologic studies: A fourfold rise in titer of specific antibody to RSV is diagnostic but not useful for immediate diagnosis or treatment.

Diagnostic Tests/Procedures
Respiratory Syncytial Virus Antigen by EIA *on page 435*
Respiratory Syncytial Virus Culture *on page 436*
Respiratory Syncytial Virus Serology *on page 436*

Treatment Treatment is generally supportive, with supplemental oxygen and fluid replacement as needed. Most mild to moderate cases are self-resolving. Severe cases in infants have been treated with the antiviral agent ribavirin, administered as an aerosol. Ribavirin has been shown to improve arterial blood gas values in hypoxic infants, but improvement in mortality or duration of hospitalization has not been demonstrated.

Drug Therapy
Recommended
Ribavirin *on page 660*

Selected Readings
Englund JA, Sullivan CJ, Jordan MC, et al, "Respiratory Syncytial Virus Infection in Immunocompromised Adults," *Ann Intern Med*, 1988, 109(3):203-8.
Smith DW, Frankel LR, Mathers LH, et al, "A Controlled Trial of Aerosolized Ribavirin in Infants Receiving Mechanical Ventilation for Severe Respiratory Syncytial Virus Infection," *N Engl J Med*, 1991, 325(1):24-9.

Rickettsia rickettsii

Microbiology *Rickettsia rickettsii* is the etiologic agent of Rocky Mountain spotted fever (RMSF). The organism is a small coccobacillus measuring 0.2-0.5 μm by 0.3-2.0 μm. It is an obligate intracellular bacteria. The organism can be identified in smears of infected tissue using the Gimenez method, by acridine orange, or by immunofluorescence in tissue sections. The organism does not stain well by Gram stain. The spotted fever group includes other rickettsial species that are human pathogens, specifically *R. sibirica*, the etiologic agent of North Asian tick typhus, *R. conorii*, the etiologic agent of boutonneuse fever, *R. akari*, the etiologic agent of rickettsialpox, and *R. australis*, the etiologic agent of Queensland tick typhus. The cell walls of these organisms contain lipopolysaccharide and ultrastructurally resemble those of gram-negative rods. They cannot be grown in a cell-free medium but can be isolated in cell culture.

Epidemiology Rocky Mountain spotted fever is transmitted by a tick bite. The tick serves as both vector and main reservoir for the disease. *Dermacentor andersoni* (Rocky Mountain wood tick) and *D. variabilis* (American dog tick) are the main vectors in the United States. The tick transmits *Rickettsia* to humans during feeding. The initial bite may not be symptomatic and is frequently not recommended. Infection may occur as the organisms are released from the ticks salivary gland after 4-6 hours of feeding or when the tick is crushed in an attempt to remove it from the skin. The disease is seen primarily in late spring and summer. In the southeast, most cases are observed in children; while in the western states, adults who work in forestry and related industry have the highest incidence of infection. Incidence is related to tick exposure. There have been few western cases in recent years.

Clinical Syndromes The symptoms of Rocky Mountain spotted fever (RMSF) appear 2-14 days after exposure. There is sudden onset of moderate to high fever, myalgia, severe headache, chills, and conjunctival injection. Abdominal
(Continued)

183

Rickettsia rickettsii (Continued)

symptoms which may include nausea, pain, vomiting, diarrhea, and tenderness are sometimes present. Young patients may not complain of pain. The hallmark rash is maculopapular, appearing on the extremities by the third day and involving the palms and soles of the feet thereafter. Frequently the rash is generalized. Ultimately more than 90% of patients develop a rash. Late onset or "spotless" fever may delay diagnosis. RMSF without a rash occurs more frequently in blacks and adult patients. The cases are more frequently fatal in blacks than whites, in males, and in adults. Age, glucose-6-phosphate dehydrogenase deficiency, and alcoholism are predispositions to fatal outcome. The organisms target the vascular endothelium. The damaged endothelial cells increase vascular permeability with resultant edema, hypovolemia, hypoalbuminemia, and hypotension. The local vascular injuries consume platelets with resultant thrombocytopenia, although clinical DIC is rare. Lung, kidney, CNS, GI tract, pancreas, and skeletal muscle may be symptomatically involved. The case fatality rate is 15% to 20% if specific therapy is not instituted. Overall reported mortality has been about 4% in recent years.

Diagnosis Diagnosis is based on clinical signs and symptoms. Cutaneous biopsy direct immunofluorescence to identify *R. rickettsii* in tissue is available in some institutions. Specific serologic tests confirm the diagnosis. The Weil-Felix test which relies upon cross reaction with the *Proteus* OX-19 and OX-2 antigens is nonspecific and not reliable. Culture is usually not attempted because of technical demands and the extreme infection risk to laboratory workers.

Diagnostic Tests/Procedures
Rocky Mountain Spotted Fever Serology *on page 437*
Skin Biopsy, Immunofluorescence *on page 446*

Duration of Therapy 7 days or at least 2 days after the patient becomes afebrile

Treatment Patients with severe systemic symptoms should receive supportive therapy. Pulmonary edema caused by extravasation of fluid into the alveolar spaces requires careful management as does overall fluid volume. Doxycycline and tetracycline are considered the drugs of choice. Chloramphenicol is used in pregnant women to avoid the effects of tetracycline on fetal teeth and bones. Chloramphenicol is also favored for children younger than 7 years of age. Dosages are:
Tetracycline, oral: 25-50 μg/kg/day
Doxycycline, oral: 100 μg every 12 hours
Chloramphenicol: 50-75 μg/kg/day in 4 divided doses administered every 6 hours
Ciprofloxacin, oral: 250-750 μg every 12 hours

The use of erythromycin, β-lactams, aminoglycosides, and co-trimoxazole is not indicated.

Pediatric Drug Therapy
Recommended
<7 years
Chloramphenicol *on page 531*
>7 years
Doxycycline *on page 557*
Tetracycline *on page 679*

Alternate
>7 years
Chloramphenicol *on page 531*

Adult Drug Therapy
Recommended
Doxycycline *on page 557*
Tetracycline *on page 679*

Alternate
Chloramphenicol *on page 531*
Ciprofloxacin Hydrochloride *on page 537*

Selected Readings
Salgo MP, Telzak EE, Currie B, et al, "A Focus of Rocky Mountain Spotted Fever Within New York City," *N Engl J Med*, 1988, 318(21):1345-8.
Woodward TE, "Rickettsial Diseases," *Harrison's Principles and Practice of Internal Medicine*, 13th ed, Isselbacher KJ, Braunwald E, Wilson JD, et al, eds, New York, NY: McGraw-Hill, 1994, 747-57.

Rochalimaea Species *see Bartonella* Species *on page 62*

Rotavirus

Microbiology Rotavirus is a double-stranded, nonenveloped RNA virus with two icosahedral capsids which make the virus appear as a wheel (Latin: rota) when viewed with an electron microscope. Rotavirus can be cultured but only in special cell cultures and only by special procedures. Therefore, routine culture of rotavirus is not practical. The traditional rotavirus ("typical" rotavirus) occurs worldwide, usually produces disease in young children, has a common group inner capsid antigen (VP6), and is called group A rotavirus. Nongroup A rotaviruses (groups G through F; "atypical" rotavirus) are newly described. Group B rotavirus is clinically important only in China; group C rotavirus in swine.

Epidemiology Rotaviruses are ubiquitous and are found in all parts of the world. Rotaviruses occur year round in tropical climates and mostly in the winter months in temperate climates. Rotaviruses infect humans and most animals. The most common age group affected by rotaviruses is 6 months to 2 years. Most rotaviruses which are clinically important are members of group A. Rotaviruses primarily are spread by the fecal-oral route. The incubation period for rotaviruses is less than 2 days in infants and 2-4 days in adults. Maximum shedding of rotaviruses occurs 2-5 days after the onset of diarrhea. Infant mortality due to rotavirus infection in developing countries is extremely high; in developed countries, mortality is rare. Rotavirus usually does not cause chronic disease.

Clinical Syndromes Rotavirus can cause asymptomatic to fatal disease. The most common form of rotavirus infection is sudden onset of vomiting and diarrhea. Common clinical presentations include vomiting, abdominal pain, diarrhea, and dehydration. Fever is present in ca. 50% of the cases. Rotavirus disease usually lasts 3-9 days, and hospitalization often is required. Nosocomial infections and epidemics are not uncommon.

Diagnosis Rotavirus should be in the differential diagnosis of any newborn or young child with the aforementioned clinical presentations or other form of gastroenteritis. Visualization of rotavirus by electron microscopy is considered by many experts to be the standard method of laboratory diagnosis, but the method is expensive and not widely available. Enzyme immunoassay (EIA) and latex agglutination (LA) are much more widely available and used. Detection of rotavirus antigen by EIA is by far the most practical and cost-efficient method. EIA probably is at least as sensitive as electron microscopy and is a highly recommended method.

Diagnostic Tests/Procedures
Electron Microscopic (EM) Examination for Viruses, Stool *on page 329*
Rotavirus, Direct Detection *on page 437*

Drug Therapy Comment
No antiviral agents proven effective.

Selected Readings
Christensen ML, "Human Viral Gastroenteritis," *Clin Microbiol Rev*, 1989, 2(1):51-89.
Gray LG, "Novel Viruses Associated with Gastroenteritis," *Clin Microbiol Newslett*, 1991, 13:137-40.
Offit PA and Clark HF, "Rotavirus," *Principles and Practice of Infectious Diseases*, 4th ed, Mandell GL, Bennett JE, and Dolin R, eds, New York, NY: Churchill Livingstone, 1995, 1448-55.

RSV *see* Respiratory Syncytial Virus *on page 181*
Rubeola Virus *see* Measles Virus *on page 145*

Salmonella Species
Related Information
Timing of Food Poisoning *on page 723*
Microbiology *Salmonella* species are gram-negative bacilli which are important causes of bacterial gastroenteritis, septicemia, and a nonspecific febrile illness called typhoid fever. Unfortunately, the classification system for the different *Salmonella* species is complex and confusing to most clinicians. Over 2000 separate serotypes have been identified, and, in the past and currently, each is named as if it was a species. Most experts agree that there are seven distinct subgroups of *Salmonella* (1, 2, 3a, 3b, 4, 5, and 6) each of which contain many serotypes ("species"). The main pathogens in humans are serotypes, *S. choleraesuis*, *S. typhi*, and *S. paratyphi* (all in subgroup 1).

Salmonella is an aerobic gram-negative bacillus in the family Enterobacteriaceae. It is almost always associated with disease when isolated from hu-
(Continued)

185

Salmonella Species *(Continued)*

mans, and is not considered part of the normal human flora. As with other members of this family, *Salmonella* carries the endotoxin lipopolysaccharide on its outer membrane, which is released upon cell lysis.

Epidemiology It is estimated that about 3 million new cases of salmonellosis occur each year. *Salmonella* species are found worldwide. Many are easily recovered from animals such as chickens, birds, livestock, rodents, and reptiles (turtles). Some serotypes cause disease almost exclusively in man (*S. typhi*) while others are primarily seen in animals but can cause severe disease when infecting humans (*S. choleraesuis*). Transmission is via ingestion of contaminated materials, particularly raw fruits and vegetables, oysters and other shellfish, and contaminated water. Eggs, poultry, and other dairy products are important sources. Outbreaks have been described in the summer months where children consume contaminated egg salad. Other outbreaks have been associated with pet turtles, other pets, marijuana, and, rarely, food handlers. The incubation period is about 1-3 weeks. The period of communicability lasts until all *Salmonella* have been eradicated from the stool or urine.

Clinical infection is favored when there is a high inoculum of bacteria in the ingested food, since experimental models suggest that 10^6 bacteria are needed for clinical disease. Contaminated food improperly refrigerated will allow such multiplication. Host factors are important and disease is more likely in immunocompromised individuals, sickle cell disease, or achlorhydria (gastric acid decreases the viable bacterial inoculum). Although salmonellosis can occur at any age, children are most commonly infected.

Clinical Syndromes The following are the major syndromes associated with salmonellosis. It should be emphasized that these syndromes are often overlapping.

• **Gastroenteritis:** The most common manifestation of *Salmonella* infection. After ingestion of contaminated food, the bacteria are absorbed in the terminal portion of the small intestine. The organisms then penetrate into the lamina propria of the ileocecal area. Following this, there is reticuloendothelial hypertrophy with usually a brisk host immune response. As the organisms multiply in the lymphoid follicles, polymorphonuclear leukocytes attempt to limit the infection. There is release of prostaglandins and other mediators, which stimulates cyclic AMP. This results in intestinal fluid secretion which is nonbloody. Clinically, the patient complains of nausea, vomiting, and diarrhea from several hours to several days after consumption of contaminated food. Other symptoms include fever, malaise, muscle aches, and abdominal pain. Symptoms usually resolve from several days to 1 week, even without antibiotics.

• **Sepsis syndrome:** Patients may present in flora sepsis, indistinguishable from other forms of gram-negative sepsis. Fever, confusion, hypotension, end-organ damage, and poor perfusion may all be seen. *Salmonella* bacteremia may lead to multiple metastatic foci, such as liver abscess, osteomyelitis (particularly with sickle cell disease); septic arthritis, and endocarditis. Mycotic aneurysms may develop following bacteremia, and *Salmonella* is a leading cause of infected aortic aneurysms. Bacteremia is also common in AIDS and repeated relapses with *Salmonella* are common, despite prolonged antibiotics.

• **Typhoid fever:** Also known as enteric fever, this febrile illness is caused classically by *S. typhi*. Following ingestion of the bacteria, the organisms pass into the ileocecal area where intraluminal multiplication occurs. There is a mononuclear host cell response, but the organisms remain viable within the macrophages. The bacteria are carried to the organs of the reticuloendothelial system (spleen, liver, bone marrow) by the macrophages and clinical signs of infection become apparent. Patients complain of insidious onset of fever, myalgias, headache, malaise, and constipation, corresponding to this phase of bacteremia. A pulse-temperature dissociation may be present. A characteristic rash may be seen in about 50% of patients, called "rose spots", which are 2-4 mm pink maculopapular lesions that blanch with pressure, usually on the trunk. Symptoms last for 1 or more weeks. During this time, bacteria multiply in the mesenteric lymphoid tissue, and these areas eventually exhibit necrosis and bleeding. There are microperforations of the abdominal wall. *Salmonella* spreads from the liver through the gallbladder and eventually back into the intestines. This phase of intestinal reinfection is characterized by prominent gastrointestinal symptoms including diarrhea. Overall, fatality with treatment is less than 2%. A similar, but milder syndrome, can occur with *S. paratyphi*, called paratyphoid fever.

ORGANISMS

- **Chronic carrier state:** Following infection with *S. typhi*, up to 5% of patients will excrete the bacteria for over 1 year. Such patients are termed chronic carriers and are asymptomatic. Millions of viable bacteria are present in the biliary tree and are shed into the bile and into the feces. Urinary carriage can also occur, particularly in patients who are co-infected with *Schistosoma haematobium*. The chronic carrier state is less important for other *Salmonella* species, where the carriage rate is less than 1%.

Diagnosis Laboratory confirmation is generally required, since the major syndromes are seldom distinctive enough to be diagnosed solely on clinical criteria. *Salmonella* grows readily on most media under standard aerobic conditions. Cultures from blood, joint aspirations, and cerebrospinal fluid can be plated on routine media. Specimens which are likely to contain other organisms, such as stool or sputum, require selective media, and the laboratory should be appropriately notified. Recovery of *Salmonella* from the stool is the most common means of establishing the diagnosis, and enrichment media are available to maximize the yield. Other laboratory findings may suggest salmonellosis, including a profound leukopenia often seen with typhoid fever.

Recent antimicrobial therapy may render blood and stool cultures negative. In such cases, proctoscopy with biopsy and culture of ulcerations may establish the diagnosis in the enterocolitis syndrome. Serologic tests are not particularly useful in this instance. When typhoid fever is suspected but the patient has already received antimicrobial agents, bone marrow biopsies, as well as skin biopsies of any rose spots, may yield *Salmonella typhi* in culture. Serologic studies are more helpful in diagnosing typhoid fever, but greater than 50% of patients will fail to show the expected rise in agglutinins against the typhoid O antigen.

Diagnostic Tests/Procedures
Blood Culture, Aerobic and Anaerobic *on page 271*
Bone Marrow Culture, Routine *on page 281*
Stool Culture *on page 448*

Treatment Note: *Salmonella* species resistant to multiple antimicrobials are increasing in frequency. *In vitro* susceptibility studies should be performed, particularly in severe cases. Treatment guidelines vary with the type of syndrome, as follows:

Enterocolitis: The majority of cases are self-resolving and do not need antibiotics. Clinical trials have demonstrated that a variety of antibiotics fail to influence the course of mild infections and may prolong excretion of the organisms. For severe cases, or in the immunosuppressed host, a number of antibiotics are usually effective, including ampicillin, chloramphenicol, co-trimoxazole, and third generation cephalosporins.

Typhoid fever: Cases should be treated promptly. Chloramphenicol and ampicillin are effective and have been the most extensively studied. Recent studies show that ciprofloxacin is highly active. Third generation cephalosporins and co-trimoxazole is useful in organisms that are resistant to standard agents.

Bacteremia: Ampicillin, chloramphenicol, co-trimoxazole, and third generation cephalosporins are all effective. However, chloramphenicol should be avoided in endocarditis or mycotic aneurysms. Ciprofloxacin is effective in treating recurrent *Salmonella* bacteremia in AIDS.

Chronic carriage: Ampicillin or amoxicillin for 6 weeks, although elapses are common if there is underlying gallbladder disease cholecystectomy may be an option with repeated relapses. Ciprofloxacin may also be effective.

Drug Therapy
Recommended
Cephalosporins, 3rd Generation *on page 528*
Alternate
Ampicillin *on page 495*
Co-trimoxazole *on page 545*
Chloramphenicol *on page 531*
Ciprofloxacin Hydrochloride *on page 537*

Selected Readings
Levine WC, Buehler JW, Bean NH, et al, "Epidemiology of Nontyphoidal *Salmonella* Bacteremia During the Human Immunodeficiency Virus Epidemic," *J Infect Dis*, 1991, 164(1):81-7.
"Outbreaks of *Salmonella enteritidis* Gastroenteritis – California 1993," *MMWR Morb Mortal Wkly Rep*, 1993, 42(41):793-7.

Sarcoptes scabiei

Microbiology *Sarcoptes scabiei*, or the human mite, is the causative agent of scabies, a common parasitic infestation of the skin. *Sarcoptes scabiei* is an ectoparasite of humans belonging to the class *Arachnida*. It tends to form skin "burrows" several millimeters wide within the stratum corneum of the epidermis. The fertilized female deposits its eggs in these skin burrows, and the larvae exit after several days to become adults weeks later. The adult is about 0.3 mm long.

Epidemiology Scabies is distributed worldwide. The incidence in the United States has been increasing since the 1970s. The reservoir resides in humans, although animal mites can sometimes cause brief human disease. Transmission is person to person by direct contact. Occasionally, transmission may occur when there is contact with heavily contaminated clothing or bedsheets. The incubation period varies from several days to weeks. Infected individuals remain communicable until all the ova and mites are eradicated from the skin.

Clinical Syndromes

- **Human scabies:** Patients present with intense itching, usually in the interdigital web spaces, along the "belt line," the genital region, the periumbilical area, and also on the wrists, elbows, knees, and feet. Additional areas are common in children, including the hands and face. On physical examination, the characteristic burrows may be seen, appearing linear and several millimeters wide, often in the interdigital spaces. Atypical presentations of scabies may occur, including vesicles and bullae in infants, eczematous eruptions, and urticaria. A variant known as "nodular scabies" has been described in which there are small, brown, intensely pruritic nodules usually on the penis and scrotum. An unusual manifestation of severe scabies called "Norwegian scabies" has been seen in immunocompromised individuals and patients with Down syndrome. The skin is diffusely scaling and thickened as a result of infestation of thousands of mites. Secondary bacterial infections of the skin may occur in all forms of scabies.
- **Animal scabies:** This is due to *Sarcoptes scabiei* var. *canis*, carried on some dogs. The clinical presentation is similar to human scabies although burrows are not present.

Diagnosis Infestation with scabies is often suspected when an individual presents with pruritic papules, or an otherwise compatible clinical history. Some patients may present because of a recent history of contact. It should be noted that scabies often imitates other skin lesions, and thus a broad differential diagnosis should be entertained if the linear burrows are not demonstrated. Other diagnostic considerations include impetigo, insect bites, drug eruptions, varicella, eczema, and others.

The linear burrows of the mite can be further demonstrated by applying blue ink over a possible burrow. The ink is drawn into the defect and when excess ink is wiped off with an alcohol pad, the ink within the burrow remains. This and other suspicious areas should covered with oil, the area should be scraped with a sterile blade, the scrapings should be placed into oil on a microscope slide, and the preparation should be examined with a microscope.

Diagnostic Tests/Procedures
Arthropod Identification *on page 268*

Treatment For adults and older children: Lindane 1% lotion or cream is applied to all skin areas from the neck to the toes then washed off after 8-12 hours. During the treatment period, the medication should be reapplied to the hands after routine handwashing; failure to do so may result in treatment failure since the hands are often infected. Lindane is contraindicated for pregnant or lactating women. Of note, lindane has been associated with central nervous system toxicity, particularly when an underlying skin disorder was present to allow greater than normal systemic absorption of drug. The regimen described here is generally safe. The alternative regimen is crotamiton (10%) applied as a thin smear from the neck down and left on for 1 day. A second application is done the following day, then washed off 24 hours later. Crotamiton should be used in individuals with extensive dermatitis.

For children younger than 2 years of age, infants, and pregnant women, crotamiton should be used instead of lindane. Treatment should be administered to sexual partners and close contacts in the same house. Other principles of management include cleaning all potentially contaminated clothes (dry cleaning or machine washing and drying in the hot cycle), prescribing medications for pruritus (Atarax®, diphenhydramine, topical corticosteroids and others), and treating secondary bacterial infections of the skin with antistaphylococcal antibiotics.

Drug Therapy
Recommended

Lindane *on page 599*
Permethrin *on page 640*

Schistosoma mansoni

Synonyms Blood Fluke

Microbiology *Schistosoma mansoni* also known as the blood fluke, is a common parasite in South America, the Caribbean, and Africa. The organism causes schistosomiasis (bilharziasis) with diverse clinical manifestations ranging from a mild dermatitis to a fulminant dysentery with bloody stools.

S. mansoni is a parasite classified as a trematode (fluke). As with other trematodes, it appears flat, fleshy, and has a leaf shape. There are two muscular suckers, the oral type being the beginning of an incomplete digestive system and the ventral sucker being an organ of attachment. Unlike other trematodes, *S. mansoni* is not a hermaphrodite and there are separate male and female worms. The intermediate host of *S. mansoni* is the snail, which is necessary for the parasite to complete its life cycle.

The life cycle of the organism begins when the infective forms called cercariae are liberated from the snail. These ciliated, free-swimming organisms travel through fresh water until they reach the human host. The cercariae are able to penetrate intact skin. Following this they enter the circulation and mature in the intrahepatic porta blood. During this developmental period, the parasites coat themselves with a substance that prevents the host from recognizing them immunologically. This remarkable defense explains the mechanism whereby cases of chronic infection have lasted for decades. After 3 weeks of maturation the adult migrates to the mesenteric veins, specifically the small branches of the inferior mesenteric vein near the lower colon. Fertilization occurs in these vessels and eventually eggs are released into the environment, to begin the cycle again.

Epidemiology *S. mansoni* is common in South America (Brazil, Venezuela), the Caribbean (West Indies, Puerto Rico), and Africa. Travelers or immigrants from these areas are the main source for cases seen in the United States. The reservoir for *S. mansoni* is the human, although primates, marsupials, and rodents can also serve as hosts. As noted, transmission occurs when there is skin penetration of the parasite larvae in stool-contaminated waters. The incubation period is 4-6 weeks after skin penetration. There is no defined period of communicability since the parasite is not transmitted person to person. However, ova may be recovered from stools for years.

Clinical Syndromes

- **Asymptomatic infection:** Occurs commonly.
- **Dermatitis:** Following skin penetration by the larvae, a brisk local allergic reaction may be seen, with pruritus, maculopapular lesions, and edema.
- **Cough:** when migrating worms reach the lungs.
- **Mesenteric adenitis:** When the adults begin to lay eggs in the mesenteric vessels, a febrile illness often results. There is abdominal pain, liver tenderness, and malaise. Eventually, the area may become walled off in a foreign-body type reaction, and fibrosis and abscess formation may be seen. Characteristically, there is bloody diarrhea.
- **Chronic infection:** After infection has become established, the patient over time may develop ascites, massive hepatosplenomegaly, lymphadenopathy, white granulomas on the liver called pseudotubercles. Extraintestinal infections may be seen, eggs may be recovered from the spinal cord, lungs, and other areas. Fibrosis is also seen at these other sites. Severe neurologic disease results from the presence of eggs in the spinal cord and brain.

Diagnosis Schistosomiasis is suspected in an individual who resides in an endemic area, or a traveler who has recently returned from such an area who presents with a compatible clinical history. Routine laboratory studies may be helpful, with elevated liver function tests and peripheral blood eosinophilia seen.

The stool examination is critical in confirming the diagnosis. Large eggs 115-175 μm long are seen in established cases. Rectal biopsy may also be considered if serial stool exams are negative but clinical suspicion remains high. The biopsy may reveal the egg tracks laid by the worms in the rectal vessels.

Diagnostic Tests/Procedures

Ova and Parasites, Stool *on page 416*
Ova and Parasites, Urine or Aspirates *on page 419*

(Continued)

Schistosoma mansoni (Continued)

Treatment Asymptomatic cases do not necessarily require treatment. The drugs used have potential toxicities and the situation must be weighed by the physician. The same applies to mild infections; the nature of the patient's immune status must be considered also. Moderate or severe cases respond to praziquantel.

Drug Therapy
Recommended

Praziquantel *on page 650*

Oxamniquine *on page 628*

Selected Readings

Mahmoud AA, "Trematodes (Schistosomiasis) and Other Flukes," *Principles and Practice of Infectious Diseases*, 4th ed, Mandell GL, Bennett JE, and Dolin R, eds, New York, NY: Churchill Livingstone, 1995, 2538-44.

"Schistosomiasis in U.S. Peace Corps Volunteers – Malawi, 1992," *MMWR Morb Mortal Wkly Rep*, 1993, 42(29):565-70.

Scrimgeour EM and Gajdusek DC, "Involvement of the Central Nervous System in *Schistosoma mansoni* and *S. haematobium* Infection: A Review," *Brain*, 1985, 108(Pt 4):1023-38.

Tsang VC and Wilkins PP, "Immunodiagnosis of Schistosomiasis: Screen With FAST-ELISA and Confirm With Immunoblot," *Clin Lab Med*, 1991, 11(4):1029-39.

Serratia Species

Microbiology *Serratia* species are gram-negative rods which are important causes of nosocomial infection and are only rarely associated with community-acquired infections in normal hosts.

Serratia species are moderate-sized aerobic gram-negative bacilli which belong to the large family Enterobacteriaceae. The organisms cannot be identified on the basis of morphologic appearance on Gram stain alone and are indistinguishable from other Enterobacteriaceae. *Serratia* species are related to such gram-negative bacilli as *Klebsiella*, *Enterobacter*, and *Hafnia* (all belonging to the tribe Klebsielleae). There are several distinct species of *Serratia*, but most human disease is caused by *Serratia marcescens*. Rarely, *Serratia liquefaciens* has been isolated in serious infections. Laboratory identification is generally straightforward. It is unique in that it is the only member of the Enterobacteriaceae to produce extracellular DNase. Special requests for isolation of *Serratia* are not necessary because the organism is not fastidious in its growth requirements. Most clinical isolates will exhibit growth after overnight incubation; the appearance of colonies may be delayed (or completely inhibited) if the patient is receiving antibiotic therapy. *Serratia marcescens* shares several potential virulence factors with other Enterobacteriaceae, including endotoxin, the lipopolysaccharide associated with the outer membrane of the bacteria. When cell lysis occurs (as with antibiotic therapy), the LPS is released into the host and can lead to such inflammatory responses as fever, leukopenia or leukocytosis, hypotension, and disseminated intravascular coagulation. Thus, LPS is regarded as an important mediator of the sepsis syndrome.

Epidemiology In contrast to the other members of the Enterobacteriaceae family, *Serratia* tends to colonize the respiratory and urinary tracts of hospitalized adults more so than the gastrointestinal tract. This colonization probably does not hold true for neonates, in whom the gastrointestinal tract is an important source of the organism. An outbreak of *Serratia marcescens* was reported in a neonatal intensive care unit in 1982; a gastrointestinal reservoir was found to be important. Nosocomial transmission can occur by several routes, the most frequent being hand-to-hand spread via nurses, physicians, and other health care workers. *Serratia marcescens* has also been associated with hospital outbreaks caused by contaminated respiratory equipment used for inhalational therapy, bronchoscopes, antiseptic fluids, intravenous fluids, scalp-vein needles, peritoneal dialysis catheters, and others. Community-acquired infections with *Serratia* are unusual, and the organism is mainly a nosocomial pathogen. In the 1970s, *Serratia marcescens* was identified as an important cause of endocarditis in intravenous heroin users.

Clinical Syndromes

- **Lower respiratory tract infection:** Nosocomial *Serratia* infections are seen in debilitated, ventilator-dependent patients. *Serratia* and other gram-negative bacilli can asymptomatically colonize the upper respiratory tract of hospitalized patients. Thus, the recovery of *Serratia* from a sputum or tracheal aspirate culture does not necessarily indicate a significant infection. The diagnosis of a nosocomial pneumonia still rests on standard criteria such as the presence of purulence (many leukocytes) on the Gram stain of sputum, the presence of a pulmonary infiltrate, and signs of systemic inflammation in the patient. **A positive sputum culture alone is not sufficient justification for initiating antibiotic therapy**.

- **Urinary tract infection:** This infection is also seen in hospitalized patients, often with indwelling Foley catheters. However, *Serratia* may also harmlessly colonize the urine of patients with chronic bladder catheters without causing disease. The decision to initiate antibiotics in such patients should be based on the clinical situation (the presence of pyuria on urinalysis, suprapubic pain, fever, etc). Even the finding of large quantity of *Serratia* in a urine culture ($> 10^5$ colony forming units/mL) by itself does not automatically indicate the need for antibiotic therapy.

- **Hospital-associated bacteremias:** *Serratia* may be recovered from blood cultures in association with a known focus of infection (eg, catheter infection) or may be a "primary bacteremia" with no clear source. Bacteremia may follow instrumentation of the gastrointestinal or urinary tracts.

- **Surgical wound infections**

Diagnosis The clinical presentations of the various nosocomial infections caused by *Serratia marcescens* are not distinctive, and laboratory isolation of the organism is necessary.

Diagnostic Tests/Procedures
Aerobic Culture, Appropriate Site *on page 244*
Gram Stain *on page 352*

Treatment *Serratia* species present a challenging therapeutic problem. High level drug resistance has been described in some hospital isolates. Preliminary data suggest that the popular third generation cephalosporins may act to select mutants of *Serratia* that are resistant to a wide variety of antibiotics, including both cephalosporins and extended spectrum penicillins. These "stably derepressed mutants" are becoming more common in intensive care units and pose a significant and growing problem. Consultation with the infectious disease service may be useful in such cases.

Drug Therapy
Recommended
Penicillins, Extended Spectrum *on page 637*
Cephalosporins, 3rd Generation *on page 528*
Alternate
Imipenem/Cilastatin *on page 586*
Aztreonam *on page 501*

Selected Readings
Campbell JR, Diacovo T, and Baker CJ, "*Serratia marcescens* Meningitis in Neonates," *Pediatr Infect Dis J*, 1992, 11(10):881-6.
Heltberg O, Skov F, Gerner-Smidt P, et al, "Nosocomial Epidemic of *Serratia marcescens* Septicemia Ascribed to Contaminated Blood Transfusion Bags," *Transfusion*, 1993, 33(3):221-7.
Sokalski SJ, Jewell MA, Asmus-Shillington AC, et al, "An Outbreak of *Serratia marcescens* in 14 Adult Cardiac Surgical Patients Associated With 12-Lead Electrocardiogram Bulbs," *Arch Intern Med*, 1992, 152(4):841-4.

Shigella Species

Related Information
Timing of Food Poisoning *on page 723*

Microbiology *Shigella* species are gram-negative rods which cause a severe diarrheal syndrome, called shigellosis or bacillary dysentery. *Shigella* species belong to the family Enterobacteriaceae and is, for all practical purposes, biochemically and genetically identical to *E. coli*. Four species of *Shigella* have been identified: *S. dysenteriae*, *S. flexneri*, *S. boydii*, and *S. sonnei*. There are approximately 40 serotypes. *Shigella sonnei* is most common in the industrial world and accounts for about 64% of the cases in the United States. *S. flexneri* is seen primarily in underdeveloped countries. Shigellosis can be seen following ingestion of as few as 200 organisms.

Epidemiology Infection with *Shigella* sp is primarily a problem in the pediatric population, with most infections in the 1-4 year age group. Outbreaks of epidemic proportions have been described in day care centers and nurseries. The reservoir for the bacteria is in humans. Transmission is by direct or indirect fecal-oral transmission from patient or carrier. Hand transmission is important. Less commonly, transmission occurs by consumption of contaminated water, milk, and food. The organism is able to produce outbreaks in areas of poor sanitation, in part due to the low number of organisms required to produce disease. Shigellosis is the most communicable of the bacterial diarrheas.

(Continued)

Shigella Species *(Continued)*

Clinical Syndromes *Shigella* species invade the intestinal mucosa wherein they multiply and cause local tissue damage. The organisms rarely penetrate beyond the mucosa, and thus the isolation in blood cultures is unusual, even with the toxic patient. Mucosal ulcerations are common. Some strains are known to elaborate a toxin (the shiga-toxin), which contributes to mucosal destruction and probably causes the watery diarrhea seen initially.

- **Dysentery:** Initially, the patient complains of acute onset of fever, abdominal cramping, and large volumes of very watery diarrhea. This phase is enterotoxin mediated and reflects small bowel involvement. Within 24-48 hours, the fever resolves but the diarrhea turns frankly bloody, with mucous and pus in the stools as well. Fecal urgency and tenesmus are common. This phase reflects direct colonic invasion. This two phased "descending infection" is suggestive of dysentery. Diarrhea and abdominal pain are almost universally present, but the other symptoms may be absent. Physical examination is variable and patients may be comfortable or frankly toxic. Rectal examination is often painful due to friable and inflamed rectal mucosa. The course may be complicated from dehydration from diarrhea and vomiting, particularly in the elderly and in infants. Normally, the infection is self limited and resolves within about 1 week even without antibiotics. Complications are unusual and include febrile seizures (particularly in infants), septicemia, and the hemolytic uremic syndrome (usually from the shiga-toxin from *S. dysenteriae* 1).

- **Reactive arthritis:** Following dysentery from *Shigella*, a postinfectious arthropathy resembling Reiter's syndrome has been described, particularly in patients who are HLA-B27 positive.

Diagnosis Dysentery from *Shigella* should be suspected in any patient presenting with fever and bloody diarrhea. A history of a "descending infection" as described above is further suggestive. However, the differential diagnosis of fever with bloody diarrhea is broad and includes salmonellosis, *Campylobacter* enteritis, infection with *E. coli* 0157:H7, and inflammatory bowel disease. The WBC count may show either a leukocytosis, leukopenia, or be normal.

There are two important laboratory tests indicated in suspected cases.

1. Stool exam for fecal leukocytes: Numerous white blood cells will be present during the colonic phase of the infection. Note that this is not diagnostic for *Shigella* infections; it indicates that the colonic mucosa is inflamed, from whatever cause. The finding of sheets of fecal leukocytes on smear narrows the differential diagnosis of infectious diarrheas considerably.

2. Stool culture for *Shigella*: Recovery of the organism from stool is more easily performed early in the illness when the concentration in the stool is highest. Samples should be brought to the laboratory as soon as possible to maximize viability, and specific culture for *Shigella* sp should be requested.

Diagnostic Tests/Procedures
Fecal Leukocyte Stain *on page 334*
Stool Culture *on page 448*

Treatment Many cases of *Shigella* dysentery are self-resolving. Some have suggested that antibiotics be reserved for severe cases, but this does not eliminate the reservoir for infection in the community. Antibiotics have been shown to shorten the period of excretion of the organism in the feces, as well as decreasing morbidity. The antibiotic of choice is co-trimoxazole for both children and adults. However, some strains are resistant to co-trimoxazole, particularly in Africa and Southeast Asia, and *in vitro* susceptibility testing should be performed on all isolates. The quinolones have been effective for shigellosis in clinical trials and are useful alternatives. Antimotility agents such as opiates, paregoric, and diphenoxylate (Lomotil®) should be avoided because of the potential for worsening the dysentery and for predisposing to toxic megacolon.

Pediatric Drug Therapy
Recommended
Co-trimoxazole *on page 545*
Alternate
Ampicillin *on page 495*
Cephalosporins, 3rd Generation *on page 528*

Adult Drug Therapy
Recommended
Ciprofloxacin Hydrochloride *on page 537*
Co-trimoxazole *on page 545*

Alternate
Ampicillin *on page 495*
Cephalosporins, 3rd Generation *on page 528*
Fluoroquinolones *on page 571*

Selected Readings

Ashkenazi S, Amir J, Waisman Y, et al, "A Randomized, Double-Blind Study Comparing Cefixime and Trimethoprim-Sulfamethoxazole in the Treatment of Childhood Shigellosis," *J Pediatr*, 1993, 123(5):817-21.

Baskin DH, Lax JD, and Barenberg D, "*Shigella* Bacteremia in Patients With the Acquired Immune Deficiency Syndrome," *Am J Gastroenterol*, 1987, 82(4):338-41.

Bennish ML, "Potentially Lethal Complications of Shigellosis," *Rev Infect Dis*, 1991, 13(Suppl 4):S319-24.

Halpern Z, Dan M, Giladi M, et al, "Shigellosis in Adults: Epidemiologic, Clinical, and Laboratory Features," *Medicine (Baltimore)*, 1989, 68(4):210-7.

Salam MA and Bennish ML, "Antimicrobial Therapy for Shigellosis," *Rev Infect Dis*, 1991, 13(Suppl 4):S332-41.

Tauxe RV, Puhr ND, Wells JG, et al, "Antimicrobial Resistance of *Shigella* Isolates in the USA: The Importance of International Travelers," *J Infect Dis*, 1990, 162(5):1107-11.

Sporothrix schenckii

Microbiology *Sporothrix schenckii* is a saprophytic fungus widely dispersed in the soil, on the surface of many plants, and in decaying vegetable matter. The organism is a thermally dimorphic fungus, meaning that it exists in either a yeast or a mold form depending on the temperature. At room temperature, it exists in a mold form, but at warmer temperatures, it grows as a budding yeast. In clinical specimens such as biopsies of skin lesions, *Sporothrix schenckii* appears as a round or oval budding yeast; organisms may be difficult to find in clinical specimens and when present, may have variable size and shape. Thus, culture confirmation of *Sporothrix schenckii* is important. The organism grows relatively well on a variety of fungal media used routinely in microbiology laboratories.

Epidemiology *Sporothrix schenckii* is the causative agent of sporotrichosis or "gardener's disease". Typically, the organism is inoculated directly into the hand or face of a person handling plants or soil containing the organism. *S. schenckii* can be cultured from rose thorns, hay, compost material, mulch, and other decaying plant matter. It is important to obtain a detailed occupational and recreational history in suspected cases of sporotrichosis; individuals at risk include gardeners (particularly those handling roses), florists, landscapers, farmers, loggers, and others. Individuals who are infected with *S. schenckii* generally have a normal immune system. Although zoonotic transmission has been reported, it is much rarer then traumatic implantation of the organism. Several cases have been reported of veterinarians acquiring sporotrichosis from infected cats even without an associated penetrating injury.

The largest documented U.S. outbreak of sporotrichosis occurred in 1988. The outbreak was linked to Wisconsin-grown sphagnum moss used in packing evergreen tree seedlings; 84 individuals from 15 states developed cutaneous sporotrichosis. The attack rate was 17% in New York State, where 13 cases were reported from 109 forestry workers who had handled evergreen seedlings and moss. As expected, the attack rates were highest in those workers spending more time directly exposed to the moss. Although cultures of sphagnum moss from the Wisconsin supplier were negative for *Sporothrix schenckii*, the organism was cultured from multiple samples of the moss obtained from the tree nursery in Pennsylvania thought to be the main source of the outbreak. Several tree-handling procedures at this nursery may have contributed to the outbreak, such as the use of 3-year-old moss to pack seedlings, use of a pond water system to keep the moss wet, use of a polymer gel on the root system of the seedlings, and lengthy storage of moss-packed seedlings prior to shipping. This outbreak emphasized the need for wearing protective gloves and long-sleeved shirts in persons handling evergreens and similar plants.

Clinical Syndromes Sporotrichosis is divided into cutaneous and extracutaneous forms.

- **Cutaneous sporotrichosis:** This occurs when the organism is inoculated into the subcutaneous tissues following a minor trauma to the extremities or face. The incubation period is variable, from 1 week to several months. Cutaneous sporotrichosis can be classified as either plaque sporotrichosis or lymphocutaneous sporotrichosis. In plaque sporotrichosis, a small red plaque develops on the extremity at the original site of inoculation of the organism. The plaque is nontender and may increase in size but no additional lesions develop. In lymphocutaneous sporotrichosis, the disease begins with a single papular lesion, but in time, multiple similar lesions appear

(Continued)

Sporothrix schenckii (Continued)

more proximally following the path of lymphatic drainage. These lesions often change from painless papules to ulcers which drain pus or sero-sanguinous fluid. Interestingly, although new lesions form by lymphangitic spread, axillary (or inguinal) lymph nodes are seldom involved. Both forms of cutaneous sporotrichosis tend to be very chronic if left untreated.

When examined by light microscopy, the skin lesions in cutaneous sporo-trichosis show multinucleated giant cells and epithelioid cells consistent with granulomas; thus, sporotrichosis should be considered in the differen-tial diagnosis of any granulomatous process on an extremity or the face. It is important to note that organisms may not be seen on a single skin biop-sy and additional biopsies may be necessary. The finding of an "asteroid body" on histologic section of a skin biopsy is highly suggestive of sporo-trichosis but is not reliably present in all biopsies. The asteroid is a fungal organism surrounded by several "rays" that stain with periodic acid-Schiff (PAS). A recent study using electron microscopy suggested that an aster-oid body is composed of crystalline products of disintegrated host cells deposited around a central fungal cell.

A number of clinical entities should be considered in the differential diag-nosis of cutaneous sporotrichosis. Some can be eliminated on the basis of epidemiology alone. Diseases to consider include:
- *Mycobacterium marinum*
- *Mycobacterium kansasii*
- pyoderma gangrenosum
- *Nocardia brasiliensis*
- *Leischmania* species
- foreign body granulomas
- blastomycosis
- dermatologic diseases (especially with plaque sporotrichosis)

- **Extracutaneous sporotrichosis:** A variety of rare, extracutaneous forms have been described. The most common is osteoarticular sporotrichosis which involves the knee, elbow, wrist, or ankle. There is rarely a history of a plant or thorn injury and typically no skin lesions are present. Patients may present with either single joint involvement or a polyarticular syn-drome. The onset is indolent, and the joint develops tenderness, warmth, effusions, and sometimes draining sinuses. Osteoarticular sporotrichosis is a very difficult diagnosis to make; one study reported that it usually took over 2 years to make the correct diagnosis. Other forms of sporotrichosis include:
  - Pulmonary sporotrichosis: Only a few cases have been reported. Pa-tients present with a chronic cavitary pneumonia, usually in an upper lobe. The disease mimics tuberculosis and histoplasmosis. One recent report suggested that the Papanicolaou stain of sputum may be help-ful in making this rare diagnosis.
  - Ocular disease: This usually results from penetrating ocular injury to the conjunctica or surrounding tissues. Eighteen cases of sporotrichoid endophthalmitis have been reported, with only two cases associated with trauma; most have required enucleation.
  - Meningitis: This rare complication has been reported in a few immuno-competent individuals. In one study of meningeal sporotrichosis in 7 patients, the cerebrospinal fluid was frequently negative on both stain and fungal culture initially; repeated lumbar punctures were necessary over a 3- to 11-month period before the organism was cultured.
  - Disseminated sporotrichosis: Patients present with multiple skin lesions involving two or more extremities. Blood cultures using the lysis-centrifugation method have been reported positive for *Sporothrix sc-henckii* in some cases.

- **Sporotrichosis and AIDS:** Systemic sporotrichosis has been reported in patients with advanced HIV infection but remains an infrequent complica-tion. A number of sites of infection have been reported including the lung, liver, spleen, intestine, bone, eye, joints, and disseminated cutaneous le-sions. Recently, a case of meningitis was reported in a patient with known cutaneous sporotrichosis and a CD4 cell count of 56/mm^3. Again, the cere-brospinal fluid was sterile over a 5-month period. The skin lesions respond-ed to a prolonged course of amphotericin B and fluconazole, but the me-ningeal symptoms worsened on therapy, and on autopsy, *S. schenckii* was found infiltrating into the meninges and brain parenchyma.

Diagnosis The clinical suspicion of sporotrichosis should be confirmed microbiologically because of the number of conditions which can mimic the cutaneous lesions. Cultures of appropriate specimens such as skin biopsies, joint fluid, and bursal fluid will frequently recover the organism. *S. schenckii* is difficult to identify on fungal stains of biopsy specimens or KOH preparations since the organism burden is often low. Cultures of exudates from ulcerative skin lesions are often low-yield. Blood cultures, urine cultures, and sputum are only rarely positive. As noted earlier, cerebrospinal fluid is frequently negative in meningeal sporotrichosis, and multiple samples over time are necessary.

Specific IgG antibodies to *S. schenckii* are available at specialty laboratories but are of limited usefulness. Demonstration of IgG synthesis against the organism in cerebrospinal fluid may be a useful means of diagnosing meningeal sporotrichosis when routine cultures are negative (see Penn et al reference).

Diagnostic Tests/Procedures

Fungus Culture, Body Fluid *on page 341*
Fungus Culture, Cerebrospinal Fluid *on page 342*
Fungus Culture, Skin *on page 343*

Treatment Recently, antifungal susceptibility of *Sporothrix schenckii* to several agents has become available in specialized centers (eg, Dr. Michael Rinaldi, Fungus Testing Laboratory, University Health Science Center, San Antonio, TX). This may be useful in severe or refractory cases. The treatment of choice for cutaneous sporotrichosis is a saturated solution of potassium iodide (SSKI). The mechanism of action of SSKI is obscure. The dose is initiated at 5 drops of SSKI 3 times/day in juice and steadily increased to 40 drops 3 times/day. Toxicity of the medication is common and includes gastrointestinal distress and lacrimation; the dose should be lowered if these symptoms occur. Drug rash is also relatively common, but the medication can usually be continued safely. Local heat is useful in cutaneous disease and can be used either as an adjunctive measure or in patients intolerant of SSKI. The azole antifungal agents may have some activity against *S. schenckii*. Ketoconazole and fluconazole have limited or no activity; itraconazole has *in vitro* activity although the *in vivo* experience is limited.

Extracutaneous sporotrichosis is best treated with amphotericin B. Prolonged courses are usually necessary, and osteoarticular sporotrichosis often requires over 2 g amphotericin. Pulmonary and meningeal sporotrichosis are even more difficult to treat, and a specialist in Infectious Diseases should be consulted.

Drug Therapy
Recommended

Cutaneous sporotrichosis
  Potassium Iodide *on page 648*
Extracutaneous sporotrichosis
  Amphotericin B *on page 493*

Selected Readings
Coles FB, Schuchat A, Hibbs JR, et al, "A Multistate Outbreak of Sporotrichosis Associated With Sphagnum Moss," *Am J Epidemiol*, 1992, 136(4):475-87.

Keiser P and Whittle D, "Sporotrichosis in Human Immunodeficiency Virus-Infected Patients: Report of a Case," *Rev Infect Dis*, 1991, 13(5):1027-8.

Penn CC, Goldstein E, and Bartholomew WR, "*Sporothrix schenckii* Meningitis in a Patient With AIDS," *Clin Infect Dis*, 1992, 15(4):741-3.

Rex JH, "*Sporothrix schenckii*," *Principles and Practice of Infectious Diseases*, 4th ed, Mandell GL, Bennett JE, and Dolin R, eds, New York, NY: Churchill Livingstone, 1995, 2321-4.

Roberts GD and Larsh HW, "The Serologic Diagnosis of Extracutaneous Sporotrichosis," *Am J Clin Pathol*, 1971, 56(5):597-600.

SRGPC *see Streptococcus*-Related Gram-Positive Cocci
on page 212

Staphylococcus aureus, Methicillin-Resistant

Synonyms MRSA

Microbiology Staphylococci derives its name from the Greek word staphyle meaning "bunch of grapes". On Gram stain, staphylococci are gram-positive cocci, 0.7-1.2 μm, nonspore forming, occurring singly, in pairs, in short 4-5 cocci chains or clusters. Staphylococci grow rapidly both as an aerobe and anaerobe on blood agar. The colonies are sharply defined, smooth, and 1-4 mm in diameter. Staphylococci are catalase-positive and differ from micrococci by the following: anaerobic acid production from glucose, sensitivity <200 mg/mL lysostaphin, and production of acid from glycerol in the presence of 0.4 mg/mL
(Continued)

Staphylococcus aureus, **Methicillin-Resistant**
(Continued)

erythromycin.

Staphylococcus aureus may have a golden pigmentation secondary to carotenoid and produce β-hemolysis on horse, sheep, or human blood agar after an incubation of 24-48 hours. *Staphylococcus epidermidis* and coagulase-negative staph (CNS) are often used interchangeably but recognize that there are over 30 species of CNS of which *S. epidermidis* is the most common. It is important to distinguish three clinically relevant species: *S. aureus*, *S. epidermidis*, and *S. saprophyticus*. See table.

Major Tests for the Differentiation of Human Staphylococci

Test	Staph aureus	Staph epidermidis	Staph saprophyticus
Coagulase	+	—	—
Acid production by mannitol	+	—	+/—
DNAse	+	—	—
Novobiocin resistance	—	—	+
Anaerobic growth	+	+	—
Hemolysis	+	—	—

From Waldvogel FA, "*Staphylococcus aureus* (Including Toxic Shock Syndrome),"*Principals and Practice of Infectious Diseases*, 3rd ed, Mandell GL, Douglas R Jr, and Bennett JE, eds, New York, NY: Churchill Livingstone, 1990, 1490.

Epidemiology Colonization of health care workers with MRSA is uncommon. The two major modes of transmission of MRSA is via an infected or colonized patient, or dissemination through an infected or colonized health care worker; typically MRSA is transmitted on the hands of a health care worker after contact with an infected patient.

MRSA is not a marker for virulence nor spreading, and MRSA has not been shown to spontaneously evolve from MSSA to MRSA during the course of antibiotic therapy. Resistance to methicillin occurs predominantly by intrinsic resistance (penicillin-binding proteins) which is transmitted chromosomally. Five percent to 20% are also resistant to erythromycin, lincomycin, and clindamycin. Rifampin cannot be used alone secondary to a high one-step mutation rate to resistance.

Although universal precautions have been adopted and must be followed by all health care personnel, incidence of MRSA continues to rise. The goal of all facilities is ablation of widespread colonization and is difficult to achieve. Contact isolation is recommended.

Clinical Syndromes
- **Localized:** Most common type of infection usually secondary to poor personal hygiene, minor trauma, or diminished skin integrity (ie, eczema, psoriasis)

  Folliculitis – Typically clears with local antiseptic.

  Furuncle – Deep seated infection around a hair follicle beginning as a painful, red nodule then becoming a hot, painful, raised indurated lesion 1-2 cm long, over several days. Predilection for the face, neck, axillae, and buttocks.

  Carbuncle – Deep seated infection of multiple hair follicles that coalesce and spread into the subcutaneous tissue, frequently associated with sinus tracts. Need to exclude septicemia and/or septic thrombophlebitis. If recurrent, should evaluate for underlying phagocytic or metabolic dysfunction.

  Impetigo – Typically affects children on exposed areas. Approximately 10% due to *Streptococcus pyogenes* and 10% due to combined staph/strep infections. Begins as a red macule which progresses to a vesicle then to crust. May be confused with HSV and varicella. The bullous form may respond to topical mupirocin or oral antistaphylococcal agents. Nonbullous form usually responds to oral or intramuscular penicillin.

Hydradenitis suppurative – Recurrent pyogenic abscess of apocrine sweat glands, especially axillary, perineal, and genital. Mimics LGV. Usually requires incision and drainage, as well as oral antibiotics.

Mastitis – Occurs in 1% to 3% of nursing mothers. Requires oral antibiotics. Continued nursing is controversial.

Wound infections – Usually occurs 2 days after surgery. May need to explore wound. Requires oral antibiotics 7-10 days. May need I.V. antibiotics 4-6 weeks for underlying prosthesis.

Spreading pyodermas – Surgical intervention needed if necrotizing fasciitis.

- **Pneumonia:** Most frequently occurs a few days after influenza; mortality is 30% to 50%. Acquired via inhalation or hematogenous route. Approximately one-third develop empyemas. Patients present with chest pain, fever, shortness of breath, tachypnea, and a pleural effusion which requires drainage. May be associated with bronchiectasis or obstructive bronchogenic cancer. Hematogenous route usually secondary to right-sided endocarditis, infected intravascular device, or septic phlebitis.

- **Toxic shock syndrome caused by TSST 1 (toxin 1):** Typically occurs in young woman ages 15-25 using tampons. Starts abruptly during menses. Present with fever, profound refractory hypotension, erythroderma with desquamation, multiorgan involvement with profuse diarrhea, mental confusion. Approximately 50% will have elevated creatine kinase, decreased platelets, and leukocytosis. May be seen secondary to surgical wound packages, as well as associated with disseminated staph infections. Mortality is approximately 3%.

- **Staphylococcal scalded skin syndrome (SSSS):** Most commonly occurs in children and neonates; epidemics in neonatal nurseries and day care centers. Usually caused by phage type 2. Starts abruptly with perioral erythema with sunburn-like rash rapidly turning bright red spreading to bullae in 2-3 days and desquamating within 5 days. Positive Nikolsky sign. Recovery in 10 days. Need to exclude toxic epidermal neurolysis and Kawasaki mucocutaneous disease (culture-negative, Nikolsky-negative).

- **Food poisoning:** Usually caused by ingestion of heat stable enterotoxin B. Second most common cause of acute food poisoning. May occur by person-to-person transmission. Incubation 2-6 hours after ingestion of toxin contained in custard filled bakery goods, canned foods, processed meats, potato salads, and ice cream. Patients present with acute salivation, nausea, vomiting progressing to abdominal cramps, and watery, nonbloody diarrhea (risk of dehydration).

- **Musculoskeletal:** Frequent cause of osteomyelitis, septic arthritis, septic bursitis, and, less frequently, pyomyositis. Blood cultures positive in approximately 50% of these cases of osteomyelitis. Need bone biopsy for definitive diagnosis. Typically hematogenous or secondary to local trauma with contiguous infection. Sternoclavicular joint usually follows septic thrombosis of upper limb and often associated with IVDA. Septic arthritis usually secondary to complication of septicemia, rheumatoid arthritis, or prepubertal trauma. (Knee > hip > elbow > shoulder.)

- **Septicemia/endocarditis:** Associated with age extremes, cardiovascular disease, decompensated diabetes, heroin addicts. Mortality remains high (40% to 60%) despite antimicrobial therapy. One-third of patients have no focus for infection. Overall incidence of endocarditis with *S. aureus* infection is 10%. *S. aureus* is the second most common cause of native valve endocarditis and continues to rise in incidence in bacteremias thought secondary to IVDA and use of long-term indwelling catheters.

Diagnosis It is not possible to distinguish MRSA from MSSA clinically. Susceptibility testing should be performed on all *S. aureus* isolates.

Diagnostic Tests/Procedures

Aerobic Culture, Appropriate Site *on page 244*

Gram Stain *on page 352*

Treatment MRSA is characteristically resistant to penicillins, antistaphylococcal penicillin, erythromycin, lincomycin, clindamycin; somewhat resistant to aminoglycosides and chloramphenicol and sensitive to vancomycin and teicoplanin (not available in U.S.). MRSA will not respond clinically to cephalosporins, even though MRSA often **are susceptible *in vitro***. Both quinolones and teicoplanin have been shown to effective in short-term use, but recent studies show acquired resistance with long-term use. Doxycycline and cotrimoxazole may be used in non life-threatening infections if susceptible by *in vitro* testing. Prevention of spread to the other patients is critically important.

ORGANISMS

Drug Therapy
Recommended
Vancomycin Hydrochloride *on page 691*
or
Vancomycin Hydrochloride *on page 691*
used in combination with
Gentamicin Sulfate *on page 575*
or
Vancomycin Hydrochloride *on page 691*
used in combination with
Rifampin *on page 662*

Alternate
The following drug may be used only if susceptible:
Co-trimoxazole *on page 545*
Doxycycline *on page 557*

Selected Readings
Duckworth GJ, "Diagnosis and Management of Methicillin-Resistant *Staphylococcus aureus* Infection," *BMJ*, 1993, 307(6911):1049-52.

Mulligan ME, Murray-Leisure KA, Ribner BS, et al, "Methicillin-Resistant *Staphylococcus aureus*: A Consensus Review of the Microbiology, Pathogenesis, and Epidemiology With Implications for Prevention and Management," *Am J Med*, 1993, 94(3):313-28.

Staphylococcus aureus, Methicillin-Susceptible
Synonyms MSSA

Microbiology Staphylococci derives its name from the Greek word staphyle meaning "bunch of grapes". On Gram stain, staphylococci are gram-positive cocci, 0.7-1.2 μm, nonspore forming, occurring singly, in pairs, in short 4-5 cocci chains or clusters. Staphylococci grow rapidly both as an aerobe and anaerobe on blood agar. The colonies are sharply defined, smooth, and 1-4 mm in diameter. Staphylococci are catalase-positive and differ from micrococci by the following: anaerobic acid production from glucose, sensitivity <200 mg/mL lysostaphin, and production of acid from glycerol in the presence of 0.4 mg/mL erythromycin.

Staphylococcus aureus may have a golden pigmentation secondary to carotenoid and produce β-hemolysis on horse, sheep, or human blood agar after an incubation of 24-48 hours. *Staphylococcus epidermidis* and coagulase-negative staph (CNS) are often used interchangeably but recognize that there are over 30 species of CNS of which *S. epidermidis* is the most common. It is important to distinguish three clinically relevant species: *S. aureus*, *S. epidermidis*, and *S. saprophyticus*. See table in *Staphylococcus aureus*, Methicillin-Resistant.

Epidemiology It is estimated that 20% to 40% of the population are persistent asymptomatic nasal carriers. The carrier state is clinically relevant in that carriers have a higher rate of staphylococci infections as compared to noncarriers. Neonates may be colonized in the perianal area, umbilical stumps, skin, and gastrointestinal tract. Adults are colonized in the anterior nares, skin, and less frequently, vagina. There is an increase carrier rate among hospital personnel, diabetics receiving insulin, hemodialysis patients, and I.V. drug users.

The portal of entry is typically the skin. Patients with chemotaxis defects (ie, Chédiak-Higashi, Wiskott-Aldrich), opsonization defects (ie, complement deficiencies), and staphylocidal defects of polymorphonuclear cells (ie, chronic granulomatous disease) are at increased risk.

Eighty percent to 90% of community-acquired staphylococci are resistant to penicillin. One of the more common forms of resistance is through the production of beta-lactamase, an extracellular enzyme coded for by plasmids that inactivate penicillin by interrupting the β-lactam ring. These organisms are still susceptible to antistaphylococcal penicillins and first generation cephalosporins.

Clinical Syndromes
- **Localized:** Most common type of infection usually secondary to poor personal hygiene, minor trauma, or diminished skin integrity (ie, eczema, psoriasis)

    Folliculitis – Typically clears with local antiseptic.

    Furuncle – Deep seated infection around a hair follicle beginning as a painful, red nodule then becoming a hot, painful, raised indurated lesion 1-2 cm long, over several days. Predilection for the face, neck, axillae, and buttocks.

    Carbuncle – Deep seated infection of multiple hair follicles that coalesce and spread into the subcutaneous tissue, frequently associated with sinus tracts. Need to exclude septicemia and/or septic thrombophlebitis. If recurrent, should evaluate for underlying phagocytic or metabolic dysfunction.

Impetigo – Typically affects children on exposed areas. Approximately 10% due to *Streptococcus pyogenes* and 10% due to combined staph/strep infections. Begins as a red macule which progresses to a vesicle then to crust. May be confused with HSV and varicella. The bullous form may respond to topical mupirocin or oral antistaphylococcal agents. Nonbullous form usually responds to oral or intramuscular penicillin.

Hydradenitis suppurative – Recurrent pyogenic abscess of apocrine sweat glands, especially axillary, perineal, and genital. Mimics LGV. Usually requires incision and drainage, as well as oral antibiotics.

Mastitis – Occurs in 1% to 3% of nursing mothers. Requires oral antibiotics. Continued nursing is controversial.

Wound infections – Usually occurs 2 days after surgery. May need to explore wound. Requires oral antibiotics 7-10 days. May need I.V. antibiotics 4-6 weeks for underlying prosthesis.

Spreading pyodermas – Surgical intervention needed if necrotizing fasciitis.

- **Pneumonia:** Most frequently occurs a few days after influenza; mortality is 30% to 50%. Acquired via inhalation or hematogenous route. Approximately one-third develop empyemas. Patients present with chest pain, fever, shortness of breath, tachypnea, and a pleural effusion which requires drainage. May be associated with bronchiectasis or obstructive bronchogenic cancer. Hematogenous route usually secondary to right-sided endocarditis, infected intravascular device, or septic phlebitis.

- **Toxic shock syndrome caused by TSST 1 (toxin 1):** Typically occurs in young woman ages 15-25 using tampons. Starts abruptly during menses. Present with fever, profound refractory hypotension, erythroderma with desquamation, multiorgan involvement with profuse diarrhea, mental confusion. Approximately 50% will have elevated creatine kinase, decreased platelets, and leukocytosis. May be seen secondary to surgical wound packages, as well as associated with disseminated staph infections. Mortality is approximately 3%.

- **Staphylococcal scalded skin syndrome (SSSS):** Most commonly occurs in children and neonates; epidemics in neonatal nurseries and day care centers. Usually caused by phage type 2. Starts abruptly with perioral erythema with sunburn-like rash rapidly turning bright red spreading to bullae in 2-3 days and desquamating within 5 days. Positive Nikolsky sign. Recovery in 10 days. Need to exclude toxic epidermal neurolysis and Kawasaki mucocutaneous disease (culture-negative, Nikolsky-negative).

- **Food poisoning:** Usually caused by ingestion of heat stable enterotoxin B. Second most common cause of acute food poisoning. May occur by person-to-person transmission. Incubation 2-6 hours after ingestion of toxin contained in custard filled bakery goods, canned foods, processed meats, potato salads, and ice cream. Patients present with acute salivation, nausea, vomiting progressing to abdominal cramps, and watery, nonbloody diarrhea (risk of dehydration).

- **Musculoskeletal:** Frequent cause of osteomyelitis, septic arthritis, septic bursitis and less frequently pyomyositis. Blood cultures positive in approximately 50% of these cases of osteomyelitis. Need bone biopsy for definitive diagnosis. Typically hematogenous or secondary to local trauma with contiguous infection. Sternoclavicular joint usually follows septic thrombosis of upper limb and often associated with IVDA. Septic arthritis usually secondary to complication of septicemia, rheumatoid arthritis, or prepubertal trauma. (Knee > hip > elbow > shoulder.)

- **Septicemia/endocarditis:** Associated with age extremes, cardiovascular disease, decompensated diabetes, heroin addicts. Mortality remains high (40% to 60%) despite antimicrobial therapy. One-third of patients have no focus for infection. Overall incidence of endocarditis with *S. aureus* infection is 10%. *S. aureus* is the second most common cause of native valve endocarditis and continues to rise in incidence in bacteremias thought secondary to IVDA and use of long-term indwelling catheters.

Diagnosis Diagnosis is made by Gram stain and culture of appropriate site. Phage typing is a useful epidemiological tool. Antiteichoic antibodies by CIE or RIA are positive in approximately 90% of patients with endocarditis, 20% to 40% positive with bacteremia, and 0% to 60% positive with localized infections.

(Continued)

Staphylococcus aureus, **Methicillin-Susceptible**
(Continued)

Diagnostic Tests/Procedures
Aerobic Culture, Appropriate Site *on page 244*
Gram Stain *on page 352*
Teichoic Acid Antibody *on page 453*

Treatment Topical mupirocin may be useful in eradicating carrier states. Most localized infections will respond to penicillins or antistaphylococcal penicillins or first generation cephalosporins. Deep-seated infections usually require surgical intervention. Penicillin-allergic individuals may be given erythromycin, clindamycin, or tetracycline. Patients with line sepsis without septicemia usually require 5-7 days parenteral antibiotics, whereas therapy is extended 10-14 days with septicemia. Controversy exists as to the removal of the intravascular device, but most authors recommend removing the catheter. Beta-lactam regimens for at least 4-6 weeks plus an aminoglycoside during the first to second week of treatment remains the treatment of choice for left-sided *S. aureus* endocarditis. Patients with β-lactam allergies or failed therapy should be treated with vancomycin plus rifampin. Patients with right-sided endocarditis are typically treated with the same regimens, however, there have been some studies suggesting the efficiency of quinolones. Two-week parenteral regimens are currently being investigated for the treatment of uncomplicated MSSA endocarditis.

Drug Therapy
  Recommended
    Penicillins, Penicillinase-Resistant *on page 637*
  Alternate
    Cephalosporins, 1st Generation *on page 527*
    Clindamycin *on page 540*
    Vancomycin Hydrochloride *on page 691*

Selected Readings

Chambers MD, "Short-Course Combination and Oral Therapies of *Staphylococcus aureus* Endocarditis," *Infect Dis Clin North Am*, 1993, 7(1):69-80.

Mortara LA and Bayer AS, "*Staphylococcus aureus*, Bacteremia and Endocarditis. New Diagnostic and Therapeutic Concepts," *Infect Dis Clin North Am*, 1993, 7(1):53-68.

Turnidge J and Grayson L, "Optimun Treatment of Staphylococcal Infections," *Drugs*, 1993, 45(3):353-66.

Waldvogel FA, "*Staphylococcus aureus* (Including Toxic Shock Syndrome)," *Principles and Practice of Infectious Diseases*, 4th ed, Mandell GL, Bennett JE, and Dolin R, eds, New York, NY: Churchill Livingstone, 1995, 1754-77.

Williams RE and MacKie RM, "The Staphylococci - Importance of Their Control in the Management of Skin Disease," *Dermatol Clin*, 1993, 11(1):201-6.

Staphylococcus epidermidis, **Methicillin-Resistant**

Synonyms MRSE

Microbiology Staphylococci derives its name from the Greek word staphyle meaning "bunch of grapes". On Gram stain, staphylococci are gram-positive cocci, 0.7-1.2 μm, nonspore forming, occurring singly, in pairs, in short 4-5 cocci chains or clusters. Staphylococci grow rapidly both as an aerobe and anaerobe on blood agar. The colonies are sharply defined, smooth, and 1-4 mm in diameter. Staphylococci are catalase-positive and differ from micrococci by the following: anaerobic acid production from glucose, sensitivity <200 mg/mL lysostaphin, and production of acid from glycerol in the presence of 0.4 mg/mL erythromycin.

Staphylococcus aureus may have a golden pigmentation secondary to carotenoid and produce β-hemolysis on horse, sheep, or human blood agar after an incubation of 24-48 hours. *Staphylococcus epidermidis* and coagulase-negative staph (CNS) are often used interchangeably but recognize that there are over 30 species of CNS of which *S. epidermidis* is the most common. It is important to distinguish three clinically relevant species: *S. aureus, S. epidermidis*, and *S. saprophyticus*. See table in *Staphylococcus aureus*, Methicillin-Resistant.

Epidemiology Over the past 10 years, MSSE has continued to be the major cause of nosocomial bacteremia and sepsis with a mortality approaching 30%. MSSE is a normal inhabitant of the skin. It synthesizes an extracellular polysaccharide which is associated with persistence of infection, resistance to antibiotics, and a predilection for medical devices. Approximately 24,000 patients annually develop device-related septicemia with the most common being related to insertion site infections.

Thirty percent to 40% of prosthetic valve endocarditis (PVE) is due to CNS compared to 14% due to MSSA. Hickman/Broviac infections are 54% CNS as compared to 20% MSSA. Less than 6% of all pacemaker insertions result in infections, yet 40% to 50% are due to CNS secondary to contamination at the time of insertion. Similar findings are seen in prosthetic joint infections.

Typically, community-acquired infections are beta-lactam sensitive, whereas most hospital-acquired infections are multiply resistant. Resistance to antistaphylococcal beta-lactams is mediated by the mec gene which confers resistance by encoding a unique penicillin binding protein with low affinity for beta-lactam antibiotics.

Clinical Syndromes

- **Foreign body infections:** Common sites of infection with MSSE include intravascular catheters, pacemakers, prosthetic cardiac valves, vascular grafts, orthopedic appliances, artificial joints, CSF shunts, dialysis catheters, and breast implants.
- **Osteomyelitis:** Most commonly associated with sternal wound infections status post cardiac surgery, although overall frequently rare. Other mode of transmission is via hematogenous spread.
- **Native valve endocarditis:** Less common than PVE; occurs approximately 5%.
- **Urinary tract infection:** Hospital acquired secondary to manipulation or catheter placement.
- **Endophthalmitis:** Increasing significantly status post intraocular lens placement.

Diagnosis Diagnosis is made by Gram stain and culture with sensitivities of appropriate site. Semiquantitation roll technique by Dennis Maki in which catheter is rolled over surface of blood agar plate is useful in suggesting a true intravascular catheter sepsis when both blood culture grows MSSE and count >15 colonies on blood agar plate.

Diagnostic Tests/Procedures

Aerobic Culture, Appropriate Site *on page 244*
Gram Stain *on page 352*

Treatment Vancomycin remains the drug of choice for MRSE. More than 50% of all isolates are resistant to tetracycline, chloramphenicol, clindamycin, and erythromycin. MRSE is usually sensitive to rifampin and gentamicin, but resistance develops quickly and neither drug can be used as a sole agent. Although not available in the U.S., teicoplanin may be of benefit. Antimicrobial therapy for PVE should consist of vancomycin, rifampin, and/or gentamicin for 4-6 weeks. UTIs secondary to MRSE may be treated with co-trimoxazole if susceptible.

Drug Therapy
Recommended

Vancomycin Hydrochloride *on page 691*
or
Vancomycin Hydrochloride *on page 691*
used in combination with
Gentamicin Sulfate *on page 575*
or
Vancomycin Hydrochloride *on page 691*
used in combination with
Rifampin *on page 662*

Alternate
The following drug may be used only if susceptible:
Co-trimoxazole *on page 545*

Selected Readings
Christensen GD, "The 'Sticky' Problem of *Staphylococcus epidermidis* Sepsis," *Hosp Pract (Off Ed)*, 1993, 28(9A):27-36, 38.
Rupp ME and Archer GL, "Coagulase-Negative Staphylococci: Pathogens Associated With Medical Progress," *Clin Infec Dis*, 1994, 19:231-43.
Whitener C, Caputo GM, Weitekamp MR, et al, "Endocarditis Due to Coagulase-Negative Staphylococci," *Infect Dis Clin North Am*, 1993, 7(1):81-96.

Staphylococcus epidermidis, Methicillin-Susceptible
Synonyms MSSE
Microbiology Staphylococci derives its name from the Greek word staphyle meaning "bunch of grapes". On Gram stain, staphylococci are gram-positive cocci, 0.7-1.2 μm, nonspore forming, occurring singly, in pairs, in short 4-5

(Continued)

Staphylococcus epidermidis, Methicillin-Susceptible
(Continued)

cocci chains or clusters. Staphylococci grow rapidly both as an aerobe and anaerobe on blood agar. The colonies are sharply defined, smooth, and 1-4 mm in diameter. Staphylococci are catalase-positive and differ from micrococci by the following: anaerobic acid production from glucose, sensitivity <200 mg/mL lysostaphin, and production of acid from glycerol in the presence of 0.4 mg/mL erythromycin.

Staphylococcus aureus may have a golden pigmentation secondary to carotenoid and produce β-hemolysis on horse, sheep, or human blood agar after an incubation of 24-48 hours. *Staphylococcus epidermidis* and coagulase-negative staph (CNS) are often used interchangeably but recognize that there are over 30 species of CNS of which *S. epidermidis* is the most common. It is important to distinguish three clinically relevant species: *S. aureus*, *S. epidermidis*, and *S. saprophyticus*. See table in *Staphylococcus aureus*, Methicillin-Resistant.

Epidemiology Over the past 10 years, MSSE has continued to be the major cause of nosocomial bacteremia and sepsis with a mortality approaching 30%. MSSE is a normal inhabitant of the skin. It synthesizes an extracellular polysaccharide which is associated with persistence of infection, resistance to antibiotics, and a predilection for medical devices. Approximately 24,000 patients annually develop device-related septicemia with the most common being related to insertion site infections.

Thirty percent to 40% of prosthetic valve endocarditis (PVE) is due to CNS compared to 14% due to MSSA. Hickman/Broviac infections are 54% CNS as compared to 20% MSSA. Less than 6% of all pacemaker insertions result in infections, yet 40% to 50% are due to CNS secondary to contamination at the time of insertion. Similar findings are seen in prosthetic joint infections.

Typically, community-acquired infections are beta-lactam sensitive, whereas most hospital-acquired infections are multiply resistant. Resistance to antistaphylococcal beta-lactams is mediated by the mec gene which confers resistance by encoding a unique penicillin binding protein with low affinity for beta-lactam antibiotics.

Clinical Syndromes
- **Foreign body infections:** Common sites of infection with MSSE include intravascular catheters, pacemakers, prosthetic cardiac valves, vascular grafts, orthopedic appliances, artificial joints, CSF shunts, dialysis catheters, and breast implants.
- **Osteomyelitis:** Most commonly associated with sternal wound infections status post cardiac surgery, although overall frequently rare. Other mode of transmission is via hematogenous spread.
- **Native valve endocarditis:** Less common than PVE; occurs approximately 5%.
- **Urinary tract infection:** Hospital acquired secondary to manipulation or catheter placement.
- **Endophthalmitis:** Increasing significantly status post intraocular lens placement.

Diagnosis Diagnosis is made by Gram stain and culture with sensitivities of appropriate site. Semiquantitation roll technique by Dennis Maki in which catheter is rolled over surface of blood agar plate is useful in suggesting a true intravascular catheter sepsis when both blood culture grows MSSE and count >15 colonies on a blood agar plate.

Diagnostic Tests/Procedures
Aerobic Culture, Appropriate Site *on page 244*
Gram Stain *on page 352*

Treatment First choice antibiotic in MSSE infections are penicillins or antistaphylococcal penicillins (penicillinase-resistant). For most medical device infections, the medical device must be removed. Current recommendations for pacemaker infection is to remove the pacer during the second week of parenteral antibiotics before reimplantation. Sixty-seven percent of prosthetic joint infection occur during the first 2 years. If the joint is not loose, 6 weeks of parenteral antibiotics are recommended. If the joint is loose, then removal of the joint plus parenteral antibiotics for 6 weeks is recommended. For non life-threatening infections with MSSE, a first generation cephalosporin may be used. For penicillin allergic individuals, clindamycin, vancomycin, doxycycline or co-trimoxazole based on susceptibility testing may be used.

Drug Therapy
Recommended
Penicillins, Penicillinase-Resistant *on page 637*
Alternate
Cephalosporins, 1st Generation *on page 527*
Clindamycin *on page 540*
Vancomycin Hydrochloride *on page 691*
Selected Readings
Christensen GD, "The 'Sticky' Problem of *Staphylococcus epidermidis* Sepsis," *Hosp Pract (Off Ed)*, 1993, 28(9A):27-36, 38.
Rupp ME and Archer GL, "Coagulase-Negative Staphylococci: Pathogens Associated With Medical Progress," *Clin Infec Dis*, 1994, 19:231-43.
Whitener C, Caputo GM, Weitekamp MR, et al, "Endocarditis Due to Coagulase-Negative Staphylococci," *Infect Dis Clin North Am*, 1993, 7(1):81-96.

Staphylococcus saprophyticus

Microbiology Staphylococcus derives its name from the Greek word staphyle meaning "bunch of grapes". On Gram stain, staphylococci are gram-positive cocci, 0.7-1.2 μm, nonspore forming, occurring singly, in pairs, in short 4-5 cocci chains or clusters. Staphylococci grow rapidly both as an aerobe and anaerobe on blood agar. The colonies are sharply defined, smooth, and 1-4 mm in diameter. Staphylococci are catalase-positive and differ from micrococci by the following: anaerobic acid production from glucose, sensitivity <200 mg/mL lysostaphin, and production of acid from glycerol in the presence of 0.4 mg/mL erythromycin.

Staphylococcus aureus may have a golden pigmentation secondary to carotenoid and produce β-hemolysis on horse, sheep, or human blood agar after an incubation of 24-48 hours. *Staphylococcus epidermidis* and coagulase-negative staph (CNS) are often used interchangeably but recognize that there are over 30 species of CNS of which *S. epidermidis* is the most common. It is important to distinguish three clinically relevant species: *S. aureus*, *S. epidermidis*, and *S. saprophyticus*. See table in *Staphylococcus aureus*, Methicillin-Resistant.

Epidemiology *Staphylococcus saprophyticus* is a common cause of urinary tract infections (UTIs) in sexually active young women, elderly men, and children. Highest frequency occurs during late summer and early autumn; reasons unclear.

Clinical Syndromes
• **Urinary tract infection (UTI):** Present with acute dysuria, back or flank pain, and temperature <38.5°C. Hematuria and pyuria are usually present.

Diagnosis Diagnosis depends on isolation of organism from urine. Counts as low as 10^2 CFU/mL in young women with symptoms is considered significant.

Diagnostic Tests/Procedures
Urine Culture, Clean Catch *on page 470*

Treatment First choice therapy is co-trimoxazole. Controversy exists whether single dose, 3-day, 7-day, or 10-day course are equally effective. Studies suggest that for women, a 3-day course is equally effective to a 7-day course. Alternative therapies include nitrofurantoin, ampicillin, first generation cephalosporin, or quinolone based on susceptibility testing.

Drug Therapy
Recommended
Co-trimoxazole *on page 545*
Alternate
Nitrofurantoin *on page 623*
Ampicillin *on page 495*
Cephalosporins, 1st Generation *on page 527*
Fluoroquinolones *on page 571*
Selected Readings
Abrahamsson K, Hansson S, Jodal U, et al, "*Staphylococcus saprophyticus* Urinary Tract Infections in Children," *Eur J Pediatr*, 1993, 152(1):69-71.
Elder NC, "Acute Urinary Tract Infection in Women. What Kind of Antibiotic Therapy Is Optimal?" *Postgrad Med*, 1992, 91(6):159-62, 165-6, 172.

Streptococcus agalactiae

Synonyms Group B *Streptococcus*

Microbiology *Streptococcus agalactiae* is a β-hemolytic *Streptococcus* first recognized in 1938 as a cause of puerperal sepsis ("childbed fever"). By the Lancefield serogroup classification of β-hemolytic streptococci, *S. agalactiae* is also known as group B *Streptococcus*. Like other streptococci, *S. agalactiae* are gram-positive cocci that appear to form chains when grown in broth. When

(Continued)

Streptococcus agalactiae (Continued)

the organism is growing on a blood agar plate, there is an area of complete hemolysis surrounding the colony, a finding called β-hemolysis. Several streptococci are β-hemolytic including group A streptococci (*Streptococcus pyogenes*), and groups B, C, and G streptococci. *S. agalactiae* does not require special media for growth and is readily isolated from clinical specimens.

Epidemiology The spectrum of group B streptococcal infections has been changing over the past years. In the 1970s, this organism was a leading cause of neonatal meningitis and sepsis and was an important cause of maternal peripartum infections, such as postpartum endometritis and bacteremia. More recently, surveillance studies in the 1990s have shown an incidence of 3 to 4 cases of invasive *S. agalactiae* infections per 100,000 adults. The majority of these infections have appeared in nonpregnant adults. A recent report in 1993 suggested an increasing incidence of invasive group B infections in nonpregnant adults, but the reasons for this increase were unclear.

Adult groups at risk for serious group B disease include persons with AIDS, diabetes mellitus, and cancer. Newborns are also at high risk for infection, although the presence of maternal IgG antibodies to the organism correlates with protection from serious infection in the neonate. Serious *S. agalactiae* infections are uncommon in infants older than 3 months of age, even though specific antibodies usually are not present.

Clinical Syndromes

• **Asymptomatic carriage in pregnant females:** It is estimated that 15% to 25% of women are asymptomatic carriers of group B streptococci. Many such women who are carriers of group B streptococcus during pregnancy can be identified by culture of the rectum and/or vagina at approximately 26 weeks of gestation. However, the presence of group B *Streptococcus* at this time (26 weeks) does **not** predict the presence of group B *Streptococcus* **at birth**, the time when detection of the bacterium is most clinically significant. Of this group, those women who have risk factors for infant infection are candidates for preventative therapy during delivery (see Treatment below). These risk factors include premature labor, fever, premature or prolonged rupture of membranes, multiple gestations, or a history of prior group B infection in a previous neonate. Prevention of group B neonatal infections in this manner is recommended by the American College of Obstetricians and Gynecologists, and the American Academy of Pediatrics.

• **Invasive infections in neonates:** Infection is acquired during passage through a colonized birth canal. "Early onset" infections occur within 1 week and often less than 1 day. Approximately 50% of infants born to mothers with vaginal and rectal carriage of group B streptococci will themselves become colonized; however, only a small percentage will develop symptomatic infection. In general, neonates are bacteremic with this organism, and many develop pneumonia with a respiratory distress syndrome. "Late-onset" infections occur between 1 week and 3 months, and meningitis is most frequently seen.

• **Invasive infections in the adult:** Pregnancy related *S. agalactiae* infections include peripartum fever, endometritis, chorioamnionitis, often with bacteremia. In nonpregnant adults, common infections include cellulitis, diabetic ulcer infections, urinary tract infections, septic arthritis, and pneumonias. A variety of serious complications have been seen including endocarditis, pelvic abscesses, meningitis, and others.

Diagnostic Tests/Procedures

Aerobic Culture, Appropriate Site *on page 244*

Group B *Streptococcus* Antigen Test *on page 354*

Treatment Group B streptococci are susceptible to penicillins, although they exhibit less *in vitro* sensitivity than group A streptococci. Adults with invasive, localized infections such as pyelonephritis or infected joint spaces should be treated with relatively high doses of penicillin G, approximately 12 million units daily. Patients with life-threatening infections such as endocarditis should receive 18 (or more) million units of penicillin G daily.

Neonates with group B blood stream infections should also receive penicillin G. Some limited data suggest *in vitro* synergy between penicillin and gentamicin, and many pediatricians will use this combination. Therapy is usually continued 10-14 days or more due to the risk of relapse in such conditions as meningitis.

As described above, pregnant women who are found to be carriers of group B streptococci in the vagina or rectum **at the time of birth** may be candidates for antibiotic prophylaxis if an additional risk factor to the infant is identified. Prophylactic administration of ampicillin to the mother at the time of delivery has been shown to decrease the rate of infection of the newborn. Indiscriminate prophylaxis of all pregnant women who are carriers of group B streptococci is not recommended.

Drug Therapy

Recommended

Penicillin G, Parenteral *on page 633*

Alternate

Cephalosporins, 1st Generation *on page 527*
Erythromycin *on page 561*
Vancomycin Hydrochloride *on page 691*

Selected Readings

Schwartz B, Schuchat A, Oxtoby MJ, et al, "Invasive Group B Streptococcal Disease in Adults," *JAMA*, 1991, 266(8):1112-4.

Gallagher PG and Watanakunakorn C, "Group B Streptococcal Bacteremia in a Community Teaching Hospital," *Am J Med*, 1985, 78(5):795-800.

Verghese A, Mireault K, and Arbeit RD, "Group B Streptococcal Bacteremia in Men," *Rev Infect Dis*, 1986, 8(6):912-7.

***Streptococcus*, Anaerobic** *see Streptococcus*-Related Gram-Positive Cocci *on page 212*

Streptococcus anginosus *see Streptococcus*, Viridans Group *on page 213*

Streptococcus bovis

Synonyms Group D Streptococci

Applies To *Streptococcus equinus*

Microbiology *Streptococcus bovis* and *Streptococcus equinus* poses the group D lipoteichoic acid antigen in their cell walls. Since 1984, the enterococci have been classified in a separate genus (*Enterococcus*). *S. bovis* is associated with human infections while *S. equinus* is found predominantly in the alimentary tract of horses. These organisms are gram-positive cocci which appear in chains. They are β-hemolytic on rabbit blood, α-hemolytic or nonhemolytic on sheep blood. The ability to cause hemolysis on laboratory media does not correlate with clinical virulence.

Epidemiology *Streptococcus bovis* is a minor part of the normal flora of man where it is found in the genital and intestinal tracts. In sheep and cows, it inhabits the intestinal tract. Infection with *Streptococcus bovis* is correlated with colon and rectal carcinoma and hepatic dysfunction. These organisms have low intrinsic virulence.

Clinical Syndromes *Streptococcus bovis* is a cause of endocarditis and bacteremia primarily in the elderly. Eighty percent of cases occur in patients 60 years of age or older. The association with colon carcinoma is attributed to production by the tumor of transferrin-like chelators that facilitate bacterial growth. One-third of patients with *S. bovis* endocarditis are found to have an adenocarcinoma, villous adenoma, or colonic polyp. The association with liver disease may be the result of altered hepatic secretion of bile salts or immunoglobulins and compromise of the hepatic reticuloendothelial system. Bacteremia associated with *S. bovis* is polymicrobial in approximately 20% of cases.

Diagnosis The diagnosis of *S. bovis* endocarditis is established by positive blood culture in a patient with mild fever and malaise. The disease onset is usually gradual. Low grade fever, arthralgia and cardiac murmurs, splenomegaly, splinter hemorrhages, Roth spots, Osler nodes, and embolic phenomenon may also be presenting features. If *S. bovis* is recovered, a thorough search for adenocarcinoma of the colon or rectum should be undertaken.

Diagnostic Tests/Procedures

Aerobic Culture, Appropriate Site *on page 244*
Blood Culture, Aerobic and Anaerobic *on page 271*

Duration of Therapy Endocarditis: 4 weeks; nonendocarditis: 7-10 days

Treatment Differentiation between nonenterococcal group D streptococci (primarily *S. bovis*) and enterococci (now classified in separate genus *Enterococcus* including *E. faecalis*, *E. faecium*, and *E. durans*) is important in regard to antimicrobial susceptibility. *S. bovis* is sensitive to penicillin (90% have penicillin MIC <0.2 µg/mL), ampicillin, cephalothin, and clindamycin. Endocarditis due to *S. bovis* is frequently treated with parenteral penicillin G as monoth-

(Continued)

Streptococcus bovis (Continued)

erapy. *Enterococcus* species generally have much higher MICs, usually 2-4 μg/mL and are resistant to achievable levels of cephalosporins and clindamycin. Therapy for enterococci requires use of a penicillin or vancomycin in combination with an aminoglycoside. See also *Enterococcus* Species and *Streptococcus* Viridans Group.

Penicillin G, 10-20 million units/day I.V. in divided doses every 4 hours for 4 weeks for organism with an MIC ≤0.1 μg/mL. Addition of gentamicin or streptomycin may result in more rapid cure. Streptomycin dosage 7.5 mg/kg I.M. every 12 hours or gentamicin 1 mg/kg I.V. every 8 hours for the first 2 weeks of therapy with penicillin being continued for the full 4 weeks. An additional alternative in cefazolin 1-2 g I.V. or I.M. every 6-8 hours for 4 weeks.

Vancomycin, 15 μg/kg I.V. every 12 hours for 4 weeks.

Drug Therapy
Recommended
Penicillin G, Parenteral *on page 633*
Alternate
Vancomycin Hydrochloride *on page 691*
Selected Readings
Zarkin BA, Lillemoe KD, Cameron JL, et al, "The Triad of *Streptococcus bovis* Bacteremia, Colonic Pathology, and Liver Disease," *Ann Surg*, 1990, 211(6):786-92.

Streptococcus equinus see *Streptococcus bovis* on previous page

Streptococcus intermedius see *Streptococcus*, Viridans Group
on page 213

Streptococcus milleri Group see *Streptococcus*, Viridans Group
on page 213

Streptococcus mitis see *Streptococcus*, Viridans Group
on page 213

Streptococcus morbillorum see *Streptococcus*, Viridans Group
on page 213

Streptococcus mutans see *Streptococcus*, Viridans Group
on page 213

Streptococcus pneumoniae

Microbiology *Streptococcus pneumoniae* was called "the captain of the men of death" by Sir William Osler because of its lethality. It remains a leading cause of acute lobar pneumonia, otitis media, and meningitis. *Streptococcus pneumoniae* is an encapsulated gram-positive coccus. Classically, the organism appears lancet-shaped and commonly in pairs or short chains. Colonies appear circular, dimpled or mucoid, and dome shaped. They cause α-hemolysis when grown aerobically on blood agar. There are several determinants of pathogenicity:

- the polysaccharide capsule, which protects the organism from phagocytosis
- adherence, which allows colonization of epithelial cells
- enzymes, such as neuraminidase (which allows growth in mucous secretions) and proteases (which degrade IgA and facilitate colonization)
- toxins, such as pneumolysis O, which directly inhibits phagocytic activity

Epidemiology *S. pneumoniae* is a common colonizer of the nasopharynx of healthy individuals. Estimates of this carriage state range from 5% to >70% and appears more common in children. Carriage seems highest in the winter and spring months, which is also the most common period for true infection. New serotypes of *Streptococcus pneumoniae* are acquired throughout the year. When true infection occurs, it is often with a new serotype rather than the serotype associated with years of carriage. Patients with chronic bronchitis are frequently colonized in the nasopharynx and respiratory tree with pneumococcus, and purulent exacerbations of bronchitis are often associated with this organism.

Clinical Syndromes
- **Pneumonia:** Typically, pneumococcal pneumonia begins abruptly with sudden fever and shaking chills, which resolves. Pleuritic pain may be quite severe. The patient often develops a cough productive of "rusty" mucopurulent sputum. Complications include parapneumonic effusion, empyema, bacteremia, and meningitis. *Streptoccocus pneumoniae* is still the most common cause of community-acquired pneumonia in adults.

- **Otitis media:** *S. pneumoniae* is a leading cause, accounting for 35% to 50% of the cases.
- **Meningitis:** *S. pneumoniae* is the most common etiology for community-acquired meningitis in adults. Often, this is preceded by pulmonary infection or a mild upper respiratory infection. Predisposing factors include alcoholism, sickle cell disease, multiple myeloma, and general debility.
- **Bacteremia:** This may occur in 25% or more of patients with pneumococcal pneumonia and more than 80% of patients with meningitis. Endocarditis has also been described.

Diagnosis The finding of lancet-shaped gram-positive cocci in ordinarily sterile body fluids such as cerebrospinal fluid, blood, sinus aspirates, or pleural fluid is diagnostic of *S. pneumoniae* infection. However, such a finding is not necessarily diagnostic when found in expectorated sputum since respiratory colonization is common (particularly in chronic bronchitics). With respiratory secretions, it is important to note the presence of both polymorphonuclear leukocytes, as well as numerous pneumococci on Gram stain; this combination is suggestive of true infection, but physician judgment is critical.

Antigen detection techniques are widely available for identifying the soluble pneumococcal capsular polysaccharide. Latex agglutination may be used to identify *S. pneumoniae* antigens from sterile body fluids such as cerebrospinal fluid. It may be useful (but only occasionally) in patients with suspected pneumococcal meningitis who have recently been treated with antibiotics which could interfere with recovery of the organism. However, Gram stain and cultures are much more preferred to latex agglutination.

Diagnostic Tests/Procedures
Aerobic Culture, Appropriate Site *on page 244*
Bacterial Antigens, Rapid Detection Methods *on page 269*
Gram Stain *on page 352*

Treatment Penicillin is the drug of choice for *Streptoccocus pneumoniae*. Recently, strains of *S. pneumoniae* resistant to penicillin have been reported, particularly in Western Europe. The incidence of penicillin-resistance is still quite low in the United States but is a worrisome trend. Some authors have suggested using vancomycin for empiric therapy of pneumococcal meningitis until antibiotic susceptibility patterns of the specific isolate are known.

Drug Therapy
Recommended
Meningitis:
Penicillin G, Parenteral *on page 633*
Nonmeningitis:
Penicillin G, Parenteral *on page 633*
Alternate
Meningitis:
Vancomycin Hydrochloride *on page 691*
Chloramphenicol *on page 531*
Nonmeningitis:
Erythromycin *on page 561*
Vancomycin Hydrochloride *on page 691*
Cephalosporins, 1st Generation *on page 527*

Selected Readings
Austrian R, "Some Observations on the Pneumococcus and on the Current Status of Pneumococcal Disease and Its Prevention," *Rev Infect Dis*, 1981, 3(Suppl):S1-17.
Musher DM, "Infections Caused by *Streptococcus pneumoniae*: Clinical Spectrum, Pathogenesis, Immunity, and Treatment," *Clin Infect Dis*, 1992, 14(4):801-7.
Musher DM, Watson DA, and Dominguez EA, "Pneumococcal Vaccination: Work to Date and Future Prospects," *Am J Med Sci*, 1990, 300(1):45-52.
Pallares R, Gudiol F, Linares J, et al, "Risk Factors and Response to Antibiotic Therapy in Adults With Bacteremic Pneumonia Caused by Penicillin-Resistant Pneumococci," *N Engl J Med*, 1987, 317(1):18-22.

Streptococcus pyogenes

Synonyms GABHS; Group A β-Hemolytic *Streptococcus*; Group A *Streptococcus*

Microbiology *Streptococcus pyogenes* are gram-positive, spherical cocci, which frequently appear in chains. Group A refers to a specific carbohydrate (Lancefield) antigen which is part of the cell wall and is used for serogrouping streptococcal species. The M-protein, of which there are more than 100 serotypes, is associated with resistance to phagocytosis by polymorphonuclear leukocytes. M-protein acts by decreasing alternative complement pathway ac-

(Continued)

Streptococcus pyogenes (Continued)

tivation and thereby limiting deposition of C3 on the surface of the bacteria. Immunity results from the development of type specific antibodies to the M-protein. Serum antibodies are thought to be protective against invasive infection but do not prevent the carrier state. Lipoteichoic acid on the surface of group A streptococci is responsible for binding the bacteria to the epithelial cell membranes of the oropharynx initiating colonization which is the first stage in infection. The hyaluronic acid capsule also is an additional virulence factor. Extracellular products produced by group A streptococci include streptolysin O, deoxyribonuclease B (DNase B), and hyaluronidase. These antigens evoke the formation of antibodies which (when detected in serum) confirm recent streptococcal infection in cases of acute glomerulonephritis or acute rheumatic fever. In addition, DNases A, C, and D; streptolysin S; proteinase; nicotinamide adenine deaminase; streptokinase; and the pyrogenic exotoxins A, B, C, and D are produced. These exotoxins cause the rash of scarlet fever, alter the blood-brain barrier, damage organs and may cause shock, block the reticuloendothelial system, and alter T-cell function. The effects of these toxins are thought to be mediated by hypersensitivity of the host to the toxins, as well as the direct toxic effect. In culture at 35°C, *Streptococcus pyogenes* is β-hemolytic on blood agar. Streptococci are catalase-negative. Presumptive diagnosis can be made by bacitracin susceptibility followed by confirmation using agglutination or coagglutination or other rapid antigen-antibody specific tests.

Epidemiology Infections due to *Streptococcus pyogenes* are ubiquitous in temperate and semitropical areas. They are less common in the tropics. Inapparent infections are as frequent as clinical infections. Serotypes associated with acute glomerulonephritis include 1, 3, 4, 12, and 25 in association with throat infections and 2, 4, 9, 55, 57, 58, 59, and 60 in association with skin infections. M types associated with rheumatic fever include 1, 3, 5, 6,14, 18, 19, and 24. The lists are not comprehensive.

Rheumatic fever remains a major public health concern in developing countries. Strep throat occurs with a peak incidence in late winter and spring. Children and adolescents are most often affected. Outbreaks occur in school and military recruit populations. Foodborne epidemics may occur during any season. The outbreaks are most frequently associated with milk, milk products, deviled eggs, and egg salad. The reservoir for *Streptococcus pyogenes* is man; transmission is by direct or intimate contact. Transmission by hand contact or objects is rare. Nasal carriers are particularly prone to transmit the disease. Eradication of the carrier state may require several courses of antimicrobials and is difficult.

Clinical Syndromes *Streptococcus pyogenes* is a frequently encountered and ubiquitous pathogen. Acute pharyngitis ("strep throat") and impetigo or pyoderma are the most common clinical presentations. Other manifestations include septicemia, otitis, sinusitis, cellulitis, peritonsillar and retropharyngeal abscess, pneumonia, lymphangitis, gangrene, myositis, vaginitis, peripheral sepsis, perianal cellulitis, and scarlet fever. Group A streptococcal infections are associated with important nonsuppurative sequelae specifically acute glomerulonephritis, acute rheumatic fever, and rarely toxic shock-like syndrome.

Patients with streptococcal sore throat may have minimal symptoms or may develop fever, painful sore throat, exudative tonsillitis and/or pharyngitis, and anterior cervical adenopathy. The pharynx, tonsillar pillars, and soft palate may exhibit petechiae against a background of edema and erythema. Otitis media and peritonsillar abscess often complicate severe cases. Acute glomerulonephritis may follow with a mean time of 10 days. Acute rheumatic fever may follow in 7-35 days with a mean of 19 days.

Scarlet fever is characterized by a fine erythematosus rash which blanches on pressure. It has a sandpaper-like touch and is commonly seen over the neck, chest, folds of the axilla, groin, elbow, and inner thigh. It is the result of infection by a strain-producing erythrogenic toxin to which the patient is sensitive but not immune. Acute glomerulonephritis and rheumatic fever can follow.

The American Heart Association (AHA) guidelines for the diagnosis of initial attack of rheumatic fever (Jones Criteria, 1992 Update). See table.

A case definition has been developed for group A streptococcal toxic shock syndrome (TSS) which should facilitate diagnosis and may lead to the evolution of prevention strategies and more effective therapy. See Tables 1 and 2.

Diagnosis Clinical diagnosis of "strep throat" is only 30% to 60% sensitive. Throat culture is the gold standard for the diagnosis of streptococcal pharyngi-

Guidelines for the Diagnosis of Initial Attack of Rheumatic Fever
(Jones Criteria, 1992 Update)*

Major Manifestations†

Carditis
Polyarthritis
Chorea
Erythema marginatum
Subcutaneous nodules

Minor Manifestations‡

Clinical findings
    Arthralgia
    Fever
Laboratory findings
    Elevated acute phase reactants
        Erythrocyte sedimentation rate
        C-reactive protein
    Prolonged PR interval

Supporting Evidence of Antecedent Group A Streptococcal Infection§

Positive throat culture or rapid streptococcal antigen test
Elevated or rising streptococcal antibody titer

---

*If supported by evidence of preceding group A streptococcal infection, the presence of two major manifestations or of one major and two minor manifestations indicates a high probability of acute rheumatic fever.

From Diagnosis of Rheumatic Fever — Special Writing Group, "Guidelines for the Diagnosis of Rheumatic Fever," *JAMA*, 1992, 268(15):2069-73.

Table 1. Proposed Case Definition for the Streptococcal Toxic Shock Syndrome*

I. **Isolation of group A streptococci (***Streptococcus pyogenes***)**
    A. From a normally sterile site (eg, blood, cerebrospinal, pleural, or peritoneal fluid, tissue biopsy, surgical wound, etc)
    B. From a nonsterile site (eg, throat, sputum, vagina, superficial skin lesion, etc)

II. **Clinical signs of severity**
    A. Hypotension: Systolic blood pressure ≤90 mm Hg in adults or <5th percentile for age in children
                and
    B. ≥2 of the following signs:
- Renal impairment: Creatinine ≥177 μmol/L (≥2 mg/dL) for adults or greater than or equal to twice the upper limit of normal for age. In patients with pre-existing renal disease, a ≥2-fold elevation over the baseline level
- Coagulopathy: Platelets ≤100 × 10^9/L (≤100,000/mm^3) or disseminated intravascular coagulation defined by prolonged clotting times, low fibrinogen level, and the presence of fibrin degradation products
- Liver involvement: Alanine aminotransferase (ALT), aspartate aminotransferase (AST), or total bilirubin levels greater than or equal to twice the upper limit of normal for age. In patients with pre-existing liver disease, a ≥2-fold elevation over the baseline level
- Adult respiratory distress syndrome defined by acute onset of diffuse pulmonary infiltrates and hypoxemia in the absence of cardiac failure, or evidence of diffuse capillary leak manifested by acute onset of generalized edema, or pleural or peritoneal effusions with hypoalbuminemia
- A generalized erythematous macular rash that may desquamate
- Soft-tissue necrosis, including necrotizing fasciitis or myositis, or gangrene

---

*An illness fulfilling criteria IA and II (A and B) can be defined as a **definite** case. An illness fulfilling criteria IB and II (A and B) can be defined as a **probable** case if no other etiology for the illness is identified.

Streptococcus pyogenes (Continued)

Table 2. **Classification of Group A Streptococcal Infection***

I.	**Streptococcal toxic shock syndrome (streptococcal TSS):** Defined by criteria in Table 1

II.	**Other invasive infections:** Defined by isolation of group A streptococci from a **normally sterile site** in patients not meeting criteria for streptococcal TSS
	  A. Bacteremia with no identified focus
	  B. Focal infections with or without bacteremia. Includes meningitis, pneumonia, peritonitis, puerperal sepsis, osteomyelitis, septic arthritis, necrotizing fascitis, surgical wound infections, erysipeas, and cellulitis

III.	**Scarlet fever:** Defined by a scarlatina rash with evidence of group A streptococcal infection, most commonly pharyngotonsillitis

IV.	**Noninvasive infections:** Defined by the isolation of group A streptococci from a nonsterile site
	  A. Mucous membrane: Includes pharyngitis, tonsillitis, otitis media, sinusitis, vaginitis
	  B. Cutaneous: Includes impetigo

V.	**Nonsuppurative sequelae:** Defined by specific clinical findings with evidence of a recent group A streptococcal infection
	  A. Acute rheumatic fever
	  B. Acute glomerulonephritis

*Examples of conditions in each category are not inclusive.
Streptococcal Toxic Shock Syndrome Case Definition — Working Group, "Defining the Group A Streptococcal Toxic Shock Syndrome," *JAMA*, 1993, 269(3):390-1.

tis. Culture obtained during an active infection in an untreated patient is almost always positive. The culture does not distinguish between acute streptococcal infection and streptococcal carriers with viral infections. The vast majority of symptomatic sore throat patients have viral sore throat. Rapid tests for the detection of group A streptococcal antigen are specific (~95%), but sensitivity varies widely from 60% to 90%. Their sensitivity is less than that of throat culture. **A negative antigen test should be confirmed by a culture**. The organism is readily recovered by routine aerobic culture from other sites.

Diagnostic Tests/Procedures
Aerobic Culture, Appropriate Site *on page 244*
Antideoxyribonuclease-B Titer, Serum *on page 256*
Antistreptolysin O Titer, Serum *on page 263*
Gram Stain *on page 352*
Group A *Streptococcus* Antigen Test *on page 354*
Streptozyme *on page 451*
Throat Culture for Group A Beta-Hemolytic *Streptococcus*
  on page 457

Treatment Patients who have had rheumatic fever are at high risk of suffering recurrent attacks if they develop streptococcal upper respiratory infections. Even asymptomatic infections can cause recurrence, and recurrence can occur in optimally treated symptomatic infections. Thus, continuous prophylaxis with antimicrobials is recommended. This therapy should be continued into the patient's early 20s and for at least 5 years after the last recurrence. Patients who have had carditis are at relatively high risk for recurrences of carditis. Discontinuance of prophylaxis should not be undertaken without consideration of the epidemiological risk factors for the particular patient (ie, likelihood of exposure to school children, day care, military recruit, college student, etc). The American Heart Association (AHA) has recommended the following therapy:

Drug Therapy Comment Patients who have had rheumatic fever are at high risk of suffering recurrent attacks if they develop streptococcal upper respiratory infections. Even asymptomatic infections can cause recurrence, and recurrence can occur in optimally treated symptomatic infections. Thus, continuous prophylaxis with antimicrobials is recommended. This therapy should be continued into the patient's early 20's and for at least 5 years after the last recurrence. Patients who have had carditis are at relatively high risk for recur-

Primary Prevention of Rheumatic Fever
(Treatment of Streptococcal Tonsillopharyngitis)

Agent	Dose	Mode	Duration
Benzathine penicillin G	600,000 units for patients <60 lb 1,200,000 units for patients >60 lb	I.M.	Once
or			
Penicillin V (phenoxymethyl penicillin)	250 mg 3 times/day	P.O.	10 days
For individuals allergic to penicillin:			
Erythromycin estolate	20–40 mg/kg/day 2–4 times/day (maximum: 1 g/day)	P.O.	10 days
or			
Ethylsuccinate	40 mg/kg/day 2–4 times/day (maximum: 1 g/day)	P.O.	10 days

The following agents are acceptable but usually not recommended:
   Amoxicillin, dicloxacillin, oral cephalosporins, and clindamycin.
The following are not acceptable: Sulfonamides, trimethoprim, tetracyclines,
   and chloramphenicol.
From Dajani AS, Bisno AL, and Chung KJ, "Prevention of Rheumatic
Fever." *Circulation*, 1988, 78:1082–6.

Secondary Prevention of Rheumatic Fever
(Prevention of Recurrent Attacks)

Agent	Dose	Mode
Benzathine penicillin G	1,200,000 units	I.M., every 4 weeks*
or		
Penicillin V	250 mg twice daily	P.O.
or		
Sulfadiazine	0.5 g once daily for patients <60 lb 1 g once daily for patients >60 lb	P.O.
For individuals allergic to penicillin and sulfadiazine:		
Erythromycin	250 mg twice daily	P.O.

*In high-risk situations, administration every 3 weeks is advised.
From Dajani AS, Bisno AL, and Chung KJ, "Prevention of Rheumatic
Fever." *Circulation*, 1988, 78:1082–6.

rences of carditis. Discontinuance of prophylaxis should not be undertaken
without consideration of the epidemiological risk factors for the particular patient (ie, likelihood of exposure to school children, day care, military recruit, college student, etc)

Drug Therapy
Recommended
   Penicillin G, Parenteral *on page 633*
Alternate
   Erythromycin *on page 561*
   Vancomycin Hydrochloride *on page 691*
   Cephalosporins, 1st Generation *on page 527*

Selected Readings
Bisno AL, "Group A Streptococcal Infections and Acute Rheumatic Fever," *N Engl J Med*, 1991, 325(11):783-93.
Campos JM, "Laboratory Diagnosis of Group A Streptococcal Pharyngitis," *Infect Dis Clin Prac*, 1993, 2:303-7.
Centers for Disease Control, "Invasive Group A Streptococcal Infections – United Kingdom, 1994," *MMWR Morb Mortal Wkly Rep*, 1994, 43:401-2.
Dan M, Maximova S, Siegman-Igra Y, et al, "Varied Presentations of Sporadic Group A Streptococcal Bacteremia: Clinical Experience and Attempt at Classification," *Rev Infect Dis*, 1990, 12(3):537-42.

(Continued)

Streptococcus pyogenes *(Continued)*

Denny FW Jr, "Group A Streptococcal Infections – 1993," *Curr Probl Pediatr*, 1993, 23(5):179-85.

Hoge CW, Schwartz B, Talkington DF, et al, "The Changing Epidemiology of Invasive Group A Streptococcal Infections and the Emergence of Streptococcal Toxic-Shock Like Syndrome," *JAMA*, 1993, 269(3):384-9.

Schwartz B, Facklam RR, and Breiman RF, "Changing Epidemiology of Group A Streptococcal Infection in the USA," *Lancet*, 1990, 336(8724):1167-71.

Stevens DL, Tanner MH, Winship J, et al, "Severe Group A Streptococcal Infections Associated With a Toxic Shock-Like Syndrome and Scarlet Fever Toxin A," *N Engl J Med*, 1989, 321(1):1-7.

Streptococcus-Related Gram-Positive Cocci

Synonyms Anaerobic *Streptococcus*; SRGPC; *Streptococcus*, Anaerobic

Applies To Microaerophilic Streptococci; *Peptostreptococcus*

Microbiology *Streptococcus*-related gram-positive cocci (SRGPC) which are clinically important include species of the genera *Peptostreptococcus*, *Streptococcus*, and *Gemella*. SRGPC which rarely cause clinical infections include species of the genera *Peptococcus*, *Coprococcus*, *Ruminococcus*, *Sarcina*, and *Staphylococcus saccharolyticus*. *Peptostreptococcus* is the most significant pathogen and is recovered almost as frequently (~25%) as *Bacteroides fragilis* from clinical specimens. *Peptostreptococcus* and *Bacteroides* species are frequently recovered together and in combination with aerobic bacteria in abscess cavities throughout the body. The *Peptostreptococcus* species most frequently recovered include *P. magnus*, *P. asaccharolyticus*, *P. prevotii*, and *P. anaerobius*. SRGPC are speciated by biochemical and chromatographic methods in the laboratory. Reclassification of these species utilizing modern DNA, ribosomal RNA, and cell wall polysaccharide content analyses will continue.

Epidemiology SRGPC comprise a large portion of the normal flora of the mouth, intestinal tract, and vagina. Infections in humans are often the result of contamination from normal flora sites or contiguous extension of infection from colonized sites onto adjacent tissues.

Clinical Syndromes SRGPC are often recovered from abscesses, frequently in polymicrobial infections, at virtually any site in the body. More often than not, SRGPC are contaminants if isolated with other bacteria, and clinical interpretation of their presence is often difficult. Head and neck infections include infection of paranasal sinuses, brain abscess, dental abscess, lateral (pharyngomaxillary) and retropharyngeal space infections, and in Ludwig's angina (bilateral submandibular and sublingual cellulitis often, 50% to 90%, of dental origin). Thoracic infections include lung abscess and empyema. Abdominal infections include liver abscess, visceral abscess, and pelvic and perirectal abscesses. Skin and subcutaneous tissue infections often involve devitalized or necrotic skin, muscle, and subcutaneous tissue. Specific examples include anaerobic streptococcal myositis, a fulminant disease characterized by pain, marked edema, crepitant myositis, and a purulent or seropurulent exudate that on Gram stain reveals gram-positive cocci in chains. Progressive synergistic gangrene is caused by polymicrobic infection with *Staphylococcus aureus* and microaerophilic or anaerobic streptococci. The infection occurs around surgical incisions as an ulcerated lesion with surrounding gangrenous tissue. Chronic burrowing ulcer is an infection of deep soft tissue. It erodes (burrows) through subcutaneous tissue to erupt as an ulcer at a distant site.

Diagnosis Documentation of the diagnosis of infection with SRGPC requires that potentially contaminating normal flora be excluded from the cultures. Needle aspiration of loculated pus by the percutaneous route is a frequently good approach. Often Gram stain yields more information than culture because of the fastidious nature of the organisms (difficult to recover by usual laboratory methods) and the frequent polymicrobial nature of the infections.

Diagnostic Tests/Procedures

Anaerobic Culture *on page 250*

Gram Stain *on page 352*

Duration of Therapy 7-10 days

Treatment Successful therapy for anaerobic and microaerophilic streptococcal infections usually involves debridement or drainage of involved area or abscess and intravenous antimicrobial therapy usually with intravenous penicillin.

Drug Therapy

Recommended

Penicillin G, Parenteral *on page 633*

Alternate
Cephalosporins, 1st Generation *on page 527*
Clindamycin *on page 540*
Vancomycin Hydrochloride *on page 691*

Streptococcus salivarius *see Streptococcus*, Viridans Group *on this page*

***Streptococcus sanguis* I** *see Streptococcus*, Viridans Group *on this page*

***Streptococcus sanguis* II** *see Streptococcus*, Viridans Group *on this page*

Streptococcus Species
Refer To
Streptococcus agalactiae on page 203
Streptococcus bovis on page 205
Streptococcus pneumoniae on page 206
Streptococcus pyogenes on page 207
Streptococcus-Related Gram-Positive Cocci on previous page
Streptococcus, Viridans Group on this page

Streptococcus, Viridans Group
Synonyms Viridans Streptococci

Applies To *Gemella morbillorum*; *Streptococcus anginosus*; *Streptococcus intermedius*; *Streptococcus milleri* Group; *Streptococcus mitis*; *Streptococcus morbillorum*; *Streptococcus mutans*; *Streptococcus salivarius*; *Streptococcus sanguis* I; *Streptococcus sanguis* II

Microbiology Historically "viridans" or green streptococci were separated from other "β-hemolytic" strains of streptococci by their ability to produce α-hemolysis ("greening") on blood agar. Although many strains produce γ-hemolysis (nonhemolytic). More recently, antigenic, physiological, biochemical, and DNA homology techniques have resulted in more precise characterization of these organisms. The Lancefield serogroup (eg, A, B, C, D, etc) cross species lines. New species are being described and many reclassifications have been made. *S. bovis* and *S. pneumoniae* are α-hemolytic. Upon isolation of α, β, or nonhemolytic streptococci on blood agar, presumptive identification of nongroup A, B, or D can be made be resistance to bacitracin, negative hippurate or CAMP test, negative or weakly reactive bile esculin hydrolysis, negative PYR test, negative pyruvate, and failure to grow in 6.5% NaCl.

Some of these organisms are nutritionally fastidious and can require complex supplemented media. CO_2 may enhance growth. There is no correlation between serogroup and biochemical speciation. Speciation can be accomplished by biochemical testing. *S. morbillorum* has been transferred to the genus *Gemella*.

Clinical Syndromes Clinically, viridans streptococci are associated primarily with endocarditis, although infection of all tissues have been reported. *S. sanguis* I, *S. sanguis* II, and *S. mitis* are most frequently implicated in endocarditis, while *S. intermedius* is associated with noncardiac suppurative infections. *S. anginosus* and *S. constellatus* are closely related and are sometimes classified together with *S. intermedius* and *Streptococcus* MG as *Streptococcus milleri* or *S. milleri* group.

Viridans streptococci often pose a problem as they may be detected in blood culture as the result of transient insignificant bacteremia or may represent insignificant contaminants. Fifty percent of all bacterial endocarditis is due to viridans streptococci which is often diagnosed in patients with valvular heart disease. The course is subacute with cure rates in excess of 90%. Transient seeding of the blood by viridans streptococci is regarded as a commonplace occurrence. The organism has low intrinsic virulence. See table.

Diagnosis Diagnosis is usually accomplished by repeated positive blood culture or recovery of the organism in cultures from the affected site.

Diagnostic Tests/Procedures
Aerobic Culture, Appropriate Site *on page 244*
Blood Culture, Aerobic and Anaerobic *on page 271*
Gram Stain *on page 352*

Duration of Therapy Endocarditis: 4 weeks; nonendocarditis: 7-10 days

Treatment Susceptibility testing has not been standardized for fastidious CO_2-requiring *Streptococcus* species. Most isolates are reported to be sus-

Streptococcus Viridans Group

Species	Alternate Nomenclature	Lancefield Groups	Normal Human Habitat	Normal Veterinary Habitat	Human Disease	Veterinary Disease
S. acidominimus		NG, E, F		Milk, genital and intestinal tracts	Rare	—
S. anginosus, S. constellatus, S. intermedius	S. milleri	NG, A, C, F, G, K	Oropharynx, teeth surface, skin, intestinal tract		Endocarditis, suppurative infections, abcesses, bacteremia	—
S. bovis		D	Genital and intestinal tracts	Bovine and sheep — intestinal tracts	Endocarditis, bacteremia	Endocarditis
S. cremoris		N	Oropharynx	Milk	Rare	Mastitis
S. dysgalactiae	S. equisimilis	C, G, L	Upper respiratory tract, skin, vagina	Bovine and sheep	—	Mastitis
S. lactis		N	Oropharynx	Milk	Rare	Mastitis
S. mitis S. sanguis II	S. mitior	NG, A, C, F, G, H, K, M, O	Oropharynx, intestinal tract		Endocarditis, caries	—
S. morbillorum	Gemella morbillorum	NG	Intestinal and urogenital tracts		Endocarditis, suppurative infections	—
S. mutans		NG, E, F, K	Teeth surface, intestinal tract		Endocarditis, caries	—
S. pneumoniae		—	Upper respiratory tract		Common	—
S. salivarius		NG, F, H, K	Oropharynx, intestinal tract		Endocarditis	—
S. sanguis I	S. mitior	NG, C, F, H, K	Teeth surface, intestinal tract		Endocarditis, caries	—
S. suis		D (R, S, T)		Swine	Rare	Bacteremia, bone and joint infections
S. uberis		NG, E, F, K		Milk, oropharynx, skin, intestinal tract	Rare	Mastitis

Adapted from Gallis HA. "Viridans and β-Hemolytic (Non-Group A, B, and D) Streptococci," *Principles and Practice of Infectious Diseases*, Mandell GL, Douglas RG Jr, and Bennett JE, eds. New York, NY: Churchill Livingston, 1990, 1563-72.

NG = nongroupable.

ceptible to penicillin with MICs <0.06 μg/mL. Rare isolates have penicillin MICs >1.0 μg/mL. Other effective agents include cephalosporins (first and second generation), cefotaxime, clindamycin, erythromycin, and vancomycin. *In vitro* resistance to aminoglycosides is observed; however, synergy is observed *in vitro* with cell wall active agents.

Penicillin G, 10-20 million units/day I.V. in divided doses every 4 hours for 4 weeks for organisms with an MIC ≤0.1 μg/mL. Addition of gentamicin or streptomycin may result in more rapid cure. Streptomycin dosage 7.5 mg/kg I.M. every 12 hours or gentamicin 1 mg/kg I.V. every 8 hours for the first 2 weeks of therapy with penicillin being continued for the full 4 weeks. An additional alternative in cefazolin 1-2 g I.V. or I.M. every 6-8 hours for 4 weeks.

Vancomycin, 15 μg/kg I.V. every 12 hours for 4 weeks.

Drug Therapy Comment Susceptibility testing has not been standardized for fastidious CO_2 requiring *Streptococcus* species. Most isolates are reported to be susceptible to penicillin with MICs <0.06 μg/mL. Rare isolates have penicillin MICs >1.0 μg/mL. Other effective agents include cephalosporins (first and second generation), cefotaxime, clindamycin, erythromycin, and vancomycin. *In vitro* resistance to aminoglycosides is observed; however, synergy is observed *in vitro* with cell wall active agents.

Drug Therapy
Recommended
Endocarditis:
Penicillin G, Parenteral *on page 633*
or
Penicillin G, Parenteral *on page 633*
used in combination with
Gentamicin Sulfate *on page 575*
Nonendocarditis:
Penicillin G, Parenteral *on page 633*
Alternate
Endocarditis:
Vancomycin Hydrochloride *on page 691*
or
Vancomycin Hydrochloride *on page 691*
used in combination with
Gentamicin Sulfate *on page 575*
Nonendocarditis:
Cephalosporins, 1st Generation *on page 527*
Vancomycin Hydrochloride *on page 691*

Selected Readings

Bochud PY, Eggimann P, Calandra T, et al, "Bacteremia Due to Viridans *Streptococcus* in Neutropenic Patients With Cancer: Clinical Spectrum and Risk Factors," *Clin Infect Dis*, 1994, 18:25-31.

Burden AD, Oppenheim BA, Crowther D, et al, "Viridans Streptococcal Bacteremia in Patients With Haematological and Solid Malignancies," *Eur J Cancer*, 1991, 27(4):409-11.

Elting LS, Bodey GP, and Keefe BH, "Septicemia and Shock Syndrome Due to Viridans Streptococci: A Case-Control Study of Predisposing Factors," *Clin Infect Dis*, 1992, 14(6):1201-7.

Strongyloides stercoralis

Microbiology *Strongyloides stercoralis* is a small roundworm (nematode) which can cause human disease in several ways. The "direct" cycle of infection begins when the human comes in contact with soil containing the worm in its infective (filariform) larval stage. *Strongyloides* penetrates the skin and enters the circulation of the host. When the worms reach the alveolar capillaries, a pulmonary phase begins in which the parasites enter the alveoli and ascend the respiratory tract. Once in the pharynx, the organisms are swallowed. Maturation and reproduction occur in the small intestine. The fertilized adult female burrows into the mucosa of the upper small intestine and begins to lay eggs. The larvae which hatch are in a noninfectious (rhabditiform) stage; they eventually bore through the intestinal epithelium to reach the bowel lumen and are passed in the feces. The rhabditiform larvae can transform to infective filariform larvae in soil, thus completing the cycle.

In addition to this direct cycle, *Strongyloides* can also reproduce without a human host. In this "**indirect cycle**," larvae are passed into the soil, as described above. If proper environmental conditions are present, larvae mature into adult helminths capable of reproduction. After copulation, large numbers

(Continued)

Strongyloides stercoralis (Continued)

of new larvae are produced, potentially infectious to humans.

A less common but clinically important aspect of *Strongyloides* is its "**autoinfection cycle**." Instead of being passed in the stool, noninfectious larvae transform into infectious larvae in the lumen of the intestine. They can then re-enter the host circulation either by boring through the intestinal wall or penetrating the perianal skin. This "autoinfection" can cause repeated infections over the years and at times can be life-threatening because of the associated heavy worm burden ("hyperinfection syndrome").

Epidemiology *Strongyloides* infections occur worldwide. Infections are common in the tropics where the prevalence may approach 50% in some areas. In the United States, the disease is much less common, even in the southern states where the most number of cases are reported (prevalence <4%). In addition to the direct penetration of the skin, *Strongyloides* can be sexually transmitted.

Clinical Syndromes

- **Asymptomatic infection:** About 33% of infected individuals have no symptoms.
- **Abdominal pain and diarrhea (sometimes bloody):** This usually occurs as the larvae hatch in the intestinal mucosa and are passed through the lumen. Complications include ileus, weight loss, and malabsorption syndromes. Important clues to the diagnosis are concomitant peripheral eosinophilia and an urticarial skin rash.
- **Eosinophilic pneumonitis, a Löffler's-type syndrome:** This is similar to other hookworm infections which have a prominent pulmonary phase. Patients present with fever, cough, and wheezing as the larvae migrate through the pulmonary circulation and alveoli. A pruritic rash may be seen.
- **Autoinfection** (see Microbiology above): Chronic and recurrent *Strongyloides* infections can occur over months or years because of the organism's ability to autoinfect the host. These patients can present with a wide variety of symptoms, either gastrointestinal (nausea, vomiting, abdominal pain, explosive diarrhea) and/or pulmonary (wheezing, cough) depending on the phase of the parasite's life cycle. Immunocompromised individuals are at risk for life-threatening, disseminated hyperinfections with massive worm burdens. The majority of cases has been reported in organ transplant recipients and in patients with lymphoma or leukemia; in some cases, hyperinfection occurs in otherwise healthy individuals. An overwhelming pneumonitis is characteristically seen with cough, dyspnea, bronchospasm, and sputum production. Peripheral eosinophilia is common but may be absent. Other complications include bacterial sepsis, respiratory failure, bacterial meningitis, and death. The hyperinfection syndrome is an uncommon manifestation of strongyloidiasis.
- ***Strongyloides* in AIDS:** In the past, disseminated *Strongyloides* has been regarded as an AIDS-defining condition in people who are seropositive for HIV. However, it has proven a relatively uncommon occurrence even in patients from endemic areas.

Diagnosis Strongyloidiasis should be suspected in travelers or immigrants from an endemic area and presenting with diarrhea and eosinophilia. It should also be considered in the differential diagnosis of eosinophilic pneumonia (Löffler's-type syndrome) or unexplained diarrhea in an immunocompromised patient. Peripheral eosinophilia, while important, may be absent. In all cases, laboratory confirmation is essential and includes:

- Stool examination to identify the characteristic larval forms (rather than the eggs, which are rarely found). A single negative fecal exam does not rule out strongyloidiasis.
- Duodenal aspiration to identify the organism in the upper intestinal tract. This can be done as part of an upper endoscopic procedure.

Diagnostic Tests/Procedures

Ova and Parasites, Stool *on page 416*
Ova and Parasites, Urine or Aspirates *on page 419*

Treatment The drug of choice for strongyloidiasis is thiabendazole. However, it is well known that treatment failures occur with the standard drug doses for unclear reasons. A recent report has suggested that ivermectin may also be effective in people with AIDS.

Since disseminated *Strongyloides* is seen in organ transplant recipients, individuals from endemic areas awaiting transplantation should be carefully screened and treated if positive.

Drug Therapy
  Recommended
    Thiabendazole *on page 681*
    Ivermectin *on page 595*
  Selected Readings
    Gompels MM, Todd J, Peters BS, et al, "Disseminated Strongyloidiasis in AIDS: Uncommon but Important," *AIDS*, 1991, 5(3):329-32.
    Longworth DL and Weller PF, "Hyperinfection Syndrome With Strongyloidiasis," *Curr Clin Top Infect Dis*, 1986, 10:1-26.
    Torres JR, Isturiz R, Murillo J, et al, "Efficacy of Ivermectin in the Treatment of Strongyloidiasis Complicating AIDS," *Clin Infect Dis*, 1993, 17(5):900-2.

Tapeworms *see* Cestodes *on page 75*

Timing of Food Poisoning *see page 723*

T-*Mycoplasma* *see* Ureaplasma urealyticum *on page 225*

Toxoplasma gondii

Synonyms Toxo

Microbiology *Toxoplasma gondii* is a sporozoan of the order Coccidia and suborder *Eimeria*. The three forms of *T. gondii* are trophozoites (previously referred as tachyzoites), tissue cysts, and oocysts. The trophozoite is crescent to oval shape, 4 x 8 μm in size, and stains with both Wright and Giemsa stains. The trophozoite invades all nucleated cells, resides in vacuoles, and reproduces to form cysts. Tissue cysts measure 10-200 μm and may contain up to 3000 organisms. These cysts may remain dormant for years and can become reactivated. The organisms stain PAS positive, but the cyst wall itself stains very weakly positive. The oocysts measure 10-12 μm and are produced only in cats. All three forms are pathogenic to humans.

Epidemiology *Toxoplasma* infects nearly all animals and birds. It is the most widely distributed of all intracellular parasites. Prior to the AIDS epidemic, the majority of cases were benign and self-limited. There are still approximately 3000 cases of congenital toxoplasmosis reported per year with an average of 0.6 cases per 1000 pregnancies in the United States. Toxoplasmosis is the most common focal CNS infection in AIDS. It is estimated that 5% to 10% of AIDS patients have toxoplasmosis although 25% to 50% of AIDS patients will have positive IgG titers indicating previous exposure suggesting that reactivation plays an important role. In heart, but not renal or liver, transplantation, 50% of the seronegative recipients who receive seropositive donor hearts develop toxoplasmosis with a mortality rate exceeding 75%. Bone marrow transplant patients appear to be at increased risk of reactivation.

Humans become infected by ingesting the cysts either through contamination with cat feces or undercooked meat, especially pork and lamb, or through direct inoculation via blood transfusions, laboratory accidents, or congenital transmission. After ingestion of the cysts, digestive enzymes disrupt the cyst wall and release viable organisms that invade the mucosa and disseminate.

Clinical Syndromes
  • **Asymptomatic lymphadenitis:** Eighty percent to 90% of patients present with asymptomatic cervical lymphadenitis.
  • **Mononucleosis syndrome:** Some patients may present with fever, malaise, myalgias, sore throat, maculopapular rash, and hepatosplenomegaly which is self-limited and often confused with viral illnesses such as EBV. Rarely, patients develop myocarditis or pneumonitis.
  • **Congenital:** Pregnant women who acquire toxoplasmosis during the first trimester have a 25% risk of fetal transmission resulting in spontaneous abortions, stillborns, or severe disease. Sixty-five percent of infants born to women infected during the third trimester have subclinical infection with ultimately 85% developing chorioretinitis or neurological sequelae. The number of congenital cases continues to decline probably because of increased awareness of food and cat hygiene during pregnancy.
  • **Ocular:** Vast majority of chorioretinitis is due to congenital toxoplasmosis. Patients in their second or third decade of life present with blurred vision, scotoma, eye pain, and photophobia. Fundoscopic examination reveals characteristic exudative retinal lesions. Typically bilateral in congenital toxoplasmosis and unilateral in acquired infection.
  • **Encephalitis:** Increased incidence in homosexual AIDS patients. Patients present with headache, seizures, disorientation, fever, and focal neurological deficits depending on size, location, and number of lesions. MRI is more sensitive than CT. *Toxoplasma* typically appears as multiple small lesions

(Continued)

217

ORGANISMS

Toxoplasma gondii (Continued)

with predilection for corticomedullary junction and basal ganglia, whereas lymphoma usually presents with a large solitary lesion with subependymal spread or ventricular encasement. Differential diagnosis of CNS mass lesions in AIDS is toxoplasmosis 50% to 70%, primary CNS lymphoma 20% to 30%, progressive multifocal leukoencephalopathy 10% to 20%, and, less frequently, Kaposi sarcoma, tuberculosis, fungal, or herpes. Serological test may be of limited value given 3% false-negative and increased seropositivity in AIDS.

Diagnosis Diagnosis depends on serological tests and biopsy. Ocular *Toxoplasma* is diagnosed by clinical examination. Biopsy material reveals trophozoites.

Diagnostic Tests/Procedures
Brain Biopsy *on page 285*
Lymph Node Biopsy *on page 395*
Muscle Biopsy *on page 403*
Toxoplasma Antigen by ELISA *on page 459*
Toxoplasma Serology *on page 459*

Treatment Treatment should consist of sulfadiazine 1-1.5 g every 6 hours plus pyrimethamine 50-100 mg everyday plus leucovorin. If intolerant of sulfa, may substitute with clindamycin 450-600 mg every 6 hours. Ninety percent of patients will show clinical or radiographic improvement within 10-14 days of therapy. AIDS patients with mass lesions should be treated empirically; and if no response, then a brain biopsy is recommended. Dapsone, atovaquone, and clarithromycin have been shown to have moderate effects. Patients must be continued on suppressive therapy to avoid reactivation. Preventive measures include avoidance of cat feces, and freezing at -20°C, thawing, and heating to >60°C to destroy cysts in contaminated meats.

Drug Therapy
Recommended
Pyrimethamine *on page 653*
  used in combination with
Sulfadiazine *on page 671*

Alternate
Clindamycin *on page 540*
  used in combination with
Pyrimethamine *on page 653*

Selected Readings
Joiner KA and Dubremetz JF, "*Toxoplasma gondii*: A Protozoan for the Nineties," *Infect Immun*, 1993, 61(4):1169-72.
McCabe R and Chirurgi V, "Issues in Toxoplasmosis," *Infect Dis Clin North Am*, 1993, 7(3):587-604.
Wong SY and Remington JS, "Toxoplasmosis in Pregnancy," *Clin Infect Dis*, 1994, 18(6):853-61.

Treponema pallidum
Related Information
HIV Clinical Practice Guidelines *on page 765-774*

Microbiology *Treponema pallidum* (subspecies *pallidum*) is a thin, gram-negative bacterium which belongs to the order Spirochaetales. It is one of the clinically important spirochetes and is thus related to such agents as *Borrelia burgdorferi* (the cause of Lyme disease) and *Leptospira* (the cause of leptospirosis). *T. pallidum* is the etiologic agent of syphilis. The organism is thin, long, helical, and coiled and is difficult to see by light microscopy. Visualization of the organism in clinical specimens requires special techniques other than the Gram stain or Giemsa stain. There are no clinically available culture systems for *T. pallidum*, and microbiologic identification of the organism depends on such techniques as darkfield microscopy, direct fluorescent antibody stains, silver stains, and serologic tests.

Epidemiology Syphilis occurs exclusively in humans. The vast majority of cases are acquired via sexual contact with an infected person. Other modes of acquisition include congenital transmission to the newborn and blood transfusion, but these are much less common.

Despite public health measures the incidence of syphilis has continued to increase to epidemic proportions. In the United States, the number of syphilis cases increased dramatically in the late 1980s, with a near doubling of total reported cases. In 1992, there were over 120,000 reported cases of syphilis (at all stages), but this number grossly underestimates the true number of infections since many cases are undiagnosed. In many urban areas in the U.S., the number of syphilis cases has increased dramatically despite a lower incidence in the homosexual community, the population previously at highest risk. In large part, this change in the at-risk population is due to the increased use of crack cocaine and the exchange of sex for drugs. Sex partners are almost impossible to locate in some urban areas and a substantial number of crack users have undiagnosed syphilis. Currently, the groups at highest risk for syphilis are black, heterosexual men and black, heterosexual women. There has also been an increase in the number of cases of congenital syphilis corresponding roughly to the increase in primary and secondary syphilis in heterosexual women.

Sexual partner notification remains an important part of infection control measures. About 50% of partners named by an actively infected individual will also have syphilis; many partners will either be actively infected themselves or will have incubating syphilis.

Clinical Syndromes Syphilis commonly presents in one of several stages: primary, secondary, latent (early latent and late latent), or tertiary syphilis. However, it should be remembered that syphilis has been called "the great mimic" in medical literature because of its protean manifestations and tendency to mimic other diseases.

- **Primary syphilis:** This is an important cause of the common clinical syndrome of "genital ulceration with regional lymphadenopathy". This syndrome is caused by syphilis, primary herpes simplex virus infection, lymphogranuloma venereum, donovanosis, and chancroid. It may be difficult for the clinician to diagnose this on the basis of clinical findings alone. The hallmark of primary syphilis is the genital chancre. The syphilitic chancre is typically a single, painless ulcer with raised and indurated borders. The base of the ulcer is clean, usually without purulence. Up to one-third of syphilitic ulcers, however, may be mildly painful. The chancre can be found on the penis, rectum, anal verge, mouth, labia, or cervix. In the absence of treatment, chancres persist for up to 6 weeks. In addition, inguinal lymphadenopathy is present in the majority of cases of primary syphilis (about 80%). The onset of adenopathy usually occurs at the same time as the genital lesion. Characteristically, the adenopathy is painless (like the chancre), and the nodes are firm. In 70% of cases, the adenopathy is bilateral. Constitutional symptoms are usually absent in primary syphilis. In some individuals, primary syphilis goes unnoticed, especially if the chancre is small and painless. The chancre is teeming with live and active organisms and is an excellent source of material (serum and lymphatic fluid) for a darkfield examination.

- **Secondary syphilis:** In the absence of specific therapy for primary syphilis, further clinical manifestations may develop. Secondary syphilis may occur up to 2 years after initial infection. In secondary syphilis, there is evidence of a systemic illness and often the diagnosis may be difficult to make. The manifestations of secondary syphilis are protean. The most common finding is a skin rash, which is present in about 90% of cases. This rash may be macular, papular, papulosquamous, pustular, or nonspecific. The rash of secondary syphilis is somewhat unique in that it often involves the palms of the hands and soles of the feet; only a limited number of infectious and noninfectious conditions cause a rash in this distribution. In secondary syphilis, mouth or throat lesions are present in about one-third of cases, and the original genital chancre may still be present in some (15% to 20%). Hair loss can be an important clue to the diagnosis; involvement of the hair follicles (follicular syphilides) causes areas of alopecia. Condylomata lata are large fleshy papular lesions that may form in the perianal and genital areas and are characteristic of secondary syphilis. Constitutional symptoms such as fevers, myalgias, and weight loss are also common. There may be evidence of central nervous system involvement in a number of cases; about 1% to 2% may present with acute meningitis, both clinically and by cerebrospinal fluid analysis. A larger number (up to 40%) may have asymptomatic abnormalities in the spinal fluid. The Centers for Disease Control have stated that a routine lumbar puncture in secondary lues is not indicated. However, if there is evidence of auditory, cranial nerve, meningeal, or ocular manifestations of syphilis, a lumbar puncture and careful ophthalmologic exam (including slit-lamp) should be performed. A variety of unusual manifestations of secondary syphilis have been well-described including nephropathy, hepatitis, arthritis, colitis, and others.

(Continued)

Treponema pallidum (Continued)

- **Latent syphilis:** The natural history of untreated secondary syphilis is that the illness resolves spontaneously after 3-12 weeks, although viable organisms persist. In the absence of specific treatment, patients enter a stage of "latency". These patients have no symptoms related to syphilis, and the only clue for the diagnosis of latent infection is a positive serologic test for syphilis. It is important for the physician to perform a careful history and physical examination looking for signs and symptoms of tertiary syphilis; only then should patients be classified as truly "latent". Patients are classified as having "early latent" disease if they are asymptomatic and have acquired infection within the past year. Those with no symptoms and infection of longer than 1 year's duration are said to have "late latent" syphilis. In the asymptomatic patient with a positive serology, it may sometimes be difficult to distinguish early from late latent disease.

  The role of lumbar puncture in latent syphilis has recently been addressed by the Centers for Disease Control. The yield of spinal fluid analysis in detecting unsuspected tertiary syphilis in a patient who appears to have only latent syphilis is low. Lumbar puncture should be considered in the following situations:
  -patients with neurologic abnormalities
  -evidence of other syphilitic disease, such as aortitis, gummas, iritis
  -treatment failure
  -concomitant HIV infection
  -RPR or VDRL titer $> 1:32$, unless infected less than 1 year
  -if treatment with antibiotics other than penicillin is anticipated

- **Tertiary syphilis:** This includes the following:
  -asymptomatic neurosyphilis
  -symptomatic neurosyphilis, or tabes dorsalis
  -cardiovascular syphilis
  -syphilitic uveitis
  -late benign syphilis (gummas)

- **Syphilis and AIDS:** Syphilis in the HIV-infected individual can be highly aggressive. Patients progress from primary to tertiary syphilis over several years, as opposed to several decades in the non-HIV infected individual. When the clinical findings suggest syphilis (at any stage) but the standard serologic tests are negative, the diagnosis should be pursued with a biopsy, darkfield exam, or DFA antibody staining. Treatment of syphilis in the AIDS patient is no different; penicillin should be used if at all possible. A lumbar puncture should be considered in any patient with HIV and syphilis. A VDRL or RPR should be obtained at 1,2, 3, 6, 9, and 12 months. If the titers fail to decrease fourfold, retreat with penicillin and perform a lumbar puncture.

Diagnosis The definitive methods for diagnosing early syphilis are darkfield examination (of active lesions) and direct fluorescent antibody tests on active lesions or tissue biopsies. Serologic tests for syphilis, while commonly used, are not diagnostic. A presumptive diagnosis of active syphilis can be made using one of various serologic tests, which are classified as follows:

Nontreponemal tests: Venereal Disease Research Laboratory (VDRL), rapid plasma reagin (RPR)

Treponemal: Fluorescent treponemal antibody absorbed test (FTA-ABS), microhemagglutination assay for antibody to *Treponema pallidum* (MHA-TP), and *Treponema pallidum* immobilization test (TPI)

Both a treponemal and nontreponemal test are generally necessary to presumptively diagnose primary syphilis. As a rule, the treponemal tests stay positive for life following the initial infection, whether or not appropriate therapy has been administered. Since treponemal tests do not correlate with disease activity, they are usually reported as either positive or negative. In contrast, nontreponemal tests do correlate with the activity of disease, reaching high titers with primary infection or recent reinfection and falling over time following appropriate therapy. Nontreponemal tests are reported as quantitative titers. The adequacy of therapy can be determined using serial RPR (or VDRL) tests; ideally the same test in the same laboratory should be followed sequentially.

In primary syphilis, the VDRL is positive in about 70% of cases (treated or untreated), and the RPR is positive in about 80% of cases. Thus, it is important to realize that a substantial number of patients with a typical syphilitic chancre may have a negative nontreponemal test. In contrast, the VDRL and RPR are positive in nearly 100% of individuals with secondary syphilis, treated or untreated.

The treponemal tests may also be falsely negative in primary syphilis. The percent positive for the FTA-ABS is 85%, for the MHA-TP is 65%, and the TPI is 50%.

The sensitivity of the specific diagnostic tests for syphilis are summarized in the following table.

Diagnostic Tests in Syphilis

Test	Primary*	Secondary*	Late†
Nontreponemal			
VDRL	70	99–100	1
RPR	80	99–100	0
Treponemal			
FTA–ABS	85	100	98
TPHA or MHA–TP	65	100	95

*Treated or untreated
†Treated

Diagnostic Tests/Procedures
Darkfield Examination, Syphilis *on page 322*
FTA-ABS, Cerebrospinal Fluid *on page 335*
FTA-ABS, Serum *on page 336*
MHA-TP *on page 399*
RPR *on page 438*
VDRL, Cerebrospinal Fluid *on page 475*

Treatment The proper treatment of syphilis depends on the stage of infection. Primary, secondary, and early latent syphilis (defined as syphilis of less than 1 year's duration) are treated with benzathine penicillin G, 2.4 million units I.M. (one dose). For the penicillin-allergic patient, the alternative is doxycycline, 100 mg orally twice daily for 2 weeks.

The recommended therapy for the respective stages of syphilis are summarized in the following table.

Syphilis Therapy

Stage	Recommended	Alternative
Primary	Benzathine penicillin G I.M.: 2.4 million units x 1	Doxycycline P.O.: 100 mg twice daily for 2 weeks*
Secondary		
Early latent <1 year		
Latent >1 year	Benzathine penicillin G I.M.: 2.4 million units every week x 3	Doxycycline P.O.: 100 mg twice daily for 4 weeks*
Gummas		
Cardiovascular		
Neurosyphilis	Aqueous penicillin G I.V.: 12–24 million units/day for 14 days	Procaine penicillin I.M.: 2–4 million units/day and probenecid 500 mg 4 times/day for 10–14 days

*Avoid tetracyclines during pregnancy.

From U.S. Public Health Service Recommendations, "1993 Sexually Transmitted Diseases Treatment Guidelines," *MMWR Morbid Mortal Wkly Rep*, 1993, 42:1–102.

Drug Therapy
Recommended
Primary, secondary, latent syphilis:
Penicillin G Benzathine, Parenteral *on page 632*
Neurosyphilis:
Penicillin G, Parenteral *on page 633*
Alternate
Primary, secondary, latent syphilis:
Doxycycline *on page 557*
(Continued)

Treponema pallidum (Continued)

Neurosyphilis:

Penicillin G Procaine, Aqueous *on page 636*

Selected Readings

Hook EW 3d, "Diagnosing Neurosyphilis," *Clin Infect Dis*, 1994, 18(3):295-7.

Hook EW 3d and Marra CM, "Acquired Syphilis in Adults," *N Engl J Med*, 1992, 326(16):1060-9.

Lukehart SA and Holmes KK, "Syphilis," *Harrison's Principles of Internal Medicine*, 13th ed, Isselbacher KJ, Braunwald E, Wilson JD, et al, eds, New York, NY: McGraw-Hill, 1994, 726-36.

Musher DM "Syphilis," *Infect Dis Clin North Am*, 1987, 1(1):83-95.

Musher DM, Hamill RJ, and Baughn RE, "Effect of Human Immunodeficiency Virus (HIV) Infection on the Course of Syphilis and on the Response to Treatment," *Ann Intern Med*, 1990, 113(11):872-81.

"1993 Sexually Transmitted Diseases Treatment Guidelines. Centers for Disease Control and Prevention," *MMWR Morb Mortal Wkly Rep*, 1993, 42(RR-14):1-102.

Trichinella spiralis

Microbiology *Trichinella spiralis*, a nematode, is the infectious agent of human trichinosis. The adult male worm measures 1.5 mm in length and the adult female measures 2-4 mm. The average lifespan is 4 months. Identification is made by demonstration of the characteristic encapsulated larvae in biopsy specimens of infected muscles. The cyst wall is derived from the host cell muscle. The larva may incite an inflammatory reaction characterized by surrounding lymphocytes and eosinophils and eventual larval calcification.

Epidemiology *Trichinella* is found worldwide except Australia and several Pacific islands. Trichinosis results from consumption of undercooked pork, unsanitary cooking practices, and contaminated meats. Its reservoirs include pigs, horses, bears, and Arctic mammals. The three subspecies reflect three sylvatic cycles – arctic, temperate, and tropical.

The incidence in the United States continues to decline probably because of increased public awareness, commercial freezing, and legislature prohibiting feeding of raw garbage to swine. From 1982-1986, approximately 57 cases per year were reported with three associated deaths. From 1987-1990, 206 cases were reported to the CDC. Most of the cases reported in the U.S. are associated with improperly cooked game animals and travel to Mexico, Asia, and other endemic areas.

Trichinosis results from ingestion of encysted larvae in the contaminated meat. The acid-pepsin environment in the stomach digest the cyst wall, releasing the infectious larvae which burrow and attach to the mucosa at the base of the villi. Over a 6-10 day period, the larvae molt four times to become sexually mature adult worms which attach to the duodenal and jejunal mucosa producing between 200-1500 larvae over the next 2 weeks. The newborn or first stage larvae penetrate the gut mucosa into the lamina propria. An immunologic reaction partially mediated by IgE-mast cell system results in release of vasoactive substances that promote intestinal motility and secretion (diarrhea). The larvae then migrate into the draining lymphatics and blood vessels and have a high predilection to invade muscles of increased use and blood flow (ie, diaphragm, extraocular muscles, masseters, tongue, deltoids, and gastrocnemius). Once penetrated into the skeletal muscle, the larvae elicit a host inflammatory response which surrounds the larvae and creates granulomas and calcifications. Only larvae that encyst mature. Larvae may remain viable and infective for many years even in calcified cysts.

The severity of the symptoms is directly related to the larvae load. Patients usually remain asymptomatic with 1-10 larvae per gram muscle and systemic illness occurs with 50-100 larvae per gram.

Clinical Syndromes

- **Asymptomatic:** Ninety percent to 95% infections are asymptomatic.
- **Self-limited:** 1-2 weeks after ingestion, patients experience enteric phase associated with nonbloody diarrhea and abdominal cramps. Approximately 2-4 weeks later, patients experience fever, intense myalgia especially extraocular and masseters, periorbital edema, conjunctivitis, headache, and/or subconjunctival and subungual petechia. Ninety percent will have peripheral eosinophilia which peaks at 3-4 weeks. Absence of eosinophilia is a poor prognostic sign. Approximately 50% will have elevated CK and LDH enzymes.
- **Arctic trichinosis:** Described in northern Canada and Alaska in which patients have eaten contaminated walruses or seals. Associated with diar-

rhea lasting up to 14 weeks, mild and transitory myalgia without fever, peripheral eosinophilia, and no pathogens isolated in stools to explain etiology.

- **Myocarditis:** Incidence of approximately 5% of symptomatic patients. Typically occurs 3 weeks after larvae migration and presents with tachycardia and chest pain mimicking infarction. Patients have myocardium invasion without encystment. EKG reveals benign, reversible nonspecific EKG changes. May develop nonspecific inflammatory myocarditis predominantly eosinophilic and sometimes associated with pericarditis. Fewer than 0.1% patients die from cardiac complications (ie, congestive heart failure).
- **Pulmonary:** Up to 6% symptomatic patients may develop cough and dyspnea on exertion presumed secondary to larvae migration associated with infiltrates, hemorrhage, and allergic granulomatous reactions.
- **CNS:** Prevalence of 10% to 24% in symptomatic patients. In the first 2 weeks when larvae migration is maximal, CNS invasion can occur which appears as meningoencephalitis with delirium and confusion. Larvae encystment may result in focal neurological deficits, anal/urinary sphincter dysfunction, cranial nerve palsies especially VI and VII, seizures, vertigo, anisocoria, tinnitus, diminished auditory acuity, or ataxia. Papilledema, hemianopia, aphasia, and paresis have been reported. CNS and peripheral nerve deficits generally resolve in 4-6 months but may persist up to 10 years. May also cause eosinophilic meningitis. CT scan is usually normal but may see multiple nodular or ring enhancing lesions 3-8 mm and calcification. EEG reveals nonspecific abnormalities consistent with diffuse encephalopathy.

Diagnosis CDC case definition must fit one of two criteria:

1. Positive muscle biopsy or positive serology titer in a patient with clinical symptoms compatible with trichinosis including eosinophilia, fever, myalgias, or periorbital edema.
2. In an outbreak (at least one person must fit above criteria), must have either a positive serology titer or clinical symptoms compatible with trichinosis in a person who shared the implicated meat source.

IgM and IgE serology tests are helpful in distinguishing active from previous infection.

Diagnostic Tests/Procedures
Ova and Parasites, Stool *on page 416*
Trichinella Serology *on page 462*

Treatment Majority of symptomatic patients need supportive care only as infection is self-limited. Benzimidazole carbonates may be given. Mebendazole 200-400 mg three times/day for 3 days followed by 400-500 mg three times/day for 10 days is active against both invasive and encystment stages. Mebendazole does not cross the blood-brain barrier. Thiabendazole 25 mg/kg twice daily for 7 days is indicated to eliminate gut-dwelling adult worms. It is not effective against larval stages in tissue. Not well tolerated secondary to increased gastrointestinal side effects. Albendazole is still under investigation. Steroids (prednisone 40-60 mg daily) may reduce inflammation and is recommended in serious infections.

Overall prognosis is related to severity and intensity of initial infection as well as effectiveness of antiparasitic agents, anti-inflammatory agents, patients immune status, and whether any end-organ damage was rendered. Mortality related to pulmonary, cardiac, and CNS involvement.

All patients traveling outside the United States should receive pre-travel counseling. Smoking, microwaving, and freezing contaminated meats are not reliable means of eliminating trichinosis.

Drug Therapy Comment
Steroids used in combination with mebendazole in serious infections.

Drug Therapy
Recommended
Mebendazole *on page 604*
Alternate
Thiabendazole *on page 681*

Selected Readings
Bailey TM and Schantz PM, "Trends in the Incidence and Transmission Patterns of Trichinosis in Humans in the United States: Comparisons of the Periods 1975-1981 and 1982-1986," *Rev Infect Dis*, 1990, 12(1):5-11.

Compton SJ, Celum CL, Lee C, et al, "Trichinosis With Ventilatory Failure and Persistent Myocarditis," *Clin Infect Dis*, 1993, 16(4):500-4.

Mawhorter SD and Kazura JW, "Trichinosis of the Central Nervous System," *Semin Neurol*, 1993, 13(2):148-52.

(Continued)

Trichinella spiralis (Continued)

McAuley JB, Michelson MK, and Schantz PM, "*Trichinella* Infection in Travelers," *J Infect Dis*, 1991, 164(5):1013-6.

Trichomonas vaginalis

Microbiology *Trichomonas vaginalis* is the causative agent of trichomoniasis, a sexually transmitted vaginal infection. *Trichomonas vaginalis* is a flagellated protozoan which exists only in the trophozoite stage. It is easily visualized on wet mount slides under low power and high dry (40X).

Epidemiology The organism is transmitted by sexual intercourse, and the only known reservoir is humans. Occasional transmission can be indirect via contact with contaminated articles. The incubation period is 4-20 days. The period of communicability lasts the duration of the infection. Asymptomatic infections are common.

Clinical Syndromes

- **Vaginitis:** *Trichomonas* is a common cause of vaginitis and must be distinguished from other causes of vaginitis, such as *Candida* and *Gardnerella vaginalis* (the cause of bacterial vaginosis). Typically, there is a vaginal discharge accompanied by vulvar pruritus, dyspareunia, and dysuria. The vaginal discharge is often profuse, thin, frothy, and gray to yellow in color. On pelvic exam, there may be mild erythema of the vaginal walls and endocervix. In severe cases, there are vaginal erosions and petechiae, and occasionally a "strawberry cervix" may be seen where the endocervix is erythematous, granular, and friable. Addition of 10% KOH to the vaginal discharge liberates a fishy odor, as with bacterial vaginosis. On wet prep or Gram stain, there are many polymorphonuclear cells seen, reflecting the inflammatory nature of this form of vaginitis (as opposed to bacterial vaginosis). On wet prep, the motile trichomonads can be seen under low power and high dry, establishing the diagnosis. Asymptomatic infection is very common, and it is estimated that 50% of women carrying *Trichomonas* are asymptomatic.
- **Urethritis in males:** Infection with *Trichomonas* accounts for about 5% of cases of nongonococcal urethritis in males. This is characterized by persistent dysuria with a nonpurulent urethral discharge and may be suspected in patients who have failed the usual tetracycline regimens.
- **Prostatitis:** *Trichomonas* is a rare but reported cause of prostatitis in males.

Diagnosis The symptoms of vaginitis are not specific enough to distinguish infection with *Trichomonas* from other causes. In addition, patients may present following exposure to a sexual partner with *Trichomonas* and have no symptoms. Pelvic examination is mandatory in the female, as is a wet prep of any vaginal discharge. The finding of motile trichomonads is diagnostic. Negative wet mounts may be seen in asymptomatic women or in women who have recently douched. Gram-stained smears are useful in diagnosing bacterial vaginosis but add little to the yield for *Trichomonas* detection. Occasionally, forms resembling *Trichomonas* are incidentally found on Papanicolaou smears of the cervix. Since the cytologic smear is not the ideal procedure for identifying this organism, the patient should be promptly re-examined and a fresh wet mount obtained to confirm the presence of the protozoan. Culture techniques for *Trichomonas* are available in some specialized laboratories but is not usually necessary.

Prostatic and urethral secretions may similarly be examined for motile trichomonads. This may be a reasonable procedure in symptomatic males with persistent symptoms of urethritis where gonorrhea and *Chlamydia* have been excluded. Occasionally, the organism can be visualized in spun urine sediment.

Diagnostic Tests/Procedures

Trichomonas Preparation on page 462

Treatment Both symptomatic and asymptomatic individuals should be treated, the latter to decrease the incidence of reinfection from a sexual partner. The recommended regimen is metronidazole 2 g orally as a single dose. Alternatively, metronidazole can be given as 500 mg orally twice daily for 7 days. If failure occurs on the single dose regimen, the patient should be given the full 7-day regimen. In refractory cases, a patient may be given up to 2 g orally daily for 3-5 consecutive days. Such cases warrant consultation with an infectious disease specialist and *in vitro* testing of the isolate in culture for metronidazole resistance.

The sexual partners should be treated with either the 2 g single dose regimen or the 500 mg twice a day regimen for 7 days. During pregnancy, metronida-

ORGANISMS

zole is contraindicated based on data suggesting the drug is mutagenic in rodents. No other agent is reliable, although some authors have suggested clotrimazole intravaginally if necessary in the first trimester. During the second or third trimester of pregnancy, severe cases may be treated with a single 2 g dose at the discretion of the physician.

Drug Therapy Comment

Treat sexual partners as well.

Drug Therapy
Recommended

Metronidazole *on page 610*

Selected Readings

Krieger JN, Tam MR, Stevens CE, et al, "Diagnosis of Trichomoniasis. Comparison of Conventional Wet-Mount Examination With Cytologic Studies, Cultures, and Monoclonal Antibody Staining of Direct Specimens," *JAMA*, 1988, 259(8):1223-7.

Lossick JG, "The Diagnosis of Trichomoniasis," *JAMA*, 1988, 259(8):1230.

Lossick JG and Kent HL, "Trichomoniasis: Trends in Diagnosis and Management," *Am J Obstet Gynecol*, 1991, 165(4):1217-22.

Sears SD and O'Hare J, "*In vitro* Susceptibility of *Trichomonas vaginalis* to 50 Antimicrobial Agents," *Antimicrob Agents Chemother*, 1988, 32(1):144-6.

Sugarman B and Mummaw N, "Effects of Antimicrobial Agents on Growth and Chemotaxis of *Trichomonas vaginalis*," *Antimicrob Agents Chemother*, 1988, 32(9):1323-6.

Wolner-Hanssen P, Krieger JN, Stevens CE, et al, "Clinical Manifestations of Vaginal Trichomoniasis," *JAMA*, 1989, 261(4):571-6.

"1993 Sexually Transmitted Diseases Treatment Guidelines. Centers for Disease Control and Prevention," *MMWR Morb Mortal Wkly Rep*, 1993, 42(RR-14):1-102.

Tubercle Bacillus *see Mycobacterium tuberculosis on page 155*

TWAR *see Chlamydia pneumoniae on page 76*

Ureaplasma urealyticum

Synonyms T-*Mycoplasma*

Microbiology *Ureaplasma urealyticum* is a potential human pathogen formerly known as T-*Mycoplasma* (the "T" standing for tiny). The organism belongs to the *Mycoplasma* group (class: Mollicutes; order: Mycoplasmatales; family: Mycoplasmataceae, genus: *Ureaplasma*). As with other mycoplasmas, *Ureaplasma* is one of the smallest free-living organisms in existence, intermediate in size between viruses and bacteria. Important points regarding its microbiology include the organism is very difficult to see using standard light microscopy, the organism picks up the Gram stain poorly, the lack of a cell wall makes the organism resistant to beta-lactam antibiotics, and *Ureaplasma* demonstrates complex nutritional requirements necessitating special medium for optimal growth in culture.

Because of the fastidious nature of *Ureaplasma*, it is important to consult with the microbiology laboratory prior to obtaining cultures, particularly if important body fluids are sent (such as blood cultures, cerebrospinal fluid, synovial fluid, etc). Specimen collection is important; both the proper transport media (eg, 2 SP, Sp-4) and proper swabs (eg, calcium alginate, wire loops, and others) must be used. The organism can occasionally grow in routine blood culture media and blood agar plates, but the yield is low.

Epidemiology Infants: *Ureaplasma* is a common colonizer of the urogenital tract in infants. The organism can be cultured from the genital tract of roughly 33% of female infants. In most cases, the organism is acquired from the mother as the newborn passes through an infected birth canal. Male infants are colonized less frequently. After 2 years, the rate of colonization for both sexes decreases significantly, but some children have persistently positive genital tract cultures. Colonization rates are higher in sexually abused children.

Adults: Colonization of the adult urogenital tract is also quite common, but the pathogenesis is usually from sexual contact. Studies have shown that *Ureaplasma* can be cultured from the cervix and vagina in 40% to 80% of sexually active women, nearly all being asymptomatic. Risk factors for colonization include multiple sexual partners, lower socioeconomic status, and perhaps black race. Adults who are sexually inexperienced have low rates of colonization. Thus, the finding of a positive urogenital culture for *Ureaplasma* must be interpreted cautiously since in many cases the organism is a harmless commensal.

Clinical Syndromes *Ureaplasma* has been associated with a variety of diseases, but many of these associations are supported only at the case report level and remain controversial. The evidence for causality can be divided as follows:

(Continued)

Ureaplasma urealyticum (Continued)

Good evidence supporting the role of *Ureaplasma urealyticum*:

- **Nongonococcal urethritis (NGU) in the adult male:** The etiologic role of *Ureaplasma* in this common syndrome is supported by evidence from animal models and human volunteer studies. In addition, a small number of placebo-controlled antibiotic trials in males with urethritis has demonstrated improvement in urethral symptoms in the group receiving tetracyclines. The number of NGU cases caused by *Ureaplasma* is unknown.

- **Postpartum bacteremia:** *Ureaplasma* has been isolated from blood cultures in case reports of women with postpartum fever following vaginal delivery. Bloodstream infections with *Ureaplasma* have also been reported following abortions. The role of this organism in postpartum or postabortal fever is still unclear since blood cultures for *Ureaplasma* are rarely obtained.

- **Urethroprostatitis:** *Ureaplasma* appears to be a cause of acute urethroprostatitis in rare cases. There is no evidence to date proving *Ureaplasma* as a cause of chronic urethroprostatitis.

- **Epididymitis:** A single case report has shown *Ureaplasma* to be a likely causative pathogen in an acute case of epididymitis.

- **Septic arthritis:** An unusual septic arthritis due to *Ureaplasma urealyticum* has been described in patients with underlying hypogammaglobulinemia. Joint aspirations have yielded the organism in pure culture. Other clinical features that have accompanied the septic arthritis include subcutaneous abscesses and chronic cystitis. Septic arthritis due to *Ureaplasma* has also been reported in renal transplant patients. Important clinical clues to this syndrome include an immunocompromised host, synovial fluid on arthrocentesis that is "culture-negative" on routine testing, evidence of joint destruction without macroscopic purulence in the joint, and lack of improvement on conventional antibiotic therapy.

- **Chorioamnionitis:** Women who carry *Ureaplasma* in the urogenital tract chronically may potentially develop colonization of the endometrium during pregnancy. Cases have been described where *U. urealyticum* has been repeatedly isolated from amniotic fluid containing inflammatory cells. Symptoms may or may not be present. A low-grade chronic amnionitis has been described and may be associated with premature spontaneous labor and delivery.

- **Respiratory infection in newborns:** Increasing evidence has shown that *Ureaplasma* is a potential cause of congenital pneumonia, probably from acquisition *in utero*. Premature, low-birth weight infants appear to be at risk. The clinical spectrum of respiratory infection has ranged from asymptomatic colonization of the airways to overwhelming pneumonia with acute respiratory distress syndrome. In some cases, endotracheal aspirates, lung biopsies, and lung tissue at autopsy have all yielded pure cultures of *Ureaplasma* with histologic evidence of pneumonia. Blood cultures and cerebrospinal fluid may also be positive for *Ureaplasma*. However, it is important to note that *Ureaplasma* is frequently a harmless colonizer of the airways, and the diagnosis of ureaplasmal pneumonia must be made cautiously.

- **Chronic respiratory disease in neonates:** *Ureaplasma* has been implicated as a risk factor for bronchopulmonary dysplasia, based on limited evidence.

- **Newborn meningitis:** Several studies suggest that *Ureaplasma* may be an important but under-recognized cause of meningitis in premature infants. A fulminant meningitis with intraventricular hemorrhage has been described, but there may also be a more chronic and indolent form. This remains a controversial topic.

Limited evidence supporting the role of *Ureaplasma urealyticum*:

- **Pelvic inflammatory disease**
- **Renal calculi**
- **Reiter's syndrome**
- **Infertility**
- **Repeated spontaneous abortions**
- **Pyelonephritis**

Diagnosis Isolation of the organism from the appropriate site or body fluid is essential for confirming the diagnosis, since the clinical syndromes described above are not specific for *Ureaplasma*. The main errors in diagnosis are failure to consider this organism in the differential diagnosis of a disease syndrome, improper specimen collection, and failure to ask the laboratory to specifically culture for *Ureaplasma* (or *Mycoplasma*). Routine culturing techniques can occasionally yield the organism, but this is not recommended. Serologic testing has limited usefulness. The polymerase chain reaction using the 16S rRNA gene sequence has been described but is currently only a research tool.

Another potential error is confusing colonization of *Ureaplasma* at a body site with true disease. Several of the clinical syndromes described above are only loosely associated with the particular disease entity. There is a risk for overdiagnosis and overtreatment.

Diagnostic Tests/Procedures
Genital Culture for *Ureaplasma urealyticum on page 350*

Treatment Because *Ureaplasma* has no cell wall, it is resistant to penicillins, cephalosporins, sulfonamides, and other cell wall-active antibiotics. The organism is often resistant *in vitro* to aminoglycosides, clindamycin, and chloramphenicol. About 90% of *Ureaplasma* strains are sensitive to the tetracyclines, and these are the drugs of choice. Tetracycline resistance has been described and is likely to increase; most strains of tetracycline-resistant *Ureaplasma* remain sensitive to erythromycin. Recent *in vitro* studies have shown a potential role for the quinolones (particularly sparfloxacin), but little clinical data is available yet.

A difficult situation arises when there is life-threatening *Ureaplasma* infection in the newborn. Tetracyclines are generally contraindicated in this age group, but some have reported the use of intravenous doxycycline in severe neonatal meningitis. Erythromycin is the drug of choice in patients younger than 8 years of age, but the penetration into the spinal fluid is poor. Consultation with an infectious disease specialist may be warranted in these cases.

Pediatric Drug Therapy
Recommended
Erythromycin *on page 561*
Alternate
>7 years
Tetracycline *on page 679*

Adult Drug Therapy
Recommended
Erythromycin *on page 561*
Tetracycline *on page 679*
Doxycycline *on page 557*
Alternate
Clarithromycin *on page 539*
Azithromycin Dihydrate *on page 500*

Selected Readings
Cassell GH, Waites KB, Watson HL, et al, "*Ureaplasma urealyticum* Intrauterine Infection: Role in Prematurity and Disease in Newborns," *Clin Microbiol Rev*, 1993, 6(1):69-87.
Forgacs P, Kundsin RB, Margles SW, et al, "A Case of *Ureaplasma urealyticum* Septic Arthritis in a Patient With Hypogammaglobulinemia," *Clin Infect Dis*, 1993, 16(2):293-4.
Taylor-Robinson D, "*Ureaplasma urealyticum* (T-strain *Mycoplasma*) and *Mycoplasma hominis*," *Principles and Practice of Infectious Diseases*, 4th ed, Mandell GL, Bennett JE, and Dolin R, eds, New York, NY: Churchill Livingstone, 1995, 1713-8.
Valencia GB, Banzon F, Cummings M, et al, "*Mycoplasma hominis* and *Ureaplasma urealyticum* in Neonates With Suspected Infection," *Pediatr Infect Dis J*, 1993, 12(7):571-3.
Waites KB, Crouse DT, and Cassell GH, "Antibiotic Susceptibilities and Therapeutic Options for *Ureaplasma urealyticum* Infections in Neonates," *Pediatr Infect Dis J*, 1992, 11(1):23-9.

Vaccines *see page 706*

Varicella-Zoster Virus
Related Information
Immunization Guidelines *on page 710-717*
Synonyms VZV
Microbiology VZV is the cause of two different clinical entities, chickenpox (also called varicella) and shingles (also called zoster or herpes zoster).
Epidemiology Chickenpox (varicella): Approximately 3 million cases of primary chickenpox occur annually, leading to over 500,000 physician visits. Most cases occur in the late winter and spring. Humans are the only known reservoir for VZV. Transmission is probably via respiratory secretions, although this point has been difficult to substantiate. Intimate contact between a susceptible host (who is seronegative) and an individual actively shedding virus is necessary for transmission. Chickenpox still remains predominantly a pediatric
(Continued)

Varicella-Zoster Virus *(Continued)*

disease, with >90% of all cases reported in children younger than the age of 3. Household contacts of infected children are at high risk for varicella. The estimated secondary attack rate in susceptible family members is about 90%; the secondary attack rate in susceptible school mates approaches 40%. The incubation period between exposure and clinical disease is about 14 days, with a range of 10-20 days. Patients can be infectious and spread virus to others for about 2 days prior to the appearance of any skin rash. Patients remain infectious until all skin vesicles have crusted over (5 days or more).

Shingles (zoster): This is also a common disorder, with nearly 10% of the general population afflicted at some time. Almost 1.5 million physician office visits are for management of shingles. Shingles is predominantly a disease of the elderly, although immunocompromised patients are accounting for an increasing fraction. Cases appear sporadically in the population rather than in clusters, due to the pathogenesis of the disease. Herpes zoster results from reactivation of VZV which has remained latent in dorsal root ganglia of peripheral or cranial nerves since the original episode of chickenpox. The factors that govern both latency and reactivation are still under study, but clearly host immune competency is important. Shingles is not spread from one individual to another in the same manner as chickenpox, although the lesions of herpes zoster do contain active VZV and can potentially infect susceptible individuals.

Clinical Syndromes

- **Chickenpox in the normal child:** In the otherwise healthy child, chickenpox is generally a benign, self-limited infection. Typically, the child presents with fever, malaise, and a new generalized skin eruption. The skin rash is distinctive and consists of hundreds of discrete circular lesions. An individual lesion will pass through several stages over time: lesions first appear as vesicles with clear fluid ("dew drops"), then vesicles containing purulent fluid (pustules), then ruptured pustules, and then hard scabs. New vesicles continue to emerge for several days as older ones reach the scab stage. Thus, the rash of chickenpox characteristically has lesions in all stages of evolution at any single point in time. Patients complain of fatigue, pruritus, and anorexia. Lesions can be found in nearly all areas of the skin, and in some cases, the mucous membranes as well. The disease remains active for about 5 days. Complications are unusual in healthy children. Secondary bacterial infection of excoriated skin lesions is the most common complication in children. A variety of unusual neurologic syndromes has been reported in association with chickenpox including cerebellar ataxia (characterized by vertigo, abnormal gait, fever, and vomiting; usually resolves over weeks without treatment), encephalitis (characterized by confusion, personality changes, and seizures; a particularly worrisome complication, with up to 20% of cases resulting in death), cerebral angiitis, meningitis, and Reye's syndrome (particularly if aspirin is given). In clinical trials, acyclovir has demonstrated a statistically significant benefit in normal children (2-12 years of age) with chickenpox. This benefit, however, is small. New lesion formation was decreased from 2.5 days to 2 days, and the number of lesions was decreased from 350 to 300. Acyclovir did not alter the rate of serious complications or spread of infection within the family. The U.S. Food and Drug Administration has supported the use of acyclovir in this setting. The cost-benefit ratio of routine acyclovir use in normal children is likely to be low, since the disease is usually benign. Supportive care remains the mainstay of treatment.

- **Chickenpox in the healthy adult:** About 10% of adults do not acquire VZV infection in childhood and thus remain susceptible to primary infection later in life. Infection in the adult is more severe than in childhood, with varicella pneumonitis a significant concern. Data derived from studies of military recruits suggest that varicella pneumonia may be underdiagnosed. Pulmonary infiltrates were found on chest x-ray in 16% of all recruits with primary varicella, most of whom had no respiratory complaints.

  Perinatal varicella can occur when a pregnant woman develops chickenpox. This is unusual because most adult females are seropositive and immune. Maternal varicella can result in transmission to the fetus, especially if maternal infection occurs several days before delivery. The fetus may be born with visceral VZV dissemination, central nervous system abnormalities, skin scarring and other defects collectively called the congenital varicella syndrome. Potentially infected neonates are candidates for varicella zoster immune globulin (with or without antiviral drugs).

Clinical trials examining chickenpox in normal adolescents and adults have shown acyclovir to be effective when administered within 24 hours of symptoms. The treatment effect demonstrated in this older age group is greater than similar studies in children. The U.S. FDA has also approved the use of oral acyclovir for chickenpox in healthy adults and teenagers. Pregnant women who contract varicella pneumonia are frequently given intravenous acyclovir because of the high mortality of this complication in pregnancy. Newborns with perinatal varicella probably benefit from acyclovir, although formal data to support this practice are limited.

- **Chickenpox in the immunocompromised host:** Morbidity and mortality are high in this population, with >50% of children suffering visceral complications. Mortality approaches 20% overall. Most reported cases of life-threatening varicella have been described in leukemic children. Other risk groups include patients with solid tumors, lymphoproliferative malignancies, and organ transplant recipients. The skin rash tends to be more severe, with delayed time to crusting of lesions. Pneumonitis, hepatitis, and encephalitis are common.

  HIV-infected children who develop chickenpox are also at risk for serious disease. In addition to the visceral complications as noted above, these children are at risk for an unusual, chronic form of the infection, where recurrent vesicular eruptions take place. Several clinical trials have been performed to examine the efficacy of antiviral agents in this setting. Acyclovir decreased the incidence of varicella pneumonia but did not alter the natural history of skin lesions. Intravenous acyclovir has been recommended for both adults and children who are immunosuppressed.

- **Shingles in the normal host:** Most cases of shingles occur in normal individuals aged 60-90 years old, although cases have been reported in all age groups including children. Reactivation of VZV is heralded by localized pain along a dermatomal distribution, the phase of "acute neuritis." After 2-3 days of pain, the skin erupts with papules and vesicles along the same unilateral dermatomal distribution. As with primary varicella, the skin lesions evolve from fluid filled vesicles into pustules and later scabs. The number of skin lesions is variable. Pain can be quite severe and may require narcotics. New lesions continue to form over 3-5 days. The disease stays active for about 1 week, but complete healing requires several additional weeks, particularly in the elderly.

  Selective involvement of the ophthalmic branch of the trigeminal nerve (cranial nerve V) is called herpes zoster ophthalmicus. Keratitis, uveitis, and other ocular complications may result in visual loss if untreated. Involvement of the geniculate ganglion results in the Ramsay Hunt syndrome – vesicles in the external auditory canal, facial palsy, and loss of taste in the anterior two-thirds of the tongue. Other serious complications of herpes zoster in the normal host include cutaneous dissemination and aseptic meningitis. Unlike chickenpox, visceral complications such as pneumonitis and hepatitis are rare. The most common complication of herpes zoster is postherpetic neuralgia, particularly problematic in the elderly. The incidence of this is unclear. Pain persists in the involved dermatome for months after the skin eruption has resolved. Narcotics are only partially helpful, and patients may be quite disabled from the pain; nerve blocks have been attempted with variable success.

  Several clinical trials have been conducted to evaluate the efficacy of acyclovir in herpes zoster in the normal adult. Acyclovir improved the healing time of skin lesions (only by 24 hours) but had a variable and often negligible effect on postherpetic neuralgia. This is an important limitation because postherpetic neuralgia is the most commonly encountered complication and a particularly frustrating problem for physicians. The U.S. FDA has recommended licensure of acyclovir in this setting, but other experts believe the benefit of acyclovir to be small and decisions regarding treatment should by made on a case-by-case basis. Certainly herpes zoster ophthalmicus and other complications warrant prompt treatment.

- **Herpes zoster in the immunocompromised host:** Severe herpes zoster has been described in patients with lymphoma, leukemia, organ transplant recipients, solid malignancies, and those receiving chemotherapy or chronic corticosteroids. Skin lesions frequently extend beyond the original dermatomal distribution. The period of new lesion formation may continue for weeks, and healing is delayed. Generalized skin dissemination has been observed in nearly 25% of patients. One-half of those patients with cutane-

(Continued)

Varicella-Zoster Virus *(Continued)*

ous dissemination will progress to visceral dissemination. In HIV-infected individuals, herpes zoster is also severe and potentially life-threatening. Often multiple dermatomes are involved, and recurrences are common. A chronic form of herpes zoster has been described in patients with advanced AIDS.

Acyclovir has been shown to clearly benefit the immunocompromised host. It is generally given intravenously for 7 days or more. Chronic suppressive doses of oral acyclovir have been given to HIV-infected patients with recurrent herpes zoster. Acyclovir-resistant VZV has been isolated from some individuals on chronic therapy, but this appears to still be uncommon.

Diagnostic Tests/Procedures

Herpes Cytology *on page 362*

Varicella-Zoster Virus Culture *on page 473*

Varicella-Zoster Virus Serology *on page 474*

Virus, Direct Detection by Fluorescent Antibody *on page 480*

Drug Therapy
Recommended

Acyclovir *on page 484*

Selected Readings

Dunkle LM, Arvin AM, Whitley RJ, et al, "A Controlled Trial of Acyclovir for Chickenpox in Normal Children," *N Engl J Med*, 1991, 325(22):1539-44.

Straus SE, Ostrove JM, Inchauspé G, "Varicella-Zoster Virus Infections. Biology, Natural History, Treatment, and Prevention," *Ann Intern Med*, 1988, 108(2):221-37.

Wallace MR, Bowler WA, Murray NB, et al, "Treatment of Adult Varicella with Oral Acyclovir. A Randomized, Placebo-Controlled Trial," *Ann Intern Med*, 1992, 117(5):358-63.

Watson PN and Evans RJ, "Postherpetic Neuralgia: A Review," *Arch Neurol*, 1986, 43(8):836-40.

Wood MJ, Johnson RW, McKendrick MW, et al, "A Randomized Trial of Acyclovir for 7 Days or 21 Days With and Without Prednisolone for Treatment of Acute Herpes Zoster," *N Engl J Med*, 1994, 330(13):896-900.

Vibrio cholerae

Related Information

Timing of Food Poisoning *on page 723*

Microbiology *Vibrio cholerae* is an oxidase-positive, fermentative, gram-negative rod that can have a comma-shaped appearance on initial isolation. *V. cholerae* can be subdivided by the production of endotoxin and agglutination in 0-1 antisera with the nomenclature of *V. cholerae* 0-1, atypical or nontoxigenic 0-1, or non-0-1. The serogroup 0-1 can further be subdivided into the El Tor and Classic cholera biotypes which can be further subdivided into a variety of serotypes. The major virulence factor of *V. cholerae* is the extracellular enterotoxin produced by the 0-1 strain, although nontoxin producing organisms have been implicated in some outbreaks.

V. cholerae is a facultative anaerobe which grows best at a pH of 7.0 and at a wide temperature range (18°C to 37°C). *Vibrio* species can be differentiated from other gram-negative bacilli by their sensitivity to 0129 and may be speciated by a variety of biochemical tests.

Epidemiology Cholera is usually spread by contamination of water and food by infected feces, with fecal contamination of water being the principal vehicle of transmission. Person-to-person transmission is less common due to the large organism load necessary for infection. Asymptomatic carriers play a minor role in cholera outbreaks. Outbreaks may be seasonally dependent based on either temperature or rainfall. Transmission by food can be eliminated by thorough cooking. Adequate sanitation is the best means of cholera prevention.

There have been several pandemics of cholera reported since 1817, originating in Bengal and subsequently spreading to a variety of geographic locations, responsible for hundreds of thousands of deaths. The latest pandemic originated in Indonesia in 1961 and moved to the Western hemisphere. In 1991, a cholera outbreak in Peru and 20 other countries in the Western hemisphere accounted for over 600,000 cases with 5000 deaths caused by El Tor 0-1.

Clinical Syndromes After a 2- to 5-day incubation period, classic cholera is characterized by an abrupt onset of vomiting and profuse watery diarrhea with flecks of mucus (rice water stool). Fluid losses can be significant (up to 20 L/day). Hypovolemic shock and metabolic acidosis can cause death within a few hours of onset, especially in children. Mortality, in untreated cases, is as high as 60%. Milder forms of the disease also occur, especially with the non-0-1 cholera.

ORGANISMS

Diagnosis Organisms can be identified by darkfield microscopy showing large numbers of comma-shaped organisms with significant motility. However, this test is relatively insensitive and is nonspecific. Thiosulfate-citrate-bile salt-sucrose agar (TCBS) or alkaline peptone broth are used to facilitate growth and identification. Positive identification depends on serologic and biochemical testing.

Diagnostic Tests/Procedures
  Fecal Leukocyte Stain *on page 334*
  Stool Culture, Uncommon Organisms *on page 451*

Treatment Early and rapid replacement of fluid and electrolytes can decrease the mortality to <1%. Oral rehydration is usually successful, but in severe cases, intravenous replacement is required. When fluid and electrolyte imbalances are corrected, cholera is a short, self-limiting disease lasting a few days. According to the *MMWR*, doxycycline, tetracycline, co-trimoxazole, erythromycin, and furazolidone have all demonstrated effectiveness in decreasing the diarrhea and bacterial shedding in this disease. The usual recommendation is doxycycline 300 mg as a single dose for adults, and co-trimoxazole 5 mg/kg, twice daily for 3 days.

Pediatric Drug Therapy
Recommended
  <7 years
    Co-trimoxazole *on page 545*
  >7 years
    Tetracycline *on page 679*
    Doxycycline *on page 557*
Alternate
  >7 years
    Co-trimoxazole *on page 545*

Adult Drug Therapy
Recommended
  Doxycycline *on page 557*
  Tetracycline *on page 679*
Alternate
  Co-trimoxazole *on page 545*

Selected Readings
"Cholera Associated with International Travel, 1992," *MMWR Morb Mortal Wkly Rep*, 1992, 41(36):664-7.

Falkow S and Mekalanos J, "The Enteric Bacilli and Vibrios," *Microbiology*, 4th ed, Davis BD, Dulbecco R, Eisen HN, et al, eds, Philadelphia, PA: JB Lippincott Co, 1990, 561-87.

Johnston JM, Becker SF, McFarland LM, "*Vibrio vulnificus*: Man and the Sea," *JAMA*, 1985, 253(19):2850-3.

Levine WC and Griffin PM, "*Vibrio* Infections on the Gulf Coast: The Results of a First Year of Regional Surveillance. Gulf Coast *Vibrio* Working Group," *J Infect Dis*, 1993, 167(2):479-83.

Rabbani GH, "Cholera," *J Clin Gastroenterol*, 1986, 15(3):507-28.

Tacket CO, Brenner F, Blake PA, "Clinical Features and an Epidemiological Study of *Vibrio vulnificus* Infections," *J Infect Dis*, 1984, 149(4):558-61.

"Update: Cholera -- Western Hemisphere, and Recommendations for Treatment of Cholera," *MMWR Morb Mortal Wkly Rep*, 1991, 40(32):562-5.

"*Vibrio vulnificus* Infections Associated With Raw Oyster Consumption – Florida, 1981-1992," *MMWR Morb Mortal Wkly Rep*, 1993, 42(21):405-7.

Zwadyk P, "Vibrionaceae," *Zinsser Microbiology*, 20th ed, Joklik WK, Willett HP, Amos DB, et al, eds, Norwalk, CT: Appleton & Lange, 1992, 566-76.

Viridans Streptococci *see Streptococcus*, Viridans Group *on page 213*

VZV *see Varicella-Zoster Virus on page 227*

Xanthomonas maltophilia

Synonyms *Maltophilia*

Microbiology *Xanthomonas maltophilia* is a lactose-negative, oxidase-negative, nonfermenting, aerobic, gram-negative bacillus with polar flagella. The organism grows well on common laboratory media as characteristic gray, nonhemolytic colonies.

Epidemiology *Xanthomonas maltophilia* is ubiquitous and is considered opportunistic, usually nosocomial, pathogens. The increasing presence of this organism is most likely due to antimicrobial selective pressure and the increase in debilitated patients. Virulence factors for *Xanthomonas maltophilia* have not been extensively investigated.

(Continued)

Xanthomonas maltophilia (Continued)

Clinical Syndromes *Xanthomonas maltophilia* can infect any tissue or organ system including blood, lung, heart, urinary tract, or musculoskeletal system. Syndromes caused by *Xanthomonas maltophilia* are usually indistinguishable from those caused by the Enterobacteriaceae. Organisms are often grown as part of mixed cultures; therefore, distinguishing colonization from true infection is often difficult.

Diagnosis The only way a diagnosis of *Xanthomonas maltophilia* infection can be made is by identification of the organism through culture in a patient with a relevant clinical syndrome. No special media or conditions are necessary to grow this organism.

Diagnostic Tests/Procedures

Aerobic Culture, Appropriate Site *on page 244*
Blood Culture, Aerobic and Anaerobic *on page 271*
Gram Stain *on page 352*

Treatment *Xanthomonas maltophilia* is resistant to a wide variety of antimicrobial agents. The organism is almost always resistant to imipenem, and often resistant to extended spectrum penicillins, cephalosporins and the fluoroquinolones. *Xanthomonas maltophilia* is almost universally susceptible to cotrimoxazole with alternative therapies dependent on susceptibility testing.

Drug Therapy

Recommended

Co-trimoxazole *on page 545*

Alternate

Fluoroquinolones *on page 571*
Ticarcillin and Clavulanate Potassium *on page 682*
Consider alternate agents only if susceptible.

Selected Readings

Elting LS and Bodey GP, "Septicemia Due to *Xanthomonas* Species and Non-Aeruginosa *Pseudomonas* Species: Increasing Incidence of Catheter-Related Infections," *Medicine (Baltimore)*, 1990, 69(5):296-306.

Marshall WF, Keating MR, Anhalt JP, et al, "*Xanthomonas maltophilia*: An Emerging Nosocomial Pathogen," *Mayo Clin Proc*, 1989, 64(9):1097-104.

Murray PR, Drew WL, Kobayashi GS, et al, eds, "Pseudomonadaceae," *Medical Microbiology*, St Louis, MO: CV Mosby Co, 1990, 119-26.

Yersinia enterocolitica

Microbiology *Yersinia enterocolitica* is a gram-negative bacillus named in honor of the French bacteriologist Alexander Yersin, who discovered *Yersinia pestis* (the cause of plague) in 1894. *Y. enterocolitica* is an unusual cause of enterocolitis, terminal ileitis mimicking acute appendicitis, and septicemia. The organism is an aerobic gram-negative rod, nonlactose fermenting, which is motile at 25°C. It is unusual in that it grows better at somewhat cooler temperatures than do other pathogenic gram-negative rods (25°C to 32°C). It also is able to grow well at 4°C, which is the basis for CEM.

Epidemiology *Yersinia enterocolitica* is endemic in many animals which serve as reservoirs: cattle, pigs, dogs, cats, and others. The usual route of human infection is via ingestion of contaminated food, milk, and water. There have been three major foodborne epidemics in the United States: June 1982 – outbreak in several states linked to consumption of milk pasteurized at a plant in Memphis, Tennessee; 172 positive cultures from cases in Tennessee, Arkansas, and Mississippi, where patients presented with diarrhea, fever, abdominal pain. It also included 24 cases of extraintestinal infections including throat, blood, urinary tract, central nervous system, and wounds; 1976 – contaminated chocolate milk in New York State; 1982 – contaminated tofu in Washington state.

Clinical Syndromes

- **Enterocolitis:** *Yersinia enterocolitica* is a rare cause of enterocolitis. The severity of symptoms can be quite variable and can range from mild fever, diarrhea and abdominal pain, to fulminant colitis with spiking fevers and rectal bleeding.

- **Mesenteric adenopathy with or without terminal ileitis:** This form of *Yersinia* infection is known to mimic acute appendicitis. Patients present with right lower quadrant pain, fever, and leukocytosis. Upon laparotomy the appendix is normal but enlarged mesenteric lymph nodes are palpable and when cultured will yield the organism. This has been described primarily in adolescents, although cases have been reported in adults.

- **Polyarthritis:** This has been described as the sole manifestation of *Yersinia enterocolitica* infection or as a secondary manifestation of gastrointestinal infection. Well documented cases have been described in Scandinavia, where up to 30% of cases develop erythema nodosum, and 10% to 30% develop polyarthritis (especially associated with HLA-B27 haplotype). *Yersinia* antigens have recently been found in synovial joint cells from patients suffering from reactive arthritis following *Yersinia* infection.

- **Liver abscess:** *Yersinia* is a rare but reported cause of liver abscess in the absence of typical enterocolitis symptoms.
- **Ascending infection of an extremity:** Recently, cases of infections of the hand and upper extremity due to *Yersinia enterocolitica* have been described. These infections occurred in adults preparing contaminated chitterlings (pig intestines) with local inoculation into the hand via small cuts.
- **Septicemia:** *Yersinia* is an unusual cause of community-acquired septicemia but may occur following ingestion of heavily contaminated food. Risk factors for septicemia are cirrhosis, malignancy, diabetes mellitus, and patients with iron overload syndromes (such as hemachromatosis, frequent blood transfusions). Typically, there is fever, myalgias, confusion, and possibly hypotension. Symptoms of enterocolitis, such as diarrhea and abdominal pain, may be completely absent, adding to the diagnostic confusion. Elevated liver enzymes and muscle enzymes may occur. Blood cultures are often positive for the organism.
- **Miscellaneous:** Other manifestations of *Yersinia* infection include osteomyelitis, meningitis, pharyngitis (without enterocolitis), and intra-abdominal abscess.

Diagnosis In the absence of an outbreak, the diagnosis of enterocolitis due to *Yersinia* is difficult to make on clinical grounds alone. Thus, laboratory confirmation is important in most cases. Appropriate specimens for culture include stool, blood, lymph node, pharyngeal exudates, ascites fluid, and cerebrospinal fluid. Joint aspiration fluid may be sent for *Yersinia* culture in the appropriate clinical setting (ie, reactive polyarthritis following a diarrheal illness), but the yield is extremely low. The laboratory should be notified if a stool specimen is being examined for *Yersinia*. Serologic tests for specific antibody production to *Yersinia enterocolitica* are available in some laboratories.

Diagnostic Tests/Procedures
Aerobic Culture, Appropriate Site *on page 244*
Stool Culture, Uncommon Organisms *on page 451*

Treatment Many cases of enterocolitis and mesenteric adenitis secondary to *Yersinia* are self-resolving, and the role of antibiotics is unclear. Patients with *Yersinia* septicemia, however, definitely require antibiotic therapy since the mortality approaches 50%. The organism is susceptible *in vitro* to a number of agents, including third generation cephalosporins, piperacillin, co-trimoxazole, and aminoglycosides. Most isolates are resistant to penicillin, ampicillin, and first generation cephalosporins. The optimal drug regimen *in vivo* has not been defined in the literature. For serious infections, it seems reasonable to treat initially with a combination (eg, third generation cephalosporin and aminoglycoside) until the patient has stabilized.

Adult Drug Therapy
Recommended
Severe infection
Cephalosporins, 3rd Generation *on page 528*
used in combination with
Aminoglycosides *on page 489*

Selected Readings
Bottone E and Sheehan DJ, "*Yersinia enterocolitica*: Guidelines for Serologic Diagnosis of Human Infections," *Rev Infect Dis*, 1983, 5(5):898-906.
Centers for Disease Control, "*Yersinia enterocolitica* Bacteremia and Endotoxin Shock Associated With Red Blood Cell Transfusions – United States, 1991," *JAMA*, 1991, 256(17):2174-5.
Cohen JI and Rodday P, "*Yersinia enterocolitica* Bacteremia in a Patient With the Acquired Immunodeficiency Syndrome," *Am J Med*, 1989, 86(2):254-5.
Cover TL and Aber RC, "*Yersinia enterocolitica*," *N Engl J Med*, 1989, 321(1):16-24.
Gayraud M, Mollaret HH, et al, "Antibiotic Treatment of *Yersinia enterocolitica* Septicemia: A Retrospective Review of 43 Cases," *Clin Infect Dis*, 1993, 17(3):405-10.
Granfors K, Jalkanen S, von Essen R, et al, "*Yersinia* Antigens in Synovial Fluid Cells From Patients With Reactive Arthritis," *N Engl J Med*, 1989, 320(4):216-21.
Naqvi SH, Swierkosz EM, and Gerard J, "Presentation of *Yersinia enterocolitica* Enteritis in Children," *Pediatr Infect Dis J*, 1993, 12(5):386-9.

Yersinia pestis

Microbiology *Yersinia pestis* is the etiological agent of plague. All of the 11 species of *Yersinia* are aerobic, gram-negative rods, are well established members of the family Enterobacteriaceae, and have been isolated from human
(Continued)

ORGANISMS

Yersinia pestis (Continued)

clinical specimens. At least three species of *Yersinia* are unequivocal human pathogens: *Y. pestis*, *Y. enterocolitica*, and *Y. pseudotuberculosis*.

Epidemiology *Yersinia pestis* infections are rare in the United States. From 1970 to 1991, 295 cases were reported to the Center for Disease Control and Prevention. Plague occurs worldwide; most cases occur in Asia and Africa. In the United States, plague occurs (rarely) in New Mexico, Arizona, California, Utah, and Colorado. Yersinioses are zoonotic infections that usually affect rodents, small animals, and birds. Rats are the natural reservoir of *Y. pestis* in areas of urban ("city") plague; small animals such as ground squirrels, wood rats, rabbits, and cats are the natural reservoirs of *Y. pestis* in areas of sylvatic ("country") plague. Humans are accidental hosts of *Yersinia* species. Humans become infected with the bacterium after being bitten by fleas of the aforementioned animals, or, much less commonly, by handling infected animals or inhaling aerosolized *Y. pestis* generated by a person with pulmonary plague.

Clinical Syndromes Plague: Plague presents in many different and protean clinical forms: bubonic, septicemic, pneumonic, cutaneous, and meningitis. After an incubation period of 2-8 days, most patients with **bubonic plague**, the most common form, experience fever, chills, headache, aches, extreme exhaustion, and lymphadenitis. At the same time, extremely painful bubos develop in the groin, axilla, or neck. These patients have overwhelming numbers of bacteria in their blood. Patients with **septicemic plague** also have tremendous numbers of bacteria in their blood; however, these patients have a more septic presentation, and bubos usually are not present. **Pneumonic plague** is a complication of bubonic plague and is characterized by cough, chest pain, difficulty breathing, and hemoptysis; bubos might or might not be present. Pneumonic plague, if not treated immediately, has a very high mortality rate and can be rapidly fatal within 1 day. The natural progression of plague is from the bubonic, to the septicemic, to the pneumonic forms. The overall mortality rate for untreated cases of plague is 50% to 60%.

Diagnosis Diagnosis of plague is mainly a clinical diagnosis. Laboratories must be notified if *Y. pestis* is suspected as an etiological agent because many laboratories do not routinely suspect *Y. pestis* or culture clinical specimens for *Y. pestis* because special media and techniques easily can be used to enhance isolation of the bacterium and because the colonial morphology of *Y. pestis* is not typical of many other gram-negative rods. Culture is the most productive test for the laboratory diagnosis of plague. *Yersinia pestis* is not fastidious and grows well on blood agar media and many enteric media. Many commercial bacterial identification systems do not include *Y. pestis* in their databases. The most appropriate clinical specimens for culture include blood, biopsy or aspirate of bubo, sputum, cerebrospinal fluid, and cutaneous biopsy.

Diagnostic Tests/Procedures
Aerobic Culture, Appropriate Site *on page 244*
Blood Culture, Aerobic and Anaerobic *on page 271*

Treatment Supportive care is essential. The antibiotic of choice is streptomycin. Gentamicin, tetracyclines, and chloramphenicol are all effective alternatives. Timely treatment can potentially reduce mortality from plague to 10%.

Travelers to endemic areas are generally at low risk for developing infection. The CDC does, however, recommend the following precautions: avoid rat-infested areas; generous use of insect repellents and insecticides including body, clothing, and bedding application; avoid handling sick or dead animals. The CDC also recommends the use of prophylactic antibiotics if the risk of exposure is high. Tetracycline or doxycycline should be used in adults, and sulfonamides used for children less than 8 years of age. Plague vaccine requires multiple dosing over several months for protection and is therefore not recommended for immediate protection during outbreaks.

Drug Therapy
Recommended
Streptomycin Sulfate *on page 669*
Alternate
Gentamicin Sulfate *on page 575*
Tetracycline *on page 679*
Doxycycline *on page 557*
Chloramphenicol *on page 531*

Selected Readings
Butler TB, "*Yersinia* Infections: Centennial of the Discovery of the Plague Bacillus," *Clin Infect Dis*, 1994, 19:655-63.

Butler TB, "*Yersinia* Species (Including Plague)," *Principles and Practice of Infectious Diseases*, 4th ed, Mandell GL, Bennett JE, and Dolin R, eds, New York, NY: Churchill Livingstone, 1995, 2070-8.

Centers for Disease Control, "Human Plague – India, 1994," *MMWR Morb Mortal Wkly Rep*, 1994, 43(38):689-91.

Centers for Disease Control, "Human Plague – United States, 1993-1994," *MMWR Morb Mortal Wkly Rep*, 1994, 43(13):242-3.

Craven RB, Maupin GO, Beard ML, et al, "Reported Cases of Human Plague Infections in the United States, 1970-1991," *J Med Entomol*, 1993, 30(4):758-61.

Crook LD and Tempest B, "Plague. A Review of 27 Cases," *Arch Intern Med*, 1992, 152(6):1253-6.

LABORATORY DIAGNOSIS

Abdomen, CT *see* Computed Transaxial Tomography, Abdomen
Studies *on page 306*

Abdominal Paracentesis *see* Paracentesis *on page 420*

Abscess Aerobic and Anaerobic Culture

Related Information

Antimicrobial Susceptibility Testing, Aerobic and Facultatively Anaerobic Organisms *on page 259*

Antimicrobial Susceptibility Testing, Anaerobic Bacteria
on page 260

Genital Culture *on page 349*

Wound Culture *on page 480*

Applies To Aerobic Culture, Abscess; Anaerobic Culture, Abscess

Test Includes Culture for aerobic and facultative anaerobic organisms. Culture for anaerobic organisms usually must be specifically requested and may require a separate specimen.

Patient Preparation Aseptic preparation of the aspiration site. The overlying and adjacent areas must be carefully decontaminated to eliminate isolation of potentially contaminating anaerobes which colonize the skin surface.

Special Instructions The laboratory should be informed of the specific site of specimen, age of patient, current antibiotic therapy, clinical diagnosis, and time of collection.

Clinical Symptoms Suggestive
of Anaerobic Infection

Foul-smelling discharge

Location of infection in proximity to a mucosal surface

Necrotic tissue, gangrene, pseudomembrane formation

Gas in tissues or discharges

Endocarditis with negative routine blood cultures

Infection associated with malignancy or other process producing tissue destruction

Infection related to the use of aminoglycosides (oral, parenteral, or topical)

Septic thrombophlebitis

Bacteremic picture with jaundice

Infection resulting from human or other bites

Black discoloration of blood-containing exudates (may fluoresce red under ultraviolet light in *B. melaninogenicus* infections)

Presence of "sulfur granules" in discharges (actinomycosis)

Classical clinical features of gas gangrene

Clinical setting suggestive for anaerobic infection (septic abortion, infection after gastrointestinal surgery, genitourinary surgery, etc)

From Bartlett JG, "Anaerobic Bacterial Infections of the Lung," *Chest,* 1987, 91:901-9, with permission.

Specimen Fluid, pus, abscess wall tissue, or other material properly obtained from an abscess for optimal yield. Specimens for anaerobic culture should be accompanied by a specimen for aerobic culture from the same site. Aspirated fluid is acceptable for anaerobic culture if it is submitted in a properly capped syringe or an approved anaerobic transport device.

Container Anaerobic transport container swab with anaerobic transport medium and aerobic transport media or swab may be used if aspirated fluid is not available. However, swabs always provide inferior specimens.

Collection Specimens are to be collected from a prepared site using sterile technique. Contamination with normal flora from skin, rectum, vaginal tract, all mucus membranes, or other body surfaces must be avoided. Some anaerobes will be killed by contact with oxygen for only a few seconds. Ideally, pus obtained by needle aspiration through an intact surface, which has been aseptically prepared, is put directly into an anaerobic transport device or transported directly to the laboratory in the original syringe. Sampling of open lesions is enhanced by deep aspiration using a sterile needle and syringe. Curettings of the base of an open lesion may also provide a good yield. If irrigation is necessary, nonbacteriostatic sterile normal saline may be used. Pulmonary samples may be obtained by transtracheal percutaneous needle aspiration by physicians trained in this procedure or by use of a special sheathed catheter. If swabs must be used, two should be collected; one for culture and one for Gram stain. Specimens collected and transported in syringes should be transported to the laboratory within 30 minutes of collection.

Storage Instructions If syringe is used to transport specimen to the laboratory, all air should be expelled, and the needle removed.

Causes for Rejection Specimens which have been exposed to air, refrigerated, or delayed in transit have a less-than-optimal yield. Specimens from sites which have anaerobic bacteria as normal flora (eg, throat, feces, colostomy stoma, rectal swabs, bronchial washes, cervical-vaginal mucosal swabs, sputums, skin and superficial wounds, voided or catheterized urine) **are not** acceptable for anaerobic culture because of contamination by the normal flora.

Turnaround Time Cultures showing no bacterial growth can generally be reported after 2-3 days. However, initial growth may not appear for up to 7 days. Complete reports of cultures with anaerobic bacteria may take as long as 2 weeks after receipt of culture, depending upon the nature and number of the organisms isolated.

Reference Range No growth of anaerobic bacteria

Use Determine microbial etiology of the abscess and provide a guide for therapy

Limitations The only sources for specimens with established validity for meaningful anaerobic culture in patients with pleuropulmonary infections are blood, pleural fluid, transtracheal aspirates, transthoracic pulmonary aspirates, specimens obtained at thoracotomy, and fiberoptic bronchoscopic aspirates using the protected brush or sheathed catheter. Aspirated pleural fluid is preferred for patients with empyema. Blood cultures yield positive results in less than 5% of cases of anaerobic pulmonary infection.

Mycobacterium sp or *Nocardia* sp which may cause abscesses will **not** be recovered even if present, since extended incubation periods, aerobic incubation, and special media are necessary for their isolation. Cultures for these organisms should be specifically requested.

Contraindications Bronchoscopically obtained specimens are extremely poor specimens because the instrument becomes contaminated by organisms normally contaminating the oropharynx during insertion. Culture of specimens from sites harboring endogenous anaerobic organisms or contaminated by endogenous organisms (usually sites at or contiguous with any mucus membrane) usually will be misleading with regard to etiology and selection of appropriate therapy.

Additional Information In open wounds, anaerobic organisms may play an etiologic role, whereas aerobes may represent superficial contamination. Serious anaerobic infections are often due to mixed flora which are pathologic synergists. Anaerobes frequently recovered from closed postoperative wound infections include *Bacteroides fragilis*, approximately 50%; *Bacteroides* sp, approximately 25%; *Peptostreptococcus* sp, approximately 15%; and *Fusobacterium* sp, approximately 25%. Anaerobes are seldom recovered in pure culture (10% to 15% of cultures). Aerobes and facultative anaerobes when present are frequently found in lesser numbers than the anaerobes. Anaerobic infection is most commonly associated with operations involving opening or manipulating the bowel, mucus membranes, or a hollow viscus (eg, appendectomy, cholecystectomy, colectomy, gastrectomy, bile duct exploration, etc). The ratio of anaerobes to facultative anaerobes is normally about 10:1 in the mouth, vagina, and sebaceous glands and at least 1000:1 in the colon.

Selected Readings

Brook I, "A 12 Year Study of Aerobic and Anaerobic Bacteria in Intra-abdominal and Postsurgical Abdominal Wound Infections," *Surg Gynecol Obstet*, 1989, 169(5):387-92.

Styrt B and Gorbach SL, "Recent Developments in the Understanding of the Pathogenesis and Treatment of Anaerobic Infections," *N Engl J Med*, 1989, 321(4):240-6.

Swenson RM, "Rationale for the Identification and Susceptibility Testing of Anaerobic Bacteria," *Rev Infect Dis*, 1986, 8(5):809-13.

Acid-Fast Stain

Related Information

Mycobacteria Culture, Cerebrospinal Fluid *on page 405*
Mycobacteria Culture, Sputum *on page 406*

Synonyms AFB Smear; Atypical *Mycobacterium* Smear; Kinyoun Stain; *Mycobacterium* Smear; TB Smear; Ziehl-Neelsen Stain

(Continued)

Acid-Fast Stain *(Continued)*

Applies To Auramine-Rhodamine Stain; Fluorochrome Stain

Test Includes Acid-fast stain. For diagnosis, acid-fast stain and culture are usually ordered together. For monitoring therapy, stain alone may be sufficient.

Abstract Acid-fast bacilli are so called because they are surrounded by a waxy envelope that is resistant to destaining by acid-alcohol. Either heat (classic Ziehl-Neelsen) or a detergent (Tergitol Kinyoun method) is required to allow the stain to penetrate the cell wall. Once stained, acid-fast bacteria resist decolorization, whereas other bacteria are destained with acid-alcohol.

Patient Preparation Same as for mycobacteria culture of given site

Special Instructions The laboratory should be informed of the source of the specimen. Specimens may be divided for fungus culture and stain (KOH) preparation, mycobacteria culture and acid-fast smear, and routine bacterial culture and Gram stain only if the specimen is accompanied by appropriate requests for these procedures and if the specimen is of adequate volume for all tests requested.

Specimen The appropriate specimen for an acid-fast smear is the same as for culture: See specific site mycobacteria culture listings for details.

Container Same as for culture of specific site

Collection See specific mycobacteria culture listings for specific site.

Causes for Rejection Insufficient specimen volume, specimen received on a swab

Turnaround Time Routine: 24-48 hours; stat (if available): 2 hours

Reference Range No mycobacteria identified. Positive smears usually are reported in a quantitative manner such as a number of bacilli per field or entire smear.

Use Determine presence of mycobacteria, monitor the course of antimycobacterial therapy. Establish the diagnosis of mycobacterial infection in undiagnosed granulomatous disease, fever of unknown origin (FUO), and in patients suspected of having a defect in cellular immunity, eg, AIDS, lymphoma, etc.

Limitations Cultures are more sensitive than smears; therefore, the smear may be negative when culture is positive. Fluorochrome stains (auramine-rhodamine) are more sensitive than carbolfuchsin stains. Nonpathogenic acid-fast bacilli can be present as normal flora. Culture is necessary to determine the specific species of *Mycobacterium* present, however a presumptive determination of whether *Mycobacterium tuberculosis* or mycobacteria other than *M. tuberculosis* (formerly called "atypical mycobacteria") are present can be made. DNA probes, which are more sensitive and specific than smears for the diagnosis of mycobacterial infection are now in use in some laboratories.

Methodology Acid-fast stain of concentrated or unconcentrated specimen

Additional Information A stat acid-fast smear can be performed by some laboratories upon special request. However, concentration procedures are not usually performed on a stat basis. Very active infection is required to produce a positive without concentration. In extrapulmonary tuberculosis, the acid-fast stain can be useful in yielding a rapid diagnosis. Routine acid-fast staining and culturing of CSF for AFB is rarely, if ever, productive. However, positive smears have been reported from CSF in 67% of cases of culture-proven tuberculous meningitis, lymph nodes biopsy in 80% of miliary tuberculosis cases, 75% peritoneal biopsies in peritonitis, and urine in 80% of the cases of renal tuberculosis.

Acid-fast stains performed on gastric aspirates and urine when positive are reliable indicators of true mycobacterial disease. However, tap water can contain *M. gordonae* and can be responsible for false-positive results. Klotz and Penn have reported the sensitivity, compared to culture, as approximately 30% for gastric aspirates and approximately 50% for urine. False-positives were negligible, less than 1%.

The sensitivity and specificity of acid-fast staining for the diagnosis of pulmonary mycobacteria tuberculosis infection in a large prospective study was 53.1% and 99.8%, respectively, and 81.5% and 98.4%, respectively, for culture.

Selected Readings
Gordin F and Slutkin G, "The Validity of Acid-Fast Smears in the Diagnosis of Pulmonary Tuberculosis," *Arch Pathol Lab Med*, 1990, 114(10):1025-7.

Klotz SA and Penn RL, "Acid-Fast Staining of Urine and Gastric Contents is an Excellent Indicator of Mycobacterial Disease," *Am Rev Respir Dis*, 1987, 136(5):1197-8.

Levy H, Feldman C, Sacho H, et al, "A Re-evaluation of Sputum Microscopy and Culture in the Diagnosis of Pulmonary Tuberculosis," *Chest*, 1989, 95(6):1193-7.

LABORATORY DIAGNOSIS

Morris A, Reller LB, Salfinger M, et al, "Mycobacteria in Stool Specimens: The Nonvalue of Smears for Predicting Culture Results," *J Clin Microbiol*, 1993, 31(5):1385-7.

Murray PR, Elmore C, and Krogstad DJ, "The Acid-Fast Stain: A Specific and Predictive Test for Mycobacterial Disease," *Ann Intern Med*, 1980, 92(4):512-3.

Acid-Fast Stain, Modified, *Cryptosporidium* see *Cryptosporidium*
Diagnostic Procedures, Stool *on page 314*

Acid-Fast Stain, Modified, *Nocardia* Species

Related Information

Actinomyces Culture, All Sites *on next page*

Gram Stain *on page 352*

Nocardia Culture, All Sites *on page 415*

Synonyms Hank's Stain; *Nocardia* Species Modified Acid-Fast Stain

Test Includes Modified acid-fast stain. Culture generally must be ordered specifically as such. The recovery of *Nocardia* sp usually requires special culture techniques.

Abstract Infections with *Nocardia* sp may resemble many other more common diseases. Because therapy differs, it is important to establish a definitive diagnosis, preferably by culture. The diagnosis of nocardiosis should be considered in unexplained cavitary lung disease, granulomatous lung disease of an established cause not responsive to appropriate therapy, brain abscess particularly in the presence of cavitary lung disease, alveolar proteinosis, with mycetoma, and in any patient in whom a disseminated granulomatous disease is considered.

Specimen Appropriate preparation, specimen and container for smear is the same as for culture

Causes for Rejection Insufficient specimen volume, specimen received on a dry swab

Reference Range No acid-fast organisms seen

Use Determine the presence or absence of *Nocardia* sp which are usually, but not invariably, acid-fast when stained by the modified acid-fast stain. *Actinomyces* and *Streptomyces* sp which may be microscopically similar to *Nocardia* on Gram stain, are negative with the modified acid-fast stain. Establish the etiology of maduromycosis and of fever of unknown origin in patients with suspected defects of cellular immunity (eg, AIDS, Hodgkin's disease, lymphoma, and so forth).

Limitations *Nocardia* sp do not always stain acid-fast by this method; consequently, the presence of branching, gram-positive bacilli on Gram stain suggests that Gram stain might have greater sensitivity. *Nocardia* sp, however, cannot be distinguished from *Actinomyces* sp and other closely related organisms by Gram stain. Organisms from clinical material are more likely to be "modified acid-fast" than those from culture.

Methodology Kinyoun stain followed by relatively less severe decolorization with 3% acid alcohol (940 mL of 95% ethanol and 60 mL of concentrated HCl). If clumps or granules are observed, they should be crushed between two glass slides and examined microscopically.

Additional Information Nocardiosis has also been reported with lupus, rheumatoid arthritis, and liver disease. Aggressive diagnostic procedures are often necessary to obtain appropriate specimen for definitive diagnosis. Organisms consistent with *Nocardia* sp can be identified presumptively on Gram stain and modified acid-fast stain pending more definitive diagnosis by culture. Examination of sputum with *Nocardia* may show thin, crooked, weakly to strongly gram-positive, modified acid-fast positive, irregularly staining or beaded filaments. Opaque or pigmented sulfur granules may occasionally be present in direct smear of pus. Colonization without apparent infection may occur.

Selected Readings

Beaman BL and Beaman L, "*Nocardia* Species: Host-Parasite Relationships," *Clin Microbiol Rev*, 1994, 7(2):213-64.

Javaly K, Horowitz HW, and Wormser GP, "Nocardiosis in Patients With Human Immunodeficiency Virus Infection. Report of 2 Cases and Review of the Literature," *Medicine (Baltimore)*, 1992, 71(3):128-38.

Koneman EW, Allen SD, Janda WM, et al, *Color Atlas and Textbook of Diagnostic Microbiology*, 4th ed, Philadelphia, PA: JB Lippincott Co, 1992, 505.

McNeil MM and Brown JM, "The Medically Important Aerobic Actinomycetes: Epidemiology and Microbiology," *Clin Microbiol Rev*, 1994, 7(3):357-417.

Osoagbaka OU and Njoku-Obi AN, "Presumptive Diagnosis of Pulmonary Nocardiosis: Value of Sputum Microscopy," *J Appl Bacteriol*, 1987, 63(1):27-38.

Wilson JP, Turner HR, Kirchner KA, et al, "Nocardial Infections in Renal Transplant Recipients," *Medicine (Baltimore)*, 1989, 68(1):38-57.

LABORATORY DIAGNOSIS

Acromioclavicular Joint, Left or Right, X-ray *see* Bone Films
on page 277

Actinomyces Culture, All Sites
Related Information
Acid-Fast Stain, Modified, *Nocardia* Species *on previous page*
Gram Stain *on page 352*
Nocardia Culture, All Sites *on page 415*

Applies To Intrauterine Device Culture; IUD Culture; Sulfur Granule, Culture

Test Includes Anaerobic culture for *Actinomyces* sp and direct microscopic examination of Gram stain for sulfur granules and gram-positive branching bacilli

Abstract Actinomycosis is a chronic progressive suppurative disease characterized by the formation of multiple abscesses, draining sinuses, and dense fibrosis. The classic presentations include cervicofacial, thoracic, abdominal, and pelvic infections.

Patient Preparation Cleanse the skin around the opening of a draining sinus with an alcohol swab, allow to dry, and obtain the specimen from as deep within the sinus as possible. Submit aspirated material or tissue. Do not submit a swab specimen.

Special Instructions In tissues, *Actinomyces* sp produce chronic suppuration with formation of multiple draining sinuses. Examination of material from such sinuses often reveals tangled masses of filamentous elements and granules called sulfur granules. The presence of sulfur granules is highly suggestive of *Actinomyces* infection. If actinomycosis is suspected clinically, the laboratory should be informed. The specific site of specimen, current antibiotic therapy, and clinical diagnosis should be provided.

Specimen Exudate, material from draining sinus

Container Anaerobic specimen transport medium

Collection *Actinomyces* sp are fastidious anaerobic organisms. It is, therefore, essential that the specimen be placed into the appropriate anaerobic transport tube and delivered to the laboratory as quickly as possible. If a syringe is used, expel all air before transferring into the tube. Swabs invariably collect poor specimens, but if used, should be transported in anaerobic transport medium. With a draining sinus, obtain the specimen by aspirating as far into the sinus as possible.

Storage Instructions Specimens should be transported immediately to the laboratory and processed as soon as possible.

Causes for Rejection Specimens exposed to air, specimens which have been refrigerated or have an excessive delay in transit, have a less than optimal yield. Specimens from sites which have anaerobic bacteria as normal flora (eg, throat, feces, colostomy stoma, rectal swabs, bronchial washes, cervical-vaginal mucosal swabs, sputums, skin and superficial wounds, voided or catheterized urine), may **not** be acceptable for anaerobic culture because of contamination by the normal flora.

Turnaround Time Preliminary reports are usually available after 7 days. Cultures with no growth may be reported after 14 days.

Reference Range No *Actinomyces* isolated. *A. israelii* is a normal inhabitant of the mouth, oropharynx, and gastrointestinal tract.

Use Detect infections due to *Actinomyces* sp; establish the etiology of granulomatous disease, chronic draining sinus, and fever of unknown origin (FUO) particularly in immunocompromised patients

Limitations Inform the laboratory that actinomycosis is clinically suspected, to ensure that cultures will be incubated long enough to permit recovery of *Actinomyces* sp; *Actinomyces* sp are relatively slow growing and will often fail to grow in the period in which most laboratories incubate routine cultures. Additionally, even when incubated appropriately, recovery of *Actinomyces* sp may be hindered by overgrowth with obligate and facultative anaerobic bacteria.

Methodology Anaerobic culture including thioglycolate broth media

Additional Information If granules are detected on the gauze pad covering a draining sinus, submit the granules to the laboratory. A Gram stain and culture should be performed on such granules. On smear branching gram-positive rods may be found. They may be similar in appearance to other actinomycetes including species of *Nocardia*, *Streptomyces*, and also *Mycobacterium*. Actinomycetes are not stained by the modified acid-fast stain used for *Nocardia* sp. Several species of *Actinomyces* are responsible for human infection. *Actinomyces israelii* is the most significant. *A. naeslundii*, *A. odontolyticus*, *A. viscosus*, and *Arachnia propionica* also have been reported as human pathogens.

Pelvic and perirectal infections have been associated with intrauterine devices (IUDs). A classic presentation of actinomycosis is as a painless lump in the jaw. *Actinomyces* may be found in rare instances of recurrent ventral hernia following appendectomy for appendicitis. The diagnosis of actinomycosis in many settings requires consideration of the possibility followed by persistence on the part of laboratory personnel.

Selected Readings

Bellingan GJ, "Disseminated Actinomycosis," *BMJ*, 1990, 301(6764):1323-4.

Feder HM Jr, "Actinomycosis Manifesting as an Acute Painless Lump of the Jaw," *Pediatrics*, 1990, 85(5):858-64.

Holtz HA, Lavery DP, and Kapila R, "Actinomycetales Infection in the Acquired Immunodeficiency Syndrome," *Ann Intern Med*, 1985, 102:203-5.

Levine LA and Doyle CJ, "Retroperitoneal Actinomycosis: A Case Report and Review of the Literature," *J Urol*, 1988, 140(2):367-9.

Nahass RG, Scholz P, Mackenzie JW, et al, "Chronic Constrictive Pericarditis, A Case Report and Review of the Literature," *Arch Intern Med*, 1989, 149(5):1202-3.

Persson E, "Genital Actinomycosis and *Actinomyces israelii* in the Female Genital Tract," *Adv Contracept*, 1987, 3:115-23, (review).

Acute Phase Reactant *see* C-Reactive Protein *on page 311*

Adenovirus Antibody Titer
Related Information

Adenovirus Culture *on this page*

Special Instructions Acute and convalescent sera should be tested simultaneously.

Specimen Serum

Container Red top tube or serum separator tube

Sampling Time Acute and convalescent sera drawn 12-21 days apart

Reference Range A fourfold increase in titer of paired sera is indicative of a virus infection. Titers suggestive of no previous exposure are usually ≤1:16.

Use Establish the diagnosis of adenovirus infection; can be useful in differential diagnosis of respiratory ailments, hemorrhagic cystitis, and keratoconjunctivitis

Limitations The specific adenovirus serotype responsible for infection and the distinction between IgG and IgM titers cannot be determined by complement fixation test. Complement fixation tests are of low sensitivity, particularly in children.

Methodology Complement fixation (CF), hemagglutination inhibition (HAI), enzyme-linked immunosorbent assay (ELISA), serum neutralization, indirect immunofluorescent assay (IFA)

Additional Information There are 41 different types of adenovirus, and many infections are both asymptomatic and persistent. Thus, serologic evidence of adenovirus, and even isolation of an adenovirus from a patient, may be coincidental rather than the cause of the patient's present complaints.

Selected Readings

Bryan JA, "The Serologic Diagnosis of Viral Infections," *Arch Pathol Lab Med*, 1987, 111(11):1015-23.

Hierholzer JC, "Adenoviruses," *Manual of Clinical Laboratory Immunology*, 4th ed, Rose NR, de Macario EC, Fahey JL, et al, eds, Washington, DC: American Society for Microbiology, 1992, 590-5.

Adenovirus Culture
Related Information

Adenovirus Antibody Titer *on this page*

Viral Culture, Throat *on page 479*

Test Includes Culture for adenovirus only; adenovirus usually is detected in a routine/general virus culture

Specimen Midstream urine, stool, nasopharyngeal secretions, eye exudates, throat swab or tissue

Container Sterile container. Swabs should be placed into cold viral transport medium.

Storage Instructions Keep specimens cold and moist. Adenoviruses are more stabile than are most other viruses; however, specimens should not be stored or refrigerated for long periods of time. Specimens should be delivered immediately to the clinical laboratory.

Causes for Rejection Dry specimen, specimen not in proper viral transport medium, specimen not refrigerated during transport, specimen fixed in formalin

Turnaround Time Variable (1-14 days) and depends on culture method used and amount of virus in the specimen

(Continued)

Adenovirus Culture *(Continued)*

Reference Range No virus isolated

Use Aid in the diagnosis of disease caused by adenovirus (eg, conjunctivitis, cystitis, pneumonia, and pharyngoconjunctivitis)

Limitations Rule out or identify adenovirus **only**

Methodology Inoculation of specimen into cell cultures, incubation of cell cultures, observation of characteristic cytopathic effect, and identification by fluorescent monoclonal antibody

Additional Information Adenoviruses can be the etiologic agent of respiratory infections in children up to 6 years of age and of ocular infections in both children and adults. Adenovirus respiratory infections can mimic pertussis. Serology to detect adenovirus antibodies is often helpful in establishing a diagnosis.

Selected Readings

Hierholzer JC, "Adenoviruses," *Manual of Clinical Microbiology*, 5th ed, Balows A, Hausler WJ Jr, Herrmann KL, et al, eds, Washington, DC: American Society for Microbiology, 1991, 896-903.

Hierholzer JC, "Adenoviruses – A Spectrum of Human Diseases," *Clin Microbiol Newslett*, 1992, 14(15):113-20.

Hierholzer JC, "Adenoviruses in the Immunocompromised Host," *Clin Microbiol Rev*, 1992, 5(3):262-74.

ADNase-B *see* Antideoxyribonuclease-B Titer, Serum
on page 256

Aerobic Blood Culture *see* Blood Culture, Aerobic and Anaerobic
on page 271

Aerobic Culture, Abscess *see* Abscess Aerobic and Anaerobic
Culture *on page 238*

Aerobic Culture, Appropriate Site

Refer To

Aerobic Culture, Body Fluid *on this page*
Aerobic Culture, Cerebrospinal Fluid *on next page*
Aerobic Culture, Sputum *on page 246*

Aerobic Culture, Body Fluid

Related Information

Anaerobic Culture *on page 250*

Synonyms Body Fluid Culture, Routine

Applies To Ascitic Fluid Culture; Bone Marrow Culture; Culture, Biopsy; Joint Fluid Culture; Pericardial Fluid Culture; Peritoneal Fluid Culture; Pleural Fluid Culture; Surgical Specimen Culture; Synovial Fluid Culture

Test Includes Aerobic culture of biopsy or body fluid specimens

Patient Preparation Aseptic preparation of biopsy site

Special Instructions The laboratory should be informed of the specific source of the specimen, age of patient, current antibiotic therapy, and clinical diagnosis. Specimens may be divided for fungus culture and stain, mycobacteria culture and acid-fast stain, and routine bacterial culture and Gram stain only if the specimen is of adequate volume for all tests requested.

Specimen Surgical tissue, bone marrow, biopsy material from normally sterile site or aseptically aspirated body fluid

Container Sterile container with lid, no preservative. Bone marrow aspirates and body fluids may be directly inoculated into blood culture media. Contact the laboratory and obtain approval before inoculating fluids into blood culture media.

Collection Do **not** submit fluid collected with a swab. This type of specimen is rarely productive. The portion of the fluid specimen submitted for culture should be separated (utilizing sterile technique) from the portion submitted for histopathology.

Storage Instructions The specimen should be transported immediately to the laboratory.

Causes for Rejection Specimens in fixative, specimens collected on swabs, specimens having an excess transit time to the laboratory. Specimens which have been refrigerated have a less than optimal yield.

Turnaround Time Preliminary reports are available at 24 hours. Cultures with no growth are reported after 48 hours. Reports on specimens from which pathogens are isolated require a minimum of 48 hours for completion.

Reference Range No growth

Use Isolate and identify aerobic organisms causing infections in tissue

Limitations If anaerobes are suspected submit a properly collected specimen. See Anaerobic Culture, and Abscess Aerobic and Anaerobic Culture listings. If mycobacteria or fungi are suspected see Mycobacteria Culture, Biopsy or Body Fluid, or Fungus Culture, Body Fluid for detailed instructions.

Methodology Aerobic culture

Additional Information The specimen should be obtained before empiric antimicrobial therapy is started.

Selected Readings
Gorbach SL, "Treatment of Intra-abdominal Infection," *Am J Med*, 1984, 76(5A):107-10.

Aerobic Culture, Cerebrospinal Fluid

Related Information
Cerebrospinal Fluid Analysis *on page 288*

Synonyms Cerebrospinal Fluid Aerobic Culture

Applies To Ventricular Fluid Culture

Test Includes Aerobic culture and Gram stain (stat) if requested. Gram stain, cell count, differential, glucose, and protein levels are usually requested. Additional fluid if available may be used for additional cultures and other diagnostic tests such as those for bacterial or cryptococcal antigen and/or for acid-fast stain.

Abstract The major tests to be performed on the CSF for meningitis are the Gram stain and the bacteriologic culture. The "gold standard" for the diagnosis of bacterial meningitis is the isolation of a bacterium from the cerebrospinal fluid. Diagnosis of meningitis is made by blood culture and examination and culture of CSF.

Patient Preparation Aseptic preparation of the aspiration site

Special Instructions The laboratory should be informed of the specific source of specimen, age of patient, current antibiotic therapy, clinical diagnosis, and time of collection.

Specimen Cerebrospinal fluid

Container Sterile CSF tube

Collection Tubes should be numbered 1, 2, 3 with tube #1 representing the first portion of the sample collected. Contamination with normal flora from skin or other body surfaces must be avoided. The second or third tube collected during lumbar puncture is most suitable for culture, as skin contaminants from the puncture usually are washed out with fluid collected in the first two tubes. Since blood cultures are often positive in subjects with bacterial meningitis, blood cultures should be requested as well. Peripheral blood white cell count and differential are usually abnormal in patients with meningitis and represent an important part of the clinical investigation.

Storage Instructions The specimen should be transported immediately to the laboratory. If the specimen cannot be processed immediately, it should be kept at room temperature or placed in an incubator. Refrigeration inhibits viability of certain anaerobic organisms and may prevent the recovery of the common aerobic pathogens *Streptococcus pneumoniae*, *Neisseria meningitidis*, and *Haemophilus influenzae*.

Turnaround Time Preliminary reports are usually available at 24 hours. Cultures with no growth can be reported after 72 hours. Reports of cultures from which pathogens are isolated require a minimum of 48 hours for completion.

Reference Range No growth

Use Isolate and identify pathogenic organisms causing meningitis, shunt infection, brain abscess, subdural empyema, cerebral or spinal epidural abscess, bacterial endocarditis with embolism. The time honored Gram stain and aerobic CSF cultures in suspected bacterial meningitis are fundamental to appropriate diagnosis and treatment.

Limitations Cultures may be negative in partially treated cases of meningitis. Gram stain is the single most useful laboratory test to diagnose bacterial meningitis. However, Gram stains should be interpreted with care. Gram-positive organisms may decolorize (ie, stain gram-negative in partially treated cases). Acridine orange stain (AO) may have better sensitivity than Gram stain in detecting the presence of organisms in partially treated cases of meningitis but it is not at all widely used.

Methodology Aerobic culture

Additional Information See Cerebrospinal Fluid Analysis for table of laboratory values of components of CSF from healthy persons and from persons with

(Continued)

Aerobic Culture, Cerebrospinal Fluid *(Continued)*

meningitis. *Haemophilus influenzae*, *Neisseria meningitidis*, and *Streptococcus pneumoniae*, the most commonly isolated pathogens, can be serotyped if requested. Infections of cerebrospinal fluid shunts pose a difficult clinical problem. Organisms cultured include coagulase-negative staphylococci, *S. aureus*, *Streptococcus*, viridans group, enterococci, and *H. influenzae*. Culture of CSF or shunt fluid is diagnostic. Simultaneous blood cultures are rarely positive. Removal of the catheter and later replacement are frequently required to eradicate the infection. Susceptibility testing will be performed if indicated.

Selected Readings
Feigin RD, McCracken GH Jr, and Klein JO, "Diagnosis and Management of Meningitis," *Pediatr Infect Dis J*, 1992, 11(9):785-814.

Gray LD and Fedorko DP, "Laboratory Diagnosis of Bacterial Meningitis," *Clin Microbiol Rev*, 1992, 5(2):130-45.

Greenlee JE, "Approach to Diagnosis of Meningitis – Cerebrospinal Fluid Evaluation," *Infect Dis Clin North Am*, 1990, 4(4):583-98.

Wenger JD, Hightower AW, Facklam RR, et al, "Bacterial Meningitis in the United States, 1986: Report of a Multistate Surveillance Study," *J Infect Dis*, 1990, 162(6):1316-23.

Aerobic Culture, Sputum

Related Information
Anaerobic Culture *on page 250*
Legionella pneumophila Culture *on page 381*
Mycoplasma pneumoniae Diagnostic Procedures *on page 408*

Synonyms Sputum Culture, Aerobic

Applies To Bronchial Washings Culture; Bronchoscopy Culture; Percutaneous Transtracheal Culture Routine; Tracheal Aspirate Culture; Transtracheal Aspirate Culture

Test Includes Culture of aerobic organisms and usually Gram stain

Patient Preparation The patient should be instructed to remove dentures, rinse mouth, and gargle with water. The patient should then be instructed to cough deeply and expectorate sputum into proper container.

Special Instructions The laboratory should be informed of the specific site of specimen, the age of patient, current antibiotic therapy, clinical diagnosis, and time of collection.

Specimen Sputum, first morning specimen preferred; tracheal aspiration, bronchoscopy specimen, or transtracheal aspirate

Container Sputum container, sputum trap, sterile tracheal aspirate, or bronchoscopy aspirate tube

Collection Specimen collected, at time of bronchoscopy, by aspiration or by transtracheal aspiration by a physician skilled in the procedure. The specimen should be transported to laboratory within 1 hour of collection for processing.

Storage Instructions Refrigerate if the specimen cannot be promptly processed.

Causes for Rejection Specimens spilled or leaking onto the outside of the container pose excessive risk to laboratory personnel and may not be acceptable to the laboratory.

Turnaround Time Preliminary reports are usually available at 24 hours. Cultures with no growth or normal flora are usually reported after 48 hours. Reports on specimens from which pathogens are isolated require at least 48 hours for completion.

Reference Range Normal upper respiratory flora. Tracheal aspirate and bronchoscopy specimens usually are contaminated with normal oral flora. Transtracheal aspiration: no growth.

Use Isolate and identify potentially pathogenic organisms present in the lower respiratory tract. Presence or absence of normal upper respiratory flora is often reported.

Limitations An adequate sputum specimen should contain many neutrophils and few to no squamous epithelial cells, which are indicative of contamination with saliva. Results obtained by culture without evaluation for contamination may be noncontributory or misleading. A carefully collected and Gram stained specimen with neutrophils and gram-positive lancet-shaped diplococci can provide strong support for a clinical diagnosis of pneumococcal pneumonia.

In bronchoscopy and aspirated specimens reduction of contamination may be accomplished by a head-down position to reduce gravitational flow of saliva, when combined with quantitative culture techniques. Oral contamination may successfully be reduced by using a protected brush (PBC) catheter. The use of the PBC and bronchoalveolar lavage increases the overall diagnostic yield. Quantitation aids interpretation. Qualitatively, a bronchial washing is no better than sputum. If anaerobic bacteria are suspected in a transtracheal aspiration, a properly collected specimen for anaerobic culture should be submitted.

Methodology Aerobic culture following appropriate specimen selection. The most important step in the evaluation of a specimen is to be certain that the secretions that are examined are the product of the inflammatory process in the bronchi and not oropharyngeal material. All laboratories should perform this step.

Bacterial Species Recovered From Sputa in 103 Acute Bronchitic Exacerbations

	Number	Percent of All Types Cultured	Percent of Sputa Cultured
H. influenzae	41	24.0	39.8
H. parainfluenzae	29	17.0	28.2
S. pneumoniae	34	19.9	33.0
M. catarrhalis	19	11.1	18.4
N. meningitidis	5	2.9	4.9
K. pneumoniae	8	4.7	7.8
P. aeruginosa	4	2.3	3.9
Other possible pathogens	14	8.2	13.6
Unlikely pathogens	17	9.9	16.5

From Chodosh S, "Acute Bacterial Exacerbations in Bronchitis and Asthma, *Am J Med,* 1987, 82(Suppl 4A):154–63, with permission.

Additional Information See table. Potential pathogens recovered by usual sputum culture methods include: *Staphylococcus aureus, Haemophilus influenzae, Streptococcus pneumoniae, Neisseria meningitidis, Haemophilus parainfluenzae, Pseudomonas aeruginosa, Escherichia coli, Proteus* sp, *Moraxella catarrhalis, Bacteroides fragilis,* and rarely many other organisms. *Haemophilus* sp and *Neisseria* sp may not be isolated and identified by routine procedures. Thus, if their presence is clinically suspected, specific isolation procedures should be requested.

Organisms such as *Bordetella pertussis, Chlamydia pneumoniae Corynebacterium diphtheriae, Legionella pneumophila, Mycoplasma pneumoniae,* and *Mycobacterium tuberculosis* require special laboratory tests for isolation. Clinical suspicion of involvement by these agents should be communicated to the laboratory. See also listings for the specific agents.

The critical criteria for the diagnosis of acute bacterial infection of the bronchi are obtained from examination and culture of the sputum. The presence of bacteria in numbers greater than when the patient's condition is stable and a significant increase (ie, doubling) in the numbers of neutrophils present are essential laboratory criteria for the diagnosis of an acute bronchitic exacerbation. Gram stain results more closely reflect the clinical outcome and along with the criterion of the number of neutrophils in the sputum should be laboratory basis for determining success. Other commonly recognized agents causing pneumonia are listed in the following tables.

Selected Readings
Bartlett JG, Brewer NS, and Ryan KJ, "Laboratory Diagnosis of Lower Respiratory Tract Infections," *Cumitech 7,* Washington, DC: American Society for Microbiology, 1978.

Boerner DF and Zwadyk P, "The Value of the Sputum Gram's Stain in Community-Acquired Pneumonia," *JAMA,* 1982, 247(5):642-5.

Stratton CW, "Bacterial Pneumonias - An Overview With Emphasis on Pathogenesis, Diagnosis, and Treatment," *Heart Lung,* 1986, 15(3):226-44.

Community–Acquired Bacterial Pneumonias: Frequency of Various Pathogens	%
Streptococcus pneumoniae	40–60
Haemophilus influenzae	2.5–20
Gram–negative bacilli	6–37
Staphylococcus aureus	2–10
Anaerobic infections	5–10
Legionella	0–22.5
Mycoplasma pneumoniae	5–15

Nosocomial Pneumonias: Frequency of Various Pathogens	%
Klebsiella	13
Pseudomonas aeruginosa	10–12
Staphylococcus aureus	3–10.6
Escherichia coli	4–7.2
Enterobacter	6.2
Group D Streptococcus	1.3
Proteus and Providencia	6
Serratia	3.5
Pneumococcus	10–20
Aspiration pneumonia anaerobic pneumonia*	5–25
Legionella*	0–15

*The specific incidence of pneumonias caused by Mycoplasma, Legionella, and anaerobes is difficult to document because of the technical problems in isolating the organisms.

From Verghese A and Berk SL, "Bacterial Pneumonia in the Elderly Medicine," 1983, 62:271–85, with permission.

Spectrum of Frequent Etiologic Agents in Pneumonia

Aerobic Bacteria	Anaerobes	Fungi
Gram-positive aerobes Streptococcus pneumoniae Staphylococcus aureus Streptococcus pyogenes Gram-negative aerobes Haemophilus influenzae Legionella pneumophila Escherichia coli Klebsiella pneumoniae Pseudomonas aeruginosa	Bacteroides melaninogenicus Fusobacterium Peptostreptococcus Bacteroides fragilis Actinomyces israelii	Aspergillus Coccidioides immitis Histoplasma capsulatum Blastomyces dermatitidis Cryptococcus neoformans Zygomycetes

Viruses	Parasites	Other
Respiratory syncytial virus Parainfluenza virus Influenza virus Adenovirus Enterovirus Rhinovirus Measles virus Varicella-zoster virus Rickettsia Coxiella burnetii Cytomegalovirus	Pneumocystis carinii Ascaris lumbricoides Toxocara canisand catis Filaria Strongyloides stercoralis Hookworms Paragonimus Echinococcus Schistosomes	Mycoplasma pneumoniae Chlamydia trachomatis Chlamydia psittaci Mycobacterium tuberculosis ChlamydiaTWAR strains Nocardia

From Cohen GJ, "Management of Infections of the Lower Respiratory Tract in Children," Pediatr Infect Dis, 1987, 6:317-23, with permission.

Aerobic Culture, Tissue see Biopsy Culture, Routine on page 270

AFB Culture, Biopsy see Mycobacteria Culture, Biopsy or Body Fluid on page 404

AFB Culture, Bronchial Aspirate see Mycobacteria Culture, Sputum on page 406

AFB Culture, Gastric Aspirate *see* Mycobacteria Culture, Sputum
on page 406

AFB Culture, Sputum *see* Mycobacteria Culture, Sputum
on page 406

AFB Smear *see* Acid-Fast Stain *on page 239*

AIDS Antigen *see* p24 Antigen *on page 420*

AIDS Blood Culture *see* Blood Culture, Mycobacteria
on page 276

AIDS Virus Culture *see* Human Immunodeficiency Virus Culture
on page 370

Amebiasis Serological Test *see* Entamoeba histolytica Serology
on page 330

Amikacin

Related Information
Antibiotic Level, Serum *on page 255*

Synonyms Amikin®

Applies To Kanamycin (Kantrex®)

Abstract Aminoglycoside antibiotics, including amikacin, are used primarily to treat infections caused by aerobic gram-negative bacilli. Amikacin has a narrow therapeutic window. Its use in life-threatening infections makes it mandatory that effective levels be achieved without overdosing.

Specimen Serum

Container Red top tube or serum separator tube

Collection Not more than 30 minutes before the next dose for trough level; for peak level draw 15-30 minutes after completion of infusion or 45-75 minutes following intramuscular injection. Specify dosage, time of dosage, and all other co-administered antimicrobials. For send outs, ship specimen frozen in plastic vial on dry ice.

Storage Instructions Separate serum within 1 hour of collection, refrigerate or freeze until assayed.

Reference Range Therapeutic: peak: 15-25 μg/mL (SI: 26-43 μmol/L) (depends in part on the minimal inhibitory concentration of the drug against the organism being treated); trough: <10 μg/mL (SI: <17 μmol/L).

Critical Values Toxic: peak: >35 μg/mL (SI: >60 μmol/L); trough: >10 μg/mL (SI: >17 μmol/L)

Use Peak levels are necessary to assure adequate therapeutic levels for organism being treated. Trough levels are necessary to reduce the likelihood of nephrotoxicity.

Limitations High peak levels may not have strong correlation with toxicity.

Methodology High performance liquid chromatography (HPLC), fluorescence polarization immunoassay (FPIA), enzyme immunoassay (EIA)

Additional Information Amikacin is cleared by the kidney and accumulates in renal tubular cells. **Nephrotoxicity** is most closely related to the length of time that trough levels exceed 10 μg/mL (SI: >17 μmol/L). Creatinine levels should be monitored every 2-3 days as an indicator of impending renal toxicity. The initial toxic result is nonoliguric renal failure that is usually reversible if the drug is discontinued. Continued administration of amikacin may produce oliguric renal failure. Nephrotoxicity may occur in as many as 10% to 25% of patients receiving aminoglycosides; most of this toxicity can be avoided by monitoring levels and adjusting dosing schedules accordingly.

Aminoglycosides may also cause irreversible **ototoxicity** that manifests itself clinically as hearing loss. Aminoglycoside ototoxicity is relatively uncommon and clinical trials in which levels were carefully monitored and dosing adjusted failed to show a correlation between auditory toxicity and plasma aminoglycoside levels. In situations where dosing is not adjusted, however, sustained high levels may be associated with ototoxicity. This association is far from clear cut, and new once-daily dosing regimens (and associated high peak serum concentrations) that fail to enhance toxicity further complicate the understanding of this issue.

Selected Readings
Edson RS and Terrell CL, "The Aminoglycosides," *Mayo Clin Proc*, 1991, 66(11):1158-64.

Porter WH, "Therapeutic Drug Monitoring," *Clin Chem*, Taylor EH, ed, New York, NY: John Wiley and Sons, 1989, 217-48.

Amikin® *see* Amikacin *on previous page*

Amphotericin B

Synonyms Fungizone®

Abstract Amphotericin B is a clinically useful but highly toxic antifungal agent. Newer, less toxic agents are available. However, for many serious fungal infections, amphotericin B is still used despite its toxicity.

Specimen Serum

Container Red top tube or serum separator tube

Reference Range Therapeutic range: 1.0-2.0 μg/mL (SI: 1.0-2.2 μmol/L)

Use Monitor serum levels for potential toxicity and correlation with *in vitro* susceptibility data

Limitations Assays for amphotericin B are performed only in a few reference laboratories. In routine clinical use it is probably more prudent to follow creatinine, potassium, bicarbonate, and magnesium concentrations and the CBC, than to perform amphotericin B assays.

Methodology High performance liquid chromatography (HPLC), bioassay

Additional Information Amphotericin B therapy frequently induces fever, chills, nausea, and reversible bone marrow suppression.

Additionally, approximately 80% of patients develop increased creatinine concentrations, and occasional patients show an acute deterioration in **renal function**; when creatinine levels exceed 3.0 μg/mL it is advisable to withhold amphotericin B for several days and resume therapy at a lower dose.

Because the pharmacokinetics and biodistribution of the drug are not clearly defined, it may be useful to correlate serum levels with desired concentrations determined by *in vitro* susceptibility testing. Susceptibility testing, however, is not widely available, is not well standardized, and may not accurately predict clinical response. Amphotericin B can increase digitalis toxicity and decrease the anti-*Candida* effect of miconazole, and its toxicities are additive with those of aminoglycosides.

Selected Readings

Bodey GP, "Topical and Systemic Antifungal Agents," *Med Clin North Am*, 1988, 72(3):637-59.

Drutz DJ, "Newer Antifungal Agents and Their Use, Including an Update on Amphotericin B and Flucytosine," *Curr Clin Top Infect Dis*, Remington JS and Swartz MN, eds, New York, NY: McGraw-Hill Book Co, 1982, 3:97-135.

Terrell CL and Hughes CE, "Antifungal Agents Used for Deep-Seated Mycotic Infections," *Mayo Clin Proc*, 1992, 67(1):69-91.

Anaerobic Bacterial Susceptibility *see* Antimicrobial Susceptibility Testing, Anaerobic Bacteria *on page 260*

Anaerobic Blood Culture *see* Blood Culture, Aerobic and Anaerobic *on page 271*

Anaerobic Culture

Related Information

Aerobic Culture, Body Fluid *on page 244*

Aerobic Culture, Sputum *on page 246*

Biopsy Culture, Routine *on page 270*

Applies To Biopsy Culture, Anaerobic; Body Fluid Anaerobic Culture; Bronchial Aspirate Anaerobic Culture; Cerebrospinal Fluid Anaerobic Culture; Cyst Culture, Anaerobic; Surgical Specimen Anaerobic Culture; Tissue Anaerobic Culture; Transtracheal Aspirate Anaerobic Culture

Test Includes Isolation and identification of anaerobic organisms; susceptibility testing may be performed if clinically warranted.

Patient Preparation Sterile preparation of the site

Special Instructions The following information will assist the laboratory in the proper processing of the specimen: specific site of specimen, current antibiotic therapy, age and sex of patient, collection time and date, and clinical diagnosis.

Specimen Surgical tissue, biopsy material from normally sterile site, aspirated fluids, etc. Specimen for anaerobic culture should be accompanied by a specimen for aerobic culture from the same site.

Container Fluids: anaerobic transport container or original syringe; tissue: sterile container, no preservative

Collection Specimens are to be collected from a prepared site using sterile technique. Contamination with normal flora from skin, rectum, vagina, or other body surfaces **must** be avoided.

Storage Instructions Transport specimen to the laboratory within 30 minutes. Do not refrigerate. Refrigeration inhibits viability of certain anaerobic organisms and also the common important aerobic pathogens *Neisseria meningitidis*, *Streptococcus pneumoniae*, and *Haemophilus influenzae*.

Causes for Rejection Specimen not received in appropriate transport container or sterile container, specimen in fixative. Specimens delayed in transport to the laboratory and specimens which have been refrigerated have a less than optimal yield. Specimens from unacceptable sites (see above) may not be acceptable for anaerobic culture because of contamination by the normal flora.

Turnaround Time Cultures showing no bacterial growth will be reported after 2 days. Complete reports of cultures with anaerobic bacteria may take as long as 2 weeks after receipt of culture depending upon the nature and number of the organisms isolated.

Reference Range No growth of anaerobic bacteria

Use Anaerobic cultures are indicated particularly when suspected infections are related to mucus membranes, gastrointestinal tract, pelvic organs, associated with malignancy, related to use of aminoglycosides, or occur in a setting where the diagnosis of gas gangrene or actinomycosis is considered. Anaerobic culture is especially indicated when an exudate has a foul odor or if the exudate has a grayish discoloration and is hemorrhagic. Frequently more than one organism is recovered from an anaerobic infection.

Limitations Specimens received in anaerobic transport containers are less-than-optimal for aerobic or fungal cultures.

Contraindications Specimens absolutely contraindicated for anaerobic culture include the following: oral, GI, skin, urogenital, throat, sputum, bronchial wash, bowel contents, void urine, vaginal, cervical, material adjacent to a mucus membrane, and surface material from a wound or decubitus.

Additional Information Biopsy culture is particularly useful in establishing the diagnosis of anaerobic osteomyelitis, clostridial myonecrosis, intracranial actinomycosis and pleuropulmonary infections. In cases of osteomyelitis, biopsy is mandatory. Anaerobic infections of soft tissue include the following: anaerobic cellulitis, necrotizing fasciitis, clostridial myonecrosis (gas gangrene), anaerobic streptococcal myositis or myonecrosis, synergistic nonclostridial anaerobic myonecrosis, and infected vascular gangrene. These infections, particularly clostridial myonecrosis, necrotizing fasciitis, and nonclostridial anaerobic myonecrosis, may be fulminant and are frequently characterized by the presence of gas and foul smelling necrotic tissue. Empiric therapy based on likely pathogens should be instituted as soon as appropriate cultures are collected.

Oral contamination of bronchial aspirates can be minimized by using a telescoping double catheter with a plug to protect the brush. Even by this method, many anaerobes might not survive transit to the laboratory because of aeration of specimens and transport to the laboratory in an inappropriate transport device. Because of difficulty in interpretation, the usefulness of bronchial aspirate anaerobic cultures collected in the usual manner by routine bronchoscopy (ie, contaminated with oral flora), has been questioned. Pleuropulmonary infections caused by anaerobic organisms are most often secondary to aspiration of oropharyngeal contents. They may also be caused by septic emboli or from intra-abdominal infections (ie, subphrenic abscess, diverticulitis, appendicitis, etc). Community-acquired aspiration pneumonia, necrotizing pneumonia with multiple small abscesses, frank lung abscess, and pulmonary empyema yield significant anaerobes, 60% to 95% of cases, if appropriate culture technique is employed. The characteristic foul smelling odor of an anaerobic infection may not be present early in the course.

Selected Readings

Allen SD and Siders JA, "An Approach to the Diagnosis of Anaerobic Pleuropulmonary Infection," *Clin Lab Med*, 1982, 2(2):285-303.

Bartlett JG, Alexander J, Mayhew J, et al, "Should Fiberoptic Bronchoscopy Aspirates be Cultured?" *Am Rev Respir Dis*, 1976, 114(1):73-8.

Finegold SM, "Anaerobic Bacteria: General Concepts," *Principles and Practice of Infectious Diseases*, 4th ed, Mandell GL, Bennett JE and Dolin R, eds, New York, NY: Churchill Livingstone, 1995, 2156-73.

Finegold SM, "Anaerobic Infections," *Surg Clin North Am*, 1980, 60(1):49-64.

Willis AR, "Anaerobic Bacterial Diseases Now and Then. Where Do We Go From Here?" *Rev Infect Dis*, 1984, 6(Suppl 1):S293-9.

Anaerobic Culture, Abscess *see* Abscess Aerobic and Anaerobic Culture *on page 238*

Ancobon® *see* Flucytosine *on page 335*

Anergy Control Panel *see* Anergy Skin Test Battery
on this page

Anergy Skin Test Battery

Related Information

Fungal Skin Testing *on page 337*

Tuberculin Skin Testing, Intracutaneous *on page 463*

Synonyms Anergy Control Panel; Anergy Skin Testing; Delayed Reaction Intracutaneous Tests; Skin Test Battery

Test Includes Injection of several common antigenic substances into the skin, such as *Candida*, *Trichophyton*, and mumps antigens. Anergy skin testing is an *in vivo* means of evaluating the cell-mediated immune system. Skin injection sites are examined at 24, 48, and 72 hours. The development of local erythema and induration indicates an adequate delayed hypersensitivity response, and implies competent T-cell function. Failure to respond to any skin test antigen is termed cutaneous anergy, and is seen in a variety of systemic disorders.

Patient Preparation Procedure and risks are explained to the patient. No specific skin preparation is necessary. However, those patients with generalized skin disease, such as psoriasis, should be examined beforehand to ensure that there are suitable areas of normal appearing skin. Although testing need not be performed by a physician, one should be immediately available in the event of a systemic reaction.

Aftercare If no adverse reaction has occurred within 30 minutes, patient may be discharged from the testing center. Test sites should be kept reasonably clean for 72 hours. No restrictions on bathing are necessary. Patient should contact physician if severe local reactions develop, extensive erythema beyond the test site occurs, or if fever, dyspnea, or lightheadedness develops.

Special Instructions Requisition should include a list of all current medications, with attention to corticosteroids or other immunosuppressive agents.

Complications Anergy skin testing is generally quite safe. However, as with other forms of skin testing, immediate local reactions to antigens are distinctly unusual but possible. These reactions are usually IgE-mediated and lead to an immediate wheal and flare reaction. Rarely, serious local reactions have been reported to various antigens commonly included in the test battery; these include vesiculation, skin necrosis, and extensive erythema. Systemic reactions have been reported only on an individual case basis.

Equipment Antigens used for anergy testing are commercially prepared liquid extracts of a variety of foreign substances. These antigens are chosen because ubiquitous exposure to these substances is expected in the general population. Thus, in any randomly selected subgroup, a high rate of delayed hypersensitivity skin reactions would be anticipated. Commonly used bacterial antigens include streptococcal antigen (derived from *Streptococcus* group CH 46A), *Proteus* antigen (often from *Proteus mirabilis* IM 2104 strain), and in some centers, tuberculin is also included. Fungal antigens frequently employed include *Candida* antigen (derived from *Candida albicans* strain 2111), *Trichophyton* antigen (from *Trichophyton mentagrophytes*), and frequently histoplasmin is used (from *Histoplasma capsulatum*). Toxoids are also included in the test battery, usually tetanus toxoid (from *Clostridium tetani*, Harvard strain 401) and diphtheria toxoid (from *Corynebacterium diphtheriae*). Mumps skin test antigen is a viral antigen derived from inactivated mumps virus cultured in chick embryo. The choice of antigens and total number employed has yet to be standardized. Most test centers use less than five antigens in their routine battery, but considerable variation exists, with the total number ranging from 1-11. In studies, 90% of 750 hospitalized patients reacted to one or more of the following: mumps, *Candida*, *Trichophyton*, and tuberculin. Increasing the total number of antigens improved the rate of skin reactions by only 1%. With respect to the individual selection of antigens, a representative battery might therefore include mumps, *Candida*, and *Trichophyton*; this combination is commonly seen in practice. However, in one literature review, more than thirty different antigens were found to be in routine use at major centers. Disposable plastic or glass tuberculin syringes, 0.5-1 mL are also required, along with 26- or 27-gauge short ($\frac{1}{4}$" to $\frac{1}{2}$") beveled needles, some alcohol pads, and gauze. An alternative anergy testing technique has been developed in recent years to address the aforementioned lack of standardization in antigen selection and number. Termed the Multitest® CMI system, seven standardized antigens and one control are simultaneously injected by means of a multiple puncture device. Antigens used in the system are tetanus toxoid, diphtheria toxoid, streptococcal antigen, *Proteus*, tuberculin, *Candida*, and *Trichophyton*. This device obviates the need for separate syringes, needles, and antigens.

Technique Traditional method: Antigens are injected separately. Antigens are individually drawn up into tuberculin syringes immediately prior to testing. The volar aspects of the arms or forearms are the preferred test sites. Only normal appearing skin should be used. Sites are prepared with alcohol swabs. Using a 26- or 27-gauge needle, each antigen is injected intradermally at a 45° angle, bevel down. A small bleb approximately 2-3 mm in diameter should be raised; usually an injected volume of 0.05 mL is sufficient. Care should be taken to avoid deeper subcutaneous injections. Each antigen is separately planted in this fashion with adequate spacing between injection sites (>2 cm).

Multipuncture method: Antigens are placed simultaneous by means of the Multitest® CMI device. Seven antigens and one glycerol control are standardized with respect to selection and concentration and are preloaded onto this disposable plastic device. A different antigen coats each of seven multiple puncture heads, which are spaced approximately 2 cm apart, in two parallel rows of four. The skin over the forearm is held taut. The device is then oriented per manufacturer's instructions ("T" bar towards the head) and applied to the skin with a rocking motion. Each head must sufficiently puncture the skin.

Regardless of technique, all tests sites should be examined immediately and at 24, 48, and 72 hours. Date and time of injection must be recorded. The precise location, identity, and concentration of each antigen should be recorded, most often in a pictorial format or standardized table. It may be helpful to circle and label each antigen with a waterproof pen directly onto the skin, but this must not replace formal notations in the medical chart.

Data Acquired The transverse diameter of induration at each test site should be carefully measured by both inspection and palpation. Results are recorded in millimeters at the appropriate 24-hour intervals. Areas of erythema are also measured but play a minor role in most grading schemes.

Reference Range Normal individuals should demonstrate a positive skin reaction to one or more test antigens.

Critical Values A positive skin test is usually defined as the presence of induration and accompanying erythema ≥5 mm in transverse diameter at an injection site at 24, 48, or 72 hours. Immediate skin reactions (ie, within minutes) are due to mechanisms other than cellular immunity and do not define a positive test. When the Multitest® CMI system is used, induration ≥2 mm in transverse diameter is considered significant. This disparity in definition between the intradermal and multiple puncture technique results from a variety of technical factors including volume of antigen introduced, depth of skin penetration, etc. A state of anergy is defined as an inability to mount an appropriate delayed hypersensitivity response. In clinical practice this is manifested as a complete absence of reactivity to a skin test battery of at least four to five antigens. Some authorities require repetition of the test battery at least once before labeling a patient "anergic". Normal individuals are expected to develop a positive skin test in response to at least one antigen, barring technical error. Anergy may be present as a generalized defect in T-cell function, as in sarcoidosis, AIDS, or tuberculosis, or as a specific defect in cellular immunity, as in mucocutaneous candidiasis where T-cell response to *Candida* is selectively deficient. There are numerous causes of anergy and may be categorized as follows:

- infections: bacterial, tuberculosis, disseminated fungal infections, viral (influenza, mumps, mononucleosis, hepatitis, and others), parasitic
- congenital: cell-mediated deficiency (DiGeorge syndrome), combined cellular and humoral deficiency (Nezelof's, Wiskott-Aldrich syndrome, etc)
- acquired/iatrogenic: neoplasms (solid tumors, lymphomas, leukemias), medications (corticosteroids, antineoplastic agents, methotrexate, and others), AIDS
- rheumatic diseases: rheumatoid arthritis, lupus, Behçet's disease
- miscellaneous: uremia, diabetes mellitus, inflammatory bowel disease, sarcoidosis, extremes of age, malnutrition

However, anergy skin testing by itself does not distinguish amongst these conditions from a diagnostic viewpoint. Clinically, anergy testing is most useful in evaluating the patient who presents with chronic or recurrent infections, or infection with unusual organisms. In such cases, formal evaluation of the immune system may be warranted. This may include assessment of all four major components of the immune system: cell-mediated (T-cell) immunity, antibody-mediated (B-cell) immunity, phagocytic system (polymorphonuclear leuko-

(Continued)

Anergy Skin Test Battery *(Continued)*

cytes, macrophages), and complement. Often a careful history and physical, with attention to infectious diseases, will identify the particular component deficiency. Anergy testing is an appropriate and recommended screening procedure for suspected deficiencies in cell-mediated immunity, often characterized by fungal, mycobacterial, or disseminated viral infections (eg, varicella-zoster, cytomegalovirus, herpes simplex virus). Among the many laboratory tests available to evaluate host defense, anergy testing is rightfully obtained soon after the history and physical (along with a complete blood count with differential) but prior to more elaborate *in vitro* investigation of T-cell function. These latter tests include T-cell surface marker studies, T-cell subsets, and response to mitogens (such as pokeweed mitogen, phytohemagglutinin, concanavalin A). Some individuals demonstrate partial or inconclusive responses to skin testing. This is seen as a "borderline" skin induration diameter (ie, 1-4 mm) or as a poor reactivity rate when a large antigen battery is employed (ie, one positive reaction out of ten tested). These patients have sometimes been called "hypoergic," which implies a partially impaired delayed hypersensitivity response. The clinical significance of this phenomenon is unclear at present.

Use
- Objectively demonstrate cutaneous anergy in cases of suspected cellular immune system deficiency (T-cell dysfunction); often this procedure is performed as part of an initial immune system assessment, but may also be repeated in a serial fashion in cases of protracted or chronic illness
- Serve as a "control" skin test accompanying the tuberculin skin test (or other specific antigen tests); this allows more accurate interpretation of a negative tuberculin test; patients with generalized cutaneous anergy predictably fail to react to injected tuberculin despite prior exposure to *M. tuberculosis*
- Establish the presence of cutaneous anergy prior to more extensive *in vitro* evaluation of lymphocyte and monocyte function
- Less commonly, to help predict postoperative morbidity and mortality, especially in the patient with sepsis
- Occasionally, to provide general prognostic information in patients with cancer

Limitations "Traditional" skin test battery limitations, mentioned previously, include variation in selection and total number of antigens used as well as a lack of standardization of antigen potency. However, some practitioners consider the inability to select and interchange antigens in the Multitest® CMI system a major drawback. False-positive reactions may occur:
- when an immediate wheal and flare is interpreted as delayed hypersensitivity
- when intradermal bleeding is interpreted as erythema
- when dermographism is present

False-negative reactions may be caused by:
- lack of antigen potency
- subcutaneous injection
- inadequate dose or concentration
- incomplete skin puncture by the Multitest® device
- attenuated skin response, as in atopic dermatitis

Contraindications
- Prior systemic reaction to any antigen included in the skin test battery; alternate antigens may be substituted in most cases
- Known hypersensitivity to a stabilizer or diluent used in commercial antigen preparations; for example, mumps skin test antigen is derived from virus incubated in chicken embryo and preserved in thimerosal. Patients should therefore be questioned regarding feather and egg allergy as well as sensitivity to thimerosal prior to administering mumps antigen. Depending on the particular antigens selected, published manufacturer's warnings should be reviewed and potential hypersensitivity reactions avoided.

Selected Readings
Gordin FM, Hartigan PM, Klimas NG, et al, "Delayed-Type Hypersensitivity Skin Tests are an Independent Predictor of Human Immunodeficiency Virus Disease Progression," *J Infect Dis*, 1994, 169(4):893-7.

Kniker WT, Anderson CT, McBryde JL, et al, "Multitest CMI for Standardized Measurement of Delayed Cutaneous Hypersensitivity and Cell-Mediated Immunity. Normal Values and Proposed Scoring System for Healthy Adults in the U.S.A.," *Ann Allergy*, 1984, 52(2):75-82.

Anergy Skin Testing *see* Anergy Skin Test Battery *on page 252*

Animal and Human Bites Guidelines *see page 736*

Ankle Arthrogram *see* Arthrogram *on page 267*

Ankle, Left or Right, X-ray *see* Bone Films *on page 277*

Anti-B19 Parvovirus IgG Antibodies *see* Parvovirus B19 Serology *on page 425*

Anti-B19 Parvovirus IgM Antibodies *see* Parvovirus B19 Serology *on page 425*

Antibacterial Activity, Serum *see* Serum Bactericidal Test *on page 441*

Antibiotic-Associated Colitis Toxin Test *see* Clostridium difficile Toxin Assay *on page 300*

Antibiotic Level, Serum
Related Information
Amikacin *on page 249*
Chloramphenicol Serum Level *on page 299*
Flucytosine *on page 335*
Gentamicin *on page 351*
Tobramycin *on page 458*
Vancomycin *on page 473*

Synonyms Antimicrobial Assay

Abstract Assays for antimicrobial agents in serum are performed for two primary reasons: 1. to ensure therapeutic levels, and 2. to monitor for potentially toxic levels. In most situations, it is not necessary to monitor antimicrobial levels because serum levels are relatively predictable based on dosing; *in vitro* susceptibility testing uses those predictable levels to determine clinical efficacy. Similarly, toxicity is not always related to serum levels. It may be more appropriate to monitor for toxicity by following determinants of hematologic, renal, or hepatic function. In certain situations however (eg, aminoglycoside antibiotics which have a narrow therapeutic range and a high potential for toxicity), it is essential to follow serum levels.

Specimen Serum

Container Red top tube or serum separator tube

Sampling Time Peak: 30 minutes after 30 minute I.V. infusion; 1 hour after I.M. dose. Trough: immediately prior to next dose.

Collection Keep frozen if not assayed immediately.

Causes for Rejection Incomplete clinical information (eg, specific antimicrobial, dosage and schedule, other concurrent antimicrobials)

Reference Range Therapeutic range depends on agent being tested for, and minimal inhibitory concentration of drug against organism. Selected ranges in µg/mL are presented as a guide only.

Antibiotic Level, Serum

Drug	Peak		Trough	
	µg/mL	SI: µmol/L	µg/mL	SI: µmol/L
Amikacin	15–25	26–43	<10	<17
Chloramphenicol	25	77		
Flucytosine	100	775		
Gentamicin	4–10	8–21	<2	<4
Netilmicin	4–8	8.0–17.0	1–2	0.7–1.4
Streptomycin	5–20	9–34	<5	<9
Tobramycin	4–10	8–21	<2	<4
Vancomycin	20–40	13.6–27.2	5–10	3.4–6.8

Selected ranges in µg/mL are presented as a guide only.

Possible Panic Range See entries on aminoglycoside drugs (eg, Gentamicin and Tobramycin).

(Continued)

Antibiotic Level, Serum *(Continued)*

Use Evaluate adequacy of serum antibiotic level; detection of toxic levels

Limitations May not be technically possible in a patient taking more than one antibiotic

Methodology Bioassay: cephalosporins, clindamycin, erythromycin, metronidazole, penicillins, polymyxin, tetracycline, trimethoprim. High performance liquid chromatography: chloramphenicol, flucytosine, mezlocillin. Fluorescence polarization immunoassay (FPIA): amikacin, gentamicin, tobramycin, kanamycin, streptomycin, vancomycin, neomycin, netilmicin.

Additional Information With the increasing availability of *in vitro* sensitivity testing expressed as the minimal inhibitory or bactericidal concentration of an antibiotic, measurement of serum levels of these drugs has taken on practical clinical importance. This is especially true for agents with narrow therapeutic ranges and significant toxicity. It should be remembered, however, that in most patients, cure of infection depends on numerous host factors as well as on antibiotics. Therefore, antibiotic levels should not be relied on as the sole guide to therapy.

Selected Readings

Donowitz GR and Mandell GL, "Drug Therapy. Beta-Lactam Antibiotics," *N Engl J Med*, 1988, 318(8):490-500.

Rosenblatt JE, "Laboratory Tests Used to Guide Antimicrobial Therapy," *Mayo Clin Proc*, 1991, 66(9):942-8.

Smith AL and Opheim E, "Comparison of Methods for Clinical Quantitation of Antibiotics," *Curr Clin Top Infect Dis*, Remington JS and Swartz MN, eds, New York, NY: McGraw-Hill Book Co, 1983, 4:333-57.

Antideoxyribonuclease-B Titer, Serum

Related Information

Antistreptolysin O Titer, Serum *on page 263*

Streptozyme *on page 451*

Synonyms ADNase-B; Anti-DNase-B Titer; Antistreptococcal DNase-B Titer; Streptodornase

Specimen Serum

Container Red top tube or serum separator tube

Causes for Rejection Excessive hemolysis, chylous serum

Reference Range Preschool: $\leq$60 units; school: $\leq$170 units; adult: $\leq$85 units; A rise in titer of two or more dilution increments between acute and convalescent sera is significant.

Use Documentation of recent streptococcal infection

Limitations Normal ranges may vary in different populations

Contraindications Not valid in patients with hemorrhagic pancreatitis

Methodology Colorimetry based on hydrolysis of DNA

Additional Information Presence of antibodies to streptococcal DNase is an indicator of recent infection, especially if a rise in titer can be documented. This test has both theoretical and technical advantages over the ASO test: it is more sensitive to streptococcal pyoderma, it is not so subject to false-positives due to liver disease, and one need not worry about test invalidation due to oxidation of reagents.

Anti-DNase-B Titer *see* Antideoxyribonuclease-B Titer, Serum *on this page*

Antifungal Susceptibility Testing

Synonyms Fungi, Susceptibility Testing; Susceptibility Testing, Fungi

Test Includes Broth dilution, agar dilution and disc diffusion testing of antifungal agents. Results may be quantitative or qualitative.

Special Instructions Consult the laboratory to determine availability and choice of methods.

Specimen Pure isolate of the organism

Causes for Rejection Organism disposed of prior to request for testing.

Reference Range See table on following pages

Use Determine susceptibility of isolated fungi to available therapeutic agents, predict probable clinical response, explain observed or suspected therapeutic failures, determine if primary or secondary resistance is present

Limitations This test procedure is usually available only from specialized laboratories. Methods for fungal susceptibility testing are not as yet as standardized as for bacteria. Stability and solubility of some of the agents cause technical difficulty.

In vitro Antifungal Activities of Four Antifungal Agents Against Pathogenic Fungi*

Organism	Amphotericin B		Flucytosine (5–FC)		Miconazole		Ketoconazole
	MIC (µg/mL)	MFC (µg/mL)	MIC (µg/mL)	MFC (µg/mL)	MIC (µg/mL)	MFC (µg/mL)	MIC (µg/mL)
Filamentous fungi							
Pseudallescheria (Petriellidium) boydii	1.56–>100#	>100	Resistant		0.5§	0.05	0.1–4#
Aspergillus sp including *A. fumigatus*	0.05–8	6.25–>100	0.2–1.56#	>100	0.4–>100	0.8–>100	0.1–100
Blastomyces dermatitidis	0.05–0.2	0.1–0.4	Resistant		≤0.25	ND	0.1–2
Xylohypha bautiano	3.13–>100	3.13–>100	3.13–12.5#	12.5–>100	0.5–>64	ND	0.1–64
Coccidioides immitis	0.1–0.78	0.70–1.56	Resistant		0.25–1.0	ND	0.1–0.8
Histoplasma capsulatum	0.05–1.0	0.05–0.2	Resistant		≤0.25	ND	0.1–0.5
Phialophora sp and other dematiaceous fungi	0.05–>128	6.25–>128	Variable susceptibility	Resistant	0.05–32	ND	0.1–64
Sporothrix schenckii	1.56–12.5	3.13–>100	Resistant		1–2	ND	0.1–16
Zygomycetes	0.78–1.56	1.56–>100	Variable susceptibility	Resistant			

(Continued)

(continued)

Organism	Amphotericin B		Flucytosine (5-FC)		Miconazole		Ketoconazole
	MIC (µg/mL)	MFC (µg/mL)	MIC (µg/mL)	MFC (µg/mL)	MIC (µg/mL)	MFC (µg/mL)	MIC (µg/mL)
Pathogenic yeasts							
Cryptococcus neoformans	0.05-0.78†	0.1-12.5	0.10-100#	0.39->100	0.05-3.13	0.05-25	0.1-32
Candida albicans	0.2-0.78●	0.39-0.78	0.05-12.5#	0.10->100	0.1-2.0●	0.1-10	<0.1-128
Candida sp not C. albicans	0.2-1.56●	0.39-6.25	0.10-50#	0.20->100	<0.1-2.0	0.1->10	<0.1-64
Torulopsis glabrata	0.1-0.4	0.2-0.78	0.05-1.56	0.4->100	0.5-10	2-10	1-64
Trichosporon sp	0.78-3.13	1.56-3.13	25-100	>100	0.2-25	0.2->100	
Geotrichum sp	0.4-1.56	0.78-3.13	1.56-12.5	25->100	0.1-2	0.5->10	
Control organisms							
S. cerevisiae ATCC 36375, etc	0.1	0.2	0.05	0.10	0.20	0.39	0.20
C. pseudotropicalis ATCC 28838	0.05		0.05	0.10	0.10	0.20	0.05

*Based upon both data obtained at the Medical College of Virginia, Virginia Commonwealth University, Richmond, and a review of the literature. In vitro data for nystatin is not included because of the narrow clinical spectrum of this agent; however, most isolates of Candida species and Torulopsis species should be clinically susceptible (MIC ≤10 µg/mL) to nystatin. MFC, minimal fungicidal concentration; ND, not determined.
†Expected ranges of MICs and MFCs.
●Resistance not uncommon.
#Resistance reported but rare.
§Only limited data available.
‡In vitro susceptibility of Aspergillus sp to ketoconazole is highly species dependent.

From Shadomy S and Pfaller MA, "Laboratory Studies With Antifungal Agents: Susceptibility Tests and Quantitation in Body Fluids," Manual of Clinical Microbiology, 5th ed, Washington, DC, American Society for Microbiology, 1991, 1173-83, with permission.

Methodology Standardized methods are evolving for the susceptibility of yeasts. The availability of a choice of therapeutic agents will continue to cause laboratories to attempt to provide susceptibility data with a useful predictive value for clinicians.

Additional Information Interpretation of *in vitro* susceptibility data for antifungal drugs is hindered by the absence of standardized test criteria. Thus, it is extremely difficult to identify a clear relation between minimal inhibitory concentrations and clinical outcome. The situation appears more readily resolvable for yeast-like fungi than for filamentous fungi since the former are more easily quantified by standardized microbiologic techniques.

Selected Readings

Bennett JE, "Antifungal Agents," *Principles and Practice of Infectious Diseases*, New York, NY: John Wiley & Sons, 1985, 263-70.

Drutz DJ, "*In Vitro* Antifungal Susceptibility Testing and Measurement of Levels of Antifungal Agents in Body Fluids," *Rev Infect Dis*, 1987, 9(2):392-7.

Fromtling RA, "Overview of Medically Important Antifungal Azole Derivatives," *Clin Microbiol Rev*, 1988, 1(2):187-217.

Shadomy S and Pfaller MA, "Laboratory Studies With Antifungal Agents: Susceptibility Tests and Quantitation in Body Fluids," *Manual of Clinical Microbiology*, 5th ed, Balows A, Hausler WJ Jr, Herrmann KL, et al, eds, Washington, DC: American Society for Microbiology, 1991, 1173-83.

Anti-HCV (IgM) *see* Hepatitis C Serology *on page 360*

Antimicrobial Assay *see* Antibiotic Level, Serum *on page 255*

Antimicrobial Removal Device (ARD) Blood Culture *see* Blood Culture, Aerobic and Anaerobic *on page 271*

Antimicrobial Susceptibility Testing, Aerobic and Facultatively Anaerobic Organisms

Related Information

Abscess Aerobic and Anaerobic Culture *on page 238*

Penicillinase Test *on page 427*

Serum Bactericidal Test *on page 441*

Synonyms Kirby-Bauer Susceptibility Test; MIC; Minimum Inhibitory Concentration Susceptibility Test; Susceptibility Testing, Aerobic and Facultatively Anaerobic Organisms

Test Includes Qualitative or quantitative determination of antimicrobial susceptibility of an isolated organism

Abstract The purpose of antimicrobial susceptibility testing is to determine the degree of activity of antimicrobial agents against specific pathogens.

Specimen Viable pure culture of aerobic or facultatively anaerobic rapidly growing organism

Turnaround Time Usually 1 day after isolation of a pure culture

Reference Range As of December, 1993, the National Committee for Clinical Laboratory Standards revised interpretations of antimicrobial susceptibility testing results. The interpretation "moderately susceptible" has been eliminated. The current interpretations of results are "susceptible," "intermediate," and "resistant."

Use Determine the antimicrobial susceptibility of organisms involved in infectious processes when the susceptibility of the organism cannot be predicted from its identity

Methodology Disc diffusion, broth dilution, agar dilution, or microbroth dilution.

Additional Information Effective antimicrobial therapy is usually selected with the intent of achieving peak level 2 to 4 times the MIC at the site of infection. An antimicrobial level 10 times the MIC is usually sought in urinary tract infections. The "breakpoints" indicate clinically achievable levels and relate to MICs above which organisms are resistant and would not be expected to respond to readily achievable levels of antimicrobial therapy.

Susceptible: This category implies that an infection due to the strain may be appropriately treated with the dosage of antimicrobial agent recommended for that type of infection and infecting species, unless otherwise contraindicated.

Intermediate: This interpretation implies clinical applicability in body sites where the agent is physiologically concentrated (eg, in urine) or when a high dose of agent can be administered (eg, penicillins). In some cases "intermediate" applies to an MIC literally between a "susceptible" MIC and a "resistant" MIC. Such MICs are due to small uncontrollable technical errors/factors.

(Continued)

Antimicrobial Susceptibility Testing, Aerobic and Facultatively Anaerobic Organisms *(Continued)*

Resistant: Strains falling in this category are not inhibited by the usually achievable systemic concentrations of the agent with normal dosage schedules and/or fall in the range where specific microbial resistance mechanisms are likely (eg, beta-lactamases), and clinical efficacy has not been reliable in treatment studies. See table.

Major Mechanisms of Bacterial Antimicrobial Resistance

Enzymatic inactivation or modification of drug

- β-lactamase hydrolysis of β-lactam ring with subsequent inactivation of β-lactam antibiotics
- Modification of aminoglycosides by acetylating, adenylating, or phosphorylating enzymes
- Modification of chloramphenicol by chloramphenicol acetyltransferase

Decreased drug uptake or accumulation

- Intrinsic or acquired lack of outer membrane permeability
- Faulty or lacking antibiotic uptake and transport system
- Antibiotic efflux system (eg, tetracycline resistance)

Altered or lacking antimicrobial target

- Altered penicillin-binding proteins (β-lactam resistance)
- Altered ribosomal target (eg, aminoglycoside, macrolide, and lincomycin resistance)
- Altered enzymatic target (eg, sulfonamide, trimethoprim, rifampin, and quinolone resistance)

Circumvention of drug action consequences

- Hyperproduction of drug targets or competitive substrates (eg, sulfonamide and trimethoprim resistance)

Uncoupling of antibiotic attack and cell death

- Bacterial tolerance and survival in presence of usually bactericidal drugs (eg, β-lactams and vancomycin)

Selected Readings

Gill VJ, Witebsky FG, and MacLowry JD, "Multicategory Interpretive Reporting of Susceptibility Testing With Selected Antimicrobial Concentrations. Ten Years of Laboratory and Clinical Experience," *Clin Lab Med*, 1989, 9(2):221-38.

Hindler JA and Thrupp LD, "Interpretive Guidelines for Antimicrobial Susceptibility Test Results: What Do They Mean?" *Clin Microbiol Newslett*, 1989, 17:129-36.

"Methods for Dilution Antimicrobial Susceptibility Tests for Bacteria Which Grow Aerobically – Third Edition; Approved Standard. Document M7-A3," Vol 13, Villanova, PA: National Committee for Laboratory Standards, 1993.

"Performance Standards for Antimicrobial Disk Susceptibility Tests –Fifth Edition; Approved Standard. Document M2-A5," Vol 13, Villanova, PA: National Committee for Laboratory Standards, 1993.

Rosenblatt JE, "Laboratory Tests Used to Guide Antimicrobial Therapy," *Mayo Clin Proc*, 1991, 66(9):942-8.

Antimicrobial Susceptibility Testing, Anaerobic Bacteria

Related Information

Abscess Aerobic and Anaerobic Culture *on page 238*
Penicillinase Test *on page 427*

Synonyms Anaerobic Bacterial Susceptibility; MIC, Anaerobic Bacteria; Susceptibility Testing, Antimicrobial, Anaerobic Bacteria

Special Instructions The laboratory should be consulted regarding appropriateness and scope of anaerobic susceptibility testing in a particular clinical setting.

Specimen Viable pure culture of anaerobic organism

Turnaround Time 2-5 days from time organism is isolated and identified

Typical Sensitivities of Important Anaerobic Pathogens to Major Classes of Antibiotics

Antibiotic	B. fragilis Group	B. melanino-genicus Group	Fusobacterium	Clostridium	Propioni-bacterium	Actinomyces	Peptostrepto-coccus
Penicillin G	– to +	– to +++	++	+ to ++	+++	+++	+++
Antipseudomonal penicillins	++ to +++	+ to +++	+++	+++	+++	+++	+++
Cefoxitin	++	+++	++ to +++	– to ++	+++	+++	+++
Imipenem–cilastatin	+++	+++	++	+++	+++	+++	+++
Combinations of beta–lactam and beta–lactamase inhibitor	+++	+++	+++	+++	+++	+++	+++
Clindamycin	++ to +++	+++	+++	++	+++	+++	+++
Chloramphenicol	+++	+++	+++	+++	+++	+++	+++
Metronidazole	+++	+++	+++	+++	–	–	++ to +++

– denotes that <50% of the strains were susceptible.
+ denotes that 50% to 70% of the strains were susceptible.
++ denote that 70% to 90% of the strains were susceptible.
+++ denote that >90% of the strains were susceptible.

From Styrt B and Gorbach SL, "Recent Developments in the Understanding of the Pathogenesis and Treatment of Anaerobic Infections," N Engl J Med, 1989, Part I, 321:240–6 and Part II, 321:298–302, (review), with permission.

(Continued)

Antimicrobial Susceptibility Testing, Anaerobic Bacteria *(Continued)*

Reference Range See table on previous page.

Use Susceptibility test results are usually reported on anaerobic bacterial isolates only on special request to the laboratory. Susceptibility testing of anaerobes is not usually performed. It may be indicated for individual patient isolates when the selection of therapeutic agents is critical. This situation may occur because of failure of empiric therapy or because of lack of response to empiric therapy. Difficulty in making empiric decisions due to lack of precedent, specific infections which may be appropriate for the determination of anaerobic susceptibility include brain abscess, endocarditis, osteomyelitis, joint infection, infection of prosthetic devices or vascular grafts.

Limitations Breakpoints are not well defined or universally accepted for categorization of susceptible and resistant. Methods are still being developed to standardize testing, reporting, and interpretation of anaerobic susceptibility tests for the broth disc elution and microdilution methods. Anaerobic infections are frequently mixed involving aerobic and anaerobic flora, thus, the predictive value of an anaerobic susceptibility test for a successful clinical outcome may be limited by the complexity of the clinical infection.

Contraindications Anaerobe isolate from patient is not available or fails to give adequate growth for susceptibility testing.

Methodology Broth disc elution, broth microdilution, and agar dilution technique; beta-lactamase testing

Additional Information At present, routine susceptibility testing of anaerobic isolates is not recommended. Infections involving anaerobes frequently contain mixed flora and appropriate drainage rather than antimicrobial therapy seems to be the most crucial factor in the successful treatment of these infections.

Indications for anaerobic susceptibility testing include:

- determination of susceptibility of anaerobes to new antimicrobial agents
- monitoring susceptibility patterns by geographic area
- monitoring susceptibility patterns in local hospitals
- assisting in the management of selected individual patients.

Many anaerobes grow so slowly that by the time isolation and susceptibility testing is completed (6-14 days), the results are of little clinical value. Most anaerobes have very predictable *in vitro* susceptibility patterns that appear to have changed little over the years. For these reasons, many laboratories perform anaerobic susceptibility testing only on anaerobic isolates from blood, pleural fluid, peritoneal fluid, and CSF. In cases of chronic anaerobic infections (septic arthritis, osteomyelitis, etc), susceptibility testing may be done by special request. The physician should contact the laboratory regarding the specific antibiotic(s) to be tested and the testing method (broth disk, MICs, etc) available.

Organisms that are recognized as virulent (ie, *Bacteroides fragilis* group, pigmented *Bacteroides* sp, *Bacteroides gracilis*, certain *Fusobacterium*, *Clostridium perfringens*, and *Clostridium ramosus*) may also be considered for testing.

Selected Readings

Finegold SM, "Susceptibility Testing of Anaerobic Bacteria," *J Clin Microbiol*, 1988, 26(7):1253-6.

Rosenblatt JE, "Susceptibility Testing of Anaerobic Bacteria," *Clin Lab Med*, 1989, 9(2):239-54, (review).

Styrt B and Gorbach SL, "Recent Developments in the Understanding of the Pathogenesis and Treatment of Anaerobic Infections," *N Engl J Med*, 1989, Part I, 321(4):240-6 and Part II, 321(5):298-302.

Zebransky RJ, "Revisiting Anaerobe Susceptibility Testing," *Clin Microbiol Newslett*, 1989, 11:185-92.

Antimycobacterial Susceptibility Testing

Related Information

Mycobacteria Culture, Biopsy or Body Fluid *on page 404*

Synonyms Mycobacteria, Susceptibility Testing; Susceptibility Testing, Mycobacteria

Test Includes Panel of antimycobacterial agents tested against isolates at appropriate concentrations

Specimen Pure isolate of an organism

Causes for Rejection Specimen not available for testing.

Turnaround Time 4-6 weeks after organism is isolated

Use Determine the susceptibility of the isolated organism to a panel of antimycobacterial agents

Limitations Susceptibilities cannot be reported if the organism fails to grow on test media.

Methodology Agar dilution. Some laboratories use the Bactec® broth system to determine susceptibility to some antimycobacterial agents. The CDC recommends this broth method. See table.

Antimicrobials Commonly Used for Mycobacterial Susceptibility Testing

Antituberculosis Drugs	
Primary	**Secondary**
Ethambutol	Capreomycin
Isoniazid	Ciprofloxacin
Pyrazinamide	Cycloserine
Rifampin	Ethionamide
Streptomycin	Kanamycin

Other Mycobacterial Isolates*	
Primary	**Secondary**
Amikacin	Azithromycin
Ciprofloxacin	Clarithromycin
Ethambutol	Clofazimine
Isoniazid	Doxycycline
Rifampin	
Streptomycin	
Sulfonamides	
Tobramycin	

*Drug regimens will depend on the mycobacterial species identified.

From Wolinsky E, "Mycobacterial Diseases Other Than Tuberculosis," *Clin Infect Dis*, 1992, 15:1-12, with permission.

Additional Information Susceptibilities are performed on the first organism isolated from a patient, and at 3-6 month intervals if that organism continues to be isolated while the patient is on therapy. Susceptibility tests should be performed in patients with recurrent tuberculosis as resistant strains are common in recurrent infection. Failure to take all drugs in a multidrug regimen can lead to a shift toward resistant organisms and treatment failure. Atypical or environmental mycobacteria, particularly stains of the *M. avium* complex, have variable susceptibility within species. Frequently, they are resistant to oral therapy.

Selected Readings
Heifets L, "Qualitative and Quantitative Drug Susceptibility Tests in Mycobacteriology," *Am Rev Respir Dis*, 1988, 137(5):1217-22.

Swenson JM, Wallace RJ Jr, Silcox VA, et al, "Antimicrobial Susceptibility of Five Subgroups of *Mycobacterium fortuitum* and *Mycobacterium chelonae*," *Antimicrob Agents Chemother*, 1985, 28(6):807-11.

Van Scoy RE and Wilkowske CJ, "Antituberculous Agents," *Mayo Clin Proc.* 1992, 67(2):179-87.

Wallace RJ Jr, Swenson JM, Silcox VA, et al, "Treatment of Nonpulmonary Infections Due to *Mycobacterium fortuitum* and *Mycobacterium chelonei* Based on *In Vitro* Susceptibilities," *J Infect Dis*, 1985, 152(3):500-14.

Antistreptococcal DNase-B Titer *see* Antideoxyribonuclease-B Titer, Serum *on page 256*

Antistreptolysin O Titer, Serum
Related Information
Antideoxyribonuclease-B Titer, Serum *on page 256*
Streptozyme *on page 451*
Synonyms ASO
Specimen Serum
Container Red top tube or serum separator tube
Causes for Rejection Excessive hemolysis
(Continued)

263

LABORATORY DIAGNOSIS

Antistreptolysin O Titer, Serum *(Continued)*

Reference Range Less than 2 years of age: usually <50 Todd units; 2-5 years: <100 Todd units; 5-19 years: <166 Todd units; adults: <125 Todd units. A rise in titer of four or more dilution increments from acute to convalescent specimens is considered to be significant regardless of the magnitude of the titer. For a single specimen, ASO titers ≤166 Todd units are considered normal, but higher titers may be "normal" in demographic groups, or may be associated with chronic pharyngeal carriage.

Use Document streptococcal infection. A marked rise in titer or a persistently elevated titer indicates that a *Streptococcus* infection or poststreptococcal sequelae are present. Elevated titers are seen in 80% to 85% of patients with acute rheumatic fever and in 95% of patients with acute glomerulonephritis.

Limitations False-positive ASO titers can be caused by increased levels of serum beta-lipoprotein produced in liver disease and by contamination of the serum with *Bacillus cereus* and *Pseudomonas* sp. ASO is usually not formed as a result of streptococcal pyoderma. Test is subject to technical false-positives due to oxidation of reagents.

Methodology Hemolysis inhibition, latex agglutination (LA)

Additional Information Streptolysin is a cytolysin produced by group A streptococci. In an infected individual streptolysin O acts as a protein antigen, and the patient mounts an antibody response. A rise in titer begins about 1 week after infection and peaks 2-4 weeks later. In the absence of complications or reinfection, the ASO titer will usually fall to preinfection levels within 6-12 months. Both clinical and laboratory findings should be correlated in reaching a diagnosis.

Selected Readings

Ayoub EM and Harden E, "Immune Response to Streptococcal Antigens: Diagnostic Methods," *Manual of Clinical Laboratory Immunology*, 4th ed, Rose NR, de Macario EC, Fahey JL, et al, eds, Washington, DC: American Society for Microbiology, 1992, 427-34.

Escobar MR, "Hemolytic Assays: Complement Fixation and Antistreptolysin O," *Manual of Clinical Microbiology*, 5th ed, Balows A, Hausler WJ Jr, Herrmann KL, et al, eds, Washington, DC: American Society for Microbiology, 1991, 73-8.

Keren DF and Warren JS, *Diagnostic Immunology*, Baltimore, MD: Williams & Wilkins, 1992, 168-70.

ARD, Blood Culture *see* Blood Culture, Aerobic and Anaerobic *on page 271*

Arterial Line Culture *see* Intravenous Line Culture *on page 376*

Arthritis Series, X-ray *see* Bone Films *on page 277*

Arthrocentesis

Synonyms Closed Joint Aspiration; Joint Tap

Test Includes Passing a needle into a joint space and aspirating synovial fluid for diagnostic analysis

Patient Preparation Procedure and risks are explained and consent is obtained. No intravenous pain medications or sedatives are required.

Aftercare Determined by results of procedure, as outlined by physician. May range from joint immobilization with passive range of motion, as in septic arthritis, to full weight bearing, as in effusions secondary to osteoarthritis. No specific joint positioning postprocedure has been demonstrated to reduce complications.

Complications Arthrocentesis is usually a safe procedure, especially when performed on an easily accessible joint such as the knee. Potential complications include:

- iatrogenic joint space infection (if properly performed, incidence has been estimated at 1 in 15,000 cases)
- hemorrhage or hematoma formation (usually when alternative approaches are used and blood vessels are ruptured on the flexor surface of the joint)
- local pain caused by needle trauma to the periosteum
- injury to cartilage, particularly problematic due to slow repair rate
- tendon rupture
- nerve palsies

Equipment Alcohol swabs, povidone-iodine prep solution, sterile gloves and towels, gauze, and forceps. Local anesthesia with ethyl chloride vinyl spray and/or lidocaine 1% with appropriate syringes and subcutaneous needles. If the joint to be aspirated is large, use 18- or 20-gauge 1.5" needle on a 20 mL syringe (additional syringes should be available). If joint is small or effusion minimal, use 20- or 22-gauge 1.5" needle on 3 mL syringe. In this latter case, additional tubes for fluid collection will not be needed. Otherwise, use three sterile tubes for collection, the first one with either EDTA additive or a small amount of heparin. If gonococcal arthritis is suspected, obtain chocolate (Thayer-Martin) media. Glass slides and polarized microscope are necessary if crystalline arthropathy is suspected.

Technique The following description details the technique of knee arthrocentesis, a joint commonly aspirated by the generalist. Patient is instructed to lie supine and remain relaxed. Physician selects the type of approach: suprapatellar, parapatellar, or infrapatellar. The parapatellar approach is popular and effective with tense effusions. Here, the knee is placed in 20° flexion to relax the quadriceps. The preferred entry site is the midportion of the patella (approximately 2 cm superior to the inferior portion of the patella), preferably the medial aspect. This site is marked by indenting the skin with the retracted end of a ballpoint pen. The skin is prepped with alcohol first then povidone-iodine. Some clinicians prefer strict aseptic technique (5-minute scrub, masks, gowns, and drapes) whereas others do not use even sterile gloves or drapes. We prefer a middle-ground approach, using sterile gloves and drapes but foregoing masks and gowns. The use of local anesthesia also varies amongst practitioners. If the joint is tense, and anatomical landmarks easily palpable, we prefer cutaneous anesthesia with only a spray of ethyl chloride solution. Alternatively, a subcutaneous wheal of lidocaine may be raised in the usual fashion. Injection of lidocaine into deeper structures is not usually required (where it may potentially interfere with culture results because of bacteriostatic properties). Following this, the needle-on-syringe is passed through the marked skin site and advanced slowly while aspirating. A "pop" may be felt as the needle penetrates the capsule. The needle should be directed parallel to the plane of the synovial capsule if the parapatellar approach is used. Once fluid is returned, the needle should not be advanced further in order to avoid cartilage damage. Only mild suction should be used to aspirate so that trauma and hemorrhage do not occur. In general, joint effusions should be drained completely. A blind "search" with the needle (often with vigorous aspiration) is hazardous and should not be attempted. Forceps may be used to stabilize the needle if several syringe changes are required. Once completed, withdraw the needle, apply pressure, and place adhesive tape over puncture site. If persistent pain is encountered during the procedure, trauma to cartilage or periosteum is likely. Do not reflexly anesthetize these deeper tissues with lidocaine; instead, withdraw the needle and redirect it along a new plane. Correct placement of the needle in the joint space is normally painless. In the case of a "dry tap," folds of synovium may be acting as a valve obstructing the needle lumen. Reposition the needle slightly, or if there is fluid in the syringe, inject a small amount to clear the needle bevel. This problem can be avoided by using the infrapatellar approach. The technique for suprapatellar and infrapatellar aspiration has been detailed elsewhere. The suprapatellar approach is most useful in tense effusions where the suprapatellar bursa (usually in communication with the joint space) is visibly distended. While easily performed, there is a potential for sinus tract formation especially if the entry site is directly over the bursa, rather than several centimeters away. The infrapatellar approach has a low risk of cartilage damage compared with the parapatellar approach and is useful for patients with marked flexion contractures of the knee. However, clinicians may not be familiar with the technical details of this approach. Similar principles apply to aspiration of joints other than the knee.

Data Acquired A wide array of tests on synovial fluid is available. Routine tests on effusions of unknown etiology include: cell count, glucose, Gram stain and routine culture, and microscopic examination for crystals (urate, calcium, pyrophosphate dihydrate). Optional tests include: viscosity, mucin clot test, uric acid level, and culture for *Neisseria gonorrhoeae*, tuberculosis, fungi, *Mycoplasma pneumoniae*, nontuberculous, acid-fast bacteria, etc. Occasionally, ordered tests include: synovial fluid protein, LDH, cytology, rheumatoid factor, complement.

Specimen Synovial fluid

Container For small fluid volumes, send capped syringe without needle to laboratory; otherwise, fluid may be carefully transferred to sterile tubes.

Collection Tube 1: Gram stain and culture; tube 2: mucin clot, if ordered (no heparin); tube 3: (add heparin or EDTA) cell count, chemistries, crystals, additional studies. If gonococcal arthritis is suspected, chocolate (Thayer-Martin) agar should be available either at the bedside or during specimen processing in the Microbiology laboratory.

(Continued)

LABORATORY DIAGNOSIS

Arthrocentesis *(Continued)*

Storage Instructions Specimen should be hand carried to the laboratory. Delay in processing may cause spuriously low synovial fluid glucose levels or false-negative results.

Reference Range In the absence of disease, synovial fluid usually cannot be aspirated. Normal synovial fluid is clear and viscous. A drop placed between the thumb and forefinger (or two microscope slides) can form a string >2 cm long as the fingers are separated, indicating high viscosity. Similarly, the mucin clot test is performed by adding 1 mL of synovial fluid to a 5% solution of acetic acid. Normally, a firm clot forms. Both tests reflect high viscosity of synovial fluid caused by leukocyte hyaluronic acid. Cell count and differential normally reveal <200 WBCs/mm^3 with <25% neutrophils. Chemistries show protein <2 g/dL, uric acid <8 mg/dL, synovial glucose nearly equal to serum glucose, and synovial LDH less than serum LDH. Gram stain and cultures are negative (acellular).

Critical Values Abnormal synovial fluid can be divided into four diagnostic categories. Considerable overlap exists among these categories and correlation with the clinical presentation is required.

Group I synovial fluids are seen commonly in degenerative joint disease (osteoarthritis) and trauma. Fluid is clear or yellow tinged, viscous and mucin clot firm. WBC count is <200/mm^3 with <25% neutrophils (often mononuclears >50%). Chemistries including glucose are normal and microbiologic cultures are negative. This is considered a "noninflammatory" effusion. Some inflammatory conditions may at times cause a group I fluid, such as acute rheumatic fever and systemic lupus erythematosus.

Group II fluids are "inflammatory" in nature. Diseases leading to this category include: crystal-induced arthropathies (gout, CPPD or "pseudogout"), rheumatoid arthritis, connective tissue diseases (SLE, polymyositis, etc), ankylosing spondylitis and other seronegative spondyloarthropathies (Reiter's syndrome, psoriatic arthritis), and acute rheumatic fever. Synovial fluid appears opaque and turbid from cellular fragmentation. Viscosity is similar to water and the "string test" yields only short strings. Mucin clot testing results in a friable gel rather than a tight, rope-like clot. WBC counts are elevated, 5000 to 75,000/mm^3 with >50% neutrophils. Synovial glucose tends to be lower than serum glucose, especially if synovial WBCs are elevated (neutrophils consume glucose). Gram stain and cultures are negative.

Group III effusions are characteristic of septic arthritis. Fluid appears grossly turbid and may be frankly purulent. WBC count as a rule is >50,000/mm^3 and may be >1,000,000/mm^3. Differential shows preponderance of neutrophils (>90%), with the exception of tuberculous arthritis where lymphocytes may comprise 50% of leukocytes. Synovial glucose is characteristically <50% of simultaneous serum glucose and this finding strongly suggests septic arthritis. Glucose values <10 mg/dL have been reported and support classification into group III (rather than group II) in cases where WBC count is moderately elevated. However, sensitivity of low glucose levels in the septic joint is approximately 50%. Gram stain yield in group III effusions varies with the bacteria isolated. In patients with staphylococcal septic arthritis, the Gram stain is diagnostic in 75% of cases in patients with gram-negative arthritis, 50% of Gram stains are diagnostic, but with gonococcal arthritis, only 25% of Gram stains are positive. In nongonococcal septic arthritis, the bacterial culture is more helpful than the Gram stain, the former being positive in 85% to 95% of cases (provided no recent antibiotic use). However, with gonococcal arthritis, the culture is less sensitive, with only a 25% positive yield.

Group IV synovial effusions are grossly hemorrhagic. Etiologies include: systemic abnormalities (eg, excessive heparin anticoagulation, severe thrombocytopenia) and local joint pathology (eg, femur fracture, neuropathic joint).

As mentioned earlier, diagnostic groups are not mutually exclusive. Certain disease entities may fall into more than one diagnostic category. For example, synovial fluid in acute rheumatic fever may appear as either a group I or a group II effusion; neuropathic arthropathy may appear as group I or IV, and lupus-associated effusions as group I or II. In addition, an individual patient may suffer from more than one pathologic process over the course of time. For example, a joint effusion from rheumatoid arthritis (group II effusion) maybe a predisposing factor to the later development of bacterial arthritis (group III) and both may be present in the same patient. Finally, some diseases may change from one diagnostic category to another over a short time period. For example, septic arthritis in an early stage may present with a low synovial WBC count and normal glucose (group I) and only later on progress to a typical septic arthritis (group III) picture on subsequent arthrocentesis.

Use Diagnostic indications include:
- joint effusions of unknown etiology
- arthritis of unclear etiology
- all cases of suspected infectious arthritis (bacterial, fungal, tuberculous)
- confirmation of a diagnosis strongly suspected on clinical grounds, such as suspected gout in patients with podagra
- monitoring synovial fluid response to antibiotic therapy in established cases of septic arthritis

Therapeutic indications include:
- decompression of a tense, painful joint effusion
- evacuation of pus in bacterial arthritis (repeated closed drainage)
- removal of inflammatory cells and crystals in selected cases of gout or pseudogout
- intra-articular injection of corticosteroids

Contraindications
- local infection along the proposed needle entrance tract (eg, overlying cellulitis, periarticular infection)
- uncooperative patient, especially if unable to keep the joint immobile throughout procedure
- difficulty identifying boney landmarks
- a poorly accessible joint space, as in hip aspiration in the obese patient
- inability to demonstrate a joint effusion on physical examination, except when septic arthritis is strongly suspected (and effusions may be barely detectable)

In addition, some authors consider bacteremia (documented or suspected) a contraindication to arthrocentesis based on the theoretical concern of seeding a sterile joint when the entering needle ruptures surrounding capillaries. No data is available to support or refute this and clinical judgment must be individualized in each case. If infectious arthritis is suspected, arthrocentesis should be promptly performed even with documented bacteremia. However, more elective indications for the procedure, such as corticosteroid injection, should be deferred, at physician's discretion.

Additional Information Arthrocentesis is indispensable for the accurate diagnosis (or exclusion) of septic arthritis and crystal-induced arthropathy and therein lies its greatest utility. Despite the difficulties with the classification scheme described above, synovial fluid findings in both these treatable conditions is often pathognomonic. Practically, the procedure carries a low risk of complications and can be performed in minutes when an accessible joint is involved. The general physician often handles aspirations of the knee, elbow, and first metatarsal phalangeal joint. When septic arthritis is suspected in a less accessible area, such as the sacroiliac joint, aspiration should not be delayed due to a lack of familiarity. Rheumatologic or orthopedic consultation should be obtained.

Selected Readings
Gatter RA, "Arthrocentesis Technique and Intrasynovial Therapy," *Arthritis and Allied Conditions: A Textbook of Rheumatology*, 11th ed, Chapter 39, McCarty DJ, ed, Philadelphia, PA: Lea & Febiger, 1989.

Rodnan GP and Schumacher HR, "Examination of Synovial Fluid," *Primer on the Rheumatic Diseases*, 8th ed, Chapter 90, Atlanta, GA: Arthritis Foundation, 1983.

Simon RR and Brenner BE, "Orthopedic Procedures," *Emergency Medicine Procedures and Techniques*, 2nd ed, Chapter 7, Baltimore, MD: Williams & Wilkins, 1987, 192-243.

Arthrogram

Synonyms Joint Study

Applies To Ankle Arthrogram; Elbow Arthrogram; Hip Arthrogram; Knee Arthrogram; Shoulder Arthrogram; Temporomandibular Joint Arthrogram; Wrist Arthrogram

Patient Preparation Informed consent is obtained

Aftercare No strenuous activity involving the joint of interest for 24 hours.

Equipment 22-gauge needle, contrast medium, and fluoroscopic and x-ray equipment

Technique Local anesthesia is instilled at the appropriate site. A small gauge needle is inserted into the joint space. Any fluid within the joint space is aspirated and sent for appropriate chemical or bacteriologic analysis. Contrast medium and air are then inserted into the joint space under fluoroscopic guid-

(Continued)

Arthrogram *(Continued)*

ance. Radiographs and occasionally tomograms are then obtained in multiple projections.

Data Acquired Visualization of the components of the joint space including the cartilage, ligaments, menisci, and connecting bursa

Reference Range The joint space should not contain fluid. The cartilaginous surfaces and menisci should be smooth without evidence for erosions, tears, or disintegration.

Use Evaluation of any damage to the cartilage, ligaments, and bony structures composing the joint

Limitations Large joint effusions can be difficult to aspirate completely, thus resulting in dilution of the contrast material and poor visualization of the joint space structures.

Contraindications Bleeding abnormalities

Selected Readings

Resnick D, "Arthrography, Tenography and Bursography," *Diagnosis of Bone and Joint Disorders*, 2nd ed, Resnick D and Niwayama G, eds, Philadelphia, PA: WB Saunders Co, 1988, 302-444.

Arthropod Identification

Synonyms Ectoparasite Identification; Insect Identification

Applies To Bed Bugs Identification; Body Lice Identification; *Cimex* Identification; Crab Lice Identification; Deer Tick Identification; Flea Identification; Head Lice Identification; *Ixodes dammini* Identification; Lice Identification; Mite Identification; Nits Identification; *Pediculus humanus* Identification; *Phthirus pubis* Identification; Pubic Lice Identification; *Sarcoptes scabiei* Skin Scrapings Identification; Skin Scrapings for *Sarcoptes scabiei* Identification; Tick Identification

Specimen Gross arthropod, skin scrapings

Container Screw cap tube or screw cap jar

Collection Arthropods (gross) are to be submitted in alcohol (70%) or formaldehyde in tube or container with secure closure. To establish the diagnosis of scabies, skin scrapings may be collected with a scalpel and a drop of mineral oil. The liquid may be examined directly or alternatively the organism may be teased away from its burrow or papule with a needle or scalpel.

Storage Instructions Room temperature, fill the container with preservative as completely as possible to avoid damage to the specimen by air bubbles in the container

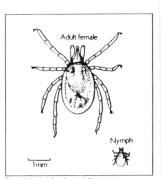

Deer tick *(Ixodes dammini)*

Turnaround Time 1-2 hours; if referral to a state or federal laboratory is required, 2-4 weeks

Reference Range No arthropod identified

Use Identify arthropods affecting humans; establish the presence of ectoparasite infestation

Methodology Macroscopic evaluation

Selected Readings

Hobbs GD and Harrell RE Jr, "Brown Recluse Spider Bites: A Common Cause of Necrotic Arachnidism," *Am J Emerg Med*, 1989, 7(3):309-12.

Nelson JA and Bouseman JK, "Human Tick-Borne Illnesses: United States," *Clin Microbiol Newslett*, 1992, 14(14):105-12.

Pratt HD and Smith JW, "Arthropods of Medical Importance," *Manual of Clinical Microbiology*, 5th ed, Balows A, Hausler WJ Jr, Herrmann KL, et al, eds, Washington, DC: American Society for Microbiology, 1991, 796-810.

Ascites Fluid Tap *see* Paracentesis *on page 420*

Ascitic Fluid Culture *see* Aerobic Culture, Body Fluid *on page 244*

Ascitic Fluid Cytology *see* Cytology, Body Fluids *on page 318*

Ascitic Fluid Fungus Culture *see* Fungus Culture, Body Fluid
on page 341

ASO *see* Antistreptolysin O Titer, Serum *on page 263*

***Aspergillus* Immunodiffusion** *see* Fungal Serology *on page 337*

Aspirates for Ova and Parasites *see* Ova and Parasites, Urine or
Aspirates *on page 419*

Atypical *Mycobacterium* Smear *see* Acid-Fast Stain
on page 239

Auramine-Rhodamine Stain *see* Acid-Fast Stain *on page 239*

Bacterial Antigens by Coagglutination *replaced by* Bacterial Antigens,
Rapid Detection Methods *on this page*

Bacterial Antigens by Counterimmunoelectrophoresis *replaced by*
Bacterial Antigens, Rapid Detection Methods *on this page*

Bacterial Antigens, Rapid Detection Methods
Related Information
Group A *Streptococcus* Antigen Test *on page 354*
Group B *Streptococcus* Antigen Test *on page 354*
Synonyms Cerebrospinal Fluid Latex Agglutination for Bacterial Antigens; Latex
Agglutination, Bacterial Antigens, Cerebrospinal Fluid
Replaces Bacterial Antigens by Coagglutination; Bacterial Antigens by Counter-
immunoelectrophoresis
Test Includes Qualitative determination of the presence of antigens of *H. in-
fluenzae*, *S. pneumoniae*, *N. meningitidis*. Test may also identify subgroups of
above organisms and may include testing for group B *Streptococcus* and *E.
coli* K1 antigen in neonates. Gram stain and culture are preferable to bacterial
antigen testing, and results of Gram stain must be coordinated with antigen
testing by knowledgeable laboratory workers.
Abstract Rapid adjunctive tests include latex agglutination, which is more sensitive than coagglutination. False-negative results occur. *Clinical Microbiology
Procedures Handbook* (Isenberg HD, ed) indicates that **these latex agglutination tests are not intended as a substitute for bacterial culture. Confirmatory diagnosis of bacterial meningitis infection is possible only with
appropriate culture procedures.** Similar observations are published by others as well. Concentration of antigen depends on variables including the number of bacteria, the duration of infection, and the presence or absence of specific antibodies which may prevent antigen detection. Several publications recognize these tests' shortcomings and describe the rapid diagnostic tests as
not essential but note that they may be helpful in establishing an etiologic diagnosis rapidly.
Patient Preparation Usual aseptic aspiration
Specimen Cerebrospinal fluid, serum, urine
Container Sterile CSF tube, red top tube, sterile urine container
Storage Instructions Keep refrigerated
Reference Range Negative
Use Detect bacterial antigens in CSF for the rapid diagnosis of meningitis. The
method may be applied to other body fluids, blood culture supernatants, and
urine (depending on the body fluid tested and the test used).
Limitations May be negative in early meningitis. **Does not replace Gram stain
and culture.** Group B *Streptococcus* and the *E. coli* K1 antigen are frequently
not tested on infants over 6 months of age. The sensitivity of the tests vary
from 55% to 100% depending on the specificity of the antibody and the concentration of antigen in the specimen. Nonspecific cross reactions occur.
False-positive reactions and nonspecific agglutination occur. Antigenic cross-
over (cross reactions) are seen, eg, *E. coli* K1 and *N. meningitidis* group B. The
sensitivity of commercial antigen detection kits remains imperfect, the sensitivity differing substantially with various organisms and in various clinical series. False-negative results occur, especially those taken early in the disease,
with low antigen load. Pneumococcal and *Haemophilus* strains not possessing
capsular antigens may not be detected by immunological techniques. Pneumococcal antigen is not detected in urine.

Many authors have stated that these tests are expensive and have, usually, no
impact on patient care. Physicians are urged to order only Gram stain and culture. These tests can be used later if stain and culture results are negative.
Counterimmunoelectrophoresis is no longer in common clinical use.
(Continued)

Bacterial Antigens, Rapid Detection Methods
(Continued)

Methodology Latex agglutination and coagglutination

Additional Information Antigen detection methods should never be substituted for culture and Gram stain. Culture and Gram stain must always have priority when only very limited quantities of CSF are available.

The rapid diagnosis of group A and group B *Streptococcus* infection is discussed specifically in Group A *Streptococcus* Screen and Group B *Streptococcus* Screen test listings.

Selected Readings

Gray LD and Fedorko DP, "Laboratory Diagnosis of Bacterial Meningitis," *Clin Microbiol Rev*, 1992, 5(2):130-45.

Greenlee JE, "Approach to Diagnosis of Meningitis – Cerebrospinal Fluid Evaluation," *Infect Dis Clin North Am*, 1990, 4(4):583-98.

Isenberg HD, "Bacterial Antigen Detection by Latex Agglutination," *Clinical Microbiology Procedures Handbook*, Washington DC: American Society for Microbiology, 1992, 2:9.2.-9.2.4.

Rodewald LE, Woodin KA, Szilágyi PG, et al, "Relevance of Common Tests of Cerebrospinal Fluid in Screening for Bacterial Meningitis," *J Pediatr*, 1991, 119(3):363-9.

Smith AL, "Bacterial Meningitis," *Pediatr Rev*, 1993, 14(1):11-8.

Bacterial Inhibitory Level, Serum *see* Serum Bactericidal Test *on page 441*

Bacterial Smear *see* Gram Stain *on page 352*

Bacteria Screen, Urine *see* Leukocyte Esterase, Urine *on page 386*

Bacteria Screen, Urine *see* Nitrite, Urine *on page 414*

Basement Membrane Antibodies *see* Skin Biopsy, Immunofluorescence *on page 446*

Bed Bugs Identification *see* Arthropod Identification *on page 268*

Beta-Hemolytic Strep Culture, Throat *see* Throat Culture for Group A Beta-Hemolytic *Streptococcus* *on page 457*

Beta-Lactamase Production Test *see* Penicillinase Test *on page 427*

Beta-Lactam Ring *see* Penicillinase Test *on page 427*

Biopsy Culture, Aerobic *see* Biopsy Culture, Routine *on this page*

Biopsy Culture, Anaerobic *see* Anaerobic Culture *on page 250*

Biopsy Culture, Fungus *see* Fungus Culture, Biopsy *on page 340*

Biopsy Culture, Routine
Related Information

Anaerobic Culture *on page 250*

Applies To Aerobic Culture, Tissue; Biopsy Culture, Aerobic; *Brucella* Culture, Tissue; Culture, Biopsy; Cyst Culture, Aerobic; Surgical Specimen Culture, Routine; Tissue Culture, *Brucella*; Tissue Culture, Routine

Patient Preparation Aseptic preparation of biopsy site

Special Instructions The following information must be provided to the laboratory and will assist the laboratory in the proper processing of the specimen; specific site of specimen, current antibiotic therapy, age and sex of patient, collection time and date, and clinical diagnosis.

Specimen Surgical tissue, bone marrow, biopsy material from normally sterile site or aseptically aspirated body fluid

Container Sterile container with lid, no preservative. Bone marrow aspirates and body fluids may be directly inoculated into blood culture media.

Collection The portion of the biopsy specimen submitted for culture should be separated from the portion submitted for histopathology by the surgeon or pathologist utilizing sterile technique.

Storage Instructions Transport specimen to the laboratory immediately.

Causes for Rejection Specimen not received in appropriate sterile container, specimen received in preservative, excessive delay in transport. If an unacceptable specimen is received the nursing station will be notified and another specimen will be requested before disposal of the original specimen.

Turnaround Time Preliminary reports are available at 24 hours. Cultures with no growth will be reported after 48 hours. Reports on specimens from which pathogens are isolated require a minimum of 48 hours for completion.

Reference Range No growth

Use Isolate and identify organisms causing infections in tissue

Limitations If anaerobes are suspected submit a properly collected specimen.

Additional Information The specimen should be obtained before empiric antimicrobial therapy is started.

Biopsy *Legionella* Culture *see Legionella pneumophila* Culture *on page 381*

Biopsy of Lung (Transbronchial) for *Pneumocystis* *see Pneumocystis carinii* Test *on page 431*

Blastomycosis Immunodiffusion *see* Fungal Serology *on page 337*

Blind Liver Biopsy *see* Liver Biopsy *on page 387*

Blood Cell Profile *see* Complete Blood Count *on page 302*

Blood Count *see* Complete Blood Count *on page 302*

Blood Culture, Aerobic and Anaerobic

Related Information

Blood Culture, Fungus *on page 275*

Blood Culture, Mycobacteria *on page 276*

Synonyms Aerobic Blood Culture; Anaerobic Blood Culture; Culture, Blood

Applies To Antimicrobial Removal Device (ARD) Blood Culture; ARD, Blood Culture; Blood Culture, Lysis Centrifugation; Blood Culture With Antimicrobial Removal Device (ARD)

Test Includes Isolation of both aerobic and anaerobic bacteria and susceptibility testing on all significant isolates

Patient Preparation The major difficulty in interpretation of blood cultures is contamination by skin flora. This difficulty can be markedly reduced by careful attention to the details of skin preparation and antisepsis prior to collection of the specimen.

After location of the vein by palpation, the venipuncture site should be vigorously scrubbed and cleansed with 70% alcohol (isopropyl or ethyl) and then swabbed in a circular motion concentrically from the center outward using tincture of iodine or a povidone iodine solution. **The iodine should be allowed to dry before the venipuncture is undertaken.** If palpation is required during the venipuncture, the glove covering the palpating finger tip should be disinfected.

In iodine sensitive patients, a double alcohol, green soap, or acetone alcohol preparation may be substituted.

Aftercare Iodine used in the skin preparation should be carefully removed from the skin after venipuncture.

Special Instructions The requisition should state current antibiotic therapy and clinical diagnosis.

Specimen Blood. The yield of positives is not increased by culturing arterial blood even in endocarditis.

Container Bottles of trypticase soy broth or other standard medium, one vented (for aerobes), one unvented (for anaerobes)

Collection A single blood culture is rarely indicated and to be discouraged unless medically necessary. More than four cultures in 24 hours is also not indicated (not necessary). Ideally, 2-3 cultures (1 hour apart) taken over 24 hours is adequate to recover bacteria causing septicemia.

Blood cultures should be drawn prior to initiation of antimicrobial therapy. If more than one culture is ordered at the same time (such should be ordered only in medically urgent situations), the specimens should be drawn from separately prepared sites. A syringe and needle, transfer set or pre-evacuated set of tubes containing culture media may be used to collect blood. Collection tubes should be held below the level of the venipuncture to avoid reflux. A sample volume of 10-20 mL (more is always better) in adults, 1-5 mL in pediatric patients is usually collected for each set.

If a syringe and needle or transfer set is used, the top of the blood culture bottles should also be aseptically prepared with alcohol only. See table on next page.

(Continued)

271

Blood Culture, Aerobic and Anaerobic *(Continued)*

Blood Culture Collection

Clinical Disease Suspected	Culture Recommendation	Rational
Sepsis, meningitis, osteomyelitis, septic arthritis, bacterial pneumonia	Two sets of cultures — one from each of two prepared sites, the second drawn after a brief time interval (1 hour if possible), then begin therapy	Assure sufficient sampling in cases of intermittent or low level bacteremia Minimize the confusion caused by a positive culture resulting from transient bacteremia or skin contamination
Fever of unknown origin, eg, occult abscess, empyema, typhoid fever, etc	Two sets of cultures — one from each of two prepared sites, the second drawn after a brief time interval (1 hour if possible). If cultures are negative after 24–48 hours, obtain two more sets, preferably prior to an anticipated temperature rise.	The additional yield after four sets of cultures is minimal
Endocarditis		
Acute	Obtain three blood culture sets within 2 hours, then begin therapy	95–99% of acute endocarditis patients (untreated) will yield a positive in one of the first three cultures
Subacute	Obtain three blood culture sets on day 1, repeat if negative after 24 hours If still negative or if the patient had prior antibiotic therapy, repeat again	Adequate sample volume despite low level bacteremia or previous therapy should result in a positive yield
Immunocompromised Host: eg, AIDS		
Septicemia, fungemia, mycobacteremia	Obtain two sets of cultures from each of two prepared sites; consider lysis concentration technique to enhance recovery for fungi and mycobacteria	Low levels of fungemia and mycobacteremia frequently encountered
Previous Antimicrobial Therapy		
Septicemia, bacteremia; monitor effect of antimicrobial therapy	Obtain two sets of cultures from each of two prepared sites; consider use of antimicrobial removal device (ARD) or increased volume >10 mL/set	Recovery of organisms is enhanced by dilution, increased sample volume, and removal of inhibiting antimicrobials

Transient bacteremia caused by brushing teeth, bowel movements, etc or by local irritations caused by scratching of the skin, may cause positive blood cultures as can contamination by skin flora at the time of collection. Interpretation of results can be enhanced by collecting blood cultures separated by time intervals (1 hour is acceptable and useful). Cultures should be taken as early as possible in the course of a febrile episode.

Storage Instructions Specimens collected in tubes with SPS (sodium polyanetholesulfonate) should be processed without delay. The specimen should be transferred to appropriate blood culture media **immediately** to avoid any possible decrease in yield due to storage or prolonged contact with SPS.

Causes for Rejection Unlabeled bottles are not acceptable.

Turnaround Time Common laboratory procedure is to issue a final culture report after 5-7 days. A preliminary culture report based upon Gram stain and primary subculture is usually available at 24 hours. Positive blood cultures must be reported immediately by telephone and followed with a written report.

Reference Range Negative

Interpretation of Positive Blood Cultures

> Virtually **any** organism, including normal flora, **can** cause bacteremia.
>
> A negative culture result does not necessarily rule out bacteremia; false–negative results occur when pathogens fail to grow.
>
> A positive culture result does not necessarily indicate bacteremia; false–positive results occur when contaminants grow.
>
> Gram–negative bacilli, anaerobes, and fungi should be considered pathogens until proven otherwise.
>
> The most difficult interpretation problem is to determine whether an organism that is usually considered normal skin flora is a true pathogen.

From Flournoy DJ and Adkins L, "Understanding the Blood Culture Report," *Am J Infect Control,* 1986, 14:41–6, with permission.

Use Isolate and identify potentially pathogenic organisms causing bacteremia, septicemia, meningitis, and other microbiologic states

Limitations Three negative sets of blood cultures in the absence of antimicrobial therapy are usually sufficient to exclude the presence of bacteremia. One set is seldom, if ever, sufficient. Prior antibiotic therapy may cause negative blood cultures or delayed growth. Blood cultures from patients suspected of having *Brucella* or *Leptospira* must be requested as special cultures. Consultation with the laboratory for special culture procedures for the recovery of these organisms prior to collecting the specimen is recommended. See the listings *Leptospira* Culture, and Blood Culture, *Brucella* for the proper method of collection of these specimens. Yeast often are isolated from routine blood cultures. However, if yeast or other fungi are specifically suspected, a separate fungal blood culture should be drawn along with each of the routine blood culture specimens. See separate listing for proper collection of Blood Fungus Culture. *Mycobacterium avium-intracellulare* (MAI) is frequently recovered from blood of immunocompromised patients particularly those with acquired immunodeficiency syndrome, AIDS. Special procedures are required for the recovery of these organisms, ie, lysis filtration concentration or use of a special mycobacteria blood culture medium. Radiometric methods facilitate the recovery of mycobacteria from blood.

Contraindications Use of a 2% iodine preparation is contraindicated in the preparation of patients sensitive to iodine. Green soap may be substituted for the iodine or alcohol acetone alone may be used.

Methodology Early subculture of aerobic bottle; visual, radiometric, or infrared monitoring. Aerobic and anaerobic culture in broth media usually with subculture to blood agar and chocolate agar. In the lysis centrifugation procedure, blood is lysed and centrifuged using a Du Pont Isolator™ tube or similar method. The sediment is divided to media appropriate for growing aerobic and anaerobic bacteria, fungi, and mycobacteria.

Additional Information Sequential blood cultures in nonendocarditis patients and using a 20 mL sample results in an 80% positive yield after the first set, a 90% yield after the second set, and a 99% yield after the third set. **Volume of blood** cultured seems to be more important than the specific culture technique being employed by the laboratory. The isolation of coagulase-negative *Staphylococcus* (CNS) poses a critical and difficult clinical dilemma. Although CNS is the most commonly isolated organism from blood cultures, only a few (6.3%) of the isolates represent "true" clinically significant bacteremia. Conversely, CNS is well recognized as a cause of infections involving prosthetic devices, cardiac valves, CSF shunts, dialysis catheters, and indwelling vascular catheters. Ultimately the physician is responsible for determining whether an organism is a contaminant or a pathogen. The decision is based on both laboratory and clinical data. Frequently this determination includes patient data (ie, patient history), physical examination, body temperatures, clinical course, and laboratory data (ie, culture results, white blood cell count, and differential). Clinical experience and judgment may play a significant role in resolving this clinical dilemma.

The use of a lysis centrifugation system or specific fungal blood culture media have been reported to increase the recovery rate and decrease the time of fun-

(Continued)

Blood Culture, Aerobic and Anaerobic *(Continued)*

gal recovery compared to traditional or biphasic blood culture systems. Recovery of mycobacteria and *Legionella* may also be enhanced by lysis filtration. In patients who have received antimicrobial drugs, four to six blood cultures may be necessary. Any organism isolated from the blood is usually tested for susceptibility. It is not recommended to culture blood while antimicrobials are present unless verification of an agent's efficacy is needed. This is confirmed with a single culture.

The use of antimicrobial removal devices (ARD) or resin bottles to attempt to increase the yield of blood cultures drawn from patients on antimicrobial therapy is controversial. Some microorganisms are occasionally not recovered with the use of ARD blood cultures. It is therefore advised that at least one culture in a series of three be requested without the use of the ARD bottles. ARD blood cultures are substantially more expensive than routine blood cultures. There is no consensus as to the effectiveness of the ARD cultures in enhancing recovery of organisms.

The diagnosis of bacterial meningitis is accomplished by blood culture, as well as culture and examination of the cerebrospinal fluid. Most children with bacterial meningitis are initially bacteremic.

Selected Readings
Aronson MD and Bor DH, "Blood Cultures," *Ann Intern Med*, 1987, 106(2):246-53.

MacLowry JD, "Clinical Microbiology of Bacteremia an Overview," *Am J Med*, 1983, 75(1B):2-6.

Reller BL, Murray PR, and MacLowry JD, "Blood Cultures II," *Cumitech 1A*, Washington, DC: American Society for Microbiology, 1982, (review).

Blood Culture, AIDS *see* Blood Culture, Mycobacteria
on page 276

Blood Culture, *Brucella*

Synonyms *Brucella* Blood Culture; Undulant Fever, Culture

Patient Preparation See preparation procedures under listing for Blood Culture, Aerobic and Anaerobic.

Special Instructions The laboratory must be informed of the request for *Brucella* blood culture. Collection time, date, age of patient, current antibiotic therapy, clinical diagnosis, and relevant history.

Specimen Blood

Container Castañeda bottle; *Brucella* broth and agar; conventional trypticase soy broth (TSB)

Collection Should be drawn prior to administration of antibiotics, and before an expected temperature rise. Follow collection procedure in Blood Culture, Aerobic and Anaerobic.

Causes for Rejection Specimens not received in appropriate bottles will have less than optimal yield.

Turnaround Time 6 weeks

Reference Range No growth

Use Establish the diagnosis of brucellosis

Limitations Blood cultures for *Brucella* are primarily useful in the early acute phase of the disease. Recovery of *Brucella* is limited by the relatively low level of bacteremia and the fastidious nature of the organism. Yield may be increased by culturing larger volumes of blood in a conventional trypticase soy broth or use of a lysis centrifugation concentration technique.

Methodology *Brucella* broth and agar, held at least 21 days with or without lysis concentration. Trypticase soy broth (TSB) cultures yield acceptable results (93% of possible isolates). Blood clot cultures utilizing a variety of methods provide no advantage over more conventional TSB cultures for the isolation of *Brucella melitensis*. The use of a lysis concentration procedure was found to be superior to the use of the Castañeda procedure (biphasic medium) for the recovery of *Brucella* from clinical specimens. *Brucella* may be recovered using the Roche Septi-Chek® system with growth observed on the chocolate section of the paddle. The organism appears as a small slow-growing white colony. It is a gram-negative coccobacillus. **The handling of cultures and specimens as well as the inhalation of dust-containing *Brucella* organisms is dangerous to laboratory workers**. A biologic safety cabinet should be used for all suspected isolates.

Additional Information Bone marrow culture and serologic testing of acute and convalescent specimens for *Brucella* antibodies may be useful when cultures of peripheral blood are negative. In animals, brucellosis has a bacteremic phase followed by localization in the reproductive tract and reticuloendothelial system. The disease is common worldwide, particularly in the countries of the former Soviet Union, Mediterranean, Latin America, and Spain. One hundred and six cases were reported in the U.S. in 1986. Most brucellosis in the U.S. occurs in abattoir workers, farmers and rarely veterinarians. Symptoms may be subclinical, subacute, acute relapsing and chronic. Undulant fever is most typical of *B. melitensis*. Symptoms may include abdominal pain and may mimic appendicitis or cholecystitis. Unpasteurized milk may be a source of infection. Risk factors raising an index of suspicion include travel, food, and occupation. Serologic confirmation of the diagnosis may be helpful.

Selected Readings

Etemadi H, Raissadt A, Pickett MJ, et al, "Isolation of *Brucella* spp. From Clinical Specimens," *J Clin Microbiol*, 1984, 20(3):586.

Finegold SM and Baron EJ, *Bailey and Scott's Diagnostic Microbiology*, 7th ed, St Louis, MO: CV Mosby Co, 1986, 440-3.

Moyer NP, Holcomb LA, and Hausler WJ Jr, "*Brucella*," *Manual of Clinical Microbiology*, 5th ed, Balows A, Hausler WJ Jr, Herrmann KL, et al, eds, Washington, DC: American Society for Microbiology, 1991, 457-62.

Blood Culture for CMV *see* Cytomegalovirus Culture, Blood *on page 320*

Blood Culture, Fungus

Related Information

Blood Culture, Aerobic and Anaerobic *on page 271*

Synonyms Fungus Blood Culture; Fungus Culture, Blood

Test Includes Routine blood culture and inoculation of specific fungal media at time of collection; identification of any fungi isolated

Patient Preparation See Blood Culture, Aerobic and Anaerobic.

Special Instructions Inform the laboratory of the specific request for fungus blood culture. The following information will assist the laboratory in the proper processing of the specimen: specific site of specimen, current antibiotic therapy, age and sex of patient, collection time and date, and clinical diagnosis.

Specimen Blood

Container Routine and special fungal blood culture media

Collection Standard blood culture collection procedures.

Storage Instructions Transport specimen to the laboratory immediately.

Turnaround Time Preliminary reports are usually available in one to two days. Negative cultures are commonly reported at 4-6 weeks.

Reference Range No fungi grown

Use Isolate and identify fungi; establish the diagnosis of fungemia, fungal endocarditis, and disseminated mycosis in immunocompromised patients, oncology patients, transplant patients, patients with leukemia and lymphoma, and patients with the acquired immunodeficiency syndrome (AIDS)

Limitations A single negative culture does not rule out the presence of fungal infection. Fungal blood cultures are most effective in isolating *Candida albicans* and *Candida glabrata* (*Torulopsis glabrata*). If other fungal species are suspected, a biopsy or bone marrow fungus culture should be considered. *Blastomyces dermatitidis* usually is not recovered from blood.

Additional Information Fungemia may complicate therapy with steroids, antineoplastic drugs, radiation therapy, broad spectrum antibiotic therapy, venous or arterial catheterization, hyperalimentation, and the acquired immunodeficiency syndrome (AIDS). Intravenous drug abusers are prone to *Candida* endocarditis. Although many fungal species including *Histoplasma capsulatum*, *Coccidioides immitis*, *Cryptococcus neoformans*, and many other unusual isolates are recoverable from blood cultures, the most common cause of fungemia is *Candida albicans* followed by other *Candida* sp including *Candida glabrata* (*Torulopsis glabrata*). In most cases fungemia represents a failure of the host defense system. Fungemia may be caused by contamination of an indwelling catheter or, in the critically ill and immunocompromised patient, contamination of the gastrointestinal and less frequently the urinary tract.

Blood Culture, *Leptospira* *see* Leptospira Culture *on page 384*

Blood Culture, Lysis Centrifugation *see* Blood Culture, Aerobic and Anaerobic *on page 271*

Blood Culture, Mycobacteria
Related Information
Blood Culture, Aerobic and Anaerobic *on page 271*
Applies To AIDS Blood Culture; Blood Culture, AIDS
Patient Preparation Usual sterile preparation
Special Instructions Request test specifically. Not part of routine blood culture. Contact the laboratory prior to collecting blood.
Specimen Blood
Container Aerobic blood culture bottle
Storage Instructions Incubate if unable to deliver to the laboratory on the day of collection.
Causes for Rejection Other bacteria present
Use Isolate mycobacteria, especially *M. avium-intracellulare*
Additional Information Mycobacterial usually are identified to genus and species, and susceptibility tests will be done usually without special request. Contact the laboratory for details and special collection instructions.

Blood Culture With Antimicrobial Removal Device (ARD) *see* Blood Culture, Aerobic and Anaerobic *on page 271*

Blood Smear for Malarial Parasites *see* Peripheral Blood Smear, Thick and Thin *on page 429*

Blood Smear for Trypanosomal/Filarial Parasites *see* Microfilariae, Peripheral Blood Preparation *on page 400*

Body Cavity Fluid Cytology *see* Cytology, Body Fluids *on page 318*

Body Fluid Anaerobic Culture *see* Anaerobic Culture *on page 250*

Body Fluid Culture, Routine *see* Aerobic Culture, Body Fluid *on page 244*

Body Fluid Fungus Culture *see* Fungus Culture, Body Fluid *on page 341*

Body Lice Identification *see* Arthropod Identification *on page 268*

Body Surface Areas of Adults and Children *see page 700*

Bone Biopsy
Applies To Percutaneous Biopsy of Musculoskeletal Lesions and Synovial Membranes
Test Includes This procedure involves the passage of a needle, either under fluoroscopic or computed tomographic guidance, into an area of bony abnormality to facilitate precise histologic and/or bacteriologic diagnosis. In many clinical situations, this procedure can establish definitive diagnosis without the disadvantages of surgery making it a useful alternative to open biopsy. In selected cases of arthritis, examination of the synovium may provide precise diagnostic clues or useful information about the nature of the arthritic process. A biopsy of the synovium can be performed through an open arthrotomy, percutaneous biopsy, or as part of an arthroscopic procedure during which the synovium can be visualized.
Patient Preparation Biopsies are performed in the Radiology Department. Skeletal biopsies are usually done under local anesthesia, with the exception of children and restless patients who are placed under general anesthesia or heavy sedation. Local anesthesia facilitates communication between the patient and the physician performing the procedure. Should the patient complain of radiating pain, the needle can be repositioned. Spinal biopsies necessitate a 24-hour hospitalization. Other anatomic areas may be biopsied on an outpatient basis. The patient should not eat on the morning of the examination. An intravenous catheter is generally placed for I.V. access and the patient is usually administered both a sedative and a medication for pain.
Specimen There are a wide variety of commercially available needles for these procedures. A needle aspiration biopsy consists of aspiration of fluid for cytologic and/or bacteriologic analysis. A core biopsy, however, requires a larger needle and allows retrieval of a core of tissue for histopathologic interpretation.
Use The need for a tissue or bacteriologic diagnosis in situations where it is desirable to forego open biopsy
Selected Readings
Bard M and Laredo JD, *Interventional Radiology in Bone and Joint*, New York, NY: Springer-Verlag Wien, 1988.

LABORATORY DIAGNOSIS

Bone Films

Applies To Acromioclavicular Joint, Left or Right, X-ray; Ankle, Left or Right, X-ray; Arthritis Series, X-ray; Calcaneus (heel), Left or Right, X-ray; Clavicle, Left or Right, X-ray; Elbow, Left or Right, X-ray; Femur, Left or Right, X-ray; Finger, Left or Right Hand, X-ray; Foot, Left or Right, X-ray; Forearm, Left or Right, X-ray; Hand, Left or Right, X-ray; Hands and Wrist Arthritis, X-ray; Hip, Left or Right, and Pelvis, X-ray; Hip, Left or Right, X-ray; Hips Arthritis, X-ray; Humerus, Left or Right, X-ray; Knee, Left or Right, X-ray; Knees Arthritis, X-ray; Patella of Knee, Left or Right, X-ray; Pelvis AP, X-ray; Pelvis Stereo, X-ray; Postreduction Films, X-ray; Scanogram, X-ray; Scapula, Left or Right, X-ray; Shoulder, Left or Right, X-ray; Shoulder Stereo, Left or Right, X-ray; Shoulder to Include Axial View, Left or Right, X-ray; Shoulders Arthritis, X-ray; Sternoclavicular Joint, Left or Right, X-ray; Thumb, Left or Right, X-ray; Tibia and Fibula, Left or Right, X-ray; Toes of Foot, Left or Right, X-ray; Wrist, Left or Right, X-ray

Test Includes Upper extremity and shoulder girdle: fingers, thumb, hands, wrists, wrists for carpal tunnel, wrists for navicular views, PA hands and wrists for arthritis, forearm, elbow, humerus, scapula, shoulder for trauma, shoulder for inflammatory process, shoulder to include axial view, clavicle, nonweight bearing and weight bearing views of acromioclavicular joints, bilateral comparison sternoclavicular joints, and postreduction films.

Lower extremity and pelvis: AP pelvis, stereo pelvis, pelvis and hips, hips for congenital deformity, hips for arthritis, femur, knee, weight bearing, knees for arthritis, knees with patellar views, knees with tunnel views, tibia-fibula, ankles, ankles with stress views, calcaneus, feet, toes.

Bony thorax: ribs, unilateral or bilateral, sternum.

Patient Preparation The parts under scrutiny should bear the lightest possible dressing. Patient must wear x-ray gown to department.

Special Instructions Requisition must state: if safe for patient to sit, stand, and move extremities. If questions of liability or compensation are known to exist in the case. If there is a question of fracture, how long ago injury occurred, and any previous fractures. In case of foreign bodies, state their nature since many are not visible on x-ray examination. If dressings, bivalved casts, and splints may be removed. If "wet reading" is desired. By appointment, call appropriate number. Send completed and signed requisition to Radiology. Comparison views on request. Specify right or left.

Use Evaluate bones for the presence of metastatic and primary neoplasms, trauma, infectious disease, degenerative and reactive processes

Limitations Metal appliances, casts and dressings containing aluminum paste, lead water, or Epsom salts obscure or obliterate all detail

Methodology The affected body part will be moved, if possible, into two or three different positions so films can be obtained.

Bone Marrow *see* Bone Marrow Aspiration and Biopsy
on this page

Bone Marrow Aspiration and Biopsy

Applies To Bone Marrow; Bone Marrow Iron Stain; Bone Marrow Sampling; Bone Marrow Trephine Biopsy; Iron Stain

Test Includes Aspiration and/or biopsy of bone marrow (BM) for microscopic analysis. Both procedures are carried out under local anesthesia at the patient's bedside. For aspiration, a specialized hollow needle is advanced into the intramedullary cavity (usually iliac crest). Approximately 0.4 mL liquid marrow and bone fragments are aspirated into a syringe, then smeared onto a slide. Frequently, a bone marrow biopsy is performed as a complementary, but separate, procedure (different equipment and site). A specialized biopsy needle (eg, Jamshidi needle) is used to obtain a core of solid cortical bone. This technique preserves the normal marrow architecture of the biopsy sample and allows for formal for histologic analysis.

Patient Preparation Technique and risks of the procedure are explained to the patient and consent is obtained. Considerable patient apprehension often accompanies this procedure and requires thorough, step-by-step explanation beforehand. If coagulopathy is known or suspected, a recent CBC and PT/PTT should be drawn. Requisition must state in advance any special studies to be performed on specimen, such as AFB stain, Congo red stain for amyloid, cytogenetics studies, etc. Contact referring physician if any questions arise or contact appropriate laboratories directly. Patients are commonly premedicated with a short-acting benzodiazepine or analgesic such as meperidine.

(Continued)
277

Bone Marrow Aspiration and Biopsy *(Continued)*

Aftercare Needle puncture site(s) are covered with a dry sterile dressing. If the bone marrow biopsy is performed from the posterior iliac crest, patient must lie on back for a full 30 minutes before being discharged. In the presence of a low-grade coagulopathy or mild thrombocytopenia, direct pressure should be applied by operator (not patient) to puncture sites until local bleeding ceases. Instruct patient to keep dressings dry. Ideally, puncture sites should be examined approximately 24 hours later by nurse or physician, but this is not always feasible.

Special Instructions This procedure requires at least two operators. The first obtains the aspiration and/or biopsy specimen in a sterile fashion (usually a physician or specialized nurse clinician) and the second immediately examines and prepares the specimen (usually a nurse or technologist from the Hematology Laboratory).

Complications Bone marrow sampling is considered a relatively safe but invasive procedure. Minor complications include local bleeding, hematoma, and discomfort at the needle puncture site. Local infection is rarely seen if proper aftercare is followed. Major complications have been reported with sternal biopsy (Bahir 1963), including fatal puncture of mediastinal structures. Historical reports of fistula formation, osteomyelitis, and profuse bleeding were associated with biopsy of what are now considered nonstandard sites, such as the tibia. Minimal complications are associated with sampling of the iliac crest, the preferred site.

Equipment Commercially assembled trays for aspiration and biopsy are widely available. These prepackaged kits typically contain a bone marrow biopsy needle (usually Jamshidi needle), aspiration needle (usually Illinois needle), various syringes (5 mL, 10 mL, 20 mL), assorted needles (18-gauge, 25-gauge), and 1% lidocaine with epinephrine for local anesthesia. Also included are gauze, sterile gloves, drapes and towels, No 11 scalpel blade, and alcohol and iodine prep. The Jamshidi needle is a large-bore (usually 11-gauge), hollow needle with a tapered tip, thin metal stylet, and wide plastic grip to allow easy needle rotation. The Illinois needle is somewhat smaller, but likewise comes with a stylet and plastic sheath for improved grip. Smaller gauge needles are available for use in the pediatric population.

Technique The procedure is performed by experienced operators only. May be carried out at the bedside if adequate lighting is available, otherwise done in a procedure room.

Aspiration: Preferred site is the posterior superior iliac spine (PSIS), alternatively the sternum. Patient is placed on his side or lies prone. Landmarks are identified by palpation – the PSIS primarily, but the anterior superior iliac spine also. A wide circular area (approximately 5" in diameter) overlying the PSIS is prepped with povidone-iodine in the usual sterile fashion. Using the 25-gauge needle and lidocaine, the skin directly over the PSIS is anesthetized. Following this, deeper structures are liberally anesthetized with the 18-gauge needle, including a several centimeter area of the periosteum. A 4 mm long skin incision is made over the PSIS by means of the No 11 scalpel blade, then extended deeper through fatty tissues down to the anesthetized periosteum. The Illinois aspiration needle (with stylet in place) is advanced through this soft tissue incision and firmly into the cortex of the PSIS, using a constant rotary motion of the needle ("drilling"). Once the needle has penetrated approximately 1 cm into the marrow cavity, the stylet is removed and a 10 mL syringe is attached to the open (distal) end of the aspiration needle. At least 4-5 mL marrow is aspirated using firm suction. This volume is adequate for most routine hematologic studies, but larger volumes are usually needed for fungal or tuberculous cultures, cytogenetics, cell markers, etc. This step often causes the most patient discomfort. After aspiration, the syringe is detached and immediately handed over to the technologist in order to prevent the specimen from clotting (aspiration needle is still in the PSIS). The technologist examines the specimen grossly for marrow particles, which may be visible to the naked eye. If present, this signifies that an adequate marrow specimen has likely been obtained; if absent, the aspiration needle is redirected slightly and the previous listed steps repeated. After completion, the needle is removed and direct pressure applied.

Biopsy: May be carried out immediately following aspiration, while patient is still under local anesthesia. Preferred site is again the PSIS; however, unlike bone marrow aspiration, biopsy is never obtained from the sternum. A Jamshidi biopsy needle is passed through the same skin and soft tissue incision used for aspiration (alternatively, a completely new site may be used). However, a separate hole in the PSIS must be made. Once into the cortical bone, the needle is advanced using a pronounced clockwise/counterclockwise rotary motion. The needle is oriented along an imaginary line connecting the PSIS and the anterior superior iliac spine, forcing a slight angle of the needle with respect to the skin. The needle should **not** be advanced perpendicular to the skin; this results in poor quality biopsies (often with mostly cartilage). The stylet is then removed. The "drilling" is continued until the needle is at least 2 cm deep into the cortex. This may be estimated by periodically replacing the stylet into the needle and noting the distance the stylet protrudes. The biopsy core is subsequently "sheared off" by the following maneuvers:

- needle is rotated a full 10 turns clockwise then 10 turns counterclockwise
- needle is withdrawn slightly and redirected at a different angle
- needle is readvanced
- steps 1-3 are repeated (until the core is sheared off). The needle is withdrawn, again using rotary motions so as not to lose the core. The blunt obturator or "push wire" is passed through the sharp tip of the Jamshidi needle and the specimen pushed gently out of the needle base and onto a sterile gauze. The technologist immediately makes imprints of the core then places the specimen in fixative.

The techniques for aspiration and biopsy outlined are generally agreed upon in major textbooks. However, some clinicians strongly believe that bone marrow biopsy should always **precede** aspiration, despite the "textbook" recommendations. They argue that artifacts in the core biopsy may be induced by aspiration.

Specimen The bone marrow aspirate is immediately examined for visible bone spicules. The presence of these small spicules suggests an adequate specimen. Direct smears of the aspirate fluid are prepared by the technologist at the bedside. These smears consist of marrow particles and free marrow cells spread onto coverslips. This technique helps to preserve the cytologic appearance of individual blood cells. Bone marrow biopsy samples are handled differently. In many institutions, touch preparations are made first, before specimen fixation. The marrow specimen is touched gently to a clean glass slide in several places, without smearing. These "touch preps" are allowed to air-dry and subsequently undergo routine staining. This technique also helps preserve cytologic detail. Once the touch preparations are completed, the remainder of the specimen is placed in a fixative such as formalin or Zenker's solution. The specimen is then processed according to individual laboratory protocol (for example, overnight fixation, decalcification, wash steps, dehydration, and serial sectioning). Routine stains are performed on processed specimens. These include hematoxylin and eosin (H & E), Wright-Giemsa stain, and iron stain. Optional studies may be obtained at physician request such as cytogenetic analysis, flow cytometry, electron microscopy, and amyloid stains. The Hematology Laboratory must be notified in advance for these studies. Bone marrow specimens may also be submitted for microbiological analysis. Cultures may be obtained for aerobic and anaerobic bacteria, fungi (eg, *Histoplasma capsulatum*), acid-fast bacilli (eg, *Mycobacterium tuberculosis* or *Mycobacterium avium-intracellulare*), and viruses (cytomegalovirus). Fixatives should **not** be added to specimens submitted for culture. Again, it is important to notify the Microbiology Laboratory in advance for these cultures.

Reference Range The bone marrow aspirate and biopsy are reviewed by a staff pathologist or hematologist. The preliminary report on the bone marrow aspirate may often be available several hours after the procedure, on request. Normal values for bone marrow cell lines in the adult are as follows:

Granulocytes
- blasts: 0% to 1 %
- promyelocytes: 1% to 5%
- neutrophil myelocytes and metamyelocytes: 7% to 25%
- neutrophil bands and segs: 20% to 60%
- eosinophils: 0% to 3%
- basophils: 0% to 1%
- monocytes: 0% to 2%
- lymphocytes: 5% to 15%
- plasma cells: 0% to 2%

Erythrocytes
- proerythrocytes: 0% to 1%
- early erythrocytes: 1% to 4%
- late erythrocytes: 10% to 20%
- normoblasts: 5% to 10%

(Continued)

Bone Marrow Aspiration and Biopsy (Continued)

The above bone marrow differential cell counts are calculated from the bone marrow aspirate specimen. Other useful data provided by the bone marrow aspirate include:
- myeloid/erythroid ratio (normal ratio 3-4:1)
- total cells counted
- overall cellularity
- erythropoiesis
- granulopoiesis

The bone marrow biopsy provides additional information on marrow architecture (which cannot be obtained from the aspirate). When examining the biopsy specimen, the pathologist may comment on:
- gross description including size of sample
- overall cellularity
- presence of granulomas
- infiltrative marrow processes such as lymphoma, carcinoma, granulomas
- iron stores
- results of special stains

Use Bone marrow sampling is indicated in the evaluation of a wide variety of hematologic disorders, usually noted first on the CBC or peripheral smear. It is also useful in the diagnosis of systemic diseases which may potentially involve the marrow, such as infectious or granulomatous processes. Bone marrow aspiration and biopsy should be considered separate procedures, although indications often overlap. Indications for bone marrow **aspiration** include:
- evaluation of severe anemia, especially when etiology is in doubt and reticulocyte count is low
- evaluation of macrocytic anemia, to confirm the presence of megaloblastic anemia or to exclude sideroblastic anemia and normoblastic erythropoiesis
- leukopenia and/or thrombocytopenia, to differentiate excessive consumption from decreased production
- persistent leukocytosis of unknown etiology
- suspected myelodysplastic syndrome
- suspected leukemia, to confirm diagnosis and to classify subtype (FAB categorization)
- suspected immunoglobulin disorders, such as multiple myeloma, for diagnosis and staging
- evaluation of lipid storage diseases
- evaluation of suspected iron storage abnormalities
- acquisition of marrow for chromosomal analysis
- acquisition of tissue for microbiological culture (fungi, bacteria, mycobacteria, parasites)
- evaluation of response to therapy for hematologic malignancies

Bone marrow biopsy preserves the marrow architecture and is useful in evaluating systemic diseases secondarily involving the marrow. Bone marrow **biopsy** indications include:
- evaluation of pancytopenia
- evaluation of possible myelophthisic anemia (bone marrow infiltrated with leukemic cells, metastatic tumor, lymphoma, granulomas, etc)
- diagnosis and staging of solid tumors or lymphoma
- evaluation of selected cases of fever of unknown origin
- diagnosis of systemic amyloidosis when other methods have failed
- suspected cases of myelofibrosis
- evaluation of myeloproliferative syndromes (polycythemia vera, essential thrombocythemia, etc)
- failed bone marrow aspiration attempts (the so-called "dry tap")

Authorities differ on the exact indications for both bone marrow aspiration and biopsy. Some believe that most hematologic abnormalities are adequately evaluated by bone marrow aspiration alone (without biopsy). Bone marrow biopsy should not be routinely performed with aspiration, it is argued, due to the following reasons:
- diagnosis can often be made by aspiration
- significant patient discomfort accompanies biopsy
- there is needless expense and patient risk

Thus, bone marrow biopsy should only be performed if specific indications are present (as listed).

Other experts routinely include a biopsy whenever aspiration is performed. The following reasons are cited.
- Bone marrow biopsy may be diagnostic in cases where aspiration is negative or equivocal.
- It is nearly impossible to predict in advance which aspiration attempts will be technically difficult.
- Bone marrow biopsy actually causes less discomfort than aspiration in some cases.
- Cost-benefit analysis may favor the combined approach. The cost to physician, technologist, and patient may be doubled if patient is forced to undergo a separate bone marrow biopsy at a later date.

Contraindications
- uncooperative patient
- cellulitis, osteomyelitis, or radiation therapy involving the proposed site of needle entry
- severe, noncorrectable coagulopathy
- thoracic aortic aneurysm if a sternal approach is used
- Paget's disease involving the iliac bone represents a high risk situation, due to excessive bleeding at trephine biopsy site (but not necessarily a contraindication)

Selected Readings

Batjer JP, "Preparation of Optimal Bone Marrow Samples," *Lab Med*, 1979, 10:101-6.

Beckstead JH, "The Bone Marrow Biopsy: A Diagnostic Strategy," *Arch Pathol Lab Med*, 1986, 110(3):175-9.

Brynes RK, McKenna RW, and Sundberg RD, "Bone Marrow Aspiration and Trephine Biopsy: An Approach to a Thorough Study," *Am J Clin Pathol*, 1978, 70(5):753-9.

Williams WJ and Nelson DA, "Examination of the Marrow," *Hematology*, 4th ed, Chapter 3, WJ Williams, E Beutler, AJ Erslev, et al, eds, New York, NY: McGraw-Hill, 1990, 24-31.

Bone Marrow Culture *see* Aerobic Culture, Body Fluid
on page 244

Bone Marrow Culture, Routine

Synonyms Aerobic Bone Marrow Culture; Routine Bone Marrow Culture

Test Includes Culture and Gram stain if requested. Properly collected specimens must also be cultured for anaerobes.

Patient Preparation Usual sterile preparation of aspiration site.

Special Instructions Add 0.1-0.2 mL heparin 10,000 units/mL to sterile tube or Anaport vial

Specimen Bone marrow

Container Sterile tube or Anaport vial containing 0.1-0.2 mL heparin 10,000 units/mL

Collection The specimen will be divided for aerobic, fungus, anaerobic, mycobacteria cultures and smears, volume permitting if accompanied by appropriate requisitions

Storage Instructions Transport specimen to the laboratory immediately. Do not refrigerate.

Causes for Rejection Clots, inadequate volume for studies requested. Specimen will not be discarded without consultation with the attending physician.

Turnaround Time Stat Gram stain: 1 hour. Physician will be notified of all positive smears or cultures. Preliminary results are reported at 24 hours with broth held for 5-7 days.

Reference Range No growth

Use Isolate and identify etiologic agent

Bone Marrow Iron Stain *see* Bone Marrow Aspiration and Biopsy
on page 277

Bone Marrow Mycobacteria Culture *see* Mycobacteria Culture, Biopsy or Body Fluid *on page 404*

Bone Marrow Sampling *see* Bone Marrow Aspiration and Biopsy
on page 277

Bone Marrow Trephine Biopsy *see* Bone Marrow Aspiration and Biopsy *on page 277*

Bone Scan

Synonyms Bone Scintigraphy; Radionuclide Bone Scan; Whole Body Bone Scan

Applies To Bone Scan With Flow; Three-Phase Bone Scan

Test Includes The patient receives an intravenous injection of a technetium-99m (^{99m}Tc) phosphonate radiopharmaceutical which localizes in bone with in-
(Continued)

Bone Scan *(Continued)*

tensity proportional to the degree of metabolic activity present. Three hours after the injection, whole body and appropriate regional skeletal images are acquired. An initial dynamic flow study and/or early images may also be acquired if osteomyelitis, osteonecrosis, Legg-Calvé-Perthes disease, septic arthritis, or other inflammatory disease is suspected (three-phase technique).

Patient Preparation Patient should have all RIA blood work performed, or at least drawn, prior to injection of any radioactive material. The patient does not need to be fasting or NPO for this procedure. Patient should be encouraged to drink fluids during the waiting period before scanning and will be asked to void just before scanning begins.

Special Instructions Requisition must state the current patient diagnosis in order to select the most appropriate radiopharmaceutical and/or imaging technique. When ordering liver and bone scans for the same patient, schedule liver scan at least 1 day before the bone scan. *DURATION OF PROCEDURE:* 3-4.5 hours. This includes a 2-3 hour delay after tracer injection to allow adequate localization in bone. *RADIOPHARMACEUTICAL:* ^{99m}Tc phosphonate compound.

Technique The application of single-photon emission tomography (SPECT) techniques may contribute significantly to the diagnostic accuracy of this imaging study.

Causes for Rejection Other recent Nuclear Medicine procedure may interfere. If uncertain, call the Nuclear Medicine Department.

Turnaround Time A written report will be sent to the patient's chart and/or to the referring physician.

Reference Range Homogeneous and symmetric distribution of activity throughout all skeletal structures

Use Bone imaging is extremely sensitive for the detection of infection or malignancy involving any part of the skeleton. It is the most appropriate screening test for these conditions, since scan abnormalities are present long before structural defects develop radiographically. Bone scans are also accurate for localizing lesions for biopsy, excision, or debridement. Stress fractures can be diagnosed by bone scan when radiographs are completely normal.

Limitations In postoperative orthopedic patients and diabetics, additional imaging with gallium or indium-labeled white blood cells may help to confirm the presence of active infection and serve as a baseline for later comparison

Selected Readings

Datz FL, "Radionuclide Imaging of Joint Inflammation in the 90s," *J Nucl Med*, 1990, 31(5):684-7.

Gupta NC and Prezio JA, "Radionuclide Imaging in Osteomyelitis," *Semin Nucl Med*, 1988, 18(4):287-99.

Jacobson AF, Cronin EB, Stomper PC, et al, "Bone Scans With One or Two Abnormalities in Cancer Patients With No Known Metastases: Frequency and Serial Scintigraphic Behavior of Benign and Malignant Lesions," *Radiology*, 1990, 175(1):229-32.

Lusins JO, Danielski EF, and Goldsmith SJ, "Bone SPECT in Patients With Persistent Back Pain After Lumbar Spine Surgery," *J Nucl Med*, 1989, 30(4):490-6.

Matin P, "Basic Principles of Nuclear Medicine Techniques for Detection and Evaluation of Trauma and Sports Medicine Injuries," *Semin Nucl Med*, 1988, 18(2):90-112.

McDougall IR and Keeling CA, "Complications of Fractures and Their Healing," *Semin Nucl Med*, 1988, 18(2):113-25.

McNeil BJ, "Value of Bone Scanning in Neoplastic Disease," *Semin Nucl Med*, 1985, 14(4):277-86.

Palmer E, Henrikson B, McKusick K, et al, "Pain as an Indicator of Bone Metastasis," *Acta Radiol*, 1988, 29(4):445-9.

Bone Scan With Flow *see* Bone Scan *on previous page*

Bone Scintigraphy *see* Bone Scan *on previous page*

Bordetella pertussis Antibodies *see* *Bordetella pertussis* Serology *on page 284*

Bordetella pertussis Direct Fluorescent Antibody

Related Information

Bordetella pertussis Nasopharyngeal Culture *on next page*
Bordetella pertussis Serology *on page 284*

Synonyms *Bordetella pertussis* Smear; Nasopharyngeal Smear for *Bordetella pertussis*

Replaces Cough Plate Culture for Pertussis

Test Includes Fluorescent antibody stain to detect *Bordetella pertussis* on smear

Patient Preparation Patient must not be on antimicrobial therapy.

Special Instructions Laboratory supervisor should be notified 24 hours before collection of specimen so that a special isolation medium can be prepared.

Specimen Nasopharyngeal swab

Container Nasopharyngeal swab, sterile saline

Collection Swab is passed through nose gently and into nasopharynx. Stay near septum and floor of nose. Rotate and remove. Specimen must be hand transported to the laboratory immediately following collection.

Storage Instructions Do not refrigerate. Transport to the laboratory immediately.

Causes for Rejection Specimen not received in appropriate sterile container or on appropriate isolation medium, specimen more than 2 hours old. Cough plates are unacceptable.

Reference Range No *B. pertussis* detected

Use Detect and identify *B. pertussis* and *B. parapertussis*, establish diagnosis of whooping cough

Limitations Direct detection assays are always limited by the adequacy of the sample. Bacteria may be difficult to detect if there are few bacteria present in the specimen or too much mucoid material.

Contraindications Lack of clinical symptoms of pertussis; previous antibiotic therapy

Methodology Direct fluorescent antibody (DFA)

Additional Information The procedure enables early presumptive identification of *Bordetella pertussis*, the agent of whooping cough. Definitive cultural identification should be completed. There is also available a test for serum agglutinating antibodies, which if present may be titered over time to indicate exposure.

Bordetella pertussis Nasopharyngeal Culture

Related Information

Bordetella pertussis Direct Fluorescent Antibody *on previous page*
Bordetella pertussis Serology *on next page*

Synonyms Nasopharyngeal Culture for *Bordetella pertussis*; Pertussis Culture; Whooping Cough Culture

Replaces Cough Plate Culture for Pertussis; Throat Culture for *Bordetella pertussis*

Test Includes Specific culture and identification of *Bordetella pertussis* and *Bordetella parapertussis*

Patient Preparation Patient should not be on antimicrobial therapy prior to the collection of the specimen.

Special Instructions Consult the laboratory prior to collection of the specimen so that the special isolation medium can be obtained. The laboratory should be made aware of the specific request to screen for *Bordetella pertussis* with information relevant to current antibiotic therapy and current diagnosis.

Specimen Nasopharyngeal swab

Container Flexible calcium alginate swab (Calgiswab®) and Bordet-Gengou plate. Transport medium composed of half strength Oxoid charcoal agar CM19 supplemented with 40 μg/mL cephalexin and 10% hemolyzed defibrinated horse blood may be used.

Collection Shape the flexible swab into the contour of the nares. Pass the swab gently through the nose. Leave swab in place near septum and floor of nose for 15-30 seconds. Rotate and remove. The recovery of the organism depends on collecting an adequate specimen. Inoculate the plate or transport medium directly at the bedside.

The following procedure optimizes the laboratory diagnosis of pertussis.

- Collect nasopharyngeal specimens in the early stage of illness. Providing specimen collection kits facilitates the appropriate specimen collection and transportation.
- For swab collected specimens, use a transport medium consisting of half strength Oxoid charcoal agar supplemented with 10% hemolyzed, defibrinated horse blood, and 40 μg/mL cephalexin.
- Inoculate a selective primary plating medium composed of Oxoid charcoal agar, 10% defibrinated horse blood, and 40 μg/mL cephalexin. A nonselective medium without cephalexin may be used in addition to the selective medium.
- Perform direct fluorescent antibody (DFA) tests on appropriately collected nasopharyngeal secretions with *B. pertussis*- and *B. parapertussis*-conjugated antisera to facilitate an earlier diagnosis.

(Continued)

Bordetella pertussis Nasopharyngeal Culture
(Continued)

- After inoculating primary plating media, retain swabs in the original transport medium at room temperature. If cultures become overgrown with indigenous bacterial flora or fungi, use swabs to inoculate additional media.
- Identify suspicious isolates with appropriate cultural and biochemical tests. The DFA test performed on growth from isolated colonies is an excellent procedure for confirmatory or definitive identification.

Storage Instructions The specimen should not be refrigerated. It should be transported to the laboratory as soon as possible after collection.

Causes for Rejection Specimen not received on appropriate isolation medium. Excessive delay in transit to the laboratory results in less than optimal yield.

Turnaround Time Preliminary reports are generally available at 24 hours if pathogens other than *B. pertussis* are isolated. Growth of *Bordetella pertussis* takes at least 72 hours to be detected. Cultures with no growth are usually reported after 1 week. Reports on specimens from which *B. pertussis* has been isolated generally require at least 1 week for completion.

Reference Range No *B. pertussis* or *B. parapertussis* isolated

Use Isolate and identify *B. pertussis*, and *B. parapertussis*; establish the diagnosis of whooping cough

Limitations Cough plates are less reliable than nasopharyngeal specimens.

Contraindications Lack of clinical symptoms of pertussis; previous antibiotic therapy; history of vaccination is a relative contraindication

Methodology Culture on selective medium (selective chocolate agar with 10% defibrinated horse blood and 40 μg/mL cephalexin), presumptive confirmation by direct fluorescent antibody (DFA). Culture after enrichment in transport medium for 48 hours increases yield.

Additional Information Direct fluorescent antibody (DFA) procedures provide more rapid results and have been increasingly used in the diagnosis of *B. pertussis* infection. The DFA procedures are most useful in the first 2-3 weeks of the illness. DFA test detected 42 of 164 (26%) of patients who proved culture positive for *B. pertussis* and 8 of 38 (21%) of patients who proved culture positive for *B. parapertussis*. False-negatives may be caused by inadequate specimens having little cellular material (leukocytes and brush border epithelial cells).

Selected Readings
Friedman RL, "Pertussis: The Disease and New Diagnostic Methods," *Clin Microbiol Rev*, 1988, 1(4):365-76.

Halperin SA, Bortolussi R, and Wort AJ, "Evaluation of Culture, Immunofluorescence, and Serology for the Diagnosis of Pertussis," *J Clin Microbiol*, 1989, 27(4):752-7.

Young SA, Anderson GL, and Mitchell PD, "Laboratory Observations During an Outbreak of Pertussis," *Clin Microbiol Newslett*, 1987, 9:22, 176-9.

Bordetella pertussis Serology
Related Information
Bordetella pertussis Direct Fluorescent Antibody *on page 282*
Bordetella pertussis Nasopharyngeal Culture *on previous page*

Synonyms *Bordetella pertussis* Antibodies; *Bordetella pertussis* Titer; Pertussis Serology

Test Includes Enzyme-linked immunosorbent assay to detect antibodies to *Bordetella pertussis* and/or pertussis toxin

Specimen Serum

Container Red top tube

Storage Instructions Refrigerate serum at 4°C.

Reference Range Absent IgM antibody; less than fourfold rise in titer in paired sera

Use Evaluate acute infection with or immunity following vaccination for *Bordetella pertussis*

Methodology Microhemagglutination, enzyme-linked immunosorbent assay (ELISA)

Additional Information Patients with acute infection develop IgG, IgM, and IgA antibodies to febrile agglutinogens; and IgM and IgA antibodies are probably diagnostic. Following vaccination, IgG and IgM antibodies can be demonstrated, except in infants. IgA antibodies do not develop.

Selected Readings
Manclark CR, Meade BD, and Burstyn DG, "Serologic Response to *Bordetella pertussis*," *Manual of Clinical Laboratory Immunology*, 4th ed, Vol 2, Rose NR, Conway de Macario

E, Fahey JL, et al, eds, Washington, DC: American Society for Microbiology, 1986, 388-94.

Mertsola J, Ruuskanen O, Kuronen T, et al, "Serologic Diagnosis of Pertussis: Evaluation of Pertussis Toxin and Other Antigens in Enzyme-Linked Immunosorbent Assay," *J Infect Dis*, 1990, 161(5):966-71.

Tomoda T, Ogura H, and Kurashige T, "Immune Responses to *Bordetella pertussis* Infection and Vaccination," *J Infect Dis*, 1991, 163(3):559-63.

Bordetella pertussis Smear *see Bordetella pertussis* Direct Fluorescent Antibody *on page 282*

Bordetella pertussis Titer *see Bordetella pertussis* Serology *on previous page*

Borreliosis Serology *see* Lyme Disease Serology *on page 394*

Borreliosis Serology *see* Lyme Disease Serology by Western Blot *on page 394*

Botulism, Diagnostic Procedure

Synonyms *Clostridium botulinum* Toxin Identification Procedure; Infant Botulism, Toxin Identification; Sudden Death Syndrome

Abstract A neurotoxin, botulin, may be produced by *C. botulinum* in foods which have been improperly preserved. Characteristics of this type of food poisoning include vomiting and abdominal pain, disturbances of vision, motor function and secretion, mydriasis, ptosis, dry mouth, and cough.

Special Instructions The laboratory must be notified prior to obtaining specimen in order to prepare for transport of the specimen to the State Health Laboratory or Center for Disease Control.

Specimen Vomitus, serum, stool, gastric washings, cerebrospinal fluid or autopsy tissue; food samples

Container Sterile wide-mouth, leakproof, screw-cap jar; red top tube

Storage Instructions Keep refrigerated at 4°C except for unopened food samples.

Turnaround Time 3-7 days

Reference Range No toxin identified, no *Clostridium botulinum* isolated

Use Diagnose infant botulism, sudden death syndrome, floppy baby syndrome, classic botulism in adults

Limitations The toxin from *C. botulinum* binds almost irreversibly to individual nerve terminals; thus, serum and cerebrospinal fluid specimens may yield false-negative results.

Contraindications Due to the difficulty in performance of the diagnostic test and because of the extensive epidemiological studies initiated upon receipt of the specimen, State Department of Health Laboratories require specific clinical symptomatology for infant botulism. Therefore, they should be consulted early to optimize handling of the suspect case.

Methodology Toxin neutralization test in mice, isolation of *Clostridium botulinum* from feces

Additional Information The classic presentation of **infant botulism** is hypotonia (floppy baby syndrome), constipation, difficulty in feeding, and a weak cry. Some cases of sudden death syndrome have been traced to ingesting honey containing *C. botulinum*. Both *C. botulinum* and *C. butyricum* have been identified as species capable of toxin production. Autointoxication may occur from toxin production during organism growth in tissue, the intestinal tract in both adults and infants, and in wounds. Botulism has been reported with cocaine-associated sinusitis.

Selected Readings

Hatheway CL, "Toxigenic Clostridia," *Clin Microbiol Rev*, 1990, 3(1):66-98.

Schmidt RD and Schmidt TW, "Infant Botulism: A Case Series and Review of the Literature," *J Emerg Med*, 1992, 10(6):713-8.

Wigginton JM and Thill P, "Infant Botulism. A Review of the Literature," *Clin Pediatr Phila*, 1993, 32(11):669-74.

Brain Biopsy

Related Information

Rabies *on page 433*

Test Includes Routine histopathologic diagnosis. Special tests are requested by physician.

Special Instructions Submit specimen in formalin for routine histology. Requisition must state operative diagnosis and source of specimen.

(Continued)

Brain Biopsy *(Continued)*

Specimen Brain tissue biopsy

Container Test tube

Collection For needle biopsies of brain, an open-end rather than side-opening needle should be used. All types of brain biopsies are best placed on saline-moistened Gelfoam®. Do not place on gauze or immerse in saline. Arrange for specimen to be in hands of neuropathologist in shortest possible time, otherwise store in refrigerator. Do not freeze.

Storage Instructions Any necessary storage should be done in formaldehyde in a closed container.

Causes for Rejection Unlabeled specimen container, insufficient material, improper fixative

Turnaround Time 24 hours to 3 weeks, depending on nature of clinical problem

Reference Range Results interpreted by neuropathologist

Use Morphologic evaluation of brain disease

Limitations The size of the tissue sample is often a limiting factor. Brain biopsy does not offer an answer in most obscure neurological diseases.

Additional Information The most commonly sought pathogens in brain biopsies are herpesvirus and *Toxoplasma*, especially in immunocompromised hosts. Special arrangements must be made for electron microscopy or immunoperoxidase studies.

Brain, CT *see* Computed Transaxial Tomography, Head Studies
on page 307

Bronchial Aspirate Anaerobic Culture *see* Anaerobic Culture
on page 250

Bronchial Aspirate Fungus Culture *see* Fungus Culture, Bronchial
Aspirate *on page 342*

Bronchial Aspiration for *Pneumocystis* *see* Pneumocystis carinii Test
on page 431

Bronchial Washings Culture *see* Aerobic Culture, Sputum
on page 246

Bronchoalveolar Lavage (BAL) *see* Fungus Culture, Bronchial
Aspirate *on page 342*

Bronchopulmonary Lavage for *Pneumocystis* *see* Pneumocystis
carinii Test *on page 431*

Bronchoscopic *Legionella* Culture *see* Legionella pneumophila
Culture *on page 381*

Bronchoscopy Culture *see* Aerobic Culture, Sputum
on page 246

Bronchoscopy, Fiberoptic

Synonyms Flexible Bronchoscopy

Test Includes Direct visual examination of upper airway, vocal cords, and tracheobronchial tree out to the fourth to sixth division bronchi. Other procedures such as washings, brush biopsy bronchoalveolar lavage, endobronchial and transbronchial biopsy are also included depending on the clinical indications.

Patient Preparation NPO after midnight for a morning bronchoscopy and NPO after light breakfast for afternoon procedures. Routine medications (especially antiasthmatic drugs) may be taken at any time with a small amount of water. Routine lab work including clotting times, BUN, CBC, and platelet count is essential to exclude a coagulopathy – especially if a biopsy is to be performed. Some measure of pulmonary function is useful (spirometry, blood gases) to assess pulmonary reserve and document bronchospasm. Premedication with a narcotic (meperidine 25-75 mg) or minor tranquilizer (diazepam 10 mg) is given parenterally 15-30 minutes before the procedure. Atropine 0.4 mg I.M. is given as a vagolytic agent at the same time unless contraindicated by the presence of arrhythmia, narrow angle glaucoma, or urinary retention.

Aftercare NPO for 2 hours or longer after the procedure until the gag reflex is fully recovered. Because of the premedication, outpatients are not allowed to drive until the following day. Transient fever and mild hemoptysis may be noted for the next 24 hours.

Equipment A fiberoptic bronchoscope and halogen or xenon light source are necessary for this airway exam. The bronchoscope is equipped with a thumb lever which allows angulation of the distal end of the instrument. A 2-2.6 mm hollow channel runs the length of the scope and allows injection of medication and aspiration of secretions for airway clearance and obtaining bronchial washings and lavage. It is also utilized for the passage of instruments, such as bronchial brushes and forceps.

Technique Procedure may be performed with the patient in supine or sitting position. Patient gargles with 2% lidocaine solution or alternatively tetracaine 2% aerosolized spray (Cetacaine®) is used to anesthetize the pharynx. The bronchoscope tip is lubricated with Xylocaine® jelly and introduced transnasally or transorally with the use of a bite block. Lidocaine 2% solution is then injected through the bronchoscopic channel in 2 mL aliquots for anesthesia of the vocal cords and entire tracheobronchial tree. Lidocaine has definite toxicity (seizures and respiratory arrest) and the total dosage should generally not exceed 400 mg. The duration of action generally lasts 20-30 minutes. Once adequate anesthesia has been obtained, a detailed visual examination is performed. Subsequently other procedures such as biopsies, washings, and brushings can be carried out.

Data Acquired This examination provides information regarding the patency and normality of the central airways. It is used as a vehicle for sampling the airways and lung parenchyma itself via brushing and biopsy techniques.

Specimen Bronchial washings, brushings, biopsy, or lavage

Container Formalin jars, mucous specimen containers, slides in 95% alcohol

Turnaround Time Reports: Written in chart at time of procedure.

Reference Range Normal endobronchial examination.

Use The major utility is in the assessment of malignant disease, early diagnosis of carcinoma, assessment of operability, transbronchial or endobronchial lung biopsy, hemoptysis (not massive), persistent chronic cough, removal of foreign bodies (minor role), and diagnosis of lung infections especially in immunocompromised hosts. Other uses include difficult endotracheal intubation.

Limitations Limited usefulness in retrieving foreign bodies and the management of massive hemoptysis.

Contraindications Asthma, severe hypoxemia, serious arrhythmia unstable angina pectoris, recent myocardial infarction, and poor patient cooperation. All of these are only relative contraindications and vary depending on the clinical situation and experience of the bronchoscopist. When bronchoscopy involves biopsy procedures, coagulopathies or bleeding tendencies are contraindications.

Additional Information The procedure is markedly safe. Large reviews have shown that approximately 50% of the life-threatening complications are associated with premedication or topical anesthesia. The risk seems highest in patients with underlying cardiac disease and the elderly. Patients with underlying bronchospastic disease are particularly prone to bronchospasm and laryngospasm and thus should be under optimal treatment before undertaking bronchoscopy. A drop in pO_2 of approximately 20 mm Hg occurs, and therefore supplemental oxygen administration is indicated. Transient fever and pneumonia occur in a small number of patients. Bleeding can occur from the nose or tracheobronchial tree although this complication is mainly associated with transbronchial biopsy.

Selected Readings

Ackart RS, Foreman DR, and Klayton RJ, "Fiberoptic Bronchoscopy in Outpatient Facilities, 1982," *Arch Intern Med*, 1983, 143(1):30-1.

Fulkerson WJ, "Current Concepts. Fiberoptic Bronchoscopy," *N Engl J Med*, 1984, 311(8):511-15.

Ikeda S, *Atlas of Flexible Bronchofiberoscopy*, Baltimore, MD: University Park Press, 1974.

Lukomsky GI, Ovchinnikov AA, and Bilal A, "Complications of Bronchoscopy: Comparison of Rigid Bronchoscopy Under General Anesthesia in Flexible Bronchoscopy Under Topical Anesthesia," *Chest*, 1981, 79(3):316-21.

Marini JJ, Pierson DJ, and Hudson LD, "Acute Lobar Atelectasis: A Prospective Comparison of Fiberoptic Bronchoscopy and Respiratory Therapy," *Am Rev Respir Dis*, 1979, 119(6):971-8.

Mitchell DM, Emerson CJ, and Collyer J, "Fiberoptic Bronchoscopy: Ten Years On," *Br Med J*, 1980, 281(6236):360-3.

Pereira W, Kovnat DM, Khan MA, et al, "Fever and Pneumonia After Flexible Fiberoptic Bronchoscopy," *Am Rev Respir Dis*, 1975, 112(1):59-64.

Perry LB, "Topical Anesthesia for Bronchoscopy," *Chest*, 1978, 73(Suppl 5):691-3.

Sackner MA, "Bronchofiberoscopy," *Am Rev Respir Dis*, 1975, 111(1):62-88.

Schnapf BM, "Oxygen Desaturation During Fiberoptic Bronchoscopy in Pediatric Patients," *Chest*, 1991, 99(3):591-4.

Sen RP and Walsh TE, "Fiberoptic Bronchoscopy for Refractory Cough," *Chest*, 1991, 99(1):33-5.

(Continued)

Bronchoscopy, Fiberoptic *(Continued)*

Trouillet JL, Guiguet M, Gibert C, et al, "Fiberoptic Bronchoscopy in Ventilated Patients. Evaluation of Cardiopulmonary Risk Under Midazolam Sedation," *Chest*, 1990, 97(4):927-33.

Bronchoscopy Fungus Culture *see* Fungus Culture, Sputum *on page 345*

Bronchoscopy Mycobacteria Culture *see* Mycobacteria Culture, Sputum *on page 406*

***Brucella* Blood Culture** *see* Blood Culture, *Brucella on page 274*

***Brucella* Culture, Tissue** *see* Biopsy Culture, Routine *on page 270*

Buffy Coat Culture for CMV *see* Cytomegalovirus Culture, Blood *on page 320*

Buffy Coat Viral Culture *see* Cytomegalovirus Culture, Blood *on page 320*

Bullous Pemphigoid Antibodies *see* Skin Biopsy, Immunofluorescence *on page 446*

C 100-3 *see* Hepatitis C Serology *on page 360*

Calcaneus (heel), Left or Right, X-ray *see* Bone Films *on page 277*

***Campylobacter pylori*, Gastric Biopsy Culture** *see* Helicobacter *pylori* Culture, Gastric Biopsy *on page 357*

***Campylobacter pylori* Urease Test and Culture** *see* Helicobacter *pylori* Culture and Urease Test *on page 356*

Casts, Urine *see* Urinalysis *on page 467*

Catheter Culture, Intravenous *see* Intravenous Line Culture *on page 376*

Catheter Tip Culture *see* Intravenous Line Culture *on page 376*

CBC *see* Complete Blood Count *on page 302*

Cefinase (Nitrocefin) Testing *see* Penicillinase Test *on page 427*

Cell Sorting Fluorescence Activation *see* Lymph Node Biopsy *on page 395*

Cephalosporinase Production Testing *see* Penicillinase Test *on page 427*

Cerebrospinal Fluid Aerobic Culture *see* Aerobic Culture, Cerebrospinal Fluid *on page 245*

Cerebrospinal Fluid Anaerobic Culture *see* Anaerobic Culture *on page 250*

Cerebrospinal Fluid Analysis
Related Information

Aerobic Culture, Cerebrospinal Fluid *on page 245*
Fungus Culture, Cerebrospinal Fluid *on page 342*
VDRL, Cerebrospinal Fluid *on page 475*
Viral Culture, Central Nervous System Symptoms *on page 476*

Synonyms CSF Analysis; Lumbar Puncture Analysis; Spinal Fluid Analysis; Spinal Tap

Test Includes Color of supernatant, turbidity, WBC/mm^3, polys/mm^3, lymphs/mm^3, RBC/mm^3, percent of crenated RBC, protein, sugar, and sometimes VDRL.

Abstract Examination of cerebrospinal fluid (CSF) contributes to diagnosis and sometimes management of infections of the central nervous system, meningitis, encephalitis, instances of vasculitis, demyelinating diseases, tumors, paraneoplastic entities, polyneuritis, instances of cerebrovascular disease, and cases of seizure disorders and confusional states.

Patient Preparation Aseptic preparation for aspiration

Special Instructions Specimen should be delivered to the laboratory **promptly**.

When a diagnosis of meningitis is considered, culture of other materials as well as culture of CSF may be helpful. Most children with bacterial meningitis are initially bacteremic, and blood cultures are of value. In neonates and small children, urine culture may be positive. Cultures and Gram stains of petechiae may provide immediate diagnosis.

Specimen Cerebrospinal fluid

Container Sterile test tubes from lumbar puncture tray

Collection Specimens of spinal fluid and blood, for culture, should be obtained prior to initiation of antibiotic treatment of meningitis. Tubes must be labeled with patient's name, date, and labeled with number indicating sequence in which tubes were obtained.

Storage Instructions Do **not** store; specimen should be processed as soon as possible.

Causes for Rejection Unlabeled tubes, insufficient specimen, clotted or refrigerated specimen, improper dispensation of specimen

Reference Range Adults: 0-5 cells/mm^3, all lymphocytes and monocytes; 0 red blood cells; protein: lumbar 15-50 mg/dL, cisternal 15-25 mg/dL, ventricular 6-15 mg/dL; glucose 50-80 mg/dL. Under 1 month: <32 cells/mm^3, 1 month to 1 year: <10 cells/mm^3, 1-4 years: <8 cells/mm^3, 5 years to puberty: <5 cells/mm^3; in the premature neonate: <29 cells/mm^3

Laboratory Values of Components of CSF From Healthy Persons and From Patients With Meningitis*

Source	CSF Laboratory Value			
	Protein (mg/dL)	Glucose (mg/dL)†	Leukocytes (per µL)	Predominant Cell Type (%)
Healthy persons newborns	15–170	34–119	0–30	
adults	15–50	40–80	0–10	Lymphocytes (63–99) Monocytes (3–37) PMN (0–15)
Adult patients with: bacterial meningitis fungal meningitis viral or aseptic meningitis	>100 Increased <100	<40 <30 Normal‡	>1000 Increased <500	PMN (>50) Lymphocytes PMN (early) and lymphocytes (late)

*Data are commonly observed values. Notable exceptions to these values and overlap of values elicited by different etiological agents are not uncommon.
PMN = polymorphonuclear leukocytes.
†CSF glucose/serum glucose ratio usually is 0.6 (adults) or 0.74–0.96 (neonates and preterm babies). In patients with bacterial meningitis, the ratios usually are <0.5 (adults) and <0.6 (neonates and preterm babies).
‡Lower than normal glucose concentrations have been observed during some non-infectious disease processes and in some patients with viral meningoencephalitis due to herpesviruses, varicella–zoster virus, mumps virus, lymphocytic choriomeningitis virus, and enteroviruses.

From Gray LD and Fedorko DP, "Laboratory Diagnosis of Bacterial Meningitis," *Clin Microbiol Rev*, 1992, 5(2):133.

Possible Panic Range Increased number of cells

Use Evaluate bacterial or viral encephalitis, meningitis, meningoencephalitis, mycobacterial or fungal infection, parasitic infestations, primary or secondary malignancy, leukemia/malignant lymphoma of CNS, trauma, vascular occlusive disease, vasculitis, heredofamilial and/or degenerative processes. The tables outline findings, including those with subdural empyema, brain abscess, ventricular empyema, cerebral epidural, abscess, spinal epidural abscess, tuberculosis, syphilis, sarcoidosis, and other entities.

The nucleated blood cell count in the cerebrospinal fluid is described as superior to any combination of the other CSF tests for bacterial meningitis. In patients who have not received antimicrobial agents, the ultimate diagnosis of bacterial meningitis is based on results of culture. The cell count and differential count are mandatory, and a Gram stain must be examined promptly in work up of possible meningitis. The CSF must be cultured; glucose and protein are necessary, as well, in the work-up for possible meningitis. **Viral infection**, as well as **bacterial meningitis**, can elicit neutrophil leukocytosis in

Initial Cerebrospinal Fluid Findings in Suppurative Diseases of the Central Nervous System and Meninges

Condition	Pressure (mm H$_2$O)	Leukocytes/mm^3	Protein (mg/dL)	Sugar (mg/dL)	Specific Findings
Acute bacterial meningitis	Usually elevated; average, 300	Several hundred to more than 60,000; usually a few thousand; occasionally fewer than 100 (especially meningococcal or early in disease); PMNs* predominate	Usually 100-500, occasionally >1000	<40 in >50% of cases	Organism usually seen on smear or culture in >90% of cases
Subdural empyema	Usually elevated; average, 300	Fewer than 100 to a few thousand; PMNs predominate	Usually 100-500	Normal	No organisms seen on smear or culture unless concurrent meningitis
Brain abscess	Usually elevated	Usually 10-200, fluid is rarely acellular; lymphocytes predominate	Usually 75-400	Normal	No organisms seen on smear or culture
Ventricular empyema (rupture of brain abscess)	Considerably elevated	Several thousand to 100,000; usually >90% PMNs	Usually several hundred	Usually <40	Organism may be seen on smear or culture
Cerebral epidural abscess	Slightly to modestly elevated	Few to several hundred or more cells; lymphocytes predominate	Usually 50-200	Normal	No organisms seen on smear or culture
Spinal epidural abscess	Usually reduced with spinal block	Usually 10-100; lymphocytes predominate	Usually several hundred	Normal	No organisms seen on smear or culture
Thrombophlebitis (often associated with subdural empyema)	Often elevated	Few to several hundred; PMNs and lymphocytes	Slightly to moderately elevated	Normal	No organisms seen on smear or culture
Bacterial endocarditis (with embolism)	Normal or slightly elevated	Few to fewer than 100; lymphocytes and PMNs	Slightly elevated	Normal	No organisms seen on smear or culture
Acute hemorrhagic encephalitis	Usually elevated	Few to more than 1000; PMNs predominate	Moderately elevated	Normal	No organisms seen on smear or culture

(continued)

Condition	Pressure (mm H₂O)	Leukocytes/mm³	Protein (mg/dL)	Sugar (mg/dL)	Specific Findings
Tuberculous infection	Usually elevated; may be low with dynamic block in advanced stages	Usually 25-100, rarely more than 500; lymphocytes predominate, except in early stages when PMNs may account for 80% of the cells	Nearly always elevated, usually 100-200; may be much higher if dynamic block	Usually reduced; <50 in 75% of cases	Acid-fast organisms may be seen on smear of protein coagulum (pellicle) or recovered from inoculated guinea pig or by culture
Cryptococcal infection	Usually elevated; average, 225	Average, 50 (0-800); lymphocytes predominate	Average, 100; usually 20-500	Reduced in >50% the cases; average 30; often higher in patients with concomitant diabetes mellitus	Organisms may be seen in India ink preparation and on culture (Sabouraud's medium); will usually grow on blood agar; may produce alcohol in cerebrospinal fluid from fermentation of glucose
Syphilis (acute)	Usually elevated	Average, 500; usually lymphocytes; rare PMNs	Average, 100; γ-globulin often high, with abnormal colloidal gold curve	Normal (rarely reduced)	Positive results of reagin test for syphilis; spirochetes not demonstrable by usual techniques of smear or culture
Sarcoidosis	Normal to considerably elevated	0 to <100 mononuclear cells	Slight to moderate elevation	Normal	No specific findings

*Polymorphonuclear leukocytes

From Feigin RD and Cherry JD, eds, *Textbook of Pediatric Infectious Diseases*, Vol 1, Philadelphia, PA: WB Saunders, 1992, 410, with permission.

Cerebrospinal Fluid Analysis *(Continued)*

blood and CSF. Seasonal curves for viral and bacterial infection go in opposite directions; although viral meningitis is a disease of midsummer, bacterial meningitis is relatively more common in the winter.

Signals of possible meningeal infection in the newborn: leukocyte count >30 cells/mm^3 with more than 60% PMNs, CSF protein >100 mg/dL, and/or CSF glucose <40% than that in blood are found with bacterial meningitis. CSF WBC counts >10 cells/mm^3 in very young infants, and >5 cells/mm^3 in older infants, and children with >1 PMN/mm^3 are abnormal. See table on previous page.

Limitations A traumatic (bloody) tap may make interpretation difficult. Normal CSF may be found early in meningitis.

Additional Information See table for laboratory values of components of CSF from healthy persons and from patients with meningitis.

More extensive testing: cytology, conventional cultures and cultures for mycobacteria, fungi, and viruses, additional chemistry and serologic determinations must usually be ordered separately.

Correction for traumatic tap: If cell counts and protein determinations are performed on CSF and blood obtained at the same time, correction for "bloody tap" can be calculated. All CSF measurements should be made from the same tube. The ratio of RBC count CSF to RBC count blood provides a factor which when multiplied by the blood WBC count or blood protein level indicates the expected level of contribution of these parameters from the blood to the spinal fluid. These contributed WBC or protein values can then be subtracted from the respective values measured in the spinal fluid. For example:

1. RBCs (CSF)/RBCs (blood) x WBCs (blood) or x protein (blood).
2. WBCs (CSF) or protein (CSF) - product calculated in 1 = true CSF WBC or true CSF protein.

If the peripheral blood is normal and traumatic tap had occurred, about 1 WBC is added to the CSF for each 700 RBCs that have been transferred into the CSF. RBC contamination from a traumatic tap does not adversely affect the laboratory diagnosis of bacterial meningitis.

Antigen detection methods cannot replace culture and Gram stain. Gram stain and culture must always have priority over antigen detection testing. A bacterial culture is the major test to be performed on cerebrospinal fluid for meningitis. It is the "gold standard" for diagnosis. A requirement for 50 or more leukocytes per µL of CSF has been proposed as justification for bacterial antigen testing. Another group found a CSF nucleated blood cell count of <6/mm^3 provided a criterion for an abbreviated CSF evaluation. There is substantial mortality and morbidity in subjects with bacterial meningitis. Neurologic sequelae are found in as many as 33% of all survivors, especially newborns and children. Especially when bacterial meningitis follows an insidious pattern, diagnostic delay may be unavoidable. Eight of 21 survivors of neonatal meningitis were normal, 8 had mild and 5 had moderate to severe sequelae in a culture-proven series.

White cell pleocytosis is found in only 33% of patients with multiple sclerosis (MS). The white count rarely exceeds 20 cells/mm^3. Most patients with MS (two-thirds) have normal total proteins. In contrast, patients with the demyelinating disease Guillain-Barré syndrome usually have no excess white cells but show elevated CSF protein of 100-500 mg/dL.

Selected Readings

Bonadio WA, Smith DS, Goddard S, et al, "Distinguishing Cerebrospinal Fluid Abnormalities in Children With Bacterial Meningitis and Traumatic Lumbar Puncture," *J Infect Dis*, 1990, 162(1):251-4.

Felgin RD and Cherry JD, *Textbook of Pediatric Infectious Diseases*, Philadelphia, PA: WB Saunders Co, 1987, 488.

Feigin RD, McCracken GH Jr, and Klein JO, "Diagnosis and Management of Meningitis," *Pediatr Infect Dis J*, 1992, 11(9):785-814.

Gray LD and Fedorko DP, "Laboratory Diagnosis of Bacterial Meningitis," *Clin Microbiol Rev*, 1992, 5(2):130-45.

Cerebrospinal Fluid Cryptococcal Latex Agglutination *see*

Cryptococcal Antigen Serology, Serum or Cerebrospinal Fluid on page 312

Cerebrospinal Fluid India Ink Preparation *see* India Ink Preparation

on page 373

Cerebrospinal Fluid Latex Agglutination for Bacterial Antigens *see* Bacterial Antigens, Rapid Detection Methods *on page 269*

Cerebrospinal Fluid Tap *see* Lumbar Puncture *on page 390*

Cerebrospinal Fluid VDRL *see* VDRL, Cerebrospinal Fluid *on page 475*

Cervical *Chlamydia* Culture *see* Chlamydia Culture *on next page*

Cervical Culture *see* Genital Culture *on page 349*

Cervical Culture for T-Strain *Mycoplasma* *see* Genital Culture for Ureaplasma urealyticum *on page 350*

Cervical Culture for *Ureaplasma urealyticum* *see* Genital Culture for Ureaplasma urealyticum *on page 350*

Cervical *Trichomonas* Smear *see* Trichomonas Preparation *on page 462*

Cervix Culture *Neisseria gonorrhoeae* *see* Neisseria gonorrhoeae Culture *on page 412*

Cervix, *Mycoplasma* Culture *see* Mycoplasma/Ureaplasma Culture *on page 410*

Chest Films

Synonyms CXR; PA; PA and Lateral CXR

Test Includes PA and lateral exposures of the chest. Sagel and his colleagues published an article in 1974 questioning the efficacy of screening examinations of the chest and whether or not lateral views should be obtained. Both medical and economic factors were considered. The study was based on a review of PA and lateral views of the chest in 10,597 examinations and reached the following conclusions.

- Routine screening for hospital admission or for surgery was not warranted for patients younger than 20 years of age.
- Lateral projection could be eliminated in routine screening of patients 20-39 years of age.
- Lateral projection should be obtained at any age when disease of the chest is suspected.
- Lateral projection should be obtained in screening examinations of patients older than 40 years of age.

Patient Preparation Remove medals, lockets, and other jewelry from neck. Arrange hair, when long, high on head so that no locks hang over chest or shoulders.

Special Instructions The chest x-ray can be modified in various ways to answer specific questions. For example, while the standard PA view of the chest is obtained in full inspiration, a pneumothorax will be more readily appreciated when the film is exposed in expiration. Decubitus films are helpful in differentiating mobile fluid in the pleural space from fluid loculations or pleural thickening. A lordotic view of the chest may be helpful in evaluating the apices. Oblique views of the chest done with 45° angulation in the right anterior oblique projection and 60° angulation in the left anterior oblique projection with barium opacifying the esophagus at the time of exposure are helpful in evaluating the size of the various cardiac chambers. A standard radiographic examination of the chest in addition to the modifications mentioned may be scheduled by calling the Radiology Department.

Use Evaluate lungs and thoracic bones for presence of metastatic and primary neoplasm, infectious disease, degenerative and reactive processes, trauma, and surgical change. The chest film is also used to evaluate the heart and great vessels.

Selected Readings

Sagel SS, Evens RG, Forrest JV, et al, "Efficacy of Routine Screening and Lateral Chest Radiographs in a Hospital-Based Population," *N Engl J Med*, 1974, 291(19):1001-4.

Chickenpox Culture *see* Varicella-Zoster Virus Culture *on page 473*

Chickenpox Titer *see* Varicella-Zoster Virus Serology *on page 474*

Chlamydia Culture

Related Information

Chlamydia pneumoniae Serology *on next page*
Chlamydia psittaci Serology *on page 296*
Chlamydia Species Serology *on page 296*
Chlamydia trachomatis by DNA Probe *on page 297*
Chlamydia trachomatis DFA Test *on page 298*
Genital Culture *on page 349*

Synonyms TRIC Agent Culture

Applies To Cervical *Chlamydia* Culture; Eye Swab *Chlamydia* Culture; Lymphogranuloma Venereum Culture; Urethral *Chlamydia* Culture

Test Includes Cell culture to detect *Chlamydia*

Special Instructions Availability and specific specimen collection requirements for *Chlamydia* cultures vary. Consult the laboratory for specific instructions, swabs, and transport materials prior to collection of the specimen.

Specimen *Chlamydia* is an intracellular organism; therefore, infected cells must be obtained by swabbing the urethra, cervix, rectum, conjunctiva, posterior nasopharynx, or throat.

Container Culturette® (Dacron) swabs should be used. Use specific *Chlamydia* transport medium.

Collection

Urethra: Remove mucous/pus by using a separate swab; discard this swab. The swab should be inserted 2-4 cm into the urethra. Use firm pressure to scrape cells from the mucosal surface. If possible repeat with second swab. Patient should not urinate within 1 hour prior to specimen collection.

Cervix: Remove mucous/pus with a Culturette® and discard this swab. Use a new swab (Culturette®) and use firm and rotating pressure to obtain specimen. May be combined with a urethral swab into same transport medium. This two-swab method is highly recommended.

Rectum: Sample anal crypts with a Culturette®.

Conjunctiva: Remove mucous and exudate with a separate swab; discard this swab. Use a Culturette® and firm pressure to scrape away epithelial cells from upper and lower lids.

Posterior nasopharynx or throat: Collect epithelial cells by using a Culturette®.

Storage Instructions Deliver inoculated transport medium **immediately** to laboratory. **Specimens must be refrigerated** during storage and transportation or frozen at -70°C if stored more than 2 days.

Turnaround Time Cultures with no growth usually will be reported after 4-7 days. Rapid culture methods for detection of *Chlamydia* require a minimum of 48 hours.

Reference Range No *Chlamydia* isolated

Use To aid in the diagnosis of infections caused by *Chlamydia* (eg, cervicitis, trachoma, conjunctivitis, pelvic inflammatory disease, pneumonia, urethritis, nongonococcal urethritis, pneumonitis, and sexually transmitted diseases).

Limitations Culture may be negative in presence of *Chlamydia* infection. Culture is probably not the gold standard for the detection of *C. trachomatis*. The sensitivity of culture probably is only 70% to 90% because *C. trachomatis* does not always survive transit to the laboratory and because sampling is often inadequate even with (multiple) swabs.

Methodology Inoculation of specimen onto McCoy cell culture and subsequent detection of *Chlamydia*-infected cells by immunofluorescence and monoclonal antibody

Additional Information This organism infects the endocervical columnar epithelial cells and will not be found in the inflammatory cells. In obtaining the specimen, clean the area of inflammatory cells and then attempt to scrape epithelial cells for culturing by using a new, separate swab. The results of cytological diagnosis of chlamydial infection of the female genital tract have been disappointing. Papanicolaou-stained cervical smears are not reliable enough to help establish or exclude the presence of *Chlamydia*. In patients with vaginal discharge or other genital tract symptomatology of unknown etiology, cervical cytology can be useful in identifying patients who should be cultured for *Chlamydia*. Direct immunofluorescence techniques and enzyme immunoassays are available to detect *Chlamydia* in clinical specimens. These methods usually provide reliable results in high-prevalence populations and detect both viable and nonviable organisms. Selection of the most efficient method for recovery of *Chlamydia* depends upon the incidence in the patient population and the local availability of the various methods. Urine culture for *Chlamydia* is not a sensitive procedure and generally should not be done. The incidence of cervical infection with *Chlamydia trachomatis* is two to three times that of gonorrhea: 4% to 9% in private office settings, 6% to 23% in family planning clinics, and 20% to 30% in sexually transmitted diseases clinics.

Culture should be the test-of-choice (i) in cases of child abuse, ascending pelvic infections, and rectal and throat infections, and (ii) when a test-for-cure is desired.

Chlamydia is a single genus and consists of the following:
- *C. trachomatis* (serotypes A-K): inclusion conjunctivitis, trachoma, and genital infections
- *C. trachomatis* (serotypes L1-L3): lymphogranuloma venereum
- *C. psittaci*: psittacosis
- *C. pneumoniae* (TWAR): respiratory infections

Serology to detect antibodies to each of the three species of *Chlamydia* is available.

Laboratory diagnosis of *C. pneumoniae* infections is not widely available; commercial tests for *C. pneumoniae* are not available. *C. pneumoniae* is responsible for approximately 10% of community-acquired pneumonias. The cells (McCoy) usually used to culture *C. trachomatis* will not reliably support the growth of *C. pneumoniae*. Recent studies have shown that other cell lines (H 292 and HEp-2) are more appropriate. However, culture using these cells is not generally available. An alternate, widely used method for the laboratory diagnosis of *C. pneumoniae* infection is serology by microimmunofluorescence. Currently, this serological test is the most sensitive and specific laboratory test for *C. pneumoniae*.

Selected Readings
Grayston JT, "*Chlamydia pneumoniae*, Strain TWAR," *Chest*, 1989, 95(3):664-9.

Grayston JT, Campbell LA, Kuo CC, et al, "A New Respiratory Tract Pathogen: *Chlamydia pneumoniae* Strain TWAR," *J Infect Dis*, 1990, 161(4):618-25.

Hipp SS and Coles FB, "The Virtues of *Chlamydia* Culture," *Clin Microbiol Newslett*, 1994, 16(5):37-9.

Le Scolea LJ Jr, "The Value of Nonculture Chlamydial Diagnostic Tests," *Clin Microbiol Newslett*, 1991, 13(3):21-4.

Lombardo JM and Gadol CL, "*Chlamydia trachomatis*: A Perfect Test?" *Clin Microbiol Newslett*, 1990, 12(13):100-2.

Schachter J, "Laboratory Aspects of Chlamydial Infections," *Adv Exp Med Biol*, 1987, 224:73-7.

Chlamydia pneumoniae Serology
Related Information
Chlamydia Culture *on previous page*
Chlamydia psittaci Serology *on next page*
Chlamydia Species Serology *on next page*
Chlamydia trachomatis by DNA Probe *on page 297*
Chlamydia trachomatis DFA Test *on page 298*

Synonyms *Chlamydia*, TWAR Strain; TWAR Strain *Chlamydia*

Test Includes Pan-reactive for trachoma, psittacosis, LGV, and TWAR

Specimen Serum

Container Red top tube or serum separator tube

Storage Instructions Separate serum and refrigerate.

Causes for Rejection Excessive hemolysis, chylous serum, inadequate labeling

Reference Range Negative. Titers <1:64 suggest no current or previous infection. A fourfold or greater increase in antibody titer in paired specimens usually provides unequivocal evidence of recent infection.

Use Evaluate possible chlamydial infection

Limitations The antigen (lipopolysaccharide) used in the test is group specific and not species specific. A very high "background" of immunity in the general population makes interpretation of results difficult.

Methodology Indirect fluorescent antibody (IFA)

Additional Information A new *Chlamydia* species, *C. pneumoniae* (TWAR strain), is a frequent cause of acute respiratory disease. *C. pneumoniae* antibody has been found in 25% to 60% of adults. The determination of species or type specific antibodies to *C. psittaci*, *C. trachomatis*, and *C. pneumoniae* (Continued)

Chlamydia pneumoniae Serology *(Continued)*

strain is complicated by cross reactive antigens or nonspecific stimulation of antichlamydial antibodies. Thus, a panel of *Chlamydia* must be tested to determine specific titers and establish the strongest reactions. The panel to differentiate *C. pneumoniae*, *C. psittaci*, and *C. trachomatis* may be requested from a microbiology reference laboratory.

Selected Readings
Grayston JT, "*Chlamydia pneumoniae*, Strain TWAR Pneumonia," *Annu Rev Med*, 1992, 43:317-23.
Hammerschlag MR, "*Chlamydia pneumoniae*: A New Respiratory Pathogen," *Infect Dis Newslett* 1992, 11(1):1-4.

***Chlamydia psittaci* Antibody** *see Chlamydia psittaci* Serology *on this page*

Chlamydia psittaci Serology
Related Information
Chlamydia Culture *on page 294*
Chlamydia pneumoniae Serology *on previous page*
Chlamydia Species Serology *on this page*
Chlamydia trachomatis by DNA Probe *on next page*
Chlamydia trachomatis DFA Test *on page 298*
Synonyms *Chlamydia psittaci* Antibody
Special Instructions Acute and convalescent samples are recommended.
Specimen Serum
Container Red top tube or serum separator tube
Reference Range Less than a fourfold increase in titer in paired sera
Use Diagnosis of psittacosis
Limitations Antibody response may be suppressed if patient has been treated with antibiotics
Methodology Complement fixation (CF), microimmunofluorescence
Additional Information Most patients with psittacosis develop high titers of complement fixing antibody and in some with the proper clinical setting a single very high titer may be strongly supportive of the diagnosis. Specific IgM antibody can sometimes be demonstrated.

To detect psittacosis antibody, an antigen specific for *C. psittaci* must be included in the test system. There may be significant antibody titers in veterinarians and patients with Reiter's syndrome.
Selected Readings
Schachter J, "*Chlamydia*," *Manual of Clinical Laboratory Immunology*, 3rd ed, Rose NR, Friedman H, and Fahey JL, eds, Washington, DC: American Society for Microbiology, 1986, 587-92.

***Chlamydia* Smear** *see* Ocular Cytology *on page 416*

Chlamydia Species Serology
Related Information
Chlamydia Culture *on page 294*
Chlamydia pneumoniae Serology *on previous page*
Chlamydia psittaci Serology *on this page*
Chlamydia trachomatis by DNA Probe *on next page*
Chlamydia trachomatis DFA Test *on page 298*
Test Includes Detection of antibody titer to *Chlamydia* species
Specimen Serum
Container Red top tube
Collection Collect acute phase blood as soon as possible after onset (no later than 1 week). Convalescent blood should be drawn 1-2 weeks after acute (no less than 2 weeks after onset).
Reference Range Negative. A fourfold increase in titer in paired sera is usually indicative of chlamydial infection. Determination of IgM antibody may be helpful in differentiating acute infection from prior exposure.
Use Evaluate possible chlamydial infection
Limitations The antigen (lipopolysaccharide) used in the test is group specific and not species specific. In cases of conjunctivitis, nongonococcal urethritis, and pneumonia of the newborn, there is usually **not** an antibody response detectable by complement fixation. A very high "background" of immunity in the general population makes interpretation of results difficult.

Methodology Complement fixation (CF), indirect fluorescence antibody (IFA), enzyme immunoassay (EIA)

Additional Information Because of the high prevalence of antibodies to *Chlamydia*, especially in patients being evaluated for urethritis or possible venereal disease, results of serologic tests must be interpreted with caution. Very high titers, rising titers, or IgM specific antibody should be sought. In a patient being evaluated for chlamydial disease of the genitourinary tract, culture as well as serology should be obtained, as well as a serologic test for syphilis and a culture for *Neisseria gonorrhoeae*.

Selected Readings

Ehret JM and Judson FN, "Genital *Chlamydia* Infections," *Clin Lab Med*, 1989, 9(3):481-500.

Miettinen A, Heinonen PK, Teisala K, et al, "Antigen-Specific Serum Antibody Response to *Chlamydia trachomatis* in Patients With Pelvic Inflammatory Disease," *J Clin Pathol*, 1990, 43(9):758-61.

Schachter J, "Chlamydiae," *Manual of Clinical Laboratory Immunology*, 4th ed, Rose NR, de Macario EC, Fahey JL, et al, eds, Washington, DC: American Society for Microbiology, 1992, 661-6.

Chlamydia trachomatis by DNA Probe

Related Information

Chlamydia Culture *on page 294*
Chlamydia pneumoniae Serology *on page 295*
Chlamydia psittaci Serology *on previous page*
Chlamydia Species Serology *on previous page*
Chlamydia trachomatis DFA Test *on next page*

Synonyms *Chlamydia trachomatis* DNA Detection Test; DNA Hybridization Test for *Chlamydia trachomatis*; DNA Test for *Chlamydia trachomatis*; PACE2®

Test Includes Direct detection of *Chlamydia trachomatis* nucleic acid in swab specimens.

Patient Preparation When taking urethral specimens the patient should not have urinated for 1 hour prior to collection.

Specimen Swab specimen collected from the genitourinary tract of a male or female patient

Container Special DNA transport medium is provided by the laboratory and should not be substituted. A kit containing a swab and special transport medium is made by Gen-Probe, Inc, and is required for this test.

Collection Currently the DNA test for *Chlamydia trachomatis* is FDA-approved only for urethral, cervical, and conjunctival specimens.

For a male the urethra is swabbed by rotating the swab 2-3 cm into the urethra. This should provide enough epithelial cells from the infected site to detect *C. trachomatis*. The swab is then placed in the transport tube for shipping to the laboratory.

For females, the Gen-Probe® kit provides two swabs. The cervix or endocervix should be swabbed and with one swab first to clean the area and the second swab is used to collect the specimen. The swab is inserted 2-3 cm into the endocervix and then rotated to collect the epithelial cells from the infected site. The swab is then put immediately into the transport tube and shipped to the laboratory.

For conjunctival specimens, use a "male" collection kit, clean away exudate with a separate swab and discard the swab, thoroughly swab the lower and upper conjunctiva each two to three times. Place the swab immediately into the transport tube with medium for transport to the laboratory.

Storage Instructions The specimens should be kept at room temperature or refrigerated. Do not freeze.

Causes for Rejection Contamination with urine; specimen frozen (which lyses the cells collected); gross blood in specimen

Turnaround Time Usually results are available within 24 hours of receipt of the specimen.

Reference Range The results of a normal test should be negative for *Chlamydia trachomatis* DNA. A sexually active, asymptomatic individual may harbor *C. trachomatis* in rates ranging from 0% to 7%.

Use This test provides for the rapid detection of *C. trachomatis* in clinical specimens.

Limitations DNA detection test cannot be done in child abuse cases. Cell culture is the only approved test in these cases. However, this test can be used to confirm positive culture results.

Methodology This test detects *C. trachomatis* ribosomal RNA directly from swab specimens. This requires denaturation of the RNA in the specimens by

(Continued)

Chlamydia trachomatis by DNA Probe *(Continued)*

heating, hybridization with a specific DNA probe and detection of bound probe after several washing steps. Detection is done by using a probe labeled with an acridenium ester which releases a burst of light when in the presence of H_2O_2.

Additional Information Approximately 4 million cases of *C. trachomatis* occur annually in the United States, and it is considered a serious sexually transmitted disease problem. The detection of *C. trachomatis* RNA provides a diagnostic test that has several advantages over the traditional culture method. The turnaround time is shorter, it is less labor intensive, and it provides an objective result that makes interpretation easier. The RNA detection test for *C. trachomatis* has been proven to have an equivalent sensitivity to the antibody-based test (EIA and fluorescent antibody detection methods) and to have a greater specificity than these tests. However, at the present time this test cannot be done exclusively if a child abuse case is involved. These cases must be detected with a cell culture test.

Selected Readings

Barnes RC, "Laboratory Diagnosis of Human Chlamydial Infections," *Clin Microbiol Rev*, 1989, 2(2):119-36.

Ehret JM and Judson FN, "Genital *Chlamydia* Infections," *Clin Lab Med*, 1989, 9(3):481-500.

Peterson EM, Oda R, Alexander R, et al, "Molecular Techniques for the Detection of *Chlamydia trachomatis*," *J Clin Microbiol*, 1989, 27(10):2359-63.

Chlamydia trachomatis DFA Test

Related Information

Chlamydia Culture *on page 294*

Chlamydia pneumoniae Serology *on page 295*

Chlamydia psittaci Serology *on page 296*

Chlamydia Species Serology *on page 296*

Chlamydia trachomatis by DNA Probe *on previous page*

Synonyms MicroTrak®

Test Includes Examination of specimen, specifically for *Chlamydia trachomatis*

Patient Preparation For urogenital specimens, patient should not urinate 1 hour prior to collection.

Special Instructions Specify specimen origin. Include all pertinent information, label slide and collection pack.

Specimen Direct smear

Container Single well (8 mm) glass slide, Dacron swabs (one large, one small), one cytobrush, methanol fixative (0.5 mL vial). These items are contained in a commonly used direct detection kit (collection pack) known as MicroTrak®.

Collection Endocervical with cytology brush: Nonpregnant women. Use large swab to remove exudate or mucous from exocervix. Insert cytobrush into cervical os past the squamocolumnar junction. Rest 2-3 seconds, rotate brush 360 degrees to gather columnar cells and withdraw brush. Do not touch vaginal walls with brush, and prepare slides immediately by rotating and twisting brush back and forth across center of slide well.

Endocervical with swab: Pregnant women. Use large swab to remove exudate or mucous from exocervix. Insert another large Dacron swab until tip is no longer visible, rotate swab 5-10 seconds, and withdraw swab. Do not touch vaginal walls and prepare slides immediately. Firmly roll one side of swab over top half of well. Turn swab over and roll other side over bottom half of slide well.

Urethral: Males. Patient should not urinate 1 hour before sampling. Remove pus or exudate with separate swab, insert small swab with wire shaft 2-4 cm into penis. Gently rotate swab to dislodge cells, rest swab 2 seconds, withdraw swab, and prepare slide immediately as above.

Rectal: Symptomatic patients only. Use large swab. Insert approximately 3 cm into anal canal. Move swab from side to side to sample crypts. If fecal contamination occurs, discard swab and obtain another specimen. Prepare slide immediately as above.

Conjunctival: Neonates, symptomatic only. Use large separate swab to gently remove pus or discharge and discard. If both eyes are sampled, swab less affected eye first. Swab inside of lower, then upper lid, and prepare slide immediately as above.

Nasopharyngeal: Neonates, symptomatic only. Use small swab or nasal aspirator. Collect specimen from posterior nasopharynx using standard collection method. If swab was used, prepare slide immediately. If nasal aspirate was collected, deliver to laboratory technician immediately for slide preparation.

All specimens: Write patient name and date on slip and outside of collection pack. Allow specimen to air dry. Lay slide flat and flood with methanol fixative. Let entire quantity evaporate. Refold pack without touching fixed specimen.

Storage Instructions Refrigerate slides at 2°C to 8°C or at room temperature (20°C to 30°C) until taken to the laboratory. Slides must be stained within 7 days of collection.

Causes for Rejection Specimen not labeled, slide received broken, less than 10 columnar or cuboidal epithelial cells on slide, slide more than 7 days old

Turnaround Time The time required to stain and examine the specimen is generally less than 1 hour. Turnaround time depends on staffing within the laboratory.

Reference Range Unsatisfactory specimen; negative or positive for *Chlamydia*

Use Aid in the diagnosis of disease caused by *Chlamydia* (eg, pneumonitis, sexually transmitted disease, inclusion conjunctivitis, trachoma, and pneumonia).

Limitations The direct detection of *C. trachomatis* is a useful tool in screening high-risk populations and in clinical situations where rapid positive results may be useful. However, the direct fluorescent antibody procedure is no more sensitive than the cell culture procedure. The number of cells on the slide can be too low for diagnosis.

Methodology Direct fluorescent antibody (DFA)

Additional Information The *Chlamydia trachomatis* direct test uses fluorescein-conjugated monoclonal antibodies (reactive with all 15 known serotypes of *C. trachomatis*) to detect elementary bodies in clinical smears. This test detects only *Chlamydia trachomatis* major outer membrane protein (MOMP); the test does not distinguish between living and dead organisms. Therefore, the test does not necessarily serve as a test-of-cure.

Chlamydia trachomatis, primarily a human pathogen, has been implicated in neonatal/infantile conjunctivitis and afebrile pneumonia. One-third to one-half of babies born vaginally to mothers with chlamydial infection of the cervix will be infected; the majority of these neonates will develop inclusion conjunctivitis and/or a respiratory tract infection that can lead to the distinctive (afebrile) pneumonia syndrome.

Conjunctivitis: Conjunctivitis in infected neonates usually occurs between the 5th and 12th day after birth. In neonates born to mothers with premature rupture of the membranes, *C. trachomatis* has been detected, in rare cases, as early as the first day following birth.

Afebrile pneumonia: Many neonatal chlamydial infections also involve the respiratory tract. Respiratory infections usually occur secondarily to inclusion conjunctivitis. Rhinitis is often a prodrome for severe lower respiratory tract involvement. Signs of chlamydial pneumonia include cough, tachypnea, inspiratory rales, and, in more severe cases, vomiting and periods of apnea.

Selected Readings
Barnes RC, "Laboratory Diagnosis of Human Chlamydial Infections," *Clin Microbiol Rev*, 1989, 2(2):119-36.

Chlamydia trachomatis DNA Detection Test *see Chlamydia trachomatis* by DNA Probe *on page 297*

Chlamydia, TWAR Strain *see Chlamydia pneumoniae* Serology *on page 295*

Chloramphenicol Serum Level

Related Information
Antibiotic Level, Serum *on page 255*

Synonyms Chloromycetin®; Mychel-S®

Abstract Chloramphenicol is an antimicrobial agent whose use has been greatly reduced in recent years because of the introduction of a wide variety of less toxic alternative agents. It is still appropriately used to treat certain rickettsial infections or penicillin-allergic patients with bacterial meningitis. Life-threatening bone marrow toxicity is not closely associated with high serum levels.

Specimen Serum

Container Red top tube or serum separator tube

Sampling Time Collect for trough level immediately before next dose; for peak level about 2 hours after oral dose, 30 minutes after I.V. dose (time to peak can be variable)

(Continued)

Chloramphenicol Serum Level (Continued)

Storage Instructions Freeze processed specimen

Reference Range Therapeutic range: 10-25 μg/mL (SI: 31-77 μmol/L), trough <5 μg/mL (SI: <15 μmol/L)

Critical Values Toxic range: >25 μg/mL (SI: >77 μmol/L)

Use Monitoring of drug therapy; monitoring for potential toxicity

Limitations Reversible dose related bone marrow depression may occur when serum/plasma concentration >25 μg/mL (SI: >77 μmol/L). Idiosyncratic bone marrow aplasia is a rare event that usually occurs weeks to months after completing therapy, but approximately 25% occur during the course of therapy. Hematologic studies should be performed before and during therapy.

Methodology High performance liquid chromatography (HPLC), gas-liquid chromatography (GLC), immunoassay

Additional Information Chloramphenicol is an extremely effective antibacterial agent which unfortunately has both idiosyncratic and dose-related toxicities. Half-life is 1.6-3.3 hours longer in infants and patients with hepatic and renal disease. The dose related toxicity is, in adults, bone marrow suppression. "Gray syndrome," a type of circulatory collapse, occurs primarily in infants whose livers are unable to metabolize chloramphenicol effectively. Idiosyncratic aplastic anemia occurs in between 1 in 20,000 and 1 in 40,000 exposures. There are a number of chloramphenicol drug interactions since chloramphenicol can inhibit hepatic microsomal metabolism, increasing the serum concentration of phenytoin, tolbutamide, and dicumarol. Phenobarbital may be elevated in the presence of chloramphenicol.

Selected Readings

Baselt RC, *Analytical Procedures for Therapeutic Drug Monitoring and Emergency Toxicology*, Davis, CA: Biomedical Publications, 1980, 71-5.

de Louvois J, Mulhall A, and Hurley R, "Comparison of Methods Available for Assay of Chloramphenicol in Clinical Specimens," *J Clin Pathol*, 1980, 33(6):575-80.

Smilack JD, Wilson WR, and Cockerill FR 3d, "Tetracyclines, Chloramphenicol, Erythromycin, Clindamycin, and Metronidazole," *Mayo Clin Proc*, 1991, 66(12):1270-80.

Chloromycetin® *see* Chloramphenicol Serum Level *on previous page*

CIE for Group B Streptococcal Antigen *see* Group B *Streptococcus* Antigen Test *on page 354*

Cimex Identification *see* Arthropod Identification *on page 268*

Clavicle, Left or Right, X-ray *see* Bone Films *on page 277*

Closed Joint Aspiration *see* Arthrocentesis *on page 264*

Clostridium botulinum Toxin Identification Procedure *see* Botulism, Diagnostic Procedure *on page 285*

Clostridium difficile Toxin Assay

Related Information

Fecal Leukocyte Stain *on page 334*

Synonyms Antibiotic-Associated Colitis Toxin Test; Pseudomembranous Colitis Toxin Assay; Toxin Assay, *Clostridium difficile*

Test Includes Toxin detection

Special Instructions When antibiotic-associated colitis is suspected a toxin assay rather than a *C. difficile* culture should be ordered on the stool.

Specimen Stool or proctoscopic specimen

Container Stool container with lids (swabs are inadequate because of small volume)

Collection Keep specimen **cold** and transport immediately to prevent deterioration of toxin. Specimens can be frozen if transportation will be delayed.

Storage Instructions If the specimen cannot be processed immediately, it should be stored under refrigeration.

Turnaround Time 1-2 days depending on the availability and on the protocol of laboratory

Reference Range Presence of toxin is indicative of disease. Isolation of organism (*C. difficile*) may occur in a small percentage of normal adults (5% to 21%) and in normal newborns. Isolation of the organism without demonstration of toxin production is a nonspecific finding because only certain isolates are toxigenic.

Use Determine the presence or absence of antibiotic related colitis caused by *C. difficile* toxin

Limitations Results given as titers are not significant as such because size/amounts of original specimens are usually not standardized. Results should be given as positive or negative, and any titer result should be interpreted as simply positive.

The latex agglutination test is simple and rapid, but it does not detect (is not specific for) toxin A, the protein thought to be primarily responsible for pseudomembranous colitis.

Methodology Latex agglutination test to detect toxin, toxin neutralization test in tissue culture (toxin), selective anaerobic culture (organism),

Additional Information Antibiotic-associated pseudomembranous colitis has been shown to result from the action of toxins produced by the organism, *C. difficile*. The disease has been associated with clindamycin but now it is recognized that pseudomembranous colitis can follow administration of virtually any antibiotic. More than 70% of cases in a large study were associated with cephalosporin therapy. The clinical spectrum of antibiotic-induced syndromes caused by *C. difficile* includes patients with symptoms of acute abdomen with little or no diarrhea, as well as cases with fulminant life-threatening diarrhea. Nosocomial transmission and reinfection with different strains occurs as do spontaneous cases without prior antimicrobial therapy. In cases where cessation of antibiotic therapy does not produce a response, specific therapy with oral vancomycin, metronidazole or oral bacitracin may be effective. The detection of the toxin (rather than culture of the organism or detection of the organism by latex agglutination) is essential in determining the etiology of this potentially fatal disease. In a recent report of 40 patients with *C. difficile*-associated diarrhea, 70% were positive in the cytotoxin assay, 78% positive in the LA test, and 90% culture positive. Fifty-three control patients had a 2%, 8%, and 4% positive rate respectively (ie, a small percentage of false-positives). A reasonable strategy might be to screen with the LA test and perform the toxin assay in cases which are positive. The routine use of culture is not appropriate because of the costs and the high rate of recovery of strains which do not produce toxin. Cytotoxin results are slightly more predictive of *C. difficile* disease than latex-positive results. Neither method alone is able either to predict or rule out all cases accurately. The organism is known to produce an enterotoxin, toxin A and a cytotoxin, toxin B. The exact role of each of these toxins, in clinical disease, remains unclear.

Selected Readings

Fekety R, and Shah AB, "Diagnosis and Treatment of *Clostridium difficile* Colitis," *JAMA*, 1993, 269(1):71-5.

Gerding DN, Olson MM, Peterson LR, et al, "*Clostridium difficile*-Associated Diarrhea and Colitis in Adults," *Arch Intern Med*, 1986, 146(1):95-100.

Kelly MT, Champagne SG, Sherlock CH, et al, "Commercial Latex Agglutination Test for Detection of *Clostridium difficile*-Associated Diarrhea," *J Clin Microbiol*, 1987, 25(7):1244-7.

Knoop FC, Owens M, and Crocker IC, "*Clostridium difficile*: Clinical Disease and Diagnosis," *Clin Microbiol Rev*, 1993, 6(3):251-65.

Lyerly DM, "Epidemiology of *Clostridium difficile* Disease," *Clin Microbiol Newslett*, 1993, 15(7):49-56.

Lyerly DM, Krivan HC, and Wilkins TD, "*Clostridium difficile*: It's Disease and Toxins," *Clin Microbiol Rev*, 1988, 1(1):1-18.

Wexler H, "Diagnosis of Antibiotic-Associated Disease Caused by *Clostridium difficile*," *Clin Microbiol Newslett*, 1989, 11:25-32.

CLO™ Test *see Helicobacter pylori* Culture and Urease Test *on page 356*

CMG *see Cystometrogram, Simple on page 315*

CMV Culture *see Cytomegalovirus Culture on page 319*

CMV Culture *see Cytomegalovirus Culture, Blood on page 320*

CMV Early Antigen FA Method *see* Cytomegalovirus Isolation, Rapid *on page 320*

CMV-IFA *see Cytomegalovirus Serology on page 321*

CMV-IFA, IgG *see Cytomegalovirus Serology on page 321*

CMV-IFA, IgM *see Cytomegalovirus Serology on page 321*

CMVS, Culture *see Urine Culture, Clean Catch on page 470*

CMV Shell Vial Method *see* Cytomegalovirus Isolation, Rapid *on page 320*

CMV Titer *see Cytomegalovirus Serology on page 321*

Coagglutination Test for Group A Streptococci *see* Group A *Streptococcus* Antigen Test *on page 354*

Coccidioides **Immunodiffusion** *see* Fungal Serology
on page 337

Cold Agglutinin Titer

Test Includes Titer of patient's serum against type O blood cells at 2°C to 8°C

Special Instructions Transport blood immediately to laboratory.

Specimen Serum

Container Red top tube or serum separator tube

Storage Instructions After clotting at 37°C, separate serum from cells if specimen is to be stored overnight in refrigerator.

Causes for Rejection Refrigeration of the specimen before separating serum from cells; specimen not allowed to clot at 37°C

Reference Range Screen: negative; titer: <1:32

Use Occasionally, the cold agglutination titer is useful in supporting the diagnosis of primary atypical pneumonia (infection with *Mycoplasma pneumoniae*). Because it is nonspecific, the test generally is not recommended. Tests for specific antibodies to *Mycoplasma pneumoniae* are much more useful and specific than are tests for cold agglutinins.

Limitations False-negatives may occur if serum is refrigerated on the clot; only half of patients with *M. pneumoniae* infection will have positive test; many positive results are associated with a wide variety of nonspecific conditions

Additional Information The i and I RBC antigens appear to be ceramide heptasaccharides and decasaccharides. The fetal i RBCs change after birth so that by 18 months red cells carry largely I. The i substance has been found in saliva, milk, amniotic fluid, ovarian cyst fluid, and serum.

The most common cause of elevated cold agglutinin in high titers is an infection with *Mycoplasma pneumoniae*. *M. pneumoniae* has I-like antigen specificity. Fifty-five percent of patients with disease have rising titers. In primary atypical *Mycoplasma pneumoniae* pneumonia, cold agglutinins are demonstrated 1 week after onset; the titer increases in 8-10 days, peaks at 12-25 days, and rapidly falls after day 30. Antibiotic therapy may interfere with antibody formation. Ninety percent of those who are severely affected or have prolonged illness will have a positive cold agglutination titer.

Cold agglutinins are usually IgM autoantibodies directed against the Ii antigens of human RBCs. These antibodies may be found in patients with cold agglutinin disease or may occur transiently following a number of acute infectious illnesses. Cold agglutinins of cold agglutinin disease are usually monoclonal IgM kappa. Cold antibodies of IgG, IgA, or IgM type directed against Ii antigens may be found in infectious mononucleosis. Antibodies reacting near physiologic temperatures are more likely to be clinically important. Detection of cold agglutinins may be useful in patients where cold blood is to be used such as in a blood cardioplegia unit.

Complete Blood Count

Synonyms Blood Cell Profile; Blood Count; CBC; Hemogram

Test Includes WBC, Hct, Hgb, differential count, RBC, WBC and RBC morphology, RBC indices, platelet estimate, platelet count, RDW, and histograms. Although RBC, WBC, and platelet histograms are not available on patient charts, they are helpful to the technologist in detecting problems with patients and quality control. Even though the histograms are not on the chart, they can be viewed in the laboratory along with the blood smear. New analyzers also provide automated 5-part white cell differentials: granulocytes, monocytes, lymphocytes, eosinophils, and basophils.

Abstract The standard automated test for evaluation of RBC, WBC, and platelets

Specimen Whole blood

Container Lavender top (EDTA) tube

Collection Mix specimen 10 times by gentle inversion. If specimen is not brought to the laboratory immediately refrigeration is required. If the anticipated delay in arrival is more than 4 hours, two blood smears should be prepared immediately after the venipuncture and submitted with the blood specimen.

Causes for Rejection Improper tube, clotted specimen, hemolyzed specimen, dilution of blood with I.V. fluid

Reference Range Accompanying tables summarize differences in red cell parameter normal ranges, note especially important age and sex variances. Refer to tables.

Red Cell Values on First Postnatal Day*

Gestational Age (wk)	24–25	26–27	28–29	30–31	32–33	34–35	36–37	Term
RBC (x 10^6/mm^3)	4.65 ±0.43	4.73 ±0.45	4.62 ±0.75	4.79 ±0.74	5.0 ±0.76	5.09 ±0.5	5.27 ±0.68	5.14 ±0.7
Hgb (g/dL)	19.4 ±1.5	19.0 ±2.5	19.3 ±1.8	19.1 ±2.2	18.5 ±2.0	19.6 ±2.1	19.2 ±1.7	19.3 ±2.2
Hct (%)	63 ±4	62 ±8	60 ±7	60 ±8	60 ±8	61 ±7	64 ±7	61 ±7.4
MCV (fL)	135 ±0.2	132 ±14.4	131 ±13.5	127 ±12.7	123 ±15.7	122 ±10.0	121 ±12.5	119 ±9.4
Retic (%)	6.0 ±0.5	9.6 ±3.2	7.5 ±2.5	5.8 ±2.0	5.0 ±1.9	3.9 ±1.6	4.2 ±1.8	3.2 ±1.4

*Mean values ± SD.

From Zaizov R and Matoth Y,[1] "Red Cell Values on the First Postnatal Day During the Last 16 Weeks of Gestation," *Amer J Hematol*, 1976, 1:2, 275–8, with permission.

Mean Hematologic Values for Full–Term Infants, Children, and Adults*

Age	Hemoglobin (g/dL)	Hematocrit (%)	RBC (10^6/mm^3)	MCV (fL)	MCH (pg)	MCHC (g/dL)
Birth (cord blood)	17.1 ±1.8	52.0 ±5	4.64 ±0.5	113 ±6	37 ±2	33 ±1
1 d	19.4 ±2.1	58.0 ±7	5.30 ±0.5	110 ±6	37 ±2	33 ±1
2–6 d	19.8 ±2.4	66.0 ±8	5.40 ±0.7	122 ±14	37 ±4	30 ±3
14–23 d	15.7 ±1.5	52.0 ±5	4.92 ±0.6	106 ±11	32 ±3	30 ±2
24–37 d	14.1 ±1.9	45.0 ±7	4.35 ±0.6	104 ±11	32 ±3	31 ±3
40–50 d	12.8 ±1.9	42.0 ±6	4.10 ±0.5	103 ±11	31 ±3	30 ±2
2–2.5 mo	11.4 ±1.1	38.0 ±4	3.75 ±0.5	101 ±10	30 ±3	30 ±2
3–3.5 mo	11.2 ±0.8	37.0 ±3	3.88 ±0.4	95 ±9	29 ±3	30 ±2
5–7 mo	11.5 ±0.7	38.0 ±3	4.21 ±0.5	91 ±9	27 ±3	30 ±2
8–10 mo	11.7 ±0.6	39.0 ±2	4.35 ±0.4	90 ±8	27 ±3	30 ±1
11–13.5 mo	11.9 ±0.6	39.0 ±2	4.44 ±0.4	88 ±7	27 ±2	30 ±1
1.5–3 y	11.8 ±0.5	39.0 ±2	4.45 ±0.4	87 ±7	27 ±2	30 ±2
5 y	12.7 ±1.0	37.0 ±3	4.65 ±0.5	80 ±4	27 ±2	34 ±1
10 y	13.2 ±1.2	39.0 ±3	4.80 ±0.5	81 ±6	28 ±3	34 ±1
Male	15.5 ±1.1	46.0 ±3.1	5.11 ±0.38	—	—	—
Female	13.7 ±1.0	40.9 ±3	4.51 ±0.36	—	—	—
Male and female	—	—	—	90.1 ±4.8	30.2 ±1.8	33.7 ±1.1

*Mean ± 1 SD.

From Johnson TR, "How Growing Up Can Alter Lab Values in Pediatric Laboratory Medicine," *Diag Med* (special issue), 1982, 5:13–8, with permission.

Mean Hematologic Values for Low–Birth–Weight Infants*

Weight and Gestational Age at Birth	Age at Testing	Hemoglobin (g/dL)	Hematocrit (%)	Reticulocytes (%)
<1500 g 28–32 wk	3 d	17.5 ± 1.5	54 ± 5	8.0 ± 3.5
	1 wk	15.5 ± 1.5	48 ± 5	3.0 ± 1.0
	2 wk	13.5 ± 1.1	42 ± 4	3.0 ± 1.0
	3 wk	11.5 ± 1.0	35 ± 4	—
	4 wk	10.0 ± 0.9	30 ± 3	6.0 ± 2.0
	6 wk	8.5 ± 0.5	25 ± 2	11.0 ± 3.5
	8 wk	8.5 ± 0.5	25 ± 2	8.5 ± 3.5
	10 wk	9.0 ± 0.5	28 ± 3	7.0 ± 3.0
1500–2000 g 32–36 wk	3 d	19.0 ± 2.0	59 ± 6	6.0 ± 2.0
	1 wk	16.5 ± 1.5	51 ± 5	3.0 ± 1.0
	2 wk	14.5 ± 1.1	44 ± 5	2.5 ± 1.0
	3 wk	13.0 ± 1.1	39 ± 4	—
	4 wk	12.0 ± 1.0	36 ± 4	3.0 ± 1.0
	6 wk	9.5 ± 0.8	28 ± 3	6.0 ± 2.0
	8 wk	9.5 ± 0.5	28 ± 3	5.0 ± 1.5
	10 wk	9.5 ± 0.5	29 ± 3	4.5 ± 1.5
2000–2500 g 36–40 wk	3 d	19.0 ± 2.0	59 ± 6	4.0 ± 1.0
	1 wk	16.5 ± 1.5	51 ± 5	3.0 ± 1.0
	2 wk	15.0 ± 1.5	45 ± 5	2.5 ± 1.0
	3 wk	14.0 ± 1.1	43 ± 4	—
	4 wk	12.5 ± 1.0	37 ± 4	2.0 ± 1.0
	6 wk	10.5 ± 0.9	31 ± 3	3.0 ± 1.0
	8 wk	10.5 ± 0.9	31 ± 3	3.0 ± 1.0
	10 wk	11.0 ± 1.0	33 ± 3	3.0 ± 1.0

*Mean ± 1 SD.

From Johnson TR, "How Growing Up Can Alter Lab Values in Pediatric Laboratory Medicine,"*Diag Med* (special issue), 1982, 5:13–8, with permission.

Critical Values Hematocrit <18% or >54%; hemoglobin <6 g/dL or >18 g/dL; WBC on admission <2500/mm^3 or >30,000/mm^3.

Use Evaluate anemia, leukemia, reaction to inflammation and infections, peripheral blood cellular characteristics, state of hydration and dehydration, polycythemia, hemolytic disease of the newborn; manage chemotherapy decisions

Limitations Hemoglobin may be falsely high if the plasma is lipemic or if the white count is >50,000 cells/mm^3. "Spun" (manual centrifuged) microhematocrits are approximately 3% higher (due to plasma trapping) compared to automated hematocrit levels. The increase is especially pronounced in cases of polycythemia (increased Hct levels) and when the cells are hypochromic and microcytic. The spun Hct level (as compared to Coulter S) may be 12% higher at Hct levels of 70% and MCV of 48 fL with decrease in change to 3% higher at Hct levels of 70% with MCV of 100 fL. Cold agglutinins (high titer) may cause spurious macrocytosis and low RBC count. This results when RBC couplets are "seen" and processed as single cells by the detection circuitry. Keeping the blood warm and warming the diluent prior to and during counting can correct this problem.

Methodology Varies considerably between institutions. Most laboratories have high capacity multichannel instruments in place (available from multiple commercial sources). The majority measure RBC and WBC parameters on the basis of changes in electrical impedance as cells and platelets are pulled through a tiny aperture. These are highly automated devices with extensive computer processing of the electrical signals after analog/digital conversion. Accuracy (with proper standardization) and precision (usually in the 0.5% to 2% range) is significantly improved over older manual and semiautomated methods. Some instruments count light impulses that are generated as cells flow across a laser beam.

Additional Information Presence of one or more of the following may be indications for further investigation: hemoglobin <10 g/dL, hemoglobin >18 g/dL, MCV >100 fL, MCV <80 fL, MCHC >37%, WBC >20,000/mm^3 WBC <2000/ mm^3, presence of sickle cells, significant spherocytosis, basophilic stippling, stomatocytes,significant schistocytosis, oval macrocytes, tear drop red blood cells, eosinophilia (>10%) monocytosis (>15%), nucleated red blood cells in other than the newborn, malarial organisms or the possibility of malarial organisms, hypersegmented (five or more nuclear segments) PMNs, agranular PMNs, Pelger-Huët anomaly, Auer rods, Döhle bodies, marked toxic granulation, mononuclears in which apparent nucleoli are prominent (blast type cells), presence of metamyelocytes, myelocytes, promyelocytes, neutropenia, presence of plasma cells, peculiar atypical lymphocytes, significant increase or decrease in platelets. Some quantitative elements of the CBC are related to each

Proposed Classification of Anemic Disorders Based on Red Cell Mean (MCV) and Heterogeneity (RDW)

MCV Low RDW Normal (microcytic homogeneous)	MCV Low RDW High (microcytic heterogeneous)	MCV Normal RDW Normal (normocytic homogeneous)	MCV Normal RDW High (normocytic heterogeneous)	MCV High RDW Normal (macrocytic homogeneous)	MCV High RDW High (macrocytic heterogeneous)
Heterozygous thalassemia*	Iron deficiency*	Normal	Mixed deficiency*	Aplastic anemia	Folate deficiency*
Chronic disease*	S/β-thalassemia	Chronic disease* chronic liver disease*†	Early iron or folate deficiency*†	Preleukemia†	Vitamin B$_{12}$ deficiency
	Hemoglobin H	Nonanemic hemoglobinopathy (eg, AS, AC)	Anemic hemoglobinopathy (eg, SS, SC)*		Immune hemolytic anemia
	Red cell fragmentation	Transfusion†	Myelofibrosis		
		Chemotherapy	Sideroblastic*		Cold agglutinins
		Chronic lymphocytic leukemia			Chronic lymphocytic leukemia, high count
		Chronic myelocytic leukemia			
		Hemorrhage			
		Hereditary spherocytosis			

*MCV alone <90% sensitive.
†RDW alone <90% sensitive.

From Bessman JD Jr, Gilmer PR, and Gardner FH. "Improved Classification of Anemias by MCV and RDW." Am J Clin Pathol, 1983, 80:324, with permission. The data for sensitivity of RDW and MCV in each disease category can be obtained from the authors.

other, normally, such that examination of the results of any individual analysis allow for the application of a simple but effective case individualized quality control maneuver. The RBC count, hemoglobin, and hematocrit may be analyzed by applying a "rule of three." If red cells are normochromic/normocytic, the RBC count times 3 should approximately equal the hemoglobin and the hemoglobin multiplied by 3 should approximate the hematocrit. If there is significant deviation from this relation, one should check for supporting abnormali-
(Continued)

Complete Blood Count *(Continued)*

ties in RBC indices and peripheral smear. The indices themselves offer a quick quality control check of the CBC. If patient transfusion can be excluded, then RBC indices should vary little consecutively from day to day. Anemias have been classified on the basis of their MCV and RDW (RBC heterogeneity). This classification has been especially helpful in the separation of iron deficiency from thalassemia. Heterozygous thalassemia has a normal RDW while RDW is high with iron deficiency.

In iron deficiency, the RDW is usually increased before the MCV decreases. Although this is somewhat controversial, it serves as an inexpensive screen for common iron deficiency anemia. See tables.

Selected Readings

Beautyman W and Bills T, "Osmotic Error in Erythrocyte Volume Determinations," *Am J Hematol*, 1982, 12(4):383-9.

England JM, Walford DM, Waters DA, et al, "Re-assessment of the Reliability of the Haematocrit," *Br J Haematol*, 1972, 23(2):247-56.

Fraser CG, Wilkinson SP, Neville RG, et al, "Biologic Variation of Common Hematologic Laboratory Quantities in the Elderly," *Am J Clin Pathol*, 1989, 92(4):465-70.

Computed Transaxial Tomography, Abdomen Studies

Synonyms Abdomen, CT; CT, Lower Abdomen; CT, Total Abdomen; CT, Upper Abdomen

Test Includes CT scan of liver, spleen, kidneys, pancreas, aorta, retroperitoneum, gastrointestinal tract, pelvis. **Note:** In some departments, a request for a CT study of the abdomen will yield a study extending inferiorly to the pubic symphysis. In others, the study will extend only to the pelvic brim.

Patient Preparation Patient's oral intake restricted to fluid only for 4 hours prior to the examination. Medication schedule should not be interrupted. Should the patient have recently undergone a barium examination of the gastrointestinal tract, a digital radiograph obtained with the scanner prior to commencement of the procedure may be helpful in excluding the presence of barium within the bowel. The latter may produce significant artifact and thus render the study nondiagnostic. Where possible, all CT scan studies of the abdomen should be performed prior to normal GI barium studies. A recent serum creatinine is requested on all patients 60 years of age and older, patients with known significant atherosclerotic disease, diabetes mellitus, or with pre-existing renal disease. Intravenous contrast material is routinely administered for this examination. Physician may opt to omit intravenous contrast. Patients undergoing a CT study of the abdomen are requested to drink approximately 450 mL of a dilute barium solution (approximately 1% barium) commencing 1 hour prior to the examination. Inclusion of the pelvis in this examination requires further patient preparation.

Special Instructions CT scan of the abdomen may be requested by a practicing physician. The abdominal area of interest should be specified along with pertinent clinical history. This will allow the diagnostic radiologist to tailor the examination for maximum diagnostic yield. For example, studies being performed for detection of renal calculi should be performed without contrast material, as the contrast, when excreted from the kidney, will mask the presence of small calculi within the collecting system. Adequate evaluation of small structures within the abdomen may require modification of technique such as thin slices or overlapping slices. A further example would be in the evaluation of the liver for primary or metastatic tumor. Maximum yield in the demonstration of such abnormalities requires examination both with and without contrast material.

Equipment This examination may be performed on any one of many commercially available computerized tomography scanners.

Technique Standard examination of the abdomen consists of 1 cm contiguous slices obtained from the dome of the diaphragm to the pelvic brim or pubic symphysis depending upon whether one groups the pelvis with the abdomen or treats it separately.

Causes for Rejection Patients with residual barium within the GI tract from a prior conventional barium study – this nondilute barium produces considerable artifact rendering the examination suboptimal and often nondiagnostic, uncooperative patients who are not candidates for sedation/anesthesia

Turnaround Time A verbal telephone report of the scan will be given to the referring physician if specified. A written report will be available.

Use Diagnosis and/or evaluation of cysts, tumors, masses, aneurysm, metastases, abscesses, and trauma. The modality is also often used for staging of known tumors.

Contraindications Patient cooperation is of the utmost importance as the examination requires the patient to remain motionless for the duration of the study. The time of the study will vary from 20-40 minutes depending on the equipment being used. Children and uncooperative adults may require sedation.

Additional Information Patients should be informed that the examination may take 45 minutes to 1 hour and that oral contrast and intravenous contrast are commonly required. If the pelvis is included with the abdominal CT study, rectal contrast material and placement of a vaginal tampon in the case of females may also be required. The patient's medical record should accompany the patient. This will furnish the radiologist with sufficient information to tailor the examination as he/she deems appropriate. For example, patients suspected of an adrenal adenoma may require thin (2 mm) slices through the adrenal glands for the detection of such an abnormality.

Selected Readings
Halvorsen RA Jr and Thompson WM, "Computed Tomographic Staging of Gastrointestinal Tract Malignancies, Part I. Esophagus and Stomach," *Invest Radiol*, 1987, 22(1):2-16.
Thompson WM and Halvorsen RA Jr, "Computed Tomographic Staging of Gastrointestinal Tract Malignancies, Part II," *Invest Radiol*, 1987, 22(2):96-105.

Computed Transaxial Tomography, Appropriate Site

Refer To
Computed Transaxial Tomography, Abdomen Studies
on previous page
Computed Transaxial Tomography, Head Studies *on this page*
Computed Transaxial Tomography, Paranasal Sinuses *on next page*
Computed Transaxial Tomography, Thorax *on next page*

Computed Transaxial Tomography, Head Studies

Synonyms Brain, CT; Head Studies, CT

Test Includes CT scan of the brain

Patient Preparation The examination should be ordered and a requisition with information pertaining to the reason for the request and the clinical history should be completed by the referring physician. If there is the slightest possibility that intravenous contrast material will be administered, the patient's oral intake should be limited to liquids for at least 4 hours prior to the examination. Care must be taken to ensure the patient does not become dehydrated and medications should not be interrupted. A recent serum creatinine is requested on patients with pre-existing renal disease, diabetes mellitus, significant atherosclerotic disease, and advancing age (60 years and older). Agitated patients and children may require sedation prior to the examination. In these cases, an order for the appropriate sedative and dose should be recently recorded within the patient's chart. Sedatives should be administered by a physician within the Radiology Department.

Equipment Any commercially available computed tomographic scanner

Technique CT scans of the head are usually obtained at 15° angulation to the orbitomeatal line, a line connecting the lateral canthus of the eye with the external auditory canal. Contiguous slices 8 or 10 mm in thickness are obtained from the vertex of the skull to the foramen magnum. The orbital roof should be included. The patient is positioned supine for the examination. The head is placed securely in a head holder. The chin is flexed comfortably towards the chest. The appropriate 15° angulation can be obtained by angulation of the gantry if necessary.

Use Evaluation of known/suspected primary or secondary neoplasm, cystic lesions, hydrocephalus, head trauma, seizure disorder, multiple sclerosis, atrophy, Alzheimer's disease, normal pressure hydrocephalus, Parkinson's disease, dementia, depression, organic brain syndrome, etc.

Contraindications Assuming a cooperative or quiescent patient, there are no absolute contraindications to a CT scan of the head. A decision must be taken, however, as to whether the study is to be done with or without intravenous contrast material. While each case must be assessed individually, the following broad guidelines may be helpful. Those studies indicated by virtue of a recent infarct, cerebrovascular accident or stroke, or those being done for assessment of atrophy, Alzheimer's disease, normal pressure hydrocephalus, Parkinson's disease, hydrocephalus, evaluation of an intraventricular shunt, assessment of ventricular size, subdural hematoma, or suspected dementia are examined without contrast material. Patients for whom the indication is

(Continued)

Computed Transaxial Tomography, Head Studies
(Continued)

headache, psychiatric condition (such as anorexia or bulimia), tumor follow-up, rule out tumor, rule out metastasis, multiple sclerosis, seizure disorders, depression, and organic brain syndrome are generally studied with contrast material. Patients in whom the indication is one of infection, abscess, meningitis, transient ischemic attack, arteriovenous malformation, remote subdural hematoma, or who have recently undergone a craniotomy and are being studied for postoperative evaluation are best studied with and without contrast material. Patients with a known diagnosis of plasmacytoma or multiple myeloma should not receive intravenous contrast material. Patients with compromised renal function may or may not benefit from intravenous contrast material. A recent serum creatinine and BUN will be helpful in deciding whether or not the latter group of patients receive contrast material.

Computed Transaxial Tomography, Paranasal Sinuses

Synonyms Paranasal Sinuses, CT; Sinuses, CT

Test Includes The examination is composed of contiguous 3-5 mm slices obtained from the inferior portion of the maxillary sinuses, cephalad to the superior extent of the frontal sinuses.

Patient Preparation Patients oral intake should be restricted to fluid for 4 hours prior to the examination. Medication schedule should not be interrupted. Administration of intravenous contrast material is at the discretion of the diagnostic radiologist. If a patient is being evaluated for trauma or inflammatory disease of the paranasal sinuses, no intravenous contrast material is usually administered. If a mass is identified in the course of the examination, or if a patient is known to have a tumor, then intravenous contrast material is usually given. Because of this, a recent serum creatinine is requested in all patients 60 years of age and older and those patients with known significant atherosclerotic disease, diabetes mellitus, or pre-existing renal disease. Children and uncooperative adults may require sedation.

Special Instructions If the nasopharynx is to be included in the examination, the study should be extended inferiorly to the hard palate or slightly below. The oral pharynx may be included by continuing to the base of the tongue. If there is a question of tumor invasion of the orbit from a sinus then coronal sections are very helpful.

Technique This examination may be performed in any one of many commercially available computerized tomographic scanners. Standard examination of the paranasal sinuses consist of 3-5 mm contiguous slices as previously described.

Turnaround Time Verbal telephone report of the scan will be given to the referring physician if specified. A written report will be available.

Use For the diagnosis and/or evaluation of tumors, masses, metastases, inflammatory conditions, and traumatic involvement. The modality is commonly used for staging of tumors.

Contraindications Patients who are not candidates for sedation/anesthesia, uncooperative patient; patient cooperation is of the utmost importance as the examination requires the patient to remain motionless for the duration of the study.

Additional Information Some departments offer a limited CT study of the paranasal sinuses which is competitive with plain film radiographs of the sinus in terms of pricing. This consists of 5 or 6 transaxial images through the sinus obtained parallel to Reid's baseline. The examination is achieved by obtaining a lateral digital image of the skull. From this the distance between the hard palate and the superior aspect of the frontal sinuses is measured. The distance is then divided by 5 or 6 to get the interslice distance. The slice thickness is 3-5 mm.

Selected Readings
Harnsberger HR, Osborn AG, and Smoker RK, "CT in the Evaluation of the Normal and Diseased Paranasal Sinuses," *Seminars in the Ultrasound, CT and MR*, 1986, 7:68-90.

Computed Transaxial Tomography, Thorax

Test Includes CT study of the chest extending from the lung apices to the posterior costophrenic sulci. The study may extend inferiorly to image the adrenal glands because they are a relatively frequent site of metastasis from primary lung carcinoma.

Patient Preparation The patients should be limited to a liquid diet for at least 4 hours prior to the CT examination. Medication schedules should be maintained. The use of intravenous contrast material may be required at the discretion of the diagnostic radiologist. Because of this, a recent serum creatinine is requested in all patients 60 years of age and older, and those patients with known significant atherosclerotic disease, diabetes mellitus, or pre-existing renal disease. In the case of children who need sedation, a recent (within 30 days) recording of the child's weight and a written order by the child's physician must be in the patient's medical record. All children should be accompanied by a responsible adult. Opacification of the esophagus with thick barium paste may be of value in some cases and administration should be at the discretion of the diagnostic radiologist.

Special Instructions The exam may be requested by a practicing physician. The area of interest must be specified along with pertinent clinical history and reason for the CT scan. The test should be complete in 10-30 minutes. Intravenous contrast material may be administered.

Equipment The examination may be performed on any number of commercially available CT scanners.

Technique A routine CT study of the chest consists of sequential 1 cm slices obtained from the apices through the posterior costophrenic sulci. The study may be extended to include the adrenal glands if a diagnosis of primary bronchogenic carcinoma is known or suspected. The technique may vary depending upon the indications for the study. The examination may be tailored by the diagnostic radiologist to answer specific questions. For example, the questionably abnormal pulmonary hilum on conventional films may require 5 mm contiguous sections subsequent to the intravenous administration of contrast material. The latter will facilitate enhancement of major vascular structures thus highlighting normal and abnormal anatomy. Similarly, densitometric evaluation of a solitary pulmonary nodule will require contiguous 2 mm slices throughout the nodule without intravenous contrast material. This maneuver will facilitate evaluation of the nodule for the presence and distribution of calcium within it. All modifications of the conventional contiguous 1 cm slice protocol throughout the chest are made at the discretion of the radiologist. The patient's medical record should accompany the patient to the department in order to ensure that the radiologist is furnished with sufficient information to tailor the examination appropriately.

Causes for Rejection Inability of the patient to cooperate is the major problem. Should the uncooperative patient not be a candidate for sedation and/or anesthesia, the study cannot be performed.

Turnaround Time A verbal telephone report of the scan will be given to the referring physician if specified. A written report will be available.

Use The examination facilitates evaluation of abnormalities of the lungs, mediastinum, pleura, and chest wall. Conventional PA and lateral views of the chest represent the basic screening tool in the identification of abnormalities involving the thorax. The axial anatomic display and superior density discrimination of computed tomography provides information pertaining to the extent of disease and more precise characterization of abnormalities initially noted on physical examination, chest films or on the barium swallow.

Contraindications Patient cooperation is of utmost importance as the examination requires the patient to remain motionless for the duration of the study. The time of the study will vary from 10-30 minutes depending on the equipment being used. Children and uncooperative adults may require sedation.

Selected Readings

Naidich DP, Zerhouni EA, Hutchins GM, et al, "Computed Tomography of the Pulmonary Parenchyma, Part 1: Distal Air-space Disease," *J Thorac Imaging*, 1985, 1(1):39-53.

Zerhouni EA, Naidich DP, Stitik FP, et al, "Computed Tomography of the Pulmonary Parenchyma, Part 2: Interstitial Disease," *J Thorac Imaging*, 1985, 1(1):54-64.

Conjunctival Smear *see* Ocular Cytology *on page 416*

Corneal Smear *see* Ocular Cytology *on page 416*

Cough Plate Culture for Pertussis *replaced by Bordetella pertussis* Direct Fluorescent Antibody *on page 282*

Cough Plate Culture for Pertussis *replaced by Bordetella pertussis* Nasopharyngeal Culture *on page 283*

Counterimmunoelectrophoresis for Group B Streptococcal Antigen *see* Group B *Streptococcus* Antigen Test *on page 354*

LABORATORY DIAGNOSIS

***Coxiella burnetii* Titer** *see* Q Fever Serology *on page 433*

Coxsackie A Virus Culture *see* Enterovirus Culture *on page 331*

Coxsackie A Virus Serology

Related Information

Enterovirus Culture *on page 331*

Specimen Serum

Container Red top tube or serum separator tube

Sampling Time Acute and convalescent sera drawn at least 14 days apart are required

Reference Range Less than a fourfold increase in titer in paired sera. Most healthy people do not have titers >1:8. Titers ≥1:32 are especially diagnostic. Titers ≤1:8 could represent cross reactions with other enteroviruses.

Use Establish the diagnosis of Coxsackie A virus infection, eg, in viral myocarditis

Limitations Neutralizing antibodies develop quickly and persist for many years after infection, making demonstration of a rise in titer difficult. There are at least 24 types/serotypes of Coxsackie A virus. Therefore, serotypes detected will depend on particular reagents used in a particular test. Consult the laboratory for serotypes detected.

Methodology Viral neutralization, complement fixation (CF)

Additional Information Coxsackie A virus produces a wide spectrum of disease including aseptic meningitis, myositis, encephalitis, respiratory illnesses, herpangina, hand-foot-and-mouth disease, rash, and generalized systemic infection. Documentation of infection by serology is difficult and diagnosis may depend on culture.

Selected Readings

Melnick JL, "Enteroviruses," *Manual of Clinical Laboratory Immunology*, 4th ed, Rose NR, de Macario EC, Fahey JL, et al, eds, Washington, DC: American Society for Microbiology, 1992, 631-3.

Coxsackie B Virus Culture *see* Enterovirus Culture *on page 331*

Coxsackie B Virus Serology

Related Information

Enterovirus Culture *on page 331*

Test Includes Coxsackie B_1, B_2, B_3, B_4, B_5, B_6 virus titers

Specimen Serum

Container Red top tube or serum separator tube

Sampling Time Acute and convalescent sera drawn 10-14 days apart are required.

Reference Range Less than a fourfold increase in titer in paired sera

Use Establish the diagnosis of Coxsackie B virus infection

Limitations Neutralizing antibodies arise quickly, last for years, and may make the demonstration of a rising titer difficult. Tests for complement fixing antibodies are insensitive and nonspecific. There are six types/serotypes of Coxsackie B virus. Consult the laboratory to determine if test detects some or all six types.

Methodology Complement fixation (CF), viral neutralization

Additional Information Coxsackie B virus causes a wide variety of clinical illness, including pleurodynia (Bornholm's disease), aseptic meningitis, carditis/myocarditis, rash, pulmonary infection, a generalized systemic infection, and several neonatal diseases and syndromes. Approximately 50% of clinical myocarditis and pericarditis is caused by Coxsackie B. Since culture is frequently unrewarding, diagnosis may depend on serologic studies.

Recently there has been interest in various viral assays for postviral fatigue syndrome. Antibody to Coxsackie B virus is not helpful in this assessment.

Selected Readings

Melnick JL, "Enteroviruses," *Manual of Clinical Laboratory Immunology*, 4th ed, Rose NR, de Macario EC, Fahey JL, et al, eds, Washington, DC: American Society for Microbiology, 1992, 631-3.

Miller NA, Carmichael HA, Calder BD, et al, "Antibody to Coxsackie B Virus in Diagnosing Postviral Fatigue Syndrome," *BMJ*, 1991, 302(6769):140-3.

Coxsackie Virus Culture, Stool *see* Viral Culture, Stool *on page 478*

Crab Lice Identification *see* Arthropod Identification
on page 268

C-Reactive Protein

Related Information

Sedimentation Rate, Erythrocyte *on page 440*
Serum Bactericidal Test *on page 441*

Synonyms Acute Phase Reactant; CRP

Specimen Serum

Container Red top tube or serum separator tube

Causes for Rejection Excessive hemolysis, chylous serum

Reference Range <8 μg/mL

Use Used similarly to erythrocyte sedimentation rate. CRP is a nonspecific acute phase reactant protein used as an indicator of infectious disease and inflammatory states, including active rheumatic fever and rheumatoid arthritis. Progressive increases correlate with increases of inflammation/injury. CRP is a more sensitive, rapidly responding indicator than is ESR. CRP may be used to detect early postoperative wound infection and to follow therapeutic response to anti-inflammatory agents.

Limitations Frozen specimens may give false-positive results; oral contraceptives may affect results

Methodology Agglutination, nephelometry, radioimmunoassay (RIA)

Additional Information CRP is a pentameric globulin with mobility near the gamma zone. It is an acute phase reactant which rises rapidly, but nonspecifically, in response to tissue injury and inflammation. It is particularly useful in detecting occult infections, acute appendicitis, particularly in leukemia and in postoperative patients. In uncomplicated postoperative recovery, CRP peaks on the third postop day, and returns to preop levels by day 7. It may also be helpful in evaluating extension or reinfarction after myocardial infarction, and in following response to therapy in rheumatic disorders. It may help to differentiate Crohn's disease (high CRP) from ulcerative colitis (low CRP), and rheumatoid arthritis (high CRP) from uncomplicated lupus (low CRP). When used to evaluate patients with arthritis, serum is the preferred specimen. There is no advantage to examining synovial fluid for CRP.

Selected Readings

Dowton SR and Colten HR, "Acute Phase Reactants in Inflammation and Infection," *Semin Hematol*, 1988, 25(2):84-90.
Van Lente F, "The Diagnostic Utility of C-Reactive Protein," *Hum Pathol*, 1982, 13(12):1061-3.

Creatinine Clearance

Related Information

Body Surface Areas of Adults and Children *on page 700*
Creatinine Clearance Estimating Methods in Patients With Stable Renal Function *on page 703-704*

Applies To GFR; Glomerular Filtration Rate

Replaces Urea Clearance; Urea Nitrogen Clearance

Test Includes Serum creatinine, urine creatinine

Patient Preparation Avoid cephalosporins. If possible, drugs should be stopped beforehand. Have patient drink water before the clearance is begun, and continue good hydration throughout the clearance.

Special Instructions Blood creatinine should be ordered at the same time. Requisition should state date and time collection started, date and time collection finished, patient's age, height, and weight.

Specimen 24-hour urine and serum; test can be done for shorter periods

Container Plastic urine container and red top tube

Collection Instruct the patient to void at 8 AM and discard the specimen. Then collect all urine including the final specimen voided at the end of the 24-hour collection period, ie, 8 AM the next morning. Keep specimen on ice during collection. Bottle must be labeled with patient's name, date and time for a 24-hour collection.

Especially for creatinine clearance, accuracy and precision of collection are important. Complete, carefully timed (usually 24-hour) collection is needed; 4-hour and 12-hour collections are acceptable.

Storage Instructions Refrigerate

Causes for Rejection No blood creatinine ordered, urine specimen not timed

(Continued)

311

Creatinine Clearance *(Continued)*

Reference Range Child: 70-140 mL/min/1.73 m² (SI: 1.17-2.33 mL/s/1.73 m²); adult male: 85-125 mL/min/1.73 m² (SI: 1.42-2.08 mL/s/1.73 m²); adult female: 75-115 mL/min/1.73 m² (SI: 1.25-1.92 mL/s/1.73 m²)

Use Renal function test to estimate glomerular filtration rate (GFR), to evaluate renal function in small or wasted subjects, to follow possible progression of renal disease, to adjust dosages of medications in which renal excretion is pivotal (eg, aminoglycosides, methotrexate, cisplatin).

Limitations Exercise may cause increased creatinine clearance. The glomerular filtration rate is substantially increased in pregnancy. Ascorbic acid, ketone bodies (acetoacetate), hydantoin, numerous cephalosporins and glucose may influence creatinine determinations. Trimethoprim, cimetidine, quinine, quinidine, procainamide reduce creatinine excretion. Icteric samples, lipemia and hemolysis may interfere with determination of creatinine.

Since tubular secretion of creatinine is fractionally more important in progressing renal failure, the creatinine clearance overestimates GFR with high serum creatinine levels.

While ingestion of meats may cause some increase in creatinine excretion, in practice this seems to make little difference. Intraindividual variation in creatinine clearance is about 15%. Males excrete more creatinine and have slightly higher clearance than females.

Methodology Jaffé reaction (alkaline picrate). The calculation for corrected creatinine clearance in mL/minute: = [(urine volume per minute x urine creatinine)/serum creatinine] x (1.73/surface area of body in square meters). Body surface area is obtained from nomograms which require age, height, and weight. See Appendix table, Body Surface Area of Adults and Children.

Additional Information Glomerular filtration rate declines about 10% per decade after age 50. Some patients with significant impairment of glomerular filtration rate have only slightly elevated serum creatinine.

Creatinine clearance is calculated on the basis of the surface area of the patient. The estimated error of determining creatinine clearance utilizing serum and 24-hour urine collection has been found to be in the range of 10% to 15%.

Any test requiring a 24-hour urine collection may also be run on this specimen, eg, protein, quantitative, 24-hour urine.

Selected Readings
Levey AS, Perrone RD, and Madias NE, "Serum Creatinine and Renal Function," *Annu Rev Med*, 1988, 39:465-90.

Luke DR, Halstenson CE, Opsahl JA, et al, "Validity of Creatinine Clearance Estimates in the Assessment of Renal Function," *Clin Pharmacol Ther*, 1990, 48(5):503-8.

Van Lente F and Suit P, "Assessment of Renal Function by Serum Creatinine and Creatinine Clearance: Glomerular Filtration Rate Estimated by Four Procedures," *Clin Chem*, 1989, 35(12):2326-30.

Creatinine Clearance Estimating Methods in Patients With Stable Renal Function *see page 703*

CRP *see* C-Reactive Protein *on previous page*

Cryptococcal Antigen Serology, Serum or Cerebrospinal Fluid

Related Information
Cryptococcus Serology *on next page*
Fungus Culture, Cerebrospinal Fluid *on page 342*
India Ink Preparation *on page 373*

Synonyms Cerebrospinal Fluid Cryptococcal Latex Agglutination; *Cryptococcus* Antigen, Blood; *Cryptococcus* Latex Antigen Agglutination; Spinal Fluid Cryptococcal Latex Agglutination

Test Includes Testing patient's serum or CSF for the presence of cryptococcal antigen (with rheumatoid factor/nonspecific control)

Abstract Cryptococcal antigen testing is the single most useful diagnostic test for cryptococcal meningitis.

Specimen Serum or cerebrospinal fluid

Container Red top tube, sterile CSF tube

Reference Range Negative

Use Establish the diagnosis of *Cryptococcus neoformans* infection

Limitations False-positive results can occur in patients with rheumatoid arthritis, but test controls usually eliminate this possibility. The test is less frequently positive in serum than in CSF. Disseminated cryptococcal infections usually result in a positive serum test. False-negatives occur.

Methodology Latex agglutination with rheumatoid factor/nonspecific control and in some laboratories pronase pretreatment.

Additional Information Presence of cryptococcal capsular polysaccharide is indicative of cryptococcosis. Samples should either be treated to remove rheumatoid factor and other interfering factors or tested to distinguish between positivity due to cryptococcal antigen and that due to interfering factors. If this distinction cannot be made the test cannot be interpreted. Pretreatment of the specimen with pronase reduces false-positives and increases the likelihood of positivity of the method.

The cryptococcal antigen test is positive in about 85% to 90% of cases of cryptococcal meningitis, while the India ink test is positive in ≤50%. The cryptococcal antigen test has been reported to be able to detect antigen in 95% of AIDS patients with cryptococcal disease. Culture of cerebrospinal fluid for fungus should be performed in patients who are suspected of having cryptococcosis.

Selected Readings

Gray LD and Roberts GD, "Experience With the Use of Pronase to Eliminate Interference Factors in the Latex Agglutination Test for Cryptococcal Antigen," *J Clin Microbiol*, 1988, 26(11):2450-1.

Greenlee JE, "Approach to Diagnosis of Meningitis – Cerebrospinal Fluid Evaluation," *Infect Dis Clin North Am*, 1990, 4(4):583-98.

Kaufman L and Reiss E, "Serodiagnosis of Fungal Diseases," *Manual of Clinical Laboratory Immunology*, 4th ed, Rose NR, de Macario EC, Fahey JL, et al, eds, Washington, DC: American Society for Microbiology, 1992, 506-28.

Cryptococcosis, IFA *see Cryptococcus* Serology *on this page*

Cryptococcosis, Indirect Fluorescent Antibody Titer *see Cryptococcus* Serology *on this page*

***Cryptococcus* Antigen, Blood** *see* Cryptococcal Antigen Serology, Serum or Cerebrospinal Fluid *on previous page*

***Cryptococcus* Latex Antigen Agglutination** *see* Cryptococcal Antigen Serology, Serum or Cerebrospinal Fluid *on previous page*

***Cryptococcus* Preparation** *see* India Ink Preparation *on page 373*

Cryptococcus Serology

Related Information

Cryptococcal Antigen Serology, Serum or Cerebrospinal Fluid
   on previous page

Synonyms Cryptococcosis, IFA; Cryptococcosis, Indirect Fluorescent Antibody Titer

Special Instructions Sequential assays may be desirable

Specimen Serum

Container Red top tube or serum separator tube

Reference Range Negative

Use Useful in the diagnosis and prognosis of cryptococcal infections

Limitations A negative test result does not rule out infection because an antibody response may be reduced by circulating antigen bound to antibody. Cross reactions of the IFA test have been reported with blastomycosis, histoplasmosis, and some other fungal infections.

Methodology Tube agglutination, indirect fluorescent antibody

Additional Information Antibody titers ≥1:2 are suggestive of infection with *Cryptococcus neoformans*. Antibody can be detected early in the course of the disease, but if the disease progresses, excess antigen may be produced and render antibodies undetectable. With effective chemotherapy, the antigen titer declines and antibody may once again be demonstrated. Antibodies may persist for long periods even after cessation of chemotherapy.

Selected Readings

Heyworth MF, "Immunology of *Giardia* and *Cryptosporidium* Infections," *J Infect Dis*, 1992, 166(3):465-72.

Kaufman L and Reiss E, "Serodiagnosis of Fungal Diseases," *Manual of Clinical Laboratory Immunology*, 4th ed, Rose NR, de Macario EC, Fahey JL, et al, eds, Washington, DC: American Society for Microbiology, 1992, 506-28.

***Cryptococcus* Stain** *see* India Ink Preparation *on page 373*

LABORATORY DIAGNOSIS

Cryptosporidium Diagnostic Procedures, Stool
Related Information
Fecal Leukocyte Stain *on page 334*

Synonyms Acid-Fast Stain, Modified, *Cryptosporidium*

Test Includes Examination of stool for the presence of *Cryptosporidium*

Special Instructions Procedures for the detection of *Cryptosporidium* in humans have recently become available in most clinical laboratories. Consult the laboratory regarding availability of the procedure and specific specimen collection instructions before collecting the specimen.

Specimen Fresh stool; stool preserved with 10% formalin or sodium acetate-acetic acid formalin preservative

Container Stool container with lid

Collection Transport fresh specimen to laboratory promptly following collection. Specimen on outside of container poses excessive risk of contamination to laboratory personnel.

Reference Range Negative

Use A part of the differential work-up of diarrhea, particularly in immunocompromised hosts and suspected AIDS patients; establish the diagnosis of cryptosporidiosis by demonstration of the oocysts

Limitations The organisms are most readily demonstrated in diarrheal stools. Forms of *Blastocystis hominis* may cause confusion if Giemsa stain is used. Most recommended procedures cannot be performed on polyvinyl alcohol (PVA) preserved specimens.

Methodology Phase contrast microscopy after floatation concentration technique (Sheather's method) is not particularly sensitive; modified acid-fast stain on air-dried smears. Auramine and carbol-fuchsin stain is used by some laboratories for screening. An immunofluorescence test is also available.

Additional Information *Cryptosporidium* is a coccidian parasite of the intestines and respiratory tract of many animals including mice, sheep, snakes, turkeys, chickens, monkeys, and domestic cats. It is a cause of severe and chronic diarrhea in patients with hypogammaglobulinemia and the acquired immune deficiency syndrome. The organism is widely recognized as a disease of the immunocompromised patient, however it can also cause disease in immunocompetent patients. Animal contact, travel to an endemic area, living in a rural environment, and day care attendance by toddlers have been recognized as risk factors for the development of cryptosporidiosis. Perinatal infection has been reported. Children are more prone to develop infection than are adults. In children, the disease is a self-limited gastroenteritis; in immunocompromised patients a profound enteropathy results. There is a seasonal variation in incidence with the highest frequency reported in summer and autumn. The organism can be demonstrated in biopsies of small bowel and colon, adherent to surface of the epithelial cells (Giemsa stain). Most therapeutic regimens for cryptosporidiosis are not successful unless immunosuppression is reversed.

Selected Readings
Baron EJ, Schenone C, and Tanenbaum B, "Comparison of Three Methods for Detection of *Cryptosporidium* Oocysts in a Low-Prevalence Population," *J Clin Microbiol*, 1989, 27(1):223-4.

Current WL, "The Biology of *Cryptosporidium*," *Am Soc Microbiol News*, 1988, 54:605-11, (review).

Current WL and Garcia LS, "Cryptosporidiosis," *Clin Microbiol Rev*, 1991, 4(3):325-58.

Petersen C, "Cryptosporidiosis in Patients Infected With the Human Immunodeficiency Virus," *Clin Infect Dis*, 1992, 15(6):903-9.

Soave R and Armstrong D, "*Cryptosporidium* and Cryptosporidiosis," *Rev Infect Dis*, 1986, 8(6):1012-23.

Crystals, Urine *see* Urinalysis *on page 467*

CSF Analysis *see* Cerebrospinal Fluid Analysis *on page 288*

CSF Fungus Culture *see* Fungus Culture, Cerebrospinal Fluid *on page 342*

CSF Mycobacteria Culture *see* Mycobacteria Culture, Cerebrospinal Fluid *on page 405*

CSF VDRL *see* VDRL, Cerebrospinal Fluid *on page 475*

CT, Lower Abdomen *see* Computed Transaxial Tomography, Abdomen Studies *on page 306*

CT, Total Abdomen *see* Computed Transaxial Tomography, Abdomen Studies *on page 306*

CT, Upper Abdomen *see* Computed Transaxial Tomography, Abdomen Studies *on page 306*

Culdocentesis *see* Cytology, Body Fluids *on page 318*

Culture, Biopsy *see* Aerobic Culture, Body Fluid *on page 244*

Culture, Biopsy *see* Biopsy Culture, Routine *on page 270*

Culture, Blood *see* Blood Culture, Aerobic and Anaerobic *on page 271*

Culture for *Leptospira* *see* Leptospira Culture *on page 384*

Culture, HSV Only *see* Herpes Simplex Virus Isolation, Rapid *on page 366*

Culture, *Legionella pneumophila* *see* Legionella pneumophila Culture *on page 381*

CXR *see* Chest Films *on page 293*

Cyst Culture, Aerobic *see* Biopsy Culture, Routine *on page 270*

Cyst Culture, Anaerobic *see* Anaerobic Culture *on page 250*

Cyst Culture, Fungus *see* Fungus Culture, Biopsy *on page 340*

Cystometrogram, Simple

Synonyms CMG; Cystometry; Filling Cystometrogram; Simple CMG; Urodynamic Testing of Bladder Function

Test Includes Bedside evaluation of urinary bladder function in selected patients with urinary incontinence or retention. The bladder is passively filled with sterile water through a transurethral Foley catheter. Intravesical pressures are measured with an open manometer as bladder volume increases. Information regarding bladder sensation, capacity, and contractility is obtained.

Patient Preparation Technique and risks of the procedure are explained to the patient and consent is obtained. Ideally, patient should be off sedatives, cholinergics, or anticholinergics prior to testing. Indwelling Foley catheters should be removed well in advance so that residual volume may be measured. No pain medications or anxiolytics are routinely necessary. Patient is asked to void, if possible, immediately prior to procedure.

Aftercare No specific postprocedure restrictions are required and previous activity level may be resumed. At physician discretion, a urinalysis (and possibly urine culture) may be ordered on follow-up, 48-72 hours later.

Special Instructions Simple cystometry may be easily performed by a trained nurse or physician assistant and in most cases does not require direct physician supervision. This is a considerable advantage over complex cystometry which is usually performed in the Urodynamics Laboratory.

Complications This procedure is considered relatively safe. The vast majority of patients tolerate simple cystometry with minimal problems. Reported complications are similar to those seen with straight catheterization, such as local urethral discomfort, hematuria, and urinary tract infection. The precise complication rate is not known, but in one study involving 171 incontinent geriatric patients, <8% developed new urinary symptoms consistent with infection and <2% required antibiotic therapy.

Equipment Standard Foley catheter or 14F red rubber catheter required. Alternatively, a 3-channel Foley catheter (often used for bladder irrigation) may be used. Also needed are a urinary catheterization tray (drapes, lubricant, iodine, gloves, syringes, etc), Y-connector, 50 mL syringe (sterile water in graduated container, sterile tubing, nonsterile measuring basin. An open manometer, such as a spinal manometer, is commonly used.

Technique Numerous minor variations in technique have been described with the choice depending on physician preference and patient logistics. In its simplest form, a manometer is not used. After voiding, patient is placed in supine position and a Foley catheter (or 14F red rubber straight catheter) is inserted transurethrally into the bladder. Residual urine volume is measured and the catheter is left in place. With the bladder empty, the patient is requested to relax completely and avoid all bladder or abdominal contractions for the remainder of the procedure. The inner piston of a 50 mL syringe is removed and the syringe tip inserted into the distal (open) end of the catheter. Using the syringe as a funnel, room temperature sterile water is infused through the syringe and catheter in 50 mL increments. The syringe is elevated so the highest level of the fluid column is always 15 cm above the symphysis pubis. Thus, fluid en-

(Continued)

315

Cystometrogram, Simple *(Continued)*

ters the bladder by gravity drainage and not forcibly by syringe pressure. After each 50 mL water, the height of the water column is observed. Patient subjectively reports first perceptible sensation of bladder fullness and first strong urge to void. When patient notes a strong voiding urge, additional volume is added in 25 mL increments until discomfort is reported or an involuntary bladder contraction occurs. A bladder contraction appears as a sharp and sustained rise in the water column despite attempted voluntary bladder relaxation (and may be seen at any time during the procedure). The procedure is terminated at this stage. This brief sequence of maneuvers has been described in several formal studies comparing simple and complex multichannel cystometry. A common and time-honored variation of this procedure requires the use of a spinal manometer. Initial steps are identical. After residual volume is measured, a Y-connector is attached to the distal end of the Foley. Through one arm of the Y-connector, sterile water in a calibrated reservoir is instilled by gravity drainage. The other arm is connected to an open spinal manometer via sterile connecting tubing. An anaeroid manometer (Lewis cystometer) may also be used. Pressure within the tubing system is "bled off" into the manometer port. As water incrementally fills the bladder, increasing intravesicular pressure is transmitted back through the tubing and is crudely estimated by the height of the water column in the manometer. A plot of bladder pressure versus volume may be constructed in this manner. Alternatively, a 3-channel Foley may be used. Again, fluid is introduced through 1-catheter channel, but in this technique the spinal manometer is connected to a physically separate channel. This allows more accurate intravesical pressure estimations. When bladder pressure is measured in the fluid in the flow channel (as in the Y-connector arrangement), several confounding variables are introduced, such as the internal resistance to fluid in the catheter. Some of these variables are eliminated by this simple maneuver.

Data Acquired
- residual volume (mL)
- threshold for sensation of bladder fullness (mL) – the volume at which patient reports first sensation of fullness
- maximum cystometric capacity (mL) – the volume at which patient describes a strong urge to void, or the volume just prior to an involuntary contraction
- bladder contractility (presence and number of involuntary bladder contractions, as defined)

If a manometer is used, additional data includes:
- pressure-volume characteristics of the bladder during filling, this is termed the cystometrogram – bladder pressure (ordinate) plotted against volume (abscissa)
- bladder compliance, defined as $\Delta V/\Delta P$ and is derived from the cystometrogram

Reference Range Approximated as follows:
- residual volume – usually minimal or no urine obtained
- threshold for sensation of bladder fullness, 100-200 mL
- maximum capacity, 400-500 mL
- bladder contractility, no involuntary contractions noted
- cystometrogram, normally divided into the following four phases: (see figure)

Phase 1: Initial pressure rise, stabilizes at the initial filling pressure or "resting pressure," normally approximately 10 cm H_2O.

Phase 2: The tonus limb, where compliance is high; pressure normally is low and remains constant as volume increases.

Phase 3: The limit of bladder elastic properties; increasing volume causes marked pressure increases. Patient normally can still voluntarily control micturition, even though maximum bladder capacity has almost been reached.

Phase 4: Voluntary voiding (not tested with simple cystometry).
- compliance – normally very high in phase two of the cystometrogram (approaching infinity)

Critical Values Residual volume: Significant postvoid residual may result from sensory neuropathy, lower motor neuron (LMN) disease, or bladder outlet resistance (functional or mechanical).

Threshold of sensation: Decreased sensation (ie, threshold >200 mL) is seen with sensory neuropathies such as diabetes mellitus, tabes dorsalis, cauda equina syndrome, or normal variant.

Maximum capacity: Decreased in a variety of disorders including upper motor neuron (UMN) disease, fibrotic bladder (eg, tuberculous interstitial cystitis), dysfunctionalized bladder, etc. Increased capacity (>500 mL) is seen with sensory neuropathy, LMN disease, chronic obstruction, bladder "training".

Contractility: Involuntary contractions at volumes less than capacity are abnormal. This condition has been called "detrusor hyperreflexia" and "uninhibited" or "unstable" bladder. Increased contractility is found in various stroke syndromes, UMN lesions, hypertrophic bladder. Contractility is absent or weak in LMN lesions, sensory neuropathies, or voluntary inhibition.

Cystometrogram: Both the pattern of the tracing (pressure vs volume) and the absolute values should be compared against a standard normal curve. Some cystometrogram patterns may be diagnostic but tracings generated from simple cystometry are crude and may be difficult to interpret.

Compliance: A noncompliant bladder may result from a variety of disorders, including bladder wall fibrosis, bladder contraction, idiopathic male enuresis.

Use The exact indications for simple cystometry are controversial. Even amongst urologists, considerable debate exists in the medical/surgical literature considering the optimal role of this procedure. Simple cystometry is useful in the patient with persistent urinary incontinence or retention felt to be secondary to impaired bladder filling or storage. Common clinical indications for this test include:
- suspected "neurogenic bladder"
- suspected detrusor motor instability, the hyperreflexive bladder
- suspected abnormalities in bladder sensation, capacity, or contractility
- the geriatric patient with persistent urinary incontinence of unclear etiology (controversial)

Simple cystometry is less useful in evaluating the following conditions:
- suspected stress urinary incontinence in the female
- suspected psychogenic urinary incontinence in the male
- suspected urinary obstruction in the male

Limitations Procedure has questionable utility in the diagnosis of voiding disorders due to structural abnormalities, such as stress urinary incontinence or prostatic hypertrophy with retention, or complex voiding disorders. By nature, passive filling of the bladder is nonphysiologic and may potentially alter measured variables (eg, bladder capacity) in yet-to-be-understood ways. Only urologic function related to the bladder is assessed. Urine flow, force, urethral function, and myoneural coordination are not tested. Numerous technical factors may lead to false-positive or false-negative results. As previously mentioned, intravesical pressure is only crudely estimated by spinal manometry and is limited by confounding factors, such as inflow tubing resistance. Phase 4 of the standard cystometrogram is not evaluated (ie, the voiding phase of

(Continued)

Cystometrogram, Simple *(Continued)*

micturition). Complex cystometry is required for this. Increases in intra-abdominal pressure will alter pressure readings. This is not controlled for adequately in this procedure. Increases in manometric pressure readings may be due to increased intravesical pressure, increased abdominal wall pressure, or both. Thus, any abdominal muscle contraction may be misinterpreted as a bladder contraction. Although the examiner may simply observe the patient's abdomen for signs of muscle contraction, this is imprecise. With complex cystometry this is avoided by simultaneously recording intravesical and anorectal pressures (which estimate intra-abdominal pressure). The cystometrogram generated by manometer readings is discontinuous and crude. Provocative measures (position changes, medications, etc) are not routinely performed. These are usually reserved for complex cystometry.

Contraindications
- patient refusal
- the demented patient with severe cognitive impairment; this procedure requires the patient to accurately report sensations of bladder filling
- inability to pass transurethral Foley catheter
- active urinary tract infection

Additional Information The main advantage of simple cystometry is its convenience and low cost in comparison with more complex urodynamic testing. It may be performed by a trained nurse in less than minutes and need not be done in a hospital setting. Thus, it has been advocated for the evaluation of the nursing home patient or the elderly clinic patient. Several studies have compared simple and complex cystometry directly. Sutherst and Brown (1984) found that simple cystometry achieved a sensitivity of 100% for bladder instability with 89% specificity (when compared with complex cystometry as a gold standard). Ouslander (1988) also showed a high degree of correlation between the two tests in terms of bladder capacity and stability. However, the role of cystometry has not been clearly defined. Some authorities believe that only a small percentage of patients with voiding disorders need to undergo cystometry. This subpopulation may be identified using statistically derived algorithms based primarily on historical and physical examination findings. Others feel that the urologic history is misleading often enough (or inaccurate in the demented geriatric patient) to justify frequent use of simple cystometry. In many cases, it is argued, management of a voiding disorder will be influenced by the objective results from cystometry. In all cases, test results must be interpreted in conjunction with the clinical suspicion.

Selected Readings
Hilton P and Stanton SL, "Algorithmic Method for Assessing Urinary Incontinence in Elderly Women," *Br Med J [Clin Res],* 1981, 282(6268):940-2.

Hinman F Jr, "Office Evaluation of Urodynamic Problems," *Urol Clin North Am,* 1979, 6(1):149-54.

Ouslander J, Leach G, Abelson S, et al, "Simple Versus Multichannel Cystometry in the Evaluation of Bladder Function in an Incontinent Geriatric Population," *J Urol,* 1988, 140(6):1482-6.

Sutherst JR and Brown MC, "Comparison of Single and Multichannel Cystometry in Diagnosing Bladder Instability," *Br Med J [Clin Res],* 1984, 288(6432):1720-2.

Tanagho EA, "Urodynamic Studies," *Smith's General Urology,* Tanagho EA and McAninch JW, eds, 12th ed, Chapter 21, Norwalk, CT: Appleton and Lange, 1988, 452-72.

Wein AJ, English WS, and Whitmore KE, "Office Urodynamics," *Urol Clin North Am,* 1988, 15(4):609-23.

Cystometry *see* Cystometrogram, Simple *on page 315*

Cytology, Body Fluids

Synonyms Body Cavity Fluid Cytology; Effusion, Cytology; Fluids, Cytology

Applies To Ascitic Fluid Cytology; Culdocentesis; Paracentesis Fluid Cytology; Pericardial Fluid Cytology; Peritoneal Fluid Cytology; Pleural Fluid Cytology; Synovial Fluid Cytology; Thoracentesis Fluid Cytology

Test Includes Cytologic evaluation of smears, cytocentrifuge preparations, filters, and cell block when indicated

Patient Preparation Patient should sign informed consent prior to procedure. Puncture site should be carefully cleaned and prepped as for any tap.

Special Instructions Add 1 mL of heparin per 100 mL of fluid anticipated (each mL of heparin contains 1000 units). Include pertinent clinical information on requisition - previous malignancy, drugs, radiation therapy, history of alcohol abuse, or infection suspected.

Specimen Fresh body fluid

Container 150 mL vacuum heparinized bottle

Collection Gently agitate the flask as fluid is collected to mix the heparin with the fluid

Storage Instructions After hours place in the refrigerator

Causes for Rejection Fixation of any type, improper labeling or requisition, gross contamination due to spillage, prolonged period (over 24 hours) at room temperature

Use To establish the presence of primary or metastatic neoplasms; aid in the diagnosis of rheumatoid pleuritis, systemic lupus erythematosus, myeloproliferative and lymphoproliferative disorders, fungal and parasitic infestation of serous cavities, and fistulas involving serous cavities. Examination of synovial fluid from a joint effusion may aid in the diagnosis of metabolic arthritis (gout or pseudogout), rheumatoid arthritis, or traumatic arthritis. Examination of effusion is more sensitive and specific than blind pleural biopsy in the diagnosis of malignant pleural disease.

Limitations Allowing fluid to stand for prolonged period before processing may cause deterioration and artifact. Cells in fluids of long duration may be degenerated on first tap and a second tap may be required after reaccumulation for best cytologic detail. Clots may contain diagnostic cells which are unavailable for sampling.

Contraindications Documented bleeding diathesis is a relative contraindication

Additional Information Fluids should be submitted **fresh, unfixed**, and **heparinized** to provide well-preserved, representative, diagnostic material. Exfoliated cells deteriorate rapidly in the effusion, both in and out of the body. The amount of heparin recommended is minimal but adequate to prevent clotting of body cavity fluids and act as a preservative, though excess amounts will not alter cytologic detail. Cytologic evaluation may include the type of neoplasm and suggest its site of origin. The more clinical information provided, especially prior malignancy, prior radiation or chemotherapy, and relevant clinical findings, the better the diagnostic yield.

Selected Readings

Dekker A and Bupp PA, "Cytology of Serous Effusions. An Investigation Into the Usefulness of Cell Blocks Versus Smears," *Am J Clin Pathol*, 1978, 70(6):855-60.

Frist B, Kahan AV, and Koss LG, "Comparison of the Diagnostic Values of Biopsies of the Pleura and Cytologic Evaluation of Pleural Fluids," *Am J Clin Pathol*, 1979, 72(1):48-51.

O'Hara MF, Cousar JB, Glick AD, et al, "Multiparameter Approach to the Diagnosis of Hematopoietic-Lymphoid Neoplasms in Body Fluids," *Diagn Cytopathol*, 1985, 1(1):33-8.

Spieler P and Gloor F, "Identification of Types and Primary Sites of Malignant Tumors by Examination of Exfoliated Tumor Cells in Serous Fluids," *Acta Cytol*, 1985, 29(5):753-67.

Wahl RW, "Curschmann's Spirals in Pleural and Peritoneal Fluids," *Acta Cytol*, 1986, 30(2):147-51.

Cytomegalovirus Culture

Related Information

Cytomegalovirus Culture, Blood *on next page*
Cytomegalovirus Isolation, Rapid *on next page*
Cytomegalovirus Serology *on page 321*

Synonyms CMV Culture; Viral Culture, Cytomegalovirus

Test Includes Culture for CMV only; CMV also is usually detected in a routine/general virus culture

Special Instructions Obtain viral transport medium from the laboratory prior to collecting the specimen.

Specimen Urine, throat, bronchoalveolar lavage, bronchial washings, lung biopsy

Container Sterile container; cold viral transport medium for swabs

Collection

Urine: A first morning clean catch urine should be submitted in a sterile screw cap container.

Throat: Rotate swab in both tonsillar crypts and against posterior oropharynx. Place swab in tube of viral transport medium, break off end of swab and tighten cap. This specimen is not particularly productive.

Storage Instructions Do not freeze specimens. Keep specimens cold and moist. Specimens should be delivered to the laboratory and handed to a technologist within 30 minutes of collection. If freezing is absolutely necessary, add an equal amount of 0.4 M sucrose-phosphate to the specimen before freezing.

Causes for Rejection Dry specimen, specimen not refrigerated during transport, specimen fixed in formalin, unlabeled specimen

(Continued)

Cytomegalovirus Culture *(Continued)*

Turnaround Time Variable (1-14 days) and depends on culture method used and amount of virus in the specimen

Reference Range No virus isolated

Use To aid in the diagnosis of disease caused by CMV (eg, viral infections, pneumonia, and organ transplant-related disease)

Methodology Inoculation of specimen into cell cultures, incubation of cultures, observation of characteristic cytopathic effect, and identification by fluorescent monoclonal antibody

Additional Information CMV infections are very common and are usually asymptomatic. CMV infections are frequently severe and life-threatening in immunocompromised patients including organ recipients and AIDS patients.

CMV is the most frequent cause of congenital viral infections in humans and occurs in about 1% of all newborns. Approximately 90% have no clinical symptoms at birth. Ten percent to 20% of these infants will develop complications before school age. Congenital infection may occur as a result of either primary or recurrent maternal infection.

Serology for the detection of cytomegalovirus is available, but the results are often of limited value unless a fourfold rise in titer can be documented.

Selected Readings

Griffiths PD and Grundy JE, "The Status of CMV as a Human Pathogen," *Epidemiol Infect*, 1988, 100(1):1-15.

Hodinka RL and Friedman HM, "Human Cytomegalovirus," *Manual of Clinical Microbiology*, 5th ed, Balows A, Hausler WJ Jr, Herrmann KL, et al, eds, Washington, DC: American Society for Microbiology, 1991, 829-37.

Landini MP, "New Approaches and Perspectives in Cytomegalovirus Diagnosis," *Prog Med Virol*, 1993, 40:157-77.

Yow MD, "CMV Infection in Young Women," *Hosp Pract (Off Ed)*, 1990, 25(3A):61-5, 69, 72-9.

Cytomegalovirus Culture, Blood

Related Information

Cytomegalovirus Culture *on previous page*

Cytomegalovirus Isolation, Rapid *on this page*

Cytomegalovirus Serology *on next page*

Synonyms Blood Culture for CMV; Buffy Coat Culture for CMV; Buffy Coat Viral Culture; CMV Culture

Test Includes Culture of buffy coat for cytomegalovirus

Specimen Blood

Container Heparinized syringe or green top (heparin) tube

Collection Heparinize a 2 mL syringe with sterile preservative-free heparin. Invert the syringe several times after the blood is drawn to mix the blood thoroughly with the heparin. As an alternative, two 10 mL heparinized tubes may be used if transport of a syringe is difficult.

Storage Instructions Do not store specimen. Transport to the laboratory immediately in sealed plastic bag with request form.

Causes for Rejection Excessive hemolysis, delay in transport, leaking syringes

Turnaround Time Positive cultures will be reported when identification is made. Negative cultures will be reported after 28 days.

Reference Range No virus isolated

Use Detect cytomegaloviremia

Limitations Yield of CMV from this specimen may be high in patients with the acquired immunodeficiency syndrome (AIDS), but significantly lower in non-AIDS patients.

Methodology Cell culture for isolation and identification by indirect fluorescent antibody (IFA)

Cytomegalovirus Isolation, Rapid

Related Information

Cytomegalovirus Culture *on previous page*

Cytomegalovirus Culture, Blood *on this page*

Cytomegalovirus Serology *on next page*

Synonyms CMV Early Antigen FA Method; CMV Shell Vial Method

Test Includes Inoculation of cell cultures in shell vials, 16-hour incubation, and immunofluorescence staining of CMV early nuclear antigen with monoclonal antibodies; conventional cell culture inoculation

Specimen Urine, bronchoalveolar lavage, blood, tracheal aspirates, appropriate autopsy and biopsy specimens

Container Sterile container; cold viral transport medium for swabs
Collection

Urine: A first morning clean catch urine should be submitted in a sterile screw cap container.

Throat: Rotate swab in both tonsillar crypts and against posterior oropharynx. Place swab in tube of viral transport medium, break off end of swab and tighten cap. This specimen is not particularly productive.

Turnaround Time Overnight to 2 days depending on method and capability of laboratory

Reference Range No CMV detected

Use Aid in the diagnosis of disease caused by CMV (eg, viral infections, pneumonia, and organ transplant-related disease)

Limitations The rapid shell vial method for the detection of CMV has been reported to be more sensitive than conventional cell culture.

Methodology Specimens are centrifuged onto cell cultures grown on coverslips in the bottoms of 1-dram shell vials. Centrifugation greatly accelerates virus attachment and penetration. After incubation, fluorescein-labeled monoclonal antibodies are applied to the infected cells to detect viral antigens that are expressed in the membranes of the cells. Characteristic fluorescent foci indicate the presence of virus.

Selected Readings

Gleaves CA, Smith TF, Shuster EA, et al, "Comparison of Standard Tube and Shell Vial Cell Culture Techniques for the Detection of Cytomegalovirus in Clinical Specimens," *J Clin Microbiol*, 1985, 21(2):217-21.

Smith TF, "Rapid Methods for the Diagnosis of Viral Infections," *Lab Med*, 1987, 18:16-20.

Cytomegalovirus Serology

Related Information

Cytomegalovirus Culture *on page 319*

Cytomegalovirus Culture, Blood *on previous page*

Cytomegalovirus Isolation, Rapid *on previous page*

Synonyms CMV-IFA; CMV Titer

Applies To CMV-IFA, IgG; CMV-IFA, IgM

Test Includes IgG and IgM testing of acute sera in neonates, patients suspected of post-transfusion CMV infection, immunosuppressed patients, and maternity cases; IgG testing of acute and convalescent sera

Specimen Serum

Container Red top tube or serum separator tube

Sampling Time Acute and convalescent sera drawn 10-14 days apart are required

Storage Instructions Store at 4°C or freeze.

Reference Range IgM <1:8 and IgG <1:16 is considered nondiagnostic. A fourfold increase in titer in paired sera drawn 10-14 days apart is usually indicative of acute infection.

Use Support the diagnosis of cytomegalovirus infection

Limitations Heterophil antibodies and presence of rheumatoid factor may cause false-positive IgM results. Fetal IgM antibody to maternal IgG may also cause false-positive results. Because of high levels of "background" antibody in adult populations, a single antibody determination is not useful. For rapid confirmation of new CMV infection, rapid shell vial culture for CMV is superior to serology.

Methodology Indirect fluorescent antibody (IFA), enzyme immunoassay (EIA)

Additional Information A single titer is rarely significant if past history is unknown. A fourfold or greater rise in CMV titer between acute and convalescent specimens is evidence of infection. A single IgM specific titer >1:8 is also excellent evidence of acute infection. CMV causes an infectious mononucleosis syndrome clinically indistinguishable from heterophil positive mononucleosis, a very common disease. Significant CMV titers are found almost universally in patients with AIDS, and CMV genome has been demonstrated in the cells of Kaposi's sarcoma. CMV is a significant cause of postcardiotomy, post-transplant and postpump hepatitis syndromes.

Although serology is a useful method to detect CMV infections, the newer shell vial culture can more reliably identify symptomatic CMV infections in immunocompromised patients.

Several new EIA tests agree well with the IFA serology and provide a more objective measure of infection status than the subjective IFA test.

Selected Readings

Bryan JA, "The Serologic Diagnosis of Viral Infections," *Arch Pathol Lab Med*, 1987, 111(11):1015-23.

(Continued)

Cytomegalovirus Serology *(Continued)*

Marsano L, Perrillo RP, Flye MW, et al, "Comparison of Culture and Serology for the Diagnosis of Cytomegalovirus Infection in Kidney and Liver Transplant Recipients," *J Infect Dis*, 1990, 161(3):454-61.

Van Enk RA, James KK, and Thompson KD, "Evaluation of Three Commercial Enzyme Immunoassays for *Toxoplasma* and Cytomegalovirus Antibodies," *Am J Clin Pathol*, 1991, 95(3):428-34.

Waner JL and Stewart JA, "Cytomegalovirus," *Manual of Clinical Laboratory Immunology*, 4th ed, Rose NR, de Macario EC, Fahey JL, et al, eds, Washington, DC: American Society for Microbiology, 1992, 563-7.

Darkfield Examination, Leptospirosis

Related Information

Leptospira Culture *on page 384*

Leptospira Serology *on page 385*

Mycoplasma pneumoniae Diagnostic Procedures *on page 408*

Synonyms Darkfield Microscopy, *Leptospira*; Leptospirosis, Darkfield Examination

Test Includes Examination of serum, urine, or CSF for organisms

Specimen Urine, serum, cerebrospinal fluid

Container Sterile plastic urine container, red top tube, or sterile CSF tube

Causes for Rejection Specimen dried out

Use Evaluate the presence of *Leptospira* to establish the diagnosis of leptospirosis. The failure to detect leptospires does not rule out their presence.

Limitations Culture for *Leptospira* is a more valuable and sensitive test. The concentration of leptospires in blood and CSF is low. Therefore, concentration by centrifugation with sodium oxalate or heparin can be useful. The incidence of false-positives is increased because fibrils and cellular extrusions can be mistaken for organisms. Extreme technical expertise is required.

Methodology A very small drop of fluid is distributed in a thin layer between a glass coverslip and slide. Positives should be confirmed by serologic or cultural methods. The typical morphology helicoidal, flexible organisms 6-20 μm long and 0.1 μm in diameter usually with semicircular hooked ends should be observed before a presumptive diagnosis is made. Artifacts are common.

Additional Information *Leptospira* are present in blood early in course of the disease (first week only). After 10-14 days they may be found in the urine. Urine must be neutral or alkaline. Culture has much greater value for diagnosis.

Darkfield microscopy is best used to demonstrate leptospires in specimens in which a high concentration of organisms is present, ie, tissue from animals (guinea pig or hamster), inoculation including blood, peritoneal fluid, or liver suspensions. Urine or kidney suspensions from swine, dogs, and domestic animals may also yield positive darkfield examination.

Selected Readings

Alexander AD, "*Leptospira*," *Manual of Clinical Microbiology*, 5th ed, Balows A, Hausler WJ Jr, Herrmann KL, et al, eds, Washington, DC: American Society for Microbiology, 1991, 554-9.

Darkfield Examination, Syphilis

Related Information

FTA-ABS, Serum *on page 336*

RPR *on page 438*

VDRL, Cerebrospinal Fluid *on page 475*

Synonyms Darkfield Microscopy, Syphilis; Syphilis, Darkfield Examination; *Treponema pallidum* Darkfield Examination

Test Includes Cleansing of chancre, procurement of specimen, and darkfield examination

Patient Preparation The surface of the chancre is cleansed and roughened by the physician with a swab or gauze moistened with saline. This removes exudate and excess bacteria contamination. Serum is then collected from the surface of the chancre using a small pipette. The serum is placed on a slide or coverslip. Alternatively, the specimen can be collected by directly touching the slide to the lesion. The object is to obtain clear serum exudate from the subsurface of the lesion. It is then examined by darkfield microscopy.

Specimen Moist serum from the base of a cleansed unhealed chancre. The youngest lesion available is best. The chance of identification of treponemes decreases with the age of the lesion as it dries and heals.

Causes for Rejection Healed chancre, previous treatment, ointment, dried up specimen

Reference Range *Treponema pallidum* has a rapid and purposeful motion as it travels across the microscopic field. The organisms appear as a tight cork-screw. The organisms are 1.0 to 1.5 times the diameter of an RBC in length.

Use Determine the presence of characteristic spirochetes in lesions suspected of being syphilis

Limitations Darkfield examination is of limited value in oral and rectal lesions because of the normal presence of other nonpathogenic spirochetes. Dry or bloody specimens render this examination worthless. The specimen should be examined within 15 minutes of collection because the organisms lose motility with decrease in temperature.

Contraindications Antibiotic therapy prior to the darkfield examination. The organisms are rapidly cleared following therapy.

Methodology Darkfield microscopy. Motile organisms are observed to rotate around their long axis and to bend, snap, and flex along their length. A smooth translational back and forth directed movement is also apparent.

Additional Information *Treponema* can be found in skin lesions and lymph nodes in secondary syphilis but are more plentiful in primary chancres. They cannot be grown in culture.

Selected Readings
Fitzgerald TJ, "*Treponema*," *Manual of Clinical Microbiology*, 5th ed, Balows A, Hausler WJ Jr, Herrmann KL, et al, eds, Washington, DC: American Society for Microbiology, 1991, 567-71.
Larsen SA, "Syphilis," *Clin Lab Med*, 1989, 9(3):545-57.

Darkfield Microscopy, *Leptospira* *see* Darkfield Examination, Leptospirosis *on previous page*

Darkfield Microscopy, Syphilis *see* Darkfield Examination, Syphilis *on previous page*

Davidsohn Differential *replaced by* Infectious Mononucleosis Serology *on page 374*

Deer Tick Identification *see* Arthropod Identification *on page 268*

Delayed Hypersensitivity Fungal Skin Tests *see* Fungal Skin Testing *on page 337*

Delayed Reaction Intracutaneous Tests *see* Anergy Skin Test Battery *on page 252*

Delta Agent Serology *see* Hepatitis D Serology *on page 361*

Delta Hepatitis Serology *see* Hepatitis D Serology *on page 361*

Dermatitis Herpetiformis Antibodies *see* Skin Biopsy, Immunofluorescence *on page 446*

Dermatophyte Fungus Culture *see* Fungus Culture, Skin *on page 343*

Direct Detection of Virus *see* Virus, Direct Detection by Fluorescent Antibody *on page 480*

Direct Fluorescent Antibody Smear for *Legionella pneumophila* *see* Legionella pneumophila Smear *on page 383*

Direct Fluorescent Antibody Test for Virus *see* Virus, Direct Detection by Fluorescent Antibody *on page 480*

Direct Immunofluorescent Studies, Biopsy *see* Immunofluorescent Studies, Biopsy *on page 372*

DNA Hybridization Test for *Chlamydia trachomatis* *see* Chlamydia trachomatis by DNA Probe *on page 297*

DNA Hybridization Test for *Neisseria gonorrhoeae* *see* Neisseria gonorrhoeae by Nucleic Acid Probe *on page 411*

DNA Probe for *Legionella* *see* Legionella DNA Probe *on page 381*

DNA Probe for Mycobacteria *see* Mycobacteria Culture, Sputum *on page 406*

DNA Test for *Chlamydia trachomatis* *see* Chlamydia trachomatis by DNA Probe *on page 297*

DNA Test for *Neisseria gonorrhoeae* *see* Neisseria gonorrhoeae by Nucleic Acid Probe *on page 411*

Eaton Agent Titer *see Mycoplasma* Serology *on page 410*

EB Nuclear Antigens *see* Epstein-Barr Virus Serology *on page 332*

EBV Culture *see* Epstein-Barr Virus Culture *on page 332*

EB Virus Titer *see* Epstein-Barr Virus Serology *on page 332*

EBV Titer *see* Epstein-Barr Virus Serology *on page 332*

Echocardiography, M-Mode

Synonyms M-Mode Echo; Unidimensional Echo

Test Includes M-mode echocardiography, the first form of cardiac ultrasound used in clinical practice, takes its name from the motion of the cardiac structures that was possible to visualize when this diagnostic method was introduced. M-mode echocardiography provides an "ice pick" view of the heart with a very high temporal and unidimensional space resolution, so that it provides an excellent method to measure chamber dimensions and to time cardiac events.

Patient Preparation No special patient preparation is required. Fasting is not necessary. The procedure can be done at any time. In scheduling patients that will have multiple cardiac diagnostic procedures it will be best to order the echocardiogram before Holter monitoring since the multiple electrodes placed on the chest for this procedure may interfere with the performance of the echocardiogram. Also, if a patient is to have a stress test on the same day, enough time (2-3 hours) should be allowed after the exercise test to perform the echocardiogram under basal conditions.

Special Instructions In most cases the M-mode echocardiogram is performed as part of a more complete cardiac ultrasound study that includes either 2-D echocardiography and/or Doppler echocardiography. The test that provides the most information should be requested, although sometimes this decision is left to the personnel in the Echo Laboratory. A complete cardiac ultrasound study takes anywhere from 60-90 minutes, the "M-mode" part of it takes approximately 30 minutes. To optimize the diagnostic yield of the echocardiogram a note relating the reason for the request should be made in the patient's chart or in a requisition form. Other useful information to be presented includes patient's age, weight, and height.

Technique A patient arriving at the Echo Laboratory is greeted by the laboratory personnel. He/she is asked about any previous experience with the procedure and is given a brief description of the test. Patient is asked to undress from the waist up and is given a gown with the opening in the front. Three electrodes for EKG monitorization are placed on the chest and the patient is asked to lie in a left lateral decubitus position. Currently, most M-mode echocardiograms are obtained by using a 2-D echocardiographic probe and selecting M-mode information from it. Briefly, the transducer is placed at the left parasternal border, the long axis view is selected, and the M-mode line is moved from the left ventricle to the mitral valve and finally to the aorta and left atrium. Recordings at these levels are registered in a strip chart recorder, a video recorder, or a page printer. These recordings become part of the report and of the Echo Laboratory file.

Reference Range Adequate interpretation of M-mode echocardiography requires knowledge of the normal values of the dimension of the cardiac chambers and great arteries (see table), and an understanding of the normal motion of the valves and different walls of the cardiac system. Distinct abnormalities can be characterized by M-mode echocardiography for many cardiovascular disorders.

Use The most common indications for this test include:
- wall thickness measurement of interventricular septum, posterior left ventricular wall and right ventricular free wall
- measurement of end-diastolic and end-systolic left ventricular internal dimensions
- percent of fractional shortening (difference between end-diastolic and end-systolic dimensions divided by end-diastolic dimension)
- measurement of right ventricular dimension; measurement of the anteroposterior diameter of the ascending aorta and left atrium.

M-mode echocardiography is **most useful** in:
- diagnosis of pericardial effusion

Normal M–Mode Echocardiographic Values

	Mean (cm)	Range (cm)
RVD	1.7	0.9–2.6
LVIDD	4.7	3.5–5.7
PLVWT	0.9	0.6–1.1
IVSWT	0.9	0.6–1.1
LA	2.9	1.9–4.0
AO	2.7	2.0–3.7
FS	36%	34%–44%

RVD = Right ventricular dimension
LVIDD = Left ventricular internal dimension in diastole
PLVWT = Posterior left ventricular wall thickness
IVSWT = Interventricular wall thickness
LA = Left atrium
AO = Aorta
FS = Fractional shortening

From Feigenbaum H, *Echocardiography,* 4th ed,
Philadelphia, PA: Lea & Febiger, 1986, with permission.

- left ventricular hypertrophy
- generalized left ventricular dysfunction
- hypertrophic obstructive cardiomyopathy
- mitral valve prolapse
- mitral stenosis
- left atrial myxoma

Contraindications There are no contraindications for M-mode echocardiography but patients with chronic obstructive lung disease or marked obesity will usually have tests of poor diagnostic quality.

Selected Readings
Sahn DJ, DeMaria A, Kisslo J, et al, "Recommendations Regarding Quantitation in M-Mode Echocardiography: Results of a Survey of Echocardiographic Measurements," *Circulation,* 1978, 58(6):1072-83.

Echovirus Culture *see* Enterovirus Culture *on page 331*

Echovirus Culture, Stool *see* Viral Culture, Stool *on page 478*

Ectoparasite Identification *see* Arthropod Identification *on page 268*

Effusion, Cytology *see* Cytology, Body Fluids *on page 318*

Ehrlichia Serology

Related Information
Rocky Mountain Spotted Fever Serology *on page 437*

Test Includes Antibody to *Ehrlichia canis*

Specimen Serum

Container Red top tube or serum separator tube

Sampling Time Acute and convalescent serum 14-21 days apart are recommended.

Storage Instructions Separate serum and refrigerate.

Causes for Rejection Inadequate labeling, excessive hemolysis, chylous serum

Use Establish the diagnosis of ehrlichiosis

Methodology Indirect fluorescent antibody (IFA)

Additional Information Newly recognized human ehrlichiosis is a disease caused by a Rickettsiaceae (*Ehrlichia*) family member which is well known for causing disease in animals. Human infection with an *Ehrlichia canis*-like organism was first described in the United States in 1986. Preliminary data suggest that human ehrlichiosis is tick-borne, and that most human cases present with symptoms suggestive of RMSF without the rash or as "spotless" RMSF. *E. canis* is found in white blood cells, in particular, polymorphonuclear leukocytes and mononuclear cells. During acute illness, intracellular inclusions (in monocytes) of *E. canis* can be observed on peripheral blood smears. IgG titers of

(Continued)

Ehrlichia Serology *(Continued)*

1:16-1:32 are considered equivocal while IgG titers ≥1:64 are indicative of *E. canis* infection. Titers which show a fourfold or greater increase in IgG or the presence of IgM against *E. canis* is indicative of recent or current infection. Serological testing for *E. canis* is performed only in research and specialty reference laboratories.

Selected Readings

Dawson JE, Anderson BE, Fishbein DB, et al, "Isolation and Characterization of an *Ehrlichia* sp From a Patient Diagnosed With Human Ehrlichiosis," *J Clin Microbiol*, 1991, 29(12):2741-5.

Eng TR, Harkess JR, Fishbein DB, et al, "Epidemiologic, Clinical, and Laboratory Findings of Human Ehrlichiosis in the United States, 1988," *JAMA*, 1990, 264(17):2251-8.

Goldman DP, Artenstein AW, and Bolan CD, "Human Ehrlichiosis: A Newly Recognized Tick-Borne Disease," *Am Fam Physician*, 1992, 46(1):199-208.

McDade JE, "Ehrlichiosis – A Disease of Animals and Humans," *J Infect Dis*, 1990, 161(4):609-17.

Rikihisa Y, "The Tribe *Ehrlichieae* and Ehrlichial Diseases," *Clin Microbiol Rev*, 1991, 4(3):286-308.

Elbow Arthrogram *see* Arthrogram *on page 267*

Elbow, Left or Right, X-ray *see* Bone Films *on page 277*

Electrodiagnostic Study *see* Electromyography *on this page*

Electromyography

Synonyms Electrodiagnostic Study; EMG

Test Includes Insertion of a needle electrode into skeletal muscle to measure electrical activity and assess physiologic function. In this procedure, percutaneous, extracellular needle electrodes are placed into a selected muscle group. Muscle action potentials (AP) are detected by these electrodes, amplified, and displayed on a cathode ray oscilloscope. In addition, fluctuations in voltage are heard as "crackles" over a loudspeaker, permitting both auditory and visual analysis of the muscle APs. Testing is performed with the muscle at rest, with a mild voluntary contraction, and with maximal muscle contraction (where recruitment pattern and interference are noted). Unlike nerve conduction studies, EMG does not involve external electrical stimulation. Muscle APs (normal or abnormal) are physiologically generated. In various diseases of the motor system, typical electrical abnormalities may be present: increased insertional activity, abnormal motor unit potentials, fibrillations, fasciculations, positive sharp waves, decreased recruitment pattern, and others. EMG assesses the integrity of upper motor neurons, lower motor neurons, the neuromuscular junction, and the muscle itself. However, EMG is seldom diagnostic of a particular disease entity. Its major use lies in differentiating between the following disease classes: primary myopathy, peripheral motor neuron disease, and disease of the neuromuscular junction. As with nerve conduction velocity studies (with which EMG is usually paired), EMG should be considered an extension of the history and physical examination.

Patient Preparation Details of procedure are reviewed with the patient. Considerable patient apprehension often accompanies "needle tests" and calm reassurance from the medical team will go far in allaying such anxieties. Aspirin products should be discontinued 5-7 days beforehand. Nonsteroidal agents should also be stopped several days in advance. Routine medications may be taken on the morning of the examination. If coagulopathy is suspected, appropriate hematologic tests should be ordered (PT/PTT, CBC, bleeding time, etc). If a primary muscle disease is suspected, creatine phosphokinase (CPK) level should be drawn prior to needle examination. Routine EMG testing may cause minor elevations in CPK up to one and one-half times baseline. However, striking elevations in CPK, as seen with polymyositis or muscular dystrophy, are not associated with EMG testing.

Aftercare No specific activity restrictions are necessary. Patient may resume previous activity level.

Special Instructions Requisition from ordering physician should include brief clinical history, tentative neurologic diagnosis, and the specific limb(s) or muscle group(s) in question. Physician should also state whether nerve conduction studies are desired, although in some centers these may be added at the neurologist's discretion.

Complications Local discomfort at the site of needle insertion is common. This is often mild in severity and has no significant sequelae. Pneumothorax has been rarely documented in the literature. This was associated with needle examination of paraspinal muscles. Transient bacteremia has been reported, but routine antibiotic prophylaxis for patients with high-risk cardiac lesions is not generally recommended.

Equipment EMG is performed in a specially equipped procedure room, usually reserved for electrodiagnostic studies. Basic instrumentation includes:

- needle electrodes; these may be monopolar (sharpened, coated steel wires), coaxial, or bipolar (two wires within a needle). These needles record electrical activity from muscle fibers directly contacting the tip, as well as fibers within a several millimeter radius.
- amplifier with filters
- cathode ray oscilloscope with the vertical axis measuring voltage, the horizontal axis measuring time. This device usually has an audio amplifier and loudspeaker, which converts APs to sound energy.
- data storage apparatus (eg, magnetic tape recorder)

Technique A brief neurologic examination is performed prior to the start of the procedure. For EMG of the extremities, patient lies recumbent on the examination table. When paraspinal muscles are tested, the patient adopts a prone position. No intravenous sedatives or pain medications are used. Local anesthesia is also not required despite the generous number of needle insertions. The skin is cleansed thoroughly with alcohol pads, as necessary. Patient is instructed to relax as much as possible. The following steps are carried out.

- Recording needle electrode is inserted percutaneously into the muscle under consideration. The initial electrical activity of the muscle, as seen on the oscilloscope screen and heard over the loudspeaker, is termed the **insertional activity**.
- Next, the needle is held stationary and the muscle action potentials during voluntary relaxation are recorded.
- Patient performs a mild, submaximal contraction of the test muscle. The summed muscle action potentials – the motor unit potential – are observed on the oscilloscope.
- Finally, a maximal muscle contraction is carried out. The compound action potentials generated during this maneuver are studied for **interference** and **recruitment pattern**.

Needle examination is, by nature, a slow and labor-intensive process. Numerous muscles must be tested individually including both symptomatic and clinically asymptomatic muscles. Within a specific muscle, several independent sites may need to be examined, particularly when the muscle has a large surface area. A number of myopathic processes are focal and sampling errors even within an individual muscle are possible (ie, disease process may effect proximal portion of a muscle, sparing distal fibers).

Normal Findings Results are interpreted by neurologist or physiatrist with preliminary impression written in chart immediately. A formal, typed report is completed several days later. The fundamental principles underlying test interpretation are as follows.

- Insertional activity: Immediately upon needle insertion, there is a brief burst of electrical activity lasting <300 msec. This "insertional activity" is heard over the loudspeaker and may be increased or decreased in various disease states.
- Electrical activity at rest: Muscle tissue is normally silent at rest. No action potentials are seen on the oscilloscope.
- Minimal muscle contraction: When a minimal contraction is performed, several motor unit potentials (MUPs) are activated. Several individual APs are normally visible on the oscilloscope at a rate of 4-5/second. The idealized configuration of a single MUP is depicted in the following figure (see normal column).
- Full voluntary contraction: As the strength of the muscle contraction increases, further muscle units are "recruited". On the oscilloscope the APs appear more disorganized and individual APs can no longer be recognized. At the peak of a contraction the "complete recruitment pattern" is seen, which represents a compilation of motor unit potentials firing asynchronously. The normal interference pattern is considered "full," that is, the amplitude of APs is high ($\leq$5 mV) and firing rate is fast (40/second).

Critical Values Abnormalities in one or more of the previously stated parameters may be seen.

Insertional activity: Increased in both neurogenic disorders (eg, lower motor nerve disease) and myogenic disorders (eg, polymyositis), and thus is consid-

(Continued)

Electromyography *(Continued)*

EMG FINDINGS

LESION / EMG Steps	NORMAL	NEUTOGENIC LESION		MYOGENIC LESION		
		Lower Motor	Upper Motor	Myopathy	Myotonia	Polymyositis
1 Insertional Activity	Normal	Increased	Normal	Normal	Myotonic Discharge	Increased
2 Spontaneous Activity	—	Fibrillation / Positive Wave	—	—	—	Fibrillation / Positive Wave
3 Motor Unit Potential	0.5-1.0 mV / 5-10 ms	Large Unit / Limited Recruitment	Normal	Small Unit / Early Recruitment	Myotonic Discharge	Small Unit / Early Recruitment
4 Interference Pattern	Full	Reduced / Fast Firing Rate	Reduced / Slow Firing Rate	Full / Low Amplitude	Full / Low Amplitude	Full / Low Amplitude

Idealized EMG findings, normal, neurogenic lesions, and myogenic lesions. Reproduced with permission from Kimura J, Chapter 13, "Types of Abnormality," *Electrodiagnosis in Diseases of Nerve and Muscle*: Principles and Practice, 2nd ed, Philadelphia, PA: FA Davis, 1989, 263.

ered nonspecific. Decreased insertional activity is less common, but may be associated with far advanced denervation or myopathy, especially when muscle is replaced by fat or collagen. A distinctive insertional pattern is seen with myotonia, an unusual neurologic disorder, and is termed "myotonic discharge".

Abnormal activity at rest: Instead of the electrical silence which characterizes the muscle at rest, spontaneous action potentials in single muscle fibers ("fibrillation potentials") may be observed in several disease states.

Fibrillations are seen 1-3 weeks after destruction of a lower motor neuron. Denervated muscle fibers develop heightened chemosensitivity and individual muscle fibers contract spontaneously. The phenomenon of "positive sharp waves" may also be seen. Fibrillations may also occur with severe polymyositis when extensive areas of necrosis interrupt nerve innervation. The naked eye is unable to perceive fibrillations.

Fasciculations represent random contractions of a full motor unit, often visible through the skin. (A motor unit is comprised of an anterior horn cell, axon, neuromuscular junction, and the numerous muscle fibers supplied by the axon.) Fasciculations may be benign, with no other EMG abnormalities observed. They may also be associated with amyotrophic lateral sclerosis, other anterior horn cell diseases, nerve root compression, herniated nucleus pulposus syndrome, acute polyneuropathy, and others.

Abnormalities in the motor unit potential (MUP): Individual motor unit potentials are distinguishable during a submaximal muscle contraction. Abnormalities in amplitude, shape (number of phases, serrations, configuration), and duration are possible. Increased MUP amplitude is seen in lower motor neuron disease but is normal in upper motor neuron disease. Decreased MUP amplitude is characteristic of polymyositis and other myopathies and duration of the MUP is also decreased.

Abnormalities in interference pattern: The normal "full recruitment" pattern seen during maximal muscle contraction is often compromised in disease states. In myogenic lesions, such as polymyositis and myotonia, the amplitude of the MUPs is significantly decreased but the recruitment pattern is normal (ie, the number of activated motor units is normal but the number of muscle fibers per motor unit is diminished). In LMN lesions, the number of motor units recruited is decreased. In severe cases of neuropathy, the maximum interference pattern resembles that of a single MUP, with individual potentials visible. Amplitude of MUPs may be normal. These findings are summarized in the previous figure.

Use In the neurologic literature, EMG has been performed in a wide variety of clinical situations, many of which are experimental or highly specialized in nature. Common indications for EMG in general practice include the following.

Evaluation of the patient with clinical features of primary muscle disease (symmetric and proximal weakness, muscle atrophy, intact sensory system, etc). Examples include:

- muscular dystrophy

- glycogen storage disease
- myotonia
- inflammatory myopathies (systemic lupus, sarcoidosis, infectious myopathies)
- polydermatomyositis
- alcoholic myopathy
- endocrine myopathies, and others

Evaluation of the patient with lower motor neuron disease, including:

- suspected peripheral nerve lesions, such as diffuse peripheral neuropathies, spinal root lesions, and trauma
- suspected disease of the anterior horn cells (characterized by asymmetric weakness, muscle atrophy, fasciculations), as in amyotrophic lateral sclerosis or poliomyelitis

Assessment of the patient with suspected upper motor neuron disease, when prior imaging studies are inconclusive. This includes occult lesions of the corticospinal tract (syringomyelia, tumor) and, less commonly, lesions of the cerebral tract (tumor, CVA). Evaluation of the patient with suspected neuromuscular junction disease (NMJ). This includes myasthenia gravis and the paraneoplastic Eaton-Lambert syndrome. Conventional EMG, as described here, is not the diagnostic test of choice for myasthenia gravis. However, other forms of EMG such as single fiber EMG and repetitive stimulation tests are highly specific for NMJ disease. Assessment of the patient with severe and persistent muscle cramps. Serial documentation of response to therapy for known cases of myopathy or neuropathy. Identification of significantly diseased muscle groups to help guide muscle biopsy (if clinical examination is not inconclusive). EMG is less useful in:

- the restless legs syndrome
- transient, self-resolving muscle cramps
- uncomplicated cases of polymyalgia rheumatica unless the diagnosis is in doubt or underlying myositis is suspected
- routine cases of fibrositis/fibromyalgia (EMG abnormalities have recently been documented in the medical literature but needle examination is not routinely indicated)

Contraindications The following situations represent relative contraindications:

- severe coagulopathy, including hemophilia and marked thrombocytopenia. It should be noted that EMG has been performed safely with platelet counts as low as 20,000/mm^3, but this is not recommended.
- systemic anticoagulation (eg, intravenous heparin, oral Coumadin®)
- patients with an unusual susceptibility to systemic infections (EMG has been known to cause transient bacteremia)
- patients undergoing a muscle biopsy after EMG require special consideration. It is well known that needle insertion and manipulation during EMG may cause local microscopic tissue damage on a traumatic basis. Histologically, this damage may be confused with a focal myopathy. Thus, some experts avoid detailed needle examinations of the specific muscle group which will be biopsied (although EMG testing of surrounding muscle groups is frequently performed).

Selected Readings

Adams RD and Victor M, *Principles of Neurology*, 4th ed, New York, NY: McGraw-Hill Book Co, 1989, 1009-27.

Aminoff MJ, *Electromyography in Clinical Practice*, 2nd ed, New York, NY: Churchill-Livingston, 1987.

Goodgold J and Eberstein A, *Electrodiagnosis of Neuromuscular Diseases*, 3rd ed, Baltimore, MD: Williams & Wilkins, 1983.

Griggs RC, Bradley WG, and Shahani B, "Approach to the Patient With Neuromuscular Disease," *Harrison's Principles of Internal Medicine*, 12th ed, Wilson JD, Braunwald E, Isselbacher KJ, et al, eds, New York, NY: McGraw-Hill Book Co, 1991, 2088-96.

Johnson EW and Wiechers D, "Electrodiagnosis," *Krusen's Handbook of Physical Medicine and Rehabilitation*, 3rd ed, Kottke FJ, Stillwell GK, and Lehmann JF, eds, Philadelphia, PA: WB Saunders Co, 1982, 56-85.

Kimura J, *Electrodiagnosis in Diseases of Nerve and Muscle: Principles and Practice*, 2nd ed, Philadelphia, PA: FA Davis Co, 1989.

Electron Microscopic (EM) Examination for Viruses, Stool

Synonyms EM Examination for Viruses; EM of Enteric Viruses; Enteric Viruses by EM; Gastrointestinal Viruses by EM

Applies To Rotavirus Detection by EM

(Continued)

329

Electron Microscopic (EM) Examination for Viruses, Stool *(Continued)*

Test Includes Direct visualization of virions

Special Instructions Laboratory must be notified prior to requesting examination of any specimen by EM.

Specimen Stool from the acute, diarrheal phase of disease

Container Sterile vial, tube, Petri dish, or stool carton

Sampling Time As soon as possible after the onset of disease

Turnaround Time Less than 1 day

Use Demonstration of viral particles (eg, rotavirus, Norwalk virus, calcivirus, astrovirus, and coronavirus) in stool specimens from patients with suspected viral gastroenteritis

Limitations Generally, EM visualization of virus particles is not as sensitive as is cell culture, except for detecting nonculturable viruses such as rotavirus. EM can detect viruses if they are present in quantities of 10^6 to 10^7 particles/mL. This sensitivity is appropriate for agents causing diarrhea but is not sufficiently sensitive for the detection of other potential pathogens.

It is often difficult to differentiate (by EM) the aforementioned viruses.

Methodology Diluted stool (either with or without being mixed with patient serum) is mixed with an electron-opaque heavy metal solution such as phosphotungstic acid. The stool solution is placed onto an electron-lucent grid support and examined by electron microscopy. Virions or virions agglutinated by specific antibodies (if present in serum) appear as a negative image against a black surrounding background.

Additional Information Very few clinical Microbiology/Virology Laboratories have access to electron microscopes.

Selected Readings
Christensen ML, "Human Viral Gastroenteritis," *Clin Microbiol Rev*, 1989, 2(1):51-89.

Drew WL, "Diagnostic Virology," *Clin Lab Med*, 1987, 7(4):721-40.

Gray LD, "Novel Viruses Associated With Gastroenteritis," *Clin Microbiol Newslett*, 1991, 13(18):137-44.

Miller SE, "Diagnostic Virology by Electron Microscopy," *Am Soc Microbiol News*, 1988, 54:475-81.

EM Examination for Viruses *see* Electron Microscopic (EM) Examination for Viruses, Stool *on previous page*

EMG *see* Electromyography *on page 326*

EM of Enteric Viruses *see* Electron Microscopic (EM) Examination for Viruses, Stool *on previous page*

Endocervical Culture *see* Genital Culture *on page 349*

Entamoeba histolytica Serology

Synonyms Amebiasis Serological Test

Patient Preparation Fasting blood sample required

Specimen Serum

Container Red top tube or serum separator tube

Reference Range IHA titer: <1:128; CF titer: <1:8; immunodiffusion test: negative

Use Diagnose systemic amebiasis

Limitations Sensitivity is highest in extraintestinal amebiasis, lower in amebic dysentery, and lowest in asymptomatic carriers. Some false-positives occur in patients with ulcerative colitis. Recently a serine-rich recombinant *Entamoeba histolytica* protein has proven to be a useful antigen to assist in the serodiagnosis of *Entamoeba* which has disseminated.

Methodology Complement fixation (CF), indirect hemagglutination (IHA), immunodiffusion (ID), indirect fluorescent antibody (IFA), enzyme immunoassay (EIA)

Additional Information Indirect hemagglutination is positive in 87% to 100% of patients with liver abscesses and more than 85% of patients with acute amebic dysentery. Fewer than 6% of uninfected individuals react in the test. Amebic serology when negative is strong evidence against amebic liver abscess. IHA titers of 1:128 or greater are considered to be clinically significant, and a fourfold rise in titer is diagnostic evidence. Although titers will decrease over time, serology may remain positive for as long as 2 years, even after curative therapy.

Selected Readings
Bruckner DA, "Amebiasis," *Clin Microbiol Rev*, 1992, 5(4):356-69.

Kagan IG and Maddison SE, "Serodiagnosis of Parasitic Diseases," *Manual of Clinical Laboratory Immunology*, 4th ed, Rose NR, de Macario EC, Fahey JL, et al, eds, Washington, DC: American Society for Microbiology, 1992, 529-43.

Maddison SE, "Serodiagnosis of Parasitic Diseases," *Clin Microbiol Rev*, 1991, 4(4):457-69.

Reed SL, "Amebiasis: An Update," *Clin Infect Dis*, 1992, 14(2):385-93.

Stanley SL Jr, Jackson TF, Reed SL, et al, "Serodiagnosis of Invasive Amebiasis Using a Recombinant *Entamoeba histolytica* Protein," *JAMA*, 1991, 266(14):1984-6.

Enteric Pathogens Culture, Routine *see* Stool Culture
on page 448

Enteric Viruses by EM *see* Electron Microscopic (EM) Examination for Viruses, Stool *on page 329*

Enterobiasis Test *see* Pinworm Preparation *on page 430*

Enterobius vermicularis Preparation *see* Pinworm Preparation
on page 430

Enterohemorrhagic E. coli, Stool Culture *see* Stool Culture, Diarrheagenic *E. coli on page 449*

Enteroinvasive E. coli, Stool Culture *see* Stool Culture, Diarrheagenic *E. coli on page 449*

Enteropathogenic E. coli, Stool Culture *see* Stool Culture, Diarrheagenic *E. coli on page 449*

Enterotoxigenic E. coli, Stool Culture *see* Stool Culture, Diarrheagenic *E. coli on page 449*

Enterovirus Culture
Related Information
Coxsackie A Virus Serology *on page 310*
Coxsackie B Virus Serology *on page 310*

Applies To Coxsackie A Virus Culture; Coxsackie B Virus Culture; Echovirus Culture; Poliovirus Culture

Test Includes Culture for Coxsackie A virus, Coxsackie B virus, echovirus, and poliovirus

Specimen Stool (best specimen), rectal swab, cerebrospinal fluid, upper and lower respiratory tract specimens, blood, throat swab (good specimen), various organs and tissues

Container Sterile container

Sampling Time It is important to obtain specimens very early in the disease; however, virus is shed in the stool for weeks.

Storage Instructions Enteroviruses are rather hardy; however, specimens should be refrigerated or placed into cold virus transport medium and delivered immediately to the clinical laboratory.

Causes for Rejection Dry specimen, specimen not in proper viral transport medium, specimen not refrigerated during transport, specimen fixed in formalin, unlabeled specimen

Turnaround Time Variable (1-4 days) and depends on culture method used and amount of virus in specimen

Reference Range No virus isolated

Use Aid in the diagnosis of disease caused by enteroviruses (eg, polio, congenital viral infections, and meningitis (aseptic))

Limitations Cell culture generally does not support the growth of Coxsackie A enteroviruses. Inoculation of suckling mice is the preferred method to isolate Coxsackie A virus.

Methodology Inoculation of specimens into cell culture, incubation, and observation of characteristic cytopathic effect. Specimens suspected of containing Coxsackie A virus are inoculated into suckling mice which are then observed for flaccid paralysis without encephalitis.

Some (usually reference) laboratories can identify specific enteroviruses by using a battery of specific enterovirus-neutralizing antibodies. These antibodies are useful in identifying and typing Coxsackie A, Coxsackie B, echovirus, and poliovirus.

Additional Information Infrequently, aseptic meningitis is caused by Coxsackie A virus types which require animal inoculation for isolation.

Selected Readings
Dowsett EG, "Human Enteroviral Infections," *J Hosp Infect*, 1988, 11(2):103-15.
(Continued)

Enterovirus Culture *(Continued)*

Menegus MA, "Enteroviruses," *Manual of Clinical Microbiology*, 5th ed, Balows A, Hausler WJ Jr, Herrmann KL, et al, eds, Washington, DC: American Society for Microbiology, 1991, 943-7.

Modlin JF and Kinney JS, "Perinatal Enterovirus Infections," *Adv Pediatr Infect Dis*, 1987, 2:57-78.

Moore M and Morens DM, "Enteroviruses, Including Polioviruses," *Textbook of Human Virology*, Belshe RB, ed, Littleton, MA: PSG Publishing Co, 1984, 407-83.

Enterovirus Culture, Stool *see* Viral Culture, Stool *on page 478*

Enzyme Immunoassay for Group A *Streptococcus* Antigen *see* Group A *Streptococcus* Antigen Test *on page 354*

EPEC, Stool Culture *see* Stool Culture, Diarrheagenic *E. coli* *on page 449*

Epstein-Barr Early Antigens *see* Epstein-Barr Virus Serology *on this page*

Epstein-Barr Viral Capsid Antigen *see* Epstein-Barr Virus Serology *on this page*

Epstein-Barr Virus Culture
Related Information
Epstein-Barr Virus Serology *on this page*
Synonyms EBV Culture
Applies To Lymph Node Culture; Lymphocyte Culture; Spleen Cell Culture
Test Includes Culture for EBV only
Special Instructions The laboratory must be notified prior to receipt of specimen.
Specimen Blood, lymph node, spleen, tumor biopsies, throat garglings (for isolation of excreted virus)
Container Green top (heparin) tube; sterile container
Storage Instructions Blood specimen can be maintained at room temperature but should be immediately transported to the laboratory. Biopsy specimen should be sent to the Virology Laboratory immediately after collection.
Causes for Rejection Dry specimen, specimen not in proper viral transport medium, specimen not refrigerated during transport, specimen fixed in formalin, unlabeled specimen, specimen not received in sterile container, excessive delay in transit to laboratory
Turnaround Time 4-6 weeks
Reference Range No growth of lymphocyte culture
Use Aid in the diagnosis of disease caused by EBV (eg, infectious mononucleosis, chronic fatigue syndrome, and Burkitt's lymphoma)
Limitations Cell culture for EBV is not diagnostically practical because it proliferates only in B lymphocytes. Cell culture requires at least 4 weeks, and the virus is ubiquitous in humans.
Methodology Virus is given opportunity to grow for 4 weeks in a lymphocyte culture. Virus-infected cells will proliferate; if virus is not present, lymphocytes will die.
Additional Information Viral serology (usually immunofluorescence) is the preferred diagnostic method. EBV persists regularly in the lymphoreticular system of EBV-infected individuals. EBV-positive lymphoblast lines can be established frequently from peripheral leukocytes and lymph node cells from those individuals.
Selected Readings
Lennette ET, "Epstein-Barr Virus," *Manual of Clinical Microbiology*, 5th ed, Balows A, Hausler WJ Jr, Herrmann KL, et al, eds, Washington, DC: American Society for Microbiology, 1991, 847-52.

Okano M, Thiele GM, Davis JR, et al, "Epstein-Barr Virus and Human Diseases: Recent Advances in Diagnosis," *Clin Microbiol Rev*, 1988, 1(3):300-12.

Epstein-Barr Virus Serology
Related Information
Epstein-Barr Virus Culture *on this page*
Infectious Mononucleosis Serology *on page 374*
Synonyms EB Virus Titer; EBV Titer
Applies To EB Nuclear Antigens; Epstein-Barr Early Antigens; Epstein-Barr Viral Capsid Antigen; VCA Titer

Test Includes Serology for several EBV antigens

Specimen Serum

Container Red top tube or serum separator tube

Reference Range Patients with no history of infectious mononucleosis: IgG anti-VCA <1:10; IgM anti-VCA <1:10; anti-EBNA: <1:5; early antigen: <1:10. Patients with previous infectious mononucleosis by history: IgG anti-VCA ≥1:10; IgM anti-VCA ≤1:10; anti-EBNA ≥1:50; early antigen <1:10. Patients with current or active infection: Many combinations of results are possible. Consult the laboratory for interpretation of specific results.

Use Diagnose Epstein-Barr virus infection, heterophil-negative mononucleosis, hereditary sex-linked lymphadenopathy

Limitations Despite much publicity, these tests are neither sensitive nor specific for chronic fatigue syndrome

Contraindications The Epstein-Barr viral test need not be done on patients who have heterophil antibodies, symptoms, physical findings, and lymphocyte morphology consistent with infectious mononucleosis. Typically, this test is performed on the ~15% of patients who are heterophil-negative and are still suspected of having infectious mononucleosis.

Methodology Indirect fluorescent antibody (IFA), enzyme-linked immunosorbent assay (ELISA)

Additional Information Epstein-Barr virus is a herpes group virus which is almost ubiquitous. It is the cause of classic infectious mononucleosis, and is causally implicated in the pathogenesis of Burkitt's lymphoma, some nasopharyngeal carcinomas, and rare hereditary lymphoproliferative disorders. The serologic response to EB virus includes antibody to early antigen, which is usually short lived, IgM and IgG antibodies to viral capsid antigen (VCA), and antibodies to nuclear antigen (EBNA).

Although most cases of infectious mononucleosis can be diagnosed on the basis of clinical findings, blood count and morphology, and a positive test for heterophil antibody, as many as 20% may be heterophil-negative, at least at presentation (heterophil may become positive when repeated in a few days). In some of these cases, a test for Epstein-Barr virus antibodies may be useful.

Of the numerous antibodies that may be assayed, viral capsid antibody is the most useful. A high presenting titer is good evidence for EB virus infection. Since titers are generally high by the time a patient is symptomatic, it may not be possible to demonstrate the fourfold rise in titer usually recommended. Even a very high titer may be due to past infection, so IgA and IgM titers should be measured to establish acute infection. Persistent absence of antibody to viral capsid is good evidence against EB virus infection.

Antibody to EB virus nuclear antigen (EBNA) usually develops 4-6 weeks after infection, so its presence early during an acute illness should lead one to consider diagnosis other than EB virus infectious mononucleosis.

Patients with nonkeratinizing squamous carcinoma of the nasopharynx may have elevated levels of IgG antibody to EB early antigen, but the rarity of this condition and the 10% to 20% false-positive rate vitiate its usefulness for screening. Such patients may also have IgA antibodies to VCA.

The most controversial use of EBV serology is in chronic fatigue syndrome, a complaint predominantly but not exclusively of young to middle-aged women, characterized by long persistent debilitating fatigue and a panoply of usually mild somatic complaints. In the initial reports of this illness, chronic infection with EBV was suggested as the cause, and EBV serology suggested as a diagnostic tool. In the past several years, although the legitimacy of a chronic fatigue syndrome seems to have been established, the inappropriateness of EBV serology for diagnosis has been realized. The high levels of EBV antibodies in the general population, their long persistence, and the poor correlation of antibody titers with symptoms combine to make EBV serology useless in diagnosing, following, or ruling out chronic fatigue syndrome.

IgG antibody to early antigen occurs in patients with Hodgkin's disease in higher titer than expected. This observation suggests the possibility that EB virus activation plays a pathogenetic role in Hodgkin's disease.

Selected Readings

Erlich KS, "Laboratory Diagnosis of Herpesvirus Infections," *Clin Lab Med*, 1987, 7(4):759-76.

Merlin T, "Chronic Mononucleosis: Pitfalls in the Laboratory Diagnosis," *Hum Pathol*, 1986, 17(1):2-8.

Sumaya CV and Jenson HB, "Epstein-Barr Virus," *Manual of Clinical Laboratory Immunology*, 4th ed, Rose NR, de Macario EC, Fahey JL, et al, eds, Washington, DC: American Society for Microbiology, 1992, 568-75.

(Continued)

Epstein-Barr Virus Serology *(Continued)*

Thiele GM and Okano M, "Diagnosis of Epstein-Barr Virus Infections in the Clinical Laboratory," *Clin Microbiol Newslett*, 1993, 15(6):41-8.

Esophageal Echo *see* Transesophageal Echocardiography
on page 460

Esterase, Leukocyte, Urine *see* Leukocyte Esterase, Urine
on page 386

Eye Smear for Cytology *see* Ocular Cytology *on page 416*

Eye Swab *Chlamydia* Culture *see* Chlamydia Culture
on page 294

FA Smear for *Legionella pneumophila* *see* Legionella *pneumophila*
Smear *on page 383*

5-FC *see* Flucytosine *on next page*

Fecal Leukocyte Stain

Related Information
Clostridium difficile Toxin Assay *on page 300*
Cryptosporidium Diagnostic Procedures, Stool *on page 314*
Stool Culture *on page 448*
Stool Culture, Diarrheagenic *E. coli on page 449*

Test Includes Methylene blue, Gram, or Wright's stain of stool smear

Patient Preparation Collect specimen prior to barium procedures if possible.

Specimen Fresh random stool, rectal swab

Container Culturette®, sealed plastic stool container

Collection Transport specimen to laboratory as soon as possible after collection, significant deterioration of the specimen occurs with prolonged storage.

Storage Instructions Refrigerate

Causes for Rejection Insufficient specimen volume. Specimens which are delayed in transit are less than optimal.

Turnaround Time 1 hour

Reference Range Few, if any, leukocytes

Use Assist in the differential diagnosis of diarrheal disease

Limitations Ten percent to 15% of stools which yield an invasive bacterial pathogen have an absence of fecal leukocytes. Many bacterial intestinal pathogens do not elicit a leukocyte response in stool. Fecal leukocytes are present in idiopathic inflammatory bowel disease.

Methodology Smear of stool (preferably mucus) with one drop methylene blue (or other stain), coverslip, and observe the presence of leukocytes.

Additional Information Conditions associated with varying degrees of fecal leukocytes, blood and/or mucus include diffuse antibiotic associated colitis, ulcerative colitis, shigellosis, *Campylobacter*, *Yersinia*, amebiasis, and some diarrheagenic *E. coli* infection. Conditions associated with an absence of fecal leukocytes include toxigenic bacterial infection, giardiasis, and viral infections. In a review the methylene blue stain for polymorpholeukocytes had a high sensitivity (85%) and specificity (88%) for bacterial diarrhea (*Shigella*, *Salmonella*, *Campylobacter*). Positive predictive value was poor (59%). Negative predictive value was 97%. In the presence of a history of abrupt onset, greater than four stools per day and no vomiting before the onset of diarrhea, the methylene blue stain for fecal polymorphonuclear leukocytes was a very effective presumptive diagnostic test for bacterial diarrhea. A positive occult blood test may also be suggestive of acute bacterial diarrhea. Neither method is sufficiently sensitive or specific to pre-empt the use of culture. Similar findings including a sensitivity of 81% and specificity 74% were observed when both tests were positive.

Selected Readings
Bishop WP and Ulshen MH, "Bacterial Gastroenteritis," *Pediatr Clin North Am*, 1988, 35(1):69-87.
Harris JC, Dupont HL, and Hornick RB, "Fecal Leukocytes in Diarrheal Illness," *Ann Intern Med*, 1972, 76(5):697-703.
Siegel D, Cohen PT, Neighbor M, et al, "Predictive Value of Stool Examination in Acute Diarrhea," *Arch Pathol Lab Med*, 1987, 111(8):715-8.

Femur, Left or Right, X-ray *see* Bone Films *on page 277*

Filarial Infestation *see* Microfilariae, Peripheral Blood Preparation
on page 400

Filariasis Peripheral Blood Preparation *see* Microfilariae, Peripheral Blood Preparation *on page 400*

Filling Cystometrogram *see* Cystometrogram, Simple *on page 315*

Finger, Left or Right Hand, X-ray *see* Bone Films *on page 277*

Flea Identification *see* Arthropod Identification *on page 268*

Flexible Bronchoscopy *see* Bronchoscopy, Fiberoptic *on page 286*

Flucytosine

Related Information
Antibiotic Level, Serum *on page 255*

Synonyms Ancobon®; 5-FC; 5-Fluorocytosine

Abstract Flucytosine is an antifungal agent often used in conjunction with amphotericin B for treatment of fungal meningitis and endocarditis. Bone marrow toxicity and hepatotoxicity are occasionally seen in patients being treated with flucytosine.

Specimen Serum

Container Red top tube

Sampling Time Peak serum levels are reached 4-6 hours after a single oral dose. During ongoing therapy, peak levels are reached 1-2 hours after successive doses.

Reference Range Therapeutic: 50-100 μg/mL (SI: 390-775 μmol/L)

Possible Panic Range 100-125 μg/mL (SI: 775-970 μmol/L)

Use Monitor for bone marrow toxicity; evaluate weekly if patient has normal renal function, more often if renal function is abnormal.

Limitations Serum levels do not correlate well with clinical toxicity. The hypothesis of serum level associated adverse effects has been inferred from case reports but has not been definitively studied.

Methodology High performance liquid chromatography (HPLC), gas chromatography/mass spectrometry (GC/MS)

Additional Information Clinical use of flucytosine is associated with significant frequency of life-threatening bone marrow suppression which occurs most often when blood levels are >100 μg/mL (SI: >775 μmol/L) for 2 or more weeks. The bone marrow suppression is usually reversible. It is most likely to occur in patients with underlying hematologic disorders or in patients undergoing myelosuppressive therapy.

Selected Readings
Bodey GP, "Topical and Systemic Antifungal Agents," *Med Clin North Am*, 1988, 72:637-59.
Gerson B, "Flucytosine," *Clin Lab Med*, 1987, 7(3):541-4.
Terrell CL and Hughes CE, "Antifungal Agents Used for Deep-Seated Mycotic Infections," *Mayo Clin Proc*, 1992, 67(1):69-91.

Fluids, Cytology *see* Cytology, Body Fluids *on page 318*

Fluorescent Rabies Antibody Test *see* Rabies *on page 433*

Fluorescent Treponemal Antibody Adsorption *see* FTA-ABS, Serum *on next page*

Fluorochrome Stain *see* Acid-Fast Stain *on page 239*

5-Fluorocytosine *see* Flucytosine *on this page*

Foot, Left or Right, X-ray *see* Bone Films *on page 277*

Forearm, Left or Right, X-ray *see* Bone Films *on page 277*

FRA Test *see* Rabies *on page 433*

FTA-ABS, Cerebrospinal Fluid

Related Information
VDRL, Cerebrospinal Fluid *on page 475*

Synonyms *Treponema pallidum* Antibodies, CSF

Test Includes CSF specimens are adsorbed (FTA – ABS) with nonpathogenic *Treponema* sp and tested.

Specimen Cerebrospinal fluid

Container Clean, sterile CSF tube

Causes for Rejection Bloody specimen

Reference Range Nonreactive

(Continued)

FTA-ABS, Cerebrospinal Fluid *(Continued)*

Use Test for the presence of *Treponema pallidum* antibodies; VDRL is preferred over the FTA when examining CSF.

Limitations The interpretation of FTA results when performed on CSF is not clearly defined. False-positive results may occur particularly if the specimen is not adsorbed prior to testing. VDRL on cerebrospinal fluid is recommended by the Center for Disease Control to help establish the diagnosis of neurosyphilis. However, while a positive CSF VDRL is strong evidence for active neurosyphilis, a negative does not rule it out. An FTA-ABS on CSF can be positive in cases of neurosyphilis when CSF VDRL is negative, but this combination of results is not common. Unfortunately, the CSF FTA-ABS test is less specific than CSF VDRL for distinguishing currently active neurosyphilis from past syphilis infection. Therefore, a correlation of the clinical facts with the serologic findings is essential for each case. One useful guide when screening for neurosyphilis is to first detect a serum FTA-ABS and/or a VDRL or RPR.

Methodology Indirect immunofluorescence of killed *Treponema* after serum adsorption of antibodies to nonpathogenic *Treponema* sp

Selected Readings
Davis LE and Schmitt JW, "Clinical Significance of Cerebrospinal Fluid Tests for Neurosyphilis," *Ann Neurol*, 1989, 25(1):50-5.

Larsen SA, Pope V, and Quan TJ, "Immunologic Methods for the Diagnosis of Spirochetal Diseases," *Manual of Clinical Laboratory Immunology*, 4th ed, Rose NR, de Macario EC, Fahey JL, et al. eds, Washington, DC: American Society for Microbiology, 1992, 467-81.

Young H, Moyes A, McMillan A, et al, "Enzyme Immunoassay for Anti-Treponemal IgG: Screening or Confirmatory Test?," *J Clin Pathol*, 1992, 45(1):37-41.

FTA-ABS, Serum

Related Information

Darkfield Examination, Syphilis *on page 322*

RPR *on page 438*

VDRL, Cerebrospinal Fluid *on page 475*

Synonyms Fluorescent Treponemal Antibody Adsorption

Applies To Serologic Test for Syphilis

Patient Preparation Patient should be fasting if possible

Specimen Serum

Container Red top tube or serum separator tube

Reference Range Nonreactive

Use Confirm presence of *Treponema pallidum* antibodies, establish the diagnosis of syphilis

Limitations FTA-ABS test for syphilis usually is positive in the treponemal diseases pinta, yaws and bejel, and falsely positive in patients with numerous diseases associated with increased or abnormal globulins, antinuclear antibodies, lupus erythematosus (beaded pattern), old age, pregnancy, and drug addiction (although drug addicts are likely to have true positives as well). As many as 2% of the general population may have a false-positive. Borderline results are inconclusive and cannot be interpreted; they may indicate a very low level of treponemal antibody or may be due to nonspecific factors. Further follow-up and serological confirmation with the treponemal immobilization test may be helpful.

Methodology Indirect immunofluorescence of killed *Treponema* after serum adsorption of antibodies to nonpathogenic *Treponema* sp

Additional Information FTA-ABS is the most sensitive test in all stages of syphilis, and is the best confirmatory test for a serum reactive to a screening test such as RPR. Occasionally, patients with ocular (uveitis) syphilis or otosyphilis will have a negative VDRL while their FTA-ABS is positive. FTA-ABS cannot be used to follow disease activity or response to treatment, because it will remain high for life. A modification of the test can detect IgM-specific antibodies, which may distinguish true congenital syphilis from placental transfer of maternal antibodies. However, tests for anti-*Treponema* IgM are not widely available. When a positive serum FTA-ABS is required before performing CSF VDRL examination, the specificity of the CSF test is markedly improved.

Although not officially recommended for testing cerebrospinal fluid, the FTA test, unabsorbed, can be performed on some spinal fluids with excellent specificity. At present this application of the test should be restricted to reference laboratories.

Selected Readings
Albright RE Jr, Christenson RH, Emlet JL, et al, "Issues in Cerebrospinal Fluid Management. CSF Venereal Disease Research Laboratory Testing," *Am J Clin Pathol*, 1991, 95(3):397-401.

Davis LE and Schmitt JW, "Clinical Significance of Cerebrospinal Fluid Tests for Neurosyphilis," *Ann Neurol*, 1989, 25(1):50-5.

Farnes SW and Setness PA, "Serologic Tests for Syphilis," *Postgrad Med*, 1990, 87(3):37-41, 45-6.

Larsen SA, Pope V, and Quan TJ, "Immunologic Methods for the Diagnosis of Spirochetal Diseases," *Manual of Clinical Laboratory Immunology*, 4th ed, Rose NR, de Macario EC, Fahey JL, et al, eds, Washington, DC: American Society for Microbiology, 1992, 467-81.

Fungal Immunodiffusion *see* Fungal Serology *on this page*

Fungal Precipitin Test *see* Fungal Serology *on this page*

Fungal Serology

Synonyms Fungal Immunodiffusion; Fungal Precipitin Test

Applies To *Aspergillus* Immunodiffusion; Blastomycosis Immunodiffusion; *Coccidioides* Immunodiffusion; Histoplasmosis Immunodiffusion

Specimen Serum

Container Red top tube or serum separator tube

Reference Range Negative or no bands identified

Use Confirm and aid in differential diagnosis of aspergillosis, blastomycosis, histoplasmosis, and coccidioidomycosis

Limitations Results reported as positive or negative; no titer is given

Contraindications Prior skin test may give a single precipitin band ("M") with histoplasmin

Methodology Immunodiffusion (ID), enzyme-linked immunosorbent assay (ELISA)

Additional Information Blastomycosis: A band of identity with the "A" reference antibody from an infected human indicates active infection or recent past infection. This detects about 80% of cases. A negative test has little value and in no way excludes the existence of blastomycosis. Cross reacting antibodies producing lines of partial identity are seen in patients with histoplasmosis and coccidioidomycosis.

Aspergillosis: Sera can be tested against a polyvalent antigen mixture, or a series of species preparations. The greater the number of bands, the greater the likelihood of either a fungus ball or invasive aspergillosis. A negative test does not rule out aspergillosis. Nonidentity bands could be due to presence of CRP. Cross reactions occur in cases of histoplasmosis, coccidioidomycosis and blastomycosis, or may indicate antibody to an *Aspergillus* species other than *Aspergillus fumigatus*. Bands due to reaction with C-reactive protein can be removed by sodium citrate.

Coccidioidomycosis: A band of identity with coccidioidin indicates infection but may be negative early. Some individuals continue to produce detectable antibodies up to 1 year after clinical recovery from active disease. A negative test does not exclude coccidioidomycosis.

Histoplasmosis: "H" and "M" precipitin bands are of diagnostic significance and if both are present indicate active infection. "H" identity bands alone are rarely seen; they are always associated with active infection. "M" identity bands alone indicate active infection, recent past infection (within the past year), or recent positive histoplasmin skin test (within past 2 months). The absence of precipitin antibodies does not rule out histoplasmosis.

Unfortunately, because of poorly standardized reagents and inherent biologic cross-reactivity, and interference from complement, the general clinical utility of measuring or detecting fungal antibodies is low. Only the detection of CSF antibodies to *Coccidioides* is truly diagnostic. For this reason, much effort is now devoted to tests for detecting fungal antigens, of which the most useful presently is the latex agglutination test for cryptococcal antigen.

Selected Readings

Drutz DJ, "Antigen Detection in Fungal Infections," *N Engl J Med*, 1986, 314(2):115-7.

Kaufman L and Reiss E, "Serodiagnosis of Fungal Diseases," *Manual of Clinical Laboratory Immunology*, 4th ed, Rose NR, de Macario EC, Fahey JL, et al, eds, Washington, DC: American Society for Microbiology, 1992, 506-28.

Tang CM and Cohen J, "Diagnosing Fungal Infections in Immunocompromised Hosts," *J Clin Pathol*, 1992, 45(1):1-5.

Fungal Skin Testing

Related Information

Anergy Skin Test Battery *on page 252*

Tuberculin Skin Testing, Intracutaneous *on page 463*

(Continued)

Fungal Skin Testing *(Continued)*

Synonyms Delayed Hypersensitivity Fungal Skin Tests; Skin Tests for Histoplasmosis, Blastomycosis, Coccidioidomycosis

Test Includes Intradermal injection of fungal antigen(s) to determine if a delayed hypersensitivity reaction is present to a given fungus. Skin test sites are examined at 24, 48, and 72 hours for induration which, if present, implies prior infection with the tested fungus.

Patient Preparation Procedure and risks are explained to the patient. No specific skin preparation is necessary. However, those patients with generalized skin disorders such as extensive psoriasis should be examined beforehand for suitable areas of normal appearing skin. If immediate hypersensitivity to the fungal antigen is even remotely suspected, physician should be in attendance.

Aftercare Fifteen to 30 minutes after injections, sites should be examined for adverse reactions ranging from the IgE wheal and flare response to systemic reactions; otherwise, close observation postprocedure is generally not necessary and patients should be instructed to keep test sites clean for 72 hours. No restrictions on bathing or cleaning injection sites are necessary.

Special Instructions Requisition should state the specific fungal antigens to be planted, as well as whether a simultaneous skin anergy panel is desired. Current medications should also be included in the requisition, with attention to corticosteroids or other immunosuppressive agents.

Complications As with other forms of skin testing, immediate IgE-mediated local reactions are possible, although unusual. Erythema, vesiculation, and skin necrosis may be seen, at times involving large areas. Systemic reactions, including anaphylaxis, have rarely been reported. Patients with infection with *Coccidioides immitis* who manifest erythema nodosum may be at an increased risk of a major systemic reaction after skin testing. However, in the vast majority of cases, fungal skin testing is safe.

Equipment Skin test materials are derived from cultures of the appropriate fungi and most are available commercially in standardized concentrations. Common fungal antigens tested include *Histoplasma capsulatum*, *Coccidioides immitis*, *Blastomyces dermatitidis* (not available commercially), *Candida*, and *Trichophyton*. Disposable plastic or glass tuberculin syringes are required along with 26- or 27-gauge short ($\frac{1}{4}$" to $\frac{1}{2}$") beveled needles.

Technique The volar aspect of the forearm is prepped with alcohol swabs. Skin test material(s) are injected intradermally so that discrete wheals are raised. Generally, 0.1 mL skin test antigen is injected, but more dilute solutions may be used if a severe reaction is anticipated. Subcutaneous injections should be avoided. Multiple fungal antigens may be injected at separate sites using this method. Test sites should be examined at 24, 48, and 72 hours. Date and time of injection should be recorded along with the location of each fungal antigen.

Data Acquired The transverse diameter of induration should be carefully measured by inspection and palpation and results recorded (in millimeters) at 24-hour intervals. Areas of erythema, however, are not as important as induration and are excluded in most grading schemes unless extensive (>10 mm).

Reference Range No induration or erythema

Critical Values A positive skin test is defined by many authorities as a diameter of induration ≥5 mm. Induration of 0-4 mm is considered negative. Alternatively, a standardized grading scale, which is popular with general delayed-type hypersensitivity skin testing, may be used:

- 0: no reaction
- 1+: erythema >10 mm and/or induration 1-5 mm
- 2+: induration 6-10 mm
- 3+: induration 11-20 mm
- 4+: induration >20 mm

The interpretation of a positive (or negative) skin test is so problematic that the clinical utility of fungal skin testing is significantly limited. A positive reaction indicates only that exposure to the relevant fungus has occurred at some time in the past, whether recent or remote. In addition, fungal infections are endemic in many areas of the United States, where >90% of the local population may be skin test positive following asymptomatic or subclinical infections (eg, histoplasmosis in the Ohio River Valley). Thus, in the individual patient with suspected active fungal infection, a positive skin test adds little new diagnostic information and fails to establish the fungus as the infecting agent. This becomes especially relevant if the patient has ever lived in a known endemic area. In the patient with pulmonary nodules, the importance of a positive test is also unclear. Some authorities consider a positive histoplasmin test in an

LABORATORY DIAGNOSIS

area of low prevalence as strong evidence for histoplasmosis. Others argue that lung nodules may still be due to bronchogenic carcinoma despite a positive histoplasmin test, and skin testing adds little to clinical decision making. Similarly, a negative skin test presents major problems in interpretation. Lack of reactivity may be seen in the following situations:

- no previous fungal infection
- previous fungal infection in an immunocompromised patient
- acute systemic fungal infection, where skin test positivity is often delayed for 2-4 weeks
- waning skin test reactivity to a given fungus, as occurs in the elderly
- technical errors in antigen placement

Even the documentation of skin test conversion (ie, negative test converting to positive or serial testing) is regarded as only indirect evidence of fungal exposure in the interim and does not necessarily imply active infection. Regarding the specific fungal antigens, the derivative of *Histoplasma capsulatum* is termed histoplasmin. An older preparation of histoplasmin cross reacted frequently with *Blastomyces* and *Coccidioides* and caused a rise in complement fixation titers to *Histoplasma*. A newer histoplasmin preparation ameliorates, but does not entirely eliminate, these problems. The histoplasmin skin test may cause a spurious increase in *Histoplasma* complement fixation titers. Since the CF serologic test is clinically more useful than the histoplasmin skin test, serologies should be drawn first in suspected cases. Coccidioidomycosis skin testing shares many of the same interpretive difficulties as histoplasmosis testing, such as waning reactivity over time, delay in test positivity during acute fungal infection, and areas of high prevalence. Two preparations of *Coccidioides* antigen are available, the older coccidioidin (derived from the mycelia phase) and Spherulin® (derived from lysed spherules). Spherulin® may have superior sensitivity and has been found to be positive in 30% more cases than coccidioidin. Although testing is not useful in the individual with suspected *Coccidioides* pneumonia, it may provide prognostic information in culture proven cases. In a classic study, patients with disseminated coccidioidomycosis had a higher survival rate if their skin test was positive (75%) compared with those who tested negative (15%). Patients with limited coccidioidomycosis almost always develop a positive test; failure to do so may predict impending disseminated disease. Use of the coccidioidin preparation may cause false-positive histoplasmosis serologic tests, but neither Spherulin® nor coccidioidin interferes with serologic tests for coccidioidomycosis. Coccidioidal skin tests are generally positive before coccidioidal serologic tests; some clinicians use this fact to justify skin testing in acute cases (despite its limited diagnostic utility). Skin tests for blastomycosis are presently of questionable value due to poor sensitivity and specificity, even in the study of epidemics. Fungal antigens derived from *Candida albicans* and *Trichophyton* are primarily used only for anergy testing because of high prevalence of positive skin tests in the general population.

Use Fungal skin testing has been applied for the following reasons:

- as an epidemiologic tool for defining geographic regions of endemic fungal infection
- as a diagnostic aid in individual cases of suspected primary fungal infection (limited usefulness)
- as a prognostic indicator in culture-proven cases of fungal infection (particularly coccidioidomycosis)
- as a component of a comprehensive cutaneous anergy panel, used to assess the integrity of a patient's cell-mediated immune system (T-cell function); this standardized panel is usually comprised of *Candida*, mumps, and *Trichophyton* antigens

Contraindications Prior systemic reaction to fungal skin testing; known immediate hypersensitivity (IgE-mediated) to the specific fungus to be tested; known immediate hypersensitivity to mercury, which is contained in some commercial preparations of *Coccidioides* antigen; the presence of erythema nodosum (high risk for adverse reaction – see following information).

Additional Information Fungal skin testing is a form of delayed hypersensitivity skin testing and as such is an assessment of cell-mediated immunity. Delayed hypersensitivity is a clinical phenomenon based on the reaction of the skin to intradermal injection of an antigen. It is a common form of immune protection against a wide range of infectious agents, including fungi. Following initial exposure to a fungus, a population of transformed T-lymphocytes is created, the so-called memory cells. When fungal antigen is introduced intradermally at a later date, these sensitized T cells are activated and initiate a cascade

(Continued)

Fungal Skin Testing *(Continued)*

involving lymphokines, neutrophils, and macrophages. Clinically this is manifested by the delayed formation of significant skin induration. Delayed hypersensitivity fungal skin testing should be differentiated from immediate hypersensitivity skin testing. The former is primarily T-cell mediated and the latter is mediated by IgE mechanisms. Skin testing for common allergies to molds or fungi is carried out using the percutaneous allergy testing method and is IgE-mediated. Similarly, skin tests for immediate hypersensitivity to *Aspergillus fumigatus* also use this method. This is commonly obtained in the evaluation of patients with suspected allergic bronchopulmonary aspergillosis.

Fungus Culture, Appropriate Site
Refer To
Fungus Culture, Biopsy *on this page*

Fungus Culture, Body Fluid *on next page*

Fungus Culture, Bronchial Aspirate *on page 342*

Fungus Culture, Cerebrospinal Fluid *on page 342*

Fungus Culture, Skin *on page 343*

Fungus Culture, Sputum *on page 345*

Fungus Culture, Urine *on page 347*

Genital Culture for *Ureaplasma urealyticum on page 350*

Fungus Culture, Biopsy
Synonyms Biopsy Culture, Fungus; Fungus Culture, Tissue

Applies To Cyst Culture, Fungus; Fungus Culture, Surgical Specimen

Patient Preparation Usual sterile preparation of biopsy site

Special Instructions The following information will assist the laboratory in the proper processing of the specimen: specific site of specimen, current antibiotic therapy, age and sex of patient, collection time and date, and clinical diagnosis.

Specimen Surgical specimen. **Swab specimens are not acceptable. Tissue must be submitted.**

Container Sterile test tube or container

Collection The portion of the biopsy submitted for culture should be separated from the portion submitted for histopathology by the surgeon or pathologist utilizing sterile technique. The laboratory should be informed of the fungal species suspected. Every effort should be made to collect the specimen early in the day so that it may be processed promptly, assuring optimal yield.

Storage Instructions Transport specimen to the laboratory immediately. Do not store or refrigerate.

Causes for Rejection Specimen in fixative solution, specimen not received in a sterile container.

Turnaround Time Physician will be notified of positive cultures. Negatives are reported after 4 weeks.

Reference Range No growth

Use Isolate and identify fungi; establish the diagnosis of fungemia, fungal endocarditis, and disseminated mycosis in immunocompromised patients, oncology patients, transplant patients, patients with leukemia and lymphoma, and patients with the acquired immunodeficiency syndrome (AIDS)

Limitations A single negative culture does not rule out the presence of fungal infection

Additional Information Optimal isolation of fungi from tissue is accomplished by processing **as much tissue as possible**. Swabs should be submitted only when adequate tissue is not available. Depending upon the geographic area *Histoplasma capsulatum*, *Blastomyces dermatitidis*, and *Coccidioides immitis*, among the deep pathogenic fungi, are most frequently isolated. Immunocompromised patients, transplant patients, and patients with acquired immunodeficiency syndrome (AIDS), are susceptible to opportunistic mycoses. The most frequently encountered are *Candida albicans*, *Cryptococcus neoformans*, and *Aspergillus* sp. The recovery of a recognized fungal pathogen from a wound culture or draining sinus is significant. Isolates such as *Candida* sp and *Aspergillus* sp are often environmental in origin and must be interpreted in the clinical context.

Selected Readings
Gray LD and Roberts GD, "Laboratory Diagnosis of Systemic Fungal Diseases," *Infect Dis Clin North Am*, 1988, 2(4):779-803.

Musial CE, Cockerill FR 3d, and Roberts GD, "Fungal Infections of the Immunocompromised Host: Clinical and Laboratory Aspects," *Clin Microbiol Rev*, 1988, 1(4):349-64.

Fungus Culture, Blood *see* Blood Culture, Fungus *on page 275*

Fungus Culture, Body Fluid
Related Information
 Sporotrichosis Serology *on page 447*
Synonyms Body Fluid Fungus Culture; Fungus Culture, Biopsy
Applies To Ascitic Fluid Fungus Culture; Fungus Culture, Bone Marrow; Fungus Culture, Surgical Specimen; Fungus Culture, Tissue; Joint Fluid Fungus Culture; Pericardial Fluid Fungus Culture; Peritoneal Fluid Fungus Culture; Pleural Fluid Fungus Culture; Surgical Specimen Fungus Culture; Synovial Fluid Fungus Culture; Thoracentesis Fluid Fungus Culture Bone Marrow Fungus Culture; Tissue Fungus Culture; Wound Fungus Culture
Patient Preparation Aseptic preparation of biopsy site or site of body fluid aspiration
Special Instructions The laboratory should be informed of the specific source of specimen. Specimens may be divided for fungus culture, mycobacteria culture and acid-fast smear, and routine bacterial culture and Gram stain only if the specimen is of adequate volume for all tests requested.
Specimen Body fluid, blood, bone marrow
Container Sterile container with lid
Collection The portion of the fluid specimen submitted for culture should be separated from the portion submitted for cytology by the surgeon or pathologist utilizing sterile technique. The laboratory should be informed of the fungal species suspected. Every effort should be made to collect the specimen early in the day so as it may be processed promptly, assuring optimal yield. Multiple daily fungal blood cultures are not necessary. Single daily cultures for 2-3 days are sufficient.
Storage Instructions Specimens should not be stored or refrigerated. The specimen should be transported to the laboratory as soon as possible after collection.
Causes for Rejection Specimen in fixative
Turnaround Time Negatives are reported after 4 weeks
Reference Range No growth
Use Isolate and identify fungi; establish the diagnosis of fungemia, fungal endocarditis, and disseminated mycosis in immunocompromised patients, oncology patients, transplant patients, patients with leukemia and lymphoma, and patients with the acquired immunodeficiency syndrome (AIDS)
Methodology Culture under aerobic conditions on several media
Additional Information Optimal isolation of fungi from fluid is accomplished by processing as much tissue as possible. **Swab specimens of body fluids should not be submitted for fungal culture.** Specimen selection tables are provided in the listings for Fungus Culture, Sputum and Fungus Culture, Skin. Depending upon the geographic area *Histoplasma capsulatum*, *Blastomyces dermatitidis*, and *Coccidioides immitis*, among the deep pathogenic fungi, are most frequently isolated, but from tissue more commonly than from fluid. Immunocompromised patients, transplant patients, and patients with acquired immunodeficiency syndrome (AIDS), are susceptible to opportunistic mycoses. The recovery of a recognized fungal pathogen from a fluid or draining sinus is significant. Isolates such as *Candida* sp and *Aspergillus* sp are often environmental in origin and must be interpreted in the clinical context.

Fungal peritonitis is clinically similar to bacterial peritonitis with pain, fever, and abdominal tenderness. Thirty-two fungal infections due to *Candida* sp (mostly *Candida albicans* and *Candida parapsilosis*), and rare single cases of *Aspergillus fumigatus* and the higher bacterium *Nocardia asteroides* have been reported in patients undergoing chronic dialysis. In a series of AIDS patients, bone marrow biopsy detected opportunistic fungal or mycobacterial infections in 20%. Eighty percent of the positive biopsies were associated with bone marrow granulomas. Fever, anemia, and neutropenia were often correlated with a positive biopsy. Neutrophil count <1000/mm³ is associated with infection by *Candida*, *Aspergillus*, *Mucor*, *Rhizopus*, *Trichosporon*, and *Fusarium* sp. T-cell defects and/or impaired cell mediated immunity is associated with infection by *Candida*, *Cryptococcus neoformans*, *Histoplasma capsulatum*, *Coccidioides immitis*, and *Aspergillus* sp. Catheterization, arterial venous, or urinary and mechanical disruption of the skin is associated with *Candida* and *Rhodotorula* sp
(Continued)

Fungus Culture, Body Fluid *(Continued)*

infections. Disruption of the natural barrier of the GI tract and respiratory tree by cytotoxic chemotherapy predispose to *Candida* sp infections.

Selected Readings

Gray LD and Roberts GD, "Laboratory Diagnosis of Systemic Fungal Diseases," *Infect Dis Clin North Am*, 1988, 2(4):779-803.

Lyons RW and Andriole VT, "Fungal Infections of the CNS," *Neurol Clin*, 1986, 4(1):159-70.

Musial CE, Cockerill FR 3d, and Roberts GD, "Fungal Infections of the Immunocompromised Host: Clinical and Laboratory Aspects," *Clin Microbiol Rev*, 1988, 1(4):349-64.

Fungus Culture, Bone Marrow *see* Fungus Culture, Body Fluid
on previous page

Fungus Culture, Bronchial Aspirate

Synonyms Bronchial Aspirate Fungus Culture; Lower Respiratory Fungus Culture

Applies To Bronchoalveolar Lavage (BAL); Fungus Culture, Tracheal Aspirate; Fungus Culture, Transtracheal Aspirate; Percutaneous Transtracheal Fungus Culture; Tracheal Aspirate Fungus Culture; Transtracheal Aspirate Fungus Culture

Test Includes Culture, Gram stain, KOH preparation

Special Instructions Requisition **must** state site of specimen

Specimen Bronchial aspirate, tracheal aspirate, transtracheal aspirate. These specimens are clinically equivalent to sputum (for microbiology purposes). **Do not submit specimen on a swab.**

Container Sterile tube, Lukens tube, or sputum container

Collection The specimen can be divided for fungus culture, mycobacteria culture and smear, and routine bacterial culture and Gram stain only if the specimen is accompanied by properly completed requisitions for these procedures and if the specimen is of adequate volume for all tests requested. Specify fungal species suspected.

Storage Instructions Specimen must be delivered to the laboratory as soon as possible. Refrigerate specimen until delivery is possible.

Causes for Rejection Specimen on outside of container, insufficient numbers of completed requisitions for the procedures requested

Turnaround Time Physicians will be notified of all positive cultures. Negative cultures are reported after 4 weeks.

Reference Range No fungi grown

Use Isolate and identify fungi

Limitations A single negative culture does not rule out presence of fungal infection

Additional Information Saprophytic fungi (especially yeast) isolated from respiratory aspirates are not uncommon. If mycobacteria are isolated, the isolate will be identified and referred for susceptibility testing on request.

Fungus Culture, Bronchoscopy *see* Fungus Culture, Sputum
on page 345

Fungus Culture, Cerebrospinal Fluid

Related Information

Cerebrospinal Fluid Analysis *on page 288*

Cryptococcal Antigen Serology, Serum or Cerebrospinal Fluid
on page 312

India Ink Preparation *on page 373*

Viral Culture, Central Nervous System Symptoms *on page 476*

Synonyms CSF Fungus Culture; Fungus Culture, CSF; Fungus Culture, Spinal Fluid; Spinal Fluid Fungus Culture

Test Includes Culture for fungi, India ink, fungus smear, and cryptococcal antigen test if requested (and depending on laboratory protocol)

Patient Preparation Aseptic preparation of aspiration site

Special Instructions The laboratory should be informed of the specific source of specimen.

Specimen Cerebrospinal fluid

Container Sterile CSF tube

Collection Tubes should be numbered 1, 2, 3 with tube #1 representing the first portion of the sample collected. Contamination with normal flora from skin or other body surfaces must be avoided. The third tube collected during lumbar puncture is most suitable for culture because skin contaminants from the puncture usually are washed out with fluid collected in the first two tubes.

Storage Instructions The specimen should be transported immediately to the laboratory. If it cannot be processed immediately, it should be kept at room temperature or placed in an incubator. Do not refrigerate.

Turnaround Time Negative cultures are usually reported after 4 weeks

Reference Range No growth

Use Isolate and identify fungi, particularly *Cryptococcus neoformans*. Diagnosis is established by detection of cryptococcal antigen.

Limitations Recovery of fungi from cerebrospinal fluid is directly related to the volume of cerebrospinal fluid available. Recovery is less than 100% on one specimen. A minimum of 10 mL is recommended. *Cryptococcus* can be mistaken for small lymphocytes in the counting chamber.

Methodology Aerobic culture of centrifuged sediment on several fungal media

Additional Information India ink preparations are not very useful (sensitivity, <50%) in identifying the presence of *Cryptococcus neoformans*, the most common fungus isolated from cerebrospinal fluid. Cryptococcal antigen titers of serum and cerebrospinal fluid provide rapid diagnosis and have greater sensitivity than India ink preparation. The diagnosis of central nervous system fungal infections is frequently complicated by the overlapping array of signs and symptoms which may accompany other clinical entities such as tuberculous meningitis, pyogenic abscess, brain tumor, hypersensitivity or allergic reactions, collagen vascular disease, leptomeningeal malignancy, chemical meningitis, meningeal inflammation secondary to contiguous suppuration, Behçet's disease, Mollaret's meningitis, and the uveomeningitic syndromes.

Especially in immunocompromised hosts, aspergillosis, mucormycosis, and candidiasis are observed. Infections with species which cause phaeohyphomycosis are described. Nocardiosis can infect the meninges. *Cryptococcus neoformans* has been isolated from up to 10% of patients with acquired immunodeficiency syndrome (AIDS).

Selected Readings

Greenlee JE, "Approach to Diagnosis of Meningitis – Cerebrospinal Fluid Evaluation," *Infect Dis Clin North Am*, 1990, 4(4):583-98.

Tunkel AR, Wispelwey B, and Scheld WM, "Pathogenesis and Pathophysiology of Meningitis," *Infect Dis Clin North Am*, 1990, 4(4):555-81.

Fungus Culture, CSF *see* Fungus Culture, Cerebrospinal Fluid *on previous page*

Fungus Culture, Dermatophytes *see* Fungus Culture, Skin *on this page*

Fungus Culture, Gastric Aspirate *see* Fungus Culture, Sputum *on page 345*

Fungus Culture, Hair *see* Fungus Culture, Skin *on this page*

Fungus Culture, Nail *see* Fungus Culture, Skin *on this page*

Fungus Culture, Skin

Related Information

KOH Preparation *on page 379*

Applies To Dermatophyte Fungus Culture; Fungus Culture, Dermatophytes; Fungus Culture, Hair; Fungus Culture, Nail; Hair Fungus Culture; Nail Fungus Culture

Patient Preparation Select fluorescent hairs or nonfluorescent hairs which are broken off and appear diseased and pluck them with sterile forceps. If diseased hair stubs are not apparent, scrape the edges of a skin lesion with a sterile scalpel. Cleanse skin lesions first with 70% alcohol to reduce bacteria and saprophytic fungi. Scrape from the outer edges of skin lesions. In infections of the nails, scrape out the friable material beneath the edge of the nails, or scrape or clip off portions of abnormal appearing nail and submit for examination and culture.

Special Instructions Careful choice of specimens for laboratory study is important. See table on following page. A Wood's lamp can occasionally be useful in the collection of specimens in tinea capitis infections because hairs infected by most members of the genus *Microsporum* frequently exhibit fluorescence under a Wood's lamp. However, in tinea capitis due to *Trichophyton* sp, infected hairs usually do not fluoresce. The laboratory should be informed of the specific site of the specimen.

(Continued)

343

Fungus Culture, Skin *(Continued)*

Selection of Specimens for the Diagnosis of Superficial Mycosis and Dermatomycosis

Diagnosis	Specimen of Choice
Superficial mycoses	
Piedra	Hair
Tinea nigra	Skin scraping
Tinea versicolor	Skin scraping
Dermatomycoses (cutaneous mycoses)	
Onychomycosis	Nail scraping
Tinea capitis	Hair (black dot)
Tinea corporis	Skin scraping
Tinea pedis	Skin scraping
Tinea cruris	Skin scraping
Candidiasis	
Thrush	Scraping of oral white patches
Diaper dermatitis	Scraping of pustules at margin
Paronychia	Scraping skin around nail
Cutaneous candidiasis	Scraping of pustules at margin
Erosio interdigitalis blastomycetia (coinfection with gram–negative rods)	Scrapings of interdigital space (routine culture also)
Congenital candidiasis	Scraping of scales, pustules and cutaneous debris, cultures of umbilical stump, mouth, urine, and stool
Mucocutaneous candidiasis	Scraping of affected area

Specimen Skin scrapings, exudates, nail clippings, whole nail, debris under nail, hair

Container Petri dish, urine container, envelope

Collection Enclose hair specimens, skin scrapings, or nail clippings or scrapings in clean paper envelopes, urine container, or Petri dish. Label the specimen with the patient's name. Enclose these envelopes in larger heavy paper envelopes. Do not put specimens in cotton-plugged tubes, because the specimen may become trapped among the cotton fibers and lost. Do not put specimen into closed containers, such as rubber-stoppered tubes, because this keeps the specimen moist and allows overgrowth of bacteria and saprophytic fungi. The laboratory should be informed of the fungal species suspected.

Storage Instructions Keep specimen at room temperature until delivered to the laboratory

Turnaround Time Cultures positive for *Candida* sp are usually reported within 1 week. Cultures positive for dermatophytes are usually reported within 2-3 weeks. Negative cultures are usually reported after 1 month. Cultures in which suspicion of systemic fungal infection has been indicated are usually reported upon becoming positive, or negative after 4 weeks.

Reference Range No growth

Use Isolate and identify fungi

Limitations A single negative specimen does not rule out fungal infections. If infection with mycobacteria or aerobic organisms cannot be excluded clinically, a separate culture should be submitted as indicated.

Methodology Aerobic culture on selective media usually including nonselective Sabouraud's agar

Additional Information *Candida* sp may colonize skin. Clinical diagnosis of *Candida* infection involves consideration of predisposing factors such as occlusion, maceration altered cutaneous barrier function. Signs of *Candida* infection include bright erythema, fragile papulopustules, and satellite lesions.

Selected Readings

Cohn MS, "Superficial Fungal Infections. Topical and Oral Treatment of Common Types," *Postgrad Med*, 1992, 91(2):239-44, 249-52.

McKay M, "Cutaneous Manifestations of Candidiasis," *Am J Obstet Gynecol*, 1988, 158(4):991-3.

Meyer RD, "Cutaneous and Mucosal Manifestations of the Deep Mycotic Infections," *Acta Derm Venereol Suppl (Stockh)*, 1986, 121:57-72.

Stein DH, "Superficial Fungal Infections," *Pediatr Clin North Am*, 1983, 30(3):545-61.

Fungus Culture, Spinal Fluid *see* Fungus Culture, Cerebrospinal Fluid on page 342

Fungus Culture, Sputum

Applies To Bronchoscopy Fungus Culture; Fungus Culture, Bronchoscopy; Fungus Culture, Gastric Aspirate; Fungus Culture, Tracheal Aspirate; Fungus Culture, Transtracheal Aspirate; Gastric Aspirate Fungus Culture; Percutaneous Transtracheal Fungus Culture; Tracheal Aspirate Fungus Culture; Transtracheal Aspirate Fungus Culture

Patient Preparation The patient should be instructed to remove dentures, rinse mouth with water and cough deeply expectorating sputum into the sputum collection cup.

Special Instructions The laboratory should be informed of the specific source of specimen and the suspected clinical diagnosis should be stated.

Specimen First morning sputum. Microbiologically, this specimen is equivalent to the following: gastric aspirate, induced sputum, aspirated sputum, bronchial aspirate, tracheal aspirate, transtracheal aspirate. See table.

Selection of Specimens for the Diagnosis of Systemic and Subcutaneous Mycosis

Diagnosis	Specimen of Choice in Order of Usefulness	Diagnosis	Specimen of Choice in Order of Usefulness
Systemic Mycoses		**Systemic Mycoses** *(continued)*	
Aspergillosis	Sputum Bronchial aspirate Biopsy (lung)	Mycomycosis/ phycomycosis	Sputum Bronchial aspirate Biopsy (lung)
Blastomycosis	Skin scrapings Abscess drainage (pus) Urine Sputum Bronchial aspirate	Paracoccidioidomycosis (South American blastomycosis)	Skin scrapings Mucosal scrapings Biopsy (lymph nodes) Sputum Bronchial aspirate
Candidiasis	Sputum Bronchial aspirate Blood Cerebrospinal fluid Urine Stool	**Subcutaneous Mycoses**	
		Chromoblastomycosis	Skin scrapings Biopsy (skin) Drainage (pus)
Coccidioidomycosis	Sputum Bronchial aspirate Cerebrospinal fluid Urine Skin scrapings Abscess drainage (pus)	Maduromycosis (mycetoma)	Drainage (pus) Abscess drainage Biopsy (lesion)
		Sporotrichosis	Drainage (pus) Abscess drainage Biopsy (skin, lymph node)
Cryptococcosis	Cerebrospinal fluid Sputum Abscess drainage (pus) Skin scraping Urine		

See Skin Fungus Culture test listing for Superficial and Cutaneous Mycoses Specimen Selection.

Container Sterile sputum cup, sputum trap, sterile tracheal aspirate tube or sterile bronchoscopy tube

Collection Every effort should be made to collect the specimen early in the day so that it may be processed by the laboratory for optimal recovery. A recommended screening procedure is three first morning specimens submitted on three successive days. The specimen can be divided for fungus culture, mycobacteria culture and smear, and routine bacterial culture and Gram stain only if the specimen is of adequate volume for all tests requested.

Storage Instructions Refrigerate the specimen if storage is in excess of 1 hour

Causes for Rejection Specimens contaminated on the outside of the container pose excessive risk to laboratory personnel and may not be acceptable to the laboratory.

(Continued)

Fungus Culture, Sputum *(Continued)*

Turnaround Time Negative cultures are reported after 4 weeks

Reference Range No growth; yeast from the oropharynx may be present.

Use Establish the presence of potentially pathogenic fungi

Limitations The yield may be reduced by bacterial overgrowth during storage or on standing; therefore, fresh sputum is preferred. A single negative culture does not rule out the presence of fungal infection. If two specimens are received simultaneously, many laboratories will pool them and process them as one specimen unless specific instructions are provided.

Methodology Culture on selective and nonselective media

Additional Information Deeply coughed sputum, transtracheal aspirate, bronchial washing or brushing, or deep tracheal aspirate are preferred specimens. Oncology patients, transplant patients, and patients with the acquired immunodeficiency syndrome (AIDS) are particularly prone to infection with fungi.

Primary fungal pulmonary infections frequently result in granulomatous disease. Classically, *Histoplasma capsulatum, Coccidioides immitis, Cryptococcus neoformans,* and *Blastomyces dermatitidis* have been implicated. The incidence was largely related to geographic exposure and many cases occurred in seemingly normal hosts. Recently increasing numbers of reports of opportunistic fungal pulmonary infections due to a wide variety of etiologic agents which are ubiquitous in the environment, are being published. Definitive diagnosis depends upon the following: presence of clinical signs of pulmonary infection including rales, rhonchi and fever, and a chest x-ray picture revealing consolidation of granuloma; laboratory isolation of a potentially significant organism from a suitable specimen; histologic documentation of tissue invasion by the isolated organism. Many lists of documented etiologic agents of pulmonary fungal disease have been reported (see table). In practice a diagnosis suf-

Common Pulmonary Fungal Infections

Endemic Fungi	Opportunistic Fungi
Histoplasma capsulatum	*Candida albicans*
Blastomyces dermatitidis	*Candida tropicalis*
Coccidioides immitis	*Aspergillus niger*
Paracoccidioides brasiliensis	*Aspergillus fumigatus*
	Mucor
	Rhizopus
	Absidia
	Cryptococcus neoformans

From Haque AK, "Pathology of Common Pulmonary Fungal Infections," *J Thorac Imaging,* 1992, 7:1–11, with permission.

ficient for therapy can frequently be established by observation of hyphae, pseudohyphae or yeast cells in tissue sections; recovery of the organism from a normally sterile site; repeated isolation of the same suspect organism from the same or different sites; seroconversion, ie, the development of an immune response to the suspected organism. *Candida* and *Aspergillus* sp are the most frequently isolated usually pathogenic organisms. However, they are frequently present as the result of contamination from the patient's normal flora or airborne sources. Their presence may represent colonization rather than invasion. Recovery of *Candida* from blood (see Blood Culture, Fungus) is a major adjunct to definitive diagnosis. Even without invasion *Aspergillus* may cause IgE-mediated asthma, allergic alveolitis cell mediated hypersensitivity, mucoid impaction, and bronchocentric granulomatosis. Fungal tracheobronchitis has recently been recognized to present as a pseudomembranous form involving the circumference of the bronchial wall or as multiple or discrete plaques. The plaques or pseudomembranes are composed of necrotic tissue exudate and fungal hyphae.

Selected Readings
Rinaldi MG, "Invasive Aspergillosis," *Rev Infect Dis,* 1983, 5(6):1061-77.

Schuyler MR, "Allergic Bronchopulmonary Aspergillosis," *Clin Chest Med,* 1983, 4(1):15-22.

Stamm AM and Dismukes WE, "Current Therapy of Pulmonary and Disseminated Fungal Diseases," *Chest,* 1983, 83(6):911-7.

Zarabi MC and Salmassi S, "Antemortem Diagnosis of Systemic Aspergillosis: Ten Year Review and Report of a Case," *South Med J,* 1984, 77(5):584-8.

Fungus Culture, Surgical Specimen *see* Fungus Culture, Biopsy
on page 340

Fungus Culture, Surgical Specimen *see* Fungus Culture, Body Fluid
on page 341

Fungus Culture, Tissue *see* Fungus Culture, Biopsy
on page 340

Fungus Culture, Tissue *see* Fungus Culture, Body Fluid
on page 341

Fungus Culture, Tracheal Aspirate *see* Fungus Culture, Bronchial
Aspirate on page 342

Fungus Culture, Tracheal Aspirate *see* Fungus Culture, Sputum
on page 345

Fungus Culture, Transtracheal Aspirate *see* Fungus Culture,
Bronchial Aspirate on page 342

Fungus Culture, Transtracheal Aspirate *see* Fungus Culture, Sputum
on page 345

Fungus Culture, Urine

Patient Preparation Usual preparation for clean catch midvoid urine specimen collection. See listing for Urine Culture, Clean Catch.

Special Instructions The laboratory should be informed of the specific source of the specimen and the fungal species suspected.

Specimen Urine

Container Sterile plastic container or tube

Collection The specimen should be transported to laboratory within 2 hours of collection if not refrigerated. The patient must be instructed to thoroughly cleanse skin and collect midstream specimen.

Causes for Rejection Unrefrigerated specimen more than 2 hours old may be subject to overgrowth and may not yield valid results

Reference Range No growth

Use Isolate and identify fungi

Limitations A single negative culture does not rule out the presence of fungal infection

Additional Information Patients with candiduria may or may not have candidemia; positive urine culture for fungi often may be followed by positive blood culture for fungi. Ascending infections occur in patients with diabetes, prolonged antimicrobial therapy, or following instrumentation. Urinary obstruction due to "fungus balls" may occur in diabetes and following renal transplantation. Candiduria associated with hematogenous infections is observed in patients with granulocytopenia, corticosteroid therapy, and with immunosuppression. The source is frequently the gastrointestinal tract or indwelling catheters particular with hyperalimentation. A blood fungus culture is useful in defining invasive disease. However, proof of invasive *Candida* infection requires direct cystoscopic or operative visualization of fungus balls, or pyelonephritis, or histological evidence of mucosa invasion. Urine is a useful specimen for culture in cryptococcosis, blastomycosis, and candidiasis. See table for fungus culture specimen selection in Sputum Fungus Culture listing. The incidence of genitourinary fungal infections is increasing. They are usually associated with broad spectrum antibiotic therapy, corticosteroid therapy, underlying general debility, and AIDS. In addition to *Candida*, opportunistic pathogens in the genitourinary tract include *Aspergillus* and *Cryptococcus*. Endemic pathogens such as *Histoplasma*, *Blastomyces*, and *Coccidioides* are also encountered.

Selected Readings
Frangos DN and Nyberg LM Jr, "Genitourinary Fungal Infections," *South Med J*, 1986, 79(4):455-9.
Roy JB, Geyer JR, and Mohr JA, "Urinary Tract Candidiasis: An Update," *Urology*, 1984, 23(6):533-7.
"Urinary Tract Candidosis," *Lancet*, 1988, 2(8618):1000-2.

Gallium Abscess Scan *see* Gallium Scan on this page

Gallium Scan

Applies To Gallium Abscess Scan; Gallium Tumor Scan; Soft Tissue Scan

Test Includes The patient receives an intravenous injection of gallium-67 citrate. Images are then acquired for some combination of 24, 48, and 72 hours after injection.

(Continued)

LABORATORY DIAGNOSIS
Gallium Scan (Continued)

Patient Preparation Patient should have all RIA blood work performed, or at least drawn, prior to injection of any radioactive material. The patient does not need to be fasting or NPO for this procedure.

Special Instructions Requisition must state the current patient diagnosis in order to select the most appropriate radiopharmaceutical and/or imaging technique. Other Nuclear Medicine procedures (bone, liver, lung) should be completed prior to gallium injection. If abdominal abscess/infection is suspected, laxatives, and/or enemas may be ordered for the patient prior to delayed imaging at 48 or 72 hours. This will help clear normal intestinal gallium activity from the colon. *DURATION OF PROCEDURE:* 24-72 hours *RADIOPHARMACEUTICAL:* Gallium-67 citrate.

Technique The application of single-photon emission tomography (SPECT) techniques may contribute significantly to the diagnostic accuracy of this imaging study.

Turnaround Time A written report will be sent to the patient's chart and/or to the referring physician.

Normal Findings Gallium will localize to some degree in liver and spleen, bone, nasopharynx, lacrimal glands, and breast tissue. There is normally some secretion of gallium into the bowel. This may require laxatives and/or enemas for the patient to evacuate this normal activity before additional imaging of possible abdominal infection or abscess. Abnormal accumulation of gallium will usually be asymmetric, increase in later images, and remain in the same location (normal bowel luminal gallium activity will transit).

Use Gallium localizes at sites of active inflammation or infection as well as in some neoplasms. Gallium imaging is very sensitive in detection of abscesses, pneumonia, pyelonephritis, active sarcoidosis, and active tuberculosis. Even in immunocompromised patients, eg, those with AIDS, gallium imaging can detect early complications such as *Pneumocystis carinii* pneumonitis. The nonspecificity of gallium activity, however, requires that correlation with other radiographic studies and clinical findings be given close attention. Gallium imaging is very useful in the differential diagnosis and staging of some neoplasms, notably Hodgkin's disease, lymphoma, hepatocellular carcinoma, bronchogenic carcinoma, melanoma, and leukemia. Recent evidence has shown a correlation of gallium localization in the lungs with the activity of disease in pulmonary fibrosis and asbestosis. Gallium is also used in addition to bone scintigraphy for detecting osteomyelitis, especially in its chronic stages. A common indication for gallium imaging is as a screening procedure for infection in fever of unknown origin (FUO).

Limitations There is variable normal excretion of gallium via the intestinal tract. This contributes to the nonspecificity of gallium imaging in suspected abdominal or pelvic infections. Previous treatment with antibiotics or high doses of steroids may decrease the inflammatory response and result in false-negative gallium imaging.

Additional Information Other isotope studies may need to be postponed up to 7 days after a gallium scan has been done due to its slow elimination from soft tissue.

Selected Readings
Bisson G, Lamoureux G, and Bégin R, "Quantitative Gallium-67 Lung Scan to Assess the Inflammatory Activity in the Pneumoconioses," *Semin Nucl Med*, 1987, 17(1):72-80.

Israel O, Front D, Epelbaum R, et al, "Residual Mass and Negative Gallium Scintigraphy in Treated Lymphoma," *J Nucl Med*, 1990, 31(3):365-8.

Maderazo EG, Hickingbotham NB, Woronick CL, et al, "The Influence of Various Factors on the Accuracy of Gallium-67 Imaging for Occult Infection," *J Nucl Med*, 1988, 29(5):608-15.

Rossleigh MA, Murray IP, Mackey DW, et al, "Pediatric Solid Tumors: Evaluation by Gallium-67 SPECT Studies," *J Nucl Med*, 1990, 31(2):168-72.

Gallium Tumor Scan see Gallium Scan *on previous page*

Garamycin® see Gentamicin *on page 351*

Gastric Aspirate Fungus Culture see Fungus Culture, Sputum *on page 345*

Gastric Aspirate Mycobacteria Culture see Mycobacteria Culture, Sputum *on page 406*

Gastric Biopsy Culture for *Helicobacter pylori* see Helicobacter pylori Culture and Urease Test *on page 356*

Gastrointestinal Viruses by EM *see* Electron Microscopic (EM) Examination for Viruses, Stool *on page 329*

GC Culture *see Neisseria gonorrhoeae* Culture *on page 412*

GC Culture, Throat *see Neisseria gonorrhoeae* Culture *on page 412*

Genital Culture

Related Information

Abscess Aerobic and Anaerobic Culture *on page 238*
Chlamydia Culture *on page 294*
Genital Culture for *Ureaplasma urealyticum on next page*
Group B *Streptococcus* Antigen Test *on page 354*
Neisseria gonorrhoeae Culture *on page 412*
Trichomonas Preparation *on page 462*

Applies To Cervical Culture; Endocervical Culture; Prostatic Fluid Culture; Vaginal Culture

Test Includes Culture for aerobic organisms, *Candida* sp, and *Neisseria gonorrhoeae. Gardnerella* and *Mobiluncus*, Gram stain, and fungal stain may require separate requests.

Special Instructions The laboratory should be informed of the specific source of specimen, age of patient, current antibiotic therapy, clinical diagnosis, and time of collection.

Specimen Swab of vagina, cervix, discharge, aspirated endocervical, endometrial, prostatic fluid, or urethral discharge. Specimens to be cultured for *N. gonorrhoeae* **must** be cultured at bedside (onto special medium at room temperature) and be in the laboratory within 30 minutes.

Container Sterile Culturette® or sterile tube

Collection The specimen should be transported to laboratory within 2 hours of collection. Refrigeration may reduce yield.

Turnaround Time Preliminary reports are usually available at 24 hours. Cultures with no growth are usually reported after 48 hours. Cultures from which pathogens are isolated usually require a minimum of 48 hours for completion.

Reference Range Normal flora; properly collected prostatic fluid and endocervical cultures are normally sterile.

Use Isolate and identify potentially pathogenic organisms. Infectious causes of abnormal vaginal discharge or vulvovaginitis include *Candida albicans, Trichomonas vaginalis, Gardnerella vaginalis, Mobiluncus* sp, *Chlamydia trachomatis*, herpes simplex virus, human papillomavirus, *Enterobius vermicularis* (pinworms), *Giardia lamblia* and other microorganisms. Normal vaginal secretions have a pH of 4.5 or less, characteristic appearance, and consist of clear mucus, epithelial cells, and have no unusual odor. Many bacterial organisms and perhaps *Candida albicans* are present in a stable symbiotic relationship. Culture may allow documentation of a change in balance of normal organism populations or detection of a specific pathogen. Also used to document presence of *Staphylococcus aureus* in cases of suspected toxic shock syndrome.

Limitations *Chlamydia* and *Ureaplasma urealyticum* are not recovered by this procedure.

Methodology Aerobic culture with selective (Thayer-Martin) and nonselective media incubated at 35°C to 37°C with CO_2

Additional Information Rapid growing aerobic organisms which predominate are usually identified. Susceptibility testing can be performed if indicated. Routine culture often includes culture for *N. gonorrhoeae, Candida albicans, Staphylococcus aureus*, group B streptococci, and *Gardnerella vaginalis.* Presence or absence of normal flora will usually be reported. Normal flora of the vagina is dependent upon age, glycogen content, pH, exogenous hormone therapy, etc. Normal vaginal flora includes anaerobes, corynebacteria, enteric gram-negative rods, enterococci, lactobacilli, *Moraxella* sp, staphylococci, streptococci (alpha and nonhemolytic), *Mycobacterium smegmatis.* The laboratory should be consulted to arrange for special toxin identification procedures if toxic shock syndrome is suspected and *Staphylococcus aureus* is recovered.

Vaginitis is one of the most commonly encountered complaints of female patients. The majority of cases (approximately 90%) are caused by *Candida, Gardnerella*, or *Trichomonas.* Diagnosis and effective treatment depend upon accurate identification of the etiologic agent, effective specific therapy, and restoration of the normal ecosystem of the vagina. Proper hygiene, dietary

(Continued)

349

Genital Culture (Continued)

control, and management of stress also are important factors in control of re-current vaginal infections.

Candida sp are frequently present as normal flora in vagina. A saline wet mount may demonstrate yeast cells, or pseudohyphae and may provide rapid diagnostic information. The most common clinical presentation is a character-istic clumpy white cottage cheese appearance with vaginal or vulvar itching. Vaginitis frequently complicates pregnancy and diabetes, and is seen with broad spectrum antibiotic therapy as well as in conditions which lower host re-sistance.

Selected Readings

Faro S, "Bacterial Vaginitis," *Clin Obstet Gynecol*, 1991, 34(3):582-6.

Sobel JD, "Vaginal Infections in Adult Women," *Med Clin North Am*, 1990, 74(6):1573-602.

Spiegel CA, "Bacterial Vaginosis," *Clin Microbiol Rev*, 1991, 4(4):485-502.

Thomason JL, Gelbart SM, and Scaglione NJ, "Bacterial Vaginosis: Current Review With In-dications for Asymptomatic Therapy," *Am J Obstet Gynecol*, 1991, 165(4 Pt 2):1210-7.

Zenilman JM, "Gonorrhea: Clinical and Public Health Issues," *Hosp Pract (Off Ed)*, 1993, 28(2A):29-35, 39-40, 43-50.

Genital Culture for *Mycoplasma* T-Strain *see* Genital Culture for *Ureaplasma urealyticum on this page*

Genital Culture for *Ureaplasma urealyticum*

Related Information

Fungus Culture, Appropriate Site *on page 340*

Genital Culture *on previous page*

Mycoplasma/*Ureaplasma* Culture *on page 410*

Neisseria gonorrhoeae Culture *on page 412*

Synonyms Genital Culture for *Mycoplasma* T-Strain; *Mycoplasma* T-Strain Cul-ture, Genital; *Ureaplasma urealyticum* Culture, Genital

Applies To Cervical Culture for T-Strain *Mycoplasma*; Cervical Culture for *Urea-plasma urealyticum*; Urethral Culture for T-Strain *Mycoplasma*

Special Instructions *Ureaplasma* and *Mycoplasma* are sensitive to delays in processing and storage. Consult the laboratory prior to collecting the speci-men for optimal handling instructions.

Specimen Culturette® swab of urethra or cervix

Container Culturette® swab

Storage Instructions Keep specimen refrigerated. **Organism is remarkably sensitive to drying**; swab must be placed promptly into Culturette® and hand delivered to the Microbiology Laboratory.

Turnaround Time 8 days if negative, up to 2 weeks if positive

Reference Range Frequently isolated from asymptomatic individuals

Use Establish the diagnosis of *Ureaplasma urealyticum* infection in suspected cases of nongonococcal urethritis and cervicitis

Limitations Culture may be negative in the presence of infection, and the pres-ence of *Ureaplasma urealyticum* or *Mycoplasma hominis* does not always indi-cate infection, although there is a significant association with symptomatic dis-ease.

Methodology Culture on selective media

Additional Information *Ureaplasma* and *Mycoplasma* can be isolated from urethral and genital swabs and from urine of sexually active individuals. Sixty percent or more of all women asymptomatically carry *U. urealyticum* in their genital tract. Usual prevalence of these organisms in patients with urethral symptoms also is high; thus, conclusions regarding the etiologic role of an iso-late in a given patient are difficult to make. *U. urealyticum* is usually associated with cases of nongonococcal urethritis.

Selected Readings

Bell TA, "*Chlamydia trachomatis*, *Mycoplasma hominis*, and *Ureaplasma urealyticum* Infec-tions of Infants," *Semin Perinatol*, 1985, 9(1):29-37.

Cassell GH, Waites KB, Watson HL, et al, "*Ureaplasma urealyticum* Intrauterine Infection: Role in Prematurity and Disease in Newborns," *Clin Microbiol Rev*, 1993, 6(1):69-87.

Taylor-Robinson D and McCormack WM, "The Genital *Mycoplasma*," *N Engl J Med*, 1980, 302(19):1003-67.

Gen-Probe® for *Neisseria gonorrhoeae* *see* Neisseria gonorrhoeae by Nucleic Acid Probe *on page 411*

Gentamicin

Related Information
Antibiotic Level, Serum *on page 255*

Synonyms Garamycin®

Abstract Aminoglycoside antibiotics, including gentamicin, are used primarily to treat infections caused by aerobic gram-negative bacilli. Additionally, when used in combination with penicillins, they may have synergistic bactericidal activity against gram-positive cocci such as *Staphylococcus aureus* and *Enterococcus*. Gentamicin has a narrow therapeutic window, and its use in life-threatening infections makes it mandatory that effective levels be achieved without overdosage.

Specimen Serum, urine

Container Red top tube, plastic urine container

Sampling Time Peak: 30-60 minutes after end of 30 minute I.V. infusion or 60 minutes post I.M. dose; trough: immediately prior to next dose. Specimens should be drawn at steady-state, usually after fifth dose, if drug given every 8 hours, or after third dose, if drug given every 12 hours.

Storage Instructions Separate within 1 hour of collection and refrigerate or freeze until assayed. Must be frozen if a β-lactam antibiotic is also present because of potential inactivation of aminoglycosides.

Reference Range Therapeutic: peak: 4-10 μg/mL (SI: 8-21 μmol/L) (depends in part on the minimal inhibitory concentration of the drug against the organism being treated); trough: <2 μg/mL (SI: <4 μmol/L)

Possible Panic Range Toxic: peak: >12 μg/mL (SI: >25 μmol/L); trough: >2 μg/mL (SI: >4 μmol/L)

Use Peak levels are necessary to assure adequate therapeutic levels for organism being treated. Trough levels are necessary to reduce the likelihood of nephrotoxicity.

Limitations High peak levels may not have strong correlation with toxicity.

Methodology Enzyme immunoassay (EIA), fluorescence polarization immunoassay (FPIA), high performance liquid chromatography (HPLC)

Additional Information Gentamicin is cleared by the kidney and accumulates in renal tubular cells. Nephrotoxicity is most closely related to the length of time that trough levels exceed 2 μg/mL (SI: >4 μmol/L). Creatinine levels should be monitored every 2-3 days as an indicator of impending renal toxicity. The initial toxic result is nonoliguric renal failure that is usually reversible if the drug is discontinued. Continued administration of gentamicin may produce oliguric renal failure. Nephrotoxicity may occur in as many as 10% to 25% of patients receiving aminoglycosides; most of this toxicity can be avoided by monitoring levels and adjusting dosing schedules accordingly.

Aminoglycosides may also cause irreversible ototoxicity that manifests itself clinically as hearing loss. Aminoglycoside ototoxicity is relatively uncommon and clinical trials where levels were carefully monitored and dosing adjusted failed to show a correlation between auditory toxicity and plasma aminoglycoside levels. In situations where dosing is not monitored and adjusted, however, sustained high levels may be associated with ototoxicity. This association is far from clear cut, and new once-daily dosing regimens (and associated high peak serum concentrations) that fail to enhance toxicity further complicate this issue.

Selected Readings
Dipersio JR, "Gentamicin and Other Aminoglycosides," *Clinical Chemistry Theory, Analysis, and Correlation*, 2nd ed, Kaplan LA and Pesce AJ, eds, St Louis, MO: CV Mosby Co, 1989, 1102-8.

Edson RS and Terrell CL, "The Aminoglycosides," *Mayo Clin Proc*, 1991, 66(11):1158-64.

Pancoast SJ, "Aminoglycoside Antibiotics in Clinical Use," *Med Clin North Am*, 1987, 72(3):581-612.

German Measles Culture *see* Rubella Virus Culture *on page 440*

German Measles Serology *see* Rubella Serology *on page 439*

GFR *see* Creatinine Clearance *on page 311*

***Giardia* Antigen** *see Giardia* Specific Antigen (GSA65) *on next page*

***Giardia* Immunoassay** *see Giardia* Specific Antigen (GSA65) *on next page*

LABORATORY DIAGNOSIS

Giardia Screen see _Giardia_ Specific Antigen (GSA65)
on this page

Giardia Specific Antigen (GSA65)

Synonyms _Giardia_ Antigen; _Giardia_ Immunoassay; _Giardia_ Screen

Test Includes A solid-phase immunoassay based on specific antibody to _Giardia_ specific antigen (GSA65)

Specimen
- Fresh random stool, collected in a clean sealable plastic container – refrigerated or frozen until testing.
- Stool in 10% formalin – refrigerated or frozen.
- Stool in Cary-Blair medium – refrigerated or frozen.
- Rectal swabs, transported in Stewart's Culturette® or Ames Charcoal Culturette®. Swabs should not be allowed to dry out.
- Stool in PVA fixative **is not** acceptable.

Reference Range Negative

Use Diagnose giardiasis; monitor effectiveness of anti-_Giardia_ therapy

Methodology Solid phase immunoassay

Additional Information A positive result indicates the presence of _Giardia_ specific antigen (GGSA65). Secretion of GSA65 is present only when _Giardia_ infection is present. GSA65 does not cross react with other enteric parasites, bacteria, or yeast. This test is more sensitive for the diagnosis of _Giardia_ than the routine ova and parasite examination. It is not a substitute for the broad screen provided by the ova and parasite examination. An equivalent screening test (immunofluorescent antibody) is available in some laboratories.

Selected Readings
Maddison SE, "Serodiagnosis of Parasitic Diseases," _Clin Microbiol Rev_, 1991, 4(4):457-69.
Wolfe MS, "Giardiasis," _Clin Microbiol Rev_, 1992, 5(1):93-100.

Glomerular Filtration Rate see Creatinine Clearance
on page 311

Gonorrhea Culture see _Neisseria gonorrhoeae_ Culture
on page 412

Gonorrhea Culture, Throat see _Neisseria gonorrhoeae_ Culture
on page 412

Gram Stain

Related Information
Acid-Fast Stain, Modified, _Nocardia_ Species on page 241
Actinomyces Culture, All Sites on page 242

Synonyms Bacterial Smear; Smear, Gram Stain

Patient Preparation Same as for routine culture of specific site

Special Instructions The laboratory should be informed of the specific site of specimen, age of patient, current antibiotic therapy, and clinical diagnosis.

Specimen Duplicate of specimen appropriate for routine culture of the specific site

Container Sterile specimen container, or sterile tube or appropriate tube for swab

Collection Collection procedure same as for routine culture of the specific site. Specimen must be collected to avoid contamination with skin, adjacent structures, and nonsterile surfaces.

Storage Instructions Same as for a culture of the specimen

Causes for Rejection Insufficient specimen volume

Turnaround Time Usually same day

Reference Range Depends on site of specimen

Use Determine presence or absence of bacteria, yeast, neutrophils, and epithelial cells; establish the presence of potentially pathogenic organisms. The Gram stain is essential in evaluation of all suspected cases of bacterial meningitis.

Limitations Organism isolation and identification will usually be performed only if culture is requested. Request for Gram stain will not lead to stain for mycobacteria (TB). For detection of tubercle bacilli, an acid-fast stain must also be requested. Certain organisms do not stain or do not stain well with Gram stain, eg, _Legionella pneumophila_ and _Campylobacter_ sp. As many as 30% of cases of bacterial meningitis have a negative Gram stain. Yield may be increased by use of the acridine orange stain (AO) particularly in cases of partially treated meningitis, but few laboratories elect to use this method. Gram stain is **not** reliable for diagnosis of cervical, rectal, pharyngeal, or asymptomatic urethral gonococcal infection, except for gonococcal urethritis in males.

Methodology Gram stain technique:

- Make a thin smear of the material for study and allow to air dry.
- Fix the material to the slide by passing the slide 3 or 4 times through the flame of a Bunsen burner so that the material does not wash off during the staining procedure. Some workers now recommend the use of alcohol for the fixation of material to be Gram stained (flood the smear with methanol or ethanol for a few minutes or warm for 10 minutes at 60°C on a slide warmer).
- Place the smear on a staining rack and overlay the surface with crystal violet solution.
- After 1 minute (less time may be used with some solutions) of exposure to the crystal violet stain, wash thoroughly with distilled water or buffer.
- Overlay the smear with Gram's iodine solution for 1 minute. Wash again with water.
- Hold the smear between the thumb and forefinger and flood the surface with acetone-alcohol decolorizer until no violet color washes off. This usually takes 1-3 seconds.
- Wash with running water and again place the smear on the staining rack. Overlay the surface with safranin counterstain for 1 minute. Wash with running water.
- Use paper towels to blot the smear dry.
- Examine the stained smear under the 100X (oil) immersion objective of the microscope. Gram-positive bacteria stain dark blue; gram-negative bacteria appear pink-red.

Additional Information Gram stains are usually scanned for the presence or absence of white blood cells (indicative of infection) and squamous epithelial cells (indicative of mucosal contamination). A sputum specimen showing more than 25 squamous epithelial cells per low powered field, regardless of the number of white blood cells, is indicative that the specimen is grossly contaminated with saliva and the culture results cannot be properly interpreted. Additional sputum specimens should be submitted to the laboratory if evidence of contamination by saliva is revealed.

The Gram stain can be a reliable indicator to guide initial antibiotic therapy in community acquired pneumonia. It is imperative that a valid sputum specimen be obtained for Gram stain. In a well designed trial, valid expectorated sputum was obtained in 41% (59 of 144 patients). The Gram stain is reliable but not infallible.

Although mycobacteria have classically been considered to be gram-positive or faintly gram-positive, they are more correctly characterized as "gram-neutral" on routine stains. A careful search for mycobacteria should be undertaken when purulent sputum without stainable organisms is encountered.

Gram stains revealing 1 bacterium per high powered (100X) field in an uncentrifuged urine specimen (or any fluid) suggest a colony count of 10^5 bacteria/mL. Bacteria in the majority of fields suggests 10^6 bacteria/mL, a level associated with significant bacteriuria.

Gram stain is the most valuable immediately available diagnostic test in bacterial meningitis. Organisms are detectable in 60% to 80% of patients who have not been treated, and in 40% to 60% of those who have been given antibiotics. Its sensitivity relates to the number of organisms present. The sensitivity of the Gram stain is greater in gram-positive infections, and is only positive in half of the instances of gram-negative meningitis. It is positive even less frequently with listeriosis meningitis or with anaerobic infections.

Culture and Gram stain should always have priority over antigen detection methods.

Selected Readings

Gleckman R, DeVita J, Hibert D, et al, "Sputum Gram Stain Assessment in Community-Acquired Bacteremic Pneumonia," *J Clin Microbiol*, 1988, 26(5):846-9.

Granoff DM, Murphy TV, Ingram DL, et al, "Use of Rapidly Generated Results in Patient Management," *Diagn Microbiol Infect Dis*, 1986, 4(3 Suppl):157S-66S.

Gray LD and Fedorko DP, "Laboratory Diagnosis of Bacterial Meningitis," *Clin Microbiol Rev*, 1992, 5(2):130-45.

Provine H and Gardner P, "The Gram Stained Smear and Its Interpretation," *Hosp Pract*, 1974, 9:85-91.

Riccardi NB and Felman YM, "Laboratory Diagnosis in the Problem of Suspected Gonococcal Infection," *JAMA*, 1979, 242(24):2703-5.

Smith AL, "Bacterial Meningitis," *Pediatr Rev*, 1993, 14:11-8.

LABORATORY DIAGNOSIS

Group A Beta-Hemolytic *Streptococcus* Culture, Throat *see* Throat Culture for Group A Beta-Hemolytic *Streptococcus* on page 457

Group A *Streptococcus* Antigen Test
Related Information
Bacterial Antigens, Rapid Detection Methods *on page 269*
Throat Culture for Group A Beta-Hemolytic *Streptococcus* *on page 457*

Synonyms Coagglutination Test for Group A Streptococci; *Streptococcus* Group A Latex Screen; Throat Swab for Group A Streptococcal Antigen

Applies To Enzyme Immunoassay for Group A *Streptococcus* Antigen

Test Includes Latex agglutination test for group A *Streptococcus* (GAS) antigen

Special Instructions Some laboratories favor submission of dry swabs for antigen testing. Consult the laboratory for their specific recommendations.

Specimen Throat swab; many laboratories request two swabs, one for culture if the rapid screen is negative. Specimens negative by this test must be cultured to confirm the negative result.

Container Rayon or Dacron swabs rather than cotton swabs enhance the chance of detection.

Collection Rigorous swabbing of the tonsillar pilars and posterior throat increases the probability of detection of streptococcal antigen.

Use Detect the presence of group A streptococcal antigen in throat specimens

Limitations Many reviews have indicated a sensitivity of 75% to 80% and a specificity of 95% to 98% for the rapid methods. Sensitivity varies between manufacturers. Some kits are capable of detecting as few as 10 colony forming units (CFUs) on culture while others require 100-1000 CFU on culture. Specimens which yield <10 colonies on culture usually are negative by rapid method. Adequate specimen collection on younger patients may be difficult, and thus, contribute to the false-negative rate. A positive result can be relied upon as a rational basis to begin therapy. **A negative result is only presumptive and a culture should be performed to reasonably exclude the diagnosis of group A streptococcal infection.** Careful attention to the details of the method and the use of appropriate controls are required to assume adequate performance. Group A streptococcal antigen disappears rapidly following antibiotic therapy. Thus a history of prior therapy should be sought when assessing pharyngitis.

Contraindications The test may become negative 4 hours after therapy has been started.

Methodology The streptococcal group carbohydrate antigen is extracted from the swab used for collection by use of acid or enzyme reagents. The extraction mixture is added to particles coated with antistreptococcal antibody. If the streptococcal antigen is present visible agglutination occurs due to antigen cross links with antibody coated latex within 10 minutes. Enzyme immunoassay methods (EIA) are also used.

Additional Information Rheumatic fever remains a concern in the United States and serious complications including sepsis, soft tissue invasion, and toxic shock-like syndrome have been reported to be increasing in frequency; therefore, timely diagnosis and early institution of appropriate therapy remains important. Timely therapy may reduce the acute symptoms and overall duration of streptococcal pharyngitis. The sequelae of poststreptococcal glomerulonephritis and rheumatic fever are diminished by early therapy.

Selected Readings
Facklam RR, "Specificity Study of Kits for Detection of Group A Streptococci Directly From Throat Swabs," *J Clin Microbiol*, 1987, 25(3):504-8.
Kaplan EL, "The Rapid Identification of Group A Beta-Hemolytic Streptococci in the Upper Respiratory Tract - Current Status," *Pediatr Clin North Am*, 1988, 35(3):535-42, (review).
Nadler HL, "Group A Strep Detection," *Diagn Clin Test*, 1989, 27:3:35-41, (review of rapid methods).
"Rapid Diagnostic Tests for Group A Streptococcal Pharyngitis," *Med Lett Drugs Ther*, 1991, 33(843):40-1.

Group B *Streptococcus* Antigen Test
Related Information
Bacterial Antigens, Rapid Detection Methods *on page 269*
Genital Culture *on page 349*

Synonyms *Streptococcus agalactiae*, Latex Screen; *Streptococcus* Group B Latex Screen

Applies To CIE for Group B Streptococcal Antigen; Counterimmunoelectrophoresis for Group B Streptococcal Antigen; Group B *Streptococcus*, Counterimmunoelectrophoresis

Test Includes Latex screen for group B beta *Streptococcus* or counterimmunoelectrophoresis (CIE)

Special Instructions The specimen should be tested as soon as possible after collection.

Specimen Cerebrospinal fluid, serum, urine, endocervical, or amniotic fluid

Container Sterile container, red top tube

Storage Instructions If the specimen cannot be tested immediately it may be stored at 2°C to 8°C for 1 day or frozen at -20°C for longer storage.

Turnaround Time 1 hour stat; 24 hours routine

Use Detect group B *Streptococcus* antigen in body fluids. Detection of group B *Streptococcus* antigen at the time of delivery is usually an indication for chemoprophylaxis.

Limitations Latex agglutination tests appear to have a slightly greater sensitivity than counterimmunoelectrophoresis (CIE) procedures. Sensitivity is relatively low, 15% to 21%, for rapid group B streptococcal antigen tests. False-positives are rare. Concentrated urine is a good specimen. Testing CSF and serum, as well as culture for the organism, should be considered to establish the definitive diagnosis.

Methodology Latex agglutination (LA), counterimmunoelectrophoresis (CIE). Polystyrene latex particles coated with antibodies specific for the group B *Streptococcus* antigen agglutinate in the presence of the homologous antigen. Controls for nonspecific agglutination of latex particles are generally used. The specimen is heat inactivated and cooled to room temperature before testing. Urine may be concentrated. The infection can be diagnosed by detection of the group B specific carbohydrate antigen of the organism's cell wall which may be present in body fluids, serum and cerebrospinal fluid and which is excreted in urine. Counterimmunoelectrophoresis is an alternate method for detection of the group B *Streptococcus* antigen but is rarely available.

Additional Information Group B *Streptococcus* is currently one of the most significant human pathogens in the neonatal period. The most common mode of acquisition by the neonate is exposure to the maternal genital flora *in utero* through ruptured membranes or by contamination during passage through the birth canal. Rapid identification of group B *Streptococcus* carriers is important in management of premature rupture of the membranes because the effectiveness of intrapartum prophylactic ampicillin may be compromised by awaiting the results of conventional cultures. Infection is manifested in two major forms, early onset septicemic infection manifest in the first few days of life and late onset meningitis which occurs during the first few months of life.

Isolates of group B *Streptococcus* resistant to erythromycin, intermediate to clindamycin, and resistant to cefoxitin, as well as strains with multiple antimicrobial resistance, have been reported. Susceptibility testing may be useful in selecting alternate antibiotic regimens.

Selected Readings

Brady K, Duff P, Schilhab JC, et al, "Reliability of a Rapid Latex Fixation Test for Detecting Group B Streptococci in the Genital Tract of Parturients at Term," *Obstet Gynecol*, 1989, 73(4):678-81.

Newton ER and Clark M, "Group B *Streptococcus* and Preterm Rupture of Membranes," *Obstet Gynecol*, 1988, 71(2):198-202.

Spence MR, "A Rapid Screening Test for the Diagnosis of Endocervical Group B Streptococci in Pregnancy: Microbiologic Results and Clinical Outcome," *Obstet Gynecol*, 1988, 71(2):284, (letter).

Stiller RJ, Blair E, Clark P, et al, "Rapid Detection of Vaginal Colonization With Group B Streptococci by Means of Latex Agglutination," *Am J Obstet Gynecol*, 1989, 160(3):566-8.

Group B *Streptococcus*, Counterimmunoelectrophoresis *see* Group B *Streptococcus* Antigen Test *on previous page*

Haemophilus influenzae Susceptibility Testing *see* Penicillinase Test *on page 427*

Hair Fungus Culture *see* Fungus Culture, Skin *on page 343*

Hand, Left or Right, X-ray *see* Bone Films *on page 277*

Hands and Wrist Arthritis, X-ray *see* Bone Films *on page 277*

Hanging Drop Mount for *Trichomonas* *see* Trichomonas Preparation *on page 462*

Hank's Stain *see* Acid-Fast Stain, Modified, *Nocardia* Species
on page 241

HCV Serology *see* Hepatitis C Serology *on page 360*

Head Lice Identification *see* Arthropod Identification
on page 268

Head Studies, CT *see* Computed Transaxial Tomography, Head
Studies *on page 307*

Helicobacter pylori Culture and Urease Test

Related Information

Helicobacter pylori Culture, Gastric Biopsy *on next page*

Synonyms *Campylobacter pylori* Urease Test and Culture; CLO™ Test; Gastric Biopsy Culture for *Helicobacter pylori*; Urease Test and Culture, *Helicobacter pylori*

Test Includes Screening for the presence of urease activity indirectly indicating the presence of *Helicobacter pylori*, culture of the organism from gastric biopsy specimens

Specimen Gastric mucosal biopsy

Container Sterile container; **no fixative** for these microbiologic tests

Storage Instructions If specimen cannot be transported immediately to the laboratory, it should be placed in 0.5 mL transport medium (normal saline).

Turnaround Time 24 hours for urease final report; up to 7 days for culture

Reference Range Negative for urease activity, negative culture, biopsy negative for gastritis and negative for *H. pylori*

Use Establish the presence and possible etiologic role of *Helicobacter pylori* in cases of chronic gastric ulcer, chronic active gastritis, and a relationship with duodenal ulcers

Limitations Culture and urease testing alone, without biopsies, may allow occult neoplasms to go undetected.

Methodology Urease test: Gastric biopsies are incubated on slightly buffered medium. A change of phenol red to alkaline (pink color) persisting more than 5 minutes is considered positive and presumptively indicative of the presence of *Helicobacter pylori* even if the organism cannot be grown in culture. Specimens negative at 30 minutes should be re-examined periodically up to 24 hours. The sensitivity of urease testing leaves something to be desired and depends on the selected gold standard. It was only 62% at 24 hours in a 1991 report. This method is also is characterized by false-positive results.

Culture: Culture media may include enriched chocolate, Thayer-Martin with antibiotics, brain heart infusion (BHI) with 7% horse blood, and Mueller-Hinton with 5% sheep blood. The organism is microaerophilic and grows best in a reduced O_2 atmosphere or in a Campy-Pak™ system at 42°C. Cultures are usually observed for 7 days before being reported as negative.

Cytology: Touch cytology preparations (ie, imprints from biopsies) may provide a rapid diagnosis and preserve the biopsy specimen for histopathology or culture.

Smear: A direct smear can be Gram stained.

Approximate sensitivities of methods for detection of *H. pylori*:
• 24-hour urease: 62%
• direct Gram stain: 69%
• culture: 90%
• histology: 93%

Additional Information *Helicobacter pylori* is a major cause of chronic active gastritis. Its importance and etiologic relationship with duodenal ulcer requires further study. Seventy-eight percent to 100% of subjects who have duodenal ulcer have *H. pylori* infection, but 3% to 70% of patients without duodenal ulcer have *H. pylori* as well. The organism may be seen in biopsies stained with Gram stain, hematoxylin-eosin (H & E), Giemsa or Warthin-Starry silver stain. It is most often recognized in biopsies of the antrum but may also be seen in the fundic mucosa, metaplastic gastric mucosa of esophagus (Barrett's esophagus), or duodenum. Biopsy may also establish the diagnosis of carcinoma or lymphoma. *H. pylori* was not found in the gastric mucosa of Meckel's diverticula. Gram stains performed by a reuse imprint technique on biopsies from both the antrum and fundus yielded positives in 100% of 32 culture positive cases.

Most peptic ulcers related to *H. pylori* infection are reported as curable.

Breath isotope methods measuring bacterial urease by detection of labeled CO_2 and serologic tests for the detection of antibody are also useful but are rarely available. The breath test is preferred as a means of documenting presence of active infection and eradication of infection after therapy in the absence of endoscopy.

The serologic tests can be very helpful but are limited because they can remain positive for months following therapy. Use of specific IgA enhances the value of serology in monitoring therapy.

Past *H. pylori* infection increases risk of carcinoma of stomach. Chronic atrophic gastritis and intestinal metaplasia are related to *H. pylori* infection, which induces as well development of lymphoid tissue in the gastric mucosa. A possible role for *H. pylori* in the development of primary malignant lymphoma of stomach has been postulated.

Selected Readings

Blaser MJ, "*Helicobacter pylori*: Its Role in Disease," *Clin Infect Dis*, 1992, 15(3):386-91.

Cover TL and Blaser MJ, "*Helicobacter pylori* and Gastroduodenal Disease," *Annu Rev Med*, 1992, 43:135-45.

Debongnie JC, Delmee M, Mainguet P, et al, "Cytology: A Simple, Rapid, Sensitive Method in the Diagnosis of *Helicobacter pylori*," *Am J Gastroenterol*, 1992, 87(1):20-3.

Dooley CP and Cohen H, "The Clinical Significance of *Campylobacter pylori*," *Ann Intern Med*, 1988, 108(1):70-9.

Hoek FJ, Noach LA, Rauws EJ, et al, "Evaluation of the Performance of Commercial Test Kits for Detection of *Helicobacter pylori* Antibodies in Serum," *J Clin Microbiol*, 1992, 30(6):1525-8.

Murry DM, "Clinical Relevance of Infection by *Helicobacter pylori*," *Clin Microbiol Newslett*, 1993, 15(5):33-7.

Perez-Perez GI and Dunn BE, "Diagnosis of *C. pylori* Infection by Serologic Methods," *Campylobacter pylori* in Gastritis and Peptic Ulcer Disease, New York, NY: Igaku-Shoin, 1989, 163-74.

Peterson WL, "*Helicobacter pylori* and Peptic Ulcer Disease," *N Engl J Med*, 1991, 324(15):1043-8.

Helicobacter pylori Culture, Gastric Biopsy

Related Information

Helicobacter pylori Culture and Urease Test *on previous page*

Synonyms *Campylobacter pylori*, Gastric Biopsy Culture

Special Instructions Notify laboratory before biopsy to obtain additional instructions and transport media.

Specimen Gastric mucosal biopsy

Container Sterile container, no fixative

Collection Special instructions from laboratory

Storage Instructions Transport specimen to the laboratory immediately. If specimen cannot be transported immediately to the laboratory it should be placed in 0.5 mL transport medium (normal saline).

Causes for Rejection Excessive delay in transport.

Reference Range No *Helicobacter pylori* detected

Use Establish the presence and possible etiologic role of *Helicobacter pylori* in cases of chronic gastric ulcer, gastritis, duodenal ulcer, dyspepsia, etc

Limitations *C. pylori* infections can be very focal. A negative culture does not rule out *C. pylori* or disease that may have been caused by *C. pylori*.

Additional Information *Helicobacter pylori* has been implicated as a factor associated with chronic gastritis. The clinical significance of the organism in regard to gastric or duodenal ulcers, dyspepsia, and gastric carcinoma remains unclear. Other factors such as pepsin, nonsteroidal anti-inflammatory agents (NSAIDs), aspirin, ischemia, stress, alcohol, and bile salts as well as *H. pylori* all may have a role in altering the material mucosal barrier. The relative etiologic role of *H. pylori* remains a subject of speculation. Large numbers of small bacteria, *Helicobacter pylori*, can be cultured from, or seen microscopically (especially with Dieterle stain) in gastric biopsies from most patients with chronic gastritis and/or peptic ulcers. They can also be found in significant numbers of asymptomatic patients who have histologic gastritis, and from some individuals with no abnormality.

Helminths, Blood Preparation *see* Microfilariae, Peripheral Blood Preparation *on page 400*

Helper Cell/Suppressor Ratio *see* T4/T8 Ratio *on page 453*

Hemoflagellates *see* Microfilariae, Peripheral Blood Preparation
on page 400

Hemogram *see* Complete Blood Count *on page 302*

Hemovac® Tip Culture *see* Intravenous Line Culture
on page 376

Hepatitis A Profile

Test Includes Determination of IgG and IgM antibody to hepatitis A virus and confirmation of all new IgM positives by repeat testing

Specimen Serum

Container Red top tube or serum separator tube

Storage Instructions Transport specimen to the laboratory immediately. Separate serum and freeze.

Reference Range IgG: negative; IgM: negative

Use Determine recent or past infection with hepatitis A virus

Methodology Radioimmunoassay (RIA) or enzyme immunoassay (EIA)

Additional Information Hepatitis A is transmitted by the fecal-oral route, usually foodborne. Its incubation period is 2-7 weeks. Hepatitis A virus is a picornavirus, and antibody is made to capsid proteins. Fecal excretion of HAV peaks before symptoms develop. If hepatitis A antibody is IgM, the hepatitis A infection is probably acute. IgM antibody develops within a week of symptom onset, peaks in 3 months, and is usually gone after 6 months. Hepatitis A antibody of IgG type is indicative of old infection, is found in almost half of adults, and is not usually clinically relevant. Many cases of hepatitis A are subclinical, particularly in children. Presence of IgG antibody to HAV does not exclude acute hepatitis B or non-A, non-B hepatitis.

Incubation	Early Acute	Acute	Recovery
Duration			
15-45 Days	0-14 Days	3-6 Months	Years

Selected Readings

Giacoia GP and Kasprisin DO, "Transfusion-Acquired Hepatitis A," *South Med J*, 1989, 82(11):1357-60.

Hollinger FB and Dreesman GR, "Hepatitis Viruses," *Manual of Clinical Laboratory Immunology*, 4th ed, Rose NR, de Macario EC, Fahey JL, et al, eds, Washington, DC: American Society for Microbiology, 1992, 634-50.

Lee HS and Vyas GN, "Diagnosis of Viral Hepatitis," *Clin Lab Med*, 1987, 7:741:57.

Mbithi JN, Springthorpe VS, Boulet JR, et al, "Survival of Hepatitis A Virus on Human Hands and Its Transfer on Contact With Animate and Inanimate Surfaces," *J Clin Microbiol*, 1992, 30(4):757-63.

Mishu B, Hadler SC, Boaz VA, et al, "Foodborne Hepatitis A: Evidence That Microwaving Reduces Risk?" *J Infect Dis*, 1990, 162(3):655-8.

Summers PL, DuBois DR, Houston Cohen WH, et al, "Solid-Phase Antibody Capture Hemadsorption Assay for Detection of Hepatitis A Virus Immunoglobulin M Antibodies," *J Clin Microbiol*, 1993, 31(5):1299-302.

Hepatitis B Profile

Related Information

Postexposure Prophylaxis for Hepatitis B *on page 719-720*

Test Includes Detection of hepatitis B surface antigen (HB$_s$Ag), antibody to hepatitis B surface antigen (anti-HB$_s$), hepatitis B core antibody (anti-HB$_c$), and confirmation of all new positives by repeat testing

Specimen Serum

Container Red top tube or serum separator tube

Storage Instructions Transport specimen to the laboratory immediately. Do not store blood.

Causes for Rejection Recently administered radioisotopes if assay performed by RIA, excessive hemolysis

Reference Range Negative

Serologic and clinical patterns observed during acute hepatitis B viral infection. From Hollinger FB and Dreesman GR, Manual of Clinical Immunology, 2nd ed, Rose NR and Friedman H, eds, Washington, DC: American Society for Microbiology, 1980, with permission.

Use Determine serological status to hepatitis B virus

Limitations Patients who are negative for HB$_s$Ag may still have acute type B viral hepatitis. There is sometimes a "window" stage when HB$_s$Ag has become negative and the patient has not yet developed the antibody (anti-HB$_s$Ag). On such occasions the anti-HB$_c$Ag (IgM) is usually positive, and the patient should be treated as potentially infectious until anti-HB$_s$Ag is detected, at which time immunity is probable. In cases with strong clinical suspicion of viral hepatitis, serologic testing should not be limited to detecting HB$_s$Ag but should include a battery of tests to evaluate different stages of acute and convalescent hepatitis. These should include a test for hepatitis A antibody (IgM), and HB$_s$Ag, HB$_s$Ab, HB$_c$Ab (IgM), and hepatitis C virus (HCV).

Presence of HB$_s$Ab is not an absolute indicator of resolved hepatitis infection, nor of protection from future infection. Since there are different serologic subtypes of hepatitis B virus, it is possible (and has been reported) for a patient to have antibody to one surface antigen type and to be acutely infected with virus of a different subtype. Thus, a patient may have coexisting HB$_s$Ag and HB$_s$Ab. Transfused individuals or hemophiliacs receiving plasma components may give false-positive tests for antibody to hepatitis B surface antigen. Individuals vaccinated with HBV vaccine will have antibodies to the surface protein.

Contraindications Patients on heparin therapy may demonstrate weak positive results.

Methodology Radioimmunoassay (RIA); enzyme immunoassay (EIA)

Additional Information Hepatitis B virus (HBV) is a DNA virus with a protein coat, surface antigen (HB$_s$Ag), and a core consisting of nucleoprotein, (HB$_c$Ag is the core antigen). There are eight different serotypes. Early in infection, HB$_s$Ag, HBV DNA, and DNA polymerase can all be detected in serum.

Transmission is parenteral, sexual or perinatal. The incubation period of hepatitis B is 2-6 months. HB$_s$Ag can be detected 1-7 weeks **before** liver enzyme elevation or the appearance of clinical symptoms. Three weeks after the onset of

(Continued)

Hepatitis B Profile *(Continued)*

acute hepatitis about 50% of the patients will still be positive for HB_sAg, while at 17 weeks only 10% are positive. The best available markers for infectivity are HB_sAg and HB_eAg. The presence of HB_sAb and HB_eAb is associated with noninfectivity. The chronic carrier state is indicated by the persistence of HB_sAg and/or HB_eAg over long periods (6 months to years) without seroconversion to the corresponding antibodies. Such a condition has the potential to lead to serious liver damage but may be an isolated asymptomatic serologic phenomenon. Persistence of HB_sAg, without anti-HB_s, with combinations of positivity of anti-HB_{core}, HB_eAg, or anti-HB_e indicate infectivity and need for investigation for chronic persistent or chronic aggressive hepatitis. Chronic carrier states are found in up to 10% of cases. Some remain healthy, but evolution to chronic persistent hepatitis, chronic active hepatitis, cirrhosis, and hepatoma represent major problems of this disease.

Prevention of hepatitis B for those at risk is available via vaccination, as well as treatment for some chronic carriers. For prophylaxis information see appendix table, Postexposure Prophylaxis for Hepatitis B.

Selected Readings

Centers for Disease Control, "Screening Donors of Blood, Plasma, Organs, Tissues, and Semen for Evidence of Hepatitis B and Hepatitis C," *Lab Med*, 1991, 22(8):555-63.

Devine P, Taswell HF, Moore SB, et al, "Passively Acquired Antibody to Hepatitis B Surface Antigen. Pitfall in Evaluating Immunity to Hepatitis B Viral Infections," *Arch Pathol Lab Med*, 1989, 113(5):529-31.

Edwards MS, "Hepatitis B Serology – Help in Interpretation," *Pediatr Clin North Am*, 1988, 35(3):503-15.

Hollinger FB and Dreesman GR, "Hepatitis Viruses," *Manual of Clinical Laboratory Immunology*, 4th ed, Rose NR, de Macario EC, Fahey JL, et al, eds, Washington, DC: American Society for Microbiology, 1992, 634-50.

Lee HS and Vyas GN, "Diagnosis of Viral Hepatitis," *Clin Lab Med*, 1987, 7:741-57.

Hepatitis C Gene Product *see* Hepatitis C Serology *on this page*

Hepatitis C Serology

Synonyms HCV Serology

Applies To Anti-HCV (IgM); C 100-3; Hepatitis C Gene Product; Non-A, non-B Hepatitis; Surrogate Tests for Non-A, Non-B Hepatitis

Test Includes Detection of antibody specific for hepatitis C in patient's serum

Abstract Most cases of post-transfusion non-A, non-B viral hepatitis are caused by HCV. Application of this test has caused a great decrease of post-transfusion hepatitis.

Patient Preparation Avoid recent administration of radioisotopes if assay is RIA

Specimen Serum

Container Red top tube

Causes for Rejection Recently administered radioisotopes if assay is RIA

Reference Range Negative

Use Differential diagnosis of acute hepatitis; screen blood units for transfusion safety

Limitations Since as many as 90% of commercial intravenous immunoglobulins test positive for hepatitis C antibody, a false-positive can result briefly after such transfusion.

Methodology Radioimmunoassay (RIA), enzyme-linked immunosorbent assay (ELISA)

Additional Information Before initiation of hepatitis B surface antigen testing in the 1970's, most significant post-transfusion hepatitis was due to hepatitis B. Following the development of sensitive and specific testing for hepatitis B, greater than 90% of post-transfusion hepatitis became so called "non-A, non-B." Hepatitis C virus is the most common cause of non-A, non-B hepatitis in the United States. Chiron Corporation has isolated a gene product (c100-3) of hepatitis C virus (HCV) and developed an assay for antibodies to it. The assay detects antibody to the flavivirus which is the etiologic agent of hepatitis C. Non-A, non-B, and non-C hepatitis can still occur, probably due to CMV, hepatitis E, and to other viruses that have not been identified.

For blood donors, hepatitis C serology correlates with surrogate tests for non-A, non-B hepatitis (ALT and anti-HB_c). Since hepatitis C serology identifies a broader group of infected individuals than surrogate testing, it reduces risk of HCV during transfusion. Studies in hemophiliacs indicate that antibody to HCV is a reliable marker of HCV. Recently, IgM anti-HCV core has been shown to be a useful acute marker for HCV infection. Transmission is by intravenous drug abuse, dialysis, and other needlesticks. Sexual transmission also occurs. Before screening for hepatitis C antibody was in place, non-A, non-B hepatitis was said to occur in as many as 10% of transfusions. With the introduction of first generation hepatitis C screening tests, the number has fallen to 1 in 3300 units. With the introduction of a more sensitive second generation hepatitis C test in 1992, safety has increased even more. Chronic carrier states develop in more than half the patients, and chronic liver disease is a major problem. Substantial risk of chronic active hepatitis and cirrhosis exists in those who develop chronic non-A, non-B hepatitis, of whom, about 80% develop anti-HCV. A risk of hepatocellular carcinoma exists for these patients, as well as a risk of liver failure. Studies are currently being done on the detection of HCV in patient's specimens using reverse transcriptase and PCR.

Selected Readings

Allain JP, Dailey SH, Laurian Y, et al, "Evidence for Persistent Hepatitis C Virus (HCV) Infection in Hemophiliacs," *J Clin Invest*, 1991, 88(5):1672-9.

Alter MJ, Hadler SC, Judson FN, et al, "Risk Factors for Acute Non-A, Non-B Hepatitis in the United States and Association With Hepatitis C Virus Infection," *JAMA*, 1990, 264(17):2231-5.

Alter MJ, Margolis HS, Krawczynski K, et al, "The Natural History of Community-Acquired Hepatitis C in the United States," *N Engl J Med*, 1992, 327(27):1899-905.

Centers for Disease Control, "Screening Donors of Blood, Plasma, Organs, Tissues, and Semen for Evidence of Hepatitis B and Hepatitis C," *Lab Med*, 1991, 22(8):555-63.

Clemens JM, Taskar S, Chau K, et al, "IgM Antibody Response in Acute Hepatitis C Viral Infection," *Blood*, 1992, 79(1):169-72.

Choo Q-L, Kuo G, Weiner AJ, et al, "Isolation of a cDNA Clone Derived From a Blood-Borne Non-A, Non-B Viral Hepatitis Genome," *Science*, 1989, 244(4902):359-62.

Dodd LG, McBride JH, Gitnick GL, et al, "Prevalence of Non-A, Non-B Hepatitis/Hepatitis C Virus Antibody in Human Immunoglobulins," *Am J Clin Pathol*, 1992, 97(1):108-13.

Dodd RY, "Hepatitis C Virus, Antibodies and Infectivity – Paradox, Pragmatism, and Policy," *Am J Clin Pathol*, 1992, 97(1):4-6, (editorial).

Gambino R, "NANB Hepatitis – A New Antibody Test for the Hepatitis C Virus," *Lab Report for Physicians*,™ 1988, 10:89-93.

Hsieh TT, Yao DS, Sheen IS, et al, "Hepatitis C Virus in Peripheral Blood Mononuclear Cells," *Am J Clin Pathol*, 1992, 98(4):392-6.

Kuo G, Choo QL, Alter HJ, et al, "An Assay for Circulating Antibodies to a Major Etiologic Virus of Human Non-A, Non-B Hepatitis," *Science*, 1989, 244(4902):362-4.

Prince AM, Brotman B, Inchauspé G, et al, "Patterns and Prevalence of Hepatitis C Virus Infection in Post-Transfusion Non-A, Non-B Hepatitis," *J Infect Dis*, 1993, 167(5):1296-301.

Richards C, Holland P, Kuramoto K, et al, "Prevalence of Antibody to Hepatitis C Virus in a Blood Donor Population," *Transfusion*, 1991, 31(2):109-13.

Seeff LB, Buskell-Bales Z, Wright EC, et al, "Long-Term Mortality After Transfusion-Associated Non-A, Non-B Hepatitis," *N Engl J Med*, 1992, 327(27):1906-11.

Hepatitis D Serology

Synonyms Delta Agent Serology; Delta Hepatitis Serology

Abstract Hepatitis D virus (HDV) was first recognized in 1977 by Rizzetto and colleagues. HDV always occurs as a simultaneous coinfection with hepatitis B (HBV). Patients coinfected with HDV and HBV have fulminant hepatitis more often than patients infected with HBV alone. Testing for serological markers of HDV should be considered when a patient shows clinical signs of acute or fulminant hepatitis.

Patient Preparation Avoid recent administration of radioisotopes

Specimen Serum

Container Red top tube

Causes for Rejection Recently administered radioisotopes

Reference Range Negative

Use Differential diagnosis of chronic, recurrent, and acute viral hepatitis

Methodology Radioimmunoassay (RIA), enzyme-linked immunosorbent assay (ELISA)

Additional Information Hepatitis D virus ("delta" agent) is an incomplete RNA virus, or viroid, that can only infect livers already infected by hepatitis B virus. It may occur, therefore, as coinfection with acute HBV hepatitis or super imposed on chronic HBV infection. It cannot occur in an HB_sAg-negative individual. IgG and IgM antibodies to HDV develop 5-7 weeks after infection. IgM antibody is most useful in distinguishing those patients with active liver disease. HDAg can be detected in serum or liver biopsies but is technically demanding and offers little to diagnosis. False-positive EIA results have been reported in patients with lipemia or high titer rheumatoid factor. Studies of liver transplants in patients with end-stage liver disease due to hepatitis B/D have shown, through serial biopsies post-transplant, that HDV viral reinfection occurs within

(Continued)

Hepatitis D Serology *(Continued)*

Superinfection

Coinfection

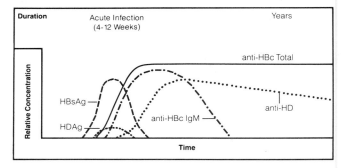

1 week but without damage. Not until HBV proliferation occurs several weeks to months later does one find histologic and clinical changes.

Selected Readings

Craig JR, "Hepatitis Delta Virus – No Longer A Defective Virus," *Am J Clin Pathol*, 1992, 98(6):552-3, (editorial).

Davies SE, Lau JY, O'Grady JG, et al, "Evidence That Hepatitis D Virus Needs Hepatitis B Virus to Cause Hepatocellular Damage," *Am J Clin Pathol*, 1992, 98(6):554-8.

Govindarajan S, Valinluck B, Lake-Bakkar G, "Evaluation of a Commercial Anti-Delta EIA Test for Detection of Antibodies to Hepatitis Delta Virus," *Am J Clin Pathol*, 1991, 95(2):240-1.

Gupta S, Govindarajan S, Cassidy WM, et al, "Acute Delta Hepatitis: Serological Diagnosis With Particular Reference to Hepatitis Delta Virus RNA," *Am J Gastroenterol*, 1991, 86(9):1227-31.

Lee HS and Vyas GN, "Diagnosis of Viral Hepatitis," *Clin Lab Med*, 1987, 7(4):741-57.

Pohl C, Baroudy BM, Bergmann KF, et al, "A Human Monoclonal Antibody That Recognizes Viral Polypeptides and *In Vitro* Translation Products of the Genome of the Hepatitis D Virus," *J Infect Dis*, 1987, 156(4):622-9.

Polish LB, Gallagher M, Fields HA, et al, "Delta Hepatitis: Molecular Biology and Clinical and Epidemiological Features," *Clin Microbiol Rev*, 1993, 6(3):211-29.

Herpes 1 and 2 *see* Herpes Simplex Antibody *on next page*

Herpes Culture *see* Herpes Simplex Virus Culture *on page 364*

Herpes Cytology
Related Information
Herpes Simplex Antibody *on next page*

Herpes Simplex Virus Culture *on page 364*

Herpes Simplex Virus, Direct Immunofluorescence *on page 365*

Herpes Simplex Virus Isolation, Rapid *on page 366*

Synonyms Herpetic Inclusion Bodies, Cytology; Inclusion Body Stain; Tzanck Smear; Viral Study, Herpes

Test Includes Preparation of cytological smears, staining of smears, and microscopic evaluation for viral inclusions

Special Instructions A stat Pap stain can be requested at the time of delivery if active herpes is suspected.

Specimen Direct scrape of lesion

Collection Firmly scrape lesion area with sterile tongue depressor, swab, scalpel, or Culturette®. Spread cellular material evenly on glass slides and fix immediately in 95% ethyl alcohol or inexpensive hairspray. Cells on a swab should be rolled onto a slide; scraped cells should be dabbed onto a slide. Cells should be obtained from a freshly unroofed lesion. Label frosted slide with patient's name. For lesions of skin or vulva, which are dry surfaces, it is helpful to moisten the lesion with saline before scraping it. **Do not air dry smears.**

Causes for Rejection Improper fixation, air drying artifact

Use To establish the presence of herpesvirus infection

Limitations Herpes inclusions may not be seen in 50% of active lesions. Viral cultures are the definitive method but may take 2 or more days.

Methodology Pap stained smear, immunoperoxidase stain for herpes viral antigen

Additional Information Diagnostic yield is increased by immunoperoxidase or immunofluorescent procedures, which become positive before characteristic viral cytopathic changes develop. Smears with a heavy inflammatory exudate may be difficult to interpret because of nonspecific staining. Smears must be done with and without the primary antibody and positive and negative controls must be run concurrently.

Selected Readings

Arvin AM and Prober CG, "Herpes Simplex Viruses," *Manual of Clinical Microbiology*, 5th ed, Balows A, Hausler WJ Jr, Herrmann KL, et al, eds, Washington, DC: American Society for Microbiology, 1991, 822-8.

Corey L and Holmes KK, "Genital Herpes Simplex Virus Infections: Current Concepts in Diagnosis, Therapy, and Prevention," *Ann Intern Med*, 1983, 98(6):973-83.

Corey L and Spear PG, "Infections With Herpes Simplex Viruses," *N Engl J Med*, 1986, 314(12):686-91 and 749-56.

Herpes Hominis 1 and 2 *see* Herpes Simplex Antibody
on this page

Herpes Simplex 1 and 2 Culture *see* Herpes Simplex Virus Culture
on next page

Herpes Simplex Antibody

Related Information

Herpes Cytology *on previous page*

Herpes Simplex Virus Culture *on next page*

Herpes Simplex Virus, Direct Immunofluorescence *on page 365*

Herpes Simplex Virus Isolation, Rapid *on page 366*

Synonyms Herpes 1 and 2; Herpes Hominis 1 and 2

Test Includes HSV 1 and 2

Specimen Serum

Container Red top tube or serum separator tube

Reference Range Interpretation depends on whether episode is initial or reinfection. IgG and IgM specific antibodies may give more useful information about an acute event.

Limitations Extensive background antibody in the population, and cross reaction of HSV 1 and HSV 2 responses make test useful only in epidemiology. The test is not generally useful except to determine rising titers.

Methodology Immunofluorescence, hemagglutination, complement fixation, enzyme immunoassay (EIA)

Additional Information A primary HSV 1 or HSV 2 infection will produce a classical rising antibody titer. However, because exposure to herpesvirus is almost universal (50% to 90% of adults have antibodies) the background of antibody makes the serologic response in any particular episode of recurrence difficult to interpret. This is made especially true by the fact the antibody to one virus type may be stimulated by infection with the heterologous virus type. Both false-positive and false-negatives are common with currently licensed en-
(Continued)

Herpes Simplex Antibody *(Continued)*

zyme immunoassays. Collecting the requisite paired sera to delineate which titers are rising or stable generally adds nothing to clinical management, and thus herpes serology cannot be recommended in routine clinical cases. However, in research settings or for epidemiologic studies serologic definition of the type of herpes infection have been worthwhile.

Herpes serology has not been proved clinically useful in determining whether caesarean delivery should be undertaken in pregnant patients with questionably active herpes. Pap smear or immunochemical demonstration of viral antigen is more useful for this. Nor is herpes serology usually helpful in the differential of a very sick infant with possible congenital herpes. Because of the fulminant course, even early IgM antibody may not be demonstrable in time to contribute to care.

Selected Readings
Ashley R, Cent A, Maggs V, et al, "Inability of Enzyme Immunoassays to Discriminate Between Infections With Herpes Simplex Virus Types 1 and 2," *Ann Intern Med*, 1991, 115(7):520-6.

Corey L, Adams HG, Brown ZA, et al, "Genital Herpes Simplex Virus Infections: Clinical Manifestations, Course, and Complications," *Ann Intern Med*, 1983, 98(6):958-72.

Corey L and Spear PG, "Infections With Herpes Simplex Viruses," *N Engl J Med*, 1986, 314(12):686-91 and 749-56.

Erlich KS, "Laboratory Diagnosis of Herpesvirus Infections," *Clin Lab Med*, 1987, 7(4):759-76.

Stewart JA, "Herpes Simplex Virus," *Manual of Clinical Laboratory Immunology*, 4th ed, Rose NR, de Macario EC, Fahey JL, et al, eds, Washington, DC: American Society for Microbiology, 1992, 554-9.

Herpes Simplex Virus Antigen Detection *see* Herpes Simplex Virus, Direct Immunofluorescence *on next page*

Herpes Simplex Virus Culture
Related Information
Herpes Cytology *on page 362*
Herpes Simplex Antibody *on previous page*
Herpes Simplex Virus, Direct Immunofluorescence *on next page*
Herpes Simplex Virus Isolation, Rapid *on page 366*

Synonyms Herpes Culture; Herpes Simplex 1 and 2 Culture; HSV 1 and 2 Culture; HSV Culture

Applies To Viral Culture, Eye; Viral Culture, Genital; Viral Culture, Skin

Test Includes Culture for HSV only; HSV also is usually detected in a routine/general virus culture

Special Instructions Special viral transport medium must be obtained from the laboratory prior to collection of specimen.

Specimen Specimen depends on type of infection:
- genital - vesicle fluid, lesion, endocervical
- conjunctivitis - conjunctival
- congenital - throat, vesicle, cerebrospinal fluid
- encephalitis - brain biopsy
- meningitis - cerebrospinal fluid
- respiratory/oral - throat, vesicle

Container Sterile container; cold viral transport medium for swabs

Collection All specimens should be kept cold and moist. As for most viral cultures, specimens should be collected in the acute stage of the disease, preferably within 3 days and no longer than 7 days after the onset of illness. Spinal fluid specimens should be submitted in the usual sterile tube; no special transport medium is necessary. All other specimens should be collected on a sterile swab as described and **the swab should be placed into cold viral transport medium immediately after collection**.

Endocervical: Swab cervix with enough force to obtain epithelial cells.

Vesicular lesion: Wash vesicles with sterile saline. Carefully open several vesicles and soak up vesicular fluid with swab. If vesicles are absent, vigorously swab base of lesion (specimen should be collected during first 3 days of eruption, because specimens collected later in the course of disease rarely yield virus).

Conjunctival: Using a moistened swab, firmly rub conjunctiva using sufficient force to obtain epithelial cells.

Throat, respiratory, oral: Rotate swab in both tonsillar crypts and against posterior oropharynx.

Storage Instructions Specimens should be delivered to the laboratory and handed to a technologist within 30 minutes of collection. Outpatient specimens: If transport is to be delayed more than 30 minutes after collection, specimen **must** be refrigerated (held at 4°C to 8°C) until it can be transported to the laboratory. Do not freeze specimen.

Causes for Rejection Dry specimen, specimen not refrigerated during transport, specimen fixed in formalin, unlabeled specimen

Turnaround Time Variable (1-14 days) and depends on culture method used and amount of virus in specimen

Reference Range No virus isolated

Use To aid in the diagnosis of HSV disease

Methodology Inoculation of specimen into cell cultures, incubation of cultures, observation of characteristic cytopathic effect, and identification by fluorescent monoclonal antibodies specific for type 1 or 2.

Additional Information HSV can only rarely be isolated from the CSF of patients with HSV 1 encephalitis. The virus is occasionally isolated from spinal fluid of patients with HSV 2 meningitis and of neonates with congenital herpes and from urine from patients with primary genital HSV infections concurrent with cystitis.

Serology for the detection of herpes simplex virus is available, but the results usually are of value only in the diagnosis of primary HSV infections. There is much cross-reaction between the antibodies to HSV 1 and HSV 2.

Selected Readings

Arvin AM and Prober CG, "Herpes Simplex Viruses," *Manual of Clinical Microbiology*, 5th ed, Balows A, Hausler WJ Jr, Herrmann KL, et al, eds, Washington, DC: American Society for Microbiology, 1991, 822-8.

Drew WL, "Diagnostic Virology," *Clin Lab Med*, 1987, 7(4):721-40.

Reichman RC, "Herpes Simplex Viruses," *Textbook of Human Virology*, Belshe RB, ed, Littleton, MA: PSG Publishing Co, 1984, 811-28.

Solomon AR, "New Diagnostic Tests for Herpes Simplex and Varicella Zoster Infections," *J Am Acad Dermatol*, 1988, 18(1 Pt 2):218-21.

Herpes Simplex Virus, Direct Detection *see* Virus, Direct Detection by Fluorescent Antibody *on page 480*

Herpes Simplex Virus, Direct Immunofluorescence

Related Information

Herpes Cytology *on page 362*

Herpes Simplex Antibody *on page 363*

Herpes Simplex Virus Culture *on previous page*

Herpes Simplex Virus Isolation, Rapid *on next page*

Synonyms Herpes Simplex Virus Antigen Detection; HSV Antigen Detection, Direct

Test Includes Direct (nonculture) detection of HSV-infected cells

Special Instructions Make more than one slide preparation

Specimen Basal cells of a freshly unroofed lesion rolled onto a clean microscope slide

Sampling Time Preferably within 3 days of lesion eruption

Collection Make a preparation of cells taken from the suspected herpetic lesion onto a plain 1" x 3" glass slide. Cells from the bottom of an ulcer or vesicle should be scraped with a swab, scalpel or curette. Swabs should be **rolled** (**not** smeared) across a small area of the slide several times, and cells scraped with a scalpel should be gently dabbed onto the slide. The best specimen is a collection of the cells at the base of an intact vesicle. Cells from a diseased cornea can also be used. **The smear should be air dried at room temperature**.

Storage Instructions Do not store the specimen. Send it to the laboratory immediately.

Causes for Rejection Insufficient quantity of specimen on slide, poorly prepared or labeled slides

Turnaround Time Less than 1 day

Reference Range No herpes simplex virus-infected cells detected

Use Rapid detection of herpes simplex virus in oral or genital lesions

Limitations Some of the variables in this test include proper collection of specimens, stage and location of lesion, and community prevalence of the disease.

The efficiency of detection of HSV material depends in great part on the collection of a sufficiently large number of intact infected cells from the lesion. It is

(Continued)

Herpes Simplex Virus, Direct Immunofluorescence
(Continued)

important to obtain cells from the base of an intact vesicle if at all possible. The presence of infected cells decreases as the lesion heals, and crusted lesions may have little or no herpes antigenic material remaining.

Methodology Immunoperoxidase or immunofluorescence staining of collected cells

Additional Information In certain situations, this direct antigen detection test can be more sensitive than cell culture; however, and in general, this test is only approximately 70% as sensitive as cell culture. In critical situations, clinicians should consider using both methods.

Air-dried preparations on slides can also be stained with Giemsa or Diff-Quik™ stains (Tzanck). Fixed preparations (usually 95% ethanol) can also be stained with the Papanicolaou or immunoperoxidase methods. Smears fixed with hairspray and subsequently stained with the Papanicolaou stain usually are excellent preparations.

Selected Readings

Arvin AM and Prober CG, "Herpes Simplex Viruses," *Manual of Clinical Microbiology*, 5th ed, Balows A, Hausler WJ Jr, Herrmann KL, et al, eds, Washington, DC: American Society for Microbiology, 1991, 822-8.

Drew WL, "Diagnostic Virology," *Clin Lab Med*, 1987, 7(4):721-40.

Smith TF, "Rapid Methods for the Diagnosis of Viral Infections," *Lab Med*, 1987, 18:16-20.

Herpes Simplex Virus Isolation, Rapid
Related Information

Herpes Cytology *on page 362*

Herpes Simplex Antibody *on page 363*

Herpes Simplex Virus Culture *on page 364*

Herpes Simplex Virus, Direct Immunofluorescence *on previous page*

Synonyms HSV Shell Vial Method, Spin Amplification

Applies To Culture, HSV Only; HSV, Rapid Isolation; Skin Culture for HSV

Test Includes Inoculation of cell cultures in shell vials, 16-hour incubation, and immunofluorescence staining for HSV 1 and 2

Specimen Swab of genital, lip, or mucous membrane lesion; vesicular fluid; biopsy

Container Sterile container; cold viral transport medium for swabs

Collection All specimens should be kept cold and moist. As for most viral cultures, specimens should be collected in the acute stage of the disease, preferably within 3 days and no longer than 7 days after the onset of illness. Spinal fluid specimens should be submitted in the usual sterile tube; no special transport medium is necessary. All other specimens should be collected on a sterile swab as described and **the swab should be placed into cold viral transport medium immediately after collection**.

Endocervical: Swab cervix with enough force to obtain epithelial cells.

Vesicular lesion: Wash vesicles with sterile saline. Carefully open several vesicles and soak up vesicular fluid with swab. If vesicles are absent, vigorously swab base of lesion (specimen should be collected during first 3 days of eruption, because specimens collected later in the course of disease rarely yield virus).

Conjunctival: Using a moistened swab, firmly rub conjunctiva using sufficient force to obtain epithelial cells.

Throat, respiratory, oral: Rotate swab in both tonsillar crypts and against posterior oropharynx.

Turnaround Time Overnight to 2 days depending on method and capability of laboratory

Reference Range No HSV detected

Use Aid in the diagnosis of disease caused by HSV

Methodology Shell vial isolation technique with direct immunofluorescent staining for HSV 1 and HSV 2. Specimens are centrifuged onto cell cultures grown on coverslips in the bottoms of 1-dram shell vials. Centrifugation greatly accelerates virus attachment and penetration. After incubation, fluorescein-labeled monoclonal antibodies are applied to the infected cells to detect viral antigens that are expressed in the membranes of the cells. Characteristic fluorescent foci indicate the presence of virus.

Additional Information The rapid shell vial culture technique for the detection of HSV 1 and 2 has been reported to be as sensitive as conventional cell culture methods.

Selected Readings
Gleaves CA, Wilson DJ, Wold AD, et al, "Detection and Serotyping of Herpes Simplex Virus in MRC-5 Cells by Use of Centrifugation and Monoclonal Antibodies 16-Hr Postinoculation," *J Clin Microbiol*, 1985, 21(1):29-32.

Smith TF, "Rapid Methods for the Diagnosis of Viral Infections," *Lab Med*, 1987, 18:16-20.

Solomon AR, "New Diagnostic Tests for Herpes Simplex and Varicella Zoster Infections," *J Am Acad Dermatol*, 1988, 18(1 Pt 2):218-21.

Herpes Zoster Serology *see* Varicella-Zoster Virus Serology *on page 474*

Herpetic Inclusion Bodies, Cytology *see* Herpes Cytology *on page 362*

HHV-6, IgM, IgG *see* Human Herpesvirus 6, IgG and IgM Antibodies, Quantitative *on page 369*

Hip Arthrogram *see* Arthrogram *on page 267*

Hip, Left or Right, and Pelvis, X-ray *see* Bone Films *on page 277*

Hip, Left or Right, X-ray *see* Bone Films *on page 277*

Hips Arthritis, X-ray *see* Bone Films *on page 277*

***Histoplasma capsulatum* Antibody and Antigen** *see* Histoplasmosis Serology *on this page*

Histoplasmosis Immunodiffusion *see* Fungal Serology *on page 337*

Histoplasmosis Serology

Applies To *Histoplasma capsulatum* Antibody and Antigen

Test Includes Reaction with yeast and mycelial antigens

Specimen Serum (antibody); urine (antigen)

Container Red top tube, plastic urine container

Collection Acute and convalescent sera are recommended, especially when acute titers are only presumptive

Reference Range Antibody: less than a fourfold change in titer between acute and convalescent samples; titers less than 1:4; negative CSF. Antigen: negative.

Use Diagnosis and prognosis of histoplasmosis

Limitations A negative result does not rule out histoplasmosis. Histoplasmin skin testing may interfere with results. Testing with both antigens must be performed. There are cross reactions with other fungi. Anticomplementary sera cannot be tested for complement fixing antibodies. The latex agglutination test gives some false-positives, and must be confirmed with another procedure.

Contraindications Previous skin testing

Methodology Complement fixation, immunodiffusion, latex agglutination, radioimmunoassay (antigen), enzyme immunoassay (EIA)

Additional Information CF titers of 1:8 or 1:16 are presumptive evidence of histoplasmosis. Titers of 1:32 or greater are highly suggestive of *H. capsulatum* infection, but cannot be relied on as the sole means of diagnosis. Complement fixation and immunodiffusion each detect about 85% of disease. H and M bands on immunodiffusion indicate active disease. Complement fixation is less sensitive to disseminated or chronic disease. The latex agglutination test detects IgM antibodies and is positive early in disease, but not in late, chronic, or recurrent infection.

Tests for fungal antigen are now available and obviate some of the problems of ordinary serology - cross reactions, decreased immune response, need for paired specimens over time. The use of enzyme immunoassay and radioimmunoassay to detect *H. capsulatum* antigen has proven to be a useful approach in the diagnosis of histoplasmosis. Antigenuria or antigenemia is excellent evidence of disseminated disease.

In addition to histoplasmosis in immunologically intact individuals, this fungal infection is a serious opportunistic infection in patients with AIDS (occasionally as its first manifestation).

Selected Readings
Drutz DJ, "Antigen Detection in Fungal Infections," *N Engl J Med*, 1986, 314(2):115-7.

Kaufman L and Reiss E, "Serodiagnosis of Fungal Diseases," *Manual of Clinical Laboratory Immunology*, 4th ed, Rose NR, de Macario EC, Fahey JL, et al, eds, Washington, DC: American Society for Microbiology, 1992, 506-28.

(Continued)

Histoplasmosis Serology *(Continued)*

Wheat LJ, Connolly-Stringfield PA, and Baker RL, "Disseminated Histoplasmosis in the Acquired Immune Deficiency Syndrome: Clinical Findings, Diagnosis and Treatment, and Review of the Literature," *Medicine (Baltimore)*, 1990, 69(6):361-74.

Wheat LJ, Kohler RB, and Tewari RP, "Diagnosis of Disseminated Histoplasmosis by Detection of *Histoplasma capsulatum* Antigen in Serum and Urine Specimens," *N Engl J Med*, 1986, 314(2):83-8.

HIV-1 Serology

Related Information

Human Immunodeficiency Virus Culture *on page 370*

p24 Antigen *on page 420*

Synonyms Human Immunodeficiency Virus Serology

Test Includes Screening test with confirmation of repeated positives

Patient Preparation In some states test may not be done or results revealed without express written or informed consent of the patient.

Special Instructions Blood and body fluid precautions must be observed

Specimen Serum

Reference Range Negative

Use Diagnosis of AIDS, exposure to HIV-1, screening of blood and blood products for transfusion

Limitations There is a 2-12 week (perhaps much longer) interval after infection before antibody becomes detectable. Positive screening tests must be confirmed by more specific follow-up procedures (usually Western blot). Antibody is not protective against disease. There are some cross reactions in some test systems due to histocompatibility antigen mismatches (in particular, antibodies to HLA-DR4). Cross-reactions have been observed to other viral antigens as well. A recent influenza vaccine resulted in reactivity against p24 antigen and give false-positive enzyme-linked immunosorbent assays.

Methodology Enzyme-linked immunosorbent assay (ELISA), Western blot, immunofluorescence (RIPA)

Additional Information Human immunodeficiency virus (HIV, formerly HTLV-III), a lentivirus, is the etiologic agent of AIDS. Acute infection, spread by blood or sexual contact, is usually followed within days by a flu-like illness, or no symptoms. During this time, HIV antigen, usually p24 core protein, may be detectable in serum. This becomes negative in 2 weeks to a month. There then follows a period of weeks to months (as long as 35 months) during which an individual is infected with HIV, which may or may not be replicating at a low rate, but screening tests for antibody to HIV are **negative**.

Present screening tests for HIV antibodies are ELISA procedures which use disrupted virus or recombinant antigen products. Different antibodies are detected. Sensitivity and specificity of these tests are both extremely high, but positive results on a screen should be repeated; if positive a second time they should be confirmed with a Western blot procedure. Because of the grave implications of a positive result, confirmation of positive results by testing a second sample may be indicated.

Some individuals may have reactive screening tests, restricted to one test system, and completely negative Western blots. This may be due to HLA antibodies reacting with residual human cell surface proteins incorporated in the test kit. False-positives have been reported in individuals who have received intravenous gamma globulin. Since these proteins are due to antibodies in the transfused gamma globulin, repeat analysis in 3 months (half-life for IgG is about 3 weeks), will show a negative or much weaker EIA result.

Western blot analysis can identify the exact viral products with which patient antibody reacts. Criteria for a positive blot include: two of the three bands for p24, gp41, and gp120/160 (Centers for Disease Control); or, one gag (p55, p24, p17), one pol (p64, p53, p31), and one env (gp41, gp120/160) (American Red Cross); or, p24, p31, and gp41 and/or gp120/160 (FDA license for Du Pont kit).

HIV antibody can be detected in postmortem specimens of blood or vitreous humor.

Although **central nervous system involvement** is extremely common in AIDS, tests to detect HIV antigen or antibody in CSF lack both sensitivity and specificity. These tests do not help in differentiating neurologic symptoms secondary to HIV infection from those due to CNS neoplasm or opportunistic infection.

Tests with greater sensitivity such as polymerase chain reaction are being developed. Application to screening programs for differing populations are extremely problematic, given the serious implications of a positive test, the lack of treatment, and the heavy legal/emotional/political encrustations of AIDS.

Selected Readings

Agbede OO, "HIV-1-Indeterminate Western Blot Results: Implications for Diagnosis and Subject Notification," *Clin Microbiol Newslett*, 1992, 14(16):121-5.

Burke DS, "Laboratory Diagnosis of Human Immunodeficiency Virus Infection," *Clin Lab Med*, 1989, 9(3):369-92.

Krieger JN, "Acquired Immunodeficiency Syndrome Antibody Testing and Precautions," *J Urol*, 1992, 147(3):713-6.

O'Gorman MR, Weber D, Landis SE, et al, "Interpretive Criteria of the Western Blot Assay for Serodiagnosis of Human Immunodeficiency Virus Type 1 Infection," *Arch Pathol Lab Med*, 1991, 115(1):26-30.

Sloand EM, Pitt E, Chiarello RJ, et al, "HIV Testing – State of the Art," *JAMA*, 1991, 266(20):2861-6.

HIV Core Antigen *see* p24 Antigen *on page 420*

HIV DNA Amplification Assay *see* Human Immunodeficiency Virus DNA Amplification *on next page*

HIV DNA PCR Test *see* Human Immunodeficiency Virus DNA Amplification *on next page*

HIV p24 Antigen *see* p24 Antigen *on page 420*

HSV 1 and 2 Culture *see* Herpes Simplex Virus Culture *on page 364*

HSV Antigen Detection, Direct *see* Herpes Simplex Virus, Direct Immunofluorescence *on page 365*

HSV Culture *see* Herpes Simplex Virus Culture *on page 364*

HSV, Rapid Isolation *see* Herpes Simplex Virus Isolation, Rapid *on page 366*

HSV Shell Vial Method, Spin Amplification *see* Herpes Simplex Virus Isolation, Rapid *on page 366*

HTLV-III Culture *see* Human Immunodeficiency Virus Culture *on next page*

Human Herpesvirus 6, IgG and IgM Antibodies, Quantitative

Synonyms HHV-6, IgM, IgG

Specimen Serum

Container Red top tube or serum separator tube

Collection Specimens should be free from bacterial contamination and hemolysis

Storage Instructions Refrigerate serum

Causes for Rejection Gross lipemia

Use IgM HHV-6 may aid in the diagnosis of acute or recent infection with HHV-6. An increase in IgG HHV-6 (fourfold titer) between acute and convalescent samples is evidence for a recent HHV-6 infection.

Methodology Indirect fluorescent antibody (IFA)

Additional Information Human herpesvirus 6 (HHV-6) has recently been identified as the agent associated with both pediatric and adult infections. Most children have been infected by age 3 years. The acute infection in children is characterized clinically by an acute febrile illness, irritability, inflammation of tympanic membranes, and (uncommonly) a rash characteristic of roseola. When acute and convalescent (4-6 weeks later) serum samples are compared, a fourfold rise in HHV-6 IgG titer is typical. It has also been thought to be the etiological agent of exanthem subitum (roseola) in children.

In adults, HHV-6 has been associated with chronic fatigue and spontaneously resolving fever resembling a mononucleosis-like illness. During the acute episode an elevated IgM HHV-6 is useful. An increase in IgG HHV-6 between acute and convalescent serum sample is consistent with a recent HHV-6 infection. There is no antiviral agents directed toward this virus.

Selected Readings

Agbede O, "Human Herpesvirus 6: A Virus in Search of a Disease," *Clin Microbiol Newslett*, 1993, 15(4):25-7.

Irving WL and Cunningham AL, "Serological Diagnosis of Infection With Human Herpesvirus Type 6," *BMJ*, 1990, 300(6718):156-9.

(Continued)

Human Herpesvirus 6, IgG and IgM Antibodies, Quantitative *(Continued)*

Oren I and Sobel JD, "Human Herpesvirus Type 6: Review," *Clin Infect Dis*, 1992, 14(3):741-6.

Pruksananonda P, Hall CB, Insel RA, et al, "Primary Human Herpesvirus 6 Infection in Young Children," *N Engl J Med*, 1992, 326(22):1445-50.

Rathore MH, "Human Herpesvirus 6," *South Med J*, 1993, 86(11):1197-205.

Human Immunodeficiency Virus Culture

Related Information

HIV-1 Serology *on page 368*

Human Immunodeficiency Virus DNA Amplification *on this page*

Synonyms AIDS Virus Culture; HTLV-III Culture

Special Instructions Request form must be complete with patient's name, hospital number, birth date, physician's name, date of collection, type of specimen, site of specimen if applicable, and appropriate clinical findings.

Specimen Blood (20-40 mL), cerebrospinal fluid (10 mL), other body fluids, biopsies. All specimens **must** be labeled with the patient's name or code and **must** be transported to the laboratory in a **sealed** plastic bag with the request form attached. Some laboratories will not accept patient names associated with HIV specimens.

Container Green top (heparin) tube for blood, sterile container for CSF and other fluids

Collection Routine venipuncture. Invert the tubes several times after drawing the blood to be sure the blood is thoroughly mixed with the heparin.

Storage Instructions Do not store the specimen. Send it to the laboratory immediately. Some laboratories require specimen to be received into the laboratory the same day the specimen is received.

Causes for Rejection Dry specimen, specimen not refrigerated during transport, specimen fixed in formalin, unlabeled specimen

Turnaround Time Positive cultures are usually reported after 2 consecutive positive reverse transcriptase assays. Blood cultures are usually incubated 4 weeks and some laboratories incubate CSF cultures 8 weeks before termination as negative.

Reference Range No virus isolated

Use To aid in the diagnosis of disease caused by HIV

Limitations A negative culture cannot be assumed to rule out the presence of the virus.

Methodology Growth of virus in lymphocyte culture and subsequent (indirect) testing for presence of virus in culture fluids by EIA reverse transcriptase assay

Additional Information Serology for the detection of HIV antibodies is available.

Selected Readings

Erice A, Sannerud KJ, Leske VL, et al, "Sensitive Microculture Method for Isolation of Human Immunodeficiency Virus Type 1 from Blood Leukocytes," *J Clin Microbiol*, 1992, 30(2):444-8.

Jackson JB, "Human Immunodeficiency Virus Type 1 Antigen and Culture Assays," *Arch Pathol Lab Med*, 1990, 114(3):249-53.

Jackson JB and Balfour HH Jr, "Practical Diagnostic Testing for Human Immunodeficiency Virus," *Clin Microbiol Rev*, 1988, 1(1):124-38.

Markham PD and Salahuddin SZ, "*In Vitro* Cultivation of Human Leukocytes: Methods for the Expression and Isolation of Human Retroviruses," *BioTechniques*, 1987, 5:432-43.

Human Immunodeficiency Virus DNA Amplification

Related Information

Human Immunodeficiency Virus Culture *on this page*

Synonyms HIV DNA Amplification Assay; HIV DNA PCR Test; Human Immunodeficiency Virus (HIV) Proviral DNA by Polymerase Chain Reaction Amplification; PCR for HIV DNA

Test Includes HIV DNA is detected by amplifying specific proviral DNA sequences from peripheral blood lymphocytes and subsequent hybridization and detection with a specific HIV DNA probe.

Abstract Human immunodeficiency virus (HIV) is the causative agent of acquired immune deficiency syndrome (AIDS). Currently, testing for HIV is based on evidence of circulating antibody to the viral proteins. Commercially available tests are remarkably accurate with a low false-positive rate (1:135,000). However, accuracy of the test is compromised during the time interval between infection and the development of antibody to HIV. The exact time to seroconversion is controversial but certain cases of accidental exposure have shown seroconversion to occur within 2-3 months. Babies born to HIV-infected mothers will be seropositive for HIV due to transplacental antibodies. Studies have shown that only 30% to 50% of babies born to HIV infected mothers are actually infected with the virus. Thus, the serologic test is unreliable for assessing HIV infection in these populations.

This virus contains an RNA genome that will incorporate into host DNA as proviral DNA. The target cells of this virus are the CD4 (T4) T-lymphocytes (helper T cells) and monocytes/macrophage populations; however, during infection, few such peripheral blood cells contain HIV. To detect the incorporated viral genome, the DNA must be amplified. This procedure specifically increases the amount of DNA within the HIV genome, and the amplified DNA product is detected by specific binding to an HIV probe. The DNA detection assay has been useful for the diagnosis of HIV in infants and for monitoring individuals with a known exposure to HIV.

Specimen Peripheral blood lymphocytes from 10-20 mL whole blood

Container Two yellow top (ACD), lavender top (EDTA), or green top (sodium heparin) tubes should be collected. Type of tube is dependent on the laboratory performing the test.

Storage Instructions Tubes of blood can be sent directly to the laboratory at ambient temperature and should arrive within 48 hours of collection.

Causes for Rejection Specimens with inadequate volume or more than 48 hours old may be rejected.

Turnaround Time 2 weeks is usually required. Turnaround time may vary with individual laboratories.

Reference Range No HIV viral DNA detected in peripheral blood lymphocytes.

Use HIV detection in patients with unusual or indeterminant HIV serology. It may also be useful in patients with immunodeficiency syndromes characterized by a negative HIV serology and Western blot tests.

Methodology DNA amplification is used, polymerase chain reaction (PCR). DNA is extracted from peripheral blood lymphocytes. The proviral HIV DNA is exponentially amplified by using specific primers that bind to regions of the HIV genome. Using a series of denaturation, annealing, and polymerization steps the original proviral DNA can be amplified 10^5 to 10^6 fold (see figure). The amplified HIV DNA is confirmed by hybridization with an HIV specific DNA probe. Hybridization with the HIV DNA probe can be detected using autoradiography or enzymatic detection procedures.

Additional Information Currently, the diagnosis of HIV infection is dependent on the detection of specific antibodies. The antibody screening test commonly used is the enzyme linked immunosorbent assay (ELISA) with a confirmatory Western blot or immunoblot. These serologic assays will identify individuals with prior exposure to HIV or passively obtained antibody such as babies born to HIV-positive mothers. In addition, serologic tests may not identify patients with recent active infection. Due to this problem, other tests have also been used to document the presence of HIV, such as viral antigen assays, viral culture, and the detection of viral DNA. Viral culture of HIV is a prolonged procedure taking 3-4 weeks; it suffers from a lack of sensitivity in that HIV cannot be consistently isolated from seropositive patients. Studies using in situ hybridization have shown that few peripheral blood mononuclear cells may actually harbor HIV proviral DNA (1 in 10,000).[3] This makes it difficult to directly assay for HIV proviral DNA. Thus, DNA amplification assays have been developed to detect HIV DNA. The assay most commonly used is the polymerase chain reaction (PCR), which can amplify a single copy of DNA by 10^5 to 10^6 fold. The PCR test for HIV DNA is useful in resolution of unsatisfactory HIV antibody test results and in determination of the status of children born to mothers with positive HIV serology without the need for viral culture.

Selected Readings

Harper ME, Marselle LM, Gallo RC, et al, "Detection of Lymphocytes Expressing Human T-Lymphotropic Virus Type III in Lymph Nodes and Peripheral Blood From Infected Individuals by In Situ Hybridization," Proc Natl Acad Sci U S A, 1986, 83(3):772-6.

Loche M and Mach B, "Identification of HIV-Infected Seronegative Individuals by a Direct Diagnostic Test Based on Hybridisation to Amplified Viral DNA," Lancet, 1988, 2(8608):418-21.

Phair JP and Wolinsky S, "Diagnosis of Infection With the Human Immunodeficiency Virus," Clin Infect Dis, 1992, 15(1):13-6.

Saiki RK, Gelfand DH, Stoffel S, et al, "Primer-Directed Enzymatic Amplification of DNA With a Thermostable DNA Polymerase," Science, 1988, 239(4839):487-91.

Sheppard HW, Dondero D, Arnon J, et al, "An Evaluation of the Polymerase Chain Reaction in HIV-1 Seronegative Men," J Acquir Immune Defic Syndr, 1991, 4(8):819-23.

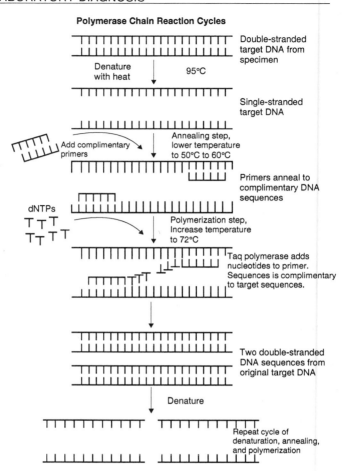

Polymerase Chain Reaction Cycles

Double-stranded target DNA from specimen

Denature with heat   95°C

Single-stranded target DNA

Add complimentary primers

Annealing step, lower temperature to 50°C to 60°C

Primers anneal to complimentary DNA sequences

dNTPs

Polymerization step, Increase temperature to 72°C

Taq polymerase adds nucleotides to primer. Sequences is complimentary to target sequences.

Two double-stranded DNA sequences from original target DNA

Denature

Repeat cycle of denaturation, annealing, and polymerization

Human Immunodeficiency Virus (HIV) Proviral DNA by Polymerase Chain Reaction Amplification *see* Human Immunodeficiency Virus DNA Amplification *on page 370*

Human Immunodeficiency Virus Serology *see* HIV-1 Serology *on page 368*

Humerus, Left or Right, X-ray *see* Bone Films *on page 277*

Hyperalimentation Line Culture *see* Intravenous Line Culture *on page 376*

IgG Antibodies to Rubella *see* Rubella Serology *on page 439*

IgM Antibodies to Rubella *see* Rubella Serology *on page 439*

Iliac Arteries Ultrasound *see* Ultrasound, Peripheral Arteries and Veins *on page 466*

Immunofluorescent Studies, Biopsy

Synonyms Direct Immunofluorescent Studies, Biopsy

Test Includes Fluorescent stains for immunoglobulins, complement, fibrin, and routine histopathology

Special Instructions Consult the pathologist prior to biopsy procedure for specific instructions. Requisition **must** state operative diagnosis and source of specimen.

Specimen Biopsy of kidney, skin, muscle, and lung submitted fresh in saline-moistened gauze as soon as possible following removal

Container Jar with gauze pad moistened with sterile saline

Collection Container must be labeled with patient's full name, and date

Storage Instructions Transport specimen to the laboratory immediately.

Causes for Rejection Specimen allowed to dry

Reference Range Negative

Use Determine the presence of tissue deposits of IgG, IgM, IgA, C_1q, C_3, albumin, fibrinogen, and kappa and lambda light chains in immunological diseases of kidney (eg, immune complex glomerulonephritis and antiglomerular basement membrane glomerulonephritis), skin (pemphigus, bullous pemphigoid, dermatitis herpetiformis, lupus erythematosus), neoplasms (plasma cell myeloma, macroglobulinemia of Waldenström, malignant lymphoma), and lung (lupus erythematosus, Goodpasture's syndrome)

Additional Information Submit additional specimen in formalin for light microscopy. Electron microscopy is commonly needed in many of the same biopsies in which fluorescence is desired, but usually requires a different fixative than does light microscopy processing.

Inclusion Body Stain *see* Herpes Cytology *on page 362*

Inclusion Conjunctivitis *see* Ocular Cytology *on page 416*

India Ink Preparation

Related Information

Cryptococcal Antigen Serology, Serum or Cerebrospinal Fluid
on page 312

Fungus Culture, Cerebrospinal Fluid *on page 342*

Synonyms Cerebrospinal Fluid India Ink Preparation; *Cryptococcus* Preparation; *Cryptococcus* Stain; Nigrosin Preparation

Patient Preparation Same as for culture of specific site

Specimen For all practical purposes, the only reasonably useful specimen is cerebrospinal fluid.

Container Sterile CSF tube

Collection The specimen may be divided for fungal culture, and mycobacteria culture and smear, and routine bacterial culture and Gram stain only if the specimen is of adequate volume for all tests requested.

Storage Instructions Do **not** refrigerate.

Causes for Rejection Insufficient specimen volume

Turnaround Time Routine: 24 hours; stat: 2 hours

Reference Range No encapsulated yeast identified

Use Establish the presence of *Cryptococcus* sp or other fungi

Limitations This technique is only 30% to 50% sensitive in cases of cryptococcal meningitis. Cultures and rapid latex agglutination (LA) methods are more sensitive than direct preparations; therefore, the India ink preparation may be negative when the culture or LA test is positive. Immunologic tests for *Cryptococcus* antigen have a sensitivity of 90% to 100%. Many laboratories have abandoned the use of the India ink preparation in favor of LA.

Methodology Wet mount with India ink (nigrosin) for contrast. Centrifugation may concentrate organisms and improve sensitivity.

Additional Information *Cryptococcus neoformans* is the most common central nervous system fungus in both normal hosts and patients with the acquired immunodeficiency syndrome (AIDS). Pigeon droppings act as a year round reservoir for dispersion of encapsulated yeast cells.

Selected Readings

Berlin L and Pincus JH, "Cryptococcal Meningitis. False-Negative Antigen Test Results and Cultures in Nonimmunosuppressed Patients," *Arch Neurol*, 1989, 46(12):1312-6.

Ellis DH and Pfeiffer TJ, "Ecology, Life Cycle, and Infectious Propagule of *Cryptococcus neoformans*," *Lancet*, 1990, 336(8720):923-5.

McGinnis MR, "Detection of Fungi in Cerebrospinal Fluid," *Am J Med*, 1983, 75(1B):129-38.

Indium-111 Labeled Leukocyte Scan *see* Indium Leukocyte Scan
on next page

Indium Leukocyte Scan

Synonyms Indium-111 Labeled Leukocyte Scan; Infection Scan; Infection Scintigraphy; Leukocyte Scintigraphy; WBC Scan; White Blood Cell Scan

Test Includes The patient receives an intravenous reinjection of radiolabeled leukocytes. The patient initially has a 60-80 mL sample of blood drawn for an *in vitro* process of labeling and separating the leukocyte component. Images are acquired at intervals between 2-24 hours after subsequent reinjection of radiolabeled cells.

Patient Preparation The patient does not need to be fasting or NPO for this procedure. Patient should have all RIA blood work performed, or at least drawn, prior to injection of any radioactive material.

Special Instructions Requisition must state the current patient diagnosis in order to select the most appropriate radiopharmaceutical and/or imaging technique. **DURATION OF PROCEDURE:** Two hours from blood draw to reinjection of labeled cells. 2-24 hours for imaging at intervals. **RADIOPHARMACEUTICAL:** Indium-111 labeled leukocytes

Causes for Rejection Other recent Nuclear Medicine procedure may interfere. If uncertain, call the Nuclear Medicine Department.

Turnaround Time A written report will be sent to the patient's chart and/or to the referring physician.

Reference Range Radiolabeled leukocytes will localize to some degree in the liver, spleen, and bone marrow. Focal accumulations in soft tissue or asymmetric uptake in bone will be seen in infected or inflamed sites. For osteomyelitis, a bone scan is usually performed first for comparison with the radiolabeled leukocyte scan findings.

Use Radiolabeled leukocyte imaging is useful either in determining the site of an occult infection or in confirming the presence or absence of infection at a suspected site. This technique has largely replaced gallium-67 imaging for acute infections because of the better image resolution and greater specificity. Some chronic infections, eg, chronic osteomyelitis, may be better imaged with gallium-67. Radiolabeled leukocyte imaging is especially helpful in detecting postoperative infection sites and in documenting lack of residual infection after a course of therapy.

Limitations Leukocyte radiolabeling is a complex process and is usually performed on-site only where there are dedicated radiopharmacy laboratories. Most commercial radiopharmacies will also provide this service locally.

Additional Information An alternative method of leukocyte radiolabeling with technetium-99m (^{99m}Tc) HMPAO is now available. Early reports show possible advantages with earlier imaging times and better sensitivity for infections in extremities with utilization of higher doses of ^{99m}Tc versus indium-111.

Selected Readings

Abreu SH, "Skeletal Uptake of Indium-111 Labeled White Blood Cells," *Semin Nucl Med*, 1989, 19(2):152-5.

Datz FL and Thorne DA, "Effect of Antibiotic Therapy on the Sensitivity of Indium-111 Labeled Leukocyte Scans," *J Nucl Med*, 1986, 27(12):1849-53.

Froelich JW and Field SA, "The Role of Indium-111 White Blood Cells in Inflammatory Bowel Disease," *Semin Nucl Med*, 1988, 18(4):300-7.

Laitinen R, Tähtinen J, Lantto T, et al, "^{99m}Tc Labeled Leukocytes in Imaging of Patients With Suspected Acute Abdominal Inflammation," *Clin Nucl Med*, 1990, 15(9):597-602.

Roddie ME, Peters AM, Danpure HJ, et al, "Inflammation: Imaging With ^{99m}Tc HMPAO-Labeled Leukocytes," *Radiology*, 1988, 166(3):767-72.

Induced Sputum Technique for *Pneumocystis* see Pneumocystis carinii Test *on page 431*

Infant Botulism, Toxin Identification see Botulism, Diagnostic Procedure *on page 285*

Infection Scan see Indium Leukocyte Scan *on this page*

Infection Scintigraphy see Indium Leukocyte Scan *on this page*

Infectious Mononucleosis Serology

Related Information

Epstein-Barr Virus Serology *on page 332*

Synonyms Monospot™ Test; Monosticon® Dri-Dot® Test; Mono Test

Replaces Davidsohn Differential; Paul-Bunnell Test

Test Includes Screening for the presence of heterophil antibodies

Specimen Serum

Container Red top tube or serum separator tube

Reference Range Negative

Use Diagnosis of infectious mononucleosis

Limitations Correlation with clinical findings is imperative since false-positive and negative results have been reported. About 15% of the adult population with infectious mononucleosis will not develop heterophil antibodies. Failure to develop heterophil antibodies occurs even more frequently in children. In these instances, patients usually are tested for specific Epstein-Barr virus antibodies. Less than 2% false-positives have been reported with Hodgkin's disease, lymphoma, acute lymphocytic leukemia, infectious hepatitis, pancreatic carcinoma, cytomegalovirus, Burkitt's lymphoma, rheumatoid arthritis, malaria, and rubella.

Overall, the Monospot™ test has 99% specificity and 86% sensitivity.

Methodology Latex agglutination (LA) and enzyme immunoassay (EIA)

Additional Information The infectious mononucleosis heterophil antibody appears in the serum of patients by the sixth to tenth day of illness. Highest titers are usually found in the second to third week. Antibody levels may remain detectable for as little as one week or persist up to a year; usual persistence is 4-8 weeks. The level of antibody activity is not correlated with the severity of disease or the degree of lymphocytosis. A positive screening or differential test in the appropriate clinical and hematologic setting is sufficient to make the diagnosis of infectious mononucleosis.

If there is clinically a mononucleosis syndrome, but the screening test is negative, a differential absorption will add nothing. Instead, consider tests for EBV specific antibodies, CMV, and toxoplasmosis antibodies.

Selected Readings
Evans AS and Niederman JC, "EBV-IgA and New Heterophile Antibody Tests in Diagnosis of Infectious Mononucleosis," *Am J Clin Pathol*, 1982, 77(5):555-60.

Fleisher GR, Collins M, and Fager S, "Limitations of Available Tests for Diagnosis of Infectious Mononucleosis," *J Clin Microbiol*, 1983, 17(4):619-24.

Horwitz CA, Henle W, Henle G, et al, "Heterophil-Negative Infectious Mononucleosis and Mononucleosis-Like Illnesses," *Am J Med*, 1977, 63(6):947-57.

Sumaya CV and Jenson HB, "Epstein-Barr Virus," *Manual of Clinical Laboratory Immunology*, 4th ed, Rose NR, de Macario EC, Fahey JL, et al, eds, Washington, DC: American Society for Microbiology, 1992, 568-75.

Influenza A and B Serology

Related Information

Influenza Virus Culture *on this page*

Test Includes IgG and IgM antibody titers

Specimen Serum

Container Red top tube or serum separator tube

Collection Acute and convalescent sera drawn 10-14 days apart are required

Reference Range Less than a fourfold increase in titer in paired sera; IgG <1:10, IgM <1:10

Use Establish the diagnosis of influenza virus infection; epidemiologic surveillance and tracking; differentiate type A from B for treatment with amantadine

Methodology Complement fixation (CF), hemagglutination inhibition (HAI), single radial immunodiffusion (RID), enzyme immunoassay (EIA)

Additional Information Influenza virus is typed by specifying a neuraminidase and hemagglutinin. Although serologic diagnosis is seldom practical (or necessary) during an influenza epidemic, serologic typing is valuable for epidemiology, and for planning therapy. Since type A influenza can be treated with amantadine, but type B cannot, this distinction may need to be made. Presence of specific IgM antibody indicates acute infection.

Selected Readings
Bryan JA, "The Serologic Diagnosis of Viral Infections," *Arch Pathol Lab Med*, 1987, 111(11):1015-23.

Rota PA, Regnery HL, and Kendal AP, "Influenza Virus," *Manual of Clinical Laboratory Immunology*, 4th ed, Rose NR, de Macario EC, Fahey JL, et al, eds, Washington, DC: American Society for Microbiology, 1992, 576-81.

Shaw MW, Arden NH, and Maassab HF, "New Aspects of Influenza Viruses," *Clin Microbiol Rev*, 1992, 5(1):74-92.

Influenza Virus Culture

Related Information

Influenza A and B Serology *on this page*

Viral Culture, Throat *on page 479*

Test Includes Concurrent culture for other respiratory viruses (parainfluenza and respiratory syncytial virus)

(Continued)

LABORATORY DIAGNOSIS

Influenza Virus Culture *(Continued)*

Specimen Throat or nasopharyngeal swab, sputum, bronchial washings, bronchoalveolar lavage

Container Sterile container; cold virus transport medium for swabs

Sampling Time Specimens should be collected within 3 days of the onset of illness.

Storage Instructions Specimens should be placed into viral transport medium and kept cold at all times. Do not freeze specimens. Specimens should be delivered immediately to the laboratory.

Causes for Rejection Dry specimen, specimen not refrigerated during transport, specimen fixed in formalin, unlabeled specimen

Turnaround Time Variable (5-14 days) and depends on culture method used and the amount of virus in the specimen

Reference Range No virus isolated

Use Isolate and identify influenza virus as an etiologic agent in cases of influenza and viral pneumonia

Methodology Inoculation of specimens into cell cultures, incubation of cultures, observation of cultures for characteristic cytopathic effect, and identification/speciation by methods such as hemadsorption and fluorescent monoclonal antibodies specific for influenza virus A or B

Additional Information The shell vial technique to rapidly (within 24 hours) detect viruses has recently been adapted to detect influenza A and B viruses. Serology for the detection of influenza antibodies is available. A commercial and rapid (less than 15 minutes) enzyme immunoassay for the detection of influenza A virus in patient specimen is available.

Selected Readings

Guenthner SH and Linneman CC, "Indirect Immunofluorescence Assay for Rapid Diagnosis of Influenza Virus," *Lab Med,* 1988, 581-3.

Harmon MW and Kendal AP, "Influenza Viruses," *Manual of Clinical Microbiology,* 5th ed, Balows A, Hausler WJ Jr, Herrmann KL, et al, eds, Washington, DC: American Society for Microbiology, 1991, 868-77.

Shaw MW, Arden NH, and Maassab HF, "New Aspects of Influenza Viruses," *Clin Microbiol Rev,* 1992, 5(1):74-92.

Van Voris LP, Young JF, Bernstein JM, et al, "Influenza Viruses," *Textbook of Human Virology,* Belshe RB, ed, Littleton, MA: PSG Publishing Co, 1984, 267-97.

Waner JL, Todd SJ, Shalaby H, et al, "Comparison of Directigen FLU-A With Viral Isolation and Direct Immunofluorescence for the Rapid Detection and Identification of Influenza A Virus," *J Clin Microbiol,* 1991, 29(3):479-82.

Influenza Virus, Direct Detection *see* Virus, Direct Detection by Fluorescent Antibody *on page 480*

Infusion Pyelogram *see* Urography *on page 472*

Insect Identification *see* Arthropod Identification *on page 268*

Intercellular Antibody Basement Membrane Antibody *see* Skin Biopsy, Immunofluorescence *on page 446*

Intrauterine Device Culture *see Actinomyces* Culture, All Sites *on page 242*

Intravenous Devices Culture *see* Intravenous Line Culture *on this page*

Intravenous Line Culture

Synonyms Arterial Line Culture; Catheter Culture, Intravenous; Catheter Tip Culture; Hemovac™ Tip Culture; Hyperalimentation Line Culture; Intravenous Devices Culture; I.V. Catheter Culture; Shunt Culture; Swan-Ganz Tip Culture; Venous Catheter Culture

Test Includes Culture of foreign body organism identification, antibiotic susceptibilities of potential pathogens

Specimen Blood and distal 2" of I.V. catheter tip collected in a sterile manner (cut with sterile scissors and at a point just below the skin line)

Container Sterile container

Collection Aseptically prepare insertion site. Remove line without contact with adjacent skin and send only intra-arterial segment. Catheter tip aseptically removed and placed in sterile container. A procedure for quantitative comparative central and peripheral blood culture is as follows:

Separate blood samples (10 mL each) are obtained in a sterile manner from a peripheral blood vessel and from the central catheter. Aseptic technique at the catheter is as follows:

• The catheter is clamped and the needle adapter removed.

376

- The end of the catheter is swabbed once with 70% isopropyl alcohol and then with an iodine solution (allow to air dry).
- A sterile needle adapter is inserted into the end of the catheter.
- The clamp is removed and 2 mL of blood is drawn through a sterile syringe to clear the catheter.
- The blood for culture is then subsequently obtained in a separate sterile syringe.
- The catheter adapter is reattached to the intravenous tubing.

The paired blood specimens are placed in separate lysis centrifugation tubes after the stopper is wiped three times with povidone-iodine. See also Blood Culture, Aerobic and Anaerobic test listing.

Storage Instructions Specimens should be transported to the laboratory within 1 hour of collection for optimal results. However, if specimens cannot be collected and delivered to the laboratory during regular hours specimen may be refrigerated overnight.

Reference Range No growth. For culture taken through a central catheter, a tenfold greater colony count than a simultaneous peripheral culture or >100 CFU/mL if only a central catheter culture is presumptive evidence of a colonized catheter. A culture of a catheter tip (rolled onto agar media) result of ≥15 CFUs also is presumptive evidence of a colonized catheter.

Use Identify a possible source of bacteremia or fungemia; particularly useful for the diagnosis of catheter related sepsis (CRS) secondary to blood-borne seedling of catheters, and CRS associated with coagulase-negative staphylococci

Limitations Culture of blood obtained from intravenous lines is fraught with problems. Blood obtained from a line is easily contaminated and interpretation of results usually is difficult.

Methodology Quantitative or semiquantitative culture with or without lysis centrifugation. A very simple and equally effective semiquantitative technique is to roll the culture tip on a blood or chocolate agar plate. Greater than 15 CFUs suggests infection; less than 15 CFUs indicates a low probability of infection.

Additional Information Infections complicating therapy with indwelling central venous catheters pose a difficult problem. Catheter-related sepsis is defined when:

- Positive blood cultures collected through the central venous catheter can show a tenfold or greater colony count compared with peripheral quantitative blood culture or >100 CFU/mL if only central venous catheter blood culture is available
- A semiquantitative catheter tip culture result of ≥15 CFU
- No obvious clinical or microbiologic source for the infection is apparent

Summary of Results of Prospective Studies Using Semiquantitative Techniques to Diagnose Vascular-Access Infections

Organism	No. With Same Organism in Semiquantitative Catheter Culture and Blood Culture
Coagulase-negative staphylococci	27
Staphylococcus aureus	26
Yeast	17
Enterobacter	7
Serratia	5
Enterococcus	5
Klebsiella	4
Streptococcus viridans group	3
Pseudomonas species	2
Proteus	2
Others Pseudomonas aeruginosa Yersinia	1 each

From Hampton A and Sheretz RJ, "Vascular-Access Infections in Hospitalized Patients," *Surg Clin North Am*, 1988, 68:57-72, with permission.

(Continued)

Intravenous Line Culture *(Continued)*

Exit site infections are defined as purulent drainage or erythema at the catheter exit site. Tunnel infection is defined as spreading cellulitis with erythema, tenderness, and swelling of the skin surrounding the subcutaneous tunnel tract of the catheter. Successful therapy of catheter-related infection with antibiotics and local care has been reported. However, catheter removal almost always is required to achieve cure. *Staphylococcus aureus* and polymicrobial infections also are more difficult to eradicate. Intraluminal culture has been reported to correlate well with catheter tip cultures (87.5% identical) while skin puncture sites are usually less frequently identical (37.5%). See table on previous page.

Selected Readings

Andremont A, Paulet R, Nitenberg G, et al, "Value of Semiquantitative Cultures of Blood Drawn Through Catheter Hubs for Estimating the Risk of Catheter Tip Colonization in Cancer Patients," *J Clin Microbiol*, 1988, 26(11):2297-9.

Henderson DK, "Bacteremia Due to Percutaneous Intravascular Devices," *Principles and Practice of Infectious Diseases*, 4th ed, Mandell GL, Bennett JE and, eds, New York, NY: Churchill Livingstone, 1995, 2587-99.

Maki DG, Weise CE, and Sarafin HW, "A Semiquantitative Culture Method for Identifying Intravenous-Catheter-Related Infection," *N Engl J Med*, 1977, 296(23):1305-9.

Widmer AF, Nettleman M, Flint K, et al, "The Clinical Impact of Culturing Central Venous Catheters. A Prospective Study," *Arch Intern Med*, 1992, 152(6):1299-302.

Intravenous Pyelogram *see* Urography *on page 472*

Iron Stain *see* Bone Marrow Aspiration and Biopsy *on page 277*

Itraconazole

Synonyms Sporanox

Abstract Itraconazole is a new orally administered antifungal agent with a broad spectrum of activity. As of this writing it has not been released in the United States, though it is available in several other countries. Similarly, its role in clinical medicine is still evolving. It appears likely that this agent will become widely accepted due to its low toxicity compared with other antifungal agents and its broad spectrum of activity. The role for monitoring of serum levels is as yet unknown in clinical care.

Specimen Serum

Container Red top tube

Sampling Time 4 hours after oral dose and approximately 1-2 weeks after therapy has begun so that a steady-state is achieved

Reference Range Therapeutic range: varies with methodology; see Additional Information below

Use May be useful to ensure therapeutic levels if poor absorption is suspected, or in cases of therapeutic failure or relapse

Limitations *In vitro* susceptibility testing of fungi against itraconazole is method dependent and may not accurately predict clinical success. Consequently, monitoring levels and adjusting dosage to attain therapeutic concentrations as determined by minimum inhibitory concentrations may not be helpful. Assays for itraconazole are performed only in a few reference laboratories.

Methodology Bioassay, high performance liquid chromatography (HPLC)

Additional Information Serum levels as determined by bioassay are approximately 10 times the levels determined by HPLC, presumably because bioassay also detects an active metabolite. Consequently therapeutic levels vary with method. Concentrations >5 μg/mL (bioassay) were predictive of therapeutic success in invasive aspergillosis, whereas serum concentrations <1 μg/mL (bioassay) predicted therapeutic failure in cases of cryptococcal meningitis. Concentrations <0.25 μg/mL (HPLC) predicted failure to prevent aspergillosis in granulocytopenic patients. Absorption is often depressed in bone marrow transplant and in AIDS patients.

Selected Readings

Bodey GP. "Topical and Systemic Antifungal Agents," *Med Clin North Am*, 1988, 72(3):637-59.

British Society for Antimicrobial Chemotherapy Working Party, "Laboratory Monitoring of Antifungal Chemotherapy," *Lancet*, 1991, 337(8757):1577-80.

Terrell CL and Hughes CE, "Antifungal Agents Used for Deep-Seated Mycotic Infections," *Mayo Clin Proc*, 1992, 67(1):69-91.

IUD Culture *see Actinomyces* Culture, All Sites *on page 242*

I.V. Catheter Culture *see* Intravenous Line Culture *on page 376*

IVP *see* Urography *on page 472*

***Ixodes dammini* Identification** *see* Arthropod Identification *on page 268*

Joint Films, Specified Site

Joint Fluid Culture *see* Aerobic Culture, Body Fluid *on page 244*

Joint Fluid Fungus Culture *see* Fungus Culture, Body Fluid *on page 341*

Joint Study *see* Arthrogram *on page 267*

Joint Tap *see* Arthrocentesis *on page 264*

Kahn Test *replaced by* RPR *on page 438*

Kanamycin (Kantrex®) *see* Amikacin *on page 249*

Ketoconazole

Synonyms Nizoral

Abstract Ketoconazole is an orally administered antifungal agent that is appropriately used for a variety of nonlife-threatening fungal infections. Determining serum levels rarely contributes significantly to patient care.

Specimen Serum

Container Red top tube

Sampling Time 2 hours after administration

Reference Range Therapeutic: 5-20 μg/mL, dependent on dose

Use Usually unnecessary. May be useful to ensure therapeutic levels if poor absorption is suspected, or in cases of therapeutic failure or relapse.

Limitations *In vitro* susceptibility testing of fungi against ketoconazole is method dependent and may not accurately predict clinical success. Consequently, monitoring levels and adjusting dosage to attain therapeutic concentrations as determined by minimum inhibitory concentrations may not be helpful. Assays for ketoconazole are performed only in a few reference laboratories.

Methodology Bioassay, high performance liquid chromatography (HPLC)

Additional Information Approximately 5% to 10% of patients receiving ketoconazole develop abnormally elevated serum transaminases, a transient and reversible state. Rarely, patients develop symptomatic hepatitis which is idiosyncratic and not dependent upon serum concentrations. Absorption is often depressed in bone marrow transplant and AIDS patients.

Selected Readings

Bodey GP, "Topical and Systemic Antifungal Agents," *Med Clin North Am*, 1988, 72(3):637-59.

British Society for Antimicrobial Chemotherapy Working Party, "Laboratory Monitoring of Antifungal Chemotherapy," *Lancet*, 1991, 337(8757):1577-80.

Terrell CL and Hughes CE, "Antifungal Agents Used for Deep-Seated Mycotic Infections," *Mayo Clin Proc*, 1992, 67(1):69-91.

Kidneys Ultrasound *see* Ultrasound, Kidneys *on page 466*

Kinyoun Stain *see* Acid-Fast Stain *on page 239*

Kirby-Bauer Susceptibility Test *see* Antimicrobial Susceptibility Testing, Aerobic and Facultatively Anaerobic Organisms *on page 259*

Kline Test *replaced by* RPR *on page 438*

Knee Arthrogram *see* Arthrogram *on page 267*

Knee, Left or Right, X-ray *see* Bone Films *on page 277*

Knees Arthritis, X-ray *see* Bone Films *on page 277*

KOH Preparation

Related Information

Fungus Culture, Skin *on page 343*

Synonyms Potassium Hydroxide Preparation

Test Includes Potassium hydroxide, (KOH) hydrolysis of proteinaceous debris, cells, etc. Microscopic examination under 10x and 40x.

Patient Preparation Same as for culture of specific site

Special Instructions The laboratory should be informed of the specific source of the specimen and the clinical diagnosis.

(Continued)

KOH Preparation *(Continued)*

Specimen Appropriate specimen for KOH preparation is a specimen composed mostly of keratin (hair, skin, nails).

Container Same as for culture of specific site

Collection The specimen may be divided for fungus culture and KOH preparation, mycobacteria culture and smear, and routine bacterial culture and Gram stain only if the specimen is of adequate volume for all tests requested.

Causes for Rejection Insufficient specimen volume

Reference Range No fungus elements identified

Use Determine presence of fungi in skin, nails, or hair

Limitations Cultures are more sensitive than smears; therefore, the KOH preparation may be negative when culture is positive. The test may require overnight incubation for complete disintegration of hair, nail, or skin debris.

Methodology 10% KOH with gentle heat, alternately 20% KOH or 10% KOH and 40% dimethyl sulfoxide (DMSO)

Additional Information See the specimen selection tables provided in the Fungus Culture, Skin and Fungus Culture, Sputum test listings. For the diagnosis of keratomycosis direct examination may have a higher yield than culture because of the presence of dead organisms in the corneal tissue.

Recent reports have emphasized the changing pattern of tinea capitis, particularly the fact that infection due to *Trichophyton tonsurans* has become increasingly common. When present it causes a less discrete, more diffuse pattern of alopecia. It is negative by Wood's light examination. The "black dot," a remnant of a broken infected hair shaft, is a good source for diagnostic material which should be sought with a magnifying glass and collected with forceps. Scale and pulled hairs are also useful specimens. Diagnostic specimens should be collected before antifungal therapy is instituted. Topic steroids should not be prescribed until fungal infection is excluded.

Selected Readings

Cohn MS, "Superficial Fungal Infections. Topical and Oral Treatment of Common Types," *Postgrad Med*, 1992, 91(2):239-44, 249-52.

Gray LD and Roberts GD, "Laboratory Diagnosis of Systemic Fungal Diseases," *Infect Dis Clin North Am*, 1988, 2(4):779-803.

Hebert AA and Burton-Esterly N, "Bacterial and Candidal Cutaneous Infections in the Neonate," *Dermatol Clin*, 1986, 4(1):3-21.

Ishibashi Y, Hommura S, and Matsumoto Y, "Direct Examination vs Culture of Biopsy Specimens for the Diagnosis of Keratomycosis," *Am J Ophthalmol*, 1987, 103(5):636-40.

Stein DH, "Superficial Fungal Infections," *Pediatr Clin North Am*, 1983, 30(3):545-61.

Latex Agglutination, Bacterial Antigens, Cerebrospinal Fluid *see* Bacterial Antigens, Rapid Detection Methods *on page 269*

LE Antibodies *see* Skin Biopsy, Immunofluorescence *on page 446*

Legionella Antigen, Urine

Related Information

Legionella pneumophila Culture *on next page*

Synonyms Urine *Legionella* Antigen

Specimen Random urine

Container Sterile specimen container

Collection Early morning specimens yield highest bacterial counts from overnight incubation in the bladder, and are the best specimens. Colony count interpretation standards are based on controlled studies from first early morning collections. Forced fluids or random specimens dilute the urine and may cause reduced colony counts. Hair from perineum will contaminate the specimen. The stream from a male may be contaminated by bacteria from beneath the prepuce. Bacteria from vaginal secretions, vulva or distal urethra may contaminate. Organisms from hands or clothing might contaminate. Receptacle must be sterile.

Males: Wash your hands thoroughly with soap and water. Rinse them well and dry with a paper towel. Tear open the towelette packages so that the towels can be easily removed with one hand as they are needed. Open the urine container. Do not touch any of the inside surfaces of the container or the lid. Pull back the foreskin to completely expose the head of the penis. Wash the head of the penis thoroughly using first one towelette then the other. Discard the used towelettes into the toilet bowl. Pass a small amount of urine into the toilet bowl, then pass a sample into the container. Do not allow the container to touch the legs or the penis. Keep your fingers away from the rim and inner surface of the container. Fill the container half full. Replace the lid on the container. The urine specimen should be refrigerated within 10 minutes of collection or taken immediately to the laboratory.

Females: Wash your hands thoroughly with soap and water. Rinse them well and dry with a paper towel. Tear open the towelette packages so that the towels can be easily removed with one hand as they are needed. Open the urine container. Do not touch any of the inside surfaces of the container or the lid. Remove your undergarments and sit on the toilet seat with your legs spread widely apart. With one hand, spread your labia apart to expose the vulva. Keep this hand in place during the washing and urinating procedure. Use one towelette to wash the vulva well passing the towelette only from front to back, not back and forth. Repeat this procedure using the second towelette. Discard the used towelettes into the toilet bowl. Begin urinating into the toilet bowl then without stopping the stream, insert the container to collect the specimen. Do not allow the container to touch the legs, vulva, or clothing. Keep your fingers away from the rim and inner surface of the container. Fill the container approximately half full. Replace the lid on the container. The urine specimen should be refrigerated within 10 minutes of collection or taken immediately to the laboratory. Apply the completed patient label to the specimen cup. Most patients, with instruction, do better with privacy than an attendant can

Catheterized specimen: Do not collect urine from the drainage bag when an indwelling catheter is in place because growth of bacteria can occur in the bag itself. Rather, clean catheter with an alcohol sponge, puncture with sterile needle, collect in sterile syringe. Catheter tips are contaminated by the urethra as they are withdrawn; do not culture them.

Storage Instructions Specimen may be refrigerated if unable to transport immediately.

Causes for Rejection Specimen received in inappropriate or unlabeled container, specimen not received on ice, contaminated specimen. If an unacceptable specimen is received, the nursing unit will be notified and another specimen requested before disposal of the original specimen.

Reference Range Negative

Use Determine the presence of *Legionella* antigen in urine

Methodology Radioimmunoassay (RIA)

Additional Information This test is sensitive and specific. However, this test should be confirmed by culture and serology for optimal chances of correct diagnosis.

***Legionella* Assay** *see Legionella DNA Probe on this page*

Legionella DNA Probe

Synonyms DNA Probe for *Legionella*; *Legionella* Assay

Specimen Respiratory secretions, sputum, bronchial washing, pleural fluid, lung biopsy

Container Sterile container

Storage Instructions Specimen should be received in the laboratory as soon as possible.

Reference Range Negative for *Legionella*

Use Determine presence of *Legionella* species

Limitations Inconclusive results can be obtained.

Methodology DNA probe

Additional Information Culture for *Legionella* is the confirmatory test and should be done on all specimens received for *Legionella* DNA probe assay. The sensitivity and specificity of the DNA probe test is 60% to 75% and 98%, respectively.

***Legionella pneumophila* Antibodies** *see Legionella Serology on page 384*

Legionella pneumophila Culture

Related Information

Aerobic Culture, Sputum *on page 246*
Legionella Antigen, Urine *on previous page*
Legionella pneumophila Smear *on page 383*

Synonyms Culture, *Legionella pneumophila*

Applies To Biopsy *Legionella* Culture; Bronchoscopic *Legionella* Culture; Pleural Fluid, *Legionella* Culture; Transtracheal Aspiration *Legionella* Culture
(Continued)

Legionella pneumophila Culture *(Continued)*

Test Includes Culture and, frequently, direct fluorescent antibody (DFA) smear for *Legionella pneumophila*

Specimen Lung tissue, other body tissue, pleural fluid, other body fluid, transtracheal aspiration, bronchoalveolar lavage, and bronchial brushing

Container Sterile container

Collection Contamination with normal flora from skin or other body surfaces should be avoided.

Turnaround Time Reports on specimens from which *Legionella* has been isolated require approximately 2-5 days.

Reference Range No growth

Use Isolate and identify *Legionella pneumophila*

Limitations Sputum (expectorated), bronchial aspirates, and other specimens having normal flora are subject to bacterial overgrowth and are not as desirable as transtracheal aspirates, pleural fluid, and biopsy material for culture. Sensitivity of cultures is relatively low (50% to 80%); however specificity is 100%. A direct fluorescent antibody smear without culture can be performed, but DFA alone is not recommended. Cross reactions with *B. fragilis*, *Pseudomonas fluorescens*, and other species occur. Newer approaches utilizing monoclonal antibodies have enhanced the yield of fluorescent procedures.

Methodology Culture on selective and nonselective media (buffered charcoal yeast extract)

Additional Information Acute and convalescent sera for *Legionella* antibodies should also be considered to increase the chance of documenting the diagnosis. A fourfold rise to a titer of 1:128 is a diagnostic standard criterion. Seroconversion may be detected in many patients in the first weeks. Seroconver-

Infections Caused by *Legionella*

Culture proven
Pneumonia
Empyema
Sinusitis
Prosthetic valve endocarditis
Wound infection
Associated with pneumonia
Bowel abscesses
Brain abscesses
Empyema
Lung abscesses
Myocarditis
Pericarditis
Peritonitis
Renal abscesses/pyelonephritis
Vascular graft infections
Strong seroepidemiological evidence
Pontiac fever
Weak seroepidemiological evidence
Encephalopathy without pneumonia
Myocarditis without pneumonia
Pericarditis without pneumonia

From Edelstein PH, "Laboratory Diagnosis of Infections Caused by *Legionella*," *Eur J Clin Microbiol*, 1987, 6:4–10, with permission.

Clinical Clues to the Diagnosis of Legionnaires' Disease

- Atypical pneumonia
- Gram's stain of respiratory secretions reveals numerous neutrophils, but few organisms
- Presence of hyponatremia (serum sodium ≤130 mmol/L)
- Failure to respond to β–lactam and aminoglycoside antibiotics
- Occurrence in hospital where potable water system is known to be contaminated with *Legionella*
- History of smoking and alcohol use
- Pleuritic chest pain
- Fever malaise, myalgia, headache

From Harrison TG and Taylor AG, "Timing of Seroconversion in Legionnaires' Disease," *Lancet*, Oct 1988, 795, with permission.

sion 0-7 days after onset, 16%; 0-14 days, 52%; 0-21 days, 66%; 0-28 days, 71%. Twenty-five percent of patients may not have diagnostic titers. Methods to detect *Legionella* antigens in urine include radioimmunoassay, enzyme immunoassay, and latex agglutination. Sensitivity of these methods can be up to 80% under ideal conditions. Consult the laboratory regarding availability and selection of the most appropriate method. Nosocomial infections have been recognized with reservoirs, water distribution systems, cooling systems, and hot water systems of hospitals being reported. Twenty species in the Legionellaceae family of bacteria have been discovered since *Legionella pneumophila* was first recognized. Thirteen species have been implicated as causes of human pneumonia. See tables on previous page.

Selected Readings

Fang GD, Yu VL, and Vickers RM, "Disease Due to the *Legionellaceae* (Other Than *Legionella pneumophila*). Historical, Microbiological, Clinical, and Epidemiological Review," *Medicine (Baltimore)*, 1989, 68(2):116-32.

Hart CA and Makin T, "*Legionella* in Hospitals: A Review," *J Hosp Infect*, 1991, 18(Suppl A):481-9.

Hoge CW and Brieman RF, "Advances in the Epidemiology and Control of *Legionella* Infections," *Epidemiol Rev*, 1991, 13:329-40.

Nguyen ML and Yu VL, "*Legionella* Infection," *Clin Chest Med*, 1991, 12(2):257-68.

Rodgers FG, "New Perspectives on *Legionella* Infections," *Infect Med*, 1994, 11(2):137, 141-7.

Legionella pneumophila Smear

Related Information

Legionella pneumophila Culture *on previous page*
Legionella Serology *on page 384*

Synonyms Direct Fluorescent Antibody Smear for *Legionella pneumophila*; FA Smear for *Legionella pneumophila*

Test Includes Direct fluorescent antibody (DFA) microscopic examination of specimen smear

Specimen Lung tissue, other body tissue, pleural fluid, other body fluid, transtracheal aspirate, sputum, bronchial washing

Container Sterile container

Collection Contamination with normal flora from skin or other body surfaces should be avoided

Causes for Rejection Saliva sent rather than sputum specimen

Reference Range No *Legionella pneumophila* seen in direct FA microscopic examination

Use Determine presence of *Legionella pneumophila* organisms in direct FA smear of specimen, providing rapid diagnosis

Limitations Staining for several serogroups may be necessary. Most methods include antibodies only to *L. pneumophilia* and not to other *Legionella* species.

Methodology Direct fluorescent antibody

Additional Information Community acquired and nosocomial infections caused by multiple serogroups of *Legionella* are increasingly recognized. Although culture is now possible on buffered charcoal yeast extract agar, the demonstration of organisms in tissue or brushings is the fastest way to make the diagnosis. It also has the advantage of applicability to specimens contaminated with other bacteria. Development of monoclonal antibodies have increased sensitivity and specificity. False-positive reaction has been reported in a case of pleuropulmonary tularemia and in cases of *Campylobacter* infection. A combination of both culture and DFA is recommended.

Selected Readings

Andersen LP and Bangsborg J, "Crossreactions Between *Legionella* and *Campylobacter* Spp," *Lancet*, 1992, 340(8813):245.

Edelstein PH, Beer KB, Sturge JC, et al, "Clinical Utility of a Monoclonal Direct Fluorescent Reagent Specific for *Legionella pneumophila*: Comparative Study With Other Reagents," *J Clin Microbiol*, 1985, 22(3):419-21.

Friedman H, Wider R, and Klein T, "Immunodiagnostic Assays for Legionellosis," *Lab Management*, 1983, 21:19-23.

Hart CA and Makin T, "*Legionella* in Hospitals: A Review," *J Hosp Infect*, 1991, 18(Suppl A):481-9.

Hicklin MD, Thomason BM, Chandler FW, et al, "Pathogenesis of Acute Legionnaires' Disease Pneumonia." *Am J Clin Pathol*, 1980, 73(4):480-7.

Roy TM, Fleming D, and Anderson WH, "Tularemic Pneumonia Mimicking Legionnaires' Disease With False-Positive Direct Fluorescent Antibody Stains for *Legionella*," *South Med J*, 1989, 82(11):1429-31.

LABORATORY DIAGNOSIS
Legionella Serology
Related Information
Legionella pneumophila Smear *on previous page*

Synonyms *Legionella pneumophila* Antibodies; Legionnaires' Disease Antibodies

Specimen Serum

Container Red top tube

Collection A convalescent sample should be obtained 10-14 days after acute sample

Reference Range Negative. Less than a fourfold change in titer between acute and convalescent samples. Less than 1:256 in a single sample.

Use Detection of antibody to *Legionella pneumophila*; support for the clinical diagnosis of Legionnaires' disease

Limitations Testing for multiple serogroups may be necessary

Methodology Indirect fluorescent antibody assay using serogroup 1: Philadelphia, Knoxville, serogroup 2: Togus, serogroup 3: Los Angeles, serogroup 4: Bloomington. A polyvalent antigen which includes serogroup 1-6 may be utilized. IgG and IgM titers may be provided. Latex agglutination may be used in some laboratories.

Additional Information A fourfold rise in titer exceeding a titer of 1:128 from the acute to convalescent phase provides evidence of recent infection. A single titer equal to or greater than 1:256 is evidence of infection at an undetermined time. However, due to the relatively high prevalence of antibodies to *Legionella pneumophila*, acute and convalescent titers are preferred to a single sample. Demonstration of a high titer in the proper clinical setting may allow timely institution of specific treatment, and may eliminate the need for an invasive procedure to obtain a specimen for culture or direct immunofluorescence. Demonstration of IgM antibody to serogroup I may allow rapid diagnosis. Recent availability of a latex agglutination test with 98.3% specificity and 97.6% sensitivity is well suited as a screening test. Serologic study is also valuable in evaluation of epidemic disease.

Selected Readings
Edelstein PH, "Detection of Antibodies to *Legionella*," *Manual of Clinical Laboratory Immunology*, 4th ed, Rose NR, de Macario EC, Fahey JL, et al, eds, Washington, DC: American Society for Microbiology, 1992, 459-66.

Holliday MG, "Use of Latex Agglutination Technique for Detecting *Legionella pneumophila* (Serogroup I) Antibodies," *J Clin Pathol*, 1990, 43(10):860-2.

Rodgers FG, "New Perspectives on *Legionella* Infections," *Infect Med*, 1994, 11(2):137, 141-7.

Legionnaires' Disease Antibodies *see Legionella* Serology *on this page*

Leptospira, Blood Culture *see Leptospira* Culture *on this page*

Leptospira Culture
Related Information
Darkfield Examination, Leptospirosis *on page 322*
Leptospira Serology *on next page*

Synonyms Culture for *Leptospira*

Applies To Blood Culture, *Leptospira*; *Leptospira*, Blood Culture

Patient Preparation Urine specimen: Thoroughly instruct patient in the proper collection technique for a midvoid urine specimen; avoid contamination with skin flora.

See also Urine Culture, Clean Catch and Blood Culture, Aerobic and Anaerobic test listings for detailed instructions.

Special Instructions The laboratory should be informed of the specific request for *Leptospira* culture, collection time, date, specific site of specimen, age of patient, current antibiotic therapy, date of onset of illness, and clinical diagnosis. Urine must be alkaline; *Leptospira* do not survive in acid urine. Repeated cultures may be required.

Specimen Urine, indicate midvoid, catheter or suprapubic puncture specimen; blood and cerebrospinal fluid may also be cultured

Container Sterile container or tube

Collection Specimen should be transported to laboratory within 1 hour of collection. For midvoid urine culture, patient should be instructed to clean skin thoroughly, do not collect first portion of stream, collect midportion of stream, and do not collect final portion of stream. Catheter or suprapubic puncture specimen may also be used.

Causes for Rejection Specimens delayed in transit to the laboratory have less than optimal value.

Turnaround Time 4-8 weeks. Consult the laboratory prior to the collection of the specimen, so that appropriate processing of the specimen can be arranged.

Reference Range No *Leptospira* isolated

Use Confirm the clinical diagnosis of leptospirosis

Limitations Specimen will be cultured for *Leptospira*; other organisms may not be identified

Contraindications Leptospiremia occurs during the septicemic acute phase of infection. This phase last 4-7 days after which organisms are not recoverable from blood. Cultures of blood should **not** be ordered after the first week of illness.

Methodology Urine or blood is inoculated onto specially prepared media containing rabbit serum or albumin and fatty acids. Incubation is for 4-6 weeks in the dark at 28°C to 29°C. Cultures are examined with darkfield or phase microscopy at weekly intervals; growth occurs 1-3 cm below the surface.

Additional Information Leptospirosis in humans is usually associated with occupational exposure. Veterinarians, dairymen, swineherds, abattoir workers, miners, fish and poultry processors and those who work in a rat-infested environment are at increased risk. During the first week of disease, the most reliable means of detecting leptospires is by direct culturing of blood or spinal fluid on appropriate media. **Urine does not become positive for *Leptospira*** until the second week of disease and then can remain positive for several months. Concentration of *Leptospira* in human urine is low and shedding may be intermittent. Therefore, repeated isolation attempts should be made. Serology (acute and early convalescent) is recommended. Darkfield examination yields many false-positives.

Selected Readings
Sperber SJ and Schleupner CJ, "Leptospirosis: A Forgotten Cause of Aseptic Meningitis and Multisystem Febrile Illness," *South Med J*, 1989, 82(10):1285-8.

Leptospira Serology

Related Information
Darkfield Examination, Leptospirosis *on page 322*
Leptospira Culture *on previous page*

Test Includes Testing of patient's serum for antibodies against *Leptospira biflexa* serovar *L. patoc*, and the following serovars of *Leptospira interrogans*: *L. copenhageni, L. canicola, L. pomona, L. autumnalis, L. grippotyphosa, L. wolffi,* and *L. djatzi*. Supplemental testing may be needed against serovars: *L. poi, L. castellonis, L. pyrogenes, L. borincana, L. szwajizak, L. bratislava, L. tarassovi, L. shermani, L. panama, L. celledoni, L. djasiman, L. cynopteri,* and *L. louisiana*.

Specimen Serum

Container Red top tube

Collection Acute and convalescent sera drawn 10-14 days apart are suggested

Causes for Rejection Inadequate labeling, excessive hemolysis, chylous serum or gross contamination of the specimen

Reference Range Negative. A fourfold increase in titer is diagnostic of infection.

Use Support the diagnosis of leptospirosis

Limitations The antigens used in the test are the ones most commonly causing disease, but there are many other serovars which might not be detected. To optimize yield, a battery of antigens are used.

Methodology Microscopic agglutination test, macroagglutination, complement fixation, hemagglutination, enzyme linked immunosorbent assay

Additional Information Leptospirosis is an acute febrile illness caused primarily by *Leptospira interrogans*, a large spirochete with over 180 serologic variants. Patients with extensive animal contact, either in the wild or with carcasses or excrement, are particularly at risk.

Although leptospires can be cultured from blood or urine during the first week of illness, this interval is often missed, and diagnosis must be based on the demonstration of rising antibody titers. Antibody appears at the end of the first week of illness and peaks at 3-4 weeks, after which it slowly disappears.

There has been an association between patients with leptospirosis and anticardiolipin antibodies which may induce vascular endothelial injury in severe cases.

(Continued)

Leptospira Serology *(Continued)*

Selected Readings

Ribeiro MA, Sakata EE, Silva MV, et al, "Antigens Involved in the Human Antibody Response to Natural Infections With *Leptospira interrogans serovar copenhageni*," *J Trop Med Hyg*, 1992, 95(4):239-45.

Rugman FP, Pinn G, Palmer MF, et al, "Anticardiolipin Antibodies in Leptospirosis," *J Clin Pathol*, 1991, 44(6):517-9.

Leptospirosis, Darkfield Examination *see* Darkfield Examination, Leptospirosis *on page 322*

Lesion Culture *see* Wound Culture *on page 480*

Leukocyte Esterase, Urine

Related Information

Nitrite, Urine *on page 414*

Synonyms Bacteria Screen, Urine; Esterase, Leukocyte, Urine

Test Includes Screening of urine for leukocyte esterase activity by dipstick; frequently a part of urinalysis

Abstract A rapid indirect test for detection of bacteriuria. It indicates presence of esterase from intact or lysed neutrophils.

Specimen Random clean catch urine; preferably midstream clean-catch collection

Container Plastic urine container

Storage Instructions If the specimen cannot be processed within 2 hours it should be refrigerated.

Causes for Rejection Improper labeling, specimen not refrigerated

Reference Range Negative

Use Detection of leukocytes in urine. Leukocyte esterase indicates the presence of either intact or lysed white blood cells and therefore can be positive when WBCs are not found on microscopic examination. The lysis of leukocytes that occurs when urine is allowed to stand intensifies the color reaction from release of esterase.

Limitations Cephalexin; cephalothin; tetracycline; large amounts of oxalic acid (eg, iced tea drinkers); high glucose and high specific gravity may decrease or suppress positive results. Albumin and ascorbic acid inhibit the method. Tetracycline may cause decreased reactivity or false-negatives. Neutropenia can cause false-negative results.

Leukocyte esterase, even combined with nitrite, should not replace microscopy and culture in symptomatic patients. Urine culture is indicated for subjects with symptoms of urinary tract infection. False-positive results from trichomonads have been controversial; however, false-positives may occur in specimens contaminated with vaginal secretions. Leukocyte esterase is unacceptable as a screen unless combined at least with nitrite testing.

Methodology Indoxyl is released by leukocyte esterase if present in the urine specimen. The substrate on the strip is indoxyl carbonic acid ester. Indoxyl is oxidized by atmospheric oxygen to indigo blue. The reaction time is 1 minute, but high sensitivity requires interpretation five minutes after immersion in the sample.

Additional Information Some institutions now perform microscopic urinalysis only on specific request or on the observation of an abnormal macroscopic finding. The principal advantage of the method is the ability to identify the presence of leukocyte esterase in dilute urine specimens and in specimens which have been subject to standing with lysis of the white cells. When combined with the nitrite test it provides sensitivity for both tests of up to 92% and specificity of 95%, respectively, either test abnormal. When false-negatives occur they are usually due to gram-positive organism bacteriuria. Some laboratories have established a screening protocol in which culture is only performed if screening with leukocyte esterase or nitrate is positive. Dipstick screening has been compared to Gram stains of unspun urine and to urine sediment microscopy and culture.

Leukocyte esterase has been used for detection of sexually transmitted disease particularly in males.

Selected Readings

High SR, Rowe JA, and Maksem JA, "Macroscopic Physiochemical Testing for Screening Urinalysis," *Lab Med*, 1988, 19:174-6.

Leukocyte Scintigraphy *see* Indium Leukocyte Scan *on page 374*

Lice Identification *see* Arthropod Identification *on page 268*

Liver Biopsy

Synonyms Blind Liver Biopsy; Needle Biopsy of the Liver; Percutaneous Liver Biopsy

Applies To Percutaneous Needle Aspiration Biopsy Under Fluoroscopic, CT, or Ultrasound Guidance; Transjugular Needle Biopsy of the Liver

Test Includes Percutaneous biopsy of liver parenchyma in a "blind" fashion (ie, not under radiologic guidance). This is carried out at the bedside under local anesthesia. A specialized, thin-bore needle is advanced between the ribs overlying the region of hepatic dullness. Several 2 cm cores of deep liver tissue are excised. Fresh specimens may be sent for gross pathologic inspection, routine light microscopy, special stains for liver storage diseases, transmission and immune electron microscopy, immunohistochemistry (using monoclonal antibodies), DNA hybridization studies, and microbiologic culture. Liver biopsy is a valuable and time-honored means of diagnosing diffuse liver parenchymal disease as well as disseminated focal disease.

Patient Preparation Procedures and risks of the procedure are explained and consent is obtained. Formal consultation with gastroenterology staff is usually required. Procedure entails overnight hospitalization in most cases but some patients may be candidates for a "same day" outpatient biopsy. This latter group is in good general health, not jaundiced, and displays no signs of liver failure (ascites, encephalopathy). They need to stay within several minutes of the hospital for 1-2 days postbiopsy and must have supervision from family or friends. Scheduling arrangements for both in-hospital and outpatient liver biopsies are handled by gastroenterology team. All aspirin products and nonsteroidal agents must be discontinued at least 5 days beforehand. If taking oral anticoagulants (Coumadin®), hospitalization is required to convert to heparin therapy before biopsy. Patient is NPO after midnight the evening prior. Daily medications may be taken on the day of procedure pending physician approval. In some hospitals, patient drinks 1-2 glasses of milk in the early AM on procedure day to empty the gallbladder. Screening laboratory studies ordered 24-48 hours in advance commonly include CBC, PT/PTT, BUN, bleeding time, and type and crossmatch for possible transfusion. Electrolytes and liver function tests are optional. If pneumonia or pleural effusion suspected on examination, PA and lateral chest x-ray is obtained. Premedication with meperidine and/or diazepam may be administered at physician discretion. This is not routine in some centers due to possible toxicity.

Aftercare Protocols are individualized for each hospital. In general, patient is monitored in a recovery area with frequent vital signs postbiopsy. If no complications are apparent, patient is transferred back to hospital room by cart. Strict bedrest is enforced for 24 hours; for the first 2 hours patient is positioned on his right side. After 5 hours, patient may be allowed to sit up. Vitals (blood pressure, pulse) are checked every 15-30 minutes for 2 hours, every 30 minutes for the next 2 hours, and then every hour for 8 hours. Following this, vitals every 4 hours are permissible. Physician should be immediately notified if hypotension, tachycardia, fever, or uncontrolled pain occurs. Diet is restricted to clear liquids for several hours, then full liquids as tolerated. Acetaminophen is usually sufficient for pain control. Some physicians recheck hematocrit 24 hours after procedure before approving hospital discharge.

Special Instructions In the appropriate high-risk patient, antibiotic prophylaxis for infective endocarditis may be considered. Little data exists regarding the risk of bacteremia, however, much less endocarditis.

Complications Based on several large series, serious morbidity has been estimated at 0.1% to 0.2%. Fatality rates have ranged from 0% to 0.17%, both figures being derived from studies involving >20,000 biopsies each. The more commonly seen complications are:

- pain – the most common adverse event, noted in ≤50% of cases. Usually it is confined to the right shoulder, probably referred pain from diaphragmatic pleura. Analgesia is required in approximately 20% of patients with acetaminophen sufficient in most cases. Symptoms resolve in 1-2 days.
- hemorrhage – minor episodes are common. Self-limited oozing from the puncture site may persist for approximately 1 minute, but with loss of only 5-10 mL blood. Significant hemorrhage is less frequent but is the most common cause of death from liver biopsy. Several series have estimated an incidence of approximately 0.2%, but Sherlock (1984) reported 40 patients out of 6379 required transfusion for intraperitoneal bleeding. She felt these statistics may even underestimate the incidence since those with se-

(Continued)

LABORATORY DIAGNOSIS
Liver Biopsy *(Continued)*

vere coagulopathies were excluded. Bleeding usually results from a tear of a distended portal or hepatic vein. Specific sites include the abdominal cavity (hemoperitoneum), liver capsule (capsular hematoma), liver parenchyma (intrahepatic hematoma), or biliary tree (hemobilia). Postulated risk factors are coagulopathy, amyloid liver, hepatocellular injury, hemangioma, and vascularized tumor. However, bleeding may be massive when no risk factors are present. Not all episodes require surgery. In a study 4 of 7532 patients needed surgical intervention while 12 others with severe hemorrhage were transfused and observed.

- bile leakage with peritonitis – associated with severe obstruction of the larger bile ducts. This is felt to result from laceration of a small, distended duct or from puncture of the gallbladder. With the widespread use of noninvasive imaging, the size of the bile ducts is known prebiopsy and the complication rate has declined.
- laceration of internal organs and viscera – right kidney, gallbladder, colon, pancreas, and others
- others: right-sided pneumothorax, arteriovenous fistula – 5.4% of all biopsies, drug toxicity

Equipment Several biopsy needles are available.

- Menghini needle – 1.9 mm diameter steel shaft with sharpened beveled tip and syringe; specimen is obtained using suction/aspiration into a 10 mL syringe. Requires only 1 second within the liver ("1-second technique") and patient need not hold his breath. Disadvantages are small samples and fragmentation of biopsy specimens.
- "Trucut" needle – disposable 2.05 mm diameter needle designed to cut out cores of tissue. Specimens are less fragmented, even in the cirrhotic liver, and thus a high success rate. However, dwell time in liver is longer (5-10 seconds), patient must cooperate more, and several steps are necessary.
- Vim-Silverman needle – sheath with inner cutting blade (similar to a "punch" biopsy). Trucut needle is a modernized Vim-Silverman.

Technique Patient lies supine in bed with right hand behind his head. Liver margins are estimated by percussion. Two approaches are popular, transthoracic (intercostal) or subcostal (anterior). With the former, biopsy site is identified along the midaxillary line in the center of hepatic dullness, usually the eighth or ninth intercostal space. This approach avoids other abdominal organs but always penetrates the pleura. With the subcostal approach, the biopsy site lies below the bottom rib anteriorly, and is used when a liver mass is easily palpable below the right costal margin. The risk of visceral laceration is higher and this approach is infrequently used; fine needle aspiration under CT guidance has become more popular. A wide area is prepped and draped in sterile fashion with operators in gowns, gloves, and masks. The skin is anesthetized with 1% lidocaine, then deeper structures are infiltrated – subcutaneous tissue, intercostal muscles, and diaphragm. Some operators make a small superficial incision with a No 11 blade at the needle entry site to facilitate needle insertion. Techniques differ with the type of biopsy needle selected. In general, the biopsy needle is advanced as far as the diaphragm (depth estimated by a finder needle). If a Menghini needle is used, suction is applied to the syringe, the needle is pushed rapidly through the pleura and into the liver parenchyma. A 2.5 cm core of liver is aspirated and needle withdrawn, all within 1 second. If other needles are used, patient may need to hold his breath at end expiration to decrease the risk of pneumothorax. Several passes of the biopsy needle are performed to minimize sampling bias.

Specimen At least 2-3 liver cores, each >2 cm in length. Initial specimen processing and transportation handled by gastroenterology team. A typical protocol would be as follows:

- tissue fixation – for light microscopy, specimen is routinely fixed in 10% buffered formalin within 1 minute. For transmission electron microscopy, 1 mm cubes of specimen are fixed immediately in glutaraldehyde with further processing in Pathology Laboratory.
- routine tissue stains including: H & E – general liver histology stain; reticulin stain – for connective tissue, especially cirrhosis, fibrosis, bridging necrosis; trichrome – fibrosis; iron stain – useful for hemosiderosis, hemochromatosis, bile pigments; diastase PAS stain – useful for alpha$_1$-antitrypsin globules, bile ducts, iron; orcein – for hepatitis B surface antigen (if present, fine granular brown material stains in hepatocytes). Also for copper-binding protein in Wilson's disease.
- cytologic preparation – fluid from aspirating syringe may be smeared on clean microscope slide, fixed, and sent to Cytology Laboratory

- microbiological culture – specimen sent without fixative in sterile container. Special stains (AFB, KOH, etc) and cultures (tuberculosis, viral, *Brucella*, parasites, fungi) as needed
- optional special stains, ie, congo red for amyloidosis, immunohistochemistry

Use Candidates for liver biopsy must be carefully selected. This procedure, by nature, is invasive and histologic findings may often be reported as "consistent with" a particular disease (without being pathognomonic) or simply "nondiagnostic". In most cases, noninvasive imaging studies such as CT scan or ultrasound are now obtained first. With these considerations in mind, indications for liver biopsy include:

- suspected cases of liver cirrhosis, in order to confirm the diagnosis pathologically; establish etiology if possible (alcohol, alpha$_1$-antitrypsin deficiency, primary biliary cirrhosis, Wilson's disease, hemochromatosis, etc); assess and stage level of activity; assess complications
- chronic hepatitis, with or without cirrhosis, to identify cases of chronic activity hepatitis (liver biopsy mandatory for diagnosis) and differentiate this entity from chronic persistent hepatitis and lobular hepatitis
- suspected liver disease in the known alcoholic patient, to confirm alcoholic liver disease, exclude alternative causes of liver disease (which may be present in ≤20% of cases), stage and assess disease activity
- diagnosis of hepatoma or metastatic neoplasms
- suspected multisystem disease with liver involvement, where traditional diagnostic techniques have not been fruitful (eg, sarcoidosis, amyloidosis, tuberculosis, glycogen storage disease)
- staging of lymphoma
- unexplained hepatomegaly
- cholestasis of unknown etiology, where prior studies for biliary obstruction are negative
- persistently elevated liver enzyme tests
- selected cases of fever of unknown origin
- selected cases of hepatitis of unknown etiology, in order to differentiate viral from drug-induced etiologies (not always possible) or to assess complications, such as cholestasis
- evaluation of response to treatment

Liver biopsy is less useful in:
- acute hepatitis A or B infection, unless the diagnosis is in question
- extrahepatic biliary obstruction, where percutaneous transhepatic cholangiography and ERCP are considered first-line procedures
- fluid-filled liver cysts detected on ultrasound or CT scan, probably more amenable to guided thin needle aspiration first

Contraindications Mahal et al (1979) noted that failure to heed accepted contraindications led directly to 22 bleeding episodes in 3800 percutaneous liver biopsies. Contraindications include:

- impaired hemostasis, accepted as prothrombin time more than 3 seconds over control, PTT more than 20 seconds over control, thrombocytopenia, and markedly prolonged bleeding time
- severe anemia (Hgb <9.5 g/dL)
- local infection near needle entry site, such as right sided pleural effusion or empyema, right lower lobe pneumonia, local cellulitis, infected ascites or peritonitis
- tense ascites (low yield technically, risk of leakage)
- high-grade extrahepatic biliary obstruction with jaundice (increased risk of bile peritonitis)
- septic cholangitis
- possible hemangioma
- possible echinococcal (hydatid) cyst
- lack of compatible blood for transfusion
- uncooperative patient

Selected Readings

Lefkowitch JH, "Pathologic Diagnosis of Liver Disease," *Hepatology: A Textbook of Liver Disease*, 2nd ed, Chapter 29, Zakim D and Boyer TD, eds, Philadelphia, PA: WB Saunders Co, 1990, 711-32.

Mahal AS, Knauer CM, and Gregory PB, "Bleeding After Liver Biopsy," *West J Med*, 1981, 134(1):11-4.

Perrault J, McGill DB, Ott BJ, et al, "Liver Biopsy: Complications in 1000 Inpatients and Outpatients," *Gastroenterology*, 1978, 78(1):103-6.

Schaffner F, "Needle Biopsy of the Liver," *Bockus Gastroenterology*, 4th ed, Chapter 49, Berk JE, ed, Philadelphia, PA: WB Saunders Co, 1985, 657-66.

(Continued)

Liver Biopsy *(Continued)*

Sherlock S, Dick R, and van Leeuwen DJ, "Liver Biopsy Today. The Royal Free Hospital Experience," *J Hepatol*, 1984, 1(1):75-85.

Sherlock S, "Needle Biopsy of the Liver," *Diseases of the Liver and Biliary System*, 7th ed, Chapter 3, Oxford, England: Blackwell Scientific Publications, 1985, 28-37.

Van Ness MM and Diehl AM, "Is Liver Biopsy Useful in the Evaluation of Patients With Chronically Elevated Liver Enzymes?" *Ann Intern Med*, 1989, 111(6):473-8.

Lower Respiratory Fungus Culture *see* Fungus Culture, Bronchial Aspirate *on page 342*

Lower Respiratory Mycobacteria Culture *see* Mycobacteria Culture, Sputum *on page 406*

LP *see* Lumbar Puncture *on this page*

Lumbar Puncture

Synonyms Cerebrospinal Fluid Tap; LP; Spinal Tap

Test Includes Collection of cerebrospinal fluid (CSF) for chemical, cellular, and microbiological analysis. Performed as a bedside procedure under local anesthesia, a needle is passed into the L4-L5 vertebral interspace and subarachnoid fluid is withdrawn.

Patient Preparation Procedure and risks are explained and consent is obtained. If patient is confused or obtunded, obtain consent from guardians. If a coagulopathy is suspected, obtain platelet count and prothrombin/partial thromboplastin time if time permits. No intravenous pain medications such as meperidine are required routinely. Likewise, sedatives or anxiolytics may serve to confuse later assessments of mental status.

Aftercare Patient should be kept at strict bedrest for a minimum of 3 hours postprocedure to minimize post-LP headache. Regarding the optimal patient positioning, opinions vary. Some authors recommend the prone position post-LP based on a study involving >1000 subjects which demonstrated a 0.5% incidence of headache in patients kept prone versus 36.5% in the supine group. The frequency of obtaining vital signs and neurologic checks after the procedure should be based on the patient's overall status. Nursing staff should be familiar with potential LP complications, especially acute deteriorations in mental status (possible tonsillar herniation), sensory deficits, leg muscle weakness, and bladder and bowel incontinence (possible expanding spinal subdural hematoma). If no complications arise, activity may later be upgraded to *ad lib* as tolerated, with physician's approval.

Complications Although a wide range of complications has been reported, LP should generally be considered a safe procedure. The most common complication is "spinal headache" with an estimated incidence of 10% to 25%. This may be minimized by using a small gauge spinal needle and placing the patient in the prone position after the procedure. Another common complication is local bleeding, the "traumatic tap," which results from needle rupture of venous plexuses surrounding the spinal sack. Incidence may be as high as 20%. As long as no coagulation defect exists, the traumatic tap is clinically insignificant and rarely leads to spinal hematoma. Immediate painful paresthesias due to nerve root irritation is another common complication (≤13%), but usually resolves upon repositioning the spinal needle. Rare complications (<1%) include persistent pain or leg paresthesias; spinal epidural, subdural or subarachnoid hematomas; arachnoiditis from tracking in povidone-iodine on the needle; local infection (epidural or subdural empyema); transient cranial nerve palsies (especially CN VI when large volumes of CSF removed); rupture of nucleus pulposus; delayed formation of intraspinal epidermoid tumors (when stylet is not used); and vagal cardiac arrest. Note that the use of anticoagulants or presence of a coagulopathy significantly increases the risk of spinal hematoma formation (≤7%). Tonsillar herniation is an infrequent but potentially lethal complication of LP which occurs in patients with increased intracranial pressure. The exact incidence is not clear. In one series of patients with papilledema and increased intracranial pressure from a variety of causes, tonsillar herniation occurred after LP in <1.2% of cases. A particularly high risk group appears to be the patient with brain abscess or subdural empyema, with an estimated 10% to 20% incidence of LP-induced herniation and death. The herniation risk in patients with brain tumor is not known, although one study (which predated head CT scans) reported neurologic deterioration following LP in only 1 of 400 brain tumor cases. In general, due to incomplete data, a variety of clinical approaches have been adopted to avoid this fatal complication (see Additional Information).

Equipment Commercial LP trays are available. Common items include iodine, alcohol pads, sterile gloves and drapes, local anesthesia (usually 1% lidocaine) with appropriate needles and syringes, four sterile collecting tubes, 3-way stopcock with connecting tubing, manometer, and spinal needle with stylette. In general, a small bore spinal needle should be used, such as a 25-gauge, due to a lower incidence of spinal headache compared with a 20- or 22-gauge needle.

Technique In all cases, perform a careful fundoscopic and neurologic exam to rule out papilledema or a focal neurologic deficit. LP is then performed in one of two ways. In the standard method, patient is placed on a firm surface in the lateral recumbent position, curled with knees down in towards the chest and neck maximally flexed. The lumbar region should be close to the edge of the bed, with the plane of the back and shoulders as perpendicular to the bed as possible. Proper positioning is by far the most important step to ensure success and usually requires one or more assistants. The L4-L5 interspace is identified by drawing an imaginary line between the two posterior iliac crests. This area is cleaned, prepped, and draped. Skin and deeper subcutaneous tissues are infiltrated with lidocaine. The spinal needle with stylette is then passed into the L4-L5 interspace along the midline, bevel upwards. The needle is angled slightly cephalad along an imaginary line between the site of entry and the umbilicus. As the needle is advanced, the stylette should be frequently withdrawn and replaced every 1-2 mm in order to identify the first drop of CSF (and avoid overpenetration). Once CSF fluid is seen in the needle hub, the manometer is immediately attached to the needle via connecting tubing. Opening pressure should be measured promptly (do not wait more than 1 minute) with the patient's legs and hips extended. If the opening pressure is elevated (>180 mm CSF), try to eliminate factors that may cause false elevations. Instruct patient to straighten his legs, breathe evenly, avoid Valsalva maneuvers, and relax his abdominal muscles. If the opening pressure remains markedly elevated, close the 3-way stopcock, collect only the CSF already in the manometer, disconnect all the tubing, reinsert stylette, and consider neurosurgical consultation. If opening pressure is normal, CSF is then collected in tubes 1-4 in sequence. Manometer is reconnected afterwards and a closing pressure recorded. Stylette is replaced and both needle and stylette removed together. Pressure is held over the puncture site. An alternate approach may be needed in the patient whose vertebral landmarks are difficult to palpate. Initially, patient is placed in a seated position with neck and spine maximally flexed, arms resting on a bedside table. The L4-L5 interspace is identified as before and the remainder of the procedure is identical. This may be used with the obese patient or the patient with ankylosing spondylitis or severe scoliosis. Variations of this procedure have been described including: a lateral approach through the paravertebral muscles, the "hanging drop" technique used by anesthesiologists for identifying entry into the subdural space, and suboccipital puncture of the cisterna magna. These techniques are not necessary in the majority of cases.

Data Acquired Estimation of spinal fluid pressure as described. CSF fluid analytic tests are ordered based on clinical suspicion. Routine tests include cell count and CSF glucose level. Optional tests (not all samples): protein, VDRL, bacterial antigen detection battery, fungal antigens (such as *Cryptococcus*), culture (bacterial, fungal, viral, tuberculous), India ink preparation for *Cryptococcus*, infectious antibody titers, Gram stain, acid-fast bacilli smear, and cytology. Specialized tests include oligoclonal bands and myelin basic protein (for multiple sclerosis). The interested reader should refer to the *Laboratory Test Handbook* for further details.

Specimen 10-12 mL maximum removed from the adult. Smaller volumes are sufficient for most routine tests (confirm with laboratory).

Container Sterile tubes, numbered 1 to 4

Collection Tube 1: CSF protein and glucose; tube 2: cell count and differential; tube 3: Gram stain and cultures; tube 4: save for optional studies

Storage Instructions Specimen should be sent to laboratory immediately, preferably hand carried by physician.

Reference Range (Adults) opening pressure: 80-180 mm of CSF in lateral recumbent position, somewhat higher in sitting position. Respiratory variation of 5-10 mm normal. Clarity: normally very clear. CSF glucose: 60% to 70% of blood glucose. This estimation does not hold for blood glucose levels >300 mg/dL where CSF glucose empirically fails to rise. CSF protein: 15-55 mg/dL. CSF cell count and differential: 0-5 mononuclear white blood cells/mm^3 (lymphocytes and monocytes). The presence of even 1 or 2 polymorphonuclear cells (PMNs) is abnormal. Red blood cells: 0. Gram stain and culture: negative.

(Continued)

Lumbar Puncture *(Continued)*

Critical Values Interpretation of CSF findings have been reviewed in detail elsewhere. As a rule, interpretation of abnormal CSF values must always be made in close conjunction with the individual patient's clinical presentation. Considerable overlap exists among the "classic" CSF patterns which are meant to characterize different disease entities. No constellation of CSF findings is entirely specific for a given disease. LP has its greatest value in the diagnosis of bacterial meningitis. A classic CSF "purulent profile" has been described for bacterial meningitis, characterized by elevated WBCs in CSF (often >500/mm^3), predominance of PMN cells on CSF differential (>5/mm^3, presumed high sensitivity, low specificity), depressed CSF glucose levels (<40 mg/dL, 58% sensitivity), low CSF glucose to blood glucose ratio (<0.3, sensitivity 70%). Gram stain of CSF is positive in most cases (60% to 90%) as is the culture (80%). However, even acute bacterial meningitis may present in an atypical fashion, with predominant CSF lymphocytosis (10%), negative Gram stain, or, rarely, normal CSF leukocyte counts. In addition, the "purulent profile" may also be seen in noninfectious conditions such as subarachnoid hemorrhage (≤20% of cases). In contrast, CSF findings in viral meningitis typically reveal < 100 WBCs/mm^3, predominantly mononuclear cells on differential, normal glucose levels, normal or elevated protein levels, and negative Gram stain. However, some overlap exists with the profile for bacterial meningitis and 10% of patients with viral meningitis may have mostly PMNs, especially early in the course. Viral cultures are positive in <50% of the cases at best and may be as low as 5% for herpes simplex virus. Thus, viral cultures have a limited role and LP is most useful clinically in ruling out bacterial meningitis. Viral meningitis rarely presents with WBC counts in CSF >1000/mm^3, CSF protein levels >100 mg/dL, or glucose <40 mg/dL. Such patients should be treated as bacterial meningitis until proven otherwise. Fungal meningitis rarely presents a normal CSF picture but the abnormalities are very nonspecific (elevated protein, depressed glucose, and lymphocytic pleocytosis). For the diagnosis of cryptococcal meningitis, the cryptococcal antigen detection test is accurate very early on. Similar nonspecific CSF profiles are seen in tuberculous meningitis and sometimes may mimic bacterial meningitis. The acid-fast smear has notoriously low sensitivity (<25%) but acid-fast bacilli culture has a 90% sensitivity. Malignancy involving the meninges (primary or metastatic) often results in a CSF picture mimicking infectious meningitis. Typically, there is a CSF leukocytosis, elevated protein, and glucose may range from normal to markedly decreased. A completely normal CSF exam essentially rules out CNS malignancy. Sensitivity of CSF cytology varies considerably among studies and varies from 60% to 90%, independent of such factors as tumor type, metastases, or primary brain site. A significant 3% false-positive rate has been reported which has limited its role as a routine staging screen for patients with malignancy. LP may be useful in diagnosing selected cases of subarachnoid hemorrhage (SAH), especially those in which head CT scan is equivocal. Interpretation of LP results may be problematic since RBCs in CSF commonly arise from a traumatic tap. The presence of xanthochromia in CSF has traditionally been associated with SAH, but has also been found in nearly one-third of traumatic taps. Similarly, a decreased RBC count from tube 1-4 has usually meant a traumatic tap but studies have shown a specificity of only 56%. Because of these limitations and potential LP complications, head CT scan has supplanted LP as the major diagnostic test in cases of suspected SAH. The diagnosis of multiple sclerosis may be supported by special CSF studies including oligoclonal banding and myelin basic protein, but sensitivity and specificity are variable. Another demyelinating condition, Guillain-Barré syndrome, is characterized by an isolated CSF protein value >200 mg/dL, with the remainder of CSF parameters normal. The absence of an elevated protein level practically excludes Guillain-Barré. In general, LP is more useful in Guillain-Barré syndrome than multiple sclerosis.

Use Practitioners vary in their threshold for performing an LP. This procedure is clearly indicated in the following clinical settings:

- clinically suspected meningitis, either acute (where procedure is emergent), subacute, or chronic; also, suspected encephalitis or meningoencephalitis
- suspected central nervous system syphilis in clearly symptomatic patients (tertiary neurosyphilis)
- evaluation of potential CNS lymphoma, meningeal leukemia, and meningeal carcinomatosis
- staging of lymphoma, previously diagnosed from another site

- clinically suspected demyelinating disease such as multiple sclerosis or Guillain-Barré syndrome
- possible cases of subarachnoid hemorrhage

CSF findings in each of these indications is fairly distinctive and LP substantially aids in clinical diagnosis. In contrast, several diseases have abnormal, but nonspecific, CSF findings and LP has low sensitivity and specificity. These include brain abscess or subdural empyema, primary brain tumor, tumors metastatic to brain, subdural or epidural hematoma, connective tissue diseases with CNS involvement (such as CNS lupus or Sjögren's syndrome). Additional studies (such as head CT scan) are necessary to confirm each of these conditions. LP should usually be delayed in favor of other more accurate and less invasive tests. Controversial indications for LP include suspected spinal epidural abscess, evaluation of the acute stroke to identify those which are hemorrhagic, evaluation of dementia (arguably to exclude neurosyphilis or chronic meningitis), evaluation of the asymptomatic patient with a positive serologic test for syphilis (to exclude asymptomatic neurosyphilis).

Limitations When a "traumatic tap" occurs (iatrogenic trauma), white blood cells may be passively transferred to the CSF. In general, for every 700 RBCs found in the CSF, 1 WBC is also expected (applies to the traumatic tap **only**).

Contraindications Procedure is contraindicated if there is a local infection at the proposed site of needle entry due to the potential for infectious seeding of meninges (several literature case reports). The presence of a severe bleeding diathesis is a relative contraindication to LP and an increased risk of spinal subdural hematoma has been demonstrated. Elevated intracranial pressure is an absolute contraindication to LP because of the risk of uncal herniation (see Complications). The presence of septicemia is **not** considered a contraindication. Retrospective studies have failed to show an increased incidence of meningitis in septic patients undergoing LP compared with septic patients who do not undergo the procedure.

Additional Information Because of the risk of tonsillar herniation following LP, controversy exists concerning the routine use of head CT scan prior to LP. Data is incomplete and several clinical approaches are available. The conservative approach is to always perform a head CT prior to LP regardless of neurologic findings, so as never to overlook an intracranial mass lesion. Other clinicians follow a more flexible approach and argue that tonsillar herniation only occurs with demonstrable papilledema or focal neurologic deficits; thus, when both of these physical signs are absent LP may be safely performed without prior head CT. A middle ground approach has been advocated where head CT scan is performed prior to LP in the following situations: papilledema, focal neurologic deficits, recent history of sinusitis or otitis media, severe and progressive headache, and deterioration of mental status. In our institution, we generally adopt the conservative approach (acute meningitis is treated empirically prior to CT and LP).

Selected Readings

Brocker RJ, "Technique to Avoid Spinal Tap Headache," *JAMA*, 1958, 68:261-3.

Chun CH, Johnson JD, Hofstetter M, et al, "Brain Abscess: A Study of 45 Consecutive Cases," *Medicine (Baltimore)*, 1986, 65(6):415-31.

Dougherty JM and Roth RM, "Cerebral Spinal Fluid," *Emerg Med Clin North Am*, 1986, 4(2):281-97.

Eng RH and Seligman SJ, "Lumbar Puncture-Induced Meningitis," *JAMA*, 1981, 245(14):1456-9.

Fishman RA, *Cerebrospinal Fluid in Diseases of the Nervous System*, Philadelphia, PA: WB Saunders Co, 1980.

Keroack MA, "The Patient With Suspected Meningitis," *Emerg Med Clin North Am*, 1987, 5(4):807-26.

Korein J, Cravisto H, and Leicach M, "Re-evaluation of Lumbar Puncture: A Study of 129 Patients With Papilledema or Intracranial Hypertension," *Neurology*, 1959, 9:290-7.

Marton KI and Gean AD, "The Spinal Tap: A New Look at an Old Test," *Ann Intern Med*, 1986, 104(6):840-8.

Reik L, "Disorders That Mimic CNS Infections," *Neurol Clin*, 1986, 4(1):223-48.

Simon R and Brenner B, "Neurosurgical Procedures," *Emergency Medicine*, Chapter 149, Baltimore, MD: Williams & Wilkins, 1982, 156-67.

Lumbar Puncture Analysis *see* Cerebrospinal Fluid Analysis
on page 288

Lupus Band Test *see* Skin Biopsy, Immunofluorescence
on page 446

Lyme Arthritis Serology *see* Lyme Disease Serology
on next page

Lyme Borreliosis Antibody by Western Blot *see* Lyme Disease
   Serology by Western Blot *on this page*

Lyme Disease Immunoblot *see* Lyme Disease Serology by Western
   Blot *on this page*

Lyme Disease Serology
Related Information
   Lyme Disease Serology by Western Blot *on this page*
Synonyms Borreliosis Serology; Lyme Arthritis Serology
Specimen Serum or cerebrospinal fluid
Container Red top tube
Reference Range Values vary among laboratories
Use Laboratory confirmation of Lyme disease
Limitations Some cases are seronegative; there are cross reactions including
   those with antibodies to EB virus, *Rickettsia*, and syphilis. There is significant
   inter- and intralaboratory variation in this assay which highlights limitations of
   currently available testing. Even the Western blot is not considered a definitive
   assay. Consequently serologic evidence should not be the sole criterion for a
   diagnosis of Lyme disease. Serology is a confirmation test and should only
   confirm a clinical diagnosis.
Methodology Enzyme immunoassay (EIA), enzyme-linked immunosorbent
   assay (ELISA), indirect immunofluorescent antibody (IFA), Western blot
Additional Information Lyme disease is a multisystem disorder. A characteristic rash and arthritis are the hallmark symptoms. It is widespread in the US
   and is caused by *Borrelia burgdorferi*, a spirochete transmitted by the bite of
   the tick *Ixodes dammini*. The disease has protean manifestations, can become
   chronic, and responds to antibiotics; prompt proper diagnosis is therefore important.

   Assay is available for IgG and IgM antibody in both serum and CSF. In early
   disease a negative assay does not exclude the diagnosis because assay sensitivity is only 40% to 60%. Antibody response may be blunted by antibiotics.
   All patients with chronic disease will have positive assays.

   Recent studies using recombinant outer surface protein A and B and flagellin
   hold out promise for better serologic testing in the near future.

   Patients may harbor *B. burgdorferi* asymptomatically and have positive serology. Some individuals may have symptoms of other illnesses incorrectly attributed to Lyme disease and be given inappropriate and ineffective treatment.

   Antibodies against Lyme disease antigens can interfere with the ANA test.
Selected Readings
   Barbour AG, "The Diagnosis of Lyme Disease: Rewards and Perils," *Ann Intern Med*, 1989,
      110(7):501-2.
   Duffey PS and Salugsugan J, "Serodiagnosis of Lyme Borreliosis," *Clin Microbiol Newslett*,
      1993, 15(11):81-5.
   Fikrig E, Huguenel ED, Berland R, et al, "Serological Diagnosis of Lyme Disease Using Re-
      combinant Outer Surface Proteins A and B and Flagellin," *J Infect Dis*, 1992,
      165(6):1127-32.
   Gill JS and Johnson RC, "Immunologic Methods for the Diagnosis of Infections by *Borrelia
      burgdorferi* (Lyme Disease)," *Manual of Clinical Laboratory Immunology*, 4th ed, Rose
      NR, de Macario EC, Fahey JL, et al, eds, Washington, DC: American Society for Microbi-
      ology, 1992, 452-8.
   Mitchell PD, "Lyme Borreliosis: A Persisting Diagnostic Dilemma," *Clin Microbiol Newslett*,
      1993, 15(8):57-9.
   Steere AC, "Lyme Disease," *N Engl J Med*, 1989, 321(9):586-96.

Lyme Disease Serology by Western Blot
Related Information
   Lyme Disease Serology *on this page*
   Nitrite, Urine *on page 414*
Synonyms Borreliosis Serology; Lyme Disease Immunoblot
Applies To Lyme Borreliosis Antibody by Western Blot
Test Includes Confirmation Lyme disease antibody test
Specimen Serum
Container Red top tube
Storage Instructions Separate and freeze serum.
Causes for Rejection Inadequate labeling, excessive hemolysis, chylous
   serum

Reference Range Normal: number of bands is defined by individual laboratory

Use Confirm positive screening tests for Lyme disease

Limitations The Western blot assay is not sensitive for detecting early Lyme disease. Its utility is for confirming stage 2 and stage 3 Lyme disease and to identify false-positive results in patients suspected of late Lyme disease. This test is performed by reference laboratories. Each laboratory designates which bands are most significant. Significant interlaboratory variation exists.

Contraindications Negative screening test for Lyme disease

Methodology Western blot technique utilizing a mixture of proteins (antigens) that are extracted from *Borrelia burgdorferi* and separated by SDS-PAGE; subsequent reaction of serum with bands/proteins.

Selected Readings

Duffey PS and Salugsugan J, "Serodiagnosis of Lyme Borreliosis," *Clin Microbiol Newslett*, 1993, 15(11):81-5.

Gill JS and Johnson RC, "Immunologic Methods for the Diagnosis of Infections by *Borrelia burgdorferi* (Lyme Disease)," *Manual of Clinical Laboratory Immunology*, 4th ed, Rose NR, de Macario EC, Fahey JL, et al, eds, Washington, DC: American Society for Microbiology, 1992, 452-8.

Mitchell PD, "Lyme Borreliosis: A Persisting Diagnostic Dilemma," *Clin Microbiol Newslett*, 1993, 15(8):57-9.

Lymph Node Biopsy

Applies To Cell Sorting Fluorescence Activation

Test Includes Microscopic examination of frozen sections, paraffin and/or plastic sections, and often, touch preparations. Immunoperoxidase studies for immunoglobulin heavy and light chains are best done on snap frozen cryostat sections rather than paraffin sections.

Special Instructions The specimen should not be placed in fixative if it can be delivered immediately to the laboratory. Diagnostic difficulties in diseases of lymph nodes are compounded by poor fixation and improper handling. Lymph node biopsies should be immediately delivered to the Histology Laboratory uncut and in a small sterile jar or Petri dish. Requests for all examinations including Microbiology should accompany the specimen. All such specimens should be brought to the immediate attention of a pathologist. Bone marrow, blood studies, and other clinical information are commonly needed for appropriate work-up.

Specimen Lymph node or other tissues suspected of harboring lymphoma, ideally submitted fresh within minutes of the biopsy

Container Sterile saline moistened sponge or Petri dish

Collection Optimal selection of site of biopsy and the lymph nodes to be biopsied enhance ultimate correct diagnosis. Supraclavicular and cervical biopsies will most likely provide diagnostic specimens. The most accessible lymph nodes are not always the best choice. The whole, intact lymph node with its capsule, and adjacent fat or other tissue provides an optimal specimen.

The proper initial triage of the tissue is of utmost importance in establishing the correct diagnosis. Usually, sufficient tissue must be available for both permanent sections and for immunophenotypic analysis of frozen sections. Tissues allocated for immunotypic studies are also suitable for genotypic studies if necessary. Routine histopathologic study remains the gold standard in diagnostic hematopathology and optimal histology begins with proper fixation. Fine nuclear detail is best achieved using B5, zinc formalin, or a Zenker's-like fixative. These fixatives are also best for cell marker analysis in paraffin section. An ever expanding selection of antibodies is useful for establishing lineage of hematopoietic cells in paraffin section (see table). However, phenotypic indicators of clonal proliferation are most reliably established in frozen section. As morphologic detail in frozen sections is intrinsically limited, every precaution to minimize artifacts must be taken. Snap freezing small, thin slices of tissue using liquid nitrogen cooled isopentane yields tissues free of freezing artifacts. Special attention to fine details of cryostat sectioning is necessary to yield interpretable results. If a frozen section evaluation is necessary to initiate a "lymphoma protocol," the tissues used for this rapid diagnosis are often unsuitable for immunophenotypic analysis. If the size of biopsy is limiting, a routine frozen section evaluation should be discouraged as freezing distorts lymphoid tissue and may result in errors in final interpretation.

If tissues are to be sent to a reference laboratory for immunotyping, three basic options are available. First, the tissues may be snap frozen and stored at -70°C or colder until such time as immunotyping is considered necessary. If facilities for proper snap freezing and storage are not available, this option should be

(Continued)

Lymphocyte Markers Useful in Paraffin Section*

	LCA CD45	EMA	LN-2 CD71w	L26 CD20	UCHL-1 CD45RO	CD3	Leu-M1 CD15	Mono Ig's	Lysozyme	KP1 CD68	CAE
Non-Hodgkin's lymphoma B-cell lymphomas†	+	–	+	+	–	–	–	+	–	–	–
T-cell lymphomas§	+	–/+	–	–	+	+	–/+	–	–	–	–
Hodgkin's disease (NS, MC, LD)	–	+/–	+	–	–	–	+	–	–	–	–
Hodgkin's disease, LP	+	+/–	+	+	–	–	–	–	–	–	–
Myeloma/plasmacytoma	–/+	–/+	–	–	–	–	–	+	–	–	–
Granulocytic sarcoma#	+/–	–	–/+	–	–	–	+/–	–	+	+	+
True histiocytic lymphoma#	+/–	–/+	–/+	–	–	–	–	–	+	+	–

Abbreviations: LCA: leukocyte common antigen; EMA: epithelial membrane antigen; Mono Ig's: monoclonal immunoglobulins; CAE: chloroacetate esterase (an enzyme cytochemical stain rather than an immunostain); Hodgkin's disease (NS, MC, LD): nodular sclerosing, mixed cellularity, and lymphocyte depleted subtypes, respectively; Hodgkin's disease, LP: lymphocyte predominate subtype.
Designated reactions: +: characteristically positive; +/–: characteristically positive but may be negative; –/+: characteristically negative but may be positive; –: characteristically negative.

Footnotes:
*Most lymphomas characteristically contain neoplastic and non-neoplastic lymphoid elements in variable proportions. Caution must be exercised in determining the phenotype of the neoplastic cells.
†Monoclonal immunoglobulins are best detected in frozen section. Large cell lymphomas and those with plasmacytic differentiation are more likely to display a convincing staining in paraffin section than other subtypes.
§T-cell clonal proliferation cannot be determined in paraffin section alone. The best phenotypic expression of clonal proliferation is aberrant expression of pan T-cell antigens which can be detected only by frozen section immunohistology, by flow cytometry using cell suspensions, or by gene rearrangement.
#Enzyme cytochemical profile using touch preparations is extremely useful in establishing these diagnoses.

Lymph Node Biopsy *(Continued)*

discouraged. Second, the tissues may be delivered in carrier media or saline soaked gauze immediately by courier to the reference laboratory, where experienced personnel will process the tissue. Third, tissues may be placed in a carrier media which may circumvent the need for immediate action for 24 hours without significantly compromising the immunologic studies.

Storage Instructions Snap frozen tissues should be maintained at -70°C or colder until immunophenotypic analysis can be performed. If the frozen tissues are to be transported to a reference laboratory, they should be shipped on dry ice, using an overnight courier if necessary. Tissues placed in carrier media should be maintained on wet ice or at room temperature and packaged in insulated containers to avoid large fluctuations in temperature during transit.

Causes for Rejection Desiccated specimen, formalin exposure, excessive freezing artifact

Use Diagnosis of various lymphadenopathies, including cat scratch disease, malignant lymphoma, and metastatic neoplasia

Limitations Formalin-fixed tissue cannot be used for culture or imprints and is suboptimal for electron microscopy.

Methodology Quality basic histology is of paramount importance in the evaluation of the lymph node biopsy. Interpretive errors are often due to deficient basic histology. Touch preparations should always be obtained and are often times invaluable for final diagnosis. Representative tissues should be allocated for immunotyping, taking the necessary precautions to minimize morphologic artifacts while maintaining maximal antigenicity. Immunoperoxidase stains on paraffin or frozen sections are accomplished according to the general procedures outlined in the test listing Immunoperoxidase Procedures. Immunologic markers on touch preparations and bone marrow smears are often best demonstrated by using an alkaline phosphatase enzyme detection system to minimize background staining. Cultures for infectious agents are sometimes indispensable.

Additional Information Correlation with peripheral blood, bone marrow, and other clinical laboratory studies is often desirable and sometimes mandatory. Flow cytometry on dissociated tissues or body fluids is often utilized instead of immunohistology for cell marker analysis. This methodology offers a more quantitative approach to cell markers but only at the critical expense of destroying the immunoarchitecture of tissues. In general, immunohistology provides the best approach for typing tissues while flow cytometry is best suited for blood, bone marrow, and other body fluids. Properly acquired and frozen tissue is suitable for gene probe analysis (gene rearrangement studies), which may be necessary to document B- or T-cell clonal proliferation in rare cases.

Selected Readings

Jaffe ES, "Surgical Pathology of the Lymph Nodes and Related Organs," *Major Problems in Pathology*, Vol 16, Philadelphia, PA: WB Saunders Co, 1985.

Knowles DM. *Neoplastic Hematopathology*, Baltimore, MD: Williams & Wilkins, 1992.

Wright DH and Isaacson PG, *Biopsy Pathology of the Lymphoreticular System*, Baltimore, MD: Williams & Wilkins, 1983.

Lymph Node Culture *see* Epstein-Barr Virus Culture
on page 332

Lymphocyte Culture *see* Epstein-Barr Virus Culture
on page 332

Lymphogranuloma Venereum Culture *see* Chlamydia Culture
on page 294

Magnetic Resonance Scan, Brain

Applies To Magnetic Resonance Scan, Head

Patient Preparation Inpatient: Patient must be able to lie quietly while the scan is performed. The patient should be screened for metallic devices by nursing personnel. (See Contraindications.) This includes metal introduced into the patient either surgically or by trauma. All metallic objects must be removed from the patient including jewelry or any other metal objects which may be in the patient's bedding. Please remove dentures or other dental appliances. I.V.s which contain no metal are fine, but infusion pumps must be removed. Oxygen tanks and metallic backboards may come with the patient but will be removed prior to the patient entering the magnet room. Oxygen may be provided in the magnet room. Trauma, ICU, or CCU patients should be accompanied by a nurse. If the patient is restless, combative, or claustrophobic, proper sedation

(Continued)

Magnetic Resonance Scan, Brain *(Continued)*

may be administered on the floor prior to the MRI, or at the MRI Center. Consult the MRI radiologists with questions on proper sedation. Outpatient: The patient should be screened for metallic devices. (See Contraindications.) If a question exists as to the patient's suitability for MRI, the MRI radiologist will assist you with your questions. If the patient is claustrophobic, oral or parenteral sedation may be necessary. If so, the patient should be accompanied by another adult to provide transportation home after the examination.

Aftercare If the patient received an MRI contrast agent (Magnevist®) and develops a delayed hypersensitivity reaction (ie, hives or shortness of breath), the referring physician or MRI radiologist should be contacted immediately.

Data Acquired Digital information with film reproduction

Use To diagnose intracranial abnormalities including tumors, ischemia, infection, multiple sclerosis or any abnormalities relating to the brain or calvarium. MRI is an excellent modality for assessment of congenital brain abnormalities or relating to the status of brain maturation in the pediatric population.

Limitations Generally, the greatest limitation of magnetic resonance imaging results from the patient's fear of the procedure. The patient must remain quiet and still for several scans, each lasting from several minutes to 10 minutes in length. Total examination time is usually 30-45 minutes and occasionally up to 1 hour. If the patient is restless during the examination, motion artifacts will be present on the images limiting their diagnostic value. If the patient is claustrophobic, mild oral sedation or occasionally parenteral sedation may be needed. Also the patient can be accompanied by a family member or friend during the examination which helps calm the patient's anxiety in many cases. Patients requiring life support equipment such as ventilators require special preparation. Please refer to Contraindications for further causes for rejection.

Contraindications Patients weighing more than 300 lb and patients unable to squeeze into the magnet cannot undergo MRI. An absolute contraindication for MRI is a cardiac pacemaker. Relative contraindications to magnetic resonance imaging include intracranial aneurysm clips, cochlear implants, insulin infusion and chemotherapy pumps, neurocutaneous stimulators and prosthetic heart valves, depending on date of manufacture and metallurgical composition. Please consult MRI physician if questions arise. Patients who have metallic foreign bodies within the eye or who have undergone recent surgery within the last 6 weeks requiring placement of a vascular surgical clip, should also not undergo MRI. The safety of MRI in pregnant patients has not been determined. In such cases, prior consultation with the MRI physician is required. Generally, patients who have undergone recent surgery not requiring vascular clips or who have had coronary artery bypass surgery in the past may undergo MRI. Patients who have shrapnel wounds or orthopedic prostheses can generally safely undergo MRI unless the metallic device is in the anatomic region to be scanned which results in degradation of the images. Patients with surgically implanted intravascular vena cava filters to prevent pulmonary embolism can usually be scanned if the device has been in place for at least 6 weeks. Patients requiring life support equipment including ventilators require special preparation. Please contact MRI physician ahead of time. Central venous lines, Swan-Ganz catheters, and nasogastric (NG) tubes usually present no problems. If the patient is positive when screened for metallic devices and you are uncertain of their significance, the MRI radiologist will provide additional information to assist you.

Methodology Unlike most conventional radiologic procedures, magnetic resonance imaging does not utilize ionizing radiation, but relies upon radio frequency or radio signals induced within the patient by the magnetic field to obtain images. There are no known biologic effects secondary to the magnetic fields currently used in clinical MRI. Prior to the scan, the patient will be asked to remove all metallic objects from their person, including loose change, hair pins, earrings, belts, etc. This is for safety reasons as the strong magnetic field could result in these and any other metal objects becoming projectiles resulting in injury to the patient or MRI personnel. Also the patient should not carry a purse or wallet into the magnetic room, as the magnetic field can permanently erase bank cards or credit cards. The magnet is open on both ends and music can be played for the patient if desired. Fresh air is constantly circulated through the magnet room and the patient is continually monitored by the MRI technologist. An intercom system is provided for communication between the patient and the technologist. For MRI of the brain, a special coil surrounds, but does not touch the patient's head. The patient will be asked to remain very still while scans are being obtained. In certain cases, an MRI contrast agent, Gado-

LABORATORY DIAGNOSIS

pentetate Dimeglumine (Magnevist®) may be necessary to increase the diagnostic accuracy of the MRI examination. This is administered intravenously, via an antecubital vein in a small volume (<20 mL). This contrast agent may be used in patients who are allergic to conventional iodinated contrast agents such as is used in IVPs or CT examination without difficulty. There are very few contraindications to its use. (See Contraindications.)

Additional Information In some cases, an MRI contrast agent (Magnevist®) may be needed to increase the diagnostic accuracy of the MRI. This contrast agent can be administered to patients with a previous history of allergies to conventional iodinated x-ray agents as it contains no iodine. Contraindications to its use include previous allergy to the contrast agent itself, renal failure, certain types of anemia, and Wilson's disease. The contrast agent is generally very safe and increases the diagnostic efficacy of the MRI.

Selected Readings
Topics in Magnetic Resonance Imaging, Rockville, MD: Aspen Publishers, Inc, 1989.

Magnetic Resonance Scan, Head *see* Magnetic Resonance Scan, Brain *on page 397*

Malarial Parasites *see* Peripheral Blood Smear, Thick and Thin *on page 429*

Malaria Smear *see* Peripheral Blood Smear, Thick and Thin *on page 429*

Mantoux Test *see* Tuberculin Skin Testing, Intracutaneous *on page 463*

Maximum Bactericidal Dilution *see* Serum Bactericidal Test *on page 441*

Mazzini *replaced by* RPR *on page 438*

MBD *see* Serum Bactericidal Test *on page 441*

Measles Antibody

Test Includes IgG and IgM levels
Specimen Serum or cerebrospinal fluid
Container Red top tube
Reference Range Less than fourfold rise in titer; absent or stable IgM titer; HI >1:10, NT >1:20 indicates immunity. Consult laboratory for more specific (custom) information.
Use Differential diagnosis of viral exanthemas, particularly in pregnant women; diagnosis of subacute sclerosing panencephalitis; document adequacy of measles immunization
Limitations Antibody sometimes present in multiple sclerosis
Methodology Hemagglutination inhibition, viral neutralization, enzyme-linked immunosorbent assay
Additional Information Measles (rubeola) is caused by a paramyxovirus. Despite vaccination programs, there have been several recent local epidemics. Revaccination appears to be of greater value at 11-12 years of age than at 4-6 years of age. Serologic study can be useful in establishing that an individual has effective immunity subsequent to vaccination. In many individuals **detectable** immunity does not persist.

In acute illness, hemagglutinating and neutralizing antibody peak two weeks after the rash appears. It is necessary to demonstrate rising titers over 2 weeks, or identify IgM antibody.

Very high serum titers in the absence of acute illness and/or high CSF titers are seen in subacute sclerosing panencephalitis.

Selected Readings
Markowitz LE, Albrecht P, Orenstein WA, et al, "Persistence of Measles Antibody After Revaccination," *J Infect Dis*, 1992, 166(1):205-8.
Wittler RR, Veit BC, McIntyre S, et al, "Measles Revaccination Response in a School-Age Population," *Pediatrics*, 1991, 88(5):1024-30.

Measles Culture, 3-Day *see* Rubella Virus Culture *on page 440*

Measles Virus, Direct Detection *see* Virus, Direct Detection by Fluorescent Antibody *on page 480*

MHA-TP

Synonyms Microhemagglutination, *Treponema pallidum*; Serologic Test for Syphilis
Applies To Syphilis Serology
(Continued)

399

MHA-TP *(Continued)*

Patient Preparation Patient should be fasting if possible

Specimen Serum

Container Red top tube

Storage Instructions Refrigerate

Reference Range Less than 1:160

Use Confirmatory serologic test for syphilis

Limitations Moderate sensitivity in early (primary) stages of syphilis. False-positives may occur in systemic lupus, infectious mononucleosis, and lepromatous leprosy.

Methodology Hemagglutination

Additional Information This is a *Treponema*-specific test and should not be used as a screening test. It is as sensitive and specific as FTA-ABS in all stages of syphilis except primary, in which it is less sensitive (but more sensitive than the VDRL). It will be positive with treponemal infections other than syphilis (bejel, pinta, yaws). Like FTA-ABS, MHA-TP once positive remains so, and cannot be used to judge effect of treatment. The test is not applicable to CSF.

Selected Readings

Hart G, "Syphilis Tests in Diagnostic and Therapeutic Decision Making," *Ann Intern Med*, 1986, 104(3):368-76.

Romanowski B, Sutherland R, Fick GH, et al, "Serologic Response to Treatment of Infectious Syphilis," *Ann Intern Med*, 1991, 114(12):1005-9.

MIC *see* Antimicrobial Susceptibility Testing, Aerobic and Facultatively Anaerobic Organisms *on page 259*

MIC, Anaerobic Bacteria *see* Antimicrobial Susceptibility Testing, Anaerobic Bacteria *on page 260*

Microfilariae, Peripheral Blood Preparation

Related Information

Peripheral Blood Smear, Thick and Thin *on page 429*

Synonyms Blood Smear for Trypanosomal/Filarial Parasites; Filariasis Peripheral Blood Preparation; Helminths, Blood Preparation; Trypanosomiasis Peripheral Blood Preparation

Applies To Filarial Infestation; Hemoflagellates; Peripheral Blood Preparation

Test Includes Examination of both thick and thin smears, wet preparation

Special Instructions If patient has traveled to an endemic area, the date of travel, the area, and the parasite suspected should be specified.

Specimen Fresh blood fingerstick

Container Slides

Collection Recommended procedure is for specimen to be obtained as follows: *Loa loa*, 10 AM – 2 PM; *Mausonella* and *Onchocerca*, anytime; *Wuchereria* and *Brugia*, 10 PM – 4 AM

Causes for Rejection Specimen clotted

Reference Range No parasites identified

Use Diagnose trypanosomiasis or microfilariasis, or parasitic infestation of blood

Limitations One negative result does not rule out the possibility of parasitic infestation. Since some species of blood parasites can be found during the day and others are nocturnal, both day and night specimens enhance identification. Most filariae generate microfilariae which can be found in peripheral blood, but *Onchocerca volvulus* and *Dipetalonema streptocerca* give rise to microfilariae which do not circulate.

Methodology Fresh wet blood film, with a coverslip, in which motile microfilariae cause agitation of adjacent red cells. Stained smears are used as well.

Additional Information Biopsy of skin and subcutaneous mass is used in diagnosis of *D. streptocerca* and *O. volvulus*. Differential diagnosis of species of circulating microfilariae requires distinction between the presence or absence of a sheath, the pattern of nuclei in the tail and sometimes the history of geographic exposure and time of sampling.

Microhemagglutination, *Treponema pallidum* *see* MHA-TP *on previous page*

Microsporidia Diagnostic Procedures

Test Includes Examination of stool, fluid, wash, or biopsy for microsporidia (*Enterocytozoon*, *Encephalitozoon*, *Nosema*, *Septata*, *Pleistophora*, and others)

Special Instructions Even though the test is relatively simple to perform, very few laboratories offer this test at this time because demand for the test is relatively low. The laboratory must be notified that microsporidia are suspected. Consult laboratory before ordering test for advice on availability of test and instructions on specimen collection.

Specimen Many different types of specimens are appropriate. The specimen must be obtained from a mucosal surface or an epithelial-lined surface (the sites of microsporidia replication) that represents the probable site of infection. In general, there are two types of specimens: those for exfoliative cytology examination and those for histological examination. Both types of specimens often are very productive. The specimen that should be collected depends on the suspected type of infection.

- Intestinal infection: direct stool smear, biliary tract biopsy, small intestine wash, small intestine mucosal biopsy
- Ocular infection: corneal scraping or swab
- Respiratory infection: sputum, BAL, transbronchial biopsy, bronchial brushing, mucosal biopsy
- Sino-nasal infection: scraping, smear, mucosal biopsy
- Urinary tract infection: concentrated urine, mucosal biopsy

Container Clean, screw-cap container appropriate for the particular specimen

Collection Appropriate for the site. Transport specimen to the laboratory as soon as possible. Biopsies should be fixed in formalin as soon as possible.

Use A part of the differential diagnostic work-up of diarrhea and other microsporidia-associated diseases in immunocompromised patients, particularly AIDS patients ; establish the diagnosis of microsporidiosis. Microsporidia have been demonstrated in immunocompetent persons.

Limitations Detection of microsporidia is entirely dependent on the adequacy of the specimen, staining and preparation of the specimen, and experience of the person who examines the specimen.

Methodology Microsporidia do not stain well with either hematoxylin, eosin, or the Papanicolaou stains. There are several good stains for microsporidia; however, not all of these stains stain the five major species of microsporidia. Microsporidia in paraffin-embedded tissues stain well with a tissue Gram stain (Brown and Hoop stain; Brown and Brenn stain). Microsporidia in plastic-embedded tissues stain well with toluidine blue and with methylene blue-azure II-basic fuchsin. Microsporidia in cytologic centrifugation, smears, and scrapings preparations usually stain well with Gram stain for specimens with little or no bacterial contamination. In these preparations, most microsporidia and bacteria are dark purple; some microsporidia are gram-negative or gram-variable. Weber's modified trichrome (chromotroph-based) stain works well with specimens with bacterial contamination; microsporidia are magenta-pink and the background (including bacteria) is blue-green. Some laboratories use Giemsa stain to stain stool smears and body fluids. Most stains cause microsporidia to appear as extremely fat bacteria which have a uniform oval shape, do not show budding, contain polar densities, and have a central clear band or area. The identification of microsporidia to species is very important in the selection of treatment. Speciation is accomplished most commonly by electron microscopy and, where available, molecular biology techniques. Cross reactions between the antibodies to the different types of microsporidia prevent serology from being clinically useful. Immunofluorescence staining techniques which include labeled antibody to specific microsporidia appear to work well in detecting microsporidia in clinical specimens and to be able to differentiate infections due to certain microsporidia. Some microsporidia have been cultured *in vitro*, but routine culture for microsporidia is not yet practical.

Selected Readings

Garcia LS, Shimuzu RY, and Brucker DA, "Detection of Microsporidial Spores in Fecal Specimens From Patients Diagnosed With Cryptosporidiosis," *J Clin Microbiol*, 1994, 32:1739-41.

Shadduck JA and Greely E, "Microsporidia and Human Infections," *Clin Microbiol Rev*, 1989, 2:158-65.

Sun T, "Microsporidiosis in the Acquired Immunodeficiency Syndrome," *Infect Dis Newslett*, 1993, 12:20-2.

Weber R and Bryan RT, "Microsporidial Infections in Immunodeficient and Immunocompetent Patients," *Clin Infect Dis*, 1994, 19:517-21.

Weber R, Bryan RT, Owen RL, et al, "Improved Light-Microscopical Detection of Microsporidia Spores in Stool and Duodenal Aspirates. The Enteric Opportunistic Infections Working Group," *N Engl J Med*, 1992, 326(3):161-6.

MicroTrak® *see* Chlamydia trachomatis DFA Test *on page 298*

Midstream Urine Culture *see* Urine Culture, Clean Catch *on page 470*

Minimum Inhibitory Concentration Susceptibility Test *see* Antimicrobial Susceptibility Testing, Aerobic and Facultatively Anaerobic Organisms *on page 259*

Mite Identification *see* Arthropod Identification *on page 268*

M-Mode Echo *see* Echocardiography, M-Mode *on page 324*

Monospot™ Test *see* Infectious Mononucleosis Serology *on page 374*

Monosticon® Dri-Dot® Test *see* Infectious Mononucleosis Serology *on page 374*

Mono Test *see* Infectious Mononucleosis Serology *on page 374*

M. pneumoniae Titer *see* Mycoplasma Serology *on page 410*

Mumps Serology
Related Information
Mumps Virus Culture *on this page*

Specimen Serum

Container Red top tube

Collection Acute and convalescent sera drawn 10-14 days apart are required.

Reference Range A fourfold or greater increase in titer is indicative of recent mumps infection in the complement fixation test; a positive IgM immunofluorescent test is indicative of infection; an increasing hemagglutination inhibition titer indicates mumps **or parainfluenza virus** infection; a positive neutralization test indicates **immunity** to mumps.

Use Support for the diagnosis of mumps virus infection; document previous exposure to mumps virus; document immunity

Limitations Several test systems are not specific for mumps

Methodology Complement fixation (CF), enzyme-linked immunosorbent assay (ELISA), immunofluorescence, hemagglutination inhibition (HAI), hemolysis-in-gel, virus neutralization

Additional Information Mumps is caused by a paramyxovirus. Serologic study may be undertaken to confirm a diagnosis in acute disease or to demonstrate established immunity. For diagnosis in an acute illness measuring the ratio of IgG to IgM antibody is simplest and fastest. Immunity depends on neutralizing antibody, which must be demonstrated in cell culture.

Selected Readings
Drew WL, "Diagnostic Virology," *Clin Lab Med*, 1987, 7(4):721-40.

Ukkonen P, Väisänen O, and Penttinen K, "Enzyme-Linked Immunosorbent Assay for Mumps and Parainfluenza Type 1 Immunoglobulin G and Immunoglobulin M Antibodies," *J Clin Microbiol*, 1980, 11(4):319-23.

Mumps Virus Culture
Related Information
Mumps Serology *on this page*

Test Includes Concurrent culture for other viruses

Specimen Saliva, urine, cerebrospinal fluid

Container Sterile container for urine and CSF; tube with cold viral transport medium for swabs

Sampling Time At or within 5 days of the onset of illness

Collection It is desirable to collect specimens as early in the disease as possible. Saliva within 2 days of onset; spinal fluid of patients with meningoencephalitis within 6 days after onset. Virus is also excreted in urine for as long as 14 days.

In young patients, saliva is collected by a suitable suction device or by swabbing, especially the area around the orifices of Stensen's duct. The swabs must immediately be placed into cold viral transport medium. Spinal fluid is obtained in the usual manner and put into a sterile tube. For urine specimens, preferably the first voided morning urine is collected in a sterile container. All specimens must immediately be placed on ice and sent to the laboratory.

Storage Instructions Specimens should be delivered immediately on ice to the laboratory.

Causes for Rejection Dry specimen, specimen not refrigerated during transport, specimen fixed in formalin, unlabeled specimen

Turnaround Time Variable (5-14 days) and depends on methods used and amount of virus in the specimen

Reference Range No virus isolated

Use Aid in the diagnosis of disease caused by mumps virus

Methodology Inoculation of specimen into cell cultures, incubation, observation of characteristic cytopathic effect, and identification by methods such as hemadsorption and fluorescent monoclonal antibodies

Additional Information Although virus isolation is the most certain means for establishing the laboratory diagnosis, serologic methods are also useful and technically easier. Demonstration of IgM antibodies in acute serum is diagnostic of primary infection.

Selected Readings

Swierkosz EM, "Mumps Virus," *Manual of Clinical Microbiology*, 5th ed, Balows A, Hausler WJ Jr, Herrmann KL, et al, eds, Washington, DC: American Society for Microbiology, 1991, 912-7.

Tolpin MD and Schauf V, "Mumps Virus," *Textbook of Human Virology*, Belshe RB, ed, Littleton, MA: PSG Publishing Co, 1984, 311-31.

Mumps Virus, Direct Detection *see* Virus, Direct Detection by Fluorescent Antibody *on page 480*

Muscle Biopsy

Synonyms Skeletal Muscle Biopsy

Test Includes Examination of muscle biopsy by histopathology. The procedure frequently includes enzyme histochemistry and electron microscopy.

Abstract Diagnosis and classification of muscle disease.

Patient Preparation Clinical data is required and should include the patient's age and sex; the pattern, severity, and tempo of the muscle involvement; relevant laboratory results (ie, CPK, ESR); electromyographic (EMG) findings; and the presence of significant related conditions (ie, dermatitis, neoplasm, steroid/AZT therapy, AIDS).

Sampling Time The biopsy should be performed early in the day as the specimen will immediately require special handling and should arrive when histotechnical personnel are available. The requisition should state a brief clinical history, pertinent laboratory findings, the biopsy site, and the name of the referring physician.

Collection Selection of muscle biopsy site: The muscle biopsies should be one that is familiar to the pathologist (ie, quadriceps, deltoid, biceps, gastrocnemius), unusual muscle groups such as oculomotor or pharyngeal muscles should be avoided as they have several unique and potentially confusing features. The biopsy should be from a muscle that is involved by the disease but has not reached "end-stage" atrophy. Injection sites, sites used for EMG, and sites near the myotendonous junction should be avoided as these biopsies will commonly exhibit artifactual changes.

Surgical technique: Except for children or exceptional adult cases, the procedure is done with local anesthesia. Ideally, the biopsied muscle should not be allowed to contract because this creates severe microscopic artifacts. To achieve an isometric specimen, it is best to use a surgical muscle clamp that prevents contraction.

If no clamp is available, pinning the muscle specimen to a tongue blade to prevent contraction may be used instead. A portion of the muscle, in continuity with that held in the clamp, should extend from the clamp so it can be cut off for freezing and histochemistry. A small piece should be placed in 1% glutaraldehyde for epon-embedding for electron microscopy, if necessary. Deliver on a saline-moistened gauze pad immediately to the Pathology Department. The moistened gauze pad is used to prevent drying. The specimen must not become saturated as this will cause severe ice crystal artifact, when the biopsy is subsequently snap frozen. The tissue should **not** be placed in fixative or frozen. It should ideally reach the Pathology Laboratory within 30 minutes to maintain enzyme activity.

Storage Instructions A small portion of the fresh material is usually stored deep frozen for possible later use as tissue for biochemical assays (eg, quantitation of glycogen, enzymes, or dystrophin levels).

Use Detect/diagnose trichinosis infection; evaluate muscle disease in terms of neurogenic atrophy, muscular dystrophies, myositis (infectious and "idiopathic," or autoimmune), endocrine myopathies, congenital myopathies, and enzyme deficiencies. Sometimes even with no observable clinical muscle disease, a muscle biopsy may shed light on a systemic condition such as systemic vasculitis.

(Continued)

403

Muscle Biopsy *(Continued)*

Methodology A portion of the clamped muscle is oriented, frozen in isopentane/liquid nitrogen, and transverse sections are obtained for H & E, trichrome, and various histochemical preparations, some of which are listed below:

- Adenosine triphosphate (ATPase): At differing pH's, used to differentiates type I, IIa, and IIb myofibers and reveals abnormal fiber type distributions and diseases that selectively involve certain myofiber types.
- Succinate dehydrogenase (SDH): Stains mitochondria and shows abnormal aggregates or loss. Nicotinamide adenine dinucleotide-tetrazolium reductase (NADH-TR) may be used for the same purpose but is less sensitive.
- Oil red O: Stains lipids to detect abnormal accumulations.
- Periodic acid-Schiff (PAS): Used to detected glycogen in glycogenoses (ie, McArdle's disease, Pompe's disease, etc).

Extra frozen sections should be obtained and held in case additional, more specific, enzyme preparations are needed (ie, cytochrome C oxidase, phosphofructokinase, phosphorylase).

The remaining muscle tissue is formalin-fixed, paraffin-embedded, and stained for H & E and trichrome. These preparations are used to detect small foci of myositis or vasculitis which may be missed on the cryostat-cut sections, which are, of necessity, much smaller.

Selected Readings

Brooke MH, "Disorders of Skeletal Muscle," *Neurology in Clinical Practice*, Bradley WG, Daroff RB, Fenichel GM, et al, eds, Boston, MA: Butterworth-Heinemann, 1991, 1843-86.

DeGirolami U, Smith TW, Chad D, et al, "Skeletal Muscle," *Principles and Practice of Surgical Pathology*, Silverberg SG, ed, New York, NY: Churchill Livingstone, 1990, 545-92.

Heffner RR Jr, "Muscle Biopsy in Neuromuscular Disorders," *Diagnostic Surgical Pathology*, Sternberg SS, ed, New York, NY: Raven Press, 1989, 119-39.

Heffner RR Jr, "Skeletal Muscle," *Histology for Pathologists*, Sternberg SS, ed, New York, NY: Raven Press, 1992, 81-108.

Plotz PH, "Not Myositis. A Series of Chance Encounters," *JAMA*, 1992, 268(15):2074-7.

Mychel-S® *see* Chloramphenicol Serum Level *on page 299*

Mycobacteria Culture, Biopsy *see* Mycobacteria Culture, Biopsy or Body Fluid *on this page*

Mycobacteria Culture, Biopsy or Body Fluid

Related Information

Antimycobacterial Susceptibility Testing *on page 262*

Mycobacteria Culture, Sputum *on page 406*

Synonyms AFB Culture, Biopsy; Mycobacteria Culture, Biopsy; TB Culture, Biopsy

Applies To Bone Marrow Mycobacteria Culture; Mycobacteria Culture, Bone Marrow; Mycobacteria Culture, Surgical Specimen; Mycobacteria Culture, Tissue; Surgical Specimen Mycobacteria Culture; Tissue Mycobacteria Culture; Wound Mycobacteria Culture

Patient Preparation Aseptic preparation of biopsy site

Special Instructions The laboratory should be informed of the specific source of specimen, age of patient, current antibiotic therapy, clinical diagnosis, and time of collection. Specimens may be divided for fungus culture and KOH preparation, mycobacteria culture and acid-fast smear, and routine bacterial culture and Gram stain only if the specimen is of adequate volume for all tests requested.

Specimen Surgical tissue, bone marrow, biopsy material; **swab specimens are never adequate**

Container Sterile, screw cap container

Collection The portion of the surgical specimen submitted for culture should be separated from the portion submitted for histopathology by the surgeon or pathologist, utilizing sterile technique

Storage Instructions The specimen should be transported to laboratory as soon as possible after collection.

Causes for Rejection Specimen in fixative

Turnaround Time Negative cultures may be be reported after 8 weeks.

Reference Range No growth

Use Isolate and identify mycobacteria; establish the etiology of granulomatous disease, fever of unknown origin (FUO) particularly in immunocompromised patients and others with subtle defects of cellular immunity

Limitations Transbronchial biopsy cultures may be of assistance in documenting the diagnosis of tuberculosis in sputum smear negative cases; however, sputum culture and bronchial washing cultures have a higher percentage of positives.

If *Mycobacterium marinum* which may cause a localized cutaneous lesion that may be nodular, verrucous, ulcerative, or sporotrichoid and which may rarely involve deeper structure is suspected, the laboratory must be notified so that the culture may be incubated at an appropriate temperature (30°C). *Mycobacterium marinum* infection occurs in patients who have been exposed to the organism following an aquatic-related exposure involving a cutaneous abrasion or penetrating injury. Common histories include exposure while cleaning aquariums or clearing barnacles.

Methodology Culture on specialized selective media, usually including Löwenstein-Jensen (LJ) and frequently Middlebrook 7H11, incubated at 35°C with 5% to 10% CO_2. (30°C if *Mycobacterium marinum* is suspected.) Mycobacteria isolated are usually definitively identified and may be tested for antimicrobial susceptibility.

Radiometric (Bactec®) and DNA probe methods are utilized by some laboratories to provide rapid detection and identification of mycobacteria.

Susceptibility testing may be required because of the often unpredictable susceptibilities of the atypical mycobacteria. Susceptibility testing of mycobacteria is frequently referred to specialized laboratories and may only be offered by specific request.

Additional Information Occult infections with **atypical** mycobacteria (not *M. tuberculosis*), particularly *Mycobacterium avium* and *Mycobacterium intracellulare*, occur in patients with acquired immune deficiency syndrome (AIDS). In some institutions, the incidence of isolation of non-*Mycobacterium tuberculosis* species, specifically *M. avium-intracellulare* (*M. avium* complex), may exceed the rate of isolation of *M. tuberculosis*. Mycobacteria have been recovered from culture of Kaposi's sarcomas and bone marrow specimens, in which the characteristic granulomatous reaction has been absent. Optimal isolation of mycobacteria from tissue is accomplished by processing as much tissue as possible for culture. Swabs should be submitted only when adequate tissue is not available. Tuberculous spondylitis represents 50% to 60% of all cases of skeletal tuberculosis. It is seen in children in developing countries and adults over 50 years of age in the United States and Europe. Frequently several vertebrae are involved and adjacent psoas muscle abscesses or paravertebral abscesses are not uncommon. Colony counts obtained from bone biopsies are low; however, greater than 90% are culture positive. The diagnosis of vertebral tuberculosis should be considered in all cases of unexplained spondylitis.

Cases of sternal wound infection and of early onset prosthetic valve endocarditis have been recognized. *M. fortuitum* is the most commonly implicated mycobacterial species in these infections. Local environmental strains rather than contaminated commercial surgical materials or devices are considered to be the source of the organisms.

Pleural effusions frequently yield positive cultures in cases of pulmonary tuberculosis. The diagnosis of peritoneal tuberculosis is difficult and is usually made at laparotomy or after a considerable delay. Tuberculosis should be considered in any patient with ascitic fluid and chronic abdominal pain.

Selected Readings
Brown JW 3d and Sanders CV, "*Mycobacterium marinum* Infections: A Problem of Recognition, Not Therapy?" *Arch Intern Med*, 1987, 147(5):817-8.
Woods GI and Washington JA, "Mycobacteria Other Than *Mycobacterium tuberculosis*: Review of Microbiologic and Clinical Aspects," *Rev Infect Dis*, 1987, 9(2):275-94.

Mycobacteria Culture, Bone Marrow *see* Mycobacteria Culture, Biopsy or Body Fluid *on previous page*

Mycobacteria Culture, Bronchial Aspirate *see* Mycobacteria Culture, Sputum *on next page*

Mycobacteria Culture, Cerebrospinal Fluid
Related Information
Acid-Fast Stain *on page 239*
Viral Culture, Central Nervous System Symptoms *on page 476*
Synonyms CSF Mycobacteria Culture; Mycobacteria Culture, CSF; Mycobacteria Culture, Spinal Fluid; Spinal Fluid Mycobacteria Culture
Test Includes Culture for mycobacteria and acid-fast stain if requested
Patient Preparation Usual sterile preparation

(Continued)

Mycobacteria Culture, Cerebrospinal Fluid *(Continued)*

Specimen Cerebrospinal fluid

Container Sterile CSF tube

Collection The specimen may be divided for fungus culture and India ink preparation, cryptococcal antigen testing, fungus smear, mycobacteria culture and smear, and routine bacterial culture and Gram stain if the specimen is of adequate volume for all tests requested. Transport specimen to the laboratory as soon as possible.

Storage Instructions Do not refrigerate.

Turnaround Time Negative cultures are often reported after 6-8 weeks.

Reference Range No growth

Use Isolate and identify mycobacteria

Limitations Culture of for *M. tuberculosis* is usually nonproductive even in cases of tuberculosis meningitis. Culture of CSF for *M. tuberculosis* should be ordered only if such is truly suspected. Recovery of mycobacteria is directly related to the volume of specimen available to the laboratory for culture. 5-10 mL is recommended for optimal yield. Recovery of organisms can require as much as 4-6 weeks.

Methodology Culture on selective media usually including Löwenstein-Jensen (LJ) and Middlebrook 7H11 broth media may also be used with or without radiometric methodology

Additional Information A culture for mycobacteria is indicated if patient is immunocompromised and the Gram stain is negative and the white cell count is elevated. Tuberculous meningitis occurs in both children and adults. Early in the course neutrophils may predominate in the CSF. Lymphocytes, mononuclear cells, and granulocytes are found later. Rarely does the cell count exceed 1000 cells/mm^3. The CSF is clear and colorless early; later, a pellicle forms on standing. Low CSF glucose, <40 mg/dL, frequently is observed as is increased protein often >300 mg/dL. Other factors raising the index of suspicion include a positive tuberculin skin test (evidence of tuberculosis outside the CNS), previous active tuberculosis, significant recent exposure to tuberculosis, and suspicion of tuberculosis on imaging procedures. Acid-fast organisms can be identified on centrifuged sediments in 60% to 80% of cases.

Untreated tuberculous meningitis can be rapidly fatal. Blacks, Hispanics, and the elderly are most frequently affected. Alcohol abuse, drug abuse, steroid therapy, head trauma, pregnancy, and AIDS all may increase risk. Despite therapy, the mortality risk is high, approximately 30%. Evaluation of contacts is recommended.

Selected Readings

Ogawa SK, Smith MA, Brennessel DJ, et al, "Tuberculous Meningitis in an Urban Medical Center," *Medicine (Baltimore)*, 1987, 66(4):317-26.

Mycobacteria Culture, CSF *see* Mycobacteria Culture, Cerebrospinal Fluid *on previous page*

Mycobacteria Culture, Gastric Aspirate *see* Mycobacteria Culture, Sputum *on this page*

Mycobacteria Culture, Spinal Fluid *see* Mycobacteria Culture, Cerebrospinal Fluid *on previous page*

Mycobacteria Culture, Sputum

Related Information

Acid-Fast Stain *on page 239*

Mycobacteria Culture, Biopsy or Body Fluid *on page 404*

Synonyms AFB Culture, Sputum; TB Culture, Sputum

Applies To AFB Culture, Bronchial Aspirate; AFB Culture, Gastric Aspirate; Bronchoscopy Mycobacteria Culture; DNA Probe for Mycobacteria; Gastric Aspirate Mycobacteria Culture; Lower Respiratory Mycobacteria Culture; Mycobacteria Culture, Bronchial Aspirate; Mycobacteria Culture, Gastric Aspirate; Mycobacteria Culture, Tracheal Aspirate; Mycobacteria Culture, Transtracheal Aspirate; Mycobacteria, DNA Probe; Percutaneous Transtracheal Mycobacteria Culture; TB Culture, Bronchial Aspirate; TB Culture, Gastric Aspirate; Tracheal Aspirate Mycobacteria Culture; Transtracheal Aspirate Mycobacteria Culture

Test Includes Mycobacteria (AFB) culture and stain

Patient Preparation The patient should be instructed to remove dentures, rinse mouth with water, and then cough deeply expectorating sputum into the sputum collection cup.

Special Instructions Early morning specimen is preferred. Since at least 5 mL of sputum (**not saliva**) is required, the specimen may be collected over a 1- to 2-hour period in order to obtain sufficient quantity. However, 24-hour specimens are unacceptable because of bacterial overgrowth.

Specimen First morning sputum or induced sputum, fasting gastric aspirate, bronchial aspirate, tracheal aspirate, transtracheal aspirate, bronchial lavage

Container Sputum cup, sputum trap, sterile tracheal aspirate tube or sterile bronchoscopy tube

Sampling Time In children, the gastric aspirate should be done early in the morning as the child awakens before the stomach empties.

Collection A recommended screening procedure is three first morning specimens submitted on three successive days. The patient should be instructed to brush his/her teeth and/or rinse mouth well with water before attempting to collect the specimen to reduce the possibility of contaminating the specimen with food particles, oropharyngeal secretions, etc. After the specimen has been collected, the specimen should be examined to make sure it contains a sufficient quantity (at least 5 mL) of thick mucus (**not saliva**). If a two part collection system has been used, only the screw cap tube should be submitted to the laboratory. (The outer container is considered contaminated and its transport through the hospital constitutes a health hazard!) The specimen should be properly labeled and accompanied by a properly completed requisition. The specimen can be divided in the laboratory for fungal, mycobacterial, and routine cultures.

Storage Instructions The specimen should be refrigerated if it cannot be promptly processed. If a gastric aspirate cannot be processed immediately the pH should be neutralized for storage until it can be processed.

Causes for Rejection Specimens contaminated on the outside of the container pose excessive risk to laboratory personnel and may not be acceptable to the laboratory.

Turnaround Time Negative cultures are reported after 6-8 weeks.

Reference Range No growth

Use Isolate and identify mycobacteria

Limitations Bronchial washings are frequently diluted with topical anesthetics and irrigating fluids which may have an inhibitory effect on mycobacterial growth. Postbronchoscopy expectorated specimens may provide a better yield of organisms in those obtained during the procedure. Gastric aspirates yield organisms in less than 50% of cases of *M. tuberculosis* infection in children. Acid-fast stain of gastric aspirate has a sensitivity of 30%. Separate Cytology specimens must be submitted.

The relative yield of mycobacteria from clinical specimens is prebronchoscopy sputum > bronchial washings > postbronchoscopy sputum > bronchial biopsy.

Methodology Culture on selective media usually including Löwenstein-Jensen (LJ) and Middlebrook 7H11 with and without antibiotics. DNA probe technology using probes complementary to the ribosomal RNA of the *M. tuberculosis* complex (*M. tuberculosis, M. bovis*, BCG, *M. africanum*, and *M. microti*), as well as to *M. avium, M. intracellulare M. kansasii* and *M. gordonae* are available for culture confirmation. The probes can provide rapid confirmation of the species of mycobacteria isolated. Mycobacteria in clinical specimens can be detected by the radiometric Bactec® system which detects production of $^{14}CO_2$ from ^{14}C labeled palmitic acid supplemented Middlebrook 7H12 medium. Detection times are more rapid than with conventional culture methods. Gas-liquid chromatography can be used to rapidly speciate mycobacteria.

Additional Information Tuberculosis decreased in incidence in the United States in the 1970s and 1980s, however, high incidence populations exist in depressed inner city areas, some rural areas, amongst new immigrants, and in HIV-positive patients. The emergence of *M. tuberculosis* and *M. avium-intracellulare* infections complicating the acquired immunodeficiency syndrome has been striking. Primary pulmonary infections are common as case defining infections. Extrapulmonary mycobacterial infections are frequent in patients with an established diagnosis of AIDS.

See also Acid-Fast Stain, and Mycobacteria Culture, Biopsy or Body Fluid listings for additional discussion of mycobacterial disease in patients with the acquired immunodeficiency syndrome (AIDS).

Implication of *M. avium-intracellulare* as a pathogen usually requires at least one of the following criteria:
- Clinical evidence of a disease process that can be explained by atypical mycobacterial infection

(Continued)

Mycobacteria Culture, Sputum *(Continued)*

- Repeated isolation of the same mycobacterial species from sputum over a period of weeks to months
- Exclusion of other possible etiologies
- Biopsy demonstrating acid-fast bacilli or diagnostic histopathologic changes

Endobronchial tuberculosis has been increasingly recognized because of its incidence in association with the acquired immunodeficiency syndrome and because it may mimic carcinoma.

Nosocomial transmission of multidrug-resistant *Mycobacterium tuberculosis* has been noted to occur from patient to patient and from patient to healthcare worker. Acid-fast bacilli isolation precautions and adherence to appropriate infection control procedures is recommended.

Selected Readings

Chaisson RE and Slutkin G, "Tuberculosis and Human Immunodeficiency Virus Infection," *J Infect Dis*, 1989, 159(1):96-100.

Inderlied CB, Kemper CA, and Bermudez LE, "The *Mycobacterium avium* Complex," *Clin Microbiol Rev*, 1993, 6(3):266-310.

Marmion BP, Williamson J, Worswick DA, et al, "Experience With Newer Techniques for the Laboratory Detection of *Mycoplasma pneumoniae* Infection: Adelaide, 1978-1992," *Clin Infect Dis*, 1993, 17(Suppl 1):S90-9.

Mehta JB and Morris F, "Impact of HIV Infection on Mycobacterial Disease," *Am Fam Physician*, 1992, 45(5):2203-11.

Pearson ML, Jereb JA, Frieden TR et al, "Nosocomial Transmission of Multidrug-Resistant *Mycobacterium tuberculosis*: A Risk to Patients and Health Care Workers," *Ann Intern Med*, 1992, 117(3):191-6.

Stratton CW, "Mycobacterial Infections Other Than Tuberculosis in the AIDS Era," *Infect Dis Newslett*, 1992, 11(12):89-96.

Wellstood SA, "Diagnostic Mycobacteriology: Current Challenges and Technologies," *Lab Med*, 1993, 24(6):357-61.

Mycobacteria Culture, Surgical Specimen *see* Mycobacteria Culture, Biopsy or Body Fluid *on page 404*

Mycobacteria Culture, Tissue *see* Mycobacteria Culture, Biopsy or Body Fluid *on page 404*

Mycobacteria Culture, Tracheal Aspirate *see* Mycobacteria Culture, Sputum *on page 406*

Mycobacteria Culture, Transtracheal Aspirate *see* Mycobacteria Culture, Sputum *on page 406*

Mycobacteria, DNA Probe *see* Mycobacteria Culture, Sputum *on page 406*

Mycobacteria, Susceptibility Testing *see* Antimycobacterial Susceptibility Testing *on page 262*

Mycobacterium Smear *see* Acid-Fast Stain *on page 239*

Mycoplasma genitalium Culture *see* Mycoplasma/Ureaplasma Culture *on page 410*

Mycoplasma hominis Culture *see* Mycoplasma/Ureaplasma Culture *on page 410*

Mycoplasma pneumoniae *see* Mycoplasma/Ureaplasma Culture *on page 410*

Mycoplasma pneumoniae Culture *see* Mycoplasma pneumoniae Diagnostic Procedures *on this page*

Mycoplasma pneumoniae Diagnostic Procedures

Related Information

Aerobic Culture, Sputum *on page 246*
Darkfield Examination, Leptospirosis *on page 322*
Mycoplasma Serology *on page 410*
Mycoplasma/Ureaplasma Culture *on page 410*

Synonyms Mycoplasma pneumoniae Culture

Test Includes Culture and identification of *Mycoplasma pneumoniae*

Abstract *Mycoplasma pneumoniae* commonly causes respiratory infections. Most involve the upper respiratory tract, but pneumonia and other manifestations can occur as well.

Specimen Throat or nasopharyngeal swabs

Collection Throat or nasopharyngeal swabs should be placed **immediately** in transport medium and sent immediately to the laboratory.

Turnaround Time 2-3 weeks

Reference Range No *Mycoplasma pneumoniae* identified

Use Aid in the diagnosis of pneumonia caused by *Mycoplasma pneumoniae*

Limitations The culture procedure is not often used because it is slow and insensitive; 2-3 weeks or more are often required for isolation and definitive identification of positive cultures.

Methodology Isolates are cultured in special broth and on special agar media and are identified by biochemical tests and ability to hemolyze erythrocytes. However, the most commonly used and currently recommended method of diagnosis is serology to measure acute and convalescent antibody levels to *M. pneumoniae*.

Additional Information *Mycoplasma pneumoniae* infection is acquired via the respiratory route from small-particle aerosols or large droplets of secretions. The organism can penetrate the mucociliary barrier of respiratory epithelium and produce cellular injury and ciliostasis which may account for the prolonged cough observed clinically. Most infections are observed in older children and young adults. Early infection in infancy or childhood may increase the severity of subsequent infections. Cold agglutinins and *Mycoplasma pneumoniae* complement fixation serology have been the mainstays of diagnosis because of the limitations and long turnaround time for cultures. However, immunofluorescence techniques and immunoassays to detect antibodies to *M. pneumoniae* are available and are the recommended diagnostic methods. DNA probes for *Mycoplasma* are not yet available for routine testing. Consult the laboratory for availability of specific tests and specific instructions for specimen collection. See table.

Mycoplasma pneumoniae Clinical Manifestations of Infection

Respiratory	Pneumonia Pharyngitis Otitis media Bullous myringitis Sinusitis Laryngotracheobronchitis Bronchiolitis Nonspecific upper respiratory symptoms
Neurologic	Meningoencephalitis Encephalitis Transverse myelitis Cranial neuropathy Poliomyelitis–like syndrome Psychosis Cerebral infarction Guillain–Barré syndrome
Cardiac	Pericarditis Myocarditis Complete heart block Congestive heart failure Myocardial infarction
Gastrointestinal	Hepatic dysfunction Pancreatitis
Hematologic	Autoimmune hemolytic anemia Bone marrow suppression Thrombocytopenia Disseminated intravascular coagulation
Musculoskeletal	Myalgias Arthralgias Arthritis
Genitourinary	Glomerulonephritis Tubulointerstitial nephritis Tubo–ovarian abscess
Immunologic	Depressed cellular immunity and neutrophil chemotaxis

From Broughton RA, "Infections Due to *Mycoplasma pneumoniae* in Childhood," *Pediatr Infect Dis J,* 1986, 71–85, with permission.

(Continued)

Mycoplasma pneumoniae Diagnostic Procedures
(Continued)

Selected Readings

Clyde WA Jr, "Clinical Overview of Typical *Mycoplasma pneumoniae* Infections," *Clin Infect Dis*, 1993, 17(Suppl 1)S32-6.

Mansel JK, Rosenow EC 3d, Smith TF, et al, "*Mycoplasma pneumoniae* Pneumonia," *Chest*, 1989, 95(3):639-46.

Martin RE and Bates JH, "Atypical Pneumonia," *Infect Dis Clin North Am*, 1991, 5(3):585-601.

"The Changing Role of Mycoplasmas in Respiratory Disease and AIDS," *Clin Infect Dis*, 1993, 17(Suppl 1):S1-315.

Wijnands GJ, "Diagnosis and Interventions in Lower Respiratory Tract Infections," *Am J Med*, 1992, 92(4SA):91S-7S.

Mycoplasma pneumoniae Titer *see Mycoplasma* Serology
on this page

Mycoplasma Serology

Related Information

Mycoplasma pneumoniae Diagnostic Procedures *on page 408*

Synonyms Eaton Agent Titer; *M. pneumoniae* Titer; *Mycoplasma pneumoniae* Titer; PPLO Titer

Specimen Serum

Container Red top tube

Collection Acute and convalescent sera drawn 10-14 days apart are required

Reference Range Negative: IgG <1:10, IgM <1:10. A fourfold increase in titer in paired sera or a single complement fixation titer >1:256 suggests infection. Contact laboratory for specific cutoff values and significant titers.

Use Support for the diagnosis of *Mycoplasma pneumoniae* infection

Limitations False-positives occur in pancreatitis.

Methodology Complement fixation, immunofluorescence, enzyme immunoassay

Additional Information *Mycoplasma pneumoniae* is the cause of the relatively common "primary atypical pneumonia." *Mycoplasma* is more difficult to culture than are bacteria; thus, serologic confirmation of the diagnosis is often desirable. The complement fixation test to detect antibody to a lipid antigen is more specific and more sensitive than is the cold agglutinin test. However, complement fixation requires paired sera, and is thus of limited clinical utility. Demonstration of specific IgG and IgM antibody by immunofluorescence is rapid, sensitive, and specific. IgM antibody indicates acute infection.

Selected Readings

Kenny GE, "Immunologic Methods for Mycoplasmas and Miscellaneous Bacteria," *Manual of Clinical Laboratory Immunology*, 4th ed, Rose NR, de Macario EC, Fahey JL, et al, eds, Washington, DC: American Society for Microbiology, 1992, 497-8.

Martin RE and Bates JH, "Atypical Pneumonia," *Infect Dis Clin North Am*, 1991, 5(3):585-601.

Smith TF, "*Mycoplasma pneumoniae* Infections: Diagnosis Based on Immunofluorescence Titer of IgG and IgM Antibodies," *Mayo Clin Proc*, 1986, 61(10):830-1.

Mycoplasma T-Strain Culture, Genital *see* Genital Culture for
Ureaplasma urealyticum on page 350

Mycoplasma/Ureaplasma Culture

Related Information

Genital Culture for *Ureaplasma urealyticum on page 350*

Mycoplasma pneumoniae Diagnostic Procedures *on page 408*

Synonyms PPLO Culture

Applies To Cervix, *Mycoplasma* Culture; *Mycoplasma genitalium* Culture; *Mycoplasma hominis* Culture; *Mycoplasma pneumoniae*; *Ureaplasma urealyticum* Culture; Urethra, *Mycoplasma* Culture; Urine, *Mycoplasma* Culture

Specimen The following specimens are appropriate: throat swabs (send two swabs), sputum, bronchial washings, tracheal aspiration, cerebrospinal fluid, heparinized blood, urethral swab, vaginal swab, cervical swab, placenta, and urine. Urine should **not** be clean catch midstream. Initial urine flow is best specimen.

Collection The laboratory **must** be contacted prior to collection for advice and for appropriate transport medium. Transport specimen to the laboratory within 1 hour. Do **not** use cotton swabs or swabs with wooden sticks.

Turnaround Time 1-6 weeks

Reference Range No *Mycoplasma* isolated

Use Isolate and identify *Mycoplasma*

Limitations Culture is frequently negative in presence of *Mycoplasma* infection.

Methodology Isolates are cultured in special broth and on special agar media and are identified by biochemical tests and ability to hemolyze erythrocytes. However, the most commonly used and currently recommended method of diagnosis is serology to measure acute and convalescent antibody levels to *M. pneumoniae*.

Additional Information *Mycoplasma pneumoniae* is the causative agent of mycoplasmal pneumonia or atypical pneumonia. This condition is generally mild, but may develop into severe illness. Other members of the *Mycoplasma* family are *M. hominis* and *Ureaplasma urealyticum*, which cause infection of the urogenital tract, namely pelvic inflammatory disease and 10% of the cases of nongonococcal urethritis. Both organisms can be isolated for identification and both respond to erythromycin and tetracycline.

Nail Fungus Culture *see* Fungus Culture, Skin *on page 343*

Nasopharyngeal Culture for *Bordetella pertussis* *see* Bordetella pertussis Nasopharyngeal Culture *on page 283*

Nasopharyngeal Smear for *Bordetella pertussis* *see* Bordetella pertussis Direct Fluorescent Antibody *on page 282*

Nebcin® *see* Tobramycin *on page 458*

Needle Biopsy of the Liver *see* Liver Biopsy *on page 387*

Negri Bodies *see* Rabies *on page 433*

Neisseria gonorrhoeae by Nucleic Acid Probe

Related Information

Neisseria gonorrhoeae Culture *on next page*

Synonyms DNA Hybridization Test for *Neisseria gonorrhoeae*; DNA Test for *Neisseria gonorrhoeae*; Gen-Probe® for *Neisseria gonorrhoeae*; *Neisseria gonorrhoeae* DNA Detection Test; PACE2®

Test Includes Direct detection of *Neisseria gonorrhoeae* nucleic acid in clinical specimens from the urogenital site. This test cannot be used in legal cases or child protection cases.

Patient Preparation When taking urethral specimens, the patient should not have urinated for 1 hour prior to collection.

Specimen Swab specimen collected from the genitourinary site of a male or female patient

Container Special transport medium is provided by the laboratory and should not be substituted. A kit containing a swab and special transport medium is made by Gen-Probe, Inc. and is recommended for this test.

Collection Currently the probe test for *Neisseria gonorrhoeae* is FDA approved only for genitourinary specimens. It has not yet been approved for testing of nongenital specimens (ie, ocular).

For a male, the urethra is swabbed by rotating the swab 2-3 cm into the urethra. This should provide enough specimen from the infected site to detect *N. gonorrhoeae* nucleic acid. The swab is then placed in the transport tube for shipment to the laboratory.

For females, the Gen-Probe® kit provides two swabs. The cervix or endocervix should be swabbed with one swab **first** to clean the area and then the **second** swab is used to collect the specimen. The swab is then put immediately into the transport tube and shipped to the laboratory. This is the same collection kit used for the *Chlamydia trachomatis* probe assay. A single swab specimen from each patient is sufficient to test for both *N. gonorrhoeae* and *C. trachomatis*.

Storage Instructions The specimens should be kept at room temperature or refrigerated. Do not freeze.

Causes for Rejection Contamination of specimen with urine

Turnaround Time Results are available within 24 hours of receipt of the specimen. However, most laboratories batch test every 2 or 3 days.

Reference Range Normal: Negative for *Neisseria gonorrhoeae* nucleic acid. A sexually active, asymptomatic female may harbor *N. gonorrhoeae* without overt clinical symptoms.

Use This test provides for the rapid detection of *N. gonorrhoeae* in clinical urogenital specimens.

(Continued)

411

Neisseria gonorrhoeae by Nucleic Acid Probe
(Continued)

Limitations Nucleic acid detection tests should not be done in child abuse cases. In these cases many laboratories perform more than one confirmatory test after culture of the isolate. The probe assay can be used to confirm the identification of organisms recovered by culture.

Methodology This test detects *N. gonorrhoeae* nucleic acid directly from swab specimens. This requires denaturation of the nucleic acid in the specimens by heating, hybridization with a specific nucleic acid probe, and detection of bound probe after several washing steps.

Additional Information Gonorrhea is a commonly reported sexually transmitted disease in the United States. The disease is manifest as acute urethritis in males and as cervicitis in females. *N. gonorrhoeae* can be isolated from asymptomatic females. Treatment of these individuals is critical because gonorrhea can result in more serious complications such as pelvic inflammatory disease, sterility, and ectopic pregnancy.

It is very important to control the spread of this disease between sexual partners, thus the use of a quick, reliable test system is essential. The DNA detection assay has a sensitivity and a specificity equal to traditional methods of organism isolation and identification. The current definitive method of detection for *N. gonorrhoeae* is the culture of the microorganism. However, this organism is fastidious and can be difficult to grow in culture when an established laboratory is not available. Loss of viability and overgrowth of contaminating microorganisms may limit recovery of *N. gonorrhoeae* by culture from clinical specimens that must be transported to a referral laboratory.

The major disadvantage of the probe method at the present time is that this test cannot be done in child abuse cases. These cases must be documented with the recovery of *N. gonorrhoeae* organism from the clinical specimen.

Selected Readings

Panke ES, Yang LI, Leist PA, et al, "Comparison of Gen-Probe DNA Probe Test and Culture for the Detection of *Neisseria gonorrhoeae* in Endocervical Specimens," *J Clin Microbiol*, 1991, 29(5):883-8.

Neisseria gonorrhoeae Culture
Related Information

Genital Culture *on page 349*

Genital Culture for *Ureaplasma urealyticum on page 350*

Neisseria gonorrhoeae by Nucleic Acid Probe *on previous page*

Penicillinase Test *on page 427*

Synonyms GC Culture; Gonorrhea Culture

Applies To Cervix Culture *Neisseria gonorrhoeae*; GC Culture, Throat; Gonorrhea Culture, Throat; Prostatic Fluid Culture *Neisseria gonorrhoeae*; Synovial Fluid Culture for *Neisseria gonorrhoeae*, Only; Throat Culture for *Neisseria gonorrhoeae*; Urethral Culture for *Neisseria gonorrhoeae*; Urine Culture, First Voided, for *Neisseria gonorrhoeae*; Vaginal Culture *Neisseria gonorrhoeae*

Patient Preparation Preparation same as for clean catch urine. See listing Urine Culture, Clean Catch for detailed information. *Neisseria gonorrhoeae* is very sensitive to lubricants and disinfectants. If possible avoid collecting urethral specimens until at least 1 hour after urinating.

Special Instructions The laboratory should be informed of the specific request for culture of *Neisseria gonorrhoeae* only, and the collection time, date, specific site of specimen, age of patient, current antibiotic therapy, and clinical diagnosis.

Specimen Body fluid, discharge, pus, swab of genital lesions, urethral discharge (best when available for men); endocervix (best when available for female); sediment of first 10 mL of centrifuged urine collected at least 2 hours after last micturition or first few drops of urine voided into a sterile cup for "first voided urine specimen" for asymptomatic males, or first void overnight urine, centrifuged.

Container Swab with transport medium or sterile container if transported to laboratory within a few minutes; otherwise, direct planting on **room temperature** transgrow medium, Jembec™, NYC, or Thayer-Martin medium

Collection

Urethral discharge: Collect male urethral discharge by endourethral swab after stripping toward the orifice to express exudate.

Rectal swab: Collect anorectal specimens from the crypts just inside the anal ring. Direct visualization with anoscopy is useful. Insert the swab past the anal

Selection of Culture Sites for the Isolation
of *Neisseria gonorrhoeae*

Culture Site	Diagnostic Sensitivity (%)
Women (nonhysterectomized) Primary site Endocervical canal	86–96
Secondary sites Vagina	55–90
Urethra	60–86
Anal canal	70–85
Oropharynx	50–70
Women (hysterectomized) Primary site Urethra	88.9
Secondary sites Vagina	55.7
Anal canal	40.7
Men (heterosexuals) Primary site Urethra	94–98 (symptomatic) 84 (asymptomatic)
Men (homosexuals) Primary sites Urethra	60–98
Anal canal	40–85
Oropharynx	50–70

From Ehret JM and Knapp JS, "Gonorrhea," *Clin Lab Med,* 1989, 9:445–80, with permission.

sphincter. Move the swab circumferentially around the anal crypts. Allow 15-30 seconds for organisms to adsorb onto the swab. Replace the swab and crush the media compartment. Prostatic fluid yields fewer positives than does culture of urethral discharge. Cultures from the urethra or vagina are indicated from females when endocervical culture is not possible.

Endocervical/cervical: Gently compress cervix between speculum blades to express any endocervical exudate. Swab in a circular pattern.

Bartholin gland: Express exudate from duct. Abscesses should be aspirated with needle and syringe.

Urethra in women: Massage the urethra against the pubic symphysis to express discharge or use endourethral swab.

Vagina: Obtain the specimen from the vaginal vault. Allow 15-30 seconds for organisms to adsorb onto the swab.

The specimen should be transported to laboratory within 1 hour of collection.

Storage Instructions Specimen **must not** be refrigerated or exposed to a cold environment. If the specimen is directly inoculated on Thayer-Martin medium it should be transported to the laboratory as soon as possible and placed directly in CO_2 incubator or candle jar.

Causes for Rejection Specimen not received in appropriate container, refrigerated specimens

Turnaround Time Preliminary reports are usually available at 24 hours. Cultures with no growth are commonly reported after 48 hours. Cultures from which *N. gonorrhoeae* is isolated require a minimum of 48 hours for completion.

Reference Range No *Neisseria gonorrhoeae* isolated

Use Isolate and identify *Neisseria gonorrhoeae*, establish the diagnosis of gonorrhea

Limitations See table. Cultures are usually screened only for *Neisseria gonorrhoeae*. No other organisms are usually identified. Overgrowth by *Proteus* and yeast may make it impossible to rule out presence of *N. gonorrhoeae*. The vancomycin in Thayer-Martin media may inhibit some stains of *N. gonorrhoeae*. Nongonococcal urethritis may be caused by *Ureaplasma urealyticum, Coryne-*
(Continued)

413

Neisseria gonorrhoeae Culture *(Continued)*

bacterium genitalium type 1, *Trichomonas vaginalis*, *Chlamydia trachomatis*, herpes simplex virus, and rarely, *Candida albicans*.

Methodology Culture on selective medium, Thayer-Martin or NYC. Nucleic acid probes, monoclonal antibodies and enzyme linked immunoassays are used as alternatives to culture in some laboratories. Advantages of the newer methods over traditional culture and smear techniques are not universally recognized.

Additional Information Thirty percent to 50% of patients infected with *N. gonorrhoeae* are also infected with *Chlamydia trachomatis*. In high prevalence populations, the recovery of *N. gonorrhoeae* is as follows: endocervix > urine sediment > anal canal > pharynx. A serologic test for syphilis (VDRL, RPR, or ART), HIV, and cervical/vaginal cytology should be considered in patients suspected of having gonorrhea.

Selected Readings
Judson FN, "Gonorrhea," *Med Clin North Am*, 1990, 74(6):1353-66.

Neisseria gonorrhoeae DNA Detection Test *see Neisseria gonorrhoeae* by Nucleic Acid Probe *on page 411*

Neisseria gonorrhoeae Susceptibility Testing *see* Penicillinase Test *on page 427*

Nigrosin Preparation *see* India Ink Preparation *on page 373*

Nitrite, Urine

Related Information

Leukocyte Esterase, Urine *on page 386*

Lyme Disease Serology by Western Blot *on page 394*

Synonyms Bacteria Screen, Urine

Test Includes This test is usually part of a routine urinalysis

Abstract A rapid method for detection of bacteriuria. A positive test indicates the presence of bacteria which reduce urinary nitrate to nitrite.

Specimen Urine, first morning specimen is preferred; random urine is acceptable; preferably midstream, clean catch collection

Container Plastic urine container

Storage Instructions If the specimen cannot be processed within 2 hours it should be refrigerated.

Reference Range Negative

Use The test is used to detect the presence of potentially significant bacteriuria; an aid to the diagnosis of cystitis, pyelonephritis, urinary tract infection

Limitations This test is not specific. The sensitivity of the nitrite test is decreased with high urine specific gravity and with high urine ascorbic acid content. False-negatives are relatively common and relate to varying retention times of urine in the bladder, varying urinary nitrate concentrations (diet dependent) and the presence and quantity of nitrate reducing organisms present. Storage of sample at room temperature for excessive periods (more than 2 hours) may lead to reduction of nitrite to nitrogen.

Some urinary tract infections are caused by organisms which do not contain reductase to convert nitrate to nitrite. These include infections caused by *Enterococcus faecalis* and other gram-positive cocci, *N. gonorrhoeae*, *M. tuberculosis*. Negative results are found when infecting organisms do not convert nitrate to nitrite. In addition, urine may not have been retained in the bladder for 4 hours or more to allow adequate reduction of nitrate to occur.

Methodology This reaction depends upon the conversion of nitrate to nitrite by the action of certain species of urinary bacteria. Nitrite from the urine reacts with p-arsanilic acid forming a diazonium compound. The diazonium compound couples with 1,2,3,4-tetrahydrobenzo(h)quinolin-3-ol.

Additional Information A positive nitrite test is strongly suggestive of urinary tract infection (ie, $\geq 10^5$ organisms/mL). Therefore, when positive, a urine culture is recommended, but urine culture is indicated in any case if the patient is symptomatic. The use of nitrate and leukocyte esterase together is more extensively discussed in the listing Leukocyte Esterase, Urine.

Selected Readings
Damato JJ, Garis J, Hawley RJ, et al, "Comparative Leukocyte Esterase-Nitrite and BAC-T-SCREEN Studies Using Single and Multiple Urine Volumes," *Arch Pathol Lab Med*, 1988, 112(5):533-5.

Nits Identification *see* Arthropod Identification *on page 268*

Nizoral *see* Ketoconazole *on page 379*

Nocardia **Culture, All Sites**

Related Information

Acid-Fast Stain, Modified, *Nocardia* Species *on page 241*
Actinomyces Culture, All Sites *on page 242*

Test Includes Culture for *Nocardia* sp and direct microscopic examination of Gram stain for branching gram-positive bacilli, modified acid-fast stain

Abstract *Nocardia asteroides, N. brasiliensis,* and *N. caviae* cause two disease entities, nocardiosis and mycetoma. The latter relates to trauma.

Special Instructions Consultation with laboratory prior to collection of the specimen is recommended when nocardiosis is suspected clinically. Culture should be specifically ordered as Culture for *Nocardia.*

Specimen Pus, tissue, cerebrospinal fluid or other body fluid, aspirate, sputum. The usual portal of entry is the lung. Swabs are vastly inferior to aspirates and/or tissue specimens.

Collection Refer to listing for culture of specific site for complete collection and storage instructions (eg, Biopsy or Body Fluid Culture, Sputum Culture, and Wound Culture).

Turnaround Time Negative cultures are reported after 2-4 weeks.

Reference Range No *Nocardia* sp isolated

Critical Values *Nocardia* sp recovered from a central nervous system specimen

Use Establish the diagnosis of nocardiosis

Limitations *Nocardia* sp will not be recovered by routine culture techniques because of its relatively slow growth. Growth of *Nocardia* may be obscured by overgrowth of other organisms in mixed culture (ie, sputum). The diagnosis may not be made unless the laboratory is advised of the clinical suspicion of nocardiosis. *Nocardia* sp are not strongly gram-positive, but their branching pattern when visible is helpful. A modified acid-fast stain (see Acid-Fast Stain, Modified, *Norcardia* Species) is needed, since *Nocardia* are weakly acid-fast and may not be found with conventional acid-fast staining. Staining may be positive when cultures fail. Repeated sputum cultures may not yield a diagnosis of pulmonary nocardiosis. Bronchoscopic biopsy, transtrachial aspiration, or fine needle biopsy is often required.

Methodology Aerobic culture on blood agar and Löwenstein-Jensen (LJ) media with no antibiotics. Recent data supports the use of *Legionella* culture media (selective and nonselective buffered charcoal yeast agar) for recovery of *Nocardia. Nocardia* sp can also be cultured on noninhibitory fungal media. Cultures are usually held for 10-30 days. Cultures for *Nocardia* often need to be decontaminated similar to the decontamination process for *Mycobacterium.*

Additional Information *Nocardia* sp are aerobic, gram-positive bacteria which are filamentous, relatively slow growing, and variably acid fast. Human infection is seen most frequently in patients whose immune systems are suppressed by HIV infection, lymphoreticular malignancy, or chemotherapy. Nocardiosis frequently affects debilitated hosts and has been implicated in cases of infections in renal transplant patients, osteomyelitis, in patients on long-term steroid therapy and with peritonsillar abscess, and in cutaneous infections. The clinical picture may be similar to that observed with systemic mycobacterial or fungal infections. Infections may be acute, subacute, or chronic; and they may be disseminated or localized to cutaneous sites or the respiratory tract. Hematogenous dissemination occurs. Metastatic infection in brain, bone, skin, or subcutaneous infection in the presence of pulmonary involvement is suggestive of nocardiosis. *Nocardia asteroides* is the species most commonly recovered from clinical specimens and is usually associated with the respiratory tract; this species is phenotypically heterogeneous, and it has been proposed that the species be considered a complex which is subdivided. *Nocardia brasiliensis* and *Nocardia caviae* also produce human infections; of the two, *Nocardia brasiliensis* is far more common. The species found in mycetoma is usually *N. brasiliensis.*

Nocardia sp are variably acid-fast and may be frequently confused with *Actinomyces* sp or saprophytic fungi in Gram stains of clinical specimens. Prognosis is dependent on early diagnosis, treatment with appropriate antimicrobials, and the course of the underlying disease. In management of high-risk patients, a strong index of suspicion for the diagnosis of nocardiosis must be maintained.

Selected Readings

Bennett JE, "Actinomycosis and Nocardiosis," *Harrison's Principles of Internal Medicine,*
(Continued)

Nocardia **Culture, All Sites** *(Continued)*

12th ed, Chapter 152, Wilson JD, Braunwald E, Isselbacher KJ, et al, eds, New York, NY: McGraw-Hill Inc, 1991, 752-3.

Chazen G, "*Nocardia*," *Infect Control*, 1987, 8:260-3.

Hellyar AG, "Experience With *Nocardia asteroides* in Renal Transplant Recipients," *J Hosp Infect*, 1988, 12(1):13-8.

Javaly K, Horowitz HW, and Wormser GP, "Nocardiosis in Patients With Human Immunodeficiency Virus Infection. Report of 2 Cases and Review of the Literature," *Medicine (Baltimore)*, 1992, 71(3):128-38.

Kalb RE, Kaplan MH, and Grossman ME, "Cutaneous Nocardiosis. Case Reports and Review," *J Am Acad Dermatol*, 1985, 13:125-33.

Kerr E, Snell H, Black BL, et al, "Isolation of *Nocardia asteroides* From Respiratory Specimens by Using Selective Buffered Charcoal-Yeast Extract Agar," *J Clin Microbiol*, 1992, 30(5):1320-2.

McNeil MM and Brown JM, "The Medically Important Aerobic Actinomycetes: Epidemiology and Microbiology," *Clin Microbiol Rev*, 1994, 7(3):357-417.

McNeil MM, Brown JM, Jarvis WR, et al, "Comparison of Species Distribution and Antimicrobial Susceptibility of Aerobic Actinomycetes From Clinical Specimens," *Rev Infect Dis*, 1990, 12(5):778-83.

Schwartz JG and Tio FO, "Nocardial Osteomyelitis: A Case Report and Review of the Literature," *Diagn Microbiol Infect Dis*, 1987, 8:37-46, (review).

Vickers RM, Rihs JD, and Yu VL, "Clinical Demonstration of Isolation of *Nocardia asteroides* on Buffered Charcoal-Yeast Extract Media," *J Clin Microbiol*, 1992, 30(1):227-8.

Wallace RJ Jr, Brown BA, Tsukamura M, et al, "Clinical and Laboratory Features of *Nocardia nova*," *J Clin Microbiol*, 1991, 29(11):2407-11.

Wilson JP, Turner HR, Kirchner KA, et al, "Nocardial Infections in Renal Transplant Recipients," *Medicine (Baltimore)*, 1989, 68(1):38-57.

Nocardia **Species Modified Acid-Fast Stain** *see* Acid-Fast Stain, Modified, *Nocardia* Species *on page 241*

Non-A, non-B Hepatitis *see* Hepatitis C Serology *on page 360*

Occult Blood, Semiquantitative, Urine *see* Urinalysis *on page 467*

Ocular Cytology

Synonyms *Chlamydia* Smear; Conjunctival Smear; Corneal Smear; Eye Smear for Cytology

Applies To Inclusion Conjunctivitis

Test Includes Papanicolaou stain and/or Giemsa stain

Specimen Direct smear of ocular lesion

Collection Swab lesion with cotton-tipped applicator or scrape with sterile ophthalmic spatula and smear on clean glass slides (2), **immediately** spray fix one slide, let other air dry. Label frosted end of slide with patient's name and date.

Causes for Rejection Inadequate fixation

Use Diagnosis of trachoma-inclusion conjunctivitis, adenovirus infection, vaccinia infection or herpetic conjunctivitis, and evaluation of possible dysplastic or malignant conjunctival lesions

Limitations The sensitivity of this test is very low. Positive results are only suggestive and should prompt subsequent culture.

Additional Information Diagnosis of viral and chlamydial infections is considerably improved by immunofluorescent and immunoperoxidase stains for organisms.

Selected Readings

Sanderson TL, Pustai W, Shelley L, et al, "Cytologic Evaluation of Ocular Lesions," *Acta Cytol*, 1980, 24(5):391-400.

Schumann GB, O'Dowd GJ, and Spinnler PA, "Eye Cytology," *Lab Med*, 1980, 11:533-40.

Ova and Parasite, Pinworm Preparation *see* Pinworm Preparation *on page 430*

Ova and Parasites, Stool

Related Information

Pinworm Preparation *on page 430*

Stool Culture *on page 448*

Synonyms Parasites, Stool; Parasitology Examination, Stool; Stool for Ova and Parasites

Test Includes Gross appearance, direct wet mounts, saline and iodine, concentration procedure, hematoxylin smear or trichrome smear

Patient Preparation Specimens obtained with a warm saline enema or Fleet Phospho(R)-Soda are acceptable. Specimens obtained with mineral oil, bismuth, or magnesium compounds are unsatisfactory. Wait 1 week or more after barium procedures before collecting stools for examination.

Aftercare Warning: Any stool collected by or from the patient may harbor pathogens which are **immediately infective.**

Specimen Fresh or preserved random stool. If pinworm is suspected, a Scotch® Tape preparation should be submitted to the laboratory instead of stool. See also Pinworm Preparation test listing.

Container Plastic stool container. The collection procedure of choice is to provide patients with containers with polyvinyl alcohol (PVA) and formalin into which they can place stool. This procedure assures that the specimen will be well preserved. Degradation of parasites during transportation to the laboratory will be markedly reduced.

Collection The specimen should be delivered within 1 hour of collection to laboratory. Direct wet preparation exams for motile trophozoite observation can be performed on stools which arrive in the laboratory not longer than 1 hour after collection. The old recommended screening procedure is the automatic ordering of three random stool specimens; one collected every other day. The current, and much more clinically relevant, recommendation is a single specimen and obtaining its result; then the ordering of additional specimens if indicated. Specimens may be preserved in polyvinyl alcohol (PVA) fixative which is suitable for the preparation of permanent stains and formalin or merthiolate-iodine-formalin (MIF), which is suitable for concentration preparations and direct examination.

Storage Instructions Liquid specimens should be brought directly to laboratory. Wet mounts can be performed immediately and the specimen placed in PVA and/or MIF preservatives to maintain ova and trophozoite states when applicable.

Causes for Rejection Because of risk to laboratory personnel, specimens sent on diaper or tissue paper, specimen contaminating outside of transport container may not be acceptable to the laboratory. Specimen containing interfering substances, eg, castor oil, bismuth, Metamucil®, barium specimens delayed in transit and those contaminated with urine will not have optimal yield.

Turnaround Time Variable, depending on method

Reference Range No parasites seen

Use Establish the diagnosis of parasitic infestation

Limitations Note: One negative result does not rule out the possibility of parasitic infestation. Stool examination for *Giardia* may be negative in early stages of infection, in patients who shed organisms cyclically, and in chronic infections. The sensitivity of microscopic methods for the detection of *Giardia* vary. Tests for *Giardia* antigen and immunofluorescence tests have a higher yield.

Contraindications Administration of barium, bismuth, Metamucil®, castor oil, mineral oil, tetracycline therapy, administration of antiamebic drugs within 1 week prior to test. Purgation contraindicated for pregnancy, ulcerative colitis, cardiovascular disease, child younger than 5 years of age, appendicitis or possible appendicitis.

Methodology Wet mount and trichrome stain after concentration, immunofluorescence (IF), counterimmunoelectrophoresis (CIE), or enzyme-linked immunosorbent assay (ELISA) for the detection of *Giardia* antigens. The use of pooled preserved specimens to contain costs is acceptable.

Additional Information Parasite exams on stool from patients hospitalized ≥3 days are rarely, if ever, productive and should not be ordered unless special circumstances exist.

Amebas and certain other parasites cannot be seen in stools containing barium. Optimal diagnostic yield is obtained by the examination of fresh, warm stool by an experienced technologist, during usual laboratory hours. Amebic cysts, *Giardia* cysts, and helminth eggs are often recovered from formed stools. Mushy or liquid stools (either normally passed or obtained by purgation) often yield trophozoites. Purgation does not enhance the yield of *Giardia*. Stools which can be processed by the laboratory in less than 1 hour need not be preserved. Mushy, loose, or watery stools which cannot reach the laboratory within 1 hour should be preserved in formalin or merthiolate-iodine-formalin (MIF) and/or polyvinyl alcohol (PVA). Formalin will preserve protozoan cysts and larvae and the eggs of helminths. It is used for concentration procedures. PVA will preserve the trophozoite stage of protozoa. A trichrome stained smear may be prepared from PVA fixed material. PVA cannot be concentrated; therefore, they should always be accompanied by a portion of the specimen in formalin. Formed stools may be preserved in formalin, or refriger-

(Continued)

417

AMEBAE							
	Entamoeba histolytica	*Entamoeba hartmanni*	*Entamoeba coli*	*Entamoeba polecki* [1]	*Endolimax nana*	*Iodamoeba bütschlii*	*Dientamoeba fragilis* [2]
Trophozoite							
Cyst							No cyst

[1]Rare, probably of animal origin
[2]Flagellate

Scale: 0   5   10 μm

Amebae found in human stool specimens.

CILIATE	COCCIDIA			BLASTOCYSTIS
Balantidium coli	*Isospora belli*	*Sarcocystis* spp.	*Cryptosporidium* spp.	*Blastocystis hominis*
Trophozoite	immature oocyst	mature oocyst	mature oocyst	
Cyst	mature oocyst	single sporocyst		

0 20 40 μm   *Scale:* 0 10 20 30 μm   *Scale:* 0 10 20 μm

Ciliate, coccidia, and *B. hominis* found in human stool specimens.

FLAGELLATES				
Trichomonas hominis	*Chilomastix mesnili*	*Giardia lamblia*	*Enteromonas hominis*	*Retortamonas intestinalis*
Trophozoite				
Cyst No cyst				

Scale: 0 5 10 μm

Flagellates found in human stool specimens. From Brooke and Melvin

418

Ova and Parasites, Stool *(Continued)*

ated in a secure container until they can be transported to the laboratory. The collection/preservation kits will preserve protozoan cysts, helminth eggs and larvae. It is meant to be sent home with the patient and mailed back to the laboratory.

Parasites commonly identified in the stool of AIDS patients include *Cryptosporidium*, *Entamoeba histolytica*, *Giardia lamblia*, and Microsporidia.

Blastocystis hominis which is commonly observed in stool of healthy and symptomatic patients is not currently deemed to be pathogenic. The current consensus is that there is no convincing proof of a causal relationship between *B. hominis* and symptoms, that there is no correlation between resolution of symptoms with therapy or with the disappearance of the organism from stool, and that treatment directed at the indication of *B. hominis* is not indicated.

In a large children's hospital study of nosocomial diarrhea rotavirus, *C. difficile*, and enteric adenovirus were recovered. Stool for ova and parasites and bacterial stool cultures yielded no pathogens.

Selected Readings

Brooke MM and Melvin DM, "Morphology of Diagnostic Stages of Intestinal Parasites of Humans," 2nd ed, *US Department of Health and Human Services*, Publication No (CDC) 84-8116. Atlanta, GA: Centers for Disease Control.

Miller RA and Minshew BH, "*Blastocystis hominis*: An Organism in Search of a Disease," *Rev Infect Dis*, 1988, 10(5):930-8.

Ova and Parasites, Urine or Aspirates

Synonyms Aspirates for Ova and Parasites; Parasites, Urine; Urine for Parasites; Urine for *Schistosoma haematobium*

Test Includes Wet preparation and concentration procedure

Special Instructions The laboratory should be informed of the parasite clinically suspected.

Specimen Freshly voided urine, sputum, aspirates, body fluid

Container Sterile urine container, sterile screw cap tube

Collection

Urine: The specimen should be less than 4 hours old and not refrigerated. The recommended screening procedure is to submit three first morning urines on successive days.

Sigmoidoscopic specimens: Mix material with 2-3 drops of PVA on a slide and allow to air dry. As an alternative, the material may be smeared on the slide and fixed immediately in Schaudinn's fixative. Please indicate on the requisition slip as sigmoidoscopic specimen and that the slide(s) has been fixed.

Material from suspected amebic abscess: Preserve in PVA fixative.

Sputum for ameba: Preserve in PVA fixative.

Sputum for nematode larvae or *Paragonimus* eggs: Preserve in formalin.

Duodenal aspirate: Centrifuge specimen if necessary (>0.5 mL) for 2 minutes at 1500 rpm. Examine sediment for motile organisms. Examination of motile organisms is best performed at the local facility. If specimen is to be sent to the laboratory, mix the sediment with 1-2 drops of PVA on a glass slide and allow to air dry. As an alternative, the material may be smeared on the slide and fixed immediately in Schaudinn's fixative.

Bone marrow aspirates: Submit alcohol fixed bone marrow films. Aspirates may also be submitted in EDTA tubes.

Storage Instructions Do **not** refrigerate. Transport to laboratory as soon as possible after collection.

Causes for Rejection Specimen more than 4 hours old, specimen sent on swab, specimen consisting entirely of saliva, specimen contaminated with urine and/or water, specimen containing interfering substances, eg, castor oil, bismuth, Metamucil®, barium (upper or lower GI); specimen refrigerated, specimen contaminated on outside of container, biopsy in formalin, specimen dried out

Turnaround Time Variable – depending upon procedure required

Reference Range No ova or parasites seen

Use Establish the diagnosis of parasitic infestation

Limitations The specimen will be examined for parasites only. One negative result does not rule out the possibility of parasitic infestation. Three specimens over 5- to 7-day period are desirable before a negative report is acceptable.

(Continued)

Ova and Parasites, Urine or Aspirates *(Continued)*

Methodology Saline preparation, iodine preparation, trichome stain

Additional Information Patient should have a geographic history consistent with schistosomiasis to warrant undertaking screening the urine.

Selected Readings

Tsang VC and Wilkins PP, "Immunodiagnosis of Schistosomiasis. Screen with FAST-ELISA and Confirm With Immunoblot," *Clin Lab Med*, 1991, 11(4):1029-39.

p24 Antigen

Related Information

HIV-1 Serology *on page 368*

Synonyms HIV Core Antigen; HIV p24 Antigen

Applies To AIDS Antigen

Special Instructions Observe strict blood and body fluid precautions. In some states written or informed patient consent is a prerequisite for the test. Results may need to be kept confidential.

Specimen Serum or cerebrospinal fluid

Container Red top tube

Reference Range Negative

Use Diagnosis of recent acute infection with HIV; may also be of prognostic significance in AIDS, if antigen becomes positive during infection, after having been negative. (Can also be used to test viral culture supernatants.)

Limitations Test is not as sensitive as culture for detecting HIV infection.

Methodology Enzyme immunoassay

Additional Information p24 antigen is a 24 kD protein product of the **gag** gene of HIV. As a viral, rather than host, product, it appears concomitant with initial infection, and then generally becomes undetectable during periods of viral latency. It reappears with renewed viral replication; the reappearance of p24 antigen in serum generally heralds progression of clinical disease in AIDS. Measuring antigen may also be useful in assessing therapy. It has not been recommended as a further screening test for blood products for transfusion. However, recent studies indicate that an acid dissociation procedure that disrupts the p24 antigen-antibody complexes can increase the sensitivity of the procedure up to fivefold. This may improve its diagnostic utility.

Selected Readings

Bollinger RC Jr, Kline RL, Francis HL, et al, "Acid Dissociation Increases the Sensitivity of p24 Antigen Detection for the Evaluation of Antiviral Therapy and Disease Progression in Asymptomatic HIV-Infected Persons," *J Infect Dis*, 1992, 165(5):913-6.

PA *see* Chest Films *on page 293*

PA and Lateral CXR *see* Chest Films *on page 293*

PACE2® *see Chlamydia trachomatis* by DNA Probe *on page 297*

PACE2® *see Neisseria gonorrhoeae* by Nucleic Acid Probe *on page 411*

Paracentesis

Synonyms Abdominal Paracentesis; Ascites Fluid Tap

Test Includes At the bedside, physician introduces a needle into the peritoneal space of a patient with free ascites, and samples the fluid for diagnostic and/or therapeutic purposes.

Patient Preparation Technique and risks of the procedure are explained. Premedications (eg, sedatives or narcotics) are not routinely required. Laboratory requisitions are completed in advance to avoid delay in fluid processing later. Prothrombin and partial thromboplastin times prior to paracentesis are ordered at physician discretion (some elect to transfuse fresh frozen plasma immediately prior to procedure if PT/PTT are prolonged).

Aftercare No special limitations exist for the patient postprocedure. If large amounts of ascites are removed (several liters), frequent blood pressure measurements are needed to monitor possible hypotension. Patients may ambulate postprocedure if vital signs remain stable. Occasionally, ascites fluid may leak persistently from the puncture site; in this instance, the patient should remain supine with the site angled directly upwards, until the leak stops spontaneously.

Special Instructions In clinical practice, paracentesis is at times performed on patients with significant hepatic encephalopathy. Additional personnel may be required for conferring with family members and for proper patient positioning during the procedure.

Complications The medical literature is divided on the incidence of complications from paracentesis. Earlier literature was more negative and tended to emphasize the possible complications, based on retrospective analysis. Some authors suggested that paracentesis itself was the cause of many cases of ascites fluid infection. A recent prospective study concluded that paracentesis is a safe procedure, carrying <1% risk of major complications and <1% risk of minor complications. No deaths or bowel perforations were seen in 229 consecutive attempts. The most feared complication is needle perforation of an abdominal viscus or solid organ such as liver or spleen. Others include: intraperitoneal hemorrhage from laceration of an umbilical vein, scrotal or penile edema, abdominal wall hematoma, contamination of ascites by nonsterile technique. Hypotension can be seen when large amounts of ascites (>1500 mL) are removed rapidly.

Equipment Sterile gloves, drapes (optional), and adequate local anesthesia (26-gauge subcutaneous needle, 2% lidocaine). In clinical practice, various needles and angiocatheters are used. A 22-gauge, 1.5" metal needle with a plastic catheter is recommended. If a thick panniculus is encountered, a 3" to 5" 22-gauge needle may be substituted. Also required are a sterile 50 mL syringe and, if large volumes of ascites are to be removed, a sterile 1 L vacuum bottles with connecting tubing.

Technique Patient empties bladder prior to procedure. Physician confirms presence of ascites by physical examination with patient in a semirecumbent position. Preferred site of entry is in the midline, inferior to the umbilicus. If a midline scar is present from prior surgery or if percussion is not reliable, an area near the flank is selected. At times, physician may request patient to assume the hand-knees position if small amounts of ascites are present. The entry site is then caudad to the umbilicus. The site is prepped with iodine solution and skin and deeper tissues are infiltrated with lidocaine. The skin is retracted caudally and the 22-gauge needle (attached to syringe) is inserted into the anesthetized area and advanced while aspirating. When ascites fluid returns freely, the needle is held in position and not advanced further (avoiding bowel trauma). Multiple aliquots (50 mL) may be obtained in this manner. For larger volumes, the syringe is removed and connecting tubing is directly attached to the 22-gauge needle to allow drainage into vacuum bottles. Once the desired amount is collected, the needle is withdrawn quickly and the caudal skin retraction is released, allowing the skin to return to its normal position. This causes the entrance and exit needle sites to form a "Z-tract" which minimizes ascites leakage.

Data Acquired Ascites fluid is routinely analyzed for cell count and differential, chemistries including LD, albumin and protein, Gram stain, bacterial culture, and cytology. Additional tests include special cultures for tuberculosis or fungi, ascites fluid pH, amylase, lipase, glucose, triglycerides, lactate, CEA, and hyaluronic acid.

Specimen When the procedure is performed therapeutically, the maximum volume of ascites that can be removed safely depends on the presence or absence of peripheral edema. It is recommended that in patients without edema, the upper limit should be 1500 mL. Patients with peripheral edema may tolerate larger volumes without hypotension (in one study, ≤5 L). When performed for diagnostic purposes, smaller volumes (50-100 mL) are adequate for routine studies. If malignancy or fastidious infection is suspected, larger volumes (>100 mL) will improve laboratory yield.

Container Lavender top tube for cell count; red top tube for routine chemistries; aerobic and anaerobic culture media bottles for bacteriology. For cytology, send sterile vacuum bottles with 5000 units of heparin added. If ascites fluid pH desired, send specimen to laboratory in an anaerobic syringe (gas bubbles removed) on ice.

Collection Some authorities recommend inoculating the bacterial culture media with ascites fluid immediately at bedside. The average concentration of bacteria in ascites fluid is very low in most cases of spontaneous peritonitis. In addition, a significant number of organisms may not survive in the time needed for specimen transport and plating in the Microbiology Laboratory. Bedside inoculation of appropriate media (standard blood culture bottles) may improve the chances of obtaining a positive bacterial culture several fold.

Reference Range Ascites fluid is traditionally categorized as either "exudative" or "transudative" based on laboratory analysis. Transudative ascites is caused for the most part by cirrhosis physiology; that is, increased portal venous pressure or decreased portal venous colloid osmotic pressure. Examples of transudates include hepatic cirrhosis, congestive heart failure, constrictive pericar-

(Continued)

Paracentesis *(Continued)*

ditis, Budd-Chiari syndrome, inferior vena caval obstruction, and nephrotic syndrome. Exudative ascites is generally noncirrhotic in its pathophysiology and may be due to peritoneal membrane permeability defects. Examples of exudates include malignancy, spontaneous bacterial peritonitis (SBP), or other ascites infections (such as tuberculosis), vasculitis, pancreatitis, myxedema.

Critical Values Transudates are characteristically "low-protein" ascites and have been defined by ascites protein <3 g/dL; exudates >3 g/dL. Exceptions are common and other laboratory tests are often used in conjunction with the protein concentration. These include (for transudates): LD <200 units/L, protein ascites/serum ratio <0.5, LD ascites/serum ratio <0.6. Values outside these ranges support the diagnosis of an exudate. The "albumin gradient," defined as serum albumin minus ascites albumin, has recently been shown to accurately identify ascites caused by portal hypertension physiology (eg, cirrhosis). An albumin gradient >1.1 is considered transudative and is due to an oncotic (albumin) pressure gradient between the systemic arterial pressure and ascites fluid, as seen with elevated portal pressures. Exudates tend to have gradients <1.1. The early diagnosis of spontaneous bacterial peritonitis (SBP) prior to bacterial culture results can frequently be made on routine analysis of ascites fluid. Patients with SBP, or other ascites fluid infections, have ascites WBC count >500/mm^3 along with many polymorphonuclear (PMN) cells on the differential (>250/mm^3). In addition, two other laboratory indices suggestive of SBP are ascites pH <7.35 and ascites lactate <25 ng/dL. The clinical utility of these last two criteria has not been as well established as the standard PMN count. Many physicians will begin empiric antibiotics on the basis of PMN >250/mm^3 alone. Gram stain of ascites fluid has low sensitivity for detecting SBP due to the low bacterial concentration, even on a centrifuged sample. Malignant ascites can be expected to have abnormal cytology in >50% of the cases. Indirect evidence of neoplasm include: grossly hemorrhagic fluid (may also be traumatic); ascites CEA >10 ng/mL with adenocarcinoma; ascites hyaluronic acid >0.25 mg/mL with mesothelioma; high ascites triglyceride levels with chronic chylous ascites (>80% of cases are lymphoma); ascites WBC count >500/mm^3 with peritoneal carcinomatosis (but PMN count low, <250/mm^3), pH <7.35, lactate <25 mg/dL. None of these values are considered diagnostic of malignancy and should be used only as supportive evidence.

Use Diagnostic indications include:
- patients with new onset of ascites
- ascites fluid of unknown etiology
- patients with clinically suspected ascites fluid infections (abdominal pain, unexplained fever, leukocytosis, declining mental status)

Therapeutic paracentesis is indicated when ascites fluid has accumulated enough to cause respiratory compromise, abdominal pain, or worsening of existing inguinal or umbilical hernias. Paracentesis should not be performed to diagnose the presence of ascites fluid. This should be known prior to the procedure (by physical examination or radiological imaging).

Limitations As described previously, the strict use of the ascites protein concentration alone in differentiating exudate from transudate has considerable potential for error. Multiple criteria should be considered, including the albumin gradient and relevant clinical findings.

Contraindications Severe coagulopathy not correctable by vitamin K, fresh frozen plasma, etc; inability of physician to demonstrate ascites fluid on physical examination; lack of patient cooperation. Recent literature suggests the following factors are **not** contraindications for paracentesis: morbid obesity, low grade coagulopathy, multiple abdominal surgical scars, and bacteremia.

Additional Information Paracentesis is a safe procedure when ascites is easily demonstrable on physical examination. When small amounts of ascites are present, a fluid wave may be difficult to demonstrate even when ≤1.5 L ascites are present. CT scan or abdominal ultrasound guided needle aspiration is particularly useful in these cases. Patients with ascites from cirrhosis may develop SBP and yet have minimal evidence of infection; some patients may be completely asymptomatic. A low threshold for performing paracentesis is recommended in this setting, despite the low-grade coagulopathy that frequently is seen.

Selected Readings

Bender MD and Ockner RK, "Ascites," *Gastrointestinal Disease*, 4th ed, Sleisenger MH and Fordtran JS, eds, Philadelphia, PA: WB Saunders Co, 1988.
Conn HO, "Bacterial Peritonitis: Spontaneous or Paracentric?" *Gastroenterology*, 1979, 77(5):1145-6.

LABORATORY DIAGNOSIS

Hoefs JC and Runyon BA, "Spontaneous Bacterial Peritonitis," *Dis Mon*, 1985, 31(9):1-48.

Kao HW, Rakov NE, Savage E, et al, "The Effect of Large Volume Paracentesis on Plasma Volume – A Cause of Hypovolemia?" *Hepatology*, 1985, 5(3):403-7.

Liebowitz HR, "Hazards of Abdominal Paracentesis in the Cirrhotic Patient," *N Y State J Med*, 1962, 62:1822-6, 1997-2004, 2223-9.

Mallory A and Schaefer JW, "Complications of Diagnostic Paracentesis in Patients With Liver Disease," *JAMA*, 1978, 239(7):628-30.

Pare P, Talbot J, and Hoefs JC, "Serum Ascites Albumin Concentration Gradient: A Physiologic Approach to the Differential Diagnosis of Ascites," *Gastroenterology*, 1983, 85(2):240-4.

Pinzello G, Simonetti RG, and Craxi A, "Spontaneous Bacterial Peritonitis: A Prospective Investigation in Predominantly Nonalcoholic Cirrhotic Patients," *Hepatology*, 1983, 3(4):545-9.

Rocco VK and Ware AJ, "Cirrhotic Ascites: Pathophysiology, Diagnosis, and Management," *Ann Intern Med*, 1986, 105(4):573-85.

Runyon BA, Umland ET, and Merlin T, "Inoculation of Blood Culture Bottles With Ascitic Fluid; Improved Detection of Spontaneous Bacterial Peritonitis," *Arch Intern Med*, 1987, 147(1):73-5.

Yang CY, Liaw YF, Chu CM, et al, "White Count, pH, and Lactate in Ascites in the Diagnosis of Spontaneous Bacterial Peritonitis," *Hepatology*, 1985, 5(1):85-90.

Paracentesis Fluid Cytology *see* Cytology, Body Fluids
on page 318

Parainfluenza 1, 2, and 3 Virus Culture *see* Parainfluenza Virus
Culture *on this page*

Parainfluenza Virus Antigen, Direct Fluorescent Antibody

Related Information
Parainfluenza Virus Serology *on next page*

Test Includes Testing of appropriate clinical materials for presence of parainfluenza virus antigen

Special Instructions Before ordering, contact laboratory to determine if this test is available. DFA test should be performed as soon as possible.

Specimen Appropriate specimens include nasopharyngeal wash (specimen of choice), respiratory secretions (next most useful), nasopharyngeal swabs (less useful), tracheal aspirates, sputum, appropriate autopsy and biopsy specimens

Collection Specimen should be received fresh, not in fixative

Reference Range Negative

Use Identification of parainfluenza antigen in clinical specimens

Methodology Direct fluorescent antibody (DFA)

Additional Information This procedure does not depend on a changing antibody titer over time, and is diagnostic for the presence of virus (although the virus may not be the cause of the clinical illness in question). There is also a nonimmunologic cytologic change, ciliocytophthoria, which may be seen in sputum cytology and suggests parainfluenza infection.

Selected Readings
Waner JL, "Parainfluenza Viruses," *Manual of Clinical Microbiology*, 5th ed, Balows A, Hausler WJ Jr, Herrmann KL, et al, eds, Washington, DC: American Society for Microbiology, 1991, 878-82.

Parainfluenza Virus Culture

Related Information
Parainfluenza Virus Serology *on next page*
Viral Culture, Throat *on page 479*

Synonyms Parainfluenza 1, 2, and 3 Virus Culture

Test Includes Concurrent culture for other respiratory viruses (influenza, adenovirus, and respiratory syncytial viruses)

Specimen Throat or nasopharyngeal swab, nasopharyngeal washes and secretions

Container Sterile container; cold viral transport medium for swabs

Collection Place swabs into cold viral transport medium and keep cold. Infants and small children: soft catheters and suction devices (syringes and suction bulbs) can be used to collect nasal secretions (best specimens) as the catheter is withdrawn from far back in the nose. Another excellent method is to introduce 3-7 mL of sterile saline into the child's posterior nasal cavity and immediately aspirate the fluid.

(Continued)

Parainfluenza Virus Culture *(Continued)*

Storage Instructions Keep specimens ice cold but **do not freeze specimens**.

Causes for Rejection Dry specimen, specimen not refrigerated during transport, specimen fixed in formalin, unlabeled specimen

Turnaround Time Variable (5-14 days) and depends on culture method and amount of virus in specimen

Reference Range No virus isolated

Use Aid in the diagnosis of disease caused by parainfluenza virus

Methodology Inoculation of specimens into cell cultures, incubation of cultures, observation of cultures for hemadsorption or characteristic cytopathic effect, and identification/speciation by fluorescent monoclonal antibodies specific for types 1, 2, or 3 or by virus neutralization

Additional Information Most virology laboratories hemadsorb all viral (especially respiratory) cultures at 14 days (prior to discarding the culture) to detect hemadsorbing viruses that have not produced cytopathic effect by that time. Positive hemadsorption tests are often reported preliminarily as "hemadsorbing virus present." This result suggests the presence of influenza, parainfluenza, measles, and/or mumps virus.

Serology for the detection of parainfluenza antibodies is available, but the results are often difficult to interpret.

Selected Readings

Waner JL, "Parainfluenza Viruses," *Manual of Clinical Microbiology*, 5th ed, Balows A, Hausler WJ Jr, Herrmann KL, et al, eds, Washington, DC: American Society for Microbiology, 1991, 878-82.

Wright PF, "Parainfluenza Viruses," *Textbook of Human Virology*, Belshe RB, ed, Littleton, MA: PSG Publishing Co, 1984, 299-309.

Parainfluenza Virus, Direct Detection *see* Virus, Direct Detection by
Fluorescent Antibody *on page 480*

Parainfluenza Virus Serology

Related Information

Parainfluenza Virus Antigen, Direct Fluorescent Antibody
on previous page

Parainfluenza Virus Culture *on previous page*

Test Includes Antibody titers to parainfluenza virus types 1, 2, and 3

Specimen Serum

Container Red top tube or serum separator tube

Sampling Time Acute and convalescent sera drawn 10-14 days apart are recommended.

Causes for Rejection Inadequate labeling, gross contamination of specimen

Reference Range A single low titer or less than a fourfold change in titer in paired sera

Use Support the diagnosis of parainfluenza virus infection

Limitations Need for convalescent specimen delays diagnosis. Heterotypic rises in parainfluenza titers may occur in infections with other viruses. Infant antibody response may be undetectable.

Methodology Complement fixation (CF), hemagglutination inhibition (HAI), enzyme-linked immunosorbent assay (ELISA)

Additional Information Since the demonstration of a fourfold rise in antibody titer requires testing a convalescent specimen, serologic diagnosis is seldom useful in clinical management of an acute illness. This is especially so since the rise may occur even in an infection caused by some other virus. Serologic studies are of value in epidemiology. Rapid diagnosis during acute illness may be accomplished by demonstrating viral antigen in smears or tissue by immunofluorescence. Since parainfluenza virus may respond to ribavirin, prompt accurate diagnosis could become important, particularly in the immunocompromised host.

Selected Readings

Mufson MA and Belshe RB, "Respiratory Syncytial Virus and the Parainfluenza Viruses," *Manual of Clinical Laboratory Immunology*, 4th ed, Rose NR, de Macario EC, Fahey JL, et al, eds, Washington, DC: American Society for Microbiology, 1992.

Sperber SJ and Hayden FG, "Antiviral Chemotherapy and Prophylaxis of Viral Respiratory Disease," *Clin Lab Med*, 1987, 7(4):869-96.

Paranasal Sinuses, CT *see* Computed Transaxial Tomography,
Paranasal Sinuses *on page 308*

Parasites, Stool *see* Ova and Parasites, Stool *on page 416*

Parasites, Urine *see* Ova and Parasites, Urine or Aspirates *on page 419*

Parasitology Examination, Stool *see* Ova and Parasites, Stool *on page 416*

Parvovirus B19 Serology

Synonyms Anti-B19 Parvovirus IgG Antibodies; Anti-B19 Parvovirus IgM Antibodies

Test Includes Assays for parvovirus B19 IgM and IgG antibodies

Specimen Blood

Container Red top tube

Storage Instructions Separate serum and freeze.

Use Diagnose parvovirus B19 infection

Methodology Radioimmunoassay (RIA) or immunoblot assay (Western blot) for the detection of IgM and IgG antibodies to parvovirus B19

Additional Information Parvovirus B19 is a DNA virus and can cause a wide spectrum of disease ranging from outbreaks of self-limiting erythema infectiosum (Fifth disease) to persistent bone marrow failure and fetal death. Intrauterine transfusion has been suggested when there is evidence of B19 parvovirus-associated hydrops and anemia. In most people the low-titer parvovirus B19 viremia, which begins approximately 1 week after exposure and lasts 7-10 days, is associated with mild symptoms and a subclinical red cell aplasia. Because the virus destroys erythroid precursor cells, which leads to a reduction in normal red blood cell production, infection with parvovirus B19 can cause a transient aplastic crisis in patients already at maximum red cell production and in those with increased red cell destruction (sickle cell disease β-thalassemia, and spherocytosis). In immunocompromised patients, parvovirus B19 infection can cause life-threatening anemia. IgM antibodies are detectable 2 weeks after exposure. IgG antibody production usually occurs 18-24 days after exposure and is probably immune-complex mediated. The presence of IgM antibodies to parvovirus B19 provide definite evidence of recent infection.

Selected Readings

Patou G and Ayliffe U, "Evaluation of Commercial Enzyme-Linked Immunosorbent Assay for Detection of B19 Parvovirus IgM and IgG," *J Clin Pathol*, 1991, 44(10):831-4.

Rodis JF, Quinn DL, Gary GW Jr, et al, "Management and Outcome of Pregnancies Complicated by Human B19 Parvovirus Infection: A Prospective Study," *Am J Obstet Gynecol*, 1991, 164(4 Pt 1):1363-4

Patella of Knee, Left or Right, X-ray *see* Bone Films *on page 277*

Paul-Bunnell Test *replaced by* Infectious Mononucleosis Serology *on page 374*

PCR for HIV DNA *see* Human Immunodeficiency Virus DNA Amplification *on page 370*

Pediculus humanus Identification *see* Arthropod Identification *on page 268*

Pelvis AP, X-ray *see* Bone Films *on page 277*

Pelvis Stereo, X-ray *see* Bone Films *on page 277*

Pemphigus Antibodies *see* Skin Biopsy, Immunofluorescence *on page 446*

Penicillin Allergy Skin Testing

Synonyms Penicillin Skin Tests; Skin Tests for Penicillin Allergy

Test Includes Skin testing patients with suspected IgE-mediated penicillin allergy. The reagents used in this procedure are derivatives of the basic benzylpenicillin molecule. They are introduced into the epidermis by a skin prick or into the dermis by an intracutaneous (intradermal) injection. An immediate wheal-and-flare reaction confirms immediate hypersensitivity (Gell and Coombs' type I reaction). This is an important procedure in clinical practice and accurately identifies those individuals at high risk for a severe allergic reaction to penicillin.

Patient Preparation In some medical centers, penicillin skin testing is permitted only after formal consultation with the allergist performing the procedure. If the procedure appears necessary, the technique, risks, and benefits should

(Continued)

Penicillin Allergy Skin Testing (Continued)

be explained to the patient. As a preliminary screening measure, the physician should perform a brief dermatologic exam to ensure adequate areas of normal-appearing skin and to identify the rare patient with dermographism. Patient should be instructed to discontinue the following medications several days prior to testing: antihistamines, tricyclic antidepressants, hydroxyzine, phenothiazines. Newer antihistamines with extended half-lives may interfere with testing for over 1 week. All medication changes should be approved by the primary physician.

Aftercare If no complications have occurred, the patient may be discharged from the testing center following completion of the test. Skin sites should be kept clean but remain uncovered. Physician should be contacted immediately if symptoms of wheezing, lightheadedness, or shortness of breath develop several hours later (the unusual case of the "late phase response").

Special Instructions If skin testing is performed by a nurse or physician-assistant, a physician should be immediately available for the rare case of anaphylactic shock. Emergency equipment must be in the testing area, including defibrillation equipment, intubation blades, lidocaine (and other cardiac medications), aqueous epinephrine for injection needles, syringes, and tourniquets.

Complications When properly performed, serious adverse reactions are unusual. The incidence of systemic reactions has been estimated at <1%, with the majority of these being mild or self-limited. Local complications are more common, but generally resolve within hours. These include subcutaneous hemorrhage, localized pruritus, and nonspecific irritant reactions. The risk of hepatitis B, local infection, or human immunodeficiency virus (HIV) transmission is diminishingly small since needles are not reused between patients. The "late response" is a rare but reported complication of allergy skin testing.

Equipment The reagents used for skin testing include:

- The "major determinant," a derivative of the benzylpenicillin molecule called benzylpenicillin-polylysine. It is standardized, commercially available, and routinely used.
- The "minor determinant mixture (MDM)," either benzylpenicillin itself or another derivative (such as penicilloate or penicilloyl-amine). The MDM has not yet been standardized and is not commercially available. Nonetheless, the MDM is widely employed by many allergists and is clinically relevant.

Both the major and minor determinants are administered in most cases. If the major determinant is used alone, 10% to 25% of allergic individuals could be missed. If the minor determinant is used alone, perhaps 5% to 10% of cases could remain undetected, including potential cases of anaphylaxis. In addition to these two reagents, positive (histamine) and negative (diluent) controls are often given. Standard tuberculin syringes, 27-gauge needles, and prick test equipment are also needed.

Technique Ideally, skin test reagents are applied first by the prick test, followed by an intradermal test if the prick test is negative. The prick test is carried out by placing a drop of the reagent in a predetermined location on the skin, usually the forearm. A small needle is passed through the drop and into the epidermis, then removed. For intracutaneous testing, each reagent is individually drawn up into a tuberculin syringe. Again, the volar aspect of the forearm is the preferred site for testing. The reagent (or control) is injected into the dermis, using a 27-gauge needle. A small bleb is raised, usually 0.01-0.02 mL.

Data Acquired Test sites are examined at 15-20 minutes for a local wheal-and-flare reaction. The largest diameter of the wheal and/or erythema is measured and recorded in millimeters.

Reference Range No wheal or erythema after the major determinant, minor determinant, and diluent control. Administration of histamine control should result in a positive skin reaction, with induration >5 mm diameter.

Critical Values For both the prick test and the intracutaneous test, a wheal >5 mm in diameter (with erythema) is considered a positive test. For proper interpretation, the patient should be questioned regarding a history of penicillin allergy. If a reasonable history of penicillin allergy is obtained, a negative skin test essentially rules out a life-threatening allergic response to therapeutic doses of penicillin. No cases of anaphylaxis have been reported in patients who are skin test negative. However, ≤3% of patients who are skin test negative may develop minor reactions while on therapy, such as rash and pruritus. In the patient who has a positive skin test and a positive history of penicillin allergy, the odds of a serious allergic reaction to penicillin therapy are quite high, perhaps 50% to 70%. If skin tests are administered to patients who provide no history of penicillin allergy, the chances of a positive test are low (about 2%). Unfortunately, anaphylaxis during penicillin therapy has been reported in this patient population, although rare. Skin testing all patients prior to beta-lactam therapy, with or without a history of penicillin allergy, is not practical or cost-effective.

Use Theoretically, all patients about to receive a beta-lactam antibiotic should be skin tested. However, it has been demonstrated that such a comprehensive testing policy has a low yield and is not cost-effective. Most authorities recommend skin testing in the following situations:

- patients with a history of penicillin allergy who require penicillin as the drug of choice (eg, treatment of central nervous system syphilis)
- patients with a history of penicillin allergy who require a beta-lactam antibiotic (eg, semisynthetic penicillin, cephalosporin)
- patients with a history of multiple "antibiotic allergies;" skin testing can determine if a beta-lactam drug is a safe treatment option.

Limitations

- This procedure detects only IgE-mediated allergic reactions. Thus, a variety of adverse drug reactions may still occur in skin test negative patients, including serum sickness, drug fever, antibiotic associated colitis, interstitial nephritis, contact dermatitis, bone marrow suppression, and others.
- A number of factors can cause false-positive and false-negative results, as seen in other forms of skin testing.
- Test results apply to penicillin-type antibiotics (natural penicillins, semisynthetic penicillins), but not to cephalosporins, aztreonam, or imipenem.

Contraindications

- Documented history of penicillin-induced anaphylaxis, Stevens-Johnson syndrome, exfoliative dermatitis, or status asthmaticus. These conditions are life-threatening and contraindicate the use of penicillins in general; thus, there is little need to skin test.
- Recent use of medications known to inhibit the IgE-mediated skin response (wheal and flare); this includes antihistamines, hydroxyzine, tricyclic antidepressants, and phenothiazines

Selected Readings

Sarti W, "Routine Use of Skin Testing for Immediate Penicillin Allergy to 6764 Patients in an Outpatient Clinic," *Ann Allergy*, 1985, 55(2):157-61.

VanArsdel PP Jr, Martonick GJ, Johnson LE, et al, "The Value of Skin Testing for Penicillin Allergy Diagnosis," *West J Med*, 1986, 144(3):311-4.

Weiss ME and Adkinson NF Jr, "β-Lactam Allergy," *Principles and Practice of Infectious Diseases*, 4th ed, Mandell GL, Bennett JE, and Dolin R, eds, New York, NY: Churchill Livingstone, 1995, 272-8.

Weiss ME and Adkinson NF, "Immediate Hypersensitivity Reactions to Penicillin and Related Antibiotics," *Clin Allergy*, 1988, 18(6):515-40.

Penicillinase-Producing Organisms Susceptibility Testing *see* Penicillinase Test *on this page*

Penicillinase Test

Related Information

Antimicrobial Susceptibility Testing, Aerobic and Facultatively Anaerobic Organisms *on page 259*

Antimicrobial Susceptibility Testing, Anaerobic Bacteria *on page 260*

Neisseria gonorrhoeae Culture *on page 412*

Synonyms Beta-Lactamase Production Test; Cefinase (Nitrocefin) Testing; Cephalosporinase Production Testing; Penicillinase-Producing Organisms Susceptibility Testing

Applies To Beta-Lactam Ring; *Haemophilus influenzae* Susceptibility Testing; *Neisseria gonorrhoeae* Susceptibility Testing

Test Includes Rapid testing of isolated bacterial colonies for the production of beta-lactamase

Abstract Certain bacteria produce enzymes that inactivate beta-lactam antibiotics. Some enzymes can hydrolyze penicillin (penicillinases); others hydrolyze cephalosporins (cephalosporinases). In either case the detection of enzyme production by bacterial isolates is essential in determination of appropriate therapy.

Specimen *Haemophilus influenzae*, *Moraxella* (*Branhamella*) *catarrhalis*, *Neisseria gonorrhoeae*, enterococci, *Staphylococcus* species or gram-negative anaerobic rods including *Bacteroides fragilis*

(Continued)

427

Penicillinase Test *(Continued)*

Use Rapid detection of beta-lactamase production from isolated colonies of *Haemophilus influenzae, Neisseria gonorrhoeae, Moraxella catarrhalis, S. aureus*, and enterococci sp. This test can be used to predict resistance to penicillins and some cephalosporins. Most isolates of *Staphylococcus aureus* produce beta-lactamases and thus, are often treated as beta-lactamase positive without testing for enzyme production.

Methodology The acidimetric method uses pH color indicators to detect increased acidity that results when the beta-lactam ring of penicillin is cleaved to yield a penicilloic acid. Penicilloic acid can also reduce iodine that can be detected as the decolorization of a starch-iodine mixture. This method is referred to as the iodometric method. The most commonly used method is the use of a chromogenic cephalosporin reagent. The hydrolysis of the beta-lactam ring results in a color change that is quickly detected. The chromogenic assay can detect both penicillinases and cephalosporinases.

Additional Information The nitrocefin method is favored for anaerobes because it can detect both the cephalosporinases produced by *Bacteroides fragilis* and *Prevotella melaninogenica* (*Bacteroides melaninogenicus*), as well as, the penicillinases produced by other anaerobes. This is also the method recommended for testing *M. catarrhalis* and *S. aureus* isolates.

Plasmid-mediated production of beta-lactamase occurs in 5% to 15% of clinical isolates of *H. influenzae* type b. However, other mechanisms of resistance have also been reported. Routine testing of *H. influenzae* for beta-lactamase production is performed by most laboratories. Strains of *N. gonorrhoeae* producing beta-lactamase have been linked to contacts of patients acquiring the infection outside the United States and in prostitutes and sexual contacts of drug users. Incidence of penicillinase-producing *N. gonorrhoeae* has increased drastically in Florida, California, and New York. Routine testing of *N. gonorrhoeae* for beta-lactamase production is not routinely necessary in many parts of the United States, but should be considered in treatment failure cases and in areas in which resistance is endemic.

Selected Readings
Bell SM and Plowman D, "Mechanisms of Ampicillin Resistance in *Haemophilus influenzae* From Respiratory Tract," *Lancet*, 1980, 1(8163):279-80.

Handsfield HH, Rice RJ, Roberts MC, et al, "Localized Outbreak of Penicillinase-Producing *Neisseria gonorrhoeae* Paradigm for Introduction and Spread of Gonorrhea in a Community," *JAMA*, 1989, 261(16):2357-61.

Rosenblatt JE, "Susceptibility Testing of Anaerobic Bacteria," *Clin Lab Med*, 1989, 9(2):239-54. (review).

Stratton CW and Cooksey RC, "Susceptibility Tests: Special Tests," *Manual of Clinical Microbiology*, 5th ed, Balows A, Hausler WJ Jr, Herrmann KL, et al, eds, Washington, DC: American Society for Microbiology, 1991, 1153-65.

Penicillin Skin Tests *see* Penicillin Allergy Skin Testing *on page 425*

Percutaneous Biopsy of Musculoskeletal Lesions and Synovial Membranes *see* Bone Biopsy *on page 276*

Percutaneous Liver Biopsy *see* Liver Biopsy *on page 387*

Percutaneous Needle Aspiration Biopsy Under Fluoroscopic, CT, or Ultrasound Guidance *see* Liver Biopsy *on page 387*

Percutaneous Transtracheal Culture Routine *see* Aerobic Culture, Sputum *on page 246*

Percutaneous Transtracheal Fungus Culture *see* Fungus Culture, Bronchial Aspirate *on page 342*

Percutaneous Transtracheal Fungus Culture *see* Fungus Culture, Sputum *on page 345*

Percutaneous Transtracheal Mycobacteria Culture *see* Mycobacteria Culture, Sputum *on page 406*

Pericardial Fluid Culture *see* Aerobic Culture, Body Fluid *on page 244*

Pericardial Fluid Cytology *see* Cytology, Body Fluids *on page 318*

Pericardial Fluid Fungus Culture *see* Fungus Culture, Body Fluid *on page 341*

Peripheral Arteries and Veins Ultrasound *see* Ultrasound, Peripheral Arteries and Veins *on page 466*

Peripheral Blood Preparation *see* Microfilariae, Peripheral Blood Preparation *on page 400*

Peripheral Blood Smear, *Bartonella* *see* Peripheral Blood Smear, Thick and Thin *on this page*

Peripheral Blood Smear, Thick and Thin
Related Information
Microfilariae, Peripheral Blood Preparation *on page 400*

Synonyms Blood Smear for Malarial Parasites; Malarial Parasites; Malaria Smear; Thin and Thick Smears, Blood

Applies To Peripheral Blood Smear, *Bartonella*

Test Includes Examination of thick and thin smears

Abstract Malaria is still one of the most common infectious disease in the world. Its rapid diagnosis in the laboratory is extremely important. Although there are not many cases in the United States, with more world travel, it can be expected to increase.

Special Instructions If the patient has traveled to a malaria-endemic area the date and area traveled should be communicated to the laboratory. Most cases of malaria seen in the U.S. are found in foreign nationals traveling in the United States.

Specimen Fresh blood – fresh fingerstick smears (two or three of each thick and thin film type) made at bedside preferred, EDTA anticoagulated blood for saponin lysis. Contact laboratory for preparation of thick and thin smears.

Container Slides and lavender top (EDTA) tube

Collection Several samples should be taken during a 24-hour period until diagnosis is established or excluded.

Causes for Rejection Specimen clotted

Reference Range No organisms identified

Use Diagnose malaria, parasitic infestation of blood; evaluate febrile disease of unknown origin

Limitations One negative result does not rule out the possibility of parasitic infestation. If protozoal, filarial, or trypanosomal infection is strongly suspected, test should be performed at least three times with samples obtained at different times in the fever cycle.

Malaria Species Infecting Human Red Cells

Plasmodium Species	Malaria	Length of Cycle (hours)
P. vivax	Tertian	45
P. falciparum	Malignant tertian	48
P. ovale	Ovale	48
P. malariae	Quartan	72

Methodology Microscopic examination of thick and thin Giemsa-stained smears. Thick films are more difficult to read and require considerable experience to interpret. Use of thick smears increases the number of cells examined in a given time period by a factor of about 12 because infected cells and organisms are concentrated. Screening by fluorescent microscopy using acridine orange and with gene probes have been described. Thin smears, although not as sensitive, are far superior for determining the species of *Plasmodium* on morphological grounds.

Additional Information Proper therapy depends upon identification of the specific variety of malaria parasite. Release of trophozoites and RBC debris results in a febrile response. Periodicity of fever correlates with type of malaria (see table). Organisms are most likely to be detected just before onset of fever which is predictable in many cases. Sampling immediately upon onset of fever is the most desirable time to obtain blood. Cases with a strong clinical history, which prove negative on initial laboratory screening, may require multiple sampling at different times in the fever cycle to document the diagnosis. Malarial parasites are destroyed in AS and SS patients. The cause of parasite death in

(Continued)

Peripheral Blood Smear, Thick and Thin *(Continued)*

Changes in Infected RBCs
Useful in Identification of Malaria Species

Plasmodium Species	Infected RBC Enlarged	Presence of Schüffner Dots	Presence of Maurer Dots	Multiple Parasites per RBC	Parasite With Double Chromatin Dots	Parasite With Sausage-Shaped Gametocytes	Usually Only Rings and Gametes Seen
P. vivax	+	+	—	Rare	Rare	—	—
P. falciparum	—	—	+	+	+	+	+
P. ovale	±	+	—	—	—	—	—
P. malariae	—	—	+	—	—	—	—

AS cells is potassium loss, in SS cells Hb S aggregates destroy the parasites by physical penetration.

Selected Readings
Krogstad DJ, Visvesvara GS, Walls KW, et al, "Blood and Tissue Protozoa," *Manual of Clinical Microbiology*, 5th ed, Balows A, Hausler WJ, Herrmann KL, et al, eds, Washington, DC: American Society for Microbiology, 1991, 727-50.

Pammenter MD, "Techniques for the Diagnosis of Malaria," *S Afr Med J*, 1988, 74(2):55-7.

Peritoneal Fluid Culture *see* Aerobic Culture, Body Fluid
on page 244

Peritoneal Fluid Cytology *see* Cytology, Body Fluids
on page 318

Peritoneal Fluid Fungus Culture *see* Fungus Culture, Body Fluid
on page 341

Pertussis Culture *see* Bordetella pertussis Nasopharyngeal Culture
on page 283

Pertussis Serology *see* Bordetella pertussis Serology
on page 284

Phthirus pubis Identification *see* Arthropod Identification
on page 268

Pinworm Preparation
Related Information
Ova and Parasites, Stool *on page 416*

Synonyms Enterobiasis Test; *Enterobius vermicularis* Preparation; Ova and Parasite, Pinworm Preparation; Scotch® Tape Test

Specimen Scotch® Tape slide preparation of perianal region

Container Scotch® Tape slide must be submitted in a covered container. Commercial kit products are also available for collection of pinworm specimens and are convenient, inexpensive, and highly recommended. **Caution**: Pinworm eggs are very infectious.

Collection The specimen is best obtained a few hours after the patient has retired (ie, 10 or 11 PM), or early in the morning before a bowel movement or bath. This collection procedure is essential if valid results are expected. Clear Scotch® Tape should be used. The nontransparent type is unsatisfactory. An 8 cm (3 in) piece of cellophane tape is placed over the end of a glass slide sticky side out. The anal folds are spread apart and the mucocutaneous junction is firmly pressed in all four quadrants. The tape is then pressed over the slide and the specimen is transported to the laboratory in a carefully sealed container. Refer to diagram on following page.

Causes for Rejection Use of nontransparent Scotch® Tape, Scotch® Tape on both sides of the slide, specimen which is not inside a covered container, use of frosted slide, tape sent sticky side up. Specimens which are not properly contained pose excessive risk to laboratory personnel and may not be acceptable to the laboratory.

Reference Range No pinworm eggs (*Enterobius vermicularis*) identified. Positives reported as few, moderate, or many eggs identified.

Use Detect cases of pinworm infestation (enterobiasis), *Enterobius vermicularis* parasitic infestation

Cellophane tape slide preparation. Attach 3'' piece of cellophane tape to undersurface of clear end of microscope slide, which has previously been identified (ground–glass end). Press sticky surface of tape against perianal skin. Then roll back tape onto slide, sticky surface down. Wash hands and nails well. From Bauer JD, *Clinical Laboratory Methods*, 9th ed, Mosby–Year Book Inc, St Louis, MO: 1982, 989, with permission.

Limitations Examination for pinworm only. One negative result does not rule out possibility of parasitic infestation. Stool specimens are not satisfactory for pinworm studies.

Contraindications Specimen collection at improper time

Additional Information The most satisfactory means of diagnosing pinworm infection is by the recovery of eggs or female worms from the perianal region. Only 5% to 10% of infected persons have demonstrable eggs in their stools. If feces is submitted for examination, only the surface should be sampled. Enterobiasis often is present in multiple family members. Therefore, it is recommended that all members of the family be tested. The responsible parent should be instructed how to collect samples using one kit per individual. Female worms or parts of them may be demonstrated on the tape by microscopic examination. Eggs, if present, may be immature, embryonated (with viable or dead larvae), or empty egg shells if the specimen is several days or more old. *Enterobius vermicularis* has been reported as a rare cause of appendicitis, salpingitis, epididymitis, and hepatic granuloma. Diagnosis at colonoscopy has also been reported.

Selected Readings
Bauer JD, "Parasitology," *Clinical Laboratory Methods*, 9th ed, St Louis, MO: CV Mosby Co, 1982, 987-9.

Pleural Fluid Culture *see* Aerobic Culture, Body Fluid
on page 244

Pleural Fluid Cytology *see* Cytology, Body Fluids *on page 318*

Pleural Fluid Fungus Culture *see* Fungus Culture, Body Fluid
on page 341

Pleural Fluid, *Legionella* Culture *see* Legionella pneumophila Culture
on page 381

Pleural Fluid "Tap" *see* Thoracentesis *on page 453*

Pneumocystis carinii Test

Applies To Biopsy of Lung (Transbronchial) for *Pneumocystis*; Bronchial Aspiration for *Pneumocystis*; Bronchopulmonary Lavage for *Pneumocystis*; Induced Sputum Technique for *Pneumocystis*; Transthoracic Needle Aspiration for *Pneumocystis*

Test Includes Methenamine silver stain; toluidine blue stain and/or Giemsa and/or Wright's stain, or monoclonal antibodies to *Pneumocystis*

Abstract Diagnosis of *Pneumocystis* pneumonia in patients with or without AIDS.

Patient Preparation Induced sputum technique: Gargle with 30 mL 3% NaCl, then inhalation of 3% NaCl mist from an ultrasonic nebulizer for 5-15 minutes.

Specimen Lung biopsy, transthoracic needle aspirate, bronchopulmonary lavage or induced sputum technique

Container Sterile jar, clean glass slides

Collection When inoculating needle aspirate on slides, single drops should be applied. They may be alcohol-fixed or allowed to air dry without spreading. Bi-
(Continued)

Pneumocystis carinii **Test** *(Continued)*

opsy specimens should be submitted in formalin. Jar must be labeled with patient's name, room number, date, and time. Slides must bear patient's name.

Causes for Rejection Inadequate specimen for diagnosis

Use Diagnosis of *Pneumocystis carinii* pneumonia, eg, in acquired immune deficiency syndrome (AIDS) and other immunocompromised conditions

Limitations *Pneumocystis* preparations applied to spontaneously expectorated sputum have an extremely low yield. In about 40% of individuals with AIDS and symptomatic pneumonia caused by other agents one may anticipate *P. carinii* in bronchoalveolar lavage fluid.

Methodology Methenamine silver stain (GMS), immunofluorescence, toluidine blue stain

Additional Information This organism is found in patients with clinical diffuse interstitial pneumonitis. Immunocompromised patients have a high incidence of *Pneumocystis carinii* infection (as high as 44% in some series). *Pneumocystis* pneumonia may be, but is not always, rapidly progressive. It may be life-threatening, so that rapid diagnosis is important to allow prompt institution of therapy. *Pneumocystis carinii* is the most frequent cause of death in children with ALL in remission, such that some institutions routinely give prophylactic trimethoprim-sulfamethoxazole to their leukemic children undergoing antineoplastic therapy. It is also the most common infection and the most common cause of death in patients with AIDS.

Selected Readings

Cameron RB, Watts JC, and Kasten BL, "*Pneumocystis carinii* Pneumonia. An Approach to Rapid Laboratory Diagnosis," *Am J Clin Pathol*, 1979, 72(1):90-3.

"Case Records of the Massachusetts General Hospital. Weekly Clinicopathological Exercises. Case 8-1987. A 44 Month-Old Girl With Fever of Unknown Origin After Repair of the Tetralogy of Fallot," *N Engl J Med*, 1987, 316(8):466-75.

Chalvardjian AM and Grawe LA, "A New Procedure for the Identification of *Pneumocystis carinii* in Tissue Sections and Smears," *J Clin Pathol*, 1963, 16:383-4.

Goodell B, Jacobs JB, Powell RD, et al, "*Pneumocystis carinii*: The Spectrum of Diffuse Interstitial Pneumonia in Patients With Neoplastic Diseases," *Ann Intern Med*, 1970, 72(3):337-40.

Kim HK and Hughes WT, "Comparison of Methods for Identification of *Pneumocystis carinii* in Pulmonary Aspirates," *Am J Clin Pathol*, 1973, 60(4):462-6.

Smith JW and Bartlett MS, "Diagnosis of *Pneumocystis* Pneumonia," *Lab Med*, 1979, 10:429.

Poliovirus Antibody *see* Poliovirus Serology *on this page*

Poliovirus Culture *see* Enterovirus Culture *on page 331*

Poliovirus Culture, Stool *see* Viral Culture, Stool *on page 478*

Poliovirus Serology

Synonyms Poliovirus Antibody

Specimen Serum

Container Red top tube

Collection Acute and convalescent sera drawn 10-14 days apart are required

Reference Range A fourfold increase in titer in paired sera is diagnostic; presence of neutralizing antibody indicates adequate immunization; normal <1:8

Use Support for the diagnosis of poliovirus infection, documentation of previous exposure to poliovirus (complement fixing antibodies); documentation of immunization (neutralizing antibodies)

Methodology Viral neutralization, complement fixation

Additional Information Poliovirus may also be cultured, producing a characteristic cytopathic effect in cell culture. Culture is more suitable than serology for diagnosis of acute infection.

Selected Readings

Melnick JL, "Enteroviruses," *Manual of Clinical Laboratory Immunology*, 4th ed, Rose NR, de Macario EC, Fahey JL, et al, eds, Washington, DC: American Society for Microbiology, 1992, 631-3.

Popliteal Ultrasound *see* Ultrasound, Peripheral Arteries and Veins *on page 466*

Postexposure Prophylaxis for Hepatitis B *see page 719*

Postreduction Films, X-ray *see* Bone Films *on page 277*

Potassium Hydroxide Preparation *see* KOH Preparation *on page 379*

PPD Test *see* Tuberculin Skin Testing, Intracutaneous
on page 463

PPLO Culture *see Mycoplasma/Ureaplasma* Culture *on page 410*

PPLO Titer *see Mycoplasma* Serology *on page 410*

Prostatic Fluid Culture *see* Genital Culture *on page 349*

Prostatic Fluid Culture *Neisseria gonorrhoeae* *see Neisseria
gonorrhoeae* Culture *on page 412*

***Proteus* OX-19** *replaced by* Rocky Mountain Spotted Fever Serology
on page 437

Pseudomembranous Colitis Toxin Assay *see Clostridium difficile*
Toxin Assay *on page 300*

Pubic Lice Identification *see* Arthropod Identification
on page 268

Purified Protein Derivative (PPD) Test *see* Tuberculin Skin Testing,
Intracutaneous *on page 463*

Q Fever Serology
Synonyms *Coxiella burnetii* Titer
Special Instructions Acute and convalescent samples are recommended.
Specimen Serum
Container Red top tube
Reference Range Titer of less than 1:2; comparison of acute and convalescent
titers is of greatest diagnostic value
Use Used to support a diagnosis of Q fever due to *Coxiella burnetii*
Limitations Reagents prepared from fresh isolates (phase I organisms) react
differently from those from multiply-passaged organism (phase II)
Methodology Complement fixation (CF), indirect fluorescent antibody (IFA)
Additional Information Q fever shows no reaction in the Weil-Felix test with
Proteus antigen, so serologic diagnosis must be based on specific rickettsial
antigen. Convalescent sera react best with phase II organism (see above), but
sera from chronic persistent infection react best with phase I organisms. Cross
reactions with *Legionella* have been described.
Selected Readings
Eisemann CS and Osterman JV, "*Rickettsia*," *Manual of Clinical Laboratory Immunology*, 3rd
ed, Rose NR, Friedman H, and Fahey JL, eds, Washington, DC: American Society for Microbiology, 1986, 847-58.
Hechemy KE, "The Immunoserology of Rickettsiae," *Manual of Clinical Laboratory Immunology*, 4th ed, Rose NR, de Macario EC, Fahey JL, et al, eds, Washington, DC: American
Society for Microbiology, 1992, 667-75.
Reimer LG, "Q Fever," *Clin Microbiol Rev*, 1993, 6(3):193-8.

Rabid Animals *see* Rabies *on this page*

Rabies
Related Information
Animal and Human Bites Guidelines *on page 736-739*
Brain Biopsy *on page 285*
Synonyms Rabid Animals
Applies To Fluorescent Rabies Antibody Test; FRA Test; Negri Bodies
Test Includes Examination of animal brain for Negri bodies or inoculation of
mice with suspension of brain tissue
Abstract Rabies has been a recognized disease in humans and animals for
more than 25 centuries. Zinke is credited with first demonstrating the virus in
1804. Unlike many other viruses, the rabies virus is capable of infecting a num-
ber of different animal species, allowing it to propagate and survive in nature.
Individuals with a high risk of contact with rabid animals (veterinarians, animal
control officers, etc) should consider vaccination against rabies.
Specimen Head of large animal or entire small animal suspected of rabies. Use
gloves and mask when handling an animal carcass suspected of rabies.
Container Sealed container
Storage Instructions Ideally, animal brain should be examined in the fresh
state. Transport using wet ice or place in absorbent material, then in two plastic bags, or, place half the brain in 50% glycerol, half in 10% formalin, depending on instructions from state laboratory. Local state laboratory must be con-
(Continued)

LABORATORY DIAGNOSIS
Rabies *(Continued)*

sulted. Rabies virus may also be demonstrated by immunofluorescence in skin biopsies of patients suspected of having rabies (*vide infra*).

Causes for Rejection Unlabeled or improperly packaged specimen

Use Diagnose rabies; evaluate animal bites

Limitations Negri bodies are found in about 90% of rabid animals.

Contraindications Formalin fixation precludes fluorescent antibody application

Methodology Fluorescent antibody examination (but Negri bodies can be seen in H & E)

Additional Information Animals at risk for rabies include skunks, raccoons, dogs, cats, bats, cattle, foxes, and to a lesser extent, jackals, wolves, coyotes, mongooses, weasels, squirrels, and any escaped wild animal. Bites of rabbits, squirrels, hamsters, guinea pigs, gerbils, chipmunks, rats, mice, and other rodents have seldom if ever resulted in human rabies in the United States and are regarded as low risk. High risk species include bats, raccoons, skunks, and foxes among wild carnivorous animals.

Domestic animals should be kept alive if possible, to be quarantined. Animal bites, when unprovoked, are more likely to transmit rabies. Survival of animal for 10 days makes rabies unlikely. Signs of rabies among wild carnivorous animals cannot be reliably interpreted and any such animal that bites or scratches a person should be killed at once and the head submitted for rabies testing.

Rabies is a zoonosis caused by a neurotropic RNA virus which occurs in saliva, central nervous system, urine, and feces. Rabies virus produces Negri bodies (viral inclusions) in neurons.

The geographic area is important. Although a dog bite along the U.S.–Mexican border is considered a rabies exposure until proven otherwise, such bites in New York or Philadelphia are reported not to require prophylaxis. Most Americans dying of rabies were exposed in foreign countries. One patient, bitten by a rabid dog in Kenya, had even had pre-exposure prophylaxis with human diploid cell vaccine. This emphasizes the **necessity for postexposure therapy in appropriate cases.** Almost all rabies follows bite exposure. However, rabies virus can (rarely) enter through nonbite exposure, such as an open wound, or by inhalation of aerosolized bat urine (eg, cave explorers) or by corneal transplantation. The following table lists location of exposure to rabid canine bites and extent of exposure as it relates to mortality rates. The proportion of cases for which the source of exposure is not known has been increasing since 1960.

Representative Mortality Rates in Nonvaccinated Individuals Following Exposure to Rabid Canines

Location of Exposure	Extent of Exposure	Mortality (%)
Face	Bites (multiple and severe)	60
Other part of head	Bites (multiple and severe)	50
Face	Bite (single)	30
Fingers/hand	Bite (severe)	15
Face	Bites (multiple and superficial)	10
Hand	Bites (multiple and superficial)	5
Trunk/legs	Scratch	3
Hands/exposed skin	Bleeding and superficial wound	2
Skin covered by clothes	Superficial wound	0.5
Recent wound	Saliva	0.1
Wounds >24 h old	Saliva	0.0

From Whitley RJ and Middlebrooks M, "Rabies," *Infections of the Central Nervous System,* Chapter 7, Scheld WM, Whitley RJ, and Durack DT, eds, New York, NY: Raven Press, 1991, 134, with permission.

Antemortem rabies virus has been isolated from human saliva, brain tissues, CSF, urine sediment, and tracheal secretions. Rabies virus may also be demonstrated by immunofluorescent rabies antibody staining of skin biopsy tissue. The most reliable and reproducible of the immunofluorescent studies that can aid in patient diagnosis is biopsy of the neck skin. A 6-8 mm full thickness wedge or punch biopsy specimen from the neck containing as many hair follicles as possible should be sampled, snap frozen, and shipped frozen at -70°C to a reference laboratory. Consult with reference laboratory for shipping instructions. False-negative results do occur especially after the development of neutralizing antibodies.

Selected Readings

Fishbein DB and Bernard KW , "Rabies Virus," *Principles and Practice of Infectious Diseases*, Mandell GL, Bennett JE, and Dolin R, eds, New York, NY: Churchill Livingstone, 1995, 1527-43.

Bussereau F, Vincent J, Coudrier D, et al, "Monoclonal Antibodies to Mokola Virus for Identification of Rabies and Rabies-Related Viruses," *J Clin Microbiol*, 1988, 26(12):2489-94.

Center for Disease Control, "Compendium of Animal Rabies Control, 1990," *MMWR Morb Mortal Wkly Rep*, 1990, 39(RR-4):1-8.

Center for Disease Control, "Human Rabies – Oregon," *MMWR Morb Mortal Wkly Rep*, 1989, 38(19):335-7.

Center for Disease Control, "Rabies Prevention – United States, 1991 – Recommendations of the Immunization Practices Advisory Committee (ACIP)," *MMWR Morb Mortal Wkly Rep*, 1991, 40(RR-3):1-19.

Dietzschold B, Tollis M, Rupprecht CE, et al, "Antigenic Variation in Rabies and Rabies-Related Viruses: Cross-Protection Independent of Glycoprotein-Mediated Virus-Neutralizing Antibody," *J Infect Dis*, 1987, 156:815.

Fishbein DB and Baer GM, "Animal Rabies: Implications for Diagnosis and Human Treatment," *Ann Intern Med*, 1988, 109(12):935-7.

Mrak, RE and Young L, "Rabies Encephalitis in a Patient With No History of Exposure," *Hum Pathol*, 1992, 24(1):109-10.

Smith JS, Fishbein DB, Rupprecht CE, et al, "Unexplained Rabies in Three Immigrants in the United States. A Virologic Investigation," *N Engl J Med*, 1991, 324(4):205-11.

Whitley RJ and Middlebrooks M, "Rabies," *Infections of the Central Nervous System*, Scheld WM, Whitley RJ, and Durack DT, eds, New York, NY: Raven Press, 1991, 134.

Rabies Virus, Direct Detection see Virus, Direct Detection by Fluorescent Antibody *on page 480*

Radionuclide Bone Scan see Bone Scan *on page 281*

Rapid Plasma Reagin Test see RPR *on page 438*

Rectal Swab Culture see Stool Culture *on page 448*

Rectal Swab Culture for Diarrheagenic, *E. coli* see Stool Culture, Diarrheagenic *E. coli on page 449*

Rectal Swab, Unusual Organism see Stool Culture, Uncommon Organisms *on page 451*

Renal Ultrasound see Ultrasound, Kidneys *on page 466*

Respiratory Syncytial Virus Antigen by EIA

Related Information

Respiratory Syncytial Virus Culture *on next page*
Respiratory Syncytial Virus Serology *on next page*

Synonyms RSV Testing

Test Includes Enzyme immunoassay for respiratory syncytial virus infection

Specimen Nasopharyngeal washes or aspirates, sputum, appropriate autopsy or biopsy specimens

Container Capped syringe

Collection Send specimen fresh, not in fixative. Tissues may be snap frozen.

Causes for Rejection Inadequate specimen

Reference Range No virus detected.

Use Identify respiratory syncytial virus, particularly in infants and young children

Limitations Inadequate specimen collection, improper sample handling/ transport or low levels of virus shedding may yield false-negative result. Accordingly, a negative result does not totally eliminate the possibility of RSV infection.

Additional Information This test allows rapid diagnosis of the presence of respiratory syncytial virus. It avoids the necessity of obtaining acute and convalescent specimens over a 2-week period. It may be particularly useful in children younger than 6 months of age, whose antibody response to infection may not be diagnostic. However, it must be remembered that showing the virus is present is not equivalent to showing that it is causing a particular disease.

Selected Readings

Hughes JH, Mann DR, and Hamparian VV, "Detection of Respiratory Syncytial Virus in Clinical Specimens by Viral Culture, Direct and Indirect Immunofluorescence, and Enzyme Immunoassay," *J Clin Microbiol*, 1988, 26(3):588-91.

(Continued)

Respiratory Syncytial Virus Antigen by EIA (Continued)

Swenson PD and Kaplan MH, "Rapid Detection of Respiratory Syncytial Virus in Nasopharyngeal Aspirates by a Commercial Enzyme Immunoassay," *J Clin Microbiol*, 1986, 23(3):485-8.

Welliver RC, "Detection, Pathogenesis, and Therapy of Respiratory Syncytial Virus Infections," *Clin Microbiol Rev*, 1988, 1(1):27-39.

Respiratory Syncytial Virus Culture

Related Information

Respiratory Syncytial Virus Antigen by EIA *on previous page*
Respiratory Syncytial Virus Serology *on this page*
Viral Culture, Throat *on page 479*

Synonyms RSV Culture

Test Includes Concurrent culture for other respiratory viruses (influenza and parainfluenza viruses)

Specimen Throat or nasopharyngeal swab, nasopharyngeal washes and secretions

Container Sterile container; cold viral transport medium for swabs

Collection Place swabs into cold viral transport medium and keep cold. Infants and small children: soft catheters and suction devices (syringes and suction bulbs) can be used to collect nasal secretions (best specimens) as the catheter is withdrawn from far back in the nose. Another excellent method is to introduce 3-7 mL of sterile saline into the child's posterior nasal cavity and immediately aspirate the fluid.

Storage Instructions Respiratory syncytial virus is extremely labile. **Do not freeze** specimens and send specimens to the laboratory **as soon as possible**.

Causes for Rejection Dry specimen, specimen not refrigerated during transport, specimen fixed in formalin, unlabeled specimen

Turnaround Time Variable (1-14 days) depending on culture method and amount of virus in specimen

Reference Range No virus isolated

Use Aid in the diagnosis of respiratory disease caused by respiratory syncytial virus

Methodology Inoculation of specimen into cell cultures, incubation of cultures, observation of cultures for characteristic cytopathic effect in 2-7 days, and identification by fluorescent monoclonal antibodies specific for respiratory syncytial virus. The use of a rapid shell viral culture technique may yield positive culture results overnight.

Additional Information Serology is available to detect antibodies to respiratory syncytial virus. Many laboratories offer enzyme immunoassay (EIA) tests for the direct detection of RSV in patient specimens. In general, these tests are very rapid, sensitive, and specific.

Selected Readings

Hughes JH, Mann DR, and Hamparian VV, "Detection of Respiratory Syncytial Virus in Clinical Specimens by Viral Culture, Direct and Indirect Immunofluorescence, and Enzyme Immunoassay," *J Clin Microbiol*, 1988, 26(3):588-91.

Welliver RC, "Detection, Pathogenesis, and Therapy of Respiratory Syncytial Virus Infections," *Clin Microbiol Rev*, 1988, 1(1):27-39.

Respiratory Syncytial Virus, Direct Detection *see* Virus, Direct Detection by Fluorescent Antibody *on page 480*

Respiratory Syncytial Virus Serology

Related Information

Respiratory Syncytial Virus Antigen by EIA *on previous page*
Respiratory Syncytial Virus Culture *on this page*

Synonyms RSV Titer

Specimen Serum

Container Red top tube

Reference Range IgG <1:5, IgM <1:5; less than fourfold rise in titer by CF

Use Establish the diagnosis of respiratory syncytial virus infection

Limitations Children less than 6 months old may not mount a diagnostic serologic response to infection

Methodology Complement fixation, enzyme linked immunosorbent assay

Additional Information Diagnosis by CF depends on demonstrating a rise in antibody titer over a 2-3 week period. As such, the test is seldom useful in planning clinical care in an acute illness. For rapid diagnosis the demonstration of viral antigen in nasopharyngeal washings or of IgM antibody is more useful.

Rhinovirus Culture *see* Viral Culture, Throat *on page 479*

***Rickettsia rickettsii* Serology** *see* Rocky Mountain Spotted Fever Serology *on this page*

Rocky Mountain Spotted Fever Serology
Related Information
Ehrlichia Serology *on page 325*
Synonyms *Rickettsia rickettsii* Serology
Replaces *Proteus* OX-19
Special Instructions Acute and convalescent specimens are recommended.
Specimen Serum
Container Red top tube
Reference Range Less than a fourfold increase in titer in paired sera; IgG <1:64, IgM <1:8
Use To establish the diagnosis of Rocky Mountain spotted fever
Limitations Cross reactions with other organism in the spotted fever group. False-positive reactions may occur during pregnancy, especially in the last two trimesters.
Methodology Complement fixation, immunofluorescence, hemagglutination, enzyme linked immunosorbent assay
Additional Information Rocky Mountain spotted fever occurs primarily in the southeastern and western United States from April through October, but is also endemic on Long Island. It is a disease of variable clinical manifestation (some cases present with few or no "spots"), and since there is good specific therapy, and serious outcome if untreated, all aids to diagnosis are important. Serologic diagnosis may be made promptly enough to direct therapy.

Hemagglutination and immunofluorescent tests are least subject to cross reactions with other *Rickettsia*. The complement fixation test can be used with different concentration of antigen to minimize cross reactions. Tests for IgM specific antibody are helpful in early disease, since they appear in 3-8 days. Patients treated with antibiotics early in illness may not develop serologic responses. A direct fluorescent test is also available to demonstrate the *Rickettsia* in tissue.

As many as 71% of patients with Rocky Mountain spotted fever also develop antibodies against cardiolipin and endothelial cells.
Selected Readings
Kaplowitz LG, Fischer JJ, and Sparling PF, "Rocky Mountain Spotted Fever: A Clinical Dilemma," *Current Clinical Topics in Infectious Disease - 2*, Remington JS and Swartz MN, eds, New York, NY: McGraw-Hill Book Co, 1981, 89-108.
Salgo MP, Telzak EE, Currie B, et al, "A Focus of Rocky Mountain Spotted Fever Within New York City," *N Engl J Med*, 1988, 318(21):1345-8.
Sexton DJ and Corey GR, "Rocky Mountain "Spotless" and "Almost Spotless" Fever: A Wolf in Sheep's Clothing," *Clin Infect Dis*, 1992, 15(3):439-48.

Rose Handlers Disease *see* Sporotrichosis Serology *on page 447*

Rotavirus Detection by EM *see* Electron Microscopic (EM) Examination for Viruses, Stool *on page 329*

Rotavirus, Direct Detection
Synonyms Rotavirus Rapid Detection
Applies To Viral Antigen Detection, Direct, Stool
Test Includes Direct (nonculture) detection of rotavirus in stool specimens
Specimen Stool from the acute, diarrheal phase of disease
Container Sterile container
Sampling Time As soon as possible after onset of disease, preferably 3 to 5 days after onset
Collection Several specimens during the course of illness should be submitted in an attempt to eliminate false-negative results.
Causes for Rejection Excessive transit time to laboratory, unlabeled specimen
Turnaround Time 1 day
Reference Range No virus detected
Use Detection of rotavirus in stools of patients suspected of having viral gastroenteritis

(Continued)

Rotavirus, Direct Detection *(Continued)*

Limitations Quality of specimens cannot be evaluated, and specimens are collected randomly.

Methodology Commercially available (and often automated) enzyme immunoassays (EIA) are the preferred diagnostic methods. Commercial kits have not been standardized.

Additional Information Rotavirus is an extremely common cause of pediatric gastroenteritis. The illness is most common in winter, is highly contagious, involves 5 to 8 days of diarrhea, and is rarely fatal. Patients should also be evaluated for possible bacterial gastroenteritis.

Selected Readings
Christensen ML, "Human Viral Gastroenteritis," *Clin Microbiol Rev*, 1989, 2(1):51-89.

Gray LD, "Novel Viruses Associated With Gastroenteritis," *Clin Microbiol Newslett*, 1991, 13(18):137-44.

Yolken RH, "Enzyme Immunoassay for the Detection of Rotavirus Antigen and Antibody," *Manual of Clinical Laboratory Immunology*, 4th ed, Rose NR, de Macario EC, Fahey JL, et al, eds, Washington, DC: American Society for Microbiology, 1992, 651-60.

Rotavirus Rapid Detection *see* Rotavirus, Direct Detection
on previous page

Routine Bone Marrow Culture *see* Bone Marrow Culture, Routine
on page 281

Routine Culture, Rectal Swab *see* Stool Culture *on page 448*

RPR

Related Information
Darkfield Examination, Syphilis *on page 322*

FTA-ABS, Serum *on page 336*

VDRL, Cerebrospinal Fluid *on page 475*

Synonyms Rapid Plasma Reagin Test; Serologic Test for Syphilis; STS; Syphilis Screening Test

Applies To Syphilis Serology

Replaces Kahn Test; Kline Test; Mazzini; VDRL; Wassermann

Test Includes Reactive specimens may be titered and/or an FTA-ABS test performed

Specimen Serum

Container Red top tube

Reference Range Negative

Use Screening test for syphilis

Limitations This is a nontreponemal test and is associated with false-positive reactions due to intercurrent infections, pregnancy, drug addiction, collagen-vascular diseases, and Gaucher's disease.

Methodology Cord agglutination test with reagin antibody

Additional Information This is a very sensitive (but nonspecific) screening test for syphilis and detects antibodies to reagin. These antibodies usually develop within 4-6 weeks of initial infection, peak during the secondary phase of disease, and then decrease. They also decrease with treatment. Greater than 90% of patients with primary syphilis will have positive tests. RPR titers are usually higher in HIV-infected patients than in those who do not have HIV infection.

Because of the many causes of false-positive tests any reactive serum should be tested by a treponemal-specific test (HAI or FTA-ABS). The RPR should not be done on cerebrospinal fluid.

False-negative tests may occur at birth in some infants with recently acquired congenital syphilis. Therefore, especially in areas where the disease is prevalent, a serologic test for syphilis should be included in evaluating febrile infants even if they had a negative screen at birth. False-negatives have also been due to the prozone effect. Therefore, pregnant women in areas with high syphilis prevalence should have dilution performed on negative screening tests.

Selected Readings
Dorfman DH and Glaser JH, "Congenital Syphilis Presenting in Infants After the Newborn Period," *N Engl J Med*, 1990, 323(19):1299-302.

Hart G, "Syphilis Tests in Diagnostic and Therapeutic Decision Making," *Ann Intern Med*, 1986, 104(3):368-76.

Huber TW, Storms S, Young P, et al, "Reactivity of Microhemagglutination, Fluorescent Treponemal Antibody Absorption, Venereal Disease Research Laboratory, and Rapid Plasma Reagin Tests in Primary Syphilis," *J Clin Microbiol*, 1983, 17(3):405-9.

RSV Culture *see* Respiratory Syncytial Virus Culture
on page 436

RSV Testing *see* Respiratory Syncytial Virus Antigen by EIA
on page 435

RSV Titer *see* Respiratory Syncytial Virus Serology *on page 436*

Rubella Antibodies *see* Rubella Serology *on this page*

Rubella Serology

Synonyms German Measles Serology; Rubella Antibodies

Applies To IgG Antibodies to Rubella; IgM Antibodies to Rubella

Test Includes Detection of serologic response to rubella infection or vaccination

Abstract German measles is a viral infection usually characterized by a macular exanthem, an incubation period of 14-21 days and lymphadenopathy, pharyngitis, and conjunctivitis. Severe transplacental infections occur in the first trimester.

Specimen Serum

Container Red top tube

Reference Range Absence of antibody indicates susceptibility to rubella. Presence of IgM antibody indicates acute infection or vaccination. Presence of IgG antibody requires interpretation.

Possible Panic Range Evidence of susceptibility in a pregnant woman recently exposed to rubella

Use Aid in diagnosis of congenital rubella infections; evaluate susceptibility to infections

Limitations Requires clinical correlation and judgment. Low levels of antibody are poorly detected by enzyme immunoassays.

Methodology Indirect fluorescent antibody (IFA), hemagglutination, enzyme-linked immunosorbent assay (ELISA), radioimmunoassay (RIA), complement fixation (CF), latex agglutination (LA), enzyme immunoassay (EIA)

Additional Information Rubella virus is the cause of German measles, usually a mild exanthem, often subclinical. However, when acquired *in utero*, rubella virus can cause the congenital rubella syndrome, and lead to fetal demise, cataracts, malformation, deafness, and mental retardation. For this reason the federal government and many states support programs to immunize women against rubella before they have children. There has been a resurgence of congenital rubella in the early 1990s and more widespread screening for rubella serology is recommended.

The role of serologic testing for antibodies to rubella is different in different clinical settings. The simplest and most straight forward application is in premarital assessment of immunity. If a woman has antibodies against rubella, even of low titer, demonstrated by any of multiple methods, she need not worry about infection during subsequent pregnancy. If she is not immune, and is not pregnant, she can receive rubella vaccine.

A second, more complex, role is in the management of a pregnant woman who has been exposed to rubella. Here the questions include susceptibility, present acute infection, and risk to the fetus. Several flowcharts are available to assess these possibilities, utilizing antibody titers, class of antibody, and changes in titer over time. Management of such a case requires individualized expert consultation. Of particular concern is that some enzyme-linked immunoassays are not as sensitive and specific as hemagglutination inhibition.

Still a third role is in the evaluation of an infant born with an illness which may be congenital rubella. Problems here include evaluating whether antibody is present, and whether it represents antibody passively acquired by transplacental passage or is indicative of true neonatal infection. In this setting determining the immunoglobulin class is particularly important; IgM antibody strongly supports congenital infection.

Selected Readings

Fayram SL, Akin S, Aarnaes SL, et al, "Determination of Immune Status in Patients With Low Antibody Titers for Rubella Virus," *J Clin Microbiol*, 1987, 25(1):178-80.

Lee SH, Ewert DF, Frederick PD, et al, "Resurgence of Congenital Rubella Syndrome in the 1990s. Report on Missed Opportunities and Failed Prevention Policies Among Women of Childbearing Age," *JAMA*, 1992, 267(19):2616-20.

Zhang T, Mauracher CA, Mitchell LA, et al, "Detection of Rubella Virus-Specific Immunoglobulin G (IgG), IgM, and IgA Antibodies by Immunoblot Assays," *J Clin Microbiol*, 1992, 30(4):824-30.

LABORATORY DIAGNOSIS

Rubella Virus Culture

Synonyms German Measles Culture; Measles Culture, 3-Day

Test Includes Isolation and identification of rubella virus in cell culture

Specimen Two throat swabs, 10 mL urine, cerebrospinal fluid, tissues, amniotic fluid

Container Sterile urine container

Sampling Time Virus is more likely to be isolated if specimen is collected within 5 days after onset of illness.

Storage Instructions Specimens should not be stored. Specimens should be delivered immediately to the laboratory. If unavoidable delays occur the specimen can be stored at 4°C for up to 3 days, but there is a loss of infectivity when culture is delayed.

Causes for Rejection Dry specimen, specimen not refrigerated during transport, specimen fixed in formalin, unlabeled specimen

Turnaround Time Positive cultures are detected in 3-7 days. Negative cultures are usually reported after 3 weeks.

Reference Range No virus isolated

Use Aid in the diagnosis of disease caused by rubella virus (eg, congenital viral infection)

Limitations Isolation of rubella virus is usually of little help in the diagnosis of rubella except in cases of severe rubella complications, epidemiological purposes, and fatality. Serological diagnosis is much more useful.

Methodology Cell culture, isolation, and confirmation/identification by antibody-specific neutralization

Additional Information The incidence of rubella has been reduced dramatically by the wide use of immunization in children. However, rubella can still occur in older people who were not vaccinated or people who have immigrated to the United States from countries where vaccination for rubella is not common. Pregnant women, who become infected with rubella, have a very high chance of the virus crossing the placenta and infecting the fetus. Congenital rubella infections have disastrous effects, causing fetal death, premature delivery, and severe congenital defects including deafness and congenital heart disease. Neonates with congenital rubella excrete rubella virus in nasopharyngeal secretions and urine for many months after birth. These children pose a risk to susceptible pregnant women. Serology is available for diagnostic purposes. Usually immune status can be determined by examining a single serum sample.

Selected Readings

Centers for Disease Control, "Increase in Rubella and Congenital Rubella Syndrome – United States, 1988-1990," *MMWR Morb Mortal Wkly Rep*, 1991, 40(6):93-9.

Chernesky MA and Mahony JB, "Rubella Virus," *Manual of Clinical Microbiology*, 5th ed, Balows A, Hausler WJ Jr, Herrmann KL, et al, eds, Washington, DC: American Society for Microbiology, 1991, 918-23.

Herrmann KL, "Rubella Virus," *Laboratory Diagnosis of Viral Infections*, Lennette EH, ed, New York, NY: Marcel Dekker Inc, 1992, 731-47.

Sabin-Feldman Dye Test *replaced by Toxoplasma* Serology *on page 459*

Sarcoptes scabiei Skin Scrapings Identification *see* Arthropod Identification *on page 268*

Scanogram, X-ray *see* Bone Films *on page 277*

Scapula, Left or Right, X-ray *see* Bone Films *on page 277*

Schlichter Test *see* Serum Bactericidal Test *on next page*

Scotch® Tape Test *see* Pinworm Preparation *on page 430*

Screening Culture for Group A Beta-Hemolytic Streptococcus *see* Throat Culture for Group A Beta-Hemolytic *Streptococcus on page 457*

Sedimentation Rate *see* Sedimentation Rate, Erythrocyte *on this page*

Sedimentation Rate, Erythrocyte

Related Information

C-Reactive Protein *on page 311*

Synonyms Sedimentation Rate; Westergren Sedimentation Rate

Abstract This test is not a very specific in measuring inflammation and infection. It is used mainly to follow management of rheumatology patients.

440

Specimen Blood

Container Blue top (sodium citrate) tube or lavender top (EDTA) tube

Collection Specimen must be received within 4 hours of collection.

Causes for Rejection Insufficient blood, clotted, hemolyzed specimen

Reference Range Male, below age 50: 0-15 mm/hour, over age 50: 0-20 mm/hour; female, below age 50: 0-25 mm/hour, over age 50: 0-30 mm/hour by Westergren method

Use Evaluate the nonspecific activity of infections, inflammatory states, autoimmune disorders, and plasma cell dyscrasias

Limitations Anemia and paraproteinemia invalidate results; some procedural methods may be associated with hazardous exposure of medical technologists to fresh whole blood.

Methodology Red cell sedimentation rate expressed in mm/hour, utilizing Westergren type sedimentation tubes

Additional Information Elevations in fibrinogen, alpha- and beta-globulins (acute phase reactants), and immunoglobulins increase the sedimentation rate of red cells through plasma. The test is important in the diagnosis of temporal arteritis, as well as its management.

Selected Readings

Bottiger LE and Svedberg CA, "Normal Erythrocyte Sedimentation Rate and Age," *Br Med J*, 1967, 2(544):85-7.

Singer JI, Buchino JJ, and Chabali R, "Selected Laboratory in Pediatric Emergency Care," *Emerg Med Clin North Am*, 1986, 4(2):377-96.

Serologic Test for Syphilis *see* MHA-TP *on page 399*

Serologic Test for Syphilis *see* RPR *on page 438*

Serologic Test for Syphilis *see* FTA-ABS, Serum *on page 336*

Serologic Test for Syphilis, CSF *see* VDRL, Cerebrospinal Fluid *on page 475*

Serum Antibacterial Titer *see* Serum Bactericidal Test *on this page*

Serum Bactericidal Level *see* Serum Bactericidal Test *on this page*

Serum Bactericidal Test

Related Information

Antimicrobial Susceptibility Testing, Aerobic and Facultatively Anaerobic Organisms *on page 259*

C-Reactive Protein *on page 311*

Synonyms Antibacterial Activity, Serum; Bacterial Inhibitory Level, Serum; Maximum Bactericidal Dilution; MBD; Schlichter Test; Serum Antibacterial Titer; Serum Bactericidal Level; Serum Inhibitory Titer; Susceptibility Testing, Schlichter Test; Susceptibility Testing, Serum Bactericidal Dilution Method

Special Instructions If a serum bactericidal test is desired, the physician **must** request that the laboratory save the patient's isolate within 48 hours of submission of the specimen for initial culture. If the isolate has not been saved, the test cannot be performed. The laboratory **must** be informed of current antibiotic therapy including date and time of last dosage, route of administration on all antimicrobial agents patient is receiving and clinical diagnosis. Time of specimen collection should be indicated on requisition.

Specimen Serum or body fluid. Bacterial isolate causing infection prepared by laboratory.

Container Red top tube; sterile tube for body fluid

Sampling Time The peak level for intravenously (I.V.) administered drugs is obtained 30-60 minutes after the drug is absorbed and distributed. The trough level is obtained within 30 minutes or less of the next dose. For intramuscularly (I.M.) administered drugs and oral drugs, the peak should be drawn later at 2-4 hours. Vancomycin peak is drawn 2 hours post dose.

Collection Specimen should be transported to laboratory within 1 hour of collection.

Storage Instructions Separate serum using aseptic technique and freeze.

Causes for Rejection Isolate discarded before request for testing.

Turnaround Time 2-3 days

Reference Range Peak bactericidal activity should be observed at ≥1:8 dilution, trough at ≥1:2

Use Determine the maximum bactericidal dilution of the serum or body fluid, MBD, which is bactericidal for the patient's infecting organism; monitor total

(Continued)

Serum Bactericidal Test *(Continued)*

therapeutic effect. Frequently used to evaluate therapy in endocarditis, osteomyelitis, and suppurative arthritis. Serum bactericidal titers of 1:8 or greater are often recommended for the optimal treatment of infective endocarditis, osteomyelitis and suppurative arthritis.

Limitations There is no universal agreement on the clinical utility and prognostic value of this test. The serum bactericidal assay has many ill-defined variables, ie, no widely accepted standard procedure, no consensus as to whether dilutions should be performed with serum or broth, the unknown inhibitory effect of serum if used as a diluent, etc. The use of pooled serum diluent may not accurately predict actual bactericidal titers in patients with abnormal protein binding.

Results will reflect the combined *in vitro* effect of all antimicrobial agents present in the patient's serum or body fluid on his/her infecting organism(s). Results are accurate to plus or minus 1 dilution, and are not necessarily equivalent to a serum assay. Maximum inhibitory concentration (MIC) may also be reported. An apparently adequate ratio may represent a highly susceptible organism responding to a relatively low blood level, or a moderately resistant organism responding to an unexpectedly high blood level. A serum inhibitory titer might suggest an adequate therapeutic level, but would give no clue to potential toxicity, when an extremely narrow margin exists between a therapeutically adequate dose and a possibly toxic one (eg, aminoglycosides).

Contraindications The bacterium isolated from patient is not available or fails to grow for the serum bactericidal test.

Methodology Serial dilution of patient's serum; each dilution is incubated with an inoculum of the patient's isolate. Subsequent steps are complicated and vary from laboratory to laboratory.

Additional Information It is preferable to perform this test with paired specimens, one obtained approximately 15 minutes before an antibiotic dose (predose trough), and one obtained 30-60 minutes after an antibiotic dose (postdose peak).

In patients with chronic osteomyelitis, the observation of peak levels <1:16 and trough levels <1:2 accurately predicted treatment failure. In acute osteomyelitis, peak levels >1:16 and trough levels >1:2 accurately predicted medical cure. The serum bactericidal test alone is not sufficient to predict outcome in endocarditis. The therapeutic outcome of endocarditis depends on many clinical factors including cardiac status, underlying medical disease, embolic complications, and clinical management of patient. In granulocytopenic patient, titers 1:8-1:16 or greater in patients on combination therapy was associated with a more favorable outcome.

The serum bactericidal test has been applied to detect antimicrobial activity in cerebrospinal fluid and joint fluid. It is also useful in determining whether serum antimicrobial activity remains adequate after a shift from parenteral to oral therapy.

Selected Readings

Jordan GW and Kawachi MM, "Analysis of Serum Bactericidal Activity in Endocarditis, Osteomyelitis, and Other Bacterial Infections," *Medicine (Baltimore)*, 1981, 60(1):49-61.

MacLowry JD, "Perspective: The Serum Dilution Test," *J Infect Dis*, 1989, 160(4):624-6.

Stratton CW, "Serum Bactericidal Test," *Clin Microbiol Rev*, 1988, 1(1):19-26.

Wolfson JS and Swartz MN, "Drug Therapy. Serum Bactericidal Activity as a Monitor of Antibiotic Therapy," *N Engl J Med*, 1985, 312(15):968-75.

Serum Inhibitory Titer *see* Serum Bactericidal Test *on previous page*

Shingles Culture *see* Varicella-Zoster Virus Culture *on page 473*

Shoulder Arthrogram *see* Arthrogram *on page 267*

Shoulder, Left or Right, X-ray *see* Bone Films *on page 277*

Shoulders Arthritis, X-ray *see* Bone Films *on page 277*

Shoulder Stereo, Left or Right, X-ray *see* Bone Films *on page 277*

Shoulder to Include Axial View, Left or Right, X-ray *see* Bone Films *on page 277*

Shunt Culture *see* Intravenous Line Culture *on page 376*

Simple CMG *see* Cystometrogram, Simple *on page 315*

Sinuses, CT *see* Computed Transaxial Tomography, Paranasal Sinuses
on page 308

Skeletal Muscle Biopsy *see* Muscle Biopsy *on page 403*

Skin Biopsy

Applies To Skin Lesions; Smears

Abstract This section deals with sampling and procurement techniques and with a selected group of diagnostic skin problems.

Container 10% neutral formalin is satisfactory for submission of most specimens, but there are special requirements for immunofluorescence and electron microscopy.

Collection Techniques for procuring skin specimens:

Shave biopsy: A technique for obtaining superficial samples of predominantly epidermal or projecting lesions by cutting them flush with the adjacent skin as illustrated in Figure 1. This technique is usually used for nonmalignant lesions but may be useful for the patch phase of mycosis fungoides. **Since shave biopsy provides the most limited specimen, a serious potential for histopathologic misdiagnosis exists, especially in regard to melanocytic lesions.**

Figure 1. Shave Biopsy

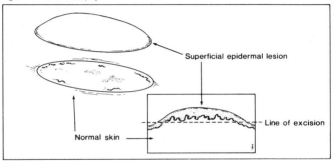

Punch biopsy: Very popular with dermatologists because it can be done easily, quickly, and repetitively at low cost in office practice. Biopsy punches, illustrated in Figure 2, range from 3-6 mm in size. The punch is pressed into the skin and rotated. It yields a plug or core of tissue which is cut from its base by scissors as the punch is withdrawn. It may be difficult to adequately sample subcutanea by punch. Punch biopsies may be submitted for culture. They may be particularly useful in the diagnosis of cutaneous myosis and mycobacterial disease. Pathologists prefer the largest possible sample.

Figure 2. Punch Biopsy

Excisional biopsy: This usually implies total removal of a skin lesion, most commonly a tumor, with a scalpel as illustrated in Figure 3. It is a preferred technique for removal of pigmented lesions and tumors.

Incisional biopsy: The removal of a portion of a lesion by scalpel as illustrated in Figure 4. It is performed when a non-neoplastic lesion (ie, necrobiosis lipoidica) is too large to be totally excised but definitive diagnosis mandates a large sample to evaluate overall architectural detail or, in the case of tumors, for which complete excision would require extensive surgery and/or would produce cosmetic deformity which would not be warranted until accurate histologic diagnosis is established.

(Continued)

Skin Biopsy *(Continued)*

Figure 3. Excisional Biopsy by Scalpel

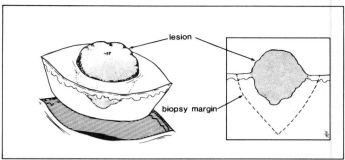

Figure 4. Incisional Biopsy by Scalpel

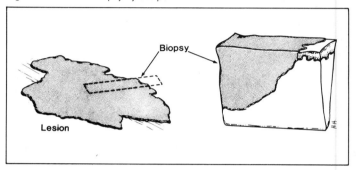

Smears and/or aspirates: Stained with Wright or Giemsa type stains may suffice to demonstrate polys or eosinophils (as in toxic erythema or pustular melanosis of newborns). Gram, acid-fast, PAS and GMS stains, and cultures are used to establish the presence of bacterial or fungal organisms. Finding multinucleated giant cells in smears in a proper clinical context suggests herpes or related viral infection. Aspirates may be adequate for cultures for bacteria, fungi, and viruses. Scrapings are often utilized in the diagnosis of dermatomycoses. Cytologic techniques (Tzanck smears) are rarely used in practice to evaluate acantholytic processes or tumors.

Storage Instructions Fixation in formalin solution or other appropriate fixative

Additional Information Selected Problems in Dermatopathology:

A. Specimens of Pigmented Lesions and Tumors
   1. In general, pigmented lesions and tumors should not be needled, aspirated, curetted, shaved or punched, but should be excised, *in toto*, whenever possible, to permit comprehensive evaluation and measurements appropriate for melanoma.

B. Specimens of Vesiculobullous Lesions
   1. If the diagnostic impression is pemphigus or pemphigoid, fresh lesions are preferred. Figure 5 illustrates appropriate biopsy technique.
   2. If the diagnostic impression is dermatitis herpetiformis, take the biopsy at the edge of the lesion (to study the change in the dermal papillae) as shown in Figure 6, rather than the lesion itself.
   3. If the diagnostic impression is epidermolysis bullosa, the clinician should be aware of the availability of four special regional reference centers in the U.S. for special studies of mechanobullous lesion.
   4. Immunofluorescent studies of vesiculobullous lesions: Vesiculobullous lesions which require biopsy should be considered for immunofluorescent studies (IF). In many laboratories, skin samples for immunofluorescent studies are separately submitted in vials of isopentane prior to snap freez-

Figure 5. Punch Biopsy: Pemphigus or Pemphigoid

Figure 6. Punch Biopsy: Dermatitis Herpetiformis

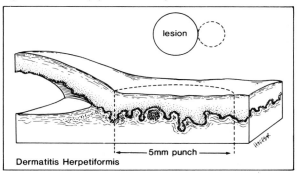

ing in liquid nitrogen by the laboratory. Some reference laboratories provide special solutions in which to store specimens for their analysis.

C. Specimens for Lupus Erythematosus (LE)
1. Direct immunofluorescence was first utilized on cutaneous biopsies in LE. The procedure (the lupus band test) was widely utilized to study SLE, DLE, and MCTD. Recent data suggests the band test is much less specific and sensitive than previously thought, that it is not clinically useful in discriminating SLE from other CT disorders or in predicting which patients with undifferentiated CT disease would develop SLE. Serologic evaluation is more sensitive, more efficient , and more cost effective in discriminating DLE and SLE.

Biopsy Site	SLE	DLE
Lesional Tissue	+	+
Uninvolved, Sun-exposed	+	–

D. Specimens of Epidermolysis Bullosa Acquisita (EBA)
1. Recent studies suggest that from 5% to 10% of patients regarded as bullous pemphigoid by routine direct immunofluorescence can be shown to be EBA based on indirect immunofluorescence on salt-split skin.

E. Special Studies for Hematopoietic Disorders
1. Special studies for T and B cells and markers for lymphocytes are considered elsewhere.

Pitfalls and artifacts to avoid: The biopsy technique should provide adequate and representative lesional tissue. Specimens should be handled gently without being crushed by forceps. Cautery of lesions may burn or coagulate tissue making pathologic diagnosis impossible. If specimens are mailed to a reference laboratory in freezing weather, they may freeze after fixation. Formation of ice crystals may render interpretation hazardous.

LABORATORY DIAGNOSIS

Skin Biopsy Antibodies *see* Skin Biopsy, Immunofluorescence *on this page*

Skin Biopsy For Bullous or Collagen Disease *see* Skin Biopsy, Immunofluorescence *on this page*

Skin Biopsy For Pemphigus *see* Skin Biopsy, Immunofluorescence *on this page*

Skin Biopsy, Immunofluorescence

Synonyms Basement Membrane Antibodies; Bullous Pemphigoid Antibodies; Dermatitis Herpetiformis Antibodies; Intercellular Antibody Basement Membrane Antibody; LE Antibodies; Lupus Band Test; Pemphigus Antibodies; Skin Biopsy Antibodies; Skin Biopsy For Bullous or Collagen Disease; Skin Biopsy For Pemphigus

Test Includes Anti-IgG, anti-IgA, anti-IgM, anti-C_3, anti-C_1q, antialbumin, antifibrinogen, antikappa and lambda light chains immunofluorescence

Specimen 3 mm skin punch biopsy and serum

Container Covered Petri dish or screw cap glass vial, red top tube for blood

Collection Take biopsies from the following sites: If pemphigus or bullous pemphigoid is suspected and fresh lesions are present, take a 3 mm biopsy at the edge of the bulla. If only old lesions are available, take biopsy from adjacent area. If dermatitis herpetiformis is suspected or both bullous pemphigoid and dermatitis herpetiformis are suspected, take not only lesion biopsy, but also biopsy of uninvolved area around lesions. Repeated biopsies are sometimes necessary to confirm dermatitis herpetiformis. If systemic lupus erythematosus or discoid LE is suspected, take biopsy of sun-exposed normal skin, preferably of the wrist, for diagnosis of SLE. Biopsies from lesions may be positive in both SLE and discoid LE while normal appearing sun-exposed skin yields positive findings in SLE only. Lesions older than 6 weeks should be biopsied in SLE. In vasculitis lesions for biopsy should be less than 24 hours old. Biopsy must be kept moist on saline soaked gauze or filter paper. Deliver to the laboratory on wet ice immediately upon completion of biopsy.

Storage Instructions Do not put specimen in formalin, Zenker's solution, or other usual fixatives. Specimen may not be stored, it must be delivered (iced or on moist saline) immediately to the laboratory. Fixation in N-ethylmaleimide requires subsequent removal of fixative and frozen section. Consult the laboratory prior to obtaining specimen.

Causes for Rejection Specimen in formalin, drying out of specimen

Reference Range No deposition of immunoglobulins, complement, or fibrinogen

Use Detect immune complexes, complement, and immunoglobulin deposition in SLE, DLE, pemphigus, bullous pemphigoid, and dermatitis herpetiformis; differential diagnosis of bullous skin diseases

Limitations Many skin lesions which may clinically resemble SLE and DLE also have deposits of Ig at the basement membrane. These include psoriasis, polymorphous light eruption, and drug eruptions.

Contraindications Specimen should not be taken from heavily keratinized body areas if possible. Failure to demonstrate IgG in some biopsies may be due to a secondary change in the tissue due to infection and inflammatory reaction.

Methodology Direct fluorescent antibody (DFA), indirect fluorescent antibody (IFA)

Additional Information Distinctive patterns of IgG, IgA, IgM, and complement components in epidermis, basement membrane, and dermal vessels may contribute to the differential diagnosis of bullous skin diseases, and discoid and systemic lupus erythematosus.

- Pemphigus: Fixation of IgG or other immunoglobulin along intercellular bridges of squamous cells; C_3 can be fixed.
- Bullous pemphigoid: Fixation of IgG and C_3 along epidermal basement membrane.
- Dermatitis herpetiformis: Fixation of IgA immunoglobulin deposits near the epidermal-dermal junction of skin adjacent to bulla.
- Lupus erythematosus: Fixation of IgG or other immunoglobulin deposits and complement along the epidermal-dermal junction. IgG, IgM, and C_3 are the most common.

Serum antibodies to the same skin components can also be demonstrated, using a tissue substrate (usually monkey or guinea pig esophagus), and these may correlate with disease activity. Steroid therapy can convert findings to negative in previously positive patients. In bullous disease antibody levels often reflect disease activity and rising titers may foretell clinical relapse.

Skin Culture for HSV *see* Herpes Simplex Virus Isolation, Rapid *on page 366*

Skin Lesions *see* Skin Biopsy *on page 443*

Skin Scrapings for *Sarcoptes scabiei* Identification *see* Arthropod Identification *on page 268*

Skin Test Battery *see* Anergy Skin Test Battery *on page 252*

Skin Tests for Histoplasmosis, Blastomycosis, Coccidioidomycosis *see* Fungal Skin Testing *on page 337*

Skin Tests for Penicillin Allergy *see* Penicillin Allergy Skin Testing *on page 425*

Smear, Gram Stain *see* Gram Stain *on page 352*

Smears *see* Skin Biopsy *on page 443*

Soft Tissue Scan *see* Gallium Scan *on page 347*

Spinal Fluid Analysis *see* Cerebrospinal Fluid Analysis *on page 288*

Spinal Fluid Cryptococcal Latex Agglutination *see* Cryptococcal Antigen Serology, Serum or Cerebrospinal Fluid *on page 312*

Spinal Fluid Fungus Culture *see* Fungus Culture, Cerebrospinal Fluid *on page 342*

Spinal Fluid Mycobacteria Culture *see* Mycobacteria Culture, Cerebrospinal Fluid *on page 405*

Spinal Fluid VDRL *see* VDRL, Cerebrospinal Fluid *on page 475*

Spinal Tap *see* Cerebrospinal Fluid Analysis *on page 288*

Spinal Tap *see* Lumbar Puncture *on page 390*

Spleen Cell Culture *see* Epstein-Barr Virus Culture *on page 332*

Sporanox *see* Itraconazole *on page 378*

***Sporothrix* Antibodies** *see* Sporotrichosis Serology *on this page*

Sporothrix schenckii *see* Sporotrichosis Serology *on this page*

Sporotrichosis Serology
Related Information
Fungus Culture, Biopsy *on page 340*
Fungus Culture, Body Fluid *on page 341*

Synonyms *Sporothrix* Antibodies

Applies To Rose Handlers Disease; *Sporothrix schenckii*

Test Includes Detection of serological response to *Sporothrix schenckii*

Abstract Sporotrichosis is a fungal disease classically beginning in a distal extremity, often at a site of inoculation, spreading proximally involving lymphatics. The organisms in tissue and in 37°C culture exist as yeast, which are often difficult or impossible to see in tissue sections. Extracutaneous disease includes monarticular arthritis. Pulmonary sporotrichosis is much less frequently found than osteoarticular infection.

Specimen Serum or cerebrospinal fluid

Container Red top tube; sterile CSF tube

Reference Range Latex agglutinating titer: <1:4; ELISA: <1:16 in serum, <1:8 in CSF

Use Diagnose sporotrichosis, especially extracutaneous disease

Limitations A negative test result does not rule out infection. Serial titers are not prognostically useful. There are occasional low titer false-positives from nonfungal disease. This test is not widely available.

Methodology Tube agglutination, latex agglutination (LA), enzyme-linked immunosorbent assay (ELISA)

Additional Information Titer ≥1:4 is presumptive evidence for sporotrichosis. Titers greater than 1:128, rising titers, and persistent elevation are common with pulmonary or systemic disease. Positive reaction in CSF is diagnostic, and is particularly useful in chronic meningitis caused by this organism, which is difficult to culture.

(Continued)

447

Sporotrichosis Serology *(Continued)*

Selected Readings

Bennett JE, "*Sporothrix schenckii*," *Principles and Practice of Infectious Diseases*, 3rd ed, Mandell GL, Douglas RG Jr, and Bennett JE, eds, New York, NY: Churchill Livingstone, 1990, 1972-5.

Scott EN, Kaufman L, Brown AC, et al, "Serologic Studies in the Diagnosis and Management of Meningitis Due to *Sporothrix schenckii*," *N Engl J Med*, 1987, 317:935-40.

Sputum Culture, Aerobic *see* Aerobic Culture, Sputum
on page 246

Sternoclavicular Joint, Left or Right, X-ray *see* Bone Films
on page 277

Stool Culture

Related Information

Fecal Leukocyte Stain *on page 334*

Ova and Parasites, Stool *on page 416*

Synonyms Enteric Pathogens Culture, Routine; Stool for Culture

Applies To Rectal Swab Culture; Routine Culture, Rectal Swab

Test Includes Screening culture for *Salmonella*, *Shigella*, *Helicobacter*, and, if requested, *Staphylococcus*.

Special Instructions The laboratory should be informed of the specific pathogen suspected if not *Salmonella*, *Shigella*, or *Campylobacter*.

Specimen Fresh random stool, rectal swab

Container Plastic stool container, Culturette®

Collection If stool is collected in a clean bedpan, it must not be contaminated with urine, residual soap, or disinfectants. Swabs of lesions of the rectal wall during proctoscopy or sigmoidoscopy are preferred.

Rectal swab: Insert the swab past the anal sphincter, move the swab circumferentially around the rectum. Allow 15-30 seconds for organisms to adsorb onto the swab. Withdraw swab, place in Culturette® tube, and crush media compartment.

Storage Instructions Refrigerate if the specimen cannot be processed promptly.

Causes for Rejection Because of risk to laboratory personnel, specimens sent on diaper or tissue paper, specimen contaminating outside of transport container may not be acceptable to the laboratory. Specimen containing interfering substances (eg, castor oil, bismuth, Metamucil®, barium), specimens delayed in transit and those contaminated with urine may not have optimal yield.

Turnaround Time Minimum 48 hours if negative

Reference Range Negative for *Salmonella*, *Shigella*, and *Campylobacter*. In endemic areas the isolation of a pathogen may not indicate the cause or only cause of diarrhea.

Use Screen for common bacterial pathogenic organisms in the stool; diagnose typhoid fever, enteric fever, bacillary dysentery, *Salmonella* infection.

Indications for stool culture include:
- Bloody diarrhea
- Fever
- Tenesmus
- Severe or persistent symptoms
- Recent travel to a third world country
- Known exposure to a bacterial agent
- Presence of fecal leukocytes

Limitations *Yersinia* species and *Vibrio* species may not be isolated unless specifically requested.

Contraindications A rectal swab culture is not as effective as a stool culture for detection of the carrier state.

Methodology Aerobic culture on selective media

Additional Information Stool cultures on patients hospitalized ≥3 days are not productive and should not be ordered unless special circumstances exist.

In enteric fever caused by *Salmonella typhi*, *S. choleraesuis*, or *S. enteritidis*, blood culture may be positive before stool cultures, and blood cultures are indicated early. Diarrhea is common in patients with the acquired immunodeficiency syndrome (AIDS). Diarrhea in AIDS is frequently caused by the classic bacterial pathogens; however, parasitic infestation is also common with

Giardia and *Cryptosporidium*. Rectal swabs are useful for the diagnosis of *Neisseria gonorrhoeae* and *Chlamydia* infections.

In acute or subacute diarrhea, three common syndromes are recognized: gastroenteritis, enteritis, and colitis (dysenteric syndrome). With colitis, patients have fecal urgency and tenesmus. Stool are frequently small in volume and contain blood, mucus, and leukocytes. External hemorrhoids are common and painful. Diarrhea of small bowel origin is indicated by the passage of few large volume stools. This is due to accumulation of fluid in the large bowel before passage. Leukocytes indicate colonic inflammation rather than a specific pathogen. Bacterial diarrhea may be present in the absence of fecal leukocytes and fecal leukocytes may be present in the absence of bacterial or parasitic agents (ie, idiopathic inflammatory bowel disease). See table. Although most bacterial diarrhea is transient (1-30 days) cases of persistent symptoms (10 months) have been reported. The etiologic agent in the reported case was *Shigella flexneri* diagnosed by culture of rectal swab. In infants younger than 1 year of age, a history of blood in the stool, more than 10 stools in 24 hours, and temperature greater than 39°C have a high probability of having bacterial diarrhea.

Diarrhea Syndromes Classified by Predominant Features

Syndrome (anatomic site)	Features	Characteristic Etiologies
Gastroenteritis (stomach)	Vomiting	Rotavirus Norwalk virus Staphylococcal food poisoning *Bacillus cereus* food poisoning
Enteritis (small bowel)	Watery diarrhea Large-volume stools, few in number	Enterotoxigenic *E. coli* *Vibrio cholerae* Any enteric microbe
Dysentery, colitis (colon)	Small-volume stools containing blood and/or mucus and many leukocytes	*Shigella* *Campylobacter* *Salmonella* Invasive *E. coli* *Plesiomonas shigelloides* *Aeromonas hydrophila* *Vibrio parahaemolyticus* *Clostridium difficile* *Entamoeba histolytica* Inflammatory bowel disease

Selected Readings

Bishop WP and Ulshen MH, "Bacterial Gastroenteritis," *Pediatr Clin North Am*, 1988, 35(1):69-87.

Farmer RG, "Infectious Causes of Diarrhea in the Differential Diagnosis of Inflammatory Bowel Disease," *Med Clin North Am*, 1990, 74(1):29-38.

Gracey M, "Bacterial Diarrhea," *J Clin Gastroenterol*, 1986, 15(1):21-37.

Guerrant RL, Wanke CA, Barrett LJ, et al, "A Cost Effective and Effective Approach to the Diagnosis and Management of Acute Infectious Diarrhea," *Bull N Y Acad Med*, 1987. 63(6):484-99.

Pickering LK, "Therapy for Acute Infectious Diarrhea in Children," *J Pediatr*, 1991, 118(4 Pt 2):S118-28.

Radetsky M, "Laboratory Evaluation of Acute Diarrhea," *Pediatr Infect Dis*, 1986, 5(2):230-8.

Stool Culture, Diarrheagenic *E. coli*

Related Information

Fecal Leukocyte Stain *on page 334*

Applies To Enterohemorrhagic *E. coli*, Stool Culture; Enteroinvasive *E. coli*, Stool Culture; Enteropathogenic *E. coli*, Stool Culture; Enterotoxigenic *E. coli*, Stool Culture; EPEC, Stool Culture; Rectal Swab Culture for Diarrheagenic, *E. coli*; Stool Culture, EPEC; Verocytotoxin Producing *E. coli*, Stool Culture

Special Instructions Routine stool culture is usually performed on all requests for enteropathogenic *E. coli*

Specimen Rectal swab, fresh stool

Container Plastic stool container, Culturette®

Collection If stool is collected in sterile bedpan, must not be contaminated with urine or residual soap or disinfectants. Swabs of lesions of the rectal wall during proctoscopy or sigmoidoscopy preferred.

Rectal swab: Insert the swab past the anal sphincter, move the swab circumferentially around the anus. Allow 15-30 seconds for organisms to adsorb onto

(Continued)

Stool Culture, Diarrheagenic *E. coli* (Continued)

the swab. Withdraw swab, place in Culturette® tube, and crush media compartment.

Storage Instructions Do not refrigerate

Causes for Rejection Because of risk to laboratory personnel, specimen sent on diaper or tissue paper, specimen contaminating outside of transport container may not be acceptable to the laboratory. Specimen containing interfering substances (eg, castor oil, bismuth, Metamucil®, barium), specimens delayed in transit, and those contaminated with urine may not have optimal yield.

Turnaround Time Preliminary report available at 24 hours; minimum 72 hours for final reports

Reference Range Normal colonic flora

Use Establish diarrheagenic *E. coli* as the cause of clinical illness

Limitations Many laboratories are not equipped to perform elaborate diagnostic procedures needed to definitively characterize diarrheagenic *E. coli*. Clinical diagnosis and exclusion of other more readily characterized pathogens form the practical basis of presumptive diagnosis of diarrheagenic *E. coli* illness.

Methodology Cultures may be screened for sorbitol-negative (colorless) colonies on sorbitol-MacConkey agar; EHEC is confirmed by serotyping. Culture filtrate can be incubated with Vero cells. Changes observed in the presence of toxin include rounding up at 36 hours and destruction of the monolayer with detachment at 72 hours. Shiga-like toxin is most frequently associated with the O157:H7 serotype.

Additional Information See table. Factors common to diarrheagenic *E. coli* include

Four Major Categories of Diarrheagenic *E. coli*

Category	Abbreviation	Clinic Manifestation
Enterotoxigenic	ETEC	Travelers diarrhea and infant diarrhea in less developed countries
Enteropathogenic	EPEC	Infant diarrhea
Enterohemorrhagic	EHEC	Hemorrhagic colitis Hemolytic uremic syndrome Thrombotic thrombocytopenia purpura
Enteroinvasive	EIEC	Dysentery

clude the presence of critical virulence factors encoded in plasmids, characteristic interaction with intestinal mucosa, production of enterotoxin or cytotoxin, and the observation that within each category the strains fall into certain O:H serotypes.

Hemorrhagic colitis can be differentiated from other causes of diarrhea by its progression from watery to bloody diarrhea over a few days time. The fecal leukocytes are markedly increased. Fever is usually absent. The disease is mediated by the production of a Shiga-like toxin which interferes with colonic brush border cells, protein synthesis, and ultimately causes cell death. Enterohemorrhagic *E. coli* (EHEC), differ from other strains of bacteria in the large amount of toxin they produce. Virtually all 0157:H7 organisms produce this toxin.

Enterotoxigenic *E. coli* (ETEC) infection is acquired by ingesting contaminated food or water. The organisms colonize the proximal small intestine and there they elaborate enterotoxins. Clinical features of ETEC infection include watery diarrhea, nausea, abdominal cramps, and low grade fever. Enterotoxigenic *E. coli* is the most common agent of travelers diarrhea. Symptoms start early in the visit, typically on day 3. The illness may typically last 3-4 days.

Enteropathogenic *E. coli* (EPEC) produce a cytotoxin similar or identical to that produced by *Shigella dysenteriae* type 1. The clinical symptoms of EPEC illness include fever, malaise, vomiting, and diarrhea with large amounts of mucus but not grossly bloody. EPEC diarrhea in infants may persist for greater than 14 days and is frequently severe.

Enteroinvasive *E. coli* (EIEC) invade and proliferate within epithelial cells and cause eventual cell death, like *Shigella*. Clinical illness is characterized by fever, severe abdominal cramps, malaise, toxemia, and watery diarrhea. The illness progresses to gross dysentery with scant stools consisting of blood and mucus. The methylene blue stain of stool reveals sheets of leukocytes.

Selected Readings

Bishop WP and Ulshen MH, "Bacterial Gastroenteritis," *Pediatr Clin North Am*, 1988, 35(1):69-87.

Doyle MP, "Pathogenic *Escherichia coli, Yersinia enterocolitica*, and *Vibrio parahaemolyticus*," *Lancet*, 1990, 336(8723):1111-5.

Griffin PM, Ostroff SM, and Tauxe RV, "Illness Associated With *Escherichia coli* 0157:H7 Infections - A Broad Clinical Spectrum," *Ann Intern Med*, 1988, 109(9):705-12.

Levine MM, "*Escherichia coli* That Cause Diarrhea: Enterotoxigenic, Enteropathogenic, Enteroinvasive, Enterohemorrhagic, and Enteroadherent," *J Infect Dis*, 1987, 155(3):377-89.

Sack RB, "Enterohemorrhagic *Escherichia coli*," *N Engl J Med*, 1987, 317(24):1535-7, (editorial).

Stool Culture, EPEC *see* Stool Culture, Diarrheagenic *E. coli*
on page 449

Stool Culture, Uncommon Organisms

Applies To Rectal Swab, Unusual Organism; *Vibrio cholerae*, Stool Culture; *Vibrio parahaemolyticus*, Stool Culture; *Yersinia enterocolitica*, Stool Culture

Special Instructions Laboratory must be contacted prior to collecting specimen

Specimen Rectal swab or fresh stool

Container Culturette® or plastic stool container

Collection If collected in sterile bedpan, must not be contaminated with urine or residual soap or disinfectants. Specimen must be less than 3 hours old.

Storage Instructions Do not refrigerate.

Causes for Rejection Specimen more than 3 hours old, rectal swabs in which the medium compartment is not broken, insufficient specimen volume, specimen contaminated with urine and/or water, specimen containing interfering substances (eg, castor oil, bismuth, Metamucil®, barium); specimen refrigerated; more than two specimens submitted to the laboratory per day; specimen not submitted as sealed swab or in a sealed plastic stool container. **Diapers are not acceptable.**

Reference Range No organisms detected.

Use Identify an etiologic agent in cases of diarrhea

Limitations Special media necessary for the isolation of these specific pathogens may have to be prepared **prior** to collection of specimen.

Stool for Culture *see* Stool Culture *on page 448*

Stool for Ova and Parasites *see* Ova and Parasites, Stool
on page 416

Strep Throat Screening Culture *see* Throat Culture for Group A Beta-Hemolytic *Streptococcus* *on page 457*

***Streptococcus agalactiae*, Latex Screen** *see* Group B *Streptococcus* Antigen Test *on page 354*

***Streptococcus* Group A Latex Screen** *see* Group A *Streptococcus* Antigen Test *on page 354*

***Streptococcus* Group B Latex Screen** *see* Group B *Streptococcus* Antigen Test *on page 354*

Streptodornase *see* Antideoxyribonuclease-B Titer, Serum
on page 256

Streptozyme

Related Information

Antideoxyribonuclease-B Titer, Serum *on page 256*

Antistreptolysin O Titer, Serum *on page 263*

Test Includes Screening for anti-NADase, anti-DNase B, antistreptokinase, antistreptolysin O (ASO), antihyaluronidase. Sheep red blood cells are sensitized with these the five streptococcal exoenzymes.

Specimen Serum

Container Red top tube

Reference Range <100 streptozyme units

Use Screening for antibodies to streptococcal antigens: NADase, DNase B, streptokinase, streptolysin O and hyaluronidase

Limitations A single determination is less useful than a series. May not be as sensitive in children as in adults.

Methodology Hemagglutination

Additional Information Streptozyme is a screening test for antibodies to sev-
(Continued)

Streptozyme *(Continued)*

eral streptococcal antigens. It has the advantages of detecting several antibodies in a single assay (although which one has been detected cannot be ascertained), of being technically quick and easy, and of being unaffected by several factors producing false-positives in the ASO test. A serially rising titer is more significant than a single determination.

A disadvantage of the test is that borderline antibody elevations, which could be clinically significant particularly in children, may not be detected.

Selected Readings

Ayoub EM and Harden E, "Immune Response to Streptococcal Antigens: Diagnostic Methods," *Manual of Clinical Laboratory Immunology*, 4th ed, Rose NR, de Macario EC, Fahey JL, et al, eds, Washington, DC: American Society for Microbiology, 1992, 427-34.

el-Kholy A, Hafez K, and Krause RM, "Specificity and Sensitivity of the Streptozyme Test for the Detection of Streptococcal Antibodies," *Appl Microbiol*, 1974, 27(4):748-52.

Klein GC and Jones WL, "Comparison of the Streptozyme Test With the Antistreptolysin O, Antideoxyribonuclease B, and Antihyaluronidase Tests," *Appl Microbiol*, 1971, 21(2):257-9.

STS *see* RPR *on page 438*

Sudden Death Syndrome *see* Botulism, Diagnostic Procedure *on page 285*

Sulfur Granule, Culture *see* Actinomyces Culture, All Sites *on page 242*

Surgical Specimen Anaerobic Culture *see* Anaerobic Culture *on page 250*

Surgical Specimen Culture *see* Aerobic Culture, Body Fluid *on page 244*

Surgical Specimen Culture, Routine *see* Biopsy Culture, Routine *on page 270*

Surgical Specimen Fungus Culture *see* Fungus Culture, Body Fluid *on page 341*

Surgical Specimen Mycobacteria Culture *see* Mycobacteria Culture, Biopsy or Body Fluid *on page 404*

Surrogate Tests for Non-A, Non-B Hepatitis *see* Hepatitis C Serology *on page 360*

Susceptibility Testing, Aerobic and Facultatively Anaerobic Organisms *see* Antimicrobial Susceptibility Testing, Aerobic and Facultatively Anaerobic Organisms *on page 259*

Susceptibility Testing, Antimicrobial, Anaerobic Bacteria *see* Antimicrobial Susceptibility Testing, Anaerobic Bacteria *on page 260*

Susceptibility Testing, Fungi *see* Antifungal Susceptibility Testing *on page 256*

Susceptibility Testing, Mycobacteria *see* Antimycobacterial Susceptibility Testing *on page 262*

Susceptibility Testing, Schlichter Test *see* Serum Bactericidal Test *on page 441*

Susceptibility Testing, Serum Bactericidal Dilution Method *see* Serum Bactericidal Test *on page 441*

Swan-Ganz Tip Culture *see* Intravenous Line Culture *on page 376*

Synovial Fluid Culture *see* Aerobic Culture, Body Fluid *on page 244*

Synovial Fluid Culture for *Neisseria gonorrhoeae*, Only *see* Neisseria gonorrhoeae Culture *on page 412*

Synovial Fluid Cytology *see* Cytology, Body Fluids *on page 318*

Synovial Fluid Fungus Culture *see* Fungus Culture, Body Fluid *on page 341*

Syphilis, Darkfield Examination *see* Darkfield Examination, Syphilis *on page 322*

Syphilis Screening Test see RPR on page 438

Syphilis Serology see MHA-TP on page 399

Syphilis Serology see RPR on page 438

T4/T8 Ratio
Synonyms Helper Cell/Suppressor Ratio
Test Includes Quantitation of T4 and T8 cells
Specimen Blood
Container Yellow top (ACD) tube or green top (heparin) tube
Collection Routine venipuncture
Storage Instructions Maintain specimen at room temperature.
Causes for Rejection Excessive hemolysis, lipemia
Use Evaluate patient with suspected AIDS
Limitations Not diagnostic for AIDS
Methodology Flow cytometry
Additional Information Normal immunity requires a balance between thymus-derived helper cells (T4) and suppressor cells (T8). The quantitation of the T4 (helper) and T8 (suppressor) is helpful in the evaluation of a patient with suspected AIDS. In AIDS, the T4 cells are severely reduced, and the T4/T8 ratio is <1.

TB Culture, Biopsy see Mycobacteria Culture, Biopsy or Body Fluid on page 404

TB Culture, Bronchial Aspirate see Mycobacteria Culture, Sputum on page 406

TB Culture, Gastric Aspirate see Mycobacteria Culture, Sputum on page 406

TB Culture, Sputum see Mycobacteria Culture, Sputum on page 406

TB Smear see Acid-Fast Stain on page 239

TEE see Transesophageal Echocardiography on page 460

Teichoic Acid Antibody
Specimen Serum
Container Red top tube
Reference Range Titer of less than or equal to 1:2. Less than a fourfold rise between acute and convalescent serum. (Reference ranges vary among laboratories.)
Use Used in assessing therapy in chronic infections caused by *Staphylococcus aureus*
Limitations Clinical utility is not well established and is equivocal. Technical variability.
Methodology Gel diffusion assay, enzyme linked immunosorbent assay
Additional Information Teichoic acid is a component of the cell wall of gram-positive bacteria. Antibodies to teichoic acid can be demonstrated in some patients with infections due to such organisms, particularly staphylococcal endocarditis and osteomyelitis. Serial determinations of teichoic acid antibodies have been used by some to assess the adequacy of therapy for these conditions, but this or other clinical applications are not yet established.
Selected Readings
Herzog C, Wood HC, Noel I, et al, "Comparison of a New Enzyme-Linked Immunosorbent Assay Method With Counterimmunoelectrophoresis for Detection of Teichoic Acid Antibodies in Sera From Patients With *Staphylococcus aureus* Infections," *J Clin Microbiol*, 1984, 19(4):511-15.
Jacob E, Durham LC, Falk MC, et al, "Antibody Response to Teichoic Acid and Peptidoglycan in *Staphylococcus aureus* Osteomyelitis," *J Clin Microbiol*, 1987, 25(1):122-7.

Temporomandibular Joint Arthrogram see Arthrogram on page 267

Thin and Thick Smears, Blood see Peripheral Blood Smear, Thick and Thin on page 429

Thoracentesis
Synonyms Pleural Fluid "Tap"
Test Includes At the bedside, a physician utilizes a needle and catheter system to withdraw fluid from a patient with radiographically demonstrable pleural effusion for diagnostic or therapeutic purposes.

(Continued)

Thoracentesis *(Continued)*

Patient Preparation Technique and risks of procedure are explained and consent is obtained. Chest x-ray is routinely performed prior to procedure, including a PA, lateral, and lateral decubitus view, and should be available for physician review. Recent prothrombin, partial thromboplastin time, and platelet count on the chart. Laboratory requisitions completed in advance. Premedication for pain (such as parenteral meperidine) is rarely required and local anesthesia during the procedure is usually sufficient.

Aftercare Immediately postprocedure, a "stat" chest x-ray is performed, usually at end-expiration. Vital signs must be monitored closely, especially if > 1 L fluid is removed. Hypoxemia is a known complication of thoracentesis and some patients may require temporary supplemented oxygen. If dyspnea or hypotension develops, physician must be contacted promptly. Otherwise, if vital signs and postprocedure chest x-ray are satisfactory, patient activity may be ad lib.

Complications Although numerous complications have been reported, diagnostic thoracentesis is generally at low risk. Complications may be classified as traumatic or nontraumatic. Nontraumatic complications are related to predictable physiologic responses and include:

- syncope
- cough
- hypotension, either immediate (vasovagal reaction) or delayed (fluid shifts)
- noncardiogenic pulmonary edema (following rapid expansion of a collapsed lung, especially on removal of large volumes of a chronic effusion)
- hypoxemia; PaO_2 may drop by 10 mm Hg within minutes and not return to baseline until the following day. Some authorities recommend supplemental oxygen routinely.

Traumatic complications are iatrogenic and include:

- pneumothorax, simple or tension (requiring chest tube); lateral decubitus radiograph demonstrating a pleural effusion <10 mm thick substantially increases the risk of pneumothorax
- hemothorax
- laceration of intercostal artery, potentially lethal
- puncture of liver or spleen
- miscellaneous, subcutaneous emphysema, air embolism, infection

Of note, the recovery of a grossly bloody pleural effusion (RBC > 100,000/mm³) does not automatically imply needle trauma since blood may be seen in several pleural diseases as well. To differentiate this, traumatic effusions tend to clot rapidly and become more clear as serial samples are withdrawn; bloody effusions from pleural disease generally are slow to clot due to defibrination over time. In doubtful cases, a hematocrit should be obtained on the bloody effusion and compared with plasma hematocrit.

Equipment Several complete thoracentesis kits are available commercially. Alternatively, individual components commonly found in most clinics and hospitals may be assembled separately. Common items include sterile drapes, iodine, alcohol pads, gauze, local anesthesia (1% lidocaine), at least four sterile tubes, syringes, and anaerobic culture media. Two red top tubes and two lavender top (EDTA containing) tubes may be used in place of the four sterile tubes. If cytologic studies are planned, heparin (1:1000) is needed as an additive. If pleural fluid pH is planned, a heparinized syringe and ice bag are needed. Several needle and catheter assemblies are available. For diagnostic thoracentesis (only 50-100 mL fluid removed), a 2" angiocatheter is convenient (18- or 20-gauge needle within catheter). For therapeutic thoracentesis with >1 L removed, a catheter within needle arrangement is effective. A 12" long plastic catheter (16-gauge) within a 14-gauge needle allows more complete pleural space drainage. Also required are liter-sized vacuum bottles and connecting tubing for collection of large volumes of fluid. Commercial thoracentesis kits represent variations of the above and are most useful when >1 L fluid is to be removed.

Technique Ideally, patient is positioned so that he is seated and leaning forward slightly, arms crossed in front and resting comfortably on a bedside table. The highest level of pleural effusion is determined on physical examination and a mark is placed one intercostal space below. The area is prepped and draped, and the skin and subcutaneous tissues are infiltrated with local anesthetic. Generally, the site is located 5-10 cm lateral to the spine, near the posterior axillary line. At this point technique varies with equipment used. If a catheter within needle is used, the needle (14-gauge) is passed bevel down over the superior aspect of the rib in the anesthetized intercostal space (avoiding the neurovascular bundle). Once the needle has penetrated the parietal pleura and fluid easily aspirated, the smaller plastic catheter (16-gauge) can be advanced its entire length into the pleural space. The needle is then completely withdrawn through the skin. Pleural fluid can be aspirated through the plastic catheter into a 50 mL syringe. Multiple samples of 50 mL may be obtained in this fashion. Alternatively, the catheter may be attached to sterile connecting tubing and fluid collected with liter-sized vacuum bottles. Once the desired amount is obtained, the catheter is pulled out completely and pressure held over the puncture site. If an angiocatheter is used (needle within catheter), the technique is similar. Immediately after collection, serum is drawn for LDH, protein, and further additional studies depending on the clinical situation (see interpretation).

Specimen For diagnostic thoracentesis, 50-100 mL is adequate for routine studies. If cytology desired, larger volumes have been recommended (100-250 mL), although occasionally as little as 5 mL have been sufficient. For therapeutic thoracentesis, removal of 1000-1500 mL is generally well tolerated.

Container Lavender top tube for cell count, red top tube for chemistries, sterile syringe adequate for transport to Microbiology Laboratory. For cytology samples add 5000-10,000 units of heparin into syringe or vacuum bottle and label. For pleural fluid pH send specimen in anaerobic syringe (air bubbles removed) on ice immediately to acute care (blood gas) laboratory.

Collection Samples should be hand carried to respective laboratories immediately.

Causes for Rejection Lack of heparin additive to cytology (or cell count, if plain glass tube used in place of lavender top tube), improper collection technique for pH (not on ice)

Normal Findings Pleural effusions are traditionally classified as either "transudates" or "exudates" based on the underlying mechanism of pleural fluid formation. This is the first and most crucial step in pleural fluid analysis. Transudates are ultrafiltrates of plasma which result from alterations in the osmotic or hydrostatic forces across pleural membranes. The pleural surface itself is usually disease-free. Examples include congestive heart failure (elevated hydrostatic pressure), nephrotic syndrome, and other hypoproteinemic states (decreased oncotic pressure), cirrhosis, myxedema, sarcoidosis, and Meig's syndrome. Exudates occur when the pleural membrane is involved in a disease process which increases pleural capillary permeability or obstructs lymphatics. Causes of exudates include pulmonary infections (pneumonia, empyema, abscess), malignancy (mesothelioma or metastases), collagen vascular diseases, pulmonary embolism, gastrointestinal diseases (pancreatitis, esophageal rupture), hemothorax, chylothorax, and miscellaneous causes such as postmyocardial infarction syndrome, uremia, and postradiation. In general, discovering a transudate allows therapy to be focused on the underlying systemic disease causing the effusion (eg, cirrhosis). Further studies of the pleural space are not necessary. Discovering an exudate, however, is more ominous and mandates additional, thorough diagnostic testing to rule out entities such as occult malignancy and pleural space infection.

Critical Values The following biochemical criteria were found by Light to accurately predict an exudate:
- pleural fluid protein to serum protein ratio >0.5
- pleural fluid LDH to serum LDH ratio >0.6
- pleural fluid LDH >200 units/L (or >two-thirds the upper limit of normal serum LDH)

Exudates satisfy one or more of these three criteria. Effusions are classified as transudates only if none of the these criteria are met. Misclassification rate is <1%, based on several prospective studies. In the past, specific gravity (SG) was used as the sole criteria for separating transudates (SG <1.016) from exudates (SG >1.016). Despite its appeal as a simple and inexpensive test, it is no longer recommended due to its high misclassification rate (≤30%). Similarly, older criteria using pleural fluid protein alone to differentiate transudates (protein <3.0 mg/dL from exudates (>3 mg/dL) carries a misclassification rate near 15% and should no longer be used.

Use The major diagnostic indication is the presence of pleural fluid of unclear etiology. In those instances where the etiology of a pleural effusion is clinically apparent, thoracentesis may be deferred at physician's discretion. For example, the patient with recurrent congestive heart failure who presents with typical left ventricular failure and pleural effusion may appropriately undergo a trial of diuresis prior to thoracentesis. The major therapeutic indication for thoracente-

(Continued)

LABORATORY DIAGNOSIS
Thoracentesis *(Continued)*

sis is respiratory compromise secondary to a large pleural effusion. Less commonly, the procedure may be used to evacuate trapped air in the pleural space (rather than fluid) as with a tension pneumothorax.

Contraindications Platelet count <50,000/mm³; severe, uncorrectable coagulopathy; effusions <10 mm thick on decubitus radiograph (or effusions not freely movable on decubitus radiograph); inability to define rib landmarks (necessary for proper needle placement); an uncooperative patient, unable to sit immobile. Other high-risk situations, not necessarily representing contraindications, include: mechanical ventilation with positive end expiratory pressure (PEEP); severe emphysema with blebs; patients who have undergone pneumonectomy with pleural effusion located on the side of the remaining lung. In these instances, ultrasound or CT guided aspiration of pleural fluid may be more prudent; a common complication such as pneumothorax could have profound consequences.

Additional Information Supplemental tests are available for more specific evaluation of the exudate. To minimize expense, test selection should be based on the differential diagnosis of an individual case. Malignant effusions are often grossly bloody with RBCs from 5000-100,000/mm³. Cytologic exam is initially positive for malignancy in approximately 60% of cases of later documented pleural malignancy; if three separate samples are sent, yield improves to 90%. Pleural fluid pH is often <7.3 and glucose is low (<60 mg/dL) in 15% of cases. In patients with empyema, enormous numbers of polymorphonuclear cells are present in pleural fluid. Parapneumonic effusions are sterile effusions secondary to pneumonia and require pleural pH measurement for optimal management. A pH <7.2, in the absence of systemic acidosis, indicates that the effusion will behave clinically like an empyema and will require chest tube drainage for resolution. Note that pleural fluid pH <7.2 may occur in other conditions (malignancy, TB, rheumatoid arthritis) which do not necessarily require tube thoracotomy. Tuberculosis effusions are characterized by WBC count >10,000/mm³ with >50% small lymphocytes. This latter finding is highly suggestive of either TB or malignancy and may warrant pleural biopsy. Mesothelial cells are absent in tuberculous effusions; some authors feel that the presence >1% mesothelial cells effectively rules out TB. AFB stains alone are initially positive in only 25% of proven cases. Rheumatoid effusions characteristically have low glucose levels and a value >30 mg/dL makes the diagnosis doubtful. Pleural pH levels are quite low (often <7). Rheumatoid factor testing on pleural fluid is nonspecific and not clinically useful. In suspected lupus effusions, the finding of lupus erythematosus (LE) cells in pleural fluid is pathognomonic for systemic lupus erythematosus. Effusions associated with both pancreatitis and esophageal rupture have similar laboratory profiles. Amylase levels are elevated >160 units/L with both esophageal rupture (salivary amylase) and pancreatitis (pancreatic amylase). Pleural fluid pH is low in both cases, and may be <7 with esophageal rupture.

Selected Readings

Brandstetter RD and Cohen RP, "Hypoxemia After Thoracentesis: A Predictable and Treatable Condition," 1979, 242(10):1060-1.

Corwin RW and Irwin RS, "Thoracentesis," *Intensive Care Med*, 3rd ed, Rippe JM, Irwin RS, Alpert JS, et al, eds, Boston, MA: Little, Brown and Co, 1985, 121-7.

Hausheer FH and Yarbro JW, "Diagnosis and Treatment of Malignant Pleural Effusion," *Semin Oncol*, 1985, 12(1):54-75.

Health and Public Policy Committee, American College of Physicians, "Diagnostic Thoracentesis and Pleural Biopsy in Pleural Diseases," *Ann Intern Med*, 1985, 103(5):799-802.

Grogan DR, Irwin RS, Channick R, et al, "Complications Associated With Thoracentesis. A Prospective, Randomized Study Comparing Three Different Methods," *Arch Intern Med*, 1990, 150(4):873-7.

Jay SJ, "Pleural Effusions: Preliminary Evaluation – Recognition of the Transudate," *Postgrad Med*, 1986, 80(5):164-7, 170-7.

Light RW, "Management of Parapneumonic Effusions," *Arch Intern Med*, 1981, 141(10):1339-41.

Light RW, Girard WM, Jenkinson SG, et al, "Parapneumonic Effusions," *Am J Med*, 1980, 69(4):507-12.

Light RW, Macgregor MI, and Luchsinger PC, "Pleural Effusions: The Diagnostic Separation of Transudates and Exudates," *Ann Intern Med*, 1972, 77(4):507-13.

McVay PA and Toy PT, "Lack of Increased Bleeding After Paracentesis and Thoracentesis in Patients With Mild Coagulation Abnormalities," *Transfusion*, 1991, 31(2):164-71.

Paradis IL and Caldwell EJ, "Diagnostic Approach to Pleural Effusion," *J Maine Med Assoc*, 1977, 68(10):378-82.

Prakash UB, "Malignant Pleural Effusions," *Postgrad Med*, 1986, 80(5):201-9.

Sahn SA, "The Differential Diagnosis of Pleural Effusions," *West J Med*, 1982, 137(2):99-108.

Thoracentesis Fluid Cytology *see* Cytology, Body Fluids
  on page 318

Thoracentesis Fluid Fungus Culture Bone Marrow Fungus Culture
  see Fungus Culture, Body Fluid *on page 341*

Three-Phase Bone Scan *see* Bone Scan *on page 281*

Throat Culture for *Bordetella pertussis* *replaced by* Bordetella
  pertussis Nasopharyngeal Culture *on page 283*

Throat Culture for Group A Beta-Hemolytic *Streptococcus*

Related Information
  Group A *Streptococcus* Antigen Test *on page 354*

Synonyms Beta-Hemolytic Strep Culture, Throat; Group A Beta-Hemolytic *Streptococcus* Culture, Throat; Screening Culture for Group A Beta-Hemolytic *Streptococcus*; Strep Throat Screening Culture

Patient Preparation Do not swab throat in cases of acute epiglottitis unless provisions to establish an alternate airway are readily available.

Special Instructions The laboratory should be informed of the specific site of specimen, age of patient, current antibiotic therapy, and clinical diagnosis.

Specimen Throat swab

Container Sterile Culturette®; Dacron or rayon swabs are acceptable.

Collection The tongue should be depressed while both tonsillar pillars and the oropharynx are swabbed. Exudates should be swabbed and the tongue and uvula should be avoided.

Turnaround Time Reports are usually available within 24 hours. Cultures with no beta-hemolytic streptococci are usually reported after 24 or 48 hours. Reports on specimens from which beta-hemolytic streptococci group A have been isolated require a minimum of 24-48 hours for completion.

Reference Range No beta-hemolytic *Streptococcus pyogenes* isolated

Use Isolate and identify group A beta-hemolytic streptococci; establish the diagnosis of strep throat

Limitations Cultures are usually screened for beta-hemolytic strep group A only. The group A designation in most laboratories is presumptive and is based on rapid commercially available tests. No other organisms are usually reported. Interpretation of throat cultures requires a significant level of experience and technical proficiency in order to avoid false-positives and false-negatives.

Methodology Culture on blood agar plate, latex agglutination screen

Additional Information *Streptococcus pyogenes* (group A beta-hemolytic strep) is generally susceptible to penicillin and its derivatives; therefore, susceptibility need not be routinely determined. The principal reason for considering an alternative drug for individual patients is allergy to penicillin. Erythromycin or a cephalosporin might be substituted in these cases. Patients allergic to penicillins may also be allergic to cephalosporins.

Use of rapid tests providing confirmation of the presence of group A streptococci is common. The sensitivity of the rapid methods is 80% to 95% in overt clinical pharyngitis. The screening method is far less sensitive in cases where concomitant cultures yield <10 colonies.

In the late 1980s, a resurgence of serious *Streptococcus pyogenes* infection was observed. Complications including rheumatic fever, sepsis, severe soft tissue invasion, and toxic shock-like syndrome (TSLS) are reported to be most common with the M1 serotype and that a unique invasive clone has become the predominant cause of severe streptococcal infections.

Selected Readings
  Cleary PP, Kaplan EL, Handley JP, et al, "Clonal Basis for Resurgence of Serious *Streptococcus pyogenes* Disease in the 1980s," *Lancet*, 1992, 339(8792):518-21.

  Kaplan EL, "The Rapid Identification of Group A Beta-Hemolytic Streptococci in the Upper Respiratory Tract," *Pediatr Clin North Am*, 1988, 35(3):535-42.

  Lieu TA, Fleisher GR, and Schwartz JS, "Cost-Effectiveness of Rapid Latex Agglutination Testing and Throat Culture for Streptococcal Pharyngitis," *Pediatrics*, 1990, 85(3):246-56.

Throat Culture for *Neisseria gonorrhoeae* *see* Neisseria gonorrhoeae Culture *on page 412*

Throat Swab for Group A Streptococcal Antigen *see* Group A *Streptococcus* Antigen Test *on page 354*

Thumb, Left or Right, X-ray *see* Bone Films *on page 277*

Tibia and Fibula, Left or Right, X-ray *see* Bone Films *on page 277*

Tick Identification *see* Arthropod Identification *on page 268*

Tissue Anaerobic Culture *see* Anaerobic Culture *on page 250*

Tissue Culture, *Brucella* *see* Biopsy Culture, Routine *on page 270*

Tissue Culture, Routine *see* Biopsy Culture, Routine *on page 270*

Tissue Fungus Culture *see* Fungus Culture, Body Fluid *on page 341*

Tissue Mycobacteria Culture *see* Mycobacteria Culture, Biopsy or Body Fluid *on page 404*

Tobramycin

Related Information
Antibiotic Level, Serum *on page 255*

Synonyms Nebcin®

Abstract Aminoglycoside antibiotics, including tobramycin, are used primarily to treat infections caused by aerobic gram-negative bacilli. Tobramycin has a narrow therapeutic window, and its use in life-threatening infections makes it mandatory that effective levels be achieved without overdosing.

Specimen Serum

Container Red top tube

Sampling Time Peak: 30 minutes after I.V. infusion; trough: immediately before next dose. Levels should be drawn at steady-state, usually 24-36 hours after starting treatment, depending on dosing schedule.

Storage Instructions Separate serum and refrigerate; must be frozen if a β-lactam is also present

Reference Range Therapeutic: peak: 4-10 μg/mL (SI: 8-21 μmol/L) (depends in part on the minimal inhibitory concentration of the drug against the organism being treated); trough: <2 μg/mL (SI: <4 μmol/L)

Possible Panic Range Toxic: peak: >12 μg/mL (SI: >25 μmol/L); trough: >2 μg/mL (SI: >4 μmol/L)

Use Peak levels are necessary to assure adequate therapeutic levels for organism being treated. Trough levels are necessary to reduce the likelihood of nephrotoxicity.

Limitations High peak levels may not have strong correlation with toxicity.

Methodology Immunoassay, fluorescence polarization immunoassay (FPIA)

Additional Information Tobramycin is cleared by the kidney, and accumulates in renal tubular cells. Nephrotoxicity is most closely related to the length of time that trough levels exceed 2 μg/mL (SI: >4 μmol/L). Creatinine levels should be monitored every 2-3 days as this serves as a useful indicator of impending renal toxicity. The initial toxic result is nonoliguric renal failure that is usually reversible if the drug is discontinued. Continued administration of tobramycin may produce oliguric renal failure. Nephrotoxicity may occur in as many as 10% to 25% of patients receiving aminoglycosides; most of this toxicity can be eliminated by monitoring levels and adjusting dosing schedules accordingly.

Aminoglycosides may also cause irreversible ototoxicity that manifests itself clinically as hearing loss. Aminoglycoside ototoxicity is relatively uncommon and clinical trials where levels were carefully monitored and dosing adjusted failed to show a correlation between auditory toxicity and plasma aminoglycoside levels. In situations where dosing is not adjusted, however, sustained high levels may be associated with ototoxicity. This association is far from clear cut, and new once-daily dosing regimens (and associated high peak serum concentrations) that fail to enhance toxicity further complicates the understanding of this issue.

Selected Readings
Edson RS and Terrell CL, "The Aminoglycosides," *Mayo Clin Proc*, 1991, 66(11):1158-64.
Gilbert DN, "Once-Daily Aminoglycoside Therapy," *Antimicrob Agents Chemother*, 1991, 35(3):399-405.

Pancoast SJ, "Aminoglycoside Antibiotics in Clinical Use," *Med Clin North Am*, 1987, 72(3):581-612.

Townsend PL, Fink MP, Stein KL, et al, "Aminoglycoside Pharmacokinetics: Dosage Requirements and Nephrotoxicity in Trauma Patients," *Crit Care Med*, 1989, 17(2):154-7.

Toes of Foot, Left or Right, X-ray *see* Bone Films *on page 277*

Toxin Assay, *Clostridium difficile* *see Clostridium difficile* Toxin Assay *on page 300*

Toxoplasma Antigen by ELISA

Related Information

Toxoplasma Serology *on this page*

Synonyms Toxoplasmosis Antibodies; Toxoplasmosis Titer

Test Includes Detection of *Toxoplasma* antigen by ELISA. IgG and IgM antibodies to *Toxoplasma gondii* may also be included. This test may also be available as a component of the TORCH serology battery.

Special Instructions Collection of convalescent specimen 10-14 days after acute specimen is collected facilitates interpretation of the results.

Specimen Serum

Container Red top tube

Storage Instructions Separate serum and refrigerate if the specimen cannot be delivered to the laboratory within 2 hours of collection.

Causes for Rejection Excessive hemolysis, chylous serum, gross contamination of the specimen.

Reference Range IgG: negative: ≤0.79; equivocal: 0.80-0.99; low positive: 1.00-2.49; midpositive: 2.50-4.59; high positive: ≥4.60. IgM: negative: ≤0.24; equivocal: 0.25-0.35; positive: ≥0.36.

Use Support the diagnosis of toxoplasmosis; document past exposure

Limitations Very limited availability

Methodology Enzyme-linked immunosorbent assay (ELISA)

Additional Information Toxoplasmosis infection in an immunocompromised patient is serious and can produce fatal cerebritis or disseminated illness. The majority of exposed individuals who are immunocompetent develop antibody without clinical disease.

Toxoplasma Serology

Related Information

Toxoplasma Antigen by ELISA *on this page*

Synonyms Toxoplasmosis Titer

Replaces Sabin-Feldman Dye Test

Test Includes IgG and IgM antibodies to *Toxoplasma*. IgA anti-*Toxoplasma* may also be available.

Special Instructions Acute and convalescent specimens are recommended.

Specimen Serum

Container Red top tube

Reference Range Titer: <1:64 by immunofluorescence; <1:256 by indirect hemagglutination; significance of titers varies by laboratory and methodology.

Use Support for the diagnosis of toxoplasmosis; documentation of past exposure and/or immunity to *Toxoplasma gondii*

Limitations Diagnosis of neonatal infection may be difficult because the clinical course of infection outstrips demonstrable antibody response

Methodology Indirect fluorescent antibody (IFA), indirect hemagglutination (IHA), enzyme-linked immunosorbent assay (ELISA)

Additional Information *Toxoplasma gondii* is endemic in cats and is excreted by them. Humans are easily exposed to cyst forms, either in caring for pets or in casual environmental contact. The majority of individuals develop antibody without any clinical disease. A self-limited lymphadenitis is the most common clinical presentation in symptomatic infection.

Congenital toxoplasmosis and infection in an immunocompromised host (AIDS) are more serious, and can produce a fatal cerebritis or disseminated illness. Congenital toxoplasmosis can now be diagnosed *in utero* by detection of IgM antibody in fetal blood.

The diagnosis of toxoplasmosis is supported by high or rising IgG antibody titer, or the demonstration of IgM antibody. The recent availability of IgA anti-*Toxoplasma* may be useful in detection of congenital toxoplasmosis. However, IgM is still the established technique.

(Continued)

Toxoplasma Serology *(Continued)*

Selected Readings

Bessieres MH, Roques C, Berrebi A, et al, "IgA Antibody Response During Acquired and Congenital Toxoplasmosis," *J Clin Pathol*, 1992, 45(7):605-8.

Daffos F, Forestier F, Capella-Pavlovsky M, et al, "Prenatal Management of 746 Pregnancies at Risk for Congenital Toxoplasmosis," *N Engl J Med*, 1988, 318(5):271-5.

Wilson M and McAuley JB, "Laboratory Diagnosis of Toxoplasmosis," *Clin Lab Med*, 1991, 11(4):923-39.

Toxoplasmosis Antibodies *see Toxoplasma* Antigen by ELISA *on previous page*

Toxoplasmosis Titer *see Toxoplasma* Antigen by ELISA *on previous page*

Toxoplasmosis Titer *see Toxoplasma* Serology *on previous page*

Tracheal Aspirate Culture *see* Aerobic Culture, Sputum *on page 246*

Tracheal Aspirate Fungus Culture *see* Fungus Culture, Bronchial Aspirate *on page 342*

Tracheal Aspirate Fungus Culture *see* Fungus Culture, Sputum *on page 345*

Tracheal Aspirate Mycobacteria Culture *see* Mycobacteria Culture, Sputum *on page 406*

Transesophageal Echocardiography

Synonyms Esophageal Echo; TEE

Test Includes Transesophageal echocardiography (TEE) has been developed to solve one of the limitations of echocardiography, that is, the poor imaging quality seen in some patients in whom the bony structures as well as increased lung interface degrade the quality of the images obtained with conventional echocardiography. By placing an echo transducer at the tip of a gastroscope and advancing it into the esophagus, the heart can be imaged from behind without any lung or chest cage interference. Additionally, the closer proximity to the heart allows for utilization of higher frequency transducers which provide higher resolution images. Transesophageal echocardiography has provided a new window through which the heart can be examined with far greater detail than was once thought possible. The mild inconvenience of having to pass a transesophageal probe has been by far outweighed by the enhanced images obtained with it. Presently, transesophageal echocardiography includes 2-D echocardiography, pulsed Doppler, and color flow imagings. Continuous wave Doppler should be incorporated in the near future.

Special Instructions To minimize the risk of aspiration, a period of 6-8 hours fasting is recommended. An intravenous line to keep a vein open for administration of I.V. antibiotics is needed, and sedation as required is advised. Patients with prosthetic valves, native valve stenosis or insufficiency, and congenital heart disease should receive I.V. antibiotic prophylaxis as recommended by the American Heart Association. After the antibiotics have been given the patient should be expected to be in the laboratory for approximately 1 hour to allow for the performance of the procedure and recovery from sedation and analgesic when used. There is no need for repeated antibiotic prophylaxis after initial dose is completed. Most patients will be able to resume full activity after the procedure, but outpatients are advised to have a companion drive them back home to minimize risks from sedation and analgesics when used.

Technique A patient arriving at the Echo Laboratory is greeted by the laboratory personnel, a fasting period of 6-8 hours is confirmed, the reasons indicated for the test are reviewed, vital signs are obtained, symptomatic status is determined, history of allergies is determined, and a detailed explanation of the procedure is made. SBE antibiotic prophylaxis is completed as recommended by the AHA. The patient is asked to undress from the waist up and is gowned with the opening in the front. Electrocardiographic and blood pressure monitorization will be made throughout the procedure. The laboratory should be prepared for cardiopulmonary resuscitation. A local anesthetic is given to the back of the throat through a spray, and a fast-acting hypnotic and analgesic is given I.V. (currently we use Versed® 0.5-2 mg I.V. and Demend® 25-100 mg I.V.). The patient is then placed on left lateral decubitus and the esophageal probe is passed. A dental suction set minimizes flow of saliva out of the mouth. Patient stays awake and comfortable throughout the procedure in most cases.

A systematic and complete study should be performed on each patient. Additionally, the area of specific concern should be evaluated with further detail. A complete study will include 2-D imaging and color flow Doppler study of all cardiac chambers, valves, and great vessels. The study is initiated with the probe placed most distally, which provides a short axis view of the left ventricle as the probe is removed a view equivalent to an apical 4-chamber is obtained. This allows for the best view of the mitral and tricuspid valves. Further removal of the probe allows for visualization of the outflow tract of the left ventricle and aortic valve, after this the left atrium atrial appendage, interatrial septum, and pulmonary veins can be studied. Finally, with further removal of the probe, the aortic arch is visualized. The color Doppler is turned on during the study to evaluate normal and abnormal flow patterns. A continuous video recording is obtained throughout the study for later study and analysis. After completion of the study, the transesophageal probe is removed and the patient is kept under observation until regaining a prestudy status.

Normal Findings Transesophageal echocardiography has provided a new window to the heart, but the operator must recognize and become familiar with the different orientation of the cardiac structures and tomographic planes as seen from a different perspective. Also, there is a limitation in the number of tomographic planes than can be obtained through TEE since the motion of the probe is somewhat limited in the esophagus. With these limitations in mind, the interpretation of images through TEE is similar to that described in the section of color Doppler echocardiography.

Use Transesophageal echocardiography currently is being used intraoperatively to follow cardiac function during cardiac and noncardiac surgery, in the intensive care units to follow and evaluate critically ill patients, and in the study of ambulatory patients to better evaluate a variety of cardiovascular disorders. Transesophageal echocardiography has been found most useful in the evaluation of prosthetic valve dysfunction, particularly mitral valve prosthesis, in the quantitation and diagnostic characterization of native mitral valve insufficiency, in the evaluation of left atrial thrombosis and masses, in the evaluation of bacterial endocarditis and its complications, and in the evaluation of intracardiac shunts.

Contraindications TEE is contraindicated in patients with esophageal obstructions or with respiratory failure if not intubated.

Selected Readings
Seward JB, Khandheria BK, Oh JK, et al, "Transesophageal Echocardiography: Technique, Anatomic Correlations, Implementation, and Clinical Applications," *Mayo Clin Proc*, 1988, 63(7):649-80.

Transjugular Needle Biopsy of the Liver *see* Liver Biopsy *on page 387*

Transthoracic Needle Aspiration for *Pneumocystis* *see* Pneumocystis carinii Test *on page 431*

Transtracheal Aspirate Anaerobic Culture *see* Anaerobic Culture *on page 250*

Transtracheal Aspirate Culture *see* Aerobic Culture, Sputum *on page 246*

Transtracheal Aspirate Fungus Culture *see* Fungus Culture, Bronchial Aspirate *on page 342*

Transtracheal Aspirate Fungus Culture *see* Fungus Culture, Sputum *on page 345*

Transtracheal Aspirate Mycobacteria Culture *see* Mycobacteria Culture, Sputum *on page 406*

Transtracheal Aspiration *Legionella* Culture *see* Legionella pneumophila Culture *on page 381*

***Treponema pallidum* Antibodies, CSF** *see* FTA-ABS, Cerebrospinal Fluid *on page 335*

***Treponema pallidum* Darkfield Examination** *see* Darkfield Examination, Syphilis *on page 322*

TRIC Agent Culture *see* Chlamydia Culture *on page 294*

***Trichinella* Antibody** *see* Trichinella Serology *on next page*

Trichinella **Serology**

Synonyms *Trichinella* Antibody; Trichinosis Serology

Applies To *Trichinella spiralis*

Specimen Serum

Container Red top tube

Reference Range Negative; Interpretation of positive results vary by method and by laboratory. Consult laboratory for specific interpretations.

Use Screen for antibodies to *Trichinella spiralis* to establish the diagnosis of trichinosis

Limitations Low titers may represent antibody from previous rather than current infection. The bentonite flocculation test cannot be used for testing lightly infected pigs. The test may have a high false-negative rate of 15% to 22% during the first period of the infection.

Methodology Bentonite flocculation test (BFT), indirect fluorescent antibody (IFA), complement fixation (CF), latex agglutination (LA), enzyme-linked immunosorbent assay (ELISA)

Additional Information The bentonite flocculation test is sensitive and specific. Antibody becomes detectable 3 weeks after infection, rises for several weeks, and then declines slowly so that most individuals will test negative in two to three years.

Immunofluorescence is more sensitive for light infection in pigs.

In humans, diagnosis can also be made by finding cysts in a muscle biopsy.

Selected Readings
Bruschi F, Tassi C, and Pozio E, "Parasite-Specific Antibody Response in *Trichinella* sp. 3 Human Infection: A One Year Follow-up," *Am J Trop Med Hyg*, 1990, 43(2):186-93.

Kagan IG, "Serodiagnosis of Parasitic Diseases," *Manual of Clinical Laboratory Immunology*, 3rd ed, Rose NR, Friedman H, and Fahey JL, eds, Washington, DC: American Society for Microbiology, 1986, 474-5.

Trichinella spiralis see *Trichinella* Serology *on this page*

Trichinosis Serology see *Trichinella* Serology *on this page*

Trichomonas **Culture** see *Trichomonas* Preparation *on this page*

Trichomonas **Pap Smear** see *Trichomonas* Preparation *on this page*

Trichomonas **Preparation**

Related Information

Genital Culture *on page 349*

Synonyms Hanging Drop Mount for *Trichomonas*; *Trichomonas vaginalis* Wet Preparation; Trich Prep; Wet Preparation for *Trichomonas vaginalis*

Applies To Cervical *Trichomonas* Smear; *Trichomonas* Culture; *Trichomonas* Pap Smear; *Trichomonas* Wet Preparation, Urine; Urethral *Trichomonas* Smear; Urine *Trichomonas* Wet Mount; Vaginal *Trichomonas* Smear

Test Includes Wet mount and microscopic examination. Pap smear and/or culture may also be performed.

Special Instructions The laboratory should be informed of the specific source of the specimen.

Specimen Vaginal, cervical, or urethral swabs, prostatic fluid, urine sediment

Container Sterile tube containing 1 mL of sterile nonbacteriostatic saline

Collection The specimen should be collected using a speculum without lubricant. The mucosa of the posterior vagina may be swabbed or the secretions may be collected with a pipette. The swab should be expressed into the saline for transport to the laboratory. The specimen should be examined as soon as possible.

Storage Instructions Transport the specimen to the laboratory as soon as possible after collection. Do not refrigerate.

Causes for Rejection Specimen dried out

Turnaround Time Same day; culture in Kupferberg's medium is examined for 5 days

Reference Range Negative: no trichomonads identified; positive: demonstration of actively motile flagellates or positive culture

Use Establish the presence of *Trichomonas vaginalis*

Limitations The specimen will be examined for *Trichomonas vaginalis* only. A separate swab (Culturette®) must be collected for culture of bacteria or fungus cultures, if required. One negative result does not rule out the possibility of *Trichomonas vaginalis* infection. The sensitivity of the wet mount procedure is low (50% to 70%); therefore, the wet mount is negative in 30% to 50% of women with trichomoniasis.

Contraindications Douching within 3 days prior to specimen collection

Methodology Wet mount microscopic examination, Pap smear, direct immunofluorescent technique with monoclonal antibody. Culture may be performed using Kupferberg's liquid medium or Hirsch charcoal agar.

Additional Information The absence of the classical yellow, frothy discharge does not exclude trichomoniasis. Culture usually yield positive results when wet preparations are negative. Cultures are the gold standard and are sensitive; however, they are expensive and have limited availability. The high rate of false-negatives, 48.4%, and false-positives observed with stained preparations (Pap smears) requires that confirmation by wet mount or culture be considered when the reported results are inconsistent with the clinical findings. Immunofluorescence tests are being adopted which have increased sensitivity. The false-positives observed when immunofluorescent methods are compared to culture may represent failure of culture in patients with few organisms. Culture is not available in many laboratories.

Trichomonas hominis

Trophozoite

Scale: 0 5 10 μm

From Brooks MM and Melvin DM, *Morphology of Diagnostic Stages of Intestinal Parasites of Humans,* 2nd ed, Atlanta, GA: U.S. Department of Health and Human Services, Publication No. 84-8116, Centers for Disease Control, 1984, with permission.

In a series of 600 "high risk" women, 88 *Trichomonas* infected patients were observed. Co-infection was noted as follows: *Ureaplasma urealyticum* 96%, *Gardnerella vaginalis* 91%, *Mycoplasma hominis* 89%, bacterial vaginosis 57%, *Neisseria gonorrhoeae* 29%, and *Chlamydia trachomatis* 15%. *Candida albicans* and other *Candida* sp are frequently implicated in vulvovaginitis. A vaginal pH above 5 is suggestive of *Trichomonas*.

In males a milky white fluid discharge and urethral irritation present for more than 4 weeks is frequently associated with urethritis caused by *T. vaginalis*.

Selected Readings

Bennett JR, "The Emergency Department Diagnosis of *Trichomonas vaginalis,*" *Ann Emerg Med,* 1989, 18(5):564-6.

Clay JC, Veeravahu M, and Smyth RW, "Practical Problems of Diagnosing Trichomoniasis in Women," *Genitourin Med,* 1988, 64(2):115-7.

Krieger JN, Tam MR, Stevens CE, et al, "Diagnosis of Trichomoniasis, Comparison of Conventional Wet-Mount Examination With Cytologic Studies, Cultures, and Monoclonal Antibody Staining of Direct Specimens," *JAMA,* 1988, 259(8):1223-7.

Pastorek JG 2d, "Common Types of Vaginitis," *Hosp Med,* 1992, 73-88.

Sobel JD, "Vaginal Infections in Adult Women," *Med Clin North Am,* 1990, 74(6):1573-602.

***Trichomonas vaginalis* Wet Preparation** *see Trichomonas* Preparation *on previous page*

***Trichomonas* Wet Preparation, Urine** *see Trichomonas* Preparation *on previous page*

Trich Prep *see Trichomonas* Preparation *on previous page*

Trypanosomiasis Peripheral Blood Preparation *see* Microfilariae, Peripheral Blood Preparation *on page 400*

Tuberculin Skin Testing *see* Tuberculin Skin Testing, Intracutaneous *on this page*

Tuberculin Skin Testing, Intracutaneous

Related Information

Anergy Skin Test Battery *on page 252*

Fungal Skin Testing *on page 337*

Synonyms Mantoux Test; PPD Test; Purified Protein Derivative (PPD) Test; Tuberculin Skin Testing

Test Includes Intradermal injection of culture extracts of *Mycobacterium tuberculosis* (MTB). This is an *in vivo* means of evaluating delayed hypersensitivity to MTB. Skin test sites are examined at 24, 48, and 72 hours for signs of induration and erythema. A positive skin test indicates prior exposure to MTB (either recent or remote), with an adequate cell-mediated immune response.

(Continued)

Tuberculin Skin Testing, Intracutaneous *(Continued)*

Patient Preparation The procedure is explained to the patient. Inquiries should be made regarding past PPD reactions. No specific skin preparation is necessary; however, patients with severe skin disease, such as psoriasis, should be examined beforehand to ensure that there are suitable areas of normal appearing skin. Although testing need not be performed by a physician, one should be immediately available for systemic reactions.

Aftercare If no adverse reaction has occurred within several minutes, the patient may be discharged from the testing center. In some centers, patients are given written instructions on measurement and recording of a positive skin reaction at home. Other centers prefer patients to return to the test center at 48 and 72 hours for formal skin test reading by a nurse or physician. Test sites should be kept clean for 72 hours. No bathing restrictions are necessary. Patient should contact physician if a severe local reaction develops or if fever and dyspnea occurs.

Special Instructions If skin testing is performed in a separate department, requisition should state:
- the strength of tuberculin test (1 TU, 5 TU, 250 TU)
- whether an anergy skin battery is also desired

Complications In general, adverse reactions are uncommon. Rare complications include fever, lymphangitis, adenopathy, and local ulcers or vesicles. If local lesions develop, these should be treated with dry sterile dressings. The use of topical ointments is optional.

Equipment Culture extracts of MTB (tuberculins) are available for injection in preparations termed "purified protein derivatives" or PPD. Commercial preparations of PPD are available in different doses, standard test dose being 5 tuberculin unit dose (5 TU). Also required are a disposable glass or plastic tuberculin syringe, a short $\frac{1}{4}$" to $\frac{1}{2}$" 26- or 27-gauge needle.

Technique The standard 5 TU tuberculin test is performed as follows. A skin site on the volar surface of the forearm is cleaned. 0.1 mL 5 TU PPD is drawn up into a tuberculin syringe and the needle is inserted bevel upwards intradermally and a discrete wheel (5-10 mL) is produced. If the test is improperly performed, a second dose can be given at an alternate location. Test sites are examined at 24, 48, and 72 hours for the presence of induration, by palpation and inspection. The largest transverse diameter of induration is measured along the long axis of the forearm. Areas of erythema are disregarded. The following should be **carefully** recorded in the chart: Strength of PPD used, date of testing, date of reading, and size of induration. The applied method described also applies to testing with nonstandard tuberculin doses (1 TU or 250 TU).

Normal Findings No reaction to the 5 TU PPD test, but a normal skin reaction to anergy skin testing. (For details see Anergy Skin Test Battery.)

Critical Values Interpretation of the tuberculin skin test is highly dependent on the background diseases of the person being tested. There is no single cutoff point for interpreting a positive or negative test. In 1990, the Centers for Disease Control recommended the following scheme for interpreting results of the 5 TU PPD test.

1. A skin reaction ≥ 5 mm is positive in those persons with:
   - HIV infection
   - chest x-ray with fibrotic lesions likely to be old healed TB
   - recent close contact with a patient with known infectious TB
2. A skin reaction of ≥ 10 mm is positive in the following groups:
   - Persons with medical risk factors known to increase the risk of active TB once infection has occurred (silicosis, diabetes mellitus, corticosteroids and other immunosuppressive therapies, hematologic disease, lymphoproliferate diseases, end-stage renal disease, intestinal bypass, postgastrectomy, carcinomas of head and neck, being 10% below ideal body weight)
   - Foreign born from areas (such as Asia, Africa, Latin America) where the prevalence of TB is high
   - Low income, high-risk minorities (blacks, hispanics, American Indians)
   - I.V. drug users
   - Residents of long-term care facilities (jails, nursing homes)
3. A skin reaction of ≥ 15 mm is positive in all other persons, including otherwise healthy persons.

Use In general, the tuberculin skin test is used to evaluate individuals with suspected MTB infection. Testing is routinely indicated in the following situations:
- patient with clinical signs and symptoms of active tuberculosis, either pulmonary or extrapulmonary

- patient with a chest radiograph compatible with past tuberculosis
- individuals who have been recently exposed to a proven (index) case of active tuberculosis; this includes close household contacts and healthcare workers with significant exposure
- individuals who have a history of tuberculosis in the remote past, never treated
- selected patients who are to start a prolonged course of steroids (or other immunosuppressives), particularly if there has been past exposure to MTB; this includes most solid organ transplantation candidates
- patients at increased risk for developing tuberculosis on the basis of their underlying disease (eg, silicosis, gastrectomy)
- routine surveillance of persons with ongoing exposure to MTB, such as nursing personnel, respiratory therapists, etc
- immigrants from areas where MTB is endemic
- epidemiologic and public health surveys (eg, nursing homes, innercity residents, etc)

Some clinicians will skin test any patient with a serious underlying illness, such as hepatitis, cirrhosis, AIDS, peptic ulcer disease, cardiomyopathy, severe pulmonary disease, end-stage renal failure, carcinoma, leukemia, and others. A positive tuberculin skin test in patients with these conditions is usually an indication for prolonged isoniazid prophylaxis.

Limitations For best results, trained personnel are necessary for administering and reading the test.

Contraindications Testing is contraindicated in the rare patient with known sensitivity to tuberculin. This includes severe local reactions (extensive erythema, vesiculations, ulcers) and anaphylaxis. Note that the development of local skin erythema (only) on a prior tuberculin skin test does not usually constitute a true hypersensitivity reaction. Some clinicians feel that the Mantoux test is contraindicated in the patient who has had a clearly documented positive PPD test in the past. The incidence and significance of this complication has not been studied formally; some physicians fear a hyperimmune local response when the patient is rechallenged with tuberculin.

Additional Information The tuberculin test is a measure of delayed (cellular) immunity to MTB. As such, a positive test indicates only exposure to MTB and does not distinguish current from past infections. False-positive tests may be seen with exposure to nontuberculous (atypical) *Mycobacterium* or previous inoculation with BCG vaccine. False-negative tests are common and can be difficult to interpret. Causes for false-negative tests relate not only to the technique of administration, but also the age and immune status of the person being tested. Insignificant reactions are commonly seen secondary to anergy from immunosuppressive therapy, neoplastic disease, various bacterial or viral infections, and vaccinations. Thus, the tuberculin test is often performed along with skin tests for common antigens, such as *Candida* and mumps, to assess possible anergic states. In addition, hypersensitivity to tuberculin may diminish gradually with age. A "booster phenomenon" has been described in the elderly whereby waning tuberculin sensitivity is augmented by repeating 5 TU skin testing at 1 week intervals. Although controversy exists concerning the interpretation of both the booster phenomenon and of the standard tuberculin test itself, this test remains an invaluable aid in diagnosing tuberculous infection.

Selected Readings

Huebner RE, Schein MF, and Bass JB Jr, "The Tuberculin Skin Test," *Clin Infect Dis*, 1993, 17(6):968-75.

Reichman LB, "Tuberculin Skin Testing, The State of the Art," *Chest*, 1979, 76(6 Suppl):764-70.

The American Thoracic Society, "The Tuberculin Skin Test," *Am Rev Respir Dis*, 1981, 124:356-63.

Snider DE Jr, "Bacille Calmette-Guérin Vaccinations and Tuberculin Skin Tests," *JAMA*, 1985, 253(23):3438-9.

Stead WW and To T, "The Significance of the Tuberculin Skin Test in Elderly Persons," *Ann Intern Med*, 1987, 107(6):837-42.

Thompson NJ, Glassroth JL, Snider DE Jr, "The Booster Phenomenon in Serial Tuberculin Testing," *Am Rev Respir Dis*, 1979, 119(4):587-97.

TWAR Strain *Chlamydia* *see Chlamydia pneumoniae* Serology
on page 295

Tzanck Smear *see* Herpes Cytology *on page 362*

UA *see* Urinalysis *on page 467*

Ultrasound, Kidneys

Synonyms Kidneys Ultrasound; Renal Ultrasound

Test Includes Kidneys

Patient Preparation The examination may be long, up to 1 hour including waiting time. An emergency examination or an unpredictably long preceding examination may result in additional delay. **Note**: Ultrasound exam to be scheduled before a barium study. If barium study was done, bowel preparation is needed before doing ultrasound examination.

Special Instructions All outpatient examinations are by appointment only. All inpatients are placed on the daily schedule as time permits and are performed as scheduled. Nonemergent examinations are given secondary priority and therefore may not be able to be performed the same day scheduled. Patients will generally be asked to stay after the examination until films are reviewed by the radiologist.

Equipment Standard B-mode real time ultrasonic imager with 2-5 MHz transducer.

Technique A gel is applied to the skin and a handheld transducer is swept across the area of interest to image the appropriate organs. Sound waves are used for the imaging and no radiation exposure is present. Images are recorded on x-ray film.

Data Acquired Longitudinal and transverse images of each kidney

Causes for Rejection Patient unable to cooperate with positioning and respiratory maneuvers; bowel gas, barium, obesity

Turnaround Time A typed report will generally be issued within 36 hours. A preliminary verbal report generally can be given to the referring physician on request.

Use Evaluation of cysts and neoplasms, calcifications, abscess, and hydronephrosis and hydroureter

Additional Information Rapid, sensitive evaluation for the presence of hydronephrosis. Useful in confirming the cystic nature of lesions. Detection of hydroureter is often problematic.

Selected Readings

Goldberg BB, *Abdominal Ultrasonography*, New York, NY: John Wiley and Sons Inc, 1984.
Grant DC, "Ultrasound of the Genitourinary Tract," *Radiology*, Taveras JT and Ferrucci JT, eds, Philadelphia, PA: JB Lippincott, 1988.

Ultrasound, Peripheral Arteries and Veins

Synonyms Iliac Arteries Ultrasound; Peripheral Arteries and Veins Ultrasound; Popliteal Ultrasound

Test Includes Peripheral arteries and/or veins

Patient Preparation The examination may be long, up to 1 hour including waiting time. An emergency examination or an unpredictably long preceding examination may result in additional delay.

Special Instructions Specific vessels of interest to be studied as well as location must be specified. All outpatient examinations are by appointment only. All inpatients are placed on the daily schedule as time permits and are performed as scheduled. Nonemergent examinations are given secondary priority and therefore may not be able to be performed the same day scheduled. Patients will generally be asked to stay after the examination until films are reviewed by the radiologist.

Equipment Standard B-mode real time ultrasonic imager with Doppler capability with 5-10 MHz transducer.

Technique A gel is applied to the skin and a handheld transducer is swept across the area of interest to image the appropriate organs. Sound waves are used for the imaging and no radiation exposure is present. Images are recorded on x-ray film.

Turnaround Time A typed report will generally be issued within 36 hours. A preliminary verbal report generally can be given to the referring physician on request.

Normal Findings Presence of appropriate flow, compressibility of venous structures

Use Determine aneurysm, cysts, pseudoaneurysm, deep vein thrombosis (DVT), arterial insufficiency

Additional Information Examination is valuable in the detection of pseudoaneurysms, aneurysms, arterial insufficiency, and deep venous thrombosis (DVT)

Undulant Fever, Culture *see* Blood Culture, *Brucella* on page 274

Unidimensional Echo *see* Echocardiography, M-Mode on page 324

Urea Clearance *replaced by* Creatinine Clearance on page 311

Urea Nitrogen Clearance *replaced by* Creatinine Clearance on page 311

***Ureaplasma urealyticum* Culture** *see Mycoplasma/Ureaplasma* Culture on page 410

***Ureaplasma urealyticum* Culture, Genital** *see* Genital Culture for *Ureaplasma urealyticum* on page 350

Urease Test and Culture, *Helicobacter pylori* *see Helicobacter pylori* Culture and Urease Test on page 356

Urethral *Chlamydia* Culture *see Chlamydia* Culture on page 294

Urethral Culture for *Neisseria gonorrhoeae* *see Neisseria gonorrhoeae* Culture on page 412

Urethral Culture for T-Strain *Mycoplasma* *see* Genital Culture for *Ureaplasma urealyticum* on page 350

Urethral *Trichomonas* Smear *see Trichomonas* Preparation on page 462

Urethra, *Mycoplasma* Culture *see Mycoplasma/Ureaplasma* Culture on page 410

Urinalysis

Synonyms UA

Applies To Casts, Urine; Crystals, Urine; Occult Blood, Semiquantitative, Urine; Urine Crystals

Test Includes Opacity, color, appearance, specific gravity, pH, protein, glucose, occult blood, ketones, bilirubin, and in some laboratories, urobilinogen and microscopic examination of urine sediment. Some laboratories include screening for leukocyte esterase and nitrite and do not perform a microscopic examination unless one of the chemical screening (macroscopic) tests is abnormal or unless a specific request for microscopic examination is made.

Abstract The examination of urine is one of the oldest practices in medicine. A carefully performed urinalysis still provides a wealth of information about the patient, both in terms of differential diagnosis, and by exclusion of many conditions when the urinalysis is "normal."

Patient Preparation Instructions should be given in method of collection. Both males and females need instruction in cleansing the urethral meatus. "Midstream collections" are performed by initiating urination into the toilet, then bringing the collection device into the urine stream to catch the midportion of the void.

Specimen Urine

Container Plastic urine container

Collection A voided specimen is usually suitable. If the specimen is likely to be contaminated by vaginal discharge or hemorrhage, a clean catch specimen is desirable. If the specimen is collected by catheter, it should be so labeled. The timing of urine collection will vary with the purpose of the test. To check for casts or renal concentration ability, a first voided morning specimen may be preferred. For screening purposes, this is also the best time, as a later and more dilute specimen may make small increases in protein, RBC, or WBC excretion harder to detect. The upright position increases protein excretion by hemodynamic factors. Mid-morning urine is likely to give the highest albumin excretion, but early morning urine is best when attempting to detect Bence Jones protein.

Storage Instructions Transport specimen to the laboratory as soon as possible after collection. If the specimen cannot be processed immediately by the laboratory it should be refrigerated. Refrigeration preserves formed elements in the urine, but may precipitate crystals not originally present.

Causes for Rejection Specimen delayed in transport, fecal contamination, decomposition, or bacterial overgrowth

Reference Range See table. **Crystals** are interpreted by the physician. Warm, freshly voided urine sediment from normal subjects almost never contains

(Continued)

467

Urinalysis *(Continued)*

crystals, despite maximal concentration. Xanthine, cystine, and uric acid crystal (and stone) formation is favored by a consistently acid urine (pH <5.5-6). Calcium oxalate and apatite stones are associated with no particular disturbance of urine pH. Calcium carbonate, calcium phosphate, and especially magnesium ammonium phosphate stones are associated with pH >7. Urine pH >7.5 may briefly follow meals (alkaline tide) but more commonly indicate systemic alkali intake (NaHCO$_3$, etc) or urine infected by bacteria which split urea to ammonia.

Urinalysis

Test	Reference Range
Specific gravity	1.003–1.029
pH	4.5–7.8
Protein	Negative
Glucose	Negative
Ketones	Negative
Bilirubin	Negative
Occult blood	Negative
Leukocyte osterase	Negative
Nitrite	Negative
Urobilinogen	0.1–1.0 EU/dL
WBCs	0–5/hpf
RBCs	male: 0–3/hpf female: 0–5/hpf
Casts	0–4/lpf hyaline
Bacteria	Negative

hpf = high power field
lpf = low power field
EU = Ehrlich units

Possible Panic Range The presence of massive amounts of oxalate crystals in fresh urine should be reported promptly to the physician, as this finding may represent ethylene glycol intoxication.

Use Screen for abnormalities of urine; diagnose and manage renal diseases, urinary tract infection, urinary tract neoplasms, systemic diseases, and inflammatory or neoplastic diseases adjacent to the urinary tract

Limitations Insufficient volume, less than 2 mL, may limit the extent of procedures performed. Metabolites of Pyridium® may interfere with the dipstick reactions by producing color interference. High vitamin C intake may cause an underestimate of glucosuria, or a false-negative nitrate test. Survival of WBCs is decreased by low osmolality, alkalinity, and lack of refrigeration. Formed elements in the urine including casts disintegrate rapidly, therefore the specimen should be analyzed as soon as possible after collection. Specific gravity is affected by glucosuria, mannitol infusion, or prior administration of iodinated contrast material for radiologic studies (IVP dye). Some brands of test strips give a "trace positive" protein indication if not stored in dry atmosphere (cap of test strip bottle not on tight). Ambient humidity exposure of the test strips over time also causes some reduction of sensitivity for occult blood and nitrate and increased sensitivity for glucose (false-positive). This can be detected by using tap water as a negative control. False-positive tests for protein can also be due to contamination of the urine by an ammonium-containing cleansing solution. Problems relevant to the sensitivity of protein detection have led to development of methods described in the listing Microalbuminuria.

Methodology The chemical portion of the urinalysis is done by test strip, with confirming chemical method for protein (sulfosalicylic acid precipitation).

Additional Information

MICROSCOPY:

Crystalluria is frequently observed in urine specimens stored at room temperature or refrigerated. Such crystals are diagnostically useful when observed in warm, fresh urine by a physician evaluating microhematuria, nephrolithiasis, or toxin ingestion.

In abundance, **calcium oxalate** and/or **hippurate crystals** may suggest ethylene glycol ingestion (especially if known to be accompanied by neurological abnormalities, appearance of drunkenness, hypertension, and a high anion gap acidosis.) Urine is usually supersaturated in calcium oxalate, often in calcium phosphate, and acid urine is often saturated in uric acid. Yet crystalluria is uncommon (in warm, fresh urine) because of the normal presence of crystal inhibitors, the lack of available nidus, and the time factor. When properly observed in fresh urine, crystals may provide a clue to the composition of renal stones even not yet passed, the nidus for such stones, or, as such, have been associated with microhematuria.

Uric acid crystals are reddish brown, rectangular, rhomboidal, or flower-like structures of narrow rectangular petals. **Ammonium urates,** in alkaline urine, are irregular blobs and crescents, sometimes resembling fragmented red cell shapes.

Calcium oxalate crystals are fairly uniform small double pyramids, base to base, which under the microscope look like little crosses on a square.

Calcium phosphate crystallizes in urine as flowers of narrow rectangular needles.

Cystine crystals, uniquely in urine, form large irregular hexagonal plates, which may dissolve if alkalinized. They occur only in the urine of subjects with cystinuria.

Calcium magnesium ammonium phosphate, or "triple phosphate," forms unique "coffin lid" angularly domed rectangles which may be present in massive quantities in alkaline urine. They usually are associated with urine infected by urea splitting bacteria which cause "infection," or "triple phosphate" stones.

Leukocyturia may indicate inflammatory disease in the genitourinary tract, including bacterial infection, glomerulonephritis, chemical injury, autoimmune diseases, or inflammatory disease adjacent to the urinary tract such as appendicitis or diverticulitis.

White cell casts indicate the renal origin of leukocytes, and are most frequently found in acute pyelonephritis. White cell casts are also found in glomerulonephritis such as lupus nephritis, and in acute and chronic interstitial nephritis. When nuclei degenerate, such leukocyte casts resemble renal tubular casts.

Red cell casts indicate renal origin of hematuria and suggest glomerulonephritis, including lupus nephritis. Red cell casts may also be found in subacute bacterial endocarditis, renal infarct, vasculitis, Goodpasture's syndrome, sickle cell disease, and in malignant hypertension. Degenerated red cell casts may be called **"hemoglobin casts"**. Orange to red casts may be found with myoglobinuria as well.

Dysmorphic red cells are observed in glomerulonephritis. "Dysmorphic" red cells refer to heterogeneous sizes, hypochromia, distorted irregular outlines and frequently small blobs extruding from the cell membrane. Phase contrast microscopy best demonstrates RBC and WBC morphology. Nonglomerular urinary red blood cells resemble peripheral circulating red blood cells. Schramek et al have used the presence or absence of dysmorphic red cells to direct the degree of work-up for hematuria and for follow-up.

Crenated RBCs provide no implication regarding RBC source.

Dark brown or smoky urine suggests a renal source of hematuria.

A **pink or red urine** suggests an extrarenal source.

Hyaline casts occur in physiologic states (eg, after exercise) and many types of renal diseases. They are best seen in phase contrast microscopy or with reduced illumination.

Renal tubular (epithelial) casts are most suggestive of tubular injury, as in acute tubular necrosis. They are also found in other disorders, including eclampsia, heavy metal poisoning, ethylene glycol intoxication, and acute allograft rejection.

Granular casts: Very finely granulated casts may be found after exercise and in a variety of glomerular and tubulointerstitial diseases.; coarse granular casts are abnormal and are present in a wide variety of renal diseases.

(Continued)

Urinalysis *(Continued)*

"Dirty brown" granular casts are typical of acute tubular necrosis.

Waxy casts are found especially in chronic renal diseases, and are associated with chronic renal failure; they occur in diabetic nephropathy, malignant hypertension, and glomerulonephritis, among other conditions. They are named for their waxy or glossy appearance. They often appear brittle and cracked.

Fatty casts are generally found in the nephrotic syndromes, diabetic nephropathy, other forms of chronic renal diseases, and glomerulonephritis. The fat droplets originate in renal tubular cells when they exceed their capacity to reabsorb protein of glomerular origin. Their inclusions have the features and significance of oval fat bodies.

Broad casts originate from dilated, chronically damaged tubules or the collecting ducts. They can be granular or waxy. Broad waxy casts are called "renal failure casts."

Spermatozoa may be seen in male urine related to recent or retrograde ejaculation. In female urine, the presence of spermatozoa may provide evidence of vaginal contamination following recent intercourse.

Automation of the urinalysis is routine in many laboratories. Some authors wish to abandon microscopic evaluation of the urine, which is not easily automated, on urine samples testing "normal" by dipstick screening. A urine sample that is normal to inspection and dipstick will be normal to microscopic exam 95% of the time.

One instrument for automating the entire urinalysis, the Yellow IRIS®, includes a module that automates the microscopic sediment exam. This has been found to be more consistent than the manual method for routine urinalysis and has increased the number of abnormal urines detected.

Selected Readings
Carlson D and Statland BE, "Automated Urinalysis," *Clin Lab Med*, 1988, 8(3):449-61.

Cohen HT and Spiegel DM, "Air-Exposed Urine Dipsticks Give False-Positive Results for Glucose and False-Negative Results for Blood," *Am J Clin Pathol*, 1991, 96(3):398-400.

Freeman JA and Beeler MF, *Laboratory Medicine/Urinalysis and Medical Microscopy*, 2nd ed, Philadelphia, PA: Lea & Febiger, 1983.

Haber MH, "Quality Assurance in Urinalysis," *Clin Lab Med*, 1988, 8(3):431-47.

Haber MH, *Urinary Sediment: A Textbook Atlas*, American Society of Clinical Pathologists, 1981.

Kiel DP and Moskowitz MA, "The Urinalysis: A Critical Appraisal," *Med Clin North Am*, 1987, 71(4):607-24.

Mariani AJ, Luangphinith S, Loo S, et al, "Dipstick Chemical Urinalysis: An Accurate Cost-Effective Screening Test," *J Urol*, 1984, 132(1):64-6.

Rizzoni G, Braggion F, and Zacchello G, "Evaluation of Glomerular and Nonglomerular Hematuria by Phase Contrast Microscopy," *J Pediatr*, 1983, 103:370-4.

Roe CE, Carlson DA, Daigneault RW, et al, "Evaluation of the Yellow IRIS™. An Automated Method for Urinalysis," *Am J Clin Pathol*, 1986, 86(5):661-5.

Schramek P, Schuster FX, Georgopoulos M, et al, "Value of Urinary Erythrocyte Morphology in Assessment of Symptomless Microhaematuria," *Lancet*, 1989, 2(8675):1316-9.

Schumann GB, "Cytodiagnostic Urinalysis for the Nephrology Practice," *Semin Nephrol*, 1986, 6(4):308-45.

Schumann GB, *Urine Sediment Examination*, Baltimore, MD: Williams and Wilkins, 1980.

Scott JH, "Abnormal Urinalysis in Appendicitis," *J Urol*, 1983, 129:1015.

Segasothy M, Lau TM, Birch DF, et al, "Immunocytologic Dissection of the Urine Sediment Using Monoclonal Antibodies," *Am J Clin Pathol*, 1988, 90(6):691-6.

Sheets C and Lyman JL, "Urinalysis," *Emerg Med Clin North Am*, 1986, 4(2):263-80.

Shenoy UA, "Current Assessment of Microhematuria and Leukocyturia," *Clin Lab Med*, 1985, 5:317-29, (review).

Wargotz ES, Hyde JE, Karcher DS, et al, "Urine Sediment Analysis by the Yellow IRIS™ Automated Urinalysis Workstation," *Am J Clin Pathol*, 1987, 88(6):746-8.

Wenz B and Lampasso JA, "Eliminating Unnecessary Urine Microscopy – Results and Performance Characteristics of an Algorithm Based on Chemical

Yager HM and Harrington JT, "Urinalysis and Urinary Electrolytes," *The Principles and Practice of Nephrology*, Chapter 28, Jacobson HR, Striker GE, and Klahr S, eds, Philadelphia, PA: BC Decker Inc, 1991, 167-77.

Urine Crystals *see* Urinalysis *on page 467*

Urine Culture *see* Urine Culture, Clean Catch *on this page*

Urine Culture, Clean Catch

Synonyms CMVS, Culture; Midstream Urine Culture; Urine Culture; Urine Culture, Midvoid Specimen

Applies To Urine Culture, Foley Catheter

Patient Preparation Thoroughly instruct patient for proper collection of "clean catch" specimen. Wash hands thoroughly. Wash penis or vulva using downward strokes four times with four soapy sponges, then once with sponge wet with warm water. Urethral meatus and perineum must be washed. Each sponge must be discarded after one use. Urinate about 30 mL (1 ounce) of urine directly into toilet or bedpan and take middle portion of urine sample. Screw cap securely on container without touching the inside rim. Apply the completed patient label to the specimen cup. Most patients, with instruction, do better with privacy than with an attendant.

Specimen Random urine

Container Plastic urine container or sterile tube

Collection Early morning specimens yield highest bacterial counts from overnight incubation in the bladder. Forced fluids dilute the urine and may cause reduced colony counts. Hair from perineum will contaminate the specimen. The stream from a male may be contaminated by bacteria from beneath the prepuce. Bacteria from vaginal secretions, vulva or distal urethra may also contaminate the specimen as may organisms from hands or clothing. Receptacle must be sterile.

Storage Instructions The specimen should be refrigerated if it cannot be promptly transported to the laboratory. A transport stabilizer may be used to preserve the specimen if refrigeration is not available.

Causes for Rejection Unrefrigerated specimen more than 2 hours old may be subject to overgrowth, may not yield valid results, and will be rejected.

Turnaround Time Preliminary reports are usually available at 24 hours. Cultures with no growth are usually reported after 24 hours. Reports on specimens from which an organism or organisms have been isolated require a minimum of 48 hours for completion.

Reference Range No growth. Significant bacteriuria is usually considered to be 10^4 CFU/mL (colony forming units). A break point of 10^2 maximizes diagnostic sensitivity. Urethral contamination particularly in women may cause colony counts of 10^3 or 10^4; thus, a breakpoint of 10^2 CFU/mL causes inclusion of a large number of normal women without significant bacteriuria.

Use Isolate and identify potentially pathogenic organisms causing urinary tract infection

Limitations Bacteria present in numbers <1000 organisms/mL may not be detected by routine methods.

Methodology Quantitative aerobic culture

Additional Information A single culture is about 80% accurate in the female; two containing the same organism with count of 10^5 or more represents 95% chance of true bacteriuria; three such specimens mean virtual certainty of true bacteriuria. Urinary tract infection is significantly higher in women who use diaphragm-spermicide contraception, perhaps secondary to increased vaginal pH and a higher frequency of vaginal colonization with *E. coli*. A single clean voided specimen from an adult male may be considered diagnostic with proper preparation and care in specimen collection. If the patient is receiving antimicrobial therapy at the time the specimen is collected, any level of bacteriuria may be significant. When more than two organisms are recovered, the likelihood of contamination is high; thus, the significance of definitive identification of the organisms and susceptibility testing in this situation is severely limited. A repeat culture with proper specimen collection patient preparation is often indicated. Periodic screening of diabetics and pregnant women for asymptomatic bacteriuria has been recommended. Cultures of specimens from Foley catheters yielding multiple organisms with high colony counts may represent colonization of the catheter and not true significant bacteriuria. Most laboratories limit the number of organisms which will be identified when recovered from urine to two and similarly do not routinely perform susceptibility tests on isolates from presumably contaminated specimens.

Failure to recover aerobic organisms from patients with pyuria or positive Gram stains of urinary sediment may indicate the presence of mycobacteria or anaerobes.

Selected Readings

Stamm WE, Counts GW, Running KR, et al, "Diagnosis of Coliform Infection in Acutely Dysuric Women," *N Engl J Med*, 1982, 307(8):462-8.

Stamm WE, Hooton TM, Johnson JR, et al, "Urinary Tract Infections: From Pathogenesis to Treatment," *J Infect Dis*, 1989, 159(3):400-6.

Urine Culture, First Voided, for *Neisseria gonorrhoeae* see

Neisseria gonorrhoeae Culture *on page 412*

Urine Culture, Foley Catheter *see* Urine Culture, Clean Catch
on page 470

Urine Culture, Midvoid Specimen *see* Urine Culture, Clean Catch
on page 470

Urine for Parasites *see* Ova and Parasites, Urine or Aspirates
on page 419

Urine for *Schistosoma haematobium* *see* Ova and Parasites, Urine or
Aspirates *on page 419*

Urine *Legionella* Antigen *see* Legionella Antigen, Urine
on page 380

Urine, *Mycoplasma* Culture *see* Mycoplasma/Ureaplasma Culture
on page 410

Urine *Trichomonas* Wet Mount *see* Trichomonas Preparation
on page 462

Urodynamic Testing of Bladder Function *see* Cystometrogram,
Simple *on page 315*

Urography

Synonyms Infusion Pyelogram; Intravenous Pyelogram; IVP

Test Includes Intravenous administration of a contrast material. The contrast material is concentrated and excreted by the kidneys. Appropriate radiographs are exposed during the concentration and excretion of the contrast material for evaluation of the morphology and function of the urinary tract.

Patient Preparation Patients are encouraged to take nothing by mouth after midnight the night before the examination. This degree of fluid restriction will not produce significant dehydration but will improve the overall quality of the examination. If the urography examination is to be performed in the afternoon, a light liquid breakfast may be consumed. Views on the necessity and the usefulness of cathartics in the preparation of patients for urography vary. Some physicians advocate the routine use of 10 oz of magnesium citrate the evening before the examination. Alternatives would include a mild laxative such as 1 ¼ oz of a standard extract of senna fruit the evening before the examination.

Aftercare Encourage hydration by fluid ingestion.

Special Instructions All patients undergoing this examination should be questioned specifically with regard to drug allergies, particularly iodine. A recent serum creatinine is requested on patients 60 years of age or older, those with significant atherosclerotic disease, those with a known diagnosis of diabetes mellitus or with known pre-existing renal disease.

Complications Reactions to contrast material and specific treatment for such reactions are beyond the scope of this handbook. An appropriately equipped emergency cart should be immediately available should resuscitation be necessary.

Equipment Overhead radiography tube with float top table. Tomographic capabilities are desirable.

Use This examination accurately demonstrates normal anatomy and a wide range of abnormalities involving the urinary tract.

Limitations Urography should be performed prior to barium studies of the gastrointestinal tract. The presence of barium within the abdomen will compromise the urographic examination.

Contraindications Allergy to iodine or a previous serious adverse reaction, advanced renal failure. A known diagnosis of multiple myeloma constitutes a relative contraindication. Every attempt should be made to hydrate patients with this diagnosis or with the diagnosis of diabetes mellitus prior to performance of a urogram as these patients run an increased risk of acute renal failure.

Selected Readings
Hattery RR, Williamson B Jr, Hartman GW, et al, "Intravenous Urographic Technique," *Radiology*, 1988, 167(3):593-9.

Miller DL, Chang R, Wells WT, et al, "Intravascular Contrast Media: Effect of Dose on Renal Function," *Radiology*, 1988, 167(3):607-11.

Vaginal Culture *see* Genital Culture *on page 349*

Vaginal Culture *Neisseria gonorrhoeae* *see* Neisseria gonorrhoeae
Culture *on page 412*

Vaginal _Trichomonas_ Smear *see* Trichomonas Preparation
on page 462

Vancocin® *see* Vancomycin *on this page*

Vancoled® *see* Vancomycin *on this page*

Vancomycin
Related Information
Antibiotic Level, Serum *on page 255*

Synonyms Vancocin®; Vancoled®

Abstract Vancomycin is an antimicrobial agent with potent activity against most gram-positive bacteria. Its use has occasionally been associated with nephrotoxicity and/or ototoxicity, though the frequency of these toxicities has decreased as vancomycin preparations have become more purified.

Specimen Serum, body fluid

Container Red top tube, sterile fluid container

Sampling Time Peak: 30 minutes following dose; trough: immediately prior to next dose

Storage Instructions Separate serum using aseptic technique and place in freezer

Causes for Rejection Specimen more than 4 hours old

Reference Range Therapeutic concentration: peak: 20-40 μg/mL (SI: 14-27 μmol/L) (depends in part on minimum inhibitory concentration of organism being treated); trough: 5-10 μg/mL (SI: 3.4-6.8 μmol/L)

Possible Panic Range Toxic: >80 μg/mL (>54 μmol/L)

Use Monitor therapeutic levels and potential toxicities, particularly in patients with impaired renal function and in patients also being treated with aminoglycoside antibiotics

Methodology High performance liquid chromatography (HPLC), gas-liquid chromatography (GLC), immunoassay

Additional Information Vancomycin is currently being used in its intravenous form to treat a variety of gram-positive bacterial infections, particularly those due to methicillin-resistant staphylococci. Additionally, otovancomycin is often used in its oral form to treat pseudomembranous colitis due to *Clostridium difficile*. When administered orally, serum vancomycin levels are undetectable due to poor absorption from the gastrointestinal tract. When administered intravenously, vancomycin may be ototoxic and nephrotoxic, though nephrotoxicity is rare with newer preparations. Ototoxicity is seen primarily in patients with extremely high serum concentrations (80-100 μg/mL; SI: 54-68 μmol/L) and rarely occurs when serum concentrations are maintained at 30 μg/mL (SI: 20 μmol/L) or lower. Both oto- and nephrotoxicity is enhanced by concurrent administration of aminoglycosides.

Selected Readings
Fogarty KA and McClain WJ, "Vancomycin: Current Perspectives and Guidelines for Use in the NICU," *Neonatal Netw*, 1989, 7(5):31-5.

Ingerman MJ and Santoro J, "Vancomycin. A New Old Agent," *Infect Dis Clin North Am*, 1989, 3(3):641-51.

Levine JF, "Vancomycin: A Review," *Med Clin North Am*, 1987, 71(6):1135-45.

Wilhelm MP, "Vancomycin," *Mayo Clin Proc*, 1991, 66(11):1165-70.

Varicella-Zoster Serology *see* Varicella-Zoster Virus Serology
on next page

Varicella-Zoster Virus Culture
Related Information
Varicella-Zoster Virus Serology *on next page*

Synonyms Chickenpox Culture; Shingles Culture

Applies To Viral Culture, Rash; Viral Culture, Skin

Test Includes Culture for VZV only; VZV also is usually detected in a routine/general virus culture

Specimen Swab specimens of the base of fresh, unroofed lesions, vesicle fluid, vesicle scrapings. In addition, acute and convalescent sera should be collected at appropriate times to document a clinically significant rise in antibody titer.

Container Cold viral transport medium

Sampling Time Specimens should be collected during the acute phase of the disease (within 3 days of lesion eruption).

Collection Unroofed lesions should be cleaned before specimens are taken. Vesicle fluid from several vesicles can be pooled and added to viral transport

(Continued)

Varicella-Zoster Virus Culture *(Continued)*

medium. Alternatively, the bases of several freshly unroofed lesions can be vigorously sampled with a sterile swab which subsequently should be placed into cold viral transport medium and sent to the laboratory as soon as possible.

Storage Instructions Keep specimens cold and moist. **Do not freeze specimens.**

Causes for Rejection Dry specimen, specimen not refrigerated during transport, specimen fixed in formalin, unlabeled specimen

Turnaround Time Variable (1-14 days) and depends on cell culture method used and amount of virus in the specimen

Reference Range No virus isolated

Use Aid in the diagnosis of disease caused by varicella-zoster virus (ie, chickenpox and shingles)

Methodology Inoculation of specimens into cell cultures, incubation of cultures, observation of characteristic cytopathic effect, and identification by fluorescent monoclonal antibody

Additional Information Varicella-zoster virus is a single virus which causes two diseases: **chickenpox** (varicella) in children and, after reactivation from latency, **shingles** (zoster) in adults.

Disease caused by VZV is usually self-limited. However, the disease can be life-threatening in pregnant persons, immunocompromised persons, and children who receive cancer therapy. In addition, congenital chickenpox can result in neonatal systemic disease and/or congenital malformations.

Serology for the detection of VZV antibodies is available. Rapid turnaround time of serological tests can be especially important in detecting the presence of antibody (prior exposure) in pregnant persons who have been exposed to persons with chickenpox because VZIg (varicella immune globulin) should be given within 3 days (maximum) of exposure.

Cell culture of VZV is considered less sensitive than direct antigen detection of VZV by immunofluorescence.

Selected Readings

Drew WL, "Diagnostic Virology," *Clin Lab Med*, 1987, 7(4):721-40.

Solomon AR, "New Diagnostic Tests for Herpes Simplex and Varicella-Zoster Infections," *J Am Acad Dermatol*, 1988, 18(1 Pt 2):218-21.

Strommen GL, Pucino F, Tight RR, et al, "Human Infection With Herpes Zoster: Etiology, Pathophysiology, Diagnosis, Clinical Course, and Treatment," *Pharmacotherapy*, 1988, 8(1):52-68.

Varicella-Zoster Virus, Direct Detection *see* Virus, Direct Detection by Fluorescent Antibody *on page 480*

Varicella-Zoster Virus Serology

Related Information

Varicella-Zoster Virus Culture *on previous page*

Synonyms Chickenpox Titer; Zoster Titer

Applies To Herpes Zoster Serology; Varicella-Zoster Serology

Special Instructions Acute and convalescent sera drawn 10-14 days apart are recommended.

Specimen Serum

Container Red top tube

Reference Range A single low titer or less than a fourfold increase in titer in paired sera by complement fixation; undetectable antibody by FAMA test

Use Establish the diagnosis of varicella-zoster infection; determine adult susceptibility to infection

Limitations Complement fixation test is insensitive and has heterologous reactions with herpesvirus

Methodology Fluorescent antibody to membrane antigen (FAMA), hemagglutination, complement fixation, enzyme linked immunosorbent assay

Additional Information Although most cases of varicella or zoster are clinically unambiguous, serology may be occasionally useful in the differential diagnosis of other blistering illnesses or when infection shows an unusual complication, such as hepatitis. It may also be important to establish whether an individual is susceptible when clinical history is unclear, or when VZIg (varicella immune globulin) may be needed, as in the immunocompromised host or cancer patient on toxic chemotherapy.

Zoster is more common with aging and may occur in the face of significant antibody titers, demonstrating that cell-mediated immunity is also significant.

Selected Readings
Landry ML, Cohen SD, Mayo DR, et al, "Comparison of Fluorescent Antibody to Membrane Antigen Test, Indirect Immunofluorescence Assay, and a Commercial Enzyme-Linked Immunosorbent Assay for Determination of Antibody to Varicella-Zoster Virus," *J Clin Microbiol*, 1987, 25(5):832-5.

Straus SE, Ostrove JM, Inchauspe G, et al, "Varicella-Zoster Virus Infections: Biology, Natural History, Treatment, and Prevention," *Ann Intern Med*, 1988, 108(2):221-36.

Weller TH, "Varicella and Herpes Zoster: Changing Concepts of the Natural History, Control, and Importance of a Not-So-Benign Virus," *N Engl J Med*, 1983, 309(22):1362-8.

VCA Titer *see* Epstein-Barr Virus Serology *on page 332*

VDRL *replaced by* RPR *on page 438*

VDRL, Cerebrospinal Fluid
Related Information
Cerebrospinal Fluid Analysis *on page 288*
Darkfield Examination, Syphilis *on page 322*
FTA-ABS, Cerebrospinal Fluid *on page 335*
FTA-ABS, Serum *on page 336*
RPR *on page 438*

Synonyms Cerebrospinal Fluid VDRL; CSF VDRL; Serologic Test for Syphilis, CSF; Spinal Fluid VDRL; VDRL, CSF

Test Includes Titer of reactive specimens

Specimen Cerebrospinal fluid

Container Clean, sterile container or glass tube

Reference Range Nonreactive

Use Test for syphilis, neurosyphilis

Limitations VDRL, CSF is the only laboratory test for neurosyphilis approved by the Center for Disease Control. It is quite specific and has acceptable sensitivity.

Methodology Flocculation test detects reagin, antibody to nontreponemal antigen

Additional Information A positive VDRL in a spinal fluid uncontaminated by serum is essentially diagnostic of neurosyphilis. However, a negative test may occur in 30% of patients with tabes dorsalis. The CSF VDRL may take years to become nonreactive after adequate therapy. In AIDS patients, serial CSF VDRL determinations may be needed when neurosyphilis is suspected. By requiring either a positive serum RPR or FTA-ABS, seropositivity of CSF VDRL could increase to 90%.

Selected Readings
Albright RE Jr, Christenson RH, Emlet JL, et al, "Issues in Cerebrospinal Fluid Management. CSF Venereal Disease Research Laboratory Testing," *Am J Clin Pathol*, 1991, 95(3):397-401.

Davis LE and Schmitt JW, "Clinical Significance of Cerebrospinal Fluid Tests for Neurosyphilis," *Ann Neurol*, 1989, 25(1):50-5.

Hart G, "Syphilis Tests in Diagnostic and Therapeutic Decision Making," *Ann Intern Med*, 1986, 104(3):368-76.

VDRL, CSF *see* VDRL, Cerebrospinal Fluid *on this page*

Venous Catheter Culture *see* Intravenous Line Culture *on page 376*

Ventricular Fluid Culture *see* Aerobic Culture, Cerebrospinal Fluid *on page 245*

Verocytotoxin Producing *E. coli*, Stool Culture *see* Stool Culture, Diarrheagenic *E. coli* *on page 449*

***Vibrio cholerae*, Stool Culture** *see* Stool Culture, Uncommon Organisms *on page 451*

***Vibrio parahaemolyticus*, Stool Culture** *see* Stool Culture, Uncommon Organisms *on page 451*

Viral Antigen Detection, Direct, Stool *see* Rotavirus, Direct Detection *on page 437*

Viral Culture, Brain *see* Viral Culture, Central Nervous System Symptoms *on next page*

Viral Culture, Bronchial Wash *see* Viral Culture, Throat *on page 479*

Viral Culture, Central Nervous System Symptoms

Related Information

Cerebrospinal Fluid Analysis *on page 288*

Fungus Culture, Cerebrospinal Fluid *on page 342*

Mycobacteria Culture, Cerebrospinal Fluid *on page 405*

Applies To Viral Culture, Brain; Viral Culture, CSF

Test Includes Isolation and identification of virus

Abstract Viral meningitis is by far the most important cause of aseptic meningitis. The latter includes multiple entities, both infectious and noninfectious. Most instances of aseptic meningitis are caused by viruses, especially enteroviruses, most often in the late summer. Subjects are usually children and young adults. Enteroviruses include polioviruses, coxsackie viruses, and echoviruses. Aseptic meningitis syndrome is characterized by an acute disease with signs and symptoms of meningeal inflammation associated with pleocytosis (usually mononuclear), variable increase in protein content, normal glucose level, and no demonstrable organism by smear and routine culture of the cerebrospinal fluid (CSF).

By definition, the cerebrospinal fluid in aseptic meningitis will show a pleocytosis of white blood cells but no growth on bacterial culture.

Specimen Cerebrospinal fluid (do not put into virus transport medium), brain biopsy, lesions, throat or throat washings, stool, urine

Container Sterile tube for CSF; sterile screw cap container for biopsy, tissue, urine, or throat washing; sterile viral transport medium for swab specimens

Sampling Time As soon as possible after the onset of illness

Collection Always consult the laboratory for specific details prior to collecting specimen. Specimen should be collected during the acute phase of the disease, as follows:

Cerebrospinal fluid: Collect 1 mL CSF aseptically in a sterile dry screw cap vial. **Keep cold and bring to laboratory immediately.**

The following may be relevant to CNS viral infection: Specimens useful for diagnosis of CNS viral infections:

Eye swab or scraping: Use a Virocult® or Culturette® swab to collect conjunctival material or take conjunctival scrapings with a fine sterile spatula and transfer the scraping to a viral transport medium. **Keep cold and bring to laboratory immediately.**

Skin lesions: Open the vesicle and absorb exudate into a dry swab, and/or vigorously scrape base of freshly exposed lesion with a swab to obtain cells which contain viruses. If enough vesicle fluid is available, aspirate the fluid with a fine gauge needle and tuberculin syringe, and place the fluid into cold viral transport medium. Use Virocult® or Culturette® swabs for specimen collection. **Keep cold and bring to laboratory immediately.** The clinical appearance of herpes zoster or the vesicles of herpes simplex may suggest the diagnosis.

Throat swab: Carefully rub the posterior wall of the nasopharynx with a dry, sterile swab. Avoid touching the tongue or buccal mucosa. Use Virocult® or Culturette® swabs for specimen collection. **Keep cold and bring to laboratory immediately.** Coxsackie, mumps, adenovirus, herpes type 1, Epstein-Barr virus may be recovered from throat washings.

Feces: Collect 4-8 g of feces (about the size of a thumbnail), and place in a clean, leakproof container. Do **not** dilute the specimen (into virus transport medium) or use preservatives. **Keep cold and bring to laboratory immediately.** Enteroviruses, adenovirus.

Urine: Collect clean-catch, midstream urine in a leakproof, sterile, plastic container. **Keep cold and bring to laboratory immediately.** Mumps virus, cytomegalovirus.

Genital swab: See skin. **Keep cold and bring to laboratory immediately.**

Storage Instructions Keep all specimens cold and moist. Transport to laboratory immediately. Enteroviruses are relatively stable from -70°C to 4°C but are labile if allowed to dry or to be at room temperature for several hours.

Causes for Rejection Dry specimen, specimen not refrigerated during transport, specimen fixed in formalin, unlabeled specimen

Turnaround Time Variable (1-14 days) and depends on culture method used and amount of virus in specimen

Reference Range No virus isolated

Use Determine etiological agent of viral CNS diseases (eg, meningitis (aseptic), meningoencephalitis, polio and encephalitis)

Limitations The CSF findings in tuberculous meningitis may simulate those of viral meningitis, especially herpes simplex and mumps.

Methodology Inoculation of specimen into cell cultures, incubation of cultures, observation of characteristic cytopathic effect, and identification/speciation by methods such as hemadsorption and fluorescent monoclonal antibodies. If specific viruses such as HSV, CMV, VZV, or adenovirus are suspected, the laboratory might be able to use rapid (1-2 days) culture (shell vial) methods to detect these viruses. Suckling mice are usually inoculated with the specimen if group A Coxsackie virus is suspected. The mice are observed for the development of flaccid paralysis. Bacterial culture, Gram stain, cell count, glucose, and protein are needed to rule out bacterial meningitis, with antigen agglutination when indicated.

Additional Information Arthropod-borne (arbo) viruses and reoviruses are not considered culturable and may be detected indirectly by viral serology.

The seasonal peak of viral meningitis in late summer is widely recognized and clinically significant in differential diagnosis. Meningitis caused by HIV, Epstein-Barr virus, CMV, or herpes simplex lacks seasonal variation. The significance of seasonal curves for viral meningitis (more frequent in summer) versus bacterial meningitis is greater than most physicians recognize.

Mumps meningitis is usually self limited and benign. As with lymphocytic choriomeningitis and herpes simplex meningoencephalitis, hypoglycorrhachia may be found.

In the differential diagnosis between viral and bacterial meningitis, much higher WBC count ($>1180 \times 10^6$/L) and protein (>220 mg/dL) may be found in many cases of bacterial meningitis. In Spanos' series, no patient with acute viral meningitis had glucose <30.6 mg/dL but 43% with acute bacterial meningitis did. Although aseptic meningitis is usually characterized by mononuclear cells, PMNs may predominate early.

Five patients with mixed viral-bacterial meningitis among 276 patients with viral and/or bacterial culture proven meningitis are described.

A high frequency of negative lumbar punctures in babies presenting with fever but without other specific findings is recognized. In a series of children with high fever, 57% of patients with bacterial meningitis and 37% of those with aseptic meningitis had vomiting. In a study of 171 children with febrile convulsions, only one had bacterial meningitis and four had aseptic meningitis.

Complications of lumbar puncture (LP) are between 0.19% and 0.43%, reaching up to 35.5% when minor complications are included. Instances of meningitis and local infection are described following LP in subjects with bacteremia, who may be at risk for meningeal seeding during the puncture.

Nonviral aseptic causes of aseptic meningitis include meningeal carcinomatosis, collagen diseases, sarcoidosis, drugs including antineoplastic agents, immunosuppressants, materials used in radiology units, Mollaret's meningitis, and many other entities.

Selected Readings

Chonmaitree T, Baldwin CD, and Lucia HL, "Role of the Virology Laboratory in Diagnosis and Management of Patients With Central Nervous System Disease," *Clin Microbiol Rev*, 1989, 2(1):1-14.

Connolly KJ and Hammer SM, "The Acute Aseptic Meningitis Syndrome," *Infect Dis Clin North Am*, 1990, 4(4):599-622.

Greenlee JE, "Approach to Diagnosis of Meningitis – Cerebrospinal Fluid Evaluation," *Infect Dis Clin North Am*, 1990, 4(4):583-98.

Hammer SM and Connolly KJ, "Viral Aseptic Meningitis in the United States: Clinical Features, Viral Etiologies, and Differential Diagnosis," *Curr Clin Top Infect Dis*, 1992, 12:1-25.

Mishu B, "A Rabies Primer for Clinicians," *Infect Dis Newslett*, 1993, 12(1):1-4.

Viral Culture, CSF *see* Viral Culture, Central Nervous System Symptoms *on previous page*

Viral Culture, Cytomegalovirus *see* Cytomegalovirus Culture *on page 319*

Viral Culture, Eye *see* Herpes Simplex Virus Culture *on page 364*

Viral Culture, Genital *see* Herpes Simplex Virus Culture *on page 364*

Viral Culture, Nasopharyngeal *see* Viral Culture, Throat *on page 479*

LABORATORY DIAGNOSIS

Viral Culture, Pulmonary Biopsy *see* Viral Culture, Throat
on next page

Viral Culture, Rash *see* Varicella-Zoster Virus Culture
on page 473

Viral Culture, Skin *see* Herpes Simplex Virus Culture
on page 364

Viral Culture, Skin *see* Varicella-Zoster Virus Culture
on page 473

Viral Culture, Stool

Applies To Adenovirus Culture, Stool; Coxsackie Virus Culture, Stool; Echovirus Culture, Stool; Enterovirus Culture, Stool; Poliovirus Culture, Stool

Test Includes Isolation and identification of viruses

Specimen Stool or rectal swab. Freshly passed stool is much more preferable than a rectal swab.

Container Stool: screw cap container. Do not use cardboard or waxed containers. Swab: cold viral transport medium

Collection Collect stools into a clean and dry container. Insert swab gently into rectum and hold there for 10-15 seconds, moisten with contents of Culturette® bulb, and send to laboratory.

Storage Instructions Keep specimens cold

Causes for Rejection Dry specimen, specimen not refrigerated during transport, specimen fixed in formalin, unlabeled specimen

Turnaround Time Variable (usually 1-14 days) and depends on cell culture methods and amount of virus in the specimen

Reference Range No virus isolated

Viruses Typically Isolated From Clinical Specimens

Specimen	Virus*
Blood	CMV, enteroviruses†,#, HSV, VZV
CSF and CNS tissues	Enteroviruses, mumps virus, HSV, CMV
Dermal lesions	HSV, VZV, adenovirus, enteroviruses
Eye	HSV, VZV, adenovirus, enteroviruses, CMV, *Chlamydia*
Genital	HSV, CMV, *Chlamydia*
Mucosal	HSV, VZV
Oral	HSV, VZV
Rectal	HSV, VZV, enterovirus
Respiratory tract upper	Adenovirus, rhinovirus, influenza, parainfluenza, enteroviruses, RSV, reovirus, HSV
lower	Adenovirus, influenza, parainfluenza, RSV, CMV•
Stool	Enteroviruses, adenoviruses, rotavirus¶
Tissues	CMV, HSV, enteroviruses
Urine	CMV, adenovirus, enteroviruses, mumps

*Abbreviations:

    HSV — herpes simplex virus
    CMV — cytomegalovirus
    VZV — varicella–zoster virus
    RSV — respiratory syncytial virus

†Enteroviruses: coxsackie virus, poliovirus, echovirus, and enterovirus.
#Occasionally isolated.
•Usually in immunocompromised hosts.
¶Antigen detection.

Use To identify carriage or excretion of a virus in stool. To isolate and identify an enterovirus which could be the cause of meningitis.

Limitations Children convalescing from upper respiratory illness or aseptic meningitis can shed virus in the stool for weeks; children recently vaccinated against polio can shed poliovirus in the stool for months after vaccination; sampling errors; presence of nonculturable, disease-causing virus (eg, encephalitis, hepatitis, and gastroenteritis viruses)

Methodology Inoculation of specimen into cell cultures, incubation of cultures, observation of characteristic cytopathic effect, and identification/speciation by methods such as hemadsorption and fluorescent monoclonal antibodies. If specific viruses such as HSV, CMV, VZV, or adenovirus are suspected, the laboratory might be able to use rapid (1-2 days) culture (shell vial) methods to detect these viruses.

Additional Information See table for viruses most likely to be isolated from stool specimens. The viruses most likely to be isolated from stool specimen are those which are extremely hardy and which do not have a lipid membrane envelope (ie, adenovirus and enterovirus (polio, coxsackie, and echoviruses)).

Selected Readings
Lennette DA, "Preparation of Specimens for Virological Examination," *Manual of Clinical Microbiology*, 5th ed, Balows A, Hausler WJ Jr, Herrmann KL, et al, eds, Washington, DC: American Society for Microbiology, 1991, 818-21.

Viral Culture, Throat

Related Information
Adenovirus Culture *on page 243*
Influenza Virus Culture *on page 375*
Parainfluenza Virus Culture *on page 423*
Respiratory Syncytial Virus Culture *on page 436*

Synonyms Viral Culture, Bronchial Wash; Viral Culture, Nasopharyngeal; Viral Culture, Pulmonary Biopsy; Viral Culture, Throat Swab

Applies To Rhinovirus Culture

Test Includes Isolation and identification of virus most likely to cause respiratory disease

Patient Preparation Local anesthesia might be necessary

Specimen Throat swab; throat washing; nasopharyngeal washing, aspirates, or secretions; sputum; bronchial washings or lavage; lung biopsy

Container Cold and sterile viral transport medium for swabs; sterile cup for feces, washings, aspirates, and sputum

Sampling Time As soon as possible after onset of illness

Collection Methods are the same as those used for collecting most respiratory specimens (see specimen). If respiratory syncytial virus or parainfluenza virus is suspected, see collection techniques in Parainfluenza Virus Culture.

Storage Instructions Keep specimen cold and moist. Transport to laboratory immediately.

Causes for Rejection Dry specimen, specimen not refrigerated during transport, specimen fixed in formalin, unlabeled specimen

Turnaround Time Variable (1-14 days) and depends on culture method and amount of virus in specimen

Reference Range No virus isolated

Use Determine etiological agent of viral respiratory infections (eg, pneumonia, pneumonitis, croup, and influenza)

Limitations Sampling errors; presence of nonculturable, disease-causing virus (eg, encephalitis, hepatitis, and gastroenteritis viruses); invasive procedures. Many persons carry and shed viruses which might not be related to the patient's illness.

Methodology Inoculation of specimen into cell cultures, incubation of cultures, observation of characteristic cytopathic effect, and identification/speciation by methods such as hemadsorption and the use of fluorescent monoclonal antibodies. If specific viruses such as HSV, CMV, VZV, or adenovirus are suspected, the laboratory might be able to use rapid (1-2 days) culture (shell vial) methods to detect these viruses. Most laboratories use hemadsorption to help determine the presence of a respiratory virus in cell culture and usually will report "hemadsorbing virus present." Some laboratories are capable of using specific virus-neutralizing antibodies to determine the particular type of virus which caused the observed hemadsorption. This final identification can require as many as several days and often is done only by reference laboratories.

Additional Information Viruses to be considered as causes of viral respiratory illness include the following: influenza virus, parainfluenza virus, rhinovirus, RSV, adenovirus, CMV, and reovirus. See table in Viral Culture, Stool test listing. Contact the virology laboratory and inform the staff if influenza or parainfluenza is suspected.

Selected Readings
Lennette DA, "Preparation of Specimens for Virological Examination," *Manual of Clinical Microbiology*, 5th ed, Balows A, Hausler WJ Jr, Herrmann KL, et al, eds, Washington, DC: American Society for Microbiology, 1991, 818-21.

(Continued)

LABORATORY DIAGNOSIS

Viral Culture, Throat *(Continued)*

Ruben FL and Cate TR, "Influenza Pneumonia," *Semin Respir Infect*, 1987, 2(2):122-9.
Welliver RC, "Detection, Pathogenesis, and Therapy of Respiratory Syncytial Virus Infections," *Clin Microbiol Rev*, 1988, 1(1):27-39.

Viral Culture, Throat Swab *see* Viral Culture, Throat
on previous page

Viral Study, Herpes *see* Herpes Cytology *on page 362*

Virus, Direct Detection by Fluorescent Antibody

Synonyms Direct Detection of Virus; Direct Fluorescent Antibody Test for Virus; Virus Fluorescent Antibody Test

Applies To Herpes Simplex Virus, Direct Detection; Influenza Virus, Direct Detection; Measles Virus, Direct Detection; Mumps Virus, Direct Detection; Parainfluenza Virus, Direct Detection; Rabies Virus, Direct Detection; Respiratory Syncytial Virus, Direct Detection; Varicella-Zoster Virus, Direct Detection

Test Includes Direct (nonculture) detection of virus-infected cells

Special Instructions Make at least four impression smears or place four frozen sections on four separate slides. Cell suspensions should be centrifuged, resuspended to slight turbidity, and applied to prewelled slides.

Specimen Impression smears of tissues, lesion scrapings and swabs, frozen sections, cell suspensions, upper respiratory tract swabs

Causes for Rejection Insufficient material, slides broken or badly scratched, fixative used on slide preparation (generally, the laboratory is responsible for fixing specimens)

Turnaround Time Less than 1 day

Reference Range No virus detected

Use Useful in the rapid diagnosis of HSV, VZV, RSV, parainfluenza, influenza, and rabies infections

Limitations Only a few viruses (HSV, VZV, RSV, influenza, parainfluenza, measles, mumps, and rabies virus) can be detected in this manner. It is possible for the test to be negative in the presence of viral infection. Expertly trained and experienced personnel, excellent quality reagents and adequate numbers of cells are required. **Contact laboratory prior to requesting test to determine if laboratory offers this/these tests.**

Methodology Monoclonal antibody reagents and immunofluorescence microscopy are used to detect viruses/viral antigens in specimen cells.

Additional Information Generally, this test is not as sensitive as cell culture.

Selected Readings

Drew WL, "Controversies in Viral Diagnosis," *Rev Infect Dis*, 1986, 8(5):814-24.
Drew WL, "Diagnostic Virology," *Clin Lab Med*, 1987, 7(4):721-40.
Smith TF, "Rapid Methods for the Diagnosis of Viral Infections," *Lab Med*, 1987, 18:16-20.

Virus Fluorescent Antibody Test *see* Virus, Direct Detection by Fluorescent Antibody *on this page*

Wassermann *replaced by* RPR *on page 438*

WBC Scan *see* Indium Leukocyte Scan *on page 374*

Westergren Sedimentation Rate *see* Sedimentation Rate, Erythrocyte *on page 440*

Wet Preparation for *Trichomonas vaginalis* *see* Trichomonas Preparation *on page 462*

White Blood Cell Scan *see* Indium Leukocyte Scan *on page 374*

Whole Body Bone Scan *see* Bone Scan *on page 281*

Whooping Cough Culture *see* Bordetella pertussis Nasopharyngeal Culture *on page 283*

Wound Culture

Related Information

Abscess Aerobic and Anaerobic Culture *on page 238*

Synonyms Lesion Culture

Test Includes Culture for aerobic organisms and usually Gram stain

Patient Preparation Sterile preparation of the aspiration site

Special Instructions The laboratory should be informed of the specific site of specimen, the age of patient, current antibiotic therapy, clinical diagnosis, and time of collection. The submission of biopsy specimens or specimens from normally sterile sites should be clearly indicated to the laboratory. Procedures for laboratory work-up of wound cultures which may contain contamination from the skin surface are different than those from sites which are expected to be sterile. Drainage cultured by aspiration away from a sinus tract may provide more useful information.

Specimen Tissue or aspirated pus/fluid properly obtained from a wound site or abscess

Container Sterile tube or screw-cap container. **Swab specimens are extremely inadequate for almost all specimens except for throat, cervix, and other small openings.**

Collection The specimen should be transported to laboratory as soon as possible after collection. Contamination with normal flora from skin, rectum, vaginal tract, or other body surfaces must be avoided.

Storage Instructions Refrigerate the specimen if it cannot be promptly processed.

Causes for Rejection Specimens delayed in transit to the laboratory may have less than optimal yields.

Turnaround Time Preliminary reports are usually available at 24 hours. Cultures with no growth are usually reported after 72 hours. Reports on specimens from which pathogens are isolated require a minimum of 48 hours for completion.

Reference Range No growth. A simultaneous Gram stain should always be performed to facilitate interpretation. Gram-negative organisms, frequently colonize wounds and mixed culture results are common.

Use Isolate and identify potentially pathogenic organisms

Limitations Only rapid-growing, nonfastidious aerobic organisms will be screened for and identified by routine methods. Often only organisms which predominate will be completely identified. Unless specifically requested by the physician or mandated by the specimen source (ie, genital specimen) fastidious organisms such as *N. gonorrhoeae* may not be isolated. Fungal and mycobacterial pathogens should be considered and appropriate cultures requested if indicated.

Contraindications Culture of contaminated open wounds which have not been cleansed or debrided

Additional Information See table. Susceptibility testing is performed if laboratory personnel determine such is appropriate; such testing is not always performed automatically when "culture and sensitivity" is ordered by a physician. If anaerobes are suspected a properly collected specimen for anaerobic culture should also be submitted.

Effective treatment of wound infection usually includes drainage, removal of foreign bodies, infected prosthetic devices, and retained foreign objects such as suture material. Suction irrigation may be helpful in resolving wound infections. Species commonly recovered from wounds include *Escherichia coli*, *Proteus* sp, *Klebsiella* sp, *Pseudomonas* sp, *Enterobacter* sp, enterococci, streptococci, staphylococci, *Bacteroides* sp, and *Clostridium* sp.

Classification of Soft–Tissue Infections

Tissue Level	Common Surgical Pathogens				
	S. pyogenes	*S. aureus*	*C. perfringens*	Mixed Bacteria	
				Staph & Strep	Enteric
Epidermis	Ecthyma contagiosum	Scalded–skin syndrome		Possibly impetigo	
Dermis and subdermis	Erysipelas/ cellulitis	Folliculitis/ abscess	Abscess/ cellulitis	Meleny's ulcer (synergistic gangrene)	Tropical ulcer
Fascial planes	Strep gangrene	Carbuncle	Fasciitis	Necrotizing fasciitis	
Muscle tissue	Strep myositis	Muscular abscess/ pyomyositis	Myonecrosis	Nonclostridial myonecrosis	

From Ahrenholz DH, "Necrotizing Soft Tissue Infections," *Surg Clin North Am*, 1988, 68:198–214, with permission.

Wound Culture *(Continued)*

Selected Readings

Erlich KS and Rumack JS, "Evaluation and Management of Nonhealing Infected Wounds in Diabetics," *Infect Med*, 1993, 10(8):21-7.

Gerding DN, Piziak VK, and Rowbotham JL, "Saving the Diabetic Foot," *Patient Care*, 1991.

Goldstein EJ, "Management of Human and Animal Bite Wounds," *J Am Acad Dermatol*, 1989, 21(6):1275-9.

Pollock AV and Evans M, "Microbiologic Prediction of Abdominal Surgical Wound Infection," *Arch Surg*, 1987, 122(1):33-7.

Wound Fungus Culture *see* Fungus Culture, Body Fluid *on page 341*

Wound Mycobacteria Culture *see* Mycobacteria Culture, Biopsy or Body Fluid *on page 404*

Wrist Arthrogram *see* Arthrogram *on page 267*

Wrist, Left or Right, X-ray *see* Bone Films *on page 277*

Yersinia enterocolitica, Stool Culture *see* Stool Culture, Uncommon Organisms *on page 451*

Ziehl-Neelsen Stain *see* Acid-Fast Stain *on page 239*

Zoster Titer *see* Varicella-Zoster Virus Serology *on page 474*

ANTIMICROBIAL THERAPY

A-200™ Pyrinate [OTC] *see* Pyrethrins *on page 653*

Acel-Immune® *see* Diphtheria and Tetanus Toxoids and Acellular Pertussis Vaccine *on page 555*

Achromycin® *see* Tetracycline *on page 679*

Achromycin® V *see* Tetracycline *on page 679*

Aciclovir *see* Acyclovir *on this page*

A-Cillin® *see* Amoxicillin Trihydrate *on page 491*

ACV *see* Acyclovir *on this page*

Acycloguanosine *see* Acyclovir *on this page*

Acyclovir (ay sye' kloe ver)
Brand Names Zovirax®
Synonyms Aciclovir; ACV; Acycloguanosine
Generic Available No
Use Treatment of initial and prophylaxis of recurrent mucosal and cutaneous herpes simplex (HSV-1 and HSV-2) infections; herpes simplex encephalitis; herpes zoster; genital herpes infection; and varicella-zoster infections in immunocompromised patients
Drug of Choice or Alternative For
Organism(s)
Herpes Simplex Virus *on page 128*
Varicella-Zoster Virus *on page 227*
Pregnancy Risk Factor C
Contraindications Hypersensitivity to acyclovir
Adverse Reactions
>10%: Headache, local inflammation at injection site
1% to 10%: Nausea, vomiting, impaired renal function, lethargy, tremors, confusion, agitation, coma, rash
<1%: Mental depression, anorexia
Toxicology In the event of an overdose, sufficient urine flow must be maintained to avoid drug precipitation within the renal tubules. Hemodialysis has resulted in up to 60% reductions in serum acyclovir levels.
Drug Interactions Increased effect with zidovudine (drowsiness, lethargy), probenecid (CNS effects)
Stability Acyclovir is incompatible with blood products and protein-containing solutions; reconstituted solution remains stable 24 hours at room temperature; do not refrigerate reconstituted solutions as they may precipitate
Mechanism of Action Inhibits DNA synthesis and viral replication by competing with deoxyguanosine triphosphate for viral DNA polymerase and being incorporated into viral DNA
Pharmacokinetics
Absorption: Oral: 15% to 30%; food does not appear to affect absorption
Distribution: Widely distributed throughout the body including brain, kidney, lungs, liver, spleen, muscle, uterus, vagina, and the CSF
Metabolism: Small percentage of hepatic elimination
Half-life:
Neonates: Terminal: 4 hours
Children 1-12 years: 2-3 hours
Adults: 3 hours
Time to peak serum concentration:
Oral: Within 1.5-2 hours
I.V.: Within 1 hour
Elimination: Primary route of elimination is the kidney; hemodialysis removes approximately 60% of dose and to a much lesser extent by peritoneal dialysis
Usual Dosage
Dosing weight should be based on the smaller of lean body weight or total body weight (see Appendix for ideal body weight calculation)
Treatment of herpes simplex virus infections:
Neonatal infection: I.V.: 1500 mg/m^2/day divided every 8 hours or 30 mg/kg/day divided every 8 hours for 10-14 days
Children and Adults: I.V.:
Mucocutaneous HSV infection: 750 mg/m^2/day divided every 8 hours or 5 mg/kg/dose every 8 hours for 5-10 days

HSV encephalitis: 1500 mg/m²/day divided every 8 hours or 10 mg/kg/dose every 8 hours for 10 days

Adults: Oral: Mucocutaneous HSV treatment: 200 mg every 4 hours while awake (5 times/day)

Prophylaxis: 200 mg 3-4 times/day or 400 mg twice daily

Topical: ½" ribbon of ointment every 3 hours (6 times/day)

Treatment of varicella-zoster virus infections:
Only to be used in serious varicella-zoster infections. May decrease infectivity of chicken pox and increase healing by 1-2 days in normal children and adults

I.V.: Children and Adults: 1500 mg/m²/day divided every 8 hours or 10 mg/kg/dose every 8 hours for 5-10 days

Oral:
Children: 10-20 mg/kg/dose (up to 800 mg) 4 times/day
Adults: 600-800 mg/dose every 4 hours while awake (5 times/day) for 7-10 days or 1000 mg every 6 hours for 5 days

Prophylaxis in immunocompromised patients:
Varicella or herpes zoster in HIV-positive patients: Oral: Adults: 400 mg 5 times/day

Bone marrow transplant recipients: I.V.: Children and Adults:
Prophylaxis in patients who are HSV-seropositive: 5 mg/kg (or 125-250 mg/m²) every 8 hours
Prophylaxis in patients who are CMV-seropositive: 10 mg/kg (or 250-500 mg/m²) every 8 hours

Dosing in renal impairment:
Oral: HSV: Cl_cr <10 mL/minute: Administer same dose every 12 hours
Oral: Varicella-zoster:
Cl_cr 10-25 mL/minute: Administer same dose every 8 hours
Cl_cr <10 mL/minute: Administer same dose every 12 hours
I.V.:
Cl_cr 25-50 mL/minute: 5-10 mg/kg/dose: Administer every 12 hours
Cl_cr 10-25 mL/minute: 5-10 mg/kg/dose: Administer every 24 hours
Cl_cr <10 mL/minute: 2.5-5 mg/kg/dose: Administer every 24 hours
Dialyzable (50% to 100%)

Overdosage Elevated serum creatinine, renal failure

Monitoring Parameters Urinalysis, BUN, serum creatinine, liver enzymes, CBC; monitor injection site for phlebitis

Reference Range Serum concentrations are not routinely monitored
Level guidelines: Pre: 0.1-1.6 μg/mL, Post: 3-10 μg/mL
Panic value: >50 μg/mL
Infusion time: 1 hour

Patient Information Recurrences of HSV tend to appear within 3 months of original infection; acyclovir is **not** a cure

Nursing Implications Infuse over 1 hour; maintain adequate hydration of patient; check infusion site for phlebitis, rotate site to prevent phlebitis; wear gloves when applying ointment for self-protection

Additional Information Sodium content of 1 g: 96.6 mg (4.2 mEq)

Dosage Forms
Capsule: 200 mg
Injection: 500 mg (10 mL); 1000 mg (20 mL)
Ointment, topical: 5% (3 g, 15 g)
Suspension, oral (banana flavor): 200 mg/5 mL (473 mL)
Tablet: 400 mg, 800 mg

Selected Readings
"Drugs for Non-HIV Viral Infections," *Med Lett Drugs Ther*, 1994, 36(919):27.
Dunkle LM, Arvin AM, Whitley RD, et al, "A Controlled Trial of Acyclovir for Chickenpox in Normal Children," *N Engl J Med*, 1991, 325(22):1539-44.
Keating MR, "Antiviral Agents," *Mayo Clin Proc*, 1992, 67(2):160-78.
Wallace MR, Bowler WA, Murray NB, et al, "Treatment of Adult Varicella With Oral Acyclovir," *Ann Intern Med*, 1992, 117(5):358-63.
Whitley RJ and Gnann JW Jr, "Acyclovir: A Decade Later," *N Engl J Med*, 1992, 327(11):782-3.

Adamantanamine Hydrochloride *see* Amantadine Hydrochloride *on next page*

Adenine Arabinoside *see* Vidarabine *on page 694*

Aerosporin® Injection *see* Polymyxin B Sulfate *on page 647*

Aftate® [OTC] *see* Tolnaftate *on page 687*

AgNO₃ *see* Silver Nitrate *on page 666*

AK-Chlor® *see* Chloramphenicol *on page 531*

AK-Tracin® Ophthalmic *see* Bacitracin *on page 503*

Amantadine Hydrochloride (a man' ta deen)

Brand Names Symadine®; Symmetrel®

Synonyms Adamantanamine Hydrochloride

Generic Available Yes

Use Prophylaxis or treatment of influenza A viral infection; also used in symptomatic parkinsonism

**Drug of Choice or Alternative For
Organism(s)**
Influenza Virus *on page 136*

Pregnancy Risk Factor C

Contraindications Hypersensitivity to amantadine hydrochloride or any component

Adverse Reactions
1% to 10%: Nausea, dizziness (lightheadedness), insomnia, depression, anxiety, irritability, hallucinations, anorexia, dry mouth, constipation, ataxia, livedo reticularis, peripheral edema, orthostatic hypotension, headache, somnolence, nervousness, dream abnormality, agitation, dry nose, diarrhea, fatigue
<1%: Congestive heart failure, psychosis, urinary retention, dyspnea, skin rash, vomiting, weakness, slurred speech, euphoria, confusion, amnesia, hyperkinesia, hypertension, decreased libido, visual disturbances, instances of convulsions, leukopenia, neutropenia, eczematoid dermatitis, oculogyric episodes

Toxicology Treatment should be directed at reducing the CNS stimulation and at maintaining cardiovascular function. Seizures can be treated with diazepam 5-10 mg I.V. every 15 minutes as needed; up to a total of 30 mg in adults (0.25-0.4 mg/kg/dose I.V. every 15 minutes as needed up to a total of 10 mg for children) while a lidocaine infusion may be required for the cardiac dysrhythmias.

Drug Interactions Additive anticholinergic effects in patients receiving drugs with anticholinergic activity; additive CNS stimulant effect with CNS stimulants

Stability Protect from freezing

Mechanism of Action As an antiviral, blocks the uncoating of influenza A virus preventing penetration of virus into host; antiparkinsonian activity may be due to its blocking the reuptake of dopamine into presynaptic neurons and causing direct stimulation of postsynaptic receptors.

Pharmacokinetics
Absorption: Well absorbed from GI tract
Distribution: To saliva, tear film, and nasal secretions; in animals, tissue (especially lung) concentrations higher than serum concentrations, crosses placenta and blood-brain barrier; excreted in breast milk
Metabolism: Not appreciable, small amounts of an acetyl metabolite identified
Half-life: 10-28 hours
Impaired renal function: 7-10 days
Time to peak serum concentration: 1-4 hours
Elimination: 80% to 90% unchanged in urine by glomerular filtration and tubular secretion

Usual Dosage
Children:
1-9 years: 4.4-8.8 mg/kg/day in 1-2 divided doses to a maximum of 150 mg/day
9-12 years: 100-200 mg/day in 1-2 divided doses
After first influenza A virus vaccine dose, amantadine prophylaxis may be administered for up to 6 weeks or until 2 weeks after the second dose of vaccine

Adults:
Influenza A viral infection: 200 mg/day in 1-2 divided doses
Prophylaxis: Minimum 10-day course of therapy following exposure or continue for 2-3 weeks after influenza A virus vaccine is given
Parkinson's disease: 100 mg twice daily

Dosing adjustment in renal impairment:
Cl$_{cr}$ 50-60 mL/minute: Administer 200 mg alternating with 100 mg/day
Cl$_{cr}$ 30-50 mL/minute: Administer 100 mg/day
Cl$_{cr}$ 20-30 mL/minute: Administer 200 mg twice weekly

Cl_{cr} 10-20 mL/minute: Administer 100 mg 3 times/week

Cl_{cr} <10 mL/minute: Administer 200 mg alternating with 100 mg every 7 days

Slightly dializable (5% to 20%)

Overdosage Nausea, vomiting, slurred speech, blurred vision, lethargy, hallucinations, seizures, myoclonic jerking

Monitoring Parameters Renal function; monitor for signs of neurotoxicity

Patient Information May impair ability to perform activities requiring mental alertness or coordination

Nursing Implications If insomnia occurs, the last daily dose should be taken several hours before retiring; assess parkinsonian symptoms prior to and throughout course of therapy

Dosage Forms

Capsule: 100 mg

Solution, oral: 50 mg/5 mL (473 mL)

Selected Readings

Arden NH, Patriarca PA, Fasano MB, et al, "The Roles of Vaccination and Amantadine Prophylaxis in Controlling an Outbreak of Influenza A (H3N2) in a Nursing Home," *Arch Intern Med*, 1988, 148(4):865-8.

Douglas RG Jr, "Prophylaxis and Treatment of Influenza," *N Engl J Med*, 1990, 322(7):443-50.

"Drugs for Non-HIV Viral Infections," *Med Lett Drugs Ther*, 1994, 36(919):27.

Keating MR, "Antiviral Agents," *Mayo Clin Proc*, 1992, 67(2):160-78.

Somani SK, Degelau J, Cooper SL, et al, "Comparison of Pharmacokinetic and Safety Profiles of Amantadine 50- and 100-mg Daily Doses in Elderly Nursing Home Residents," *Pharmacotherapy*, 1991, 11(6):460-6.

Amikacin Sulfate (am i kay' sin)

Related Information

Aminoglycoside Dosing and Monitoring *on page 721-722*

Antimicrobial Activity Against Selected Organisms *on page 757-764*

Brand Names Amikin®

Generic Available No

Use Treatment of documented gram-negative enteric infection resistant to gentamicin and tobramycin; documented infection of mycobacterial organisms susceptible to amikacin

Drug of Choice or Alternative For

Organism(s)

Mycobacterium avium-intracellulare on page 152

Pregnancy Risk Factor C

Contraindications Hypersensitivity to amikacin sulfate or any component; cross-sensitivity may exist with other aminoglycosides

Warnings/Precautions Dose and/or frequency of administration must be modified in patients with renal impairment; drug should be discontinued if signs of ototoxicity, nephrotoxicity, or hypersensitivity occurs; hearing should be tested before, during, and after treatment; aminoglycosides are associated with significant nephrotoxicity or ototoxicity; the ototoxicity is directly proportional to the amount of drug given and the duration of treatment; tinnitus or vertigo may be indications of vestibular injury and impending bilateral irreversible damage; renal damage is usually reversible

Adverse Reactions

1% to 10%: Nephrotoxicity, neurotoxicity, ototoxicity (auditory), ototoxicity (vestibular)

<1%: Skin rash, drug fever, headache, paresthesia, tremor, nausea, vomiting, eosinophilia, arthralgia, anemia, hypotension, difficulty in breathing, drowsiness, weakness

Toxicology The treatment of choice following a single acute overdose appears to be the maintenance of good urine output of at least 3 mL/kg/hour. Dialysis is of questionable value in the enhancement of aminoglycoside elimination. If required, hemodialysis is preferred over peritoneal dialysis in patients with normal renal function. Careful hydration may be all that is required to promote diuresis and, therefore, the enhancement of the drug's elimination.

Drug Interactions

Increased/prolonged effect: Depolarizing and nondepolarizing neuromuscular blocking agents

Increased toxicity: Concurrent use of amphotericin may increase nephrotoxicity

Stability Stable for 24 hours at room temperature when mixed in D_5W, $D_51/4NS$; $D_51/2NS$; NS; LR

(Continued)

Amikacin Sulfate *(Continued)*

Mechanism of Action Inhibits protein synthesis in susceptible bacteria by binding to 30S ribosomal subunits

Pharmacokinetics

Absorption: Poorly from intact GI tract; absorbed rapidly and completely after I.M. administration

Distribution: Primarily into extracellular fluid (highly hydrophilic); penetrates the blood-brain barrier when meninges are inflamed; crosses placenta

Metabolism: None

Half-life: 2-3 hours in normal adults

Time to peak serum concentration: I.M.: Within 45-120 minutes

Elimination: 94% to 98% excreted unchanged in urine via glomerular filtration; clearance dependent on renal function and age

Usual Dosage Individualization is critical because of the low therapeutic index. Use of ideal body weight (IBW) for determining the mg/kg/dose appears to be more accurate than dosing on the basis of total body weight (TBW) (see Appendix). In morbid obesity, dosage requirement may best be estimated using a dosing weight of IBW + 0.4 (TBW - IBW). Peak and trough plasma drug levels should be determined, particularly in critically ill patients with serious infections or in disease states known to significantly alter aminoglycoside pharmacokinetics (eg, cystic fibrosis, burns, or major surgery).

Neonates: I.V.:

<1200 g, 0-4 weeks: 7.5 mg/kg/dose every 12 hours

Postnatal age <7 days:

1200-2000 g: 7.5 mg/kg/dose every 12 hours

>2000 g: 10 mg/kg/dose every 12 hours

Postnatal age >7 days:

1200-2000 g: 7 mg/kg/dose every 8 hours

>2000 g: 7.5-10 mg/kg/dose every 8 hours

Infants, Children, and Adults: I.M., I.V.: 7.5 mg/kg/dose every 8 hours

Some clinicians suggest a daily dose of 15-20 mg/kg for all patients with normal renal function. This dose is at least as efficacious with similar, if not less, toxicity than conventional dosing.

Dialyzable (50% to 100%)

Overdosage Ototoxicity, nephrotoxicity, and neuromuscular toxicity

Monitoring Parameters Urinalysis, BUN, serum creatinine; be alert to ototoxicity and vestibular toxicity (nausea, vertigo, tinnitus); monitor serum concentrations regularly

Reference Range Therapeutic concentration: Peak: 25-30 μg/mL; Trough: 4-8 μg/mL. Toxic concentration: Peak: >35 μg/mL, Trough: >10 μg/mL.

Test Interactions Penicillin may decrease aminoglycoside serum concentrations *in vitro*

Patient Information Report loss of hearing, ringing or roaring in the ears, dizziness, or feeling of fullness in head

Nursing Implications Aminoglycoside levels measured from blood taken from Silastic[*] central catheters can sometimes give falsely high readings; administer I.M. injection in large muscle mass

Additional Information Sodium content of 1 g: 29.9 mg (1.3 mEq)

Dosage Forms Injection: 50 mg/mL (2 mL); 250 mg/mL (2 mL, 4 mL)

Selected Readings

Cunha BA, "Aminoglycosides: Current Role in Antimicrobial Therapy," *Pharmacotherapy*, 1988, 8(6):334-50.

Edson RS and Terrell CL, "The Aminoglycosides," *Mayo Clin Proc*, 1991, 66(11):1158-64.

Gilbert DN, "Once-Daily Aminoglycoside Therapy," *Antimicrob Agents Chemother*, 1991, 35(3):399-405.

Iseman MD, "Treatment of Multidrug-Resistant Tuberculosis," *N Engl J Med*, 1993, 329(11):784-91.

McCormack JP and Jewesson PJ, "A Critical Reevaluation of the "Therapeutic Range" of Aminoglycosides," *Clin Infect Dis*, 1992, 14(1):320-39

Van der Auwera P, "Pharmacokinetic Evaluation of Single Daily Dose Amikacin," *J Antimicrob Chemother*, 1991, 27(Suppl C):63-71.

Amikin® *see* Amikacin Sulfate *on previous page*

Aminobenzylpenicillin *see* Ampicillin *on page 495*

Aminoglycoside Dosing and Monitoring *see page 721*

Aminoglycosides
Related Information
Antimicrobial Activity Against Selected Organisms *on page 757-764*
Refer To
Amikacin Sulfate *on page 487*
Gentamicin Sulfate *on page 575*
Kanamycin Sulfate *on page 596*
Neomycin Sulfate *on page 619*
Netilmicin Sulfate *on page 620*
Streptomycin Sulfate *on page 669*
Tobramycin *on page 685*
Drug of Choice or Alternative For
Disease/Syndrome(s)
Fever, Neutropenic *on page 25*
Pneumonia, Hospital-Acquired *on page 38*
Sepsis *on page 40*
Urinary Tract Infection, Catheter-Associated *on page 44*
Organism(s)
Pseudomonas aeruginosa on page 177
Yersinia enterocolitica on page 232

Aminosalicylate Sodium (a mee noe sal i sill' ik)
Brand Names Sodium P.A.S.

Synonyms PAS

Generic Available Yes

Use Adjunctive treatment of tuberculosis used in combination with other antitubercular agents

Pregnancy Risk Factor C

Contraindications Hypersensitivity to aminosalicylate sodium

Warnings/Precautions Use with caution in patients with hepatic or renal dysfunction, patients with gastric ulcer, patients with CHF, and patients who are sodium restricted; use with caution in patients with a history of cephalosporin allergy

Adverse Reactions
1% to 10%: Nausea, vomiting, diarrhea, abdominal pain
<1%: Fever, skin eruptions, leukopenia, agranulocytosis, thrombocytopenia, hemolytic anemia, goiter with or without myxedema, jaundice, hepatitis, vasculitis

Toxicology Acute overdose results in crystalluria and renal failure, nausea, and vomiting

Mechanism of Action Aminosalicylic acid is a highly specific bacteriostatic agent active against *M. tuberculosis*. Structurally related to para-aminobenzoic acid (PABA) and its mechanism of action is thought to be similar to the sulfonamides, a competitive antagonism with PABA; disrupts plate biosynthesis in sensitive organisms

Usual Dosage Oral:
Children: 150-300 mg/kg/day in 3-4 equally divided doses
Adults: 150 mg/kg/day in 2-3 equally divided doses (usually 12-14 g/day)

Dosing adjustment in renal impairment:
Cl_{cr} 10-50 mL/minute: Administer 50% to 75% of dose
Cl_{cr} <10 mL/minute: Administer 50% of dose
Administer after hemodialysis: Dose for Cl_{cr} <10 mL/minute

Overdosage Urine can be alkalinized to prevent crystalluria and nephrotoxicity

Patient Information Notify physician if persistent sore throat, fever, unusual bleeding or bruising, persistent nausea, vomiting, or abdominal pain occurs; do not stop taking before consulting your physician; take with food or meals; do not use products that are brown or purple; store in a cool, dry place away from sunlight

Nursing Implications Do not give if discolored

Additional Information Sodium content of 1 g: 108.1 mg (4.7 mEq)

Dosage Forms Tablet: 500 mg

Selected Readings
Davidson PT and Le HQ, "Drug Treatment of Tuberculosis – 1992," *Drugs*, 1992, 43(5):651-73.
"Drugs for Tuberculosis," *Med Lett Drugs Ther*, 1993, 35(908):99-101.
Iseman MD, "Treatment of Multidrug-Resistant Tuberculosis," *N Engl J Med*, 1993, 329(11):784-91.

Amoxicillin and Clavulanate Potassium *see* Amoxicillin and Clavulanic Acid *on this page*

Amoxicillin and Clavulanic Acid

(a mox i sill' in & klav yoo lan' ick)

Related Information

Antimicrobial Activity Against Selected Organisms *on page 757-764*

Brand Names Augmentin®

Synonyms Amoxicillin and Clavulanate Potassium

Generic Available No

Use Infections caused by susceptible organisms involving the lower respiratory tract, otitis media, sinusitis, skin and skin structure, and urinary tract

Drug of Choice or Alternative For

Disease/Syndrome(s)

Bronchitis *on page 19*

Pneumonia, Community-Acquired *on page 37*

Sinusitis, Community-Acquired, Acute *on page 41*

Organism(s)

Haemophilus ducreyi on page 118

Haemophilus influenzae on page 119

Moraxella catarrhalis on page 147

Pasteurella multocida on page 170

Pregnancy Risk Factor B

Contraindications Known hypersensitivity to amoxicillin, clavulanic acid, or penicillin

Warnings/Precautions In patients with renal impairment, doses and/or frequency of administration should be modified in response to the degree of renal impairment; high percentage of patients with infectious mononucleosis have developed rash during therapy with amoxicillin; urticarial rash that appears after a few days of therapy may indicate hypersensitivity; incidence of diarrhea is higher than with amoxicillin alone; use with caution in patients with a history of cephalosporin allergy

Adverse Reactions <1%: Rash, urticaria, urticarial rash that appears after a few days of therapy may indicate hypersensitivity, nausea, vomiting, incidence of diarrhea is higher than with amoxicillin alone, vaginitis

Toxicology Neuromuscular hyperirritability or convulsive seizures; hemodialysis may be helpful to aid in the removal of the drug from the blood, otherwise most treatment is supportive or symptom directed

Drug Interactions

Decreased effect of oral contraceptives

Increased levels with probenecid; allopurinol theoretically has has an additive potential for amoxicillin rash

Stability Reconstituted oral suspension should be kept in refrigerator; discard unused suspension after 10 days

Mechanism of Action Clavulanic acid binds and inhibits beta-lactamases that inactivate amoxicillin resulting in amoxicillin having an expanded spectrum of activity. This improves activity against staphylococcal species, *H. influenzae*, *M. catarrhalis*, and *Bacteroides* species; inhibits bacterial cell wall synthesis by binding to one or more of the penicillin binding proteins (PBPs); which in turn inhibits the final transpeptidation step of peptidoglycan synthesis in bacterial cell walls, thus inhibiting cell wall biosynthesis. Bacteria eventually lyse due to ongoing activity of cell wall autolytic enzymes (autolysins and murein hydrolases) while cell wall assembly is arrested.

Pharmacokinetics

Absorption: Oral: Both amoxicillin and clavulanate are rapidly and completely absorbed

Distribution: Both distribute into pleural fluids, lungs, and peritoneal fluid; high urine concentrations are attained; also into synovial fluid, liver, prostate, muscle, and gallbladder; penetrates into middle ear effusions, maxillary sinus secretions, tonsils, sputum, and bronchial secretions; crosses the placenta; low concentrations occur in breast milk

Metabolism: Clavulanic acid is metabolized in the liver

Half-life: Children and adults with normal renal function: ~1 hour

Elimination: Amoxicillin is excreted primarily unchanged in urine

Usual Dosage Oral:

Children <40 kg: 20-40 mg (amoxicillin component)/kg/day in divided doses every 8 hours

Children >40 kg and Adults: 250-500 mg every 8 hours; maximum dose: 2 g/day

Dosing adjustment in renal impairment:
Cl$_{cr}$ 10-50 mL/minute: Administer every 12 hours
Cl$_{cr}$ <10 mL/minute: Administer every 24 hours
Moderately dialyzable (20% to 50%)

Overdosage Neuromuscular hyperirritability

Monitoring Parameters With prolonged therapy monitor renal, hepatic, and hematologic function periodically

Test Interactions May interfere with urinary glucose tests using cupric sulfate (Benedict's solution, Clinitest®); may inactivate aminoglycosides *in vitro*

Patient Information Report diarrhea promptly; entire course of medication (10-14 days) should be taken to ensure eradication of organism; females should report onset of symptoms of candidal vaginitis; may interfere with effects of oral contraceptives; pediatric drops may be placed on child's tongue or added to formula, milk, etc

Nursing Implications Assess patient at beginning and throughout therapy for infection; observe for signs and symptoms of anaphylaxis; do not give two 250 mg tablets as substitute for a 500 mg tablet (would contain too much clavulanate)

Dosage Forms
Suspension, oral (banana flavor):
125: Amoxicillin 125 mg and clavulanic acid 31.25 mg per 5 mL (75 mL, 150 mL)
250: Amoxicillin 250 mg and clavulanic acid 62.5 mg per 5 mL (75 mL, 150 mL)
Tablet:
250: Amoxicillin 250 mg and clavulanic acid 125 mg
500: Amoxicillin 500 mg and clavulanic acid 125 mg
Tablet, chewable:
125: Amoxicillin 125 mg and clavulanic acid 31.25 mg
250: Amoxicillin 250 mg and clavulanic acid 62.5 mg

Selected Readings
Donowitz GR and Mandell GL, "Beta-Lactam Antibiotics," *N Engl J Med*, 1988, 318(7):419-26 and 318(8):490-500.
Todd PA and Benefield P, "Amoxicillin/Clavulanic Acid. An Update of Its Antibacterial Activity, Pharmacokinetic Properties and Therapeutic Use," *Drugs*, 1990, 39(2):264-307.
Wright AJ and Wilkowske CJ, "The Penicillins," *Mayo Clin Proc*, 1991, 66(10):1047-63.

Amoxicillin Trihydrate (a mox i sill' in)
Related Information
Antimicrobial Activity Against Selected Organisms *on page 757-764*
Brand Names A-Cillin®; Amoxil®; Larotid®; Polymox®; Trimox®; Utimox®; Wymox®
Synonyms Amoxycillin; *p*-Hydroxyampicillin
Generic Available Yes
Use Infections caused by susceptible organisms involving the respiratory tract, otitis media, sinusitis, skin, and urinary tract; prophylaxis of bacterial endocarditis
Drug of Choice or Alternative For
Disease/Syndrome(s)
Bronchitis *on page 19*
Otitis Media, Acute *on page 35*
Pharyngitis *on page 36*
Pneumonia, Community-Acquired *on page 37*
Sinusitis, Community-Acquired, Acute *on page 41*
Urinary Tract Infection, Uncomplicated *on page 45*
Organism(s)
Haemophilus influenzae on page 119
Helicobacter pylori on page 121
Pregnancy Risk Factor B
Contraindications Hypersensitivity to amoxicillin, penicillin, or any component
Warnings/Precautions In patients with renal impairment, doses and/or frequency of administration should be modified in response to the degree of renal impairment; high percentage of patients with infectious mononucleosis have developed rash during therapy with amoxicillin; urticarial rash that appears after a few days of therapy may indicate hypersensitivity; use with caution in patients with a history of cephalosporin allergy
(Continued)

Amoxicillin Trihydrate *(Continued)*

Adverse Reactions 1% to 10%: Seizures, fever, rash (especially patients with mononucleosis), urticarial rash that appears after a few days of therapy may indicate hypersensitivity, diarrhea, superinfection

Toxicology Many beta-lactam containing antibiotics have the potential to cause neuromuscular hyperirritability or convulsive seizures. Hemodialysis may be helpful to aid in the removal of the drug from the blood, otherwise most treatment is supportive or symptom directed.

Drug Interactions
Decreased effect of oral contraceptives
Increased levels with probenecid; allopurinol theoretically has has an additive potential for amoxicillin rash

Stability Oral suspension and pediatric drops remain stable for 7 days at room temperature or 14 days if refrigerated

Mechanism of Action Inhibits bacterial cell wall synthesis by binding to one or more of the penicillin binding proteins (PBPs); which in turn inhibits the final transpeptidation step of peptidoglycan synthesis in bacterial cell walls, thus inhibiting cell wall biosynthesis. Bacteria eventually lyse due to ongoing activity of cell wall autolytic enzymes (autolysins and murein hydrolases) while cell wall assembly is arrested.

Pharmacokinetics
Absorption: Oral: Rapid and nearly complete; food does not interfere with absorption
Distribution: Widely distributed to most body fluids and bone; penetration into cells, eyes, and across normal meninges is poor
Metabolism: Partial
Half-life:
Neonates, full-term: 3.7 hours
Infants and Children: 1-2 hours
Adults: 0.7-1.4 hours
Patients with Cl_{cr} <10 mL/minute: 7-21 hours
Time to peak serum concentration:
Capsule: Within 2 hours
Suspension: Within 1 hour
Elimination: 80% unchanged in urine

Usual Dosage Oral:
Children: 25-50 mg/kg/day in divided doses every 8 hours
Subacute bacterial endocarditis prophylaxis: 50 mg/kg 1 hour before procedure and 25 mg/kg 6 hours later; not to exceed adult dosage

Adults: 250-500 mg every 8 hours; maximum dose: 2-3 g/day
Endocarditis prophylaxis: 3 g 1 hour before procedure and 1.5 g 6 hours later

Dosing adjustment in renal impairment:
Cl_{cr} of 10-50 mL/minute: Administer every 12 hours
Cl_{cr} of <10 mL/minute: Administer every 24 hours
Moderately dialyzable (20% to 50%)

Overdosage Neuromuscular sensitivity, seizures

Monitoring Parameters With prolonged therapy, monitor renal, hepatic, and hematologic function periodically

Test Interactions May interfere with urinary glucose tests using cupric sulfate (Benedict's solution, Clinitest®); may inactivate aminoglycosides *in vitro*

Patient Information Report diarrhea promptly; entire course of medication (10-14 days) should be taken to ensure eradication of organism; may interfere with oral contraceptives, females should report symptoms of vaginitis; pediatric drops may be placed on child's tongue or added to formula, milk, etc; suspension does not require refrigeration

Nursing Implications Assess patient at beginning and throughout therapy for infection; observe for signs and symptoms of anaphylaxis

Additional Information There is an increasing incidence of amoxicillin-resistant *H. influenzae* and *E. coli*; this should be taken into consideration when choosing treatment regimens

Dosage Forms
Capsule: 250 mg, 500 mg
Powder for oral suspension: 125 mg/5 mL (5 mL, 80 mL, 100 mL, 150 mL, 200 mL); 250 mg/5 mL (5 mL, 80 mL, 100 mL, 150 mL, 200 mL)
Powder for oral suspension, drops: 50 mg/mL (15 mL, 30 mL)
Tablet, chewable: 125 mg, 250 mg

Selected Readings
Donowitz GR and Mandell GL, "Beta-Lactam Antibiotics," *N Engl J Med*, 1988, 318(7):419-26 and 318(8):490-500.
Wright AJ and Wilkowske CJ, "The Penicillins," *Mayo Clin Proc*, 1991, 66(10):1047-63.

Amoxil® *see* Amoxicillin Trihydrate *on page 491*

Amoxycillin *see* Amoxicillin Trihydrate *on page 491*

Amphotericin B (am foe ter' i sin)

Brand Names Fungizone®

Synonyms Ampho

Generic Available Yes

Use Treatment of severe systemic infections and meningitis caused by susceptible fungi; fungal peritonitis; irrigant for bladder fungal infections; and topically for cutaneous and mucocutaneous candidal infections

Drug of Choice or Alternative For
Organism(s)
Aspergillus Species *on page 56*
Blastomyces dermatitidis *on page 63*
Candida Species *on page 73*
Coccidioides immitis *on page 89*
Cryptococcus neoformans *on page 94*
Dermatophytes *on page 100*
Histoplasma capsulatum *on page 130*
Mucor Species *on page 149*
Sporothrix schenckii *on page 193*

Pregnancy Risk Factor B

Contraindications Hypersensitivity to amphotericin or any component

Warnings/Precautions Because of the nephrotoxic potential of amphotericin, other nephrotoxic drugs should be avoided; BUN and serum creatinine levels should be determined every other day while therapy is increased and at least weekly thereafter. I.V. amphotericin is used primarily for the treatment of patients with progressive and potentially fatal fungal infections; topical preparations may stain clothing

Adverse Reactions
>10%: Fever, chills, nephrotoxicity, headache, anemia, hypokalemia, hypomagnesemia, anorexia, malaise, generalized pain
1% to 10%: Leukocytosis, nausea, vomiting, thrombophlebitis, hypotension, hypertension, flushing, delirium, renal tubular acidosis, bone marrow depression, renal failure, paresthesia, urinary retention, pain along lumbar nerves, arachnoiditis
<1%: Vision changes, dyspnea, maculopapular rash, anuria, acute liver failure, convulsions, hearing loss, coagulation defects, thrombocytopenia, agranulocytosis, leukopenia, cardiac arrest

Toxicology Renal dysfunction, anemia, thrombocytopenia, granulocytopenia, fever, nausea, and vomiting

Drug Interactions
Increased nephrotoxic effect of cyclosporine and aminoglycosides
Increased potassium depletion with corticosteroids; this may predispose patients receiving cardiac glycosides or skeletal muscle relaxants to toxicity secondary to hypokalemia

Stability Reconstitute **only** with sterile water without preservatives, not bacteriostatic water; amphotericin B should be further diluted in D_5W (electrolyte solutions may cause precipitation) for I.V. infusions; irrigating solutions should be diluted in sterile water. Short-term exposure (<24 hours) to light during I.V. infusion does **not** appreciably affect potency

Mechanism of Action Binds to ergosterol altering cell membrane permeability in susceptible fungi and causing leakage of cell components with subsequent cell death

Pharmacokinetics
Absorption: Poorly from GI tract
Distribution: Minimal amounts enter the aqueous humor, bile, CSF, amniotic fluid, pericardial fluid, pleural fluid and synovial fluid
Metabolism: Unknown
Half-life:
Initial: 15-48 hours
Terminal: 15 days

(Continued)

Amphotericin B *(Continued)*

Time to peak serum concentration: I.V. infusions produce peak serum levels during the first hour after a 4- to 6-hour infusion

Elimination: 2% to 5% of dose eliminated in biologically active form in urine; approximately 40% eliminated over 7-day period and may be detected in urine for at least 7 weeks after discontinued use

Usual Dosage Minimum dilution for amphotericin B infusions: 0.1 mg/mL for peripheral lines and 1 mg/mL for central lines

Infants and Children:

Test dose: I.V.: 0.1 mg/kg/dose to a maximum of 1 mg; infuse over 30-60 minutes. If the test dose is tolerated, the initial therapeutic dose is 0.25 mg/kg. The daily dose can then be gradually increased, usually in 0.25 mg/kg increments on each subsequent day until the desired daily dose is reached.

Maintenance dose: 0.25-1 mg/kg/day given once daily; infuse over 2-6 hours. Once therapy has been established, amphotericin B can be administered on an every other day basis at 1-1.5 mg/kg/dose.

I.T.: 25-100 μg every 48-72 hours; increase to 500 μg as tolerated

Adults:

Test dose: I.V.: 1 mg infused over 20-30 minutes. Institute therapy with 0.25 mg/kg administered over 2-6 hours; the daily dose can be gradually increased on subsequent days to the desired level. In patients with life-threatening infections, the full dose should be administered on day 1.

Maintenance dose: I.V.: 0.25-1 mg/kg/day or up to 1.5 mg/kg every other day; do not exceed 1.5 mg/kg/day.

I.T.: 25-300 μg every 48-72 hours; increase to 500 μg to 1 mg as tolerated

Duration of therapy varies with nature of infection: Histoplasmosis, *Cryptococcus*, or blastomycosis may be treated with total dose of 2-4 g

Children and Adults:

Bladder irrigation: 50 mg/day in 1 L of sterile water irrigation solution instilled over 24 hours for 2-7 days or until cultures are clear

Dialysate: 1-2 mg/L of peritoneal dialysis fluid either with or without low-dose I.V. amphotericin B (a total dose of 2-10 mg/kg given over 7-14 days); can be very irritating

Topical: Apply to affected areas 2-4 times/day for 1-4 weeks of therapy depending on nature and severity of infection

Dosing adjustment in renal impairment: If renal dysfunction is due to the drug, the daily total can be decreased by 50% or the dose can be given every other day; therapy may be held until creatinine concentrations begin to decline. Usual dosing is administered to patients with pre-existing renal impairment.

Overdosage Renal dysfunction, anemia, thrombocytopenia, granulocytopenia, fever, nausea, and vomiting

Monitoring Parameters Electrolytes (including magnesium), BUN, serum creatinine, liver function tests, CBC regularly; monitor input and output; monitor for signs of hypokalemia (muscle weakness, cramping, drowsiness, EKG changes, etc)

Patient Information Amphotericin cream may slightly discolor skin and stain clothing; personal hygiene is very important to help reduce the spread and recurrence of lesions; avoid covering topical applications with occlusive bandages; most skin lesions require 1-3 weeks of therapy; report any cramping, muscle weakness, or pain at or near injection site

Nursing Implications May premedicate patients with acetaminophen and diphenhydramine 30 minutes prior to the amphotericin infusion; meperidine (Demerol[®]) may help to reduce rigors; for I.V. infusion, an in-line filter (>1 micron mean pore diameter) may be used

Additional Information Renal toxicity may be minimized by sodium loading (500 mL NS or D_5 each dose), or pentoxifylline

Dosage Forms
Cream: 3% (20 g)
Lotion: 3% (30 mL)
Ointment, topical: 3% (20 g)
Powder for injection, lyophilized: 50 mg

Selected Readings
Bianco JA, Almgren J, Kern DL, et al, "Evidence That Oral Pentoxifylline Reverses Acute

Renal Dysfunction in Bone Marrow Transplant Recipients Receiving Amphotericin B and Cyclosporine," *Transplantation*, 1991, 51(4):925-7.

Branch RA, "Prevention of Amphotericin B-Induced Renal Impairment. A Review on the Use of Sodium Supplementation," *Arch Intern Med*, 1988, 148(11):2389-94.

Cruz JM, Peacock JE Jr, Loomer L, et al, "Rapid Intravenous Infusion of Amphotericin B: A Pilot Study," *Am J Med*, 1992, 93:123-30.

Gallis HA, Drew RH, and Pickard WW, "Amphotericin B: 30 Years of Clinical Experience," *Rev Infect Dis*, 1990, 12(2):308-29.

Lyman CA and Walsh TJ, "Systemically Administered Antifungal Agents. A Review of Their Clinical Pharmacology and Therapeutic Applications," *Drugs*, 1992, 44(1):9-35.

Terrell CL and Hughes CE, "Antifungal Agents Used for Deep-Seated Mycotic Infections," *Mayo Clin Proc*, 1992, 67(1):69-91.

Ampicillin (am pi sill' in)

Related Information

Antimicrobial Activity Against Selected Organisms *on page 757-764*

Brand Names Marcillin®; Omnipen®; Omnipen®-N; Polycillin®; Polycillin-N®; Principen®; Totacillin®; Totacillin®-N

Synonyms Aminobenzylpenicillin

Generic Available Yes

Use Treatment of susceptible bacterial infections

Drug of Choice or Alternative For

Disease/Syndrome(s)

Endocarditis, Subacute Native Valve *on page 23*
Meningitis, Community Acquired, Adult *on page 29*
Meningitis, Neonatal (<2 months of age) *on page 29*
Urinary Tract Infection, Catheter-Associated *on page 44*
Urinary Tract Infection, Pyelonephritis *on page 45*

Organism(s)

Actinomyces Species *on page 51*
Borrelia burgdorferi on page 68
Calymmatobacterium granulomatis on page 71
Enterococcus Species *on page 107*
Escherichia coli, Nonenterohemorrhagic *on page 113*
Gardnerella vaginalis on page 114
HACEK Group *on page 117*
Haemophilus influenzae on page 119
Listeria monocytogenes on page 143
Salmonella Species *on page 185*
Shigella Species *on page 191*
Staphylococcus saprophyticus on page 203

Pregnancy Risk Factor B

Contraindications Known hypersensitivity to ampicillin or penicillins

Warnings/Precautions In patients with renal impairment, doses and/or frequency of administration should be modified in response to the degree of renal impairment; high percentage of patients with infectious mononucleosis have developed rash during therapy with amoxicillin; urticarial rash that appears after a few days of therapy may indicate hypersensitivity; use with caution in patients with a history of cephalosporin allergy

Adverse Reactions

>10%: Diarrhea, rash, vomiting, oral candidiasis
1% to 10%: Severe abdominal or stomach cramps and pain
<1%: Penicillin encephalopathy, seizures, lymphocytic leukemia

Toxicology Many beta-lactam containing antibiotics have the potential to cause neuromuscular hyperirritability or convulsive seizures. Hemodialysis may be helpful to aid in the removal of the drug from the blood, otherwise most treatment is supportive or symptom directed.

Drug Interactions

Decreased effect of oral contraceptives
Increased levels with probenecid; allopurinol theoretically has has an additive potential for amoxicillin rash

Stability Oral suspension stable for 14 days under refrigeration; solutions for I.M. or direct I.V. should be used within 1 hour; solutions for I.V. infusion will be inactivated by dextrose at room temperature; if dextrose-containing solutions are to be used, the resultant solution will only be stable for 2 hours versus 8 hours in the 0.9% sodium chloride injection.

Mechanism of Action Inhibits bacterial cell wall synthesis by binding to one or more of the penicillin binding proteins (PBPs); which in turn inhibits the final

(Continued)

495

Ampicillin *(Continued)*

transpeptidation step of peptidoglycan synthesis in bacterial cell walls, thus inhibiting cell wall biosynthesis. Bacteria eventually lyse due to ongoing activity of cell wall autolytic enzymes (autolysins and murein hydrolases) while cell wall assembly is arrested.

Pharmacokinetics

Absorption: Oral: 50%

Distribution: Widely distributed to most body fluids and bone; penetration into CSF occurs with inflamed meninges only

Metabolism: Only partially

Half-life:

Neonates:

2-7 days: 4 hours

8-14 days: 2.8 hours

15-30 days: 1.7 hours

Children and Adults: 1-1.8 hours

Anuric patients: 8-20 hours

Elimination: ~90% excreted unchanged in urine within 24 hours

Usual Dosage I.M., I.V.:

Neonates:

Postnatal age <7 days:

<2000 g: Meningitis: 50 mg/kg/dose every 12 hours; other infections: 25 mg/kg/dose every 12 hours

>2000 g: Meningitis: 50 mg/kg/dose every 8 hours; other infections: 25 mg/kg/dose every 8 hours

Postnatal age >7 days:

<2000 g: Meningitis: 50 mg/kg/dose every 8 hours; other infections: 25 mg/kg/dose every 8 hours

>2000 g: Meningitis: 50 mg/kg/dose every 6 hours; other infections: 25 mg/kg/dose every 6 hours

Infants and Children: I.M., I.V.: 100-200 mg/kg/day in 4-6 divided doses; meningitis: 200 mg/kg/day in 4-6 divided doses; maximum dose: 12 g/day

Children: Oral: 50-100 mg/kg/day divided every 6 hours; maximum dose: 2-3 g/day

Adults:

Oral: 250-500 mg every 6 hours

I.M.: 500 mg to 1.5 g every 4-6 hours

I.V.: 500 mg to 3 g every 4-6 hours; maximum dose: 12 g/day

Sepsis/meningitis: 150-250 mg/kg/24 hours divided every 3-4 hours

Dosing adjustment in renal impairment:

Cl_{cr} 10-30 mL/minute: Administer every 8-12 hours

Cl_{cr} <10 mL/minute: Administer every 12-24 hours

Moderately dialyzable (20% to 50%)

Overdosage Neuromuscular sensitivity, seizures

Monitoring Parameters With prolonged therapy monitor renal, hepatic, and hematologic function periodically

Test Interactions May interfere with urinary glucose tests using cupric sulfate (Benedict's solution, Clinitest®); may inactivate aminoglycosides *in vitro*

Patient Information Food decreases rate and extent of absorption; take oral on an empty stomach, if possible (ie, 1 hour prior to, or 2 hours after meals); report diarrhea promptly; entire course of medication (10-14 days) should be taken to ensure eradication of organism; females should report onset of symptoms of candidal vaginitis; may interfere with the effects of oral contraceptives

Nursing Implications Ampicillin and aminoglycosides should not be mixed in the same I.V. tubing or administered concurrently

Additional Information

Sodium content of suspension (250 mg/5 mL, 5 mL): 10 mg (0.4 mEq)

Sodium content of 1 g: 66.7 mg (3 mEq)

Dosage Forms

Capsule, as anhydrous: 250 mg, 500 mg

Capsule, as trihydrate: 250 mg, 500 mg

Powder for injection, as sodium: 125 mg, 250 mg, 500 mg, 1 g, 2 g, 10 g

Powder for oral suspension, as trihydrate: 125 mg/5 mL (5 mL unit dose, 80 mL, 100 mL, 150 mL, 200 mL); 250 mg/5 mL (5 mL unit dose, 80 mL, 100 mL, 150 mL, 200 mL); 500 mg/5 mL (5 mL unit dose, 100 mL)

Powder for oral suspension, drops, as trihydrate: 100 mg/mL (20 mL)

Selected Readings

Donowitz GR and Mandell GL, "Beta-Lactam Antibiotics," *N Engl J Med*, 1988, 318(7):419-26 and 318(8):490-500.

Wright AJ and Wilkowske CJ, "The Penicillins," *Mayo Clin Proc*, 1991, 66(10):1047-63.

Ampicillin Sodium and Sulbactam Sodium

(am pi sill' in and sul bact' am)

Related Information

Antimicrobial Activity Against Selected Organisms *on page 757-764*

Brand Names Unasyn®

Synonyms Sulbactam and Ampicillin

Generic Available No

Use Treatment of susceptible bacterial infections involved with skin and skin structure, intra-abdominal infections, gynecological infections

Drug of Choice or Alternative For

Disease/Syndrome(s)

Osteomyelitis, Diabetic Foot *on page 32*

Peritonitis *on page 36*

Pneumonia, Aspiration, Community-Acquired *on page 37*

Pneumonia, Community-Acquired *on page 37*

Organism(s)

Acinetobacter Species *on page 50*

Pasteurella multocida on page 170

Pregnancy Risk Factor B

Contraindications Hypersensitivity to ampicillin, sulbactam or any component, or penicillins

Warnings/Precautions In patients with renal impairment, doses and/or frequency of administration should be modified in response to the degree of renal impairment; high percentage of patients with infectious mononucleosis have developed rash during therapy with amoxicillin; urticarial rash that appears after a few days of therapy may indicate hypersensitivity; use with caution in patients with a history of cephalosporin allergy

Adverse Reactions

>10%: Pain at injection site (I.M.)

1% to 10%: Pain at injection site (I.V.), diarrhea, rash

<1%: Chest pain, fatigue, malaise, headache, itching, nausea, vomiting, enterocolitis, pseudomembranous colitis, decreased WBC, neutrophils, platelets, hemoglobin, and hematocrit, increased liver enzymes, increased BUN and creatinine, thrombophlebitis, dysuria, hypersensitivity reactions, candidiasis, chills, hairy tongue

Toxicology Many beta-lactam containing antibiotics have the potential to cause neuromuscular hyperirritability or convulsive seizures. Hemodialysis may be helpful to aid in the removal of the drug from the blood, otherwise most treatment is supportive or symptom directed.

Drug Interactions

Decreased effect of oral contraceptives

Increased levels with probenecid; allopurinol theoretically has has an additive potential for amoxicillin/ampicillin rash

Stability I.M. and direct I.V. administration: used within 1 hour after preparation; reconstitute with sterile water for injection or 0.5% or 2% lidocaine hydrochloride injection (I.M.); sodium chloride 0.9% (NS) is the diluent of choice for I.V. piggyback use, solutions made in NS are stable up to 72 hours when refrigerated whereas dextrose solutions (same concentration) are stable for only 4 hours

Mechanism of Action The addition of sulbactam, a beta-lactamase inhibitor, to ampicillin extends the spectrum of ampicillin to include some beta-lactamase producing organisms; inhibits bacterial cell wall synthesis by binding to one or more of the penicillin binding proteins (PBPs); which in turn inhibits the final transpeptidation step of peptidoglycan synthesis in bacterial cell walls, thus inhibiting cell wall biosynthesis. Bacteria eventually lyse due to ongoing activity of cell wall autolytic enzymes (autolysins and murein hydrolases) while cell wall assembly is arrested.

Pharmacokinetics

Distribution: Widely distributed to most body fluids and bone

Half-life: Ampicillin and sulbactam are similar: 1-1.8 hours and 1-1.3 hours, respectively in normal adults

Elimination: ~75% to 85% of both drugs are excreted unchanged in urine within 8 hours following administration

(Continued)

497

Ampicillin Sodium and Sulbactam Sodium *(Continued)*

Usual Dosage Not FDA approved for children <12 years of age

Unasyn® (ampicillin/sulbactam) is a combination product. Each 3 g vial contains 2 g of ampicillin and 1 g of sulbactam. Sulbactam has very little antibacterial activity by itself, but effectively extends the spectrum of ampicillin to include beta-lactamase producing strains that are resistant to ampicillin alone. Therefore, dosage recommendations for Unasyn® are based on the ampicillin component.

Children: I.M., I.V.: 100-200 mg ampicillin/kg/day divided every 6 hours; maximum dose: 8 g ampicillin/day

Adults: I.M., I.V.: 1-2 g ampicillin every 6-8 hours; maximum dose: 8 g ampicillin/day

Dosing adjustment in renal impairment:

Cl_{cr} 15-29 mL/minute: Administer every 12 hours

Cl_{cr} 5-14 mL/minute: Administer every 24 hours

Monitoring Parameters With prolonged therapy monitor hematologic, renal and hepatic function

Test Interactions May interfere with urinary glucose tests using cupric sulfate (Benedict's solution, Clinitest®); may inactivate aminoglycosides *in vitro*

Nursing Implications Ampicillin and gentamicin should not be mixed in the same I.V. tubing or administered concurrently

Additional Information Sodium content of 1.5 g injection: 115 mg (5 mEq)

Dosage Forms Powder for injection:

1.5 g: Ampicillin sodium 1 g and sulbactam sodium 0.5 g

3 g: Ampicillin sodium 2 g and sulbactam sodium 1 g

Selected Readings

Donowitz GR and Mandell GL, "Beta-Lactam Antibiotics," *N Engl J Med*, 1988, 318(7):419-26 and 318(8):490-500.

Itokazu GS and Danziger LH, "Ampicillin-Sulbactam and Ticarcillin-Clavulanic Acid: A Comparison of Their *In Vitro* Activity and Review of Their Clinical Efficacy," *Pharmacotherapy*, 1991, 11(5):382-414.

Wright AJ and Wilkowske CJ, "The Penicillins," *Mayo Clin Proc*, 1991, 66(10):1047-63.

Ancef® *see* Cefazolin Sodium *on page 511*

Ancobon® *see* Flucytosine *on page 570*

Anocol® *see* Chloramphenicol *on page 531*

Ansamycin *see* Rifabutin *on page 661*

Antifungal, Topical

Refer To

Amphotericin B *on page 493*

Ciclopirox Olamine *on page 536*

Clotrimazole *on page 543*

Econazole Nitrate *on page 559*

Ketoconazole *on page 598*

Naftifine Hydrochloride *on page 618*

Nystatin *on page 625*

Oxiconazole Nitrate *on page 629*

Sulconazole Nitrate *on page 670*

Tolnaftate *on page 687*

Drug of Choice or Alternative For Organism(s)

Candida Species *on page 73*

Dermatophytes *on page 100*

Antimicrobial Activity Against Selected Organisms

see page 757

Antiminth® [OTC] *see* Pyrantel Pamoate *on page 651*

Antirabies Serum, Equine Origin *(an tee ray' beez)*

Synonyms ARS

Generic Available No

Use Rabies prophylaxis

Pregnancy Risk Factor C

Adverse Reactions 1% to 10%: Serum sickness, local pain, urticaria

Mechanism of Action Affords passive immunity against rabies

Usual Dosage 1000 units/55 lb in a single dose, infiltrate up to 50% of dose around the wound

Nursing Implications Take careful history of asthma, angioneurotic edema, or other allergies

Additional Information Because of a significantly lower incidence of adverse reactions, Rabies Immune Globulin, Human is preferred over Antirabies Serum Equine

Dosage Forms Injection: 125 units/mL (8 mL)

Antituberculars
Refer To
Drug of Choice or Alternative For Organism(s)

APPG *see* Penicillin G Procaine, Aqueous *on page 636*

Aqueous Procaine Penicillin G *see* Penicillin G Procaine, Aqueous *on page 636*

Ara-A *see* Vidarabine *on page 694*

Arabinofuranosyladenine *see* Vidarabine *on page 694*

Aralen® Phosphate *see* Chloroquine Phosphate *on page 534*

Aralen® Phosphate With Primaquine Phosphate *see* Chloroquine and Primaquine *on page 533*

ARS *see* Antirabies Serum, Equine Origin *on previous page*

Atabrine® *see* Quinacrine Hydrochloride *on page 655*

Atovaquone (a toe' va kwone)
Brand Names Mepron™

Generic Available No

Use Acute oral treatment of mild to moderate *Pneumocystis carinii* pneumonia (PCP) in patients who are intolerant to co-trimoxazole

Pregnancy Risk Factor C

Contraindications Life-threatening allergic reaction to the drug or formulation

Warnings/Precautions Has only been used in mild to moderate PCP; use with caution in elderly patients

Adverse Reactions
>10%: Rash, nausea, diarrhea, headache, cough, vomiting, fever, insomnia
1% to 10%: Asthenia, pruritus, oral *Monilia*, abdominal pain, constipation, dizziness, anemia, neutropenia, hyponatremia, leukopenia, elevated creatinine and BUN

Drug Interactions Possible increased toxicity with other highly protein bound drugs; however, serum concentrations of 15 μg/mL of phenytoin failed to cause an interaction

Mechanism of Action Mechanism has not been fully elucidated; may inhibit electron transport in mitochondria inhibiting metabolic enzymes

Pharmacokinetics
Absorption: Decreased significantly in single doses >750 mg; increased threefold when administered with a high fat meal (21 g of fat/meal)
Distribution: Enterohepatically recirculated
Protein binding: >99.9%
Bioavailability: ~30%
Half-life: 2.6 days
Elimination: Excreted in feces

Usual Dosage Adults: Oral: 750 mg 3 times/day with food for 21 days

Patient Information Take only prescribed dose; take each dose with a meal, preferably one with high fat content
(Continued)

Atovaquone *(Continued)*

Nursing Implications Notify physician if patient is unable to eat significant amounts of food on an ongoing basis

Dosage Forms Tablet, film coated: 250 mg

Selected Readings

Artymowicz RJ and James VE, "Atovaquone: A New Antipneumocystis Agent," *Clin Pharm*, 1993, 12(8):563-70.

Haile LG and Flaherty JF, "Atovaquone: A Review," *Ann Pharmacother*, 1993, 27(12):1488-94.

Hughes W, Leoung G, Kramer F, et al, "Comparison of Atovaquone (566C80) With Trimethoprim-Sulfamethoxazole to Treat *Pneumocystis carinii* Pneumonia in Patients With AIDS," *N Engl J Med*, 1993, 328(21):1521-7.

Attenuvax® *see* Measles Virus Vaccine, Live *on page 604*

Augmentin® *see* Amoxicillin and Clavulanic Acid *on page 490*

Avlosulfon® *see* Dapsone *on page 549*

Azactam® *see* Aztreonam *on next page*

Azidothymidine *see* Zidovudine *on page 696*

Azithromycin Dihydrate (az ith roe mye' sin)

Related Information

Antimicrobial Activity Against Selected Organisms *on page 757-764*

Brand Names Zithromax™

Generic Available No

Use Treatment of adult patients (> 16 years of age) with mild to moderate upper and lower respiratory tract, skin and skin structure, and sexually transmitted diseases caused by susceptible organisms

Drug of Choice or Alternative For

Disease/Syndrome(s)

Sinusitis, Community-Acquired, Acute *on page 41*

Urethritis, Nongonococcal *on page 44*

Organism(s)

Legionella pneumophila on page 139

Ureaplasma urealyticum on page 225

Pregnancy Risk Factor C

Contraindications Hepatic impairment, known hypersensitivity to erythromycin or its any components

Adverse Reactions

1% to 10%: Diarrhea, nausea, abdominal pain, cramping, vomiting

<1%: Thrombophlebitis, ventricular arrhythmias, fever, skin rash, eosinophilia, cholestatic jaundice, ototoxicity, hypertrophic pyloric stenosis, allergic reactions

Drug Interactions Use with caution with drugs that interact with erythromycin

Mechanism of Action Inhibits RNA-dependent protein synthesis at the chain elongation step; binds to the 50S ribosomal subunit resulting in blockage of transpeptidation

Pharmacokinetics

Absorption: Oral: Rapid; food decreases absorption by 40% to 50%

Distribution: Distributes well into skin, lungs, sputum, tonsils, and cervix; penetration into the CSF is poor

Protein binding: Variable, decreasing from 50% at 0.02 μg/mL to 7% at 2 mg/mL

Half-life: 68 hours

Time to peak: 2.5-3 hours; in elderly women, peak concentrations are increased to 30% to 50%; however no significant accumulation is seen

Elimination: Biliary excretion of unchanged drug is primary route of elimination with only 6% of unchanged drug in urine

Usual Dosage Adults: Oral: 500 mg as a single dose on day 1 followed by 250 mg day on days 2-5 (1.5 g total); the recommended dose for nongonococcal urethritis and cervicitis due to *C. trachomatis* is a single 1 g dose

Overdosage Nausea, vomiting, diarrhea, prostration

Monitoring Parameters Liver function tests

Dosage Forms Capsule: 250 mg

Selected Readings

Drew RH and Gallis HA, "Azithromycin-Spectrum of Activity, Pharmacokinetics, and Clinical Applications," *Pharmacotherapy*, 1992, 12(3): 161-73.

Goldman MP and Longworth DL, "The Role of Azithromycin and Clarithromycin in Clinical Practice," *Cleve Clin J Med*, 1993, 60(5):359-64.

AZT *see* Zidovudine *on page 696*

Azthreonam *see* Aztreonam *on this page*

Aztreonam (az' tree oh nam)
Related Information
Antimicrobial Activity Against Selected Organisms *on page 757-764*
Brand Names Azactam®
Synonyms Azthreonam
Generic Available No
Use Treatment of patients with urinary tract infection, lower respiratory tract infections, septicemia, skin/skin structure infections, intra-abdominal infections and gynecological infections caused by susceptible organisms
Drug of Choice or Alternative For
Organism(s)
Acinetobacter Species *on page 50*
Klebsiella Species *on page 137*
Serratia Species *on page 190*
Pregnancy Risk Factor B
Contraindications Hypersensitivity to aztreonam or any component
Warnings/Precautions Rare cross-allergenicity to penicillins and cephalosporins; requires dosing adjustment in renal impairment
Adverse Reactions
1% to 10%: Thrombophlebitis, pain at injection site, diarrhea, nausea, rash, vomiting
<1%: Hypotension, seizures, confusion, anaphylaxis, hepatitis, jaundice, headache, vertigo, insomnia, dizziness, tinnitus, diplopia, numb tongue, mouth ulcer, altered taste, sneezing, halitosis, vaginitis, breast tenderness, weakness, muscular aches, fever, pseudomembranous colitis, thrombocytopenia, eosinophilia, leukopenia, neutropenia, elevation of liver enzymes
Toxicology If necessary, dialysis can reduce the drug concentration in the blood
Drug Interactions Probenecid increases serum levels, aminoglycosides (synergy)
Stability Reconstituted solutions are colorless to light yellow straw and may turn pink upon standing without affecting potency; use reconstituted solutions and I.V. solutions (in NS and D_5W) within 48 hours if kept at room temperature or 7 days if kept in refrigerator; reconstituted solutions are NOT for multiple-dose use; incompatible when mixed with nafcillin, metronidazole
Mechanism of Action Inhibits bacterial cell wall synthesis by binding to one or more of the penicillin binding proteins (PBPs); which in turn inhibits the final transpeptidation step of peptidoglycan synthesis in bacterial cell walls, thus inhibiting cell wall biosynthesis. Bacteria eventually lyse due to ongoing activity of cell wall autolytic enzymes (autolysins and murein hydrolases) while cell wall assembly is arrested.
Pharmacokinetics
Absorption: I.M.: Well absorbed
Distribution: Rapidly and widely distributed to most body fluids and tissues including breast milk; crosses placenta
Metabolism: ~6% to 16% to inactive metabolites
Half-life:
Neonates <7 days, <2.5 kg: 5.5-9.9 hours
Neonates to Adults: 1.3-2.6 hours (prolonged in renal failure)
Elimination: 60% to 70% excreted unchanged in urine and partially excreted in feces
Usual Dosage All dosages are I.M. or I.V.:
Neonates:
Postnatal age <7 days:
<2000 g: 60 mg/kg/day in 2 divided doses every 12 hours
>2000 g: 90 mg/kg/day in 3 divided doses every 8 hours
Postnatal age >7 days:
<2000 g: 90 mg/kg/day in 3 divided doses every 8 hours
>2000 g: 120 mg/kg/day in 4 divided doses every 6 hours

Children >1 month: 90-120 mg/kg/day divided every 6-8 hours
Cystic fibrosis: 50 mg/kg/dose every 6-8 hours (ie, up to 200 mg/kg/day); maximum: 6-8 g/day
(Continued)

Aztreonam *(Continued)*

Adults:

Urinary tract infection: 500 mg to 1 g every 8-12 hours

Moderately severe systemic infections: 1-2 g every 8-12 hours

Severe systemic or life-threatening infections: I.V.: 2 g every 6-8 hours; maximum: 8 g/day

Dosing adjustment in renal impairment:

Cl_{cr} 10-30 mL/minute: 50% of usual dose given at the usual interval

Cl_{cr} <10 mL/minute: 25% of usual dose given at the usual interval

Moderately dialyzable (20% to 50%)

Monitoring Parameters Periodic liver function test

Test Interactions May interfere with urine glucose tests containing cupric sulfate (Benedict's solution, Clinitest®)

Nursing Implications May be administered by I.V. push over 3-5 minutes or by intermittent infusion over 20-60 minutes at a final concentration not to exceed 20 mg/mL

Additional Information Although marketed as an agent similar to aminoglycosides, aztreonam is a monobactam antimicrobial with almost pure gram-negative aerobic activity; it cannot be used for gram-positive infections; aminoglycosides are often used for synergy in gram-positive infections

Dosage Forms Powder for injection: 500 mg (15 mL, 100 mL); 1 g (15 mL, 100 mL); 2 g (15 mL, 100 mL)

Selected Readings

Brewer NS and Hellinger WC, "The Monobactams," *Mayo Clin Proc*, 1991, 66(11):1152-7.

Brogden RN and Heel RC, "Aztreonam. A Review of Its Antibacterial Activity, Pharmacokinetic Properties and Therapeutic Use," *Drugs*, 1986, 31(2):96-130.

Donowitz GR and Mandell GL, "Beta-Lactam Antibiotics," *N Engl J Med*, 1988, 318(7):419-26 and 318(8):490-500.

Baciguent® Topical [OTC] *see* Bacitracin *on next page*

Baci-IM® Injection *see* Bacitracin *on next page*

Bacillus Calmette-Guérin (BCG) Live

Brand Names TheraCys®; TICE® BCG

Synonyms BCG

Generic Available No

Use In the United States, tuberculosis control efforts are directed toward early identification, treatment of cases, and preventive therapy with isoniazid. BCG vaccine is not recommended for adults at high risk for tuberculosis in the United States. BCG vaccination may be considered for infants and children who are skin test-negative to 5 tuberculin units and who cannot be given isoniazid preventive therapy but have close contact with untreated or ineffectively treated active tuberculosis patients or who belong to groups in which other control measures have not been successful; immunotherapy for bladder cancer

Pregnancy Risk Factor C

Contraindications Tuberculin-positive individual, hypersensitivity to BCG vaccine or any component, immunocompromised and burn patients; pregnancy, unless there is unavoidable exposure to infectious tuberculosis

Warnings/Precautions Protection against tuberculosis is only relative, not permanent, nor entirely predictable; for live bacteria vaccine, proper aseptic technique and disposal of all equipment in contact with BCG vaccine as a biohazardous material is recommended

Adverse Reactions

1% to 10%: Bladder infection, flu-like syndrome, prostatitis, dysuria, urinary frequency

<1%: Skin ulceration, abscesses, hematuria, anaphylactic shock in infants, lymphadenitis

Drug Interactions Decreased effect: Antimicrobial or immunosuppressive drugs may impair response to BCG or increase risk of infection; antituberculosis drugs

Stability Refrigerate, protect from light, use within 2 (TICE® BCG) hours of mixing

Mechanism of Action Live culture preparation of Bacillus Calmette-Guérin (BCG) strain of *Mycobacterium bovis* is a substrain of Pasteur Institute strain; *M. bovis* is immunologically similar to *M. tuberculosis*, and therefore, simulates natural infection with *M. tuberculosis*, promoting cell-mediated immunity against tuberculosis. BCG live, when used intravesically for treatment of bladder carcinoma *in situ*, is thought to cause a local, chronic inflammatory response involving macrophage and leukocyte infiltration of the bladder which leads to destruction of superficial tumor cells of the urothelium.

Usual Dosage Children >1 month and Adults:

Immunization against tuberculosis (TICE® BCG): 0.2-0.3 mL percutaneous; initial lesion usually appears after 10-14 days consisting of small red papule at injection site and reaches maximum diameter of 3 mm in 4-6 weeks; conduct postvaccinal tuberculin test (ie, 5 TU of PPD) in 2-3 months; if test is negative, repeat vaccination

Immunotherapy for bladder cancer:

Intravesical treatment: Instill into bladder for 2 hours

TheraCys®: One dose diluted in 50 mL NS (preservative free) instilled into bladder once weekly for 6 weeks followed by one treatment at 3, 6, 12, 18, and 24 months after initial treatment

TICE® BCG: One dose diluted in 50 mL NS (preservative free) instilled into the bladder once weekly for 6 weeks followed by once monthly for 6-12 months

Test Interactions PPD intradermal test

Patient Information Notify physician of persistent pain on urination or blood in urine

Nursing Implications Should only be given intravesicularly or percutaneously; do not give I.V., S.C., or intradermally; can be used for bladder irrigation

Dosage Forms Powder for injection, lyophilized:

Connaught Strain (TheraCys®): 3.4 $\pm$ 3 x 10^8 CFU equivalent to approximately 27 mg

Tice Strain (TICE® BCG): 1-8 x 10^8 CFU equivalent to approximately 50 mg (2 mL)

Bacitracin (bass i tray' sin)

Brand Names AK-Tracin® Ophthalmic; Baciguent® Topical [OTC]; Baci-IM® Injection

Generic Available Yes

Use Treatment of susceptible bacterial infections (staphylococcal pneumonia and empyema); due to toxicity, systemic and irrigant uses of bacitracin should be limited to situations where less toxic alternatives would not be effective; oral administration has been successful in antibiotic-associated colitis

Pregnancy Risk Factor C

Contraindications Hypersensitivity to bacitracin or any component; I.M. use is contraindicated in patients with renal impairment

Warnings/Precautions Prolonged use may result in overgrowth of nonsusceptible organisms; I.M. use may cause renal failure due to tubular and glomerular necrosis; **do not** administer intravenously because severe thrombophlebitis occurs

Adverse Reactions 1% to 10%: Sweating, hypotension, rash, itching, anorexia, nausea, vomiting, diarrhea, blood dyscrasias, tightness of chest, swelling of lips and face, rectal itching and burning, pain

Toxicology Nephrotoxicity (parenteral); nausea, vomiting (oral)

Drug Interactions Increased toxicity: Nephrotoxic drugs; neuromuscular blocking agents and anesthetics (↑ neuromuscular blockade)

Stability Sterile powder should be stored in the refrigerator; once reconstituted, bacitracin is stable for 1 week under refrigeration (2°C to 8°C); bacitracin sterile powder should be dissolved in 0.9% sodium chloride injection containing 2% procaine hydrochloride for I.M. use; do not use diluents containing parabens

Mechanism of Action Inhibits bacterial cell wall synthesis by preventing transfer of mucopeptides into the growing cell wall

Pharmacokinetics

Duration of action: 6-8 hours

Absorption: Poor from mucous membranes and intact or denuded skin; rapidly absorbed following I.M. administration

Protein binding: Minimally bound to plasma proteins

Time to peak serum concentration: I.M.: Within 1-2 hours

Elimination: Slow elimination into urine with 10% to 40% of dose excreted within 24 hours

Usual Dosage

Do not administer I.V.

(Continued)

Bacitracin *(Continued)*

    Infants:
        <2.5 kg: 900 units/kg/day in 2-3 divided doses
        >2.5 kg: 1000 units/kg/day in 2-3 divided doses
    Children: 800-1200 units/kg/day divided every 8 hours
    Adults: Not recommended

    Antibiotic-associated colitis: Adults: Oral: 25,000 units 4 times/day for 7-10 days

    Topical: Apply 1-4 times/day to infected area

    Ophthalmic ointment: Instill $\frac{1}{4}$" to $\frac{1}{2}$" ribbon every 3-4 hours into conjunctival sac for acute infections or 2-3 times/day for mild to moderate infections for 7-10 days

    Irrigation, solution: 50-100 units/mL in normal saline, lactated Ringer's, or sterile water for irrigation; soak sponges in solution for topical compresses 1-5 times/day or as needed during surgical procedures

Monitoring Parameters I.M.: Urinalysis, renal function tests

Patient Information Ophthalmic ointment may cause blurred vision; topical bacitracin should not be used for longer than 1 week unless directed by a physician. Ophthalmic administration: Tilt head back, place medication in conjunctival sac and close eyes; apply light finger pressure on lacrimal sac for 1 minute following instillation. Do not share eye medications with others.

Nursing Implications Do **not** administer I.V.; confirm any orders for parenteral use; pH of urine should be kept >6 by using sodium bicarbonate

Additional Information 1 unit is equivalent to 0.026 mg

Dosage Forms
    Injection: 50,000 units
    Ointment:
        Ophthalmic: 500 units/g (1 g, 3.5 g, 454 g)
        Topical: 500 units/g (1.5 g, 3.75 g, 15 g, 30 g, 120 g, 454 g)

Selected Readings
Kelly CP, Pothoulakis C, and LaMont JT, "*Clostridium difficile* colitis," *N Engl J Med*, 1994, 330(4):257-62.

Bactocill® Injection *see* Oxacillin Sodium *on page 627*

Bactocill® Oral *see* Oxacillin Sodium *on page 627*

Bactrim™ *see* Co-trimoxazole *on page 545*

Bactrim™ DS *see* Co-trimoxazole *on page 545*

Bactroban® Topical *see* Mupirocin *on page 616*

BCG *see* Bacillus Calmette-Guérin (BCG) Live *on page 502*

Beepen-VK® *see* Penicillin V Potassium *on page 638*

Benzathine Benzylpenicillin *see* Penicillin G Benzathine, Parenteral *on page 632*

Benzathine Penicillin G *see* Penicillin G Benzathine, Parenteral *on page 632*

Benzene Hexachloride *see* Lindane *on page 599*

Benzylpenicillin Benzathine *see* Penicillin G Benzathine, Parenteral *on page 632*

Benzylpenicillin Potassium *see* Penicillin G, Parenteral *on page 633*

Benzylpenicillin Sodium *see* Penicillin G, Parenteral *on page 633*

Betapen®-VK *see* Penicillin V Potassium *on page 638*

Biavax®ₗₗ *see* Rubella and Mumps Vaccines, Combined *on page 664*

Biaxin™ Filmtabs® *see* Clarithromycin *on page 539*

Bicillin® C-R *see* Penicillin G Benzathine and Procaine Combined *on page 631*

Bicillin® C-R 900/300 *see* Penicillin G Benzathine and Procaine Combined *on page 631*

Bicillin® L-A *see* Penicillin G Benzathine, Parenteral *on page 632*

Biltricide® *see* Praziquantel *on page 650*

Bismuth (bis' muth)

Brand Names Devrom® [OTC]; Pepto-Bismol® [OTC]

Synonyms Bismuth Subgallate; Bismuth Subsalicylate

Generic Available Yes

Use Symptomatic treatment of mild, nonspecific diarrhea, "traveler's diarrhea"; may be part of a three-drug regimen for treatment of peptic ulcer disease associated with *Helicobacter pylori*

Drug of Choice or Alternative For
Organism(s)
Helicobacter pylori on page 121

Pregnancy Risk Factor C (D in 3rd trimester)

Contraindications Do not use salicylates in patients with influenza or chickenpox because of risk of Reye's syndrome

Adverse Reactions
>10%: Discoloration of the tongue (darkening), grayish black stools
<1%: Impaction may occur in infants and debilitated patients, anxiety, confusion, slurred speech, headache, mental depression, muscle spasms, weakness, loss of hearing, confusion, buzzing in ears

Toxicology Most toxic symptoms occur following subacute or chronic intoxications. Chelation with dimercaprol in doses of 3 mg/kg or penicillamine 100 mg/kg/day for 5 days can hasten recovery from bismuth-induced encephalopathy. When associated with methemoglobinemia, bismuth intoxications should be treated with methylene blue 1-2 mg/kg in a 1% sterile aqueous solution I.V. push over 4-6 minutes. This may be repeated within 60 minutes if necessary, up to a total dose of 7 mg/kg. Seizures usually respond to I.V. diazepam.

Drug Interactions
Decreased effect of tetracyclines
Increased toxicity of aspirin

Mechanism of Action Adsorbs extra water in large intestine, as well as toxins; forms a protective coat on the intestinal mucosa

Pharmacokinetics
Absorption: Bismuth is minimally absorbed across the GI tract while the salt (eg, salicylate) may be readily absorbed
Distribution: Locally in the gut
Protein binding: Subsalicylate: High (to albumin)
Metabolism: Following oral administration, undergoes chemical dissociation to various bismuth salts
Elimination: Fecal

Usual Dosage Oral:
Subsalicylate:
Nonspecific diarrhea:
Children: Up to 8 doses/24 hours:
3-6 years: $\frac{1}{3}$ tablet or 5 mL every 30 minutes to 1 hour as needed
6-9 years: $\frac{2}{3}$ tablet or 10 mL every 30 minutes to 1 hour as needed
9-12 years: 1 tablet or 15 mL every 30 minutes to 1 hour as needed
Adults: 2 tablets or 30 mL every 30 minutes to 1 hour as needed up to 8 doses/24 hours
Prevention of traveler's diarrhea: 2.1 g/day or 2 tablets 4 times/day before meals and at bedtime
Helicobacter (Campylobacter) pylori treatment in ulcer disease: 1 tablet with meals and 2 tablets at bedtime

Subgallate: 1-2 tablets 3 times/day with meals

Dosing comments in renal impairment: Should possibly be avoided with renal failure

Overdosage Tinnitus (subsalicylate), fever

Patient Information Chew tablet well or shake suspension well before using; may darken stools; if diarrhea persists for more than 2 days, consult a physician

Dosage Forms
Suspension, as subsalicylate: 262 mg/15 mL (240 mL)
Tablet, chewable, as subgallate: 200 mg
Tablet, chewable, as subsalicylate: 262 mg

Selected Readings
Graham DY, Lew GM, Evans DG, et al, "Effect of Triple Therapy (Antibiotics Plus Bismuth) on Duodenal Ulcer Healing," *Ann Intern Med*, 1991, 115(4):266-9.

(Continued)

Bismuth *(Continued)*

Graham DY, Lew GM, Klein PD, et al, "Effect of Treatment of *Helicobacter pylori* Infection on the Long-Term Recurrence of Gastric or Duodenal Ulcer," *Ann Intern Med*, 1992, 116(9):705-8.

Ormand JE and Talley NJ, "*Helicobacter pylori*: Controversies and an Approach to Management," *Mayo Clin Proc*, 1990, 65(3):414-26.

Bismuth Subgallate *see* Bismuth *on previous page*

Bismuth Subsalicylate *see* Bismuth *on previous page*

Botulinum Toxoid, Pentavalent Vaccine (Against Types A, B, C, D, and E Strains of *C. botulinum*)
Drug of Choice or Alternative For
Organism(s)
  Clostridium botulinum on page 83
Additional Information For advice on vaccine administration and contraindications, contact the Division of Immunization, CDC, Atlanta, GA 30333 (404-639-3356).

Capastat® Sulfate *see* Capreomycin Sulfate *on this page*

Capreomycin Sulfate (kap ree oh mye' sin)
Brand Names Capastat® Sulfate
Generic Available No
Use In conjunction with at least one other antituberculosis agent in the treatment of tuberculosis; capreomycin may also be useful (in combination) for treatment of other mycobacterial diseases
Pregnancy Risk Factor C
Contraindications Known hypersensitivity to capreomycin sulfate
Warnings/Precautions Use in patients with renal insufficiency or pre-existing auditory impairment must be undertaken with great caution, and the risk of additional eighth nerve impairment or renal injury should be weighed against the benefits to be derived from therapy. Since other parenteral antituberculous agents (eg, streptomycin) also have similar and sometimes irreversible toxic effects, particularly on eighth cranial nerve and renal function, simultaneous administration of these agents with capreomycin is not recommended. Use with nonantituberculous drugs (ie, aminoglycoside antibiotics) having ototoxic or nephrotoxic potential should be undertaken only with great caution.
Adverse Reactions
  >10%: Nephrotoxicity, ototoxicity
  1% to 10%: Eosinophilia
  <1%: Vertigo, fever, rash, leukocytosis, thrombocytopenia, pain induration, bleeding at injection site, tinnitus
Drug Interactions Increased effect/duration of nondepolarizing neuromuscular blocking agents
Mechanism of Action Capreomycin is a cyclic polypeptide antimicrobial; it is administered as a mixture of capreomycin IA and capreomycin IB. The mechanism of action of capreomycin is not well understood. Mycobacterial species that have become resistant to other agents are usually still sensitive to the action of capreomycin. However, significant cross-resistance with viomycin, kanamycin, and neomycin occurs.
Pharmacokinetics
  Half-life: 4-6 hours in patients with normal renal function
  Elimination: Excreted mainly unchanged in urine
Usual Dosage Adults: I.M.: 15 mg/kg/day up to 1 g/day for 60-120 days

  Dosing interval in renal impairment:
  Cl_{cr} >100 mL/minute: Administer 13-15 mg/kg every 24 hours
  Cl_{cr} 80-100 mL/minute: Administer 10-13 mg/kg every 24 hours
  Cl_{cr} 60-80 mL/minute: Administer 7-10 mg/kg every 24 hours
  Cl_{cr} 40-60 mL/minute: Administer 11-14 mg/kg every 48 hours
  Cl_{cr} 20-40 mL/minute: Administer 10-14 mg/kg every 72 hours
  Cl_{cr} <20 mL/minute: Administer 4-7 mg/kg every 72 hours

  Target steady-state serum concentration should be maintained at 10 μg/mL
Reference Range 10 μg/mL
Patient Information Report any hearing loss to physician immediately; do not discontinue without notifying physician

Nursing Implications Solution for injection may acquire a pale straw color and darken with time, this is not associated with a loss of potency or development of toxicity

Dosage Forms Powder for injection: 1 g (200 mg/mL; 5 mL)

Selected Readings

Davidson PT and Le HQ, "Drug Treatment of Tuberculosis – 1992," *Drugs*, 1992, 43(5):651-73.

"Drugs for Tuberculosis," *Med Lett Drugs Ther*, 1993, 35(908):99-101.

Iseman MD, "Treatment of Multidrug-Resistant Tuberculosis," *N Engl J Med*, 1993, 329(11):784-91.

Carbenicillin (kar ben i sill' in)

Related Information

Antimicrobial Activity Against Selected Organisms *on page 757-764*

Brand Names Geocillin®

Synonyms Carindacillin; Indanyl Sodium

Generic Available No

Use Treatment of urinary tract infections

Pregnancy Risk Factor B

Contraindications Hypersensitivity to carbenicillin or any component or penicillins

Warnings/Precautions Do not use in patients with severe renal impairment (Cl_{cr} <10 mL/minute); dosage modification required in patients with impaired renal and/or hepatic function; oral carbenicillin should be limited to treatment of urinary tract infections. Use with caution in patients with history of hypersensitivity to cephalosporins.

Adverse Reactions

>10%: Diarrhea

1% to 10%: Nausea, bad taste, vomiting, flatulence, glossitis

<1%: Headache, skin rash, urticaria, anemia, thrombocytopenia, leukopenia, neutropenia, eosinophilia, hyperthermia, itchy eyes, vaginitis, hypokalemia, hematuria, thrombophlebitis

Toxicology Symptoms of overdose include neuromuscular hypersensitivity, convulsions; many beta-lactam containing antibiotics have the potential to cause neuromuscular hyperirritability or convulsive seizures. Hemodialysis may be helpful to aid in the removal of the drug from the blood, otherwise most treatment is supportive or symptom directed.

Drug Interactions

Decreased effect with administration of aminoglycosides within 1 hour; may inactivate both drugs

Increased duration of half-life with probenecid

Mechanism of Action Inhibits bacterial cell wall synthesis by binding to one or more of the penicillin binding proteins (PBPs); which in turn inhibits the final transpeptidation step of peptidoglycan synthesis in bacterial cell walls, thus inhibiting cell wall biosynthesis. Bacteria eventually lyse due to ongoing activity of cell wall autolytic enzymes (autolysins and murein hydrolases) while cell wall assembly is arrested.

Pharmacokinetics

Absorption: Oral: 30% to 40%

Distribution: Crosses the placenta; small amounts appear in breast milk; distributes into bile, low concentrations attained in CSF

Half-life:

Children: 0.8-1.8 hours

Adults: 1-1.5 hours, prolonged to 10-20 hours with renal insufficiency

Time to peak serum concentration: Within 0.5-2 hours in patients with normal renal function; serum concentrations following oral absorption are inadequate for treatment of systemic infections

Elimination: ~80% to 99% excreted unchanged in urine

Usual Dosage Oral:

Children: 30-50 mg/kg/day divided every 6 hours; maximum dose: 2-3 g/day

Adults: 1-2 tablets every 6 hours for urinary tract infections or 2 tablets every 6 hours for prostatitis

Dosing interval in renal impairment:

Cl_{cr} 10-50 mL/minute: Administer every 12-24 hours

Cl_{cr} <10 mL/minute: Administer every 24-48 hours

Moderately dialyzable (20% to 50%)

(Continued)

Carbenicillin *(Continued)*

Monitoring Parameters Renal, hepatic, and hematologic function tests

Reference Range Therapeutic: Not established; Toxic: >250 μg mL (SI: >660 μmol L)

Test Interactions May interfere with urinary glucose tests using cupric sulfate (Benedict's solution, Clinitest®); may inactivate aminoglycosides *in vitro*; false-positive urine or serum proteins

Patient Information Tablets have a bitter taste; take with a full glass of water; take all medication for 7-14 days, do not skip doses; may interfere with oral contraceptives

Additional Information Sodium content of 382 mg tablet: 23 mg (1 mEq)

Dosage Forms Tablet, film coated: 382 mg

Selected Readings
Donowitz GR and Mandell GL, "Beta-Lactam Antibiotics," *N Engl J Med*, 1988, 318(7):419-26 and 318(8):490-500.
Wright AJ and Wilkowske CJ, "The Penicillins," *Mayo Clin Proc*, 1991, 66(10):1047-63.

Cardioquin® *see* Quinidine *on page 656*

Carindacillin *see* Carbenicillin *on previous page*

Ceclor® *see* Cefaclor *on this page*

Cefaclor *(sef' a klor)*

Related Information
Antimicrobial Activity Against Selected Organisms *on page 757-764*

Brand Names Ceclor®

Generic Available No

Use Infections caused by susceptible organisms involving the respiratory tract, otitis media, sinusitis, skin and skin structure, bone and joint, and urinary tract and gynecologic as well as septicemia

Drug of Choice or Alternative For
Organism(s)
Haemophilus influenzae on page 119

Pregnancy Risk Factor B

Contraindications Hypersensitivity to cefaclor or any component or other cephalosporins

Warnings/Precautions Use with caution in patients with a history of penicillin allergy especially IgE mediated reactions (eg, anaphylaxis, urticaria); use with caution in patients with a history of colitis; modify dosage in patients with severe renal impairment

Adverse Reactions
1% to 10%: Pseudomembranous colitis, diarrhea
<1%: Rash, urticaria, pruritus, nausea, eosinophilia, cholestatic jaundice, arthralgia, Stevens-Johnson syndrome, vomiting, slight elevation of AST, ALT, hemolytic anemia, neutropenia

Toxicology Many beta-lactam containing antibiotics have the potential to cause neuromuscular hyperirritability or convulsive seizures. Hemodialysis may be helpful to aid in the removal of the drug from the blood, otherwise most treatment is supportive or symptom directed.

Drug Interactions Increased levels with probenecid

Stability Refrigerate suspension after reconstitution; discard after 14 days

Mechanism of Action Inhibits bacterial cell wall synthesis by binding to one or more of the penicillin binding proteins (PBPs); which in turn inhibits the final transpeptidation step of peptidoglycan synthesis in bacterial cell walls, thus inhibiting cell wall biosynthesis. Bacteria eventually lyse due to ongoing activity of cell wall autolytic enzymes (autolysins and murein hydrolases) while cell wall assembly is arrested.

Pharmacokinetics
Absorption: Oral: Well absorbed; acid stable
Distribution: Widely distributed throughout the body and reaches therapeutic concentration in most tissues and body fluids, including synovial, pericardial, pleural, and peritoneal fluids; also bile, sputum, and urine; also bone, myocardium, gallbladder, skin and soft tissue; crosses the placenta and appears in breast milk
Half-life: 30-60 minutes (prolonged with renal impairment)
Elimination: 80% excreted unchanged in urine

age Oral:

>1 month: 20-40 mg/kg/day divided every 8-12 hours; maximum g/day (twice daily option is for treatment of otitis media or pharyngi-

-500 mg every 8 hours or daily dose can be given in 2 divided doses

justment in renal impairment: Cl$_{cr}$ <50 mL/minute: Administer se

dialyzable (20% to 50%)

Neuromuscular hypersensitivity, convulsions

ons Positive Coombs' [direct], may interfere with urinary glucose :upric sulfate (Benedict's solution, Clinitest®); false increase of e creatinine at high doses when Jaffé reaction is used

lation Chilling improves flavor (do not freeze); report diarrhea re course of medication (10-14 days) should be taken to ensure organism; may interfere with oral contraceptives, females should ns of vaginitis

ng, 500 mg
suspension (strawberry flavor): 125 mg/5 mL (75 mL, 150 mL); (50 mL, 100 mL); 250 mg/5 mL (75 mL, 150 mL); 375 mg/5 mL L)

gs
Mandell GL, "Beta-Lactam Antibiotics," *N Engl J Med*, 1988, 318(7):419-26 500.

Steckelberg JM, "Cephalosporin Antimicrobial Agents and Related *ayo Clin Proc*, 1991, 66(10):1064-73.
ohalosporins in Perspective," *DICP*, 1990, 24(1):45-51.

nohydrate (sef a drox' ill)

on
/ity Against Selected Organisms *on page 757-764*
:ef®; Ultracef®
No

usceptible bacterial infections, including those caused by olytic *Streptococcus*

tor B

Hypersensitivity to cefadroxil and cephalosporins

r and erythematous rash, dyspepsia, pseudomembranous miting, heartburn, gastritis, bloating, fatigue, chills, su-ropenia

uspension after reconstitution; discard after 14 days

n Inhibits bacterial cell wall synthesis by binding to one or binding proteins (PBPs); which in turn inhibits the final of peptidoglycan synthesis in bacterial cell walls, thus synthesis. Bacteria eventually lyse due to ongoing activi-: enzymes (autolysins and murein hydrolases) while cell ted.

dly and well absorbed from GI tract
:tributed throughout the body and reaches therapeutic st tissues and body fluids, including synovial, pericardi-neal fluids; also bile, sputum, and urine; also bone, the der, skin and soft tissue; crosses the placenta and ap-

olized
⁴ hours in renal failure
centration: Within 70-90 minutes
se excreted unchanged in urine within 8 hours

livided twice daily up to a maximum of 2 g/day
ided doses

nal impairment:
dminister every 24 hours
minister every 36 hours

ANTIMICROBIAL THERAPY

Cefadroxil Monohydrate *(Continued)*

Overdosage Neuromuscular hypersensitivity, convulsions

Test Interactions Positive Coombs' [direct], may interfere with urinary glu tests using cupric sulfate (Benedict's solution, Clinitest®)

Patient Information Report diarrhea promptly; entire course of medication 14 days) should be taken to ensure eradication of organism; may interfere oral contraceptives, females should report symptoms of vaginitis

Dosage Forms

Capsule: 500 mg

Suspension, oral: 125 mg/5 mL (50 mL, 100 mL); 250 mg/5 mL (50 ml mL); 500 mg/5 mL (50 mL, 100 mL)

Tablet: 1 g

Selected Readings

Donowitz GR and Mandell GL, "Beta-Lactam Antibiotics," *N Engl J Med*, 1988, 318(7) and 318(8):490-500.

Gustaferro CA and Steckelberg JM, "Cephalosporin Antimicrobial Agents and Compounds," *Mayo Clin Proc*, 1991, 66(10):1064-73.

Smith GH, "Oral Cephalosporins in Perspective," *DICP*, 1990, 24(1):45-51.

Cefadyl® *see Cephapirin Sodium on page 529*

Cefamandole Nafate *(sef a man' dole)*

Related Information

Antimicrobial Activity Against Selected Organisms *on page 757-764*

Brand Names Mandol®

Generic Available No

Use Treatment of susceptible bacterial infection; mainly respiratory tra and skin structure, bone and joint, urinary tract and gynecologic, sep surgical prophylaxis

Pregnancy Risk Factor B

Contraindications Hypersensitivity to cefamandole nafate or any co and cephalosporins

Adverse Reactions

1% to 10%: Diarrhea

<1%: CNS irritation, seizures, abdominal cramps, fever, rash, eosino poprothrombinemia, urticaria, leukopenia, pseudomembraneou thrombocytopenia, transient elevation of liver enzymes, cholestatic pain at injection site, superinfections

Toxicology Many beta-lactam containing antibiotics have the potentia neuromuscular hyperirritability or convulsive seizures. Hemodialysi helpful to aid in the removal of the drug from the blood, otherwise n ment is supportive or symptom directed.

Drug Interactions Increased levels with probenecid; may cause disu reaction with concomitant alcohol use

Stability After reconstitution, CO_2 gas is liberated which allows solu withdrawn without injecting air; solution is stable for 24 hours at room ture and 96 hours when refrigerated; for I.V. infusion in NS and D_5 for 24 hours at room temperature; 1 week when refrigerated or 26 w frozen

Mechanism of Action Inhibits bacterial cell wall synthesis by bindin more of the penicillin binding proteins (PBPs); which in turn inhibi transpeptidation step of peptidoglycan synthesis in bacterial cell inhibiting cell wall biosynthesis. Bacteria eventually lyse due to ong ty of cell wall autolytic enzymes (autolysins and murein hydrolases wall assembly is arrested.

Pharmacokinetics

Distribution: Well throughout the body, except CSF; poor penet with inflamed meninges

Half-life: 30-60 minutes

Time to peak serum concentration: I.M.: Within 1-2 hours

Elimination: Majority of drug excreted unchanged in urine

Usual Dosage I.M., I.V.:

Children: 100-150 mg/kg/day in divided doses every 4-6 hours

Adults: 4-12 g/24 hours divided every 4-6 hours 500-1000 mg eve

Dosing in renal impairment:

Cl_{cr} 25-50 mL/minute: 1-2 g every 8 hours

510

Cl_{cr} 10-25 mL/minute: 1 g every 8 hours
Cl_{cr} <10 mL/minute: 1 g every 12 hours
Moderately dialyzable (20% to 50%)

Overdosage Neuromuscular hypersensitivity, convulsions

Monitoring Parameters Prothrombin time

Test Interactions May interfere with urinary glucose tests using cupric sulfate (Benedict's solution, Clinitest®)

Nursing Implications Do not admix with aminoglycosides in same bottle/bag; observe for signs and symptoms of anaphylaxis during first dose

Additional Information Sodium content of 1 g: 76 mg (3.3 mEq); contains the n-methylthiotetrazole side chain

Dosage Forms Powder for injection: 500 mg, 1 g, 2 g, 10 g

Selected Readings

Donowitz GR and Mandell GL, "Beta-Lactam Antibiotics," N Engl J Med, 1988, 318(7):419-26 and 318(8):490-500.

Gentry LO, Zeluff BJ, and Cooley DA, "Antibiotic Prophylaxis in Open-Heart Surgery: A Comparison of Cefamandole, Cefuroxime, and Cefazolin," Ann Thorac Surg, 1988, 46(2):167-71.

Gustaferro CA and Steckelberg JM, "Cephalosporin Antimicrobial Agents and Related Compounds," Mayo Clin Proc, 1991, 66(10):1064-73.

Peterson CD, Lake KD, Arom KV, et al, "Antibiotic Prophylaxis in Open-Heart Surgery Patients: Comparison of Cefamandole and Cefuroxime," Drug Intell Clin Pharm, 1987, 21(9):728-32.

Cefazolin Sodium (sef a' zoe lin)

Related Information

Antimicrobial Activity Against Selected Organisms on page 757-764

Brand Names Ancef®; Kefzol®; Zolicef®

Generic Available Yes

Use Treatment of susceptible gram-positive bacilli and cocci (never enterococcus); some gram-negative bacilli including E. coli, Proteus, and Klebsiella may be susceptible; surgical prophylaxis

Drug of Choice or Alternative For
Disease/Syndrome(s)
Urinary Tract Infection, Perinephric Abscess on page 45

Pregnancy Risk Factor B

Contraindications Hypersensitivity to cefazolin sodium or any component and cephalosporins

Adverse Reactions
1% to 10%: Diarrhea
<1%: CNS irritation, seizures, abdominal cramps, fever, rash, eosinophilia, hypoprothrombinemia, urticaria, leukopenia, pseudomembraneous colitis, thrombocytopenia, transient elevation of liver enzymes, cholestatic jaundice, pain at injection site, superinfections

Toxicology Many beta-lactam containing antibiotics have the potential to cause neuromuscular hyperirritability or convulsive seizures. Hemodialysis may be helpful to aid in the removal of the drug from the blood, otherwise most treatment is supportive or symptom directed.

Drug Interactions Probenecid may decrease cephalosporin elimination

Stability Reconstituted solution is stable for 24 hours at room temperature and 96 hours when refrigerated; for I.V. infusion in NS or D_5W solution is stable for 24 hours at room temperature, 96 hours when refrigerated or 12 weeks when frozen; after freezing, thawed solution is stable for 48 hours at room temperature or 10 days when refrigerated

Mechanism of Action Inhibits bacterial cell wall synthesis by binding to one or more of the penicillin binding proteins (PBPs); which in turn inhibits the final transpeptidation step of peptidoglycan synthesis in bacterial cell walls, thus inhibiting cell wall biosynthesis. Bacteria eventually lyse due to ongoing activity of cell wall autolytic enzymes (autolysins and murein hydrolases) while cell wall assembly is arrested.

Pharmacokinetics
Distribution: Widely distributed into most body tissues and fluids including gallbladder, liver, kidneys, bone, sputum, bile, pleural and synovial fluids; CSF penetration is poor; crosses the placenta and small amounts appear in breast milk
Metabolism: Hepatic metabolism is minimal
Half-life: 90-150 minutes (prolonged with renal impairment)
Time to peak serum concentration: I.M.: Within 30 minutes to 2 hours
Elimination: 80% to 100% excreted unchanged in urine

(Continued)

Cefazolin Sodium *(Continued)*

Usual Dosage I.M., I.V.:

Neonates:

Postnatal age <7 days: 40 mg/kg/day divided every 12 hours

Postnatal age >7 days:

<2000 g: 40 mg/kg/day in 2 divided doses

>2000 g: 60 mg/kg/day in 3 divided doses

Infants and Children: 50-100 mg/kg/day in 3 divided doses; maximum dose: 6 g/day

Adults: 1-2 g every 8 hours

Dosing adjustment in renal impairment:

Cl_{cr} 10-30 mL/minute: Administer every 12 hours

Cl_{cr} <10 mL/minute: Administer every 24 hours

Moderately dialyzable (20% to 50%)

Overdosage Neuromuscular hypersensitivity, convulsions

Monitoring Parameters Renal function periodically when used in combination with other nephrotoxic drugs

Test Interactions May interfere with urinary glucose tests using cupric sulfate (Benedict's solution, Clinitest®)

Nursing Implications Do not admix with aminoglycosides in same bottle/bag; observe for signs and symptoms of anaphylaxis during first dose

Additional Information Sodium content of 1 g: 47 mg (2 mEq)

Dosage Forms

Infusion, premixed, in D_5W (frozen) (Ancef®): 500 mg (50 mL); 1 g (50 mL)

Injection (Kefzol®): 500 mg, 1 g

Powder for injection (Ancef®, Zolicef®): 250 mg, 500 mg, 1 g, 5 g, 10 g, 20 g

Selected Readings

Donowitz GR and Mandell GL, "Beta-Lactam Antibiotics," *N Engl J Med*, 1988, 318(7):419-26 and 318(8):490-500.

Gentry LO, Zeluff BJ, and Cooley DA, "Antibiotic Prophylaxis in Open-Heart Surgery: A Comparison of Cefamandole, Cefuroxime, and Cefazolin," *Ann Thorac Surg*, 1988, 46(2):167-71.

Gustaferro CA and Steckelberg JM, "Cephalosporin Antimicrobial Agents and Related Compounds," *Mayo Clin Proc*, 1991, 66(10):1064-73.

Peterson CD, Lake KD, Arom KV, et al, "Antibiotic Prophylaxis in Open-Heart Surgery Patients: Comparison of Cefamandole and Cefuroxime," *Drug Intell Clin Pharm*, 1987, 21(9):728-32.

Cefixime (sef ix' eem)

Related Information

Antimicrobial Activity Against Selected Organisms *on page 757-764*

Brand Names Suprax®

Generic Available No

Use Treatment of urinary tract infections, otitis media, respiratory infections due to susceptible organisms; outpatient therapy of soft tissue or skeletal infections due to susceptible organisms

Drug of Choice or Alternative For

Organism(s)

Neisseria gonorrhoeae on page 161

Pregnancy Risk Factor B

Contraindications Hypersensitivity to cefixime or cephalosporins

Warnings/Precautions Prolonged use may result in superinfection

Adverse Reactions

1% to 10%: Diarrhea, abdominal pain, nausea, dyspepsia, flatulence

<1%: Rash, urticaria, pruritus, headache, dizziness, thrombocytopenia, leukopenia, eosinophilia, vaginitis

Toxicology Many beta-lactam containing antibiotics have the potential to cause neuromuscular hyperirritability or convulsive seizures. Hemodialysis may be helpful to aid in the removal of the drug from the blood, otherwise most treatment is supportive or symptom directed.

Drug Interactions Probenecid may increase cefixime levels

Stability Reconstituted oral solution may be kept at room temperature without potency loss for 14 days; **do not refrigerate**

Mechanism of Action Inhibits bacterial cell wall synthesis by binding to one or more of the penicillin binding proteins (PBPs); which in turn inhibits the final transpeptidation step of peptidoglycan synthesis in bacterial cell walls, thus inhibiting cell wall biosynthesis. Bacteria eventually lyse due to ongoing activity of cell wall autolytic enzymes (autolysins and murein hydrolases) while cell wall assembly is arrested.

Pharmacokinetics
Absorption: Oral: 40% to 50%
Distribution: Widely distributed throughout the body and reaches therapeutic concentration in most tissues and body fluids, including synovial, pericardial, pleural, and peritoneal fluids; also bile, sputum, and urine; also bone, myocardium, gallbladder, and skin and soft tissue
Half-life: 3-4 hours with normal renal function and up to 11.5 hours with renal failure
Time to peak serum concentration: Within 2-6 hours
Elimination: 50% of absorbed dose excreted as active drug in urine and 10% in bile

Usual Dosage Oral:
Children: 8 mg/kg/day in 1-2 divided doses; maximum dose: 400 mg/day
Children >50 kg or >12 years and Adults: 400 mg/day in 1-2 divided doses

Dosing adjustment in renal impairment:
Cl_{cr} 21-60 mL/minute: Administer 75% of the standard dose
Cl_{cr} ≤20 mL/minute: Administer 50% of the standard dose
Moderately dialyzable (10%)

Overdosage Neuromuscular hypersensitivity, convulsions
Monitoring Parameters Renal and hepatic function periodically, with prolonged therapy
Test Interactions False-positive reaction for urine glucose using Clinitest® or Benedict's solution; false-positive Coombs' test; false-positive urine ketones
Patient Information Report diarrhea promptly; entire course of medication (10-14 days) should be taken to ensure eradication of organism; may interfere with oral contraceptives, females should report symptoms of vaginitis

Dosage Forms
Powder for oral suspension (strawberry flavor): 100 mg/5 mL (50 mL, 100 mL)
Tablet, film coated: 200 mg, 400 mg

Selected Readings
Donowitz GR and Mandell GL, "Beta-Lactam Antibiotics," *N Engl J Med*, 1988, 318(7):419-26 and 318(8):490-500.
Gustaferro CA and Steckelberg JM, "Cephalosporin Antimicrobial Agents and Related Compounds," *Mayo Clin Proc*, 1991, 66(10):1064-73.
Smith GH, "Oral Cephalosporins in Perspective," *DICP*, 1990, 24(1):45-51.

Cefizox® see Ceftizoxime Sodium *on page 522*

Cefmetazole Sodium (sef met' a zole)

Related Information
Antimicrobial Activity Against Selected Organisms *on page 757-764*
Brand Names Zefazone®
Generic Available No
Use Second generation cephalosporin, useful for susceptible aerobic and anaerobic gram-positive and gram-negative bacteria, surgical prophylaxis
Pregnancy Risk Factor B
Contraindications Hypersensitivity to cefmetazole or any component and cephalosporins

Adverse Reactions
1% to 10%: Diarrhea, nausea, rash
<1%: Epigastric pain, candidiasis, bleeding, pseudomembraneous colitis, pain at injection site, phlebitis, shock, hypotension, headache, hot flashes, dyspnea, epistaxis, respiratory distress, fever, vaginitis, alteration of color

Toxicology Many beta-lactam containing antibiotics have the potential to cause neuromuscular hyperirritability or convulsive seizures. Hemodialysis may be helpful to aid in the removal of the drug from the blood, otherwise most treatment is supportive or symptom directed.
Stability Reconstituted solution and I.V. infusion in NS or D_5W solution is stable for 24 hours at room temperature, 7 days when refrigerated or 6 weeks when frozen; after freezing, thawed solution is stable for 24 hours at room temperature or 7 days when refrigerated
Mechanism of Action Inhibits bacterial cell wall synthesis by binding to one or more of the penicillin binding proteins (PBPs); which in turn inhibits the final transpeptidation step of peptidoglycan synthesis in bacterial cell walls, thus inhibiting cell wall biosynthesis. Bacteria eventually lyse due to ongoing activity of cell wall autolytic enzymes (autolysins and murein hydrolases) while cell wall assembly is arrested.

(Continued)
513

Cefmetazole Sodium *(Continued)*

Usual Dosage Adults: I.V.:
Infections: 2 g every 6-12 hours for 5-14 days
Prophylaxis: 2 g 30-90 minutes before surgery

Dosing interval in renal impairment:
Cl_{cr} >50 mL/minute: Administer 1-2 g every 12 hours
Cl_{cr} 30-49 mL/minute: Administer 1-2 g every 16 hours
Cl_{cr} 10-29 mL/minute: Administer 1-2 g every 24 hours
Cl_{cr} <10 mL/minute: Administer 1-2 g every 48 hours

Overdosage Neuromuscular hypersensitivity, convulsions

Monitoring Parameters Prothrombin times

Patient Information Do not drink alcohol for at least 24 hours after receiving dose; report diarrhea promptly; may interfere with oral contraceptives, females should report symptoms of vaginitis

Nursing Implications Do not admix with aminoglycosides in same bottle/bag; observe for signs and symptoms of anaphylaxis during first dose

Additional Information Sodium content of 1 g: 47 mg (2 mEq); contains the n-methylthiotetrazole side chain

Dosage Forms Powder for injection: 1 g, 2 g

Selected Readings
Donowitz GR and Mandell GL, "Beta-Lactam Antibiotics," *N Engl J Med*, 1988, 318(7):419-26 and 318(8):490-500.
Gustaferro CA and Steckelberg JM, "Cephalosporin Antimicrobial Agents and Related Compounds," *Mayo Clin Proc*, 1991, 66(10):1064-73.
Jones RN, "Review of the *In vitro* Spectrum and Characteristics of Cefmetazole (CS-1170)," *J Antimicrob Chemother*, 1989, 23(Suppl D):1-12.
Plouffe JF, "Cefmetazole Versus Cefoxitin in Prevention of Infections After Abdominal Surgery," *J Antimicrob Chemother*, 1989, 23(Suppl D):85-8.

Cefobid® *see* Cefoperazone Sodium *on next page*

Cefonicid Sodium (se fon' i sid)

Related Information
Antimicrobial Activity Against Selected Organisms *on page 757-764*

Brand Names Monocid®

Generic Available No

Use Treatment of susceptible bacterial infection; mainly respiratory tract, skin and skin structure, bone and joint, urinary tract and gynecologic as well as septicemia; second generation cephalosporin

Pregnancy Risk Factor B

Contraindications Hypersensitivity to cefonicid sodium or any component and cephalosporins

Adverse Reactions
1% to 10%: Pain at injection site, increased platelets and eosinophils, liver function alterations
<1%: Fever, headache, skin rash, nausea, diarrhea, abdominal pain, pseudomembranous colitis, transient elevations in liver enzymes, BUN, or creatinine

Toxicology Many beta-lactam containing antibiotics have the potential to cause neuromuscular hyperirritability or convulsive seizures. Hemodialysis may be helpful to aid in the removal of the drug from the blood, otherwise most treatment is supportive or symptom directed.

Stability Reconstituted solution and I.V. infusion in NS or D_5W solution is stable for 24 hours at room temperature or 72 hours if refrigerated

Mechanism of Action Inhibits bacterial cell wall synthesis by binding to one or more of the penicillin binding proteins (PBPs); which in turn inhibits the final transpeptidation step of peptidoglycan synthesis in bacterial cell walls, thus inhibiting cell wall biosynthesis. Bacteria eventually lyse due to ongoing activity of cell wall autolytic enzymes (autolysins and murein hydrolases) while cell wall assembly is arrested.

Usual Dosage Adults: I.V., I.M.: 1 g every 24 hours

Dosing interval in renal impairment:
Cl_{cr} 10-20 mL/minute: 500 mg to 1 g every 48 hours
Cl_{cr} <10 mL/minute: 250 mg to 1 g every 72 hours

Overdosage Neuromuscular hypersensitivity, convulsions

Test Interactions May interfere with urinary glucose tests using cupric sulfate (Benedict's solution, Clinitest®)

Nursing Implications Do not admix with aminoglycosides in same bottle/bag; observe for signs and symptoms of anaphylaxis during first dose

Additional Information Sodium content of 1 g: 85.1 mg (3.7 mEq)

Dosage Forms Powder for injection: 500 mg, 1 g, 10 g

Selected Readings

Donowitz GR and Mandell GL, "Beta-Lactam Antibiotics," *N Engl J Med*, 1988, 318(7):419-26 and 318(8):490-500.

Gustaferro CA and Steckelberg JM, "Cephalosporin Antimicrobial Agents and Related Compounds," *Mayo Clin Proc*, 1991, 66(10):1064-73.

Cefoperazone Sodium (sef oh per' a zone)

Related Information

Antimicrobial Activity Against Selected Organisms *on page 757-764*

Brand Names Cefobid®

Generic Available No

Use Treatment of susceptible bacterial infection; mainly respiratory tract, skin and skin structure, bone and joint, urinary tract and gynecologic as well as septicemia

Pregnancy Risk Factor B

Contraindications Hypersensitivity to cefoperazone or any component and cephalosporins

Adverse Reactions

1% to 10%: Diarrhea

<1%: Maculopapular and erythematous rash, dyspepsia, pseudomembranous colitis, nausea, vomiting, bleeding, pain and induration at injection site

Toxicology Many beta-lactam containing antibiotics have the potential to cause neuromuscular hyperirritability or convulsive seizures. Hemodialysis may be helpful to aid in the removal of the drug from the blood, otherwise most treatment is supportive or symptom directed.

Drug Interactions May cause disulfiram-like reaction with concomitant alcohol use

Stability Reconstituted solution and I.V. infusion in NS or D_5W solution is stable for 24 hours at room temperature, 5 days when refrigerated or 3 weeks when frozen; after freezing, thawed solution is stable for 48 hours at room temperature or 10 days when refrigerated

Mechanism of Action Inhibits bacterial cell wall synthesis by binding to one or more of the penicillin binding proteins (PBPs); which in turn inhibits the final transpeptidation step of peptidoglycan synthesis in bacterial cell walls, thus inhibiting cell wall biosynthesis. Bacteria eventually lyse due to ongoing activity of cell wall autolytic enzymes (autolysins and murein hydrolases) while cell wall assembly is arrested.

Pharmacokinetics

Distribution: Widely distributed in most body tissues and fluids; highest concentrations in bile; low penetration in CSF; variable when meninges are inflamed; crosses placenta; small amounts into breast milk

Half-life: 2 hours

Time to peak serum concentration: I.M.: Within 1-2 hours

Elimination: Principally in bile (70% to 75%); 20% to 30% recovered unchanged in urine within 6-12 hours

Usual Dosage I.M., I.V.:

Neonates: 50 mg/kg/dose every 12 hours

Children: 100-150 mg/kg/day divided every 8-12 hours; up to 12 g/day

Adults: 2-4 g/day in divided doses every 12 hours; up to 12 g/day

Dosing adjustment in hepatic impairment: Reduce dose 50% in patients with advanced cirrhosis; maximum daily dose: 4 g

Overdosage Neuromuscular hypersensitivity, convulsions

Monitoring Parameters Prothrombin time

Test Interactions May interfere with urinary glucose tests using cupric sulfate (Benedict's solution, Clinitest®)

Nursing Implications Monitor for coagulation abnormalities and diarrhea; do not admix with aminoglycosides in same bottle/bag; observe for signs and symptoms of anaphylaxis during first dose

Additional Information Sodium content of 1 g: 34.5 mg (1.5 mEq); contains the n-methylthiotetrazole side chain

Dosage Forms

Injection, premixed, frozen: 1 g (50 mL); 2 g (50 mL)

(Continued)

Cefoperazone Sodium *(Continued)*

Powder for injection: 1 g, 2 g

Selected Readings

Donowitz GR and Mandell GL, "Beta-Lactam Antibiotics," *N Engl J Med*, 1988, 318(7):419-26 and 318(8):490-500.

Gustaferro CA and Steckelberg JM, "Cephalosporin Antimicrobial Agents and Related Compounds," *Mayo Clin Proc*, 1991, 66(10):1064-73.

Cefotan® *see* Cefotetan Disodium *on next page*

Cefotaxime Sodium (sef oh taks' eem)

Related Information

Antimicrobial Activity Against Selected Organisms *on page 757-764*

Brand Names Claforan®

Generic Available No

Use Treatment of susceptible infection in respiratory tract, skin and skin structure, bone and joint, urinary tract, gynecologic as well as septicemia, and documented or suspected meningitis

Pregnancy Risk Factor B

Contraindications Hypersensitivity to cefotaxime or any component and cephalosporins

Adverse Reactions

1% to 10%: Pain at injection site, rash, pruritus, fever, eosinophilia, colitis, diarrhea, nausea, vomiting

<1%: Headache, pseudomembranous colitis, transient neutropenia, thrombocytopenia, transient elevation of BUN, creatinine and liver enzymes, phlebitis

Toxicology Many beta-lactam containing antibiotics have the potential to cause neuromuscular hyperirritability or convulsive seizures. Hemodialysis may be helpful to aid in the removal of the drug from the blood, otherwise most treatment is supportive or symptom directed.

Drug Interactions Probenecid may increase cefotaxime levels

Stability Reconstituted solution is stable for 24 hours at room temperature and 10 days when refrigerated; for I.V. infusion in NS or D_5W solution is stable for 24 hours at room temperature, 5 days when refrigerated or 13 weeks when frozen; after freezing, thawed solution is stable for 24 hours at room temperature or 10 days when refrigerated

Mechanism of Action Inhibits bacterial cell wall synthesis by binding to one or more of the penicillin binding proteins (PBPs); which in turn inhibits the final transpeptidation step of peptidoglycan synthesis in bacterial cell walls, thus inhibiting cell wall biosynthesis. Bacteria eventually lyse due to ongoing activity of cell wall autolytic enzymes (autolysins and murein hydrolases) while cell wall assembly is arrested.

Pharmacokinetics

Distribution: Widely distributed to body tissues and fluids including aqueous humor, ascitic and prostatic fluids, and bone; penetrates CSF when meninges are inflamed; crosses the placenta and appears in breast milk

Metabolism: Partially in the liver to active metabolite, desacetylcefotaxime

Bioavailability:

Half-life:

Cefotaxime: 1-1.5 hours (prolonged with renal and/or hepatic impairment)

Desacetylcefotaxime: 1.5-1.9 hours (prolonged with renal impairment)

Cefotaxime:

Premature Neonates <1 week: 5-6 hours

Full-term Neonates <1 week: 2-3.4 hours

Time to peak serum concentration: I.M.: Within 30 minutes

Elimination: Renal excretion of parent drug and metabolites

Usual Dosage I.M., I.V.:

Neonates:

Postnatal age <7 days: 100 mg/kg/day in 2 divided doses

Postnatal age >7 days:

<1200 g: 100 mg/kg/day divided every 12 hours

>1200 g: 150 mg/kg/day in 3 divided doses

Infants and Children 1 month to 12 years:

<50 kg: 100-200 mg/kg/day in 3-4 divided doses

Meningitis: 200 mg/kg/day in 4 divided doses

>50 kg: Moderate to severe infection: 1-2 g every 6-8 hours; life-threatening infection: 2 g/dose every 4 hours; maximum dose: 12 g/day

Children >12 years and Adults: 1-2 g every 6-8 hours (up to 12 g/day)

Dosing adjustment in renal impairment:
Cl_{cr} 10-50 mL/minute: Administer every 8-12 hours
Cl_{cr} <10 mL/minute: Administer every 24 hours
Moderately dialyzable (20% to 50%)

Dosing adjustment in hepatic impairment: Moderate dosage reduction is recommended in severe liver disease

Overdosage Neuromuscular hypersensitivity, convulsions

Test Interactions False-positive Coombs' test, false-positive reaction for urine glucose tests using Clinitest® or Benedict's solution, false elevation of creatinine using Jaffé test

Nursing Implications Cefotaxime can be administered IVP over 3-5 minutes or I.V. retrograde or I.V. intermittent infusion over 15-30 minutes; do not admix with aminoglycosides in same bottle/bag; observe for signs and symptoms of anaphylaxis during first dose

Additional Information Sodium content of 1 g: 50.6 mg (2.2 mEq)

Dosage Forms
Infusion, premixed (frozen) in D_5W : 1 g (50 mL); 2 g (50 mL)
Powder for injection: 1 g, 2 g, 10 g

Selected Readings
Donowitz GR and Mandell GL, "Beta-Lactam Antibiotics," *N Engl J Med*, 1988, 318(7):419-26 and 318(8):490-500.
Gustaferro CA and Steckelberg JM, "Cephalosporin Antimicrobial Agents and Related Compounds," *Mayo Clin Proc*, 1991, 66(10):1064-73.

Cefotetan Disodium (sef' oh tee tan)

Related Information
Antimicrobial Activity Against Selected Organisms *on page 757-764*

Brand Names Cefotan®

Generic Available No

Use Treatment of susceptible bacterial infection; mainly respiratory tract, skin and skin structure, bone and joint, urinary tract and gynecologic as well as septicemia

Drug of Choice or Alternative For
Disease/Syndrome(s)
Osteomyelitis, Diabetic Foot *on page 32*
Peritonitis *on page 36*
Organism(s)
Bacteroides Species *on page 61*

Pregnancy Risk Factor B

Contraindications Hypersensitivity to cefotetan or any component and cephalosporins

Adverse Reactions
1% to 10%: Diarrhea, hypersensitivity reactions, hepatic enzyme elevation
<1%: Fever, rash, pruritus, nausea, vomiting, antibiotic-associated colitis, prolongation of bleeding time or prothrombin time, neutropenia, thrombocytopenia, phlebitis

Toxicology Many beta-lactam containing antibiotics have the potential to cause neuromuscular hyperirritability or convulsive seizures. Hemodialysis may be helpful to aid in the removal of the drug from the blood, otherwise most treatment is supportive or symptom directed.

Drug Interactions May cause disulfiram-like reaction with concomitant alcohol use

Stability Reconstituted solution is stable for 24 hours at room temperature and 96 hours when refrigerated; for I.V. infusion in NS or D_5W solution and after freezing, thawed solution is stable for 24 hours at room temperature or 96 hours when refrigerated; frozen solution is stable for 12 weeks

Mechanism of Action Inhibits bacterial cell wall synthesis by binding to one or more of the penicillin binding proteins (PBPs); which in turn inhibits the final transpeptidation step of peptidoglycan synthesis in bacterial cell walls, thus inhibiting cell wall biosynthesis. Bacteria eventually lyse due to ongoing activity of cell wall autolytic enzymes (autolysins and murein hydrolases) while cell wall assembly is arrested.

Pharmacokinetics
Distribution: Widely distributed to body tissues and fluids including bile, sputum, prostatic and peritoneal fluids; low concentrations enter CSF; crosses the placenta and appears in breast milk

(Continued)

Cefotetan Disodium *(Continued)*

Half-life: 3-5 hours

Time to peak serum concentration: I.M.: Within 1.5-3 hours

Elimination: Primarily excreted unchanged in urine with 20% excreted in bile

Usual Dosage I.M., I.V.:

Children: 40-80 mg/kg/day divided every 12 hours

Adults: 1-6 g/day in divided doses every 12 hours, 1-2 g may be given every 24 hours for urinary tract infection

Dosing adjustment in renal impairment:

Cl_{cr} 10-30 mL/minute: Administer every 24 hours

Cl_{cr} <10 mL/minute: Administer every 48 hours

Slightly dialyzable (5% to 20%)

Overdosage Neuromuscular hypersensitivity, convulsions

Test Interactions May interfere with urinary glucose tests using cupric sulfate (Benedict's solution, Clinitest®)

Nursing Implications Do not admix with aminoglycosides in same bottle/bag; observe for signs and symptoms of anaphylaxis during first dose

Additional Information Sodium content of 1 g: 34.5 mg (1.5 mEq); contains the n-methylthiotetrazole side chain

Dosage Forms Powder for injection: 1 g (10 mL, 100 mL); 2 g (20 mL, 100 mL); 10 g (100 mL)

Selected Readings

"Antimicrobial Prophylaxis in Surgery," *Med Lett Drugs Ther*, 1993, 35(906):91-4.

Donowitz GR and Mandell GL, "Beta-Lactam Antibiotics," *N Engl J Med*, 1988, 318(7):419-26 and 318(8):490-500.

Gustaferro CA and Steckelberg JM, "Cephalosporin Antimicrobial Agents and Related Compounds," *Mayo Clin Proc*, 1991, 66(10):1064-73.

Cefoxitin Sodium (se fox' i tin)

Related Information

Antimicrobial Activity Against Selected Organisms *on page 757-764*

Brand Names Mefoxin®

Generic Available No

Use Treatment of susceptible bacterial infection; mainly respiratory tract, skin and skin structure, bone and joint, urinary tract and gynecologic as well as septicemia; surgical prophylaxis; intra-abdominal infections and other mixed infections

Drug of Choice or Alternative For

Disease/Syndrome(s)

Osteomyelitis, Diabetic Foot *on page 32*

Peritonitis *on page 36*

Organism(s)

Bacteroides Species *on page 61*

Pregnancy Risk Factor B

Contraindications Hypersensitivity to cefoxitin or any component and cephalosporins

Adverse Reactions

1% to 10%: Diarrhea

<1%: Fever, rash, exfoliative dermatitis, nausea, hypotension, vomiting, dyspnea, pseudomembranous colitis, thrombophlebitis, elevations in serum creatinine and/or BUN, transient leukopenia, thrombocytopenia, anemia, eosinophilia and elevation in serum AST concentration

Toxicology Many beta-lactam containing antibiotics have the potential to cause neuromuscular hyperirritability or convulsive seizures. Hemodialysis may be helpful to aid in the removal of the drug from the blood, otherwise most treatment is supportive or symptom directed.

Drug Interactions Increased levels with probenecid

Stability Reconstituted solution is stable for 24 hours at room temperature and 48 hours when refrigerated; for I.V. infusion in NS or D_5W solution is stable for 24 hours at room temperature, 1 week when refrigerated or 26 weeks when frozen; after freezing, thawed solution is stable for 24 hours at room temperature or 5 days when refrigerated

Mechanism of Action Inhibits bacterial cell wall synthesis by binding to one or more of the penicillin binding proteins (PBPs); which in turn inhibits the final transpeptidation step of peptidoglycan synthesis in bacterial cell walls, thus inhibiting cell wall biosynthesis. Bacteria eventually lyse due to ongoing activity of cell wall autolytic enzymes (autolysins and murein hydrolases) while cell wall assembly is arrested.

Pharmacokinetics

Distribution: Widely distributed to body tissues and fluids including pleural, synovial, ascitic fluid, and bile; poorly penetrates into CSF even with inflammation of the meninges; crosses the placenta and small amounts appear in breast milk

Half-life: 45-60 minutes, increases significantly with renal insufficiency

Time to peak serum concentration: I.M.: Within 20-30 minutes

Elimination: Rapidly excreted as unchanged drug (85%) in urine

Usual Dosage I.M., I.V.:

Infants >3 months and Children:

Mild-moderate infection: 80-100 mg/kg/day in divided doses every 4-6 hours

Severe infection: 100-160 mg/kg/day in divided doses every 4-6 hours

Maximum dose: 12 g/day

Adults: 1-2 g every 6-8 hours (I.M. injection is painful)

Dosing adjustment in renal impairment:

Cl_{cr} 30-50 mL/minute: Administer every 8-12 hours

Cl_{cr} 10-30 mL/minute: Administer every 12-24 hours

Cl_{cr} <10 mL/minute: Administer every 24-48 hours

Moderately dialyzable (20% to 50%)

Overdosage Neuromuscular hypersensitivity, convulsions

Monitoring Parameters Monitor renal function periodically when used in combination with other nephrotoxic drugs

Test Interactions Positive Coombs' [direct]; false-positive urine glucose (Clinitest®), false increase in serum or urine creatinine with the Jaffé method

Nursing Implications Do not admix with aminoglycosides in same bottle/bag; observe for signs and symptoms of anaphylaxis during first dose

Additional Information Sodium content of 1 g: 53 mg (2.3 mEq)

Dosage Forms

Infusion, premixed (frozen) in D_5W: 1 g (50 mL): 2 g (50 mL)

Powder for injection: 1 g, 2 g, 10 g

Selected Readings

"Antimicrobial Prophylaxis in Surgery," *Med Lett Drugs Ther*, 1993, 35(906):91-4.

Donowitz GR and Mandell GL, "Beta-Lactam Antibiotics," *N Engl J Med*, 1988, 318(7):419-26 and 318(8):490-500.

Gustaferro CA and Steckelberg JM, "Cephalosporin Antimicrobial Agents and Related Compounds," *Mayo Clin Proc*, 1991, 66(10):1064-73.

Cefpodoxime Proxetil (sef pode ox' eem)

Related Information

Antimicrobial Activity Against Selected Organisms *on page 757-764*

Brand Names Vantin®

Generic Available No

Use Infections caused by susceptible organisms involving the respiratory tract, otitis media, sinusitis, skin and skin structure, and urinary tract and gynecologic

Pregnancy Risk Factor B

Contraindications Hypersensitivity to cefpodoxime or any components and cephalosporins

Adverse Reactions

1% to 10%: Diarrhea

<1%: Headache, diaper rash, nausea, vomiting, abdominal pain, pseudomembranous colitis, vaginal fungal infections

Stability After mixing, keep suspension in refrigerator, shake well before using; discard unused portion after 14 days

Mechanism of Action Inhibits bacterial cell wall synthesis by binding to one or more of the penicillin binding proteins (PBPs); which in turn inhibits the final transpeptidation step of peptidoglycan synthesis in bacterial cell walls, thus inhibiting cell wall biosynthesis. Bacteria eventually lyse due to ongoing activity of cell wall autolytic enzymes (autolysins and murein hydrolases) while cell wall assembly is arrested.

Pharmacokinetics

Absorption: Oral: Rapid

Half-life, elimination: 2-3 hours

Time to peak serum concentration: Oral: Within 1 hour

(Continued)

ANTIMICROBIAL THERAPY

Cefpodoxime Proxetil *(Continued)*

Usual Dosage Oral:
  Children >6 months to 12 years: 10 mg/kg/day, divided every 12 hours, for 10 days
  Adults: 100-400 mg every 12 hours, for 7-14 days
Patient Information Report diarrhea promptly; entire course of medication should be taken to ensure eradication of organism; may interfere with oral contraceptives, females should report symptoms of vaginitis
Dosage Forms
  Granules for oral suspension: 50 mg/5 mL (100 mL); 100 mg/5 mL (100 mL)
  Tablet: 100 mg, 200 mg
Selected Readings
  Adam D, Bergogne-Berezin E, and Jones RN, "Symposium on Cefpodoxime Proxetil: A New Third Generation Oral Cephalosporin," *Drugs*, 1991, 42(Suppl 3):1-66.

Cefprozil *(sef proe' zil)*

Brand Names Cefzil®
Generic Available No
Use Infections caused by susceptible organisms involving the respiratory tract, otitis media, sinusitis, skin and skin structure, and urinary tract
Pregnancy Risk Factor B
Contraindications Hypersensitivity to cefprozil or any component and cephalosporins
Adverse Reactions
  1% to 10%: Diarrhea, nausea, vomiting, abdominal pain, elevation of AST and ALT, dizziness, eosinophilia, diaper rash and superinfection, genital pruritus and vaginitis
  <1%: Rash, urticaria, headache, insomnia, confusion, elevated BUN and serum creatinine, arthralgia
Toxicology Many beta-lactam containing antibiotics have the potential to cause neuromuscular hyperirritability or convulsive seizures. Hemodialysis may be helpful to aid in the removal of the drug from the blood, otherwise most treatment is supportive or symptom directed.
Mechanism of Action Inhibits bacterial cell wall synthesis by binding to one or more of the penicillin binding proteins (PBPs); which in turn inhibits the final transpeptidation step of peptidoglycan synthesis in bacterial cell walls, thus inhibiting cell wall biosynthesis. Bacteria eventually lyse due to ongoing activity of cell wall autolytic enzymes (autolysins and murein hydrolases) while cell wall assembly is arrested.
Pharmacokinetics
  Half-life, elimination: 1-2 hours
  Time to peak serum concentration: Oral: 1-2 hours
  Elimination: Eliminated unchanged in urine
Usual Dosage Oral:
  Infants and children >6 months to 12 years: 15 mg/kg every 12 hours for 10 days
  Children >13 years and Adults: 250-500 mg every 12-24 hours for 10 days Oral:
  Dosing adjustment in renal impairment: Cl$_{cr}$ <30 mL/minute: Reduce dose by 50%
  55% reduced by hemodialysis
Overdosage Neuromuscular hypersensitivity, convulsions
Dosage Forms
  Powder for oral suspension, as anhydrous: 125 mg/5 mL (50 mL, 75 mL, 100 mL); 250 mg/5 mL (50 mL, 75 mL, 100 mL)
  Tablet, as anhydrous: 250 mg, 500 mg

Ceftazidime *(sef' tay zi deem)*

Related Information
  Antimicrobial Activity Against Selected Organisms *on page 757-764*
Brand Names Ceptaz™; Fortaz®; Pentacef™; Tazicef®; Tazidime®
Generic Available No
Use Treatment of documented susceptible *Pseudomonas aeruginosa* infection and infections due to other susceptible aerobic gram-negative organisms; empiric therapy of a febrile, granulocytopenic patient
Drug of Choice or Alternative For Disease/Syndrome(s)
  Fever, Neutropenic *on page 25*

Meningitis, Postsurgical *on page 31*
Otitis Externa, Severe (Malignant) *on page 34*
Pneumonia, Hospital-Acquired *on page 38*
Sepsis *on page 40*
Sinusitis, Hospital-Acquired *on page 41*

Organism(s)
Pseudomonas aeruginosa on page 177

Pregnancy Risk Factor B

Contraindications Hypersensitivity to ceftazidime or any component and cephalosporins

Adverse Reactions
1% to 10%: Diarrhea, pain at injection site
<1%: Fever, headache, dizziness, paresthesia, rash, angioedema, nausea, vomiting, pseudomembranous colitis, eosinophilia, thrombocytosis, transient leukopenia, hemolytic anemia, transient elevation in liver enzymes, BUN and creatinine, phlebitis, candidiasis

Toxicology Many beta-lactam containing antibiotics have the potential to cause neuromuscular hyperirritability or convulsive seizures. Hemodialysis may be helpful to aid in the removal of the drug from the blood, otherwise most treatment is supportive or symptom directed.

Drug Interactions Increased levels with probenecid; aminoglycosides: *in vitro* studies indicate additive or synergistic effect against some strains of Enterobacteriaceae and *Pseudomonas aeruginosa*

Stability Reconstituted solution and I.V. infusion in NS or D_5W solution is stable for 24 hours at room temperature, 10 days when refrigerated or 12 weeks when frozen; after freezing, thawed solution is stable for 24 hours at room temperature or 4 days when refrigerated; 96 hours under refrigeration, after mixing

Mechanism of Action Inhibits bacterial cell wall synthesis by binding to one or more of the penicillin binding proteins (PBPs); which in turn inhibits the final transpeptidation step of peptidoglycan synthesis in bacterial cell walls, thus inhibiting cell wall biosynthesis. Bacteria eventually lyse due to ongoing activity of cell wall autolytic enzymes (autolysins and murein hydrolases) while cell wall assembly is arrested.

Pharmacokinetics
Distribution: Widely distributed throughout the body including bone, bile, skin, CSF (diffuses into CSF with higher concentrations when the meninges are inflamed) endometrium, heart, pleural and lymphatic fluids; crosses placenta and distributed into amniotic fluid and milk
Half-life: 1-2 hours (prolonged with renal impairment)
Neonates <23 days: 2.2-4.7 hours
Time to peak serum concentration: I.M.: Within 60 minutes
Elimination: Eliminated by glomerular filtration with 80% to 90% of dose excreted unchanged within 24 hours

Usual Dosage
Neonates:
Postnatal age <7 days: 30-50 mg/kg/dose every 12 hours
Postnatal age >7 days: 30-50 mg/kg/dose every 8 hours

Infants and Children 1 month to 12 years: 30-50 mg/kg/dose every 8 hours; maximum dose: 6 g/day

Adults: 1-2 g every 8-12 hours (250-500 mg every 12 hours for urinary tract infections)

Dosing adjustment in renal impairment:
Cl_{cr} 30-50 mL/minute: Administer every 12 hours
Cl_{cr} 10-30 mL/minute: Administer every 24 hours
Cl_{cr} <10 mL/minute: Administer every 48 hours
Dialyzable (50% to 100%)

Overdosage Neuromuscular hypersensitivity, convulsions

Monitoring Parameters Serum creatinine with concurrent use of an aminoglycoside; a change in renal function necessitates a change in dose

Test Interactions Positive Coombs' [direct], false-positive urine glucose (Benedict's solution, Clinitest®)

Nursing Implications Any carbon dioxide bubbles that may be present in the withdrawn solution should be expelled prior to injection. Ceftazidime can be administered IVP over 3-5 minutes, or I.V. retrograde or I.V. intermittent infusion over 15-30 minutes; final concentration for I.V. administration should not
(Continued)

Ceftazidime *(Continued)*

exceed 20 mg/mL for infusions, 180 mg/mL for IVP. Do not admix with aminoglycosides in same bottle/bag; observe for signs and symptoms of anaphylaxis during first dose.

Additional Information Sodium content of 1 g: 54 mg (2.3 mEq)

Dosage Forms

Infusion, premixed (frozen):

In D_5W: 500 mg (50 mL)

In $D_{1.4}W$: 1 g (50 mL)

In $D_{3.2}W$: 2 g (50 mL)

In NS: 1 g (50 mL); 2 g (100 mL)

Powder for injection: 500 mg, 1 g, 2 g, 6 g

Selected Readings

Donowitz GR and Mandell GL, "Beta-Lactam Antibiotics," *N Engl J Med*, 1988, 318(7):419-26 and 318(8):490-500.

Gustaferro CA and Steckelberg JM, "Cephalosporin Antimicrobial Agents and Related Compounds," *Mayo Clin Proc*, 1991, 66(10):1064-73.

Vlasses PH, Bastion WA, Behal R, et al, "Ceftazidime Dosing in the Elderly: Economic Implications," *Ann Pharmacother*, 1993, 27(7-8):967-71.

Ceftin® Oral *see* Cefuroxime *on page 524*

Ceftizoxime Sodium (sef ti zox' eem)

Related Information

Antimicrobial Activity Against Selected Organisms *on page 757-764*

Brand Names Cefizox®

Generic Available No

Use Treatment of susceptible bacterial infection; mainly respiratory tract, skin and skin structure, bone and joint, urinary tract and gynecologic as well as septicemia

Pregnancy Risk Factor B

Contraindications Hypersensitivity to ceftizoxime or any component and cephalosporins

Adverse Reactions

1% to 10%: Rash, fever, pruritus, transient elevation of AST, ALT, and alkaline phosphatase; eosinophilia, thrombocytosis, pain, burning at injection site

<1%: Numbness, elevation of bilirubin, transient elevations of BUN and creatinine, anemia, leukopenia, neutropenia, thrombocytopenia, vaginitis

Toxicology Many beta-lactam containing antibiotics have the potential to cause neuromuscular hyperirritability or convulsive seizures. Hemodialysis may be helpful to aid in the removal of the drug from the blood, otherwise most treatment is supportive or symptom directed.

Drug Interactions Aminoglycosides (synergy), probenecid may increase ceftizoxime levels

Stability Reconstituted solution is stable for 24 hours at room temperature and 96 hours when refrigerated; for I.V. infusion in NS or D_5W solution is stable for 24 hours at room temperature, 96 hours when refrigerated or 12 weeks when frozen; after freezing, thawed solution is stable for 24 hours at room temperature or 10 days when refrigerated

Mechanism of Action Inhibits bacterial cell wall synthesis by binding to one or more of the penicillin binding proteins (PBPs); which in turn inhibits the final transpeptidation step of peptidoglycan synthesis in bacterial cell walls, thus inhibiting cell wall biosynthesis. Bacteria eventually lyse due to ongoing activity of cell wall autolytic enzymes (autolysins and murein hydrolases) while cell wall assembly is arrested.

Pharmacokinetics

Distribution: Widely distributed into most body tissues and fluids including gallbladder, liver, kidneys, bone, sputum, bile, and pleural and synovial fluids; has good CSF penetration; crosses placenta; small amounts excreted in breast milk

Half-life: 1.6 hours (half-life increases to 25 hours when creatinine clearances fall <10 mL/minute)

Time to peak serum concentration: I.M.: Within 30-60 minutes

Elimination: Excreted unchanged in urine

Usual Dosage I.M., I.V.:

Children ≥6 months: 50 mg/kg every 6-8 hours to 200 mg/kg/day to maximum of 12 g/24 hours

Adults: 1-2 g every 8-12 hours, up to 2 g every 4 hours or 4 g every 8 hours for life-threatening infections

Dosing adjustment in renal impairment:
Cl$_{cr}$ 10-30 mL/minute: Administer every 12 hours
Cl$_{cr}$ <10 mL/minute: Administer every 24-48 hours
Moderately dialyzable (20% to 50%)

Overdosage Neuromuscular hypersensitivity, convulsions

Test Interactions False-positive Coombs'; test, may falsely elevate creatinine values when Jaffé reaction is used, may cause false-positive results in urine glucose tests using cupric sulfate (Benedict's solution, Clinitest®)

Nursing Implications Do not admix with aminoglycosides in same bottle/bag; observe for signs and symptoms of anaphylaxis during first dose

Additional Information Sodium content of 1 g: 60 mg (2.6 mEq)

Dosage Forms
Infusion, in D$_5$W: 1 g (50 mL); 2 g (50 mL)
Powder for injection: 1 g, 2 g, 10 g

Selected Readings
Donowitz GR and Mandell GL, "Beta-Lactam Antibiotics," *N Engl J Med*, 1988, 318(7):419-26 and 318(8):490-500.
Gustaferro CA and Steckelberg JM, "Cephalosporin Antimicrobial Agents and Related Compounds," *Mayo Clin Proc*, 1991, 66(10):1064-73.

Ceftriaxone Sodium (sef try ax' one)

Related Information
Antimicrobial Activity Against Selected Organisms *on page 757-764*

Brand Names Rocephin®

Generic Available No

Use Treatment of susceptible bacterial infection; mainly respiratory tract, skin and skin structure, bone and joint, urinary tract and gynecologic as well as septicemia

Drug of Choice or Alternative For
Disease/Syndrome(s)
Arthritis, Septic *on page 18*
Meningitis, Pediatric (>2 months of age) *on page 30*
Organism(s)
Borrelia burgdorferi on page 68
Haemophilus ducreyi on page 118
Neisseria gonorrhoeae on page 161

Pregnancy Risk Factor B

Contraindications Hypersensitivity to ceftriaxone sodium or any component or other cephalosporins; do not use in hyperbilirubinemic neonates, particularly those who are premature since ceftriaxone is reported to displace bilirubin from albumin binding sites

Adverse Reactions
1% to 10%: Pain at injection site, rash, eosinophilia, thrombocytosis, leukopenia, diarrhea; elevations of SGOT (AST), SGPT (ALT), elevations of BUN
<1%: Phlebitis, pruritus, fever, chills, anemia, hemolytic anemia, neutropenia, lymphopenia, thrombocytopenia, nausea, vomiting, dysgeusia, elevations of alkaline phosphatase and bilirubin, elevation of creatinine, presence of casts in urine, headache, dizziness, moniliasis, vaginitis, diaphoresis, flushing

Toxicology Many beta-lactam containing antibiotics have the potential to cause neuromuscular hyperirritability or convulsive seizures. Hemodialysis may be helpful to aid in the removal of the drug from the blood, otherwise most treatment is supportive or symptom directed.

Drug Interactions Increased levels with probenecid; aminoglycosides (synergy)

Stability Reconstituted solution (100 mg/mL) is stable for 3 days at room temperature and 3 days when refrigerated; for I.V. infusion in NS or D$_5$W solution is stable for 3 days at room temperature, 10 days when refrigerated or 26 weeks when frozen; after freezing, thawed solution is stable for 3 days at room temperature or 10 days when refrigerated

Mechanism of Action Inhibits bacterial cell wall synthesis by binding to one or more of the penicillin binding proteins (PBPs); which in turn inhibits the final transpeptidation step of peptidoglycan synthesis in bacterial cell walls, thus inhibiting cell wall biosynthesis. Bacteria eventually lyse due to ongoing activity of cell wall autolytic enzymes (autolysins and murein hydrolases) while cell wall assembly is arrested.

Pharmacokinetics
Absorption: I.M.: Well absorbed
(Continued)

Ceftriaxone Sodium *(Continued)*

Distribution: Widely distributed throughout the body including gallbladder, lungs, bone, bile, CSF (diffuses into the CSF at higher concentrations when the meninges are inflamed); crosses placenta, reaches amniotic fluid and milk

Half-life:

Neonates:

1-4 days: 16 hours

9-30 days: 9 hours

Adults, normal renal and hepatic function: 5-9 hours

Time to peak serum concentration: I.M.: Within 1-2 hours

Elimination: Excreted unchanged in urine (33% to 65%) by glomerular filtration and in feces

Usual Dosage

Neonates: I.M., I.V.:

Postnatal age <7 days: 50 mg/kg/day given every 24 hours

Postnatal age >7 days:

<2000 g: 50 mg/kg/day given every 24 hours

>2000 g: 75 mg/kg/day given every 24 hours

Gonococcal prophylaxis: I.M.:

LBW neonates: 25-50 mg/kg as a single dose (dose not to exceed 125 mg)

Neonates: 125 mg as a single dose

Neonatal gonococcal ophthalmia: I.M.: 25-50 mg/kg/day given every 24 hours

Infants and Children: 50-100 mg/kg/day in 1-2 divided doses

Meningitis: Loading dose: 75 mg/kg may be administered at the start of therapy; then 100 mg/kg/day divided every 12 hours; maximum: 4 g/day

Chancroid, uncomplicated gonorrhea: I.M.:

<45 kg: 125 mg as a single dose

>45 kg: 250 mg as a single dose

Adults: 1-2 g every 12-24 hours depending on the type and severity of the infection; maximum dose: 4 g/day

A single I.M. dose of 125-250 mg of ceftriaxone is among the treatments of choice for gonorrhea

Dosing adjustment for renal impairment: None

Not dialyzable

Overdosage Neuromuscular hypersensitivity, convulsions

Test Interactions May falsely elevate creatinine values when Jaffé reaction is used; may cause false-positive results in urine glucose tests using cupric sulfate (Benedict's solution, Clinitest®)

Nursing Implications For I.M. injection, the maximum concentration is 250 mg/mL; ceftriaxone can be diluted with 1:1 water and 1% lidocaine for I.M. administration. Do not admix with aminoglycosides in same bottle/bag; observe for signs and symptoms of anaphylaxis during first dose.

Additional Information Sodium content of 1 g: 60 mg (2.6 mEq)

Dosage Forms

Infusion, premixed (frozen): 1 g in $D_{3.8}W$ (50 mL); 2 g in $D_{2.4}W$ (50 mL)

Powder for injection: 250 mg, 500 mg, 1 g, 2 g, 10 g

Selected Readings

Donowitz GR and Mandell GL, "Beta-Lactam Antibiotics," *N Engl J Med*, 1988, 318(7):419-26 and 318(8):490-500.

Gustaferro CA and Steckelberg JM, "Cephalosporin Antimicrobial Agents and Related Compounds," *Mayo Clin Proc*, 1991, 66(10):1064-73.

Schaad UB, Suter S, Gianella-Borradori A, et al, "A Comparison of Ceftriaxone and Cefuroxime for the Treatment of Bacterial Meningitis in Children," *N Engl J Med*, 1990, 322(3):141-7.

Cefuroxime (se fyoor ox' eem)

Related Information

Antimicrobial Activity Against Selected Organisms *on page 757-764*

Brand Names Ceftin® Oral; Kefurox® Injection; Zinacef® Injection

Generic Available No

Use Treatment of susceptible infections of the upper and lower respiratory tract, otitis media, urinary tract, skin and soft tissue, bone and joint, and sepsis

Drug of Choice or Alternative For

Disease/Syndrome(s)

Pneumonia, Community-Acquired *on page 37*

Pregnancy Risk Factor B

Contraindications Hypersensitivity to cefuroxime or any component and cephalosporins

Adverse Reactions

1% to 10%: Thrombophlebitis, decreased hemoglobin and hematocrit, eosinophilia, transient rise in SGOT (AST)/SGPT (ALT) and alkaline phosphatase

<1%: Dizziness, fever, headache, rash, nausea, vomiting, diarrhea, stomach cramps, GI bleeding, colitis, transient neutropenia and leukopenia, transient increase in liver enzymes, increase in creatinine and/or BUN, pain at the injection site, vaginitis

Toxicology Many beta-lactam containing antibiotics have the potential to cause neuromuscular hyperirritability or convulsive seizures. Hemodialysis may be helpful to aid in the removal of the drug from the blood, otherwise most treatment is supportive or symptom directed.

Drug Interactions Increased serum levels with probenecid; aminoglycosides (synergy)

Stability Reconstituted solution is stable for 24 hours at room temperature and 48 hours when refrigerated; for I.V. infusion in NS or D_5W solution is stable for 24 hours at room temperature, 7 days when refrigerated or 26 weeks when frozen; after freezing, thawed solution is stable for 24 hours at room temperature or 21 days when refrigerated

Mechanism of Action Inhibits bacterial cell wall synthesis by binding to one or more of the penicillin binding proteins (PBPs); which in turn inhibits the final transpeptidation step of peptidoglycan synthesis in bacterial cell walls, thus inhibiting cell wall biosynthesis. Bacteria eventually lyse due to ongoing activity of cell wall autolytic enzymes (autolysins and murein hydrolases) while cell wall assembly is arrested.

Pharmacokinetics

Absorption: Oral (cefuroxime axetil): Increased when given with or shortly after food or infant formula (37% to 52%)

Distribution: Widely distributed to body tissues and fluids; crosses blood-brain barrier; therapeutic concentrations achieved in CSF even when meninges are not inflamed; crosses placenta and reaches breast milk

Half-life:

Neonates:

≤3 days: 5.1-5.8 hours

6-14 days: 2-4.2 hours

3-4 weeks: 1-1.5 hours

Adults: 1-2 hours (prolonged in renal impairment)

Time to peak serum concentration: I.M.: Within 15-60 minutes

Elimination: Primarily excreted 66% to 100% as unchanged drug in urine by both glomerular filtration and tubular secretion

Usual Dosage

Neonates: 10-25 mg/kg/dose every 12 hours

Children:

Oral:

<12 years: 125 mg twice daily

>12 years: 250 mg twice daily

I.M., I.V.: 75-150 mg/kg/day divided every 8 hours; maximum dose: 9 g/day

Adults:

Oral: 125-500 mg twice daily, depending on severity of infection

I.M., I.V.: 100-150 mg/kg/day in divided doses every 6-8 hours; maximum: 6 g/24 hours

Dosing adjustment in renal impairment:

Cl_{cr} 10-20 mL/minute: Administer every 12 hours

Cl_{cr} <10 mL/minute: Administer every 24 hours

Dialyzable (25%)

Overdosage Neuromuscular hypersensitivity, convulsions

Monitoring Parameters With prolonged therapy, monitor renal, hepatic, and hematologic function periodically

Test Interactions False-positive Coombs' test; may falsely elevate creatinine values when Jaffé reaction is used; may cause false-positive results in urine glucose tests using cupric sulfate (Benedict's solution, Clinitest®)

Patient Information Report diarrhea promptly; entire course of medication should be taken to ensure eradication of organism; may interfere with oral contraceptives, females should report symptoms of vaginitis

(Continued)

ANTIMICROBIAL THERAPY
Cefuroxime *(Continued)*

Nursing Implications Do not admix with aminoglycosides in same bottle/bag; observe for signs and symptoms of anaphylaxis during first dose

Additional Information Sodium content of 1 g: 54.2 mg (2.4 mEq)

Dosage Forms

Infusion, premixed (frozen) (Zinacef®): 750 mg (50 mL); 1.5 g (50 mL)

Powder for injection, as sodium (Kefurox®, Zinacef®): 750 mg, 1.5 g, 7.5 g

Tablet, as axetil (Ceftin®): 125 mg, 250 mg, 500 mg

Selected Readings

"Antimicrobial Prophylaxis in Surgery," *Med Lett Drugs Ther*, 1993, 35(906):91-4.

Donowitz GR and Mandell GL, "Beta-Lactam Antibiotics," *N Engl J Med*, 1988, 318(7):419-26 and 318(8):490-500.

Gentry LO, Zeluff BJ, and Cooley DA, "Antibiotic Prophylaxis in Open-Heart Surgery: A Comparison of Cefamandole, Cefuroxime, and Cefazolin," *Ann Thorac Surg*, 1988, 46(2):167-71.

Gustaferro CA and Steckelberg JM, "Cephalosporin Antimicrobial Agents and Related Compounds," *Mayo Clin Proc*, 1991, 66(10):1064-73.

Peterson CD, Lake KD, Arom KV, et al, "Antibiotic Prophylaxis in Open-Heart Surgery Patients: Comparison of Cefamandole and Cefuroxime," *Drug Intell Clin Pharm*, 1987, 21(9):728-32.

Cefzil® *see* Cefprozil *on page 520*

Cephalexin Monohydrate *(sef a lex' in)*

Related Information

Antimicrobial Activity Against Selected Organisms *on page 757-764*

Brand Names Keflet®; Keflex®; Keftab®

Generic Available Yes

Use Treatment of susceptible bacterial infections of the lower respiratory tract, urinary tract, skin and soft tissue, and bone and joint

Pregnancy Risk Factor B

Contraindications Hypersensitivity to cephalexin or any component and cephalosporins

Adverse Reactions

1% to 10%: Diarrhea

<1%: Dizziness, fatigue, headache, rash, nausea, vomiting, pseudomembranous colitis, transient neutropenia, anemia, transient elevation in liver enzymes

Toxicology Many beta-lactam containing antibiotics have the potential to cause neuromuscular hyperirritability or convulsive seizures. Hemodialysis may be helpful to aid in the removal of the drug from the blood, otherwise most treatment is supportive or symptom directed.

Drug Interactions Increased levels with probenecid

Stability Refrigerate suspension after reconstitution; discard after 14 days

Mechanism of Action Inhibits bacterial cell wall synthesis by binding to one or more of the penicillin binding proteins (PBPs); which in turn inhibits the final transpeptidation step of peptidoglycan synthesis in bacterial cell walls, thus inhibiting cell wall biosynthesis. Bacteria eventually lyse due to ongoing activity of cell wall autolytic enzymes (autolysins and murein hydrolases) while cell wall assembly is arrested.

Pharmacokinetics

Absorption: Delayed in young children and may be decreased up to 50% in neonates

Distribution: Widely distributed into most body tissues and fluids, including gallbladder, liver, kidneys, bone, sputum, bile, and pleural and synovial fluids; CSF penetration is poor; crosses placenta; appears in breast milk

Half-life:

Neonates: 5 hours

Children 3-12 months: 2.5 hours

Adults: 30 minutes to 1.2 hours (prolonged with renal impairment)

Time to peak serum concentration: Oral: Within 60 minutes

Elimination: 80% to 100% excreted as unchanged drug in urine within 8 hours

Usual Dosage Oral:

Children: 25-50 mg/kg/day every 6 hours; severe infections: 50-100 mg/kg/day in divided doses every 6 hours; maximum: 3 g/24 hours

Adults: 250-1000 mg every 6 hours

Dosing adjustment in renal impairment:
Cl_{cr} 10-40 mL/minute: Administer every 8-12 hours
Cl_{cr} <10 mL/minute: Administer every 12-24 hours
Moderately dialyzable (20% to 50%)

Overdosage Neuromuscular hypersensitivity, convulsions

Monitoring Parameters With prolonged therapy monitor renal, hepatic, and hematologic function periodically

Test Interactions False-positive Coombs' test, may falsely elevate creatinine values when Jaffé reaction is used, may cause false-positive results in urine glucose tests using cupric sulfate (Benedict's solution, Clinitest®), false-positive urinary proteins and steroids

Patient Information Report diarrhea promptly; entire course of medication should be taken to ensure eradication of organism; may interfere with oral contraceptives

Nursing Implications Give on an empty stomach (ie, 1 hour prior to, or 2 hours after meals) to increase total absorption

Dosage Forms
Capsule: 250 mg, 500 mg
Powder for oral suspension: 125 mg/5 mL (5 mL unit dose, 60 mL, 100 mL, 200 mL); 250 mg/5 mL (5 mL unit dose, 100 mL, 200 mL)
Suspension, oral, pediatric: 100 mg/mL [5 mg/drop] (10 mL)
Tablet: 250 mg, 500 mg, 1 g
Tablet, as hydrochloride: 250 mg, 500 mg

Selected Readings
Donowitz GR and Mandell GL, "Beta-Lactam Antibiotics," *N Engl J Med*, 1988, 318(7):419-26 and 318(8):490-500.
Gustaferro CA and Steckelberg JM, "Cephalosporin Antimicrobial Agents and Related Compounds," *Mayo Clin Proc*, 1991, 66(10):1064-73.
Smith GH, "Oral Cephalosporins in Perspective," *DICP*, 1990, 24(1):45-51.

Cephalosporins, 1st Generation
Related Information
Antimicrobial Activity Against Selected Organisms *on page 757-764*
Refer To
Cefadroxil Monohydrate *on page 509*
Cefazolin Sodium *on page 511*
Cephalexin Monohydrate *on previous page*
Cephalothin Sodium *on next page*
Cephapirin Sodium *on page 529*
Cephradine *on page 530*
Drug of Choice or Alternative For
Disease/Syndrome(s)
Impetigo *on page 27*
Osteomyelitis, Healthy Adult *on page 33*
Osteomyelitis, Pediatric *on page 33*
Pharyngitis *on page 36*
Skin and Soft Tissue *on page 42*

Organism(s)
Escherichia coli, Nonenterohemorrhagic *on page 113*
Klebsiella Species *on page 137*
Staphylococcus aureus, Methicillin-Susceptible *on page 198*
Staphylococcus epidermidis, Methicillin-Susceptible *on page 201*
Staphylococcus saprophyticus on page 203
Streptococcus agalactiae on page 203
Streptococcus pneumoniae on page 206
Streptococcus pyogenes on page 207
Streptococcus-Related Gram-Positive Cocci *on page 212*
Streptococcus, Viridans Group *on page 213*

Cephalosporins, 2nd Generation
Related Information
Antimicrobial Activity Against Selected Organisms *on page 757-764*
Refer To
Cefaclor *on page 508*
Cefamandole Nafate *on page 510*
Cefmetazole Sodium *on page 513*
Cefonicid Sodium *on page 514*

Cefotetan Disodium *on page 517*
Cefoxitin Sodium *on page 518*
Cefpodoxime Proxetil *on page 519*
Cefprozil *on page 520*
Cefuroxime *on page 524*
Loracarbef *on page 601*

Drug of Choice or Alternative For
Disease/Syndrome(s)
Bronchitis *on page 19*
Epiglottitis *on page 24*
Otitis Media, Acute *on page 35*
Sinusitis, Community-Acquired, Acute *on page 41*

Organism(s)
Escherichia coli, Nonenterohemorrhagic *on page 113*
Haemophilus influenzae on page 119
Klebsiella Species *on page 137*
Moraxella catarrhalis on page 147

Cephalosporins, 3rd Generation
Related Information
Antimicrobial Activity Against Selected Organisms *on page 757-764*
Refer To
Cefixime *on page 512*
Cefoperazone Sodium *on page 515*
Cefotaxime Sodium *on page 516*
Ceftazidime *on page 520*
Ceftizoxime Sodium *on page 522*
Ceftriaxone Sodium *on page 523*

Drug of Choice or Alternative For
Disease/Syndrome(s)
Epiglottitis *on page 24*
Meningitis, Community Acquired, Adult *on page 29*
Meningitis, Post-Traumatic *on page 31*
Osteomyelitis, Diabetic Foot *on page 32*
Pneumonia, Community-Acquired *on page 37*
Urinary Tract Infection, Pyelonephritis *on page 45*

Organism(s)
Acinetobacter Species *on page 50*
Citrobacter Species *on page 82*
Enterobacter Species *on page 104*
Escherichia coli, Nonenterohemorrhagic *on page 113*
HACEK Group *on page 117*
Haemophilus influenzae on page 119
Klebsiella Species *on page 137*
Moraxella catarrhalis on page 147
Neisseria meningitidis on page 163
Proteus Species *on page 176*
Salmonella Species *on page 185*
Serratia Species *on page 190*
Shigella Species *on page 191*
Yersinia enterocolitica on page 232

Cephalothin Sodium (sef a' loe thin)
Related Information
Antimicrobial Activity Against Selected Organisms *on page 757-764*
Brand Names Keflin® Neutral
Generic Available Yes
Use Treatment of infections when caused by susceptible strains in respiratory, genitourinary, gastrointestinal, skin and soft tissue, bone and joint infections; septicemia
Pregnancy Risk Factor B
Contraindications Hypersensitivity to cephalothin and or other cephalosporins
Warnings/Precautions Prolonged use may result in superinfection; use with caution in patients with a history of colitis or penicillin allergy

Adverse Reactions
1% to 10%: Nausea, vomiting, diarrhea
<1%: Maculopapular and erythematous rash, dyspepsia, pseudomembranous colitis, bleeding, pain and induration at injection site

Toxicology Many beta-lactam containing antibiotics have the potential to cause neuromuscular hyperirritability or convulsive seizures. Hemodialysis may be helpful to aid in the removal of the drug from the blood, otherwise most treatment is supportive or symptom directed.

Stability Reconstituted solution is stable for 12-24 hours at room temperature and 96 hours when refrigerated; for I.V. infusion in NS or D₅W solution is stable for 24 hours at room temperature, 96 hours when refrigerated or 12 weeks when frozen; after freezing, thawed solution is stable for 24 hours at room temperature or 96 hours when refrigerated

Mechanism of Action Inhibits bacterial cell wall synthesis by binding to one or more of the penicillin binding proteins (PBPs); which in turn inhibits the final transpeptidation step of peptidoglycan synthesis in bacterial cell walls, thus inhibiting cell wall biosynthesis. Bacteria eventually lyse due to ongoing activity of cell wall autolytic enzymes (autolysins and murein hydrolases) while cell wall assembly is arrested.

Pharmacokinetics
Distribution: Crosses the placenta; small amounts appear in breast milk; does not penetrate the CSF and brain
Metabolism: Partially deacetylated in the liver and kidney
Half-life: 30-60 minutes
Time to peak serum concentration: I.M.: Within 30 minutes
Elimination: 50% to 75% of dose appearing as unchanged drug in urine

Usual Dosage I.M., I.V.:
Neonates:
Postnatal age <7 days:
<2000 g: 20 mg every 12 hours
>2000 g: 20 mg every 8 hours
Postnatal age >7 days:
<2000 g: 20 mg every 8 hours
>2000 g: 20 mg every 6 hours

Children: 75-125 mg/kg/day divided every 4-6 hours; maximum dose: 10 g in a 24-hour period

Adults: 500 mg to 2 g every 4-6 hours

Dosing adjustment in renal impairment:
Cl_cr 10-50 mL/minute: Administer every 6 hours
Cl_cr <10 mL/minute: Administer every 12 hours

Overdosage Neuromuscular hypersensitivity, convulsions

Test Interactions False-positive Coombs' test, may false elevate creatinine values when Jaffé reaction is used, may cause false-positive results in urine glucose test using cupric sulfate (Benedict's solution, Clinitest®), false-positive urinary proteins and steroids

Nursing Implications Do not admix with aminoglycosides in same bottle/bag; observe for signs and symptoms of anaphylaxis during first dose

Additional Information Sodium content of 1 g: 64.4 mg (2.8 mEq)

Dosage Forms Powder for injection: 1 g (10 mL, 100 mL); 2 g (20 mL, 100 mL); 20 g (200 mL)

Selected Readings
Donowitz GR and Mandell GL, "Beta-Lactam Antibiotics," *N Engl J Med*, 1988, 318(7):419-26 and 318(8):490-500.
Gustaferro CA and Steckelberg JM, "Cephalosporin Antimicrobial Agents and Related Compounds," *Mayo Clin Proc*, 1991, 66(10):1064-73.

Cephapirin Sodium (sef a pye' rin)
Related Information
Antimicrobial Activity Against Selected Organisms *on page 757-764*
Brand Names Cefadyl®
Generic Available No
Use Treatment of infections when caused by susceptible strains in respiratory, genitourinary, gastrointestinal, skin and soft tissue, bone and joint infections; septicemia
Pregnancy Risk Factor B
Contraindications Hypersensitivity to cephapirin sodium or any component and cephalosporins

(Continued)
529

Cephapirin Sodium *(Continued)*

Adverse Reactions
1% to 10%: Diarrhea

<1%: CNS irritation, seizures, fever, rash, urticaria, leukopenia, thrombocytopenia, transient elevation of liver enzymes

Toxicology Many beta-lactam containing antibiotics have the potential to cause neuromuscular hyperirritability or convulsive seizures. Hemodialysis may be helpful to aid in the removal of the drug from the blood, otherwise most treatment is supportive or symptom directed.

Drug Interactions Decreased elimination with probenecid

Stability Reconstituted solution is stable for 24 hours at room temperature and 10 days when refrigerated; for I.V. infusion in NS or D_5W solution is stable for 24 hours at room temperature, 10 days when refrigerated or 14 days when frozen; after freezing, thawed solution is stable for 12 hours at room temperature or 10 days when refrigerated

Mechanism of Action Inhibits bacterial cell wall synthesis by binding to one or more of the penicillin binding proteins (PBPs); which in turn inhibits the final transpeptidation step of peptidoglycan synthesis in bacterial cell walls, thus inhibiting cell wall biosynthesis. Bacteria eventually lyse due to ongoing activity of cell wall autolytic enzymes (autolysins and murein hydrolases) while cell wall assembly is arrested.

Pharmacokinetics
Distribution: Widely distributed into most body tissues and fluids including gallbladder, liver, kidneys, bone, sputum, bile, and pleural and synovial fluids; CSF penetration is poor; crosses the placenta and small amounts appear in breast milk

Metabolism: Partly in the liver, kidney and plasma to metabolites (50% active)

Half-life: 36-60 minutes

Time to peak serum concentration: I.M.: Within 30 minutes

Elimination: 60% to 85% excreted as unchanged drug in urine

Usual Dosage I.M., I.V.:
Children: 10-20 mg/kg every 6 hours up to 4 g/24 hours
Adults: 1 g every 6 hours up to 12 g/day

Dosing adjustment in renal impairment:
Cl_{cr} 10-50 mL/minute: Administer every 6-8 hours
Cl_{cr} <10 mL/minute: Administer every 12 hours

Overdosage Neuromuscular hypersensitivity, convulsions

Test Interactions False-positive Coombs' test, may falsely elevate creatinine values when Jaffé reaction is used, may cause false-positive results in urine glucose tests using cupric sulfate (Benedict's solution, Clinitest®), false-positive urinary proteins and steroids

Nursing Implications Do not admix with aminoglycosides in same bottle/bag; observe for signs and symptoms of anaphylaxis during first dose

Additional Information Sodium content of 1 g: 55.2 mg (2.4 mEq)

Dosage Forms Powder for injection: 500 mg (10 mL); 1 g (10 mL, 100 mL); 2 g (20 mL, 100 mL); 4 g (100 mL); 20 g (100 mL)

Selected Readings
Donowitz GR and Mandell GL, "Beta-Lactam Antibiotics," *N Engl J Med*, 1988, 318(7):419-26 and 318(8):490-500.

Gustaferro CA and Steckelberg JM, "Cephalosporin Antimicrobial Agents and Related Compounds," *Mayo Clin Proc*, 1991, 66(10):1064-73.

Cephradine *(sef' ra deen)*

Related Information
Antimicrobial Activity Against Selected Organisms *on page 757-764*

Brand Names Velosef®

Generic Available Yes

Use Treatment of infections when caused by susceptible strains in respiratory, genitourinary, gastrointestinal, skin and soft tissue, bone and joint infections

Pregnancy Risk Factor B

Contraindications Hypersensitivity to cephradine or any component and cephalosporins

Warnings/Precautions Prolonged use may result in superinfection; use with caution in patients with a history of colitis or penicillin allergy

Adverse Reactions
1% to 10%: Diarrhea

<1%: Rash, nausea, vomiting, pseudomembranous colitis, increased BUN and creatinine

Stability Reconstituted solution is stable for 2 hours at room temperature and 24 hours when refrigerated; for I.V. infusion in NS or D_5W solution is stable for 10 hours at room temperature, 48 hours when refrigerated or 6 weeks when frozen; after freezing, thawed solution is stable for 10 hours at room temperature or 48 hours when refrigerated

Mechanism of Action Inhibits bacterial cell wall synthesis by binding to one or more of the penicillin binding proteins (PBPs); which in turn inhibits the final transpeptidation step of peptidoglycan synthesis in bacterial cell walls, thus inhibiting cell wall biosynthesis. Bacteria eventually lyse due to ongoing activity of cell wall autolytic enzymes (autolysins and murein hydrolases) while cell wall assembly is arrested.

Pharmacokinetics

Absorption: Oral is faster than I.M. absorption, yet well absorbed from all routes

Distribution: Widely distributed into most body tissues and fluids including gallbladder, liver, kidneys, bone, sputum, bile, and pleural and synovial fluids; CSF penetration is poor; crosses the placenta and appears in breast milk

Half-life: 1-2 hours

Time to peak serum concentration: Oral, I.M.: Within 60-120 minutes

Elimination: ~80% to 90% recovered in urine as unchanged drug, within 6 hours

Usual Dosage

Children ≥9 months:

Oral: 25-50 mg/kg/day in divided doses every 6 hours

I.M., I.V.: 50-100 mg/kg/day in equally divided doses every 6 hours up to 4 g/day

Adults:

Oral: 250-500 mg every 6-12 hours

I.M., I.V.: 1 g every 6 hours

Dosing adjustment in renal impairment:

Cl_{cr} 10-50 mL/minute: Administer 50% of dose

Cl_{cr} <10 mL/minute: Administer 25% of dose

or

Cl_{cr} 25-50 mL/minute: Administer every 12 hours

Cl_{cr} 10-25 mL/minute: Administer every 24 hours

Cl_{cr} <10 mL/minute: Administer every 36 hours

Overdosage Neuromuscular hypersensitivity, convulsions

Test Interactions False-positive Coombs' test, may falsely elevate creatinine values when Jaffé reaction is used, may cause false-positive results in urine glucose tests using cupric sulfate (Benedict's solution, Clinitest®), false-positive urinary proteins and steroids

Patient Information Report diarrhea promptly; entire course of medication should be taken to ensure eradication of organism; may interfere with oral contraceptives, females should report symptoms of vaginitis

Dosage Forms

Capsule: 250 mg, 500 mg

Powder for injection: 250 mg, 500 mg, 1 g, 2 g

Suspension, oral: 125 mg/5 mL (5 mL, 100 mL, 200 mL); 250 mg/5 mL (5 mL, 100 mL, 200 mL)

Selected Readings

Donowitz GR and Mandell GL, "Beta-Lactam Antibiotics," *N Engl J Med*, 1988, 318(7):419-26 and 318(8):490-500.

Gustaferro CA and Steckelberg JM, "Cephalosporin Antimicrobial Agents and Related Compounds," *Mayo Clin Proc*, 1991, 66(10):1064-73.

Smith GH, "Oral Cephalosporins in Perspective," *DICP*, 1990, 24(1):45-51.

Ceptaz™ *see* Ceftazidime *on page 520*

Chibroxin™ Ophthalmic *see* Norfloxacin *on page 624*

Chloracol® *see* Chloramphenicol *on this page*

Chloramphenicol (klor am fen' i kole)

Related Information

Antimicrobial Activity Against Selected Organisms *on page 757-764*

Brand Names AK-Chlor®; Anocol®; Chloracol®; Chlorofair®; Chloromycetin®; Chloroptic®; Econochlor®; I-Chlor®; Ocu-Chlor®; Ophthochlor®; Spectro-Chlor®

(Continued)

Chloramphenicol *(Continued)*

Generic Available Yes

Use Treatment of infections due to organisms resistant to other less toxic antibiotics or when its penetrability into the site of infection is clinically superior to other antibiotics to which the organism is sensitive

Drug of Choice or Alternative For

Disease/Syndrome(s)

Meningitis, Community Acquired, Adult *on page 29*
Meningitis, Pediatric (>2 months of age) *on page 30*
Meningitis, Neonatal (<2 months of age) *on page 29*

Organism(s)

Bacillus anthracis on page 58
Bordetella pertussis on page 65
Calymmatobacterium granulomatis on page 71
Coxiella burnetii on page 93
Ehrlichia Species *on page 101*
Haemophilus influenzae on page 119
Neisseria meningitidis on page 163
Rickettsia rickettsii on page 183
Salmonella Species *on page 185*
Streptococcus pneumoniae on page 206
Yersinia pestis on page 233

Pregnancy Risk Factor C

Contraindications Hypersensitivity to chloramphenicol or any component

Warnings/Precautions Use with caution in patients with impaired renal or hepatic function and in neonates; reduce dose with impaired liver function; use with care in patients with glucose 6-phosphate dehydrogenase deficiency. Serious and fatal blood dyscrasias have occurred after both short-term and prolonged therapy; should not be used when less potentially toxic agents are effective; prolonged use may result in superinfection.

Adverse Reactions <1%: Optic neuritis, peripheral neuropathy, nightmares, headache, rash, diarrhea, stomatitis, enterocolitis, gray baby syndrome, bone marrow depression, aplastic anemia, nausea, vomiting

Drug Interactions

Decreased toxicity/levels with rifampin
Increased effect/toxicity/levels of chlorpropamide, phenytoin, oral anticoagulants, and phenobarbital

Stability Refrigerate ophthalmic solution; constituted solutions remain stable for 30 days; use only clear solutions; frozen solutions remain stable for 6 months

Mechanism of Action Reversibly binds to 50S ribosomal subunits of susceptible organisms preventing amino acids from being transferred to growing peptide chains thus inhibiting protein synthesis

Pharmacokinetics

Absorption: Oral: 75% to 100%; in neonates, GI absorption of chloramphenicol palmitate is slow and erratic

Distribution: Widely distributed with highest concentrations in liver and kidney; therapeutic concentrations also in CSF and brain tissue; measurable levels in pleural and ascitic fluid, bile, saliva, and aqueous and vitreous humor; readily crosses the placenta and appears in breast milk

Metabolism: Extensive in the liver (90%) to inactive metabolites, principally by glucuronidation

Half-life:

Neonates:

1-2 days: 24 hours
10-16 days: 10 hours

Adults: 1.6-3.3 hours (prolonged in hepatic insufficiency)

Time to peak serum concentration: Oral: Within 30 minutes to 3 hours

Elimination: 5% to 15% excreted as unchanged drug in urine and 4% excreted in bile

Usual Dosage

Neonates: Initial loading dose: Oral, I.V. (I.M. administration is not recommended):

Postnatal age 0-4 weeks:

<1200 g: 22 mg/kg/day every 24 hours
1200-2000 g: 25 mg/kg/day every 24 hours
Postnatal age <7 days, >2000 g: 25 mg/kg/day every 24 hours

Postnatal age 7-28 days, >2000 g: 25 mg/kg/dose every 12 hours

Meningitis: Oral, I.V.: Infants >30 days and Children: 75-100 mg/kg/day divided every 6 hours

Other infections: Oral, I.V.:
Infants and Children: 50-75 mg/kg/day divided every 6 hours; maximum daily dose: 4 g/day
Adults: 50-100 mg/kg/day in divided doses every 6 hours; maximum daily dose: 4 g/day

Dosing adjustment/comments in hepatic impairment: Avoid use in severe liver impairment as increased toxicity may occur
Slightly dialyzable (5% to 20%)

Children and Adults:
Ophthalmic: Instill 1-2 drops or 1.25 cm ($^1/_2$") of ointment every 3-4 hours; increase interval between applications after 48 hours to 2-3 times/day
Otic solution: Instill 2-3 drops into ear 3 times/day
Topical: Gently rub into the affected area 1-4 times/day
Overdosage Anemia, metabolic acidosis, hypotension, hypothermia
Monitoring Parameters CBC with reticulocyte and platelet counts, periodic liver and renal function tests
Patient Information Take on empty stomach (can take with food if GI upset)
Nursing Implications Final concentration for administration should not exceed 20 mg/mL for infusion or 100 mg/mL for IVP
Additional Information Sodium content of 1 g (injection): 51.8 mg (2.25 mEq)
Dosage Forms
Capsule: 250 mg, 500 mg
Cream: 1% (30 g)
Injection, as sodium succinate: 100 mg/mL
Ointment, ophthalmic: 1% (3.5 g)
Powder for solution, ophthalmic: 25 mg
Solution:
Ophthalmic: 0.5% (7.5 mL)
Otic: 0.5% (15 mL)
Suspension, as palmitate, oral: 150 mg/5 mL (60 mL)
Selected Readings
Smilack JD, Wilson WR, and Cockerill FR 3d, "Tetracyclines, Chloramphenicol, Erythromycin, Clindamycin, and Metronidazole," *Mayo Clin Proc*, 1991, 66(12):1270-80.
Tunkel AR, Wispelwey B, and Scheld M, "Bacterial Meningitis: Recent Advances in Pathophysiology and Treatment," *Ann Intern Med*, 1990, 112(8):610-23.

Chlorofair® *see* Chloramphenicol *on page 531*
Chloromycetin® *see* Chloramphenicol *on page 531*
Chloroptic® *see* Chloramphenicol *on page 531*

Chloroquine and Primaquine (klor' oh kwin) and (prim' a kween)
Brand Names Aralen® Phosphate With Primaquine Phosphate
Synonyms Primaquine and Chloroquine
Generic Available No
Use Prophylaxis of malaria, regardless of species, in all areas where the disease is endemic
Pregnancy Risk Factor C
Contraindications Retinal or visual field changes, known hypersensitivity to chloroquine or primaquine
Warnings/Precautions Use with caution in patients with psoriasis, porphyria, hepatic dysfunction, G-6-PD deficiency
Adverse Reactions
1% to 10%: Diarrhea, nausea
<1%: Hypotension, EKG changes, fatigue, personality changes, headache, pruritus, hair bleaching, anorexia, vomiting, stomatitis, blood dyscrasias, retinopathy, blurred vision
Toxicology Symptoms of overdose include headache, visual changes, cardiovascular collapse, seizures, abdominal cramps, vomiting, cyanosis, methemoglobinemia, leukopenia, respiratory and cardiac arrest; immediate GI decontamination is necessary; activated charcoal is effective at binding certain chemicals, and this is especially true for chloroquine; treatment is supportive; diazepam 0.1 mg/kg is effective for seizures
(Continued)

Chloroquine and Primaquine *(Continued)*

Drug Interactions
Decreased absorption if administered concomitantly with kaolin and magnesium trisilicate
Increased toxicity/levels with cimetidine

Mechanism of Action Chloroquine concentrates within parasite acid vesicles and raises internal pH resulting in inhibition of parasite growth; may involve aggregates of ferriprotoporphyrin IX acting as chloroquine receptors causing membrane damage; may also interfere with nucleoprotein synthesis. Primaquine eliminates the primary tissue exoerythrocytic forms of *P. falciparum*; disrupts mitochondria and binds to DNA.

Pharmacokinetics
Absorption: Oral: Both drugs are readily absorbed
Distribution: Concentrated in liver, spleen, kidney, heart, and brain
Metabolism: 25% of chloroquine is metabolized
Elimination: Drug may remain in tissue for 3-5 days; up to 70% excreted unchanged

Usual Dosage Oral: Start at least 1 day before entering the endemic area; continue for 8 weeks after leaving the endemic area

Children: For suggested weekly dosage (based on body weight), see table:

Weight		Chloroquine Base (mg)	Primaquine Base (mg)	Dose* (mL)
lb	kg			
10–15	4.5–6.8	20	3	2.5
16–25	7.3–11.4	40	6	5
26–35	11.8–15.9	60	9	7.5
36–45	16.4–20.5	80	12	10
46–55	20.9–25	100	15	12.5
56–100	25.4–45.4	150	22.5	$^1/_2$ tablet
100+	>45.4	300	45	1 tablet

*Dose based on liquid containing approximately 40 mg of chloroquine base and 6 mg primaquine base per 5 mL, prepared from chloroquine phosphate with primaquine phosphate tablets.

Adults: Take 1 tablet/week on the same day each week

Monitoring Parameters Periodic CBC, examination for muscular weakness and ophthalmologic examination in patients receiving prolonged therapy

Patient Information Take with meals; report any visual disturbances or difficulty in hearing or ringing in the ears; tablets are bitter tasting; may cause diarrhea, loss of appetite, nausea, stomach pain; notify physician if these become severe

Nursing Implications Periodic CBC, examination for muscular weakness, and ophthalmologic examination in patients receiving prolonged therapy

Dosage Forms Tablet: Chloroquine phosphate 500 mg [base 300 mg] and primaquine phosphate 79 mg [base 45 mg]

Selected Readings
Panisko DM and Keystone JS, "Treatment of Malaria – 1990," *Drugs*, 1990, 39(2):160-89.
Wyler DJ, "Malaria Chemoprophylaxis for the Traveler," *N Engl J Med*, 1993, 329(1):31-7.
Wyler DJ, "Malaria: Overview and Update," *Clin Infect Dis*, 1993, 16(4):449-56.

Chloroquine Phosphate *(klor' oh kwin)*

Brand Names Aralen® Phosphate

Generic Available Yes

Use Suppression or chemoprophylaxis of malaria; treatment of uncomplicated or mild-moderate malaria; extraintestinal amebiasis; rheumatoid arthritis

Drug of Choice or Alternative For
Organism(s)
Plasmodium Species *on page 172*

Pregnancy Risk Factor C

Contraindications Retinal or visual field changes; patients with psoriasis; known hypersensitivity to chloroquine

Adverse Reactions
1% to 10%: Nausea, diarrhea

<1%: Hypotension, EKG changes, fatigue, personality changes, headache, pruritus, hair bleaching, anorexia, vomiting, stomatitis, blood dyscrasias, retinopathy, blurred vision

Toxicology Activated charcoal is effective at binding certain chemicals and this is especially true for chloroquine

Drug Interactions
Decreased absorption if administered concomitantly with kaolin and magnesium trisilicate

Increased toxicity/levels with cimetidine

Mechanism of Action Binds to and inhibits DNA and RNA polymerase; interferes with metabolism and hemoglobin utilization by parasites; inhibits prostaglandin effects; chloroquine concentrates within parasite acid vesicles and raises internal pH resulting in inhibition of parasite growth; may involve aggregates of ferriprotoporphyrin IX acting as chloroquine receptors causing membrane damage; may also interfere with nucleoprotein synthesis

Pharmacokinetics
Absorption: Oral: Rapid (~89)

Distribution: Widely distributed in body tissues such as eyes, heart, kidneys, liver, and lungs where retention is prolonged; crosses the placenta; appears in breast milk

Metabolism: Partial hepatic metabolism occurs

Half-life: 3-5 days

Time to peak serum concentration: Within 1-2 hours

Elimination: ~70% excreted unchanged in urine; acidification of the urine increases elimination of drug; small amounts of drug may be present in urine months following discontinuation of therapy

Usual Dosage (Dosage expressed in terms of mg of base.) Oral:
Suppression or prophylaxis of malaria:
Children: Administer 5 mg base/kg/week on the same day each week (not to exceed 300 mg base/dose); begin 1-2 weeks prior to exposure; continue for 6-8 weeks after leaving endemic area; if suppressive therapy is not begun prior to exposure, double the initial loading dose to 10 mg base/kg and give in 2 divided doses 6 hours apart, followed by the usual dosage regimen

Adults: 300 mg/week (base) on the same day each week; begin 1-2 weeks prior to exposure; continue for 4-6 weeks after leaving endemic area; if suppressive therapy is not begun prior to exposure, double the initial loading dose to 600 mg base and give in 2 divided doses 6 hours apart, followed by the usual dosage regimen

Acute attack:
Children: 10 mg/kg on day 1, followed by 5 mg/kg 6 hours later and 5 mg/kg on days 2 and 3

Adults: 600 mg on day 1, followed by 300 mg 6 hours later, followed by 300 mg on days 2 and 3

Extraintestinal amebiasis:
Children: 10 mg/kg once daily for 2-3 weeks (up to 300 mg base/day)

Adults: 600 mg base/day for 2 days followed by 300 mg base/day for at least 2-3 weeks

Dosing adjustment in renal impairment: Cl$_{cr}$ <10 mL/minute: Administer 50% of dose

Minimally removed by hemodialysis

Overdosage Headache, visual changes, cardiovascular collapse

Monitoring Parameters Periodic CBC, examination for muscular weakness and ophthalmologic examination in patients receiving prolonged therapy

Patient Information Take with meals; report any visual disturbances or difficulty in hearing or ringing in the ears; tablets are bitter tasting

Dosage Forms Tablet: 250 mg [150 mg base]; 500 mg [300 mg base]

Selected Readings
Panisko DM and Keystone JS, "Treatment of Malaria – 1990," *Drugs*, 1990, 39(2):160-89.
Wyler DJ, "Malaria Chemoprophylaxis for the Traveler," *N Engl J Med*, 1993, 329(1):31-7.
Wyler DJ, "Malaria: Overview and Update," *Clin Infect Dis*, 1993, 16(4):449-56.

Cholera Vaccine (kol' er a)
Generic Available No

Use The World Health Organization no longer recommends cholera vaccination for travel to or from cholera-endemic areas. Some countries may still require evidence of a complete primary series or a booster dose given within 6 months

(Continued)

Cholera Vaccine *(Continued)*

of arrival. Vaccination should not be considered as an alternative to continued careful selection of foods and water. Ideally, cholera and yellow fever vaccines should be administered at least 3 weeks apart.

Pregnancy Risk Factor C

Contraindications Presence of any acute illness, history of severe systemic reaction, or allergic response following a prior dose of cholera vaccine

Warnings/Precautions There is no data on the safety of cholera vaccination during pregnancy. Use in pregnancy should reflect actual increased risk. Persons who have had severe local or systemic reactions to a previous dose should not be revaccinated. Have epinephrine (1:1000) available for immediate use.

Adverse Reactions >10%: Malaise, fever, headache, pain, swelling, tenderness, erythema, and induration at injection site

Drug Interactions Decreased effect with yellow fever vaccine; data suggests that giving both vaccines within 3 weeks of each other may decrease the response to both

Stability Refrigerate, avoid freezing

Mechanism of Action Inactivated vaccine producing active immunization

Usual Dosage

Children:

6 months to 4 years: Two 0.2 mL doses I.M./S.C. 1 week to 1 month apart; booster doses (0.2 mL I.M./S.C.) every 6 months

5-10 years: Two 0.3 mL doses I.M./S.C. or two 0.2 mL intradermal doses 1 week to 1 month apart; booster doses (0.3 mL I.M./S.C. or 0.2 mL I.D.) every 6 months

Children ≥10 years and Adults: Two 0.5 mL doses given I.M./S.C. or two 0.2 mL doses I.D. 1 week to 1 month apart; booster doses (0.5 mL I.M. or S.C. or 0.2 mL I.D.) every 6 months

Patient Information Local reactions can occur up to 7 days

Nursing Implications Defer immunization in individuals with moderate or severe febrile illness; do not give I.V.

Additional Information Inactivated bacteria vaccine

Dosage Forms Injection: Suspension of killed *Vibrio cholerae* (Inaba and Ogawa types) 8 units of each serotype per mL (1.5 mL, 20 mL)

Ciclopirox Olamine (sye kloe peer' ox)

Brand Names Loprox®

Generic Available No

Use Treatment of tinea pedis, tinea cruris, tinea corporis, cutaneous candidiasis, tinea versicolor

Pregnancy Risk Factor B

Contraindications Known hypersensitivity to ciclopirox

Warnings/Precautions For external use only; avoid contact with eyes

Adverse Reactions 1% to 10%: Irritation, redness, pain or burning; worsening of clinical condition

Mechanism of Action Inhibiting transport of essential elements in the fungal cell causing problems in synthesis of DNA, RNA and protein

Pharmacokinetics

Absorption: <2% of dose absorbed through intact skin

Distribution: To epidermis, corium (dermis), including hair, hair follicles, and sebaceous glands

Half-life: 1.7 hours

Elimination: Of the small amount of systemically absorbed drug, the majority is excreted by the kidney with small amounts excreted in feces

Usual Dosage Children >10 years and Adults: Apply twice daily, gently massage into affected areas; safety and efficacy in children <10 years have not been established

Patient Information Avoid contact with eyes; if sensitivity or irritation occurs, discontinue use

Dosage Forms

Cream, topical: 1% (15 g, 30 g, 90 g)

Lotion: 1% (30 mL)

Ciloxan™ Ophthalmic *see* Ciprofloxacin Hydrochloride
on next page

Cinobac® Pulvules® *see* Cinoxacin *on this page*

Cinoxacin (sin ox' a sin)

Brand Names Cinobac® Pulvules®

Generic Available No

Use Treatment of urinary tract infections

Pregnancy Risk Factor B

Contraindications History of convulsive disorders, hypersensitivity to cinoxacin or any component or other quinolones

Warnings/Precautions CNS stimulation may occur which may lead to tremor, restlessness, confusion, and very rarely to hallucinations or convulsive seizures. Use with caution in patients with known or suspected CNS disorders. Not recommended in children <18 years of age, ciprofloxacin (a related compound), has caused a transient arthropathy in children; prolonged use may result in superinfection; use with caution in patients with seizure disorders or renal impairment; modify dosage in patients with renal impairment

Adverse Reactions

1% to 10%: Headache, dizziness, heartburn, abdominal pain, GI bleeding, belching, flatulence, anorexia, nausea

<1%: Insomnia, confusion, diarrhea, thrombocytopenia, tinnitus, photophobia

Toxicology Symptoms of overdose include acute renal failure, seizures; GI decontamination and supportive care; diazepam for seizures; not removed by peritoneal or hemodialysis

Drug Interactions

Decreased urine levels with probenecid

Decreased absorption with aluminum-, magnesium-, calcium-containing antacids

Increased serum levels with probenecid

Mechanism of Action Inhibits microbial synthesis of DNA with resultant problems in protein synthesis

Pharmacokinetics

Absorption: Oral: Rapid and complete; food decreases peak levels by 30% but not total amount absorbed

Distribution: Crosses the placenta; concentrates in prostate tissue

Half-life: 1.5 hours, prolonged in renal impairment

Time to peak serum concentration: Oral: Within 2-3 hours

Elimination: ~60% excreted as unchanged drug in urine

Usual Dosage Children >12 years and Adults: Oral: 1 g/day in 2-4 doses for 7-14 days

Dosing interval in renal impairment:

Cl_{cr} 20-50 mL/minute: 250 mg twice daily

Cl_{cr} <20 mL/minute: 250 mg/day

Patient Information May be taken with food to minimize upset stomach; avoid antacid use; drink fluid liberally; may cause dizziness; use caution when driving or performing other tasks requiring alertness

Dosage Forms Capsule: 250 mg, 500 mg

Ciprofloxacin Hydrochloride (sip roe flox' a sin)

Related Information

Antimicrobial Activity Against Selected Organisms *on page 757-764*

Brand Names Ciloxan™ Ophthalmic; Cipro™ Injection; Cipro™ Oral

Generic Available No

Use Treatment of documented or suspected infection; documented multidrug-resistant gram-negative organisms; documented infectious diarrhea due to *Campylobacter jejuni*, *Shigella*, or *Salmonella*; osteomyelitis caused by susceptible organisms in which parenteral therapy is not feasible; used ophthalmically for treatment of corneal ulcers and conjunctivitis due to strains of microorganisms susceptible to ciprofloxacin

Drug of Choice or Alternative For

Disease/Syndrome(s)

Otitis Externa, Severe (Malignant) *on page 34*

Organism(s)

Haemophilus ducreyi on page 118

Legionella pneumophila on page 139

Mycobacterium avium-intracellulare on page 152

Neisseria gonorrhoeae on page 161

Pseudomonas aeruginosa on page 177
Rickettsia rickettsii on page 183
Salmonella Species *on page 185*
Shigella Species *on page 191*

Pregnancy Risk Factor C

Contraindications Hypersensitivity to ciprofloxacin, any component or other quinolones

Warnings/Precautions Not recommended in children <18 years of age; causes arthropathy in immature animals; CNS stimulation may occur which may lead to tremor, restlessness, confusion and very rarely to hallucinations or convulsive seizures. Use with caution in patients with known or suspected CNS disorders.

Adverse Reactions
1% to 10%: Nausea, diarrhea, vomiting, abdominal pain, headache, restlessness, rash
<1%: Tremor, dizziness, confusion, seizures, anemia, increased liver enzymes, arthralgia, acute renal failure

Drug Interactions
Decreased absorption with antacids containing aluminum, magnesium, and/or calcium by up to 98% if given at the same time
Increased toxicity/serum levels of caffeine, warfarin, cyclosporine, and theophylline; increased toxicity/levels with azlocillin, cimetidine, probenecid

Stability Refrigeration and room temperature: Prepared bags: 14 days; Premixed bags: Manufacturer expiration dating; Out of overwrap stability: 14 days

Mechanism of Action Inhibits DNA-gyrase in susceptible organisms; inhibits relaxation of supercoiled DNA and promotes breakage of double-stranded DNA

Pharmacokinetics
Absorption: Oral: Rapid from GI tract (~85%)
Distribution: Crosses the placenta; appears in breast milk; distributes widely throughout body; tissue concentrations often exceed serum concentrations especially in the kidneys, gallbladder, liver, lungs, gynecological tissue, and prostatic tissue; distributes to saliva, nasal secretions, aqueous humor, sputum, skin blister fluid, lymph, peritoneal fluid, bile, and prostatic secretions; also to skin, fat, muscle, bone, and cartilage; CSF concentrations reach 10% with noninflamed meninges and 14% to 37% with inflamed meninges
Metabolism: Partially metabolized in the liver
Half-life: 3-5 hours in patients with normal renal function
Time to peak serum concentration: Oral: Within 0.5-2 hours
Elimination: 30% to 50% excreted as unchanged drug in urine; 20% to 40% of dose excreted in feces primarily from biliary excretion

Usual Dosage
Children >18 years: Oral: 20-30 mg/kg/day in 2 divided doses; maximum dose: 1.5 g/day

Adults:
Oral: 250-750 mg every 12 hours, depending on severity of infection and susceptibility
I.V.: 200-400 mg every 12 hours depending on severity of infection
Ophthalmic: Instill 1-2 drops in eye(s) every 2 hours while awake for 2 days and 1-2 drops every 4 hours while awake for the next 5 days

Dosing adjustment in renal impairment: Cl_{cr} <30 mL/minute: Administer every 24 hours
Only small amounts of ciprofloxacin are removed by dialysis (<10%)

Monitoring Parameters Patients receiving concurrent ciprofloxacin and theophylline should have serum levels of theophylline monitored

Patient Information May be taken with food to minimize upset stomach; avoid antacid use; drink fluid liberally

Dosage Forms
Infusion, in D_5W: 400 mg (200 mL)
Infusion, in NS or D_5W: 200 mg (100 mL)
Injection: 200 mg (20 mL); 400 mg (40 mL)
Solution, ophthalmic: 3.5 mg/mL (2.5 mL, 5 mL)
Tablet: 250 mg, 500 mg, 750 mg

Selected Readings
Hooper DC and Wolfson JS, "Fluoroquinolone Antimicrobial Agents," *N Engl J Med*, 1991, 324(6):384-94.
Lomaestro BM and Bailie GR, "Quinolone-Cation Interactions: A Review," *DICP*, 1991, 25(11):1249-58.

Sanders CC, "Ciprofloxacin: *In Vitro* Activity, Mechanism of Action, and Resistance," *Rev Infect Dis*, 1988, 10(3):516-27.

Stein GE, "The 4-Quinolone Antibiotics: Past, Present, and Future," *Pharmacotherapy*, 1988, 8(6):301-14.

Walker RC and Wright AJ, "The Fluoroquinolones," *Mayo Clin Proc*, 1991, 66(12):1249-59.

Cipro™ Injection *see* Ciprofloxacin Hydrochloride *on page 537*

Cipro™ Oral *see* Ciprofloxacin Hydrochloride *on page 537*

Claforan® *see* Cefotaxime Sodium *on page 516*

Clarithromycin (kla rith' roe mye sin)

Related Information

Antimicrobial Activity Against Selected Organisms *on page 757-764*

Brand Names Biaxin™ Filmtabs®

Generic Available No

Use Active against most respiratory pathogens (eg, *S. pyogenes*, *S. pneumoniae*, *S. agalactiae*, *S. viridans*, *M. catarrhalis*, *C. trachomatis*, *Legionella* sp., *Mycoplasma pneumoniae*, *S. aureus*, *H. influenzae*). Additionally, clarithromycin has shown activity against *C. pneumoniae* (including strain TWAR) and *M. avium* infection.

Drug of Choice or Alternative For

Disease/Syndrome(s)

Sinusitis, Community-Acquired, Acute *on page 41*

Organism(s)

Legionella pneumophila on page 139

Mycobacterium avium-intracellulare on page 152

Ureaplasma urealyticum on page 225

Pregnancy Risk Factor C

Contraindications Hypersensitivity to clarithromycin, erythromycin, or any macrolide antibiotic

Warnings/Precautions In presence of severe renal impairment with or without coexisting hepatic impairment, decreased dosage or prolonged dosing interval may be appropriate; antibiotic-associated colitis has been reported with use of clarithromycin; geriatric patients experienced increased incidents of adverse effects due to known age-related decreases in renal function

Adverse Reactions

1% to 10%: Diarrhea, nausea, abnormal taste, dyspepsia, abdominal pain, headache

<1%: Ventricular tachycardia, torsade de pointes, elevated AST, alkaline phosphatase, and bilirubin, decreased white blood count, elevated prothrombin time, elevated BUN and serum creatinine

Drug Interactions Increased levels: Clarithromycin has been shown to increase serum **theophylline** levels by as much as 20%. **Carbamazepine** levels have been shown to increase after a single dose of clarithromycin. While other drug interactions (digoxin, anticoagulants, ergotamine, triazolam) known to occur with erythromycin have not been reported in clinical trials with clarithromycin, concurrent use of these drugs should be monitored closely.

Mechanism of Action Exerts its antibacterial action by binding to 50S ribosomal subunit resulting in inhibition of protein synthesis. The 14-OH metabolite of clarithromycin is twice as active as the parent compound.

Pharmacokinetics

Absorption: 50% from GI tract

Distribution: Widely distributed into most body tissues with the exception of the CNS

Metabolism: Partially converts to the microbiologically active metabolite, 14-OH clarithromycin

Half-life: 3-4 hours with a 250 mg dose and 5-7 hours with a 500 mg dose

Time to peak serum concentration: Oral: Within 2-4 hours

Elimination: ~20% to 30% of unchanged parent drug excreted in urine

Usual Dosage Safe use in children has not been established. Adults: Oral: Usual dose: 250-500 mg every 12 hours for 7-14 days

Upper respiratory tract: 250-500 mg every 12 hours for 10-14 days

Pharyngitis/tonsillitis: 250 mg every 12 hours for 10 days

Acute maxillary sinusitis: 500 mg every 12 hours for 14 days

Lower respiratory tract: 250-500 mg every 12 hours for 7-14 days

Acute exacerbation of chronic bronchitis due to:

M. catarrhalis and *S. pneumoniae*: 250 mg every 12 hours for 7-14 days

H. influenzae: 500 mg every 12 hours for 7-14 days

(Continued)

Clarithromycin *(Continued)*

Pneumonia due to *M. pneumoniae* and *S. pneumoniae*: 250 mg every 12 hours for 7-14 days

Uncomplicated skin and skin structure: 250 mg every 12 hours for 7-14 days

Dosing adjustment in severe renal impairment: Decreased doses or prolonged dosing intervals are recommended

Monitoring Parameters Monitor patients receiving clarithromycin and drugs known to interact with erythromycin (ie, theophylline, digoxin, anticoagulants, triazolam) since there are still very few studied examining drug-drug interactions with clarithromycin

Patient Information May be taken with or without meals; finish all medication; do not skip doses

Dosage Forms Tablet, film coated: 250 mg, 500 mg

Selected Readings
Barradell LB, Plosker GL, and McTavish D, "Clarithromycin. A Review of Its Pharmacological Properties and Therapeutic Use in *Mycobacterium avium-intracellulare* Complex Infection in Patients With Acquired Immune Deficiency Syndrome," *Drugs*, 1993, 46(2):289-312.
Goldman MP and Longworth DL, "The Role of Azithromycin and Clarithromycin in Clinical Practice," *Cleve Clin J Med*, 1993, 60(5):359-64.

Cleocin HCl® Oral *see* Clindamycin *on this page*

Cleocin Pediatric® Oral *see* Clindamycin *on this page*

Cleocin Phosphate® Injection *see* Clindamycin *on this page*

Cleocin T® Topical *see* Clindamycin *on this page*

Cleocin® Vaginal *see* Clindamycin *on this page*

Clindamycin *(klin da mye' sin)*

Related Information
Antimicrobial Activity Against Selected Organisms *on page 757-764*

Brand Names Cleocin HCl® Oral; Cleocin Pediatric® Oral; Cleocin Phosphate® Injection; Cleocin T® Topical; Cleocin® Vaginal

Generic Available Yes: Injection

Use Treatment of aerobic and anaerobic streptococci (except enterococci), most staphylococci, *Bacteroides* sp. and *Actinomyces*; used topically in treatment of severe acne

Drug of Choice or Alternative For
Disease/Syndrome(s)
Osteomyelitis, Diabetic Foot *on page 32*
Osteomyelitis, Healthy Adult *on page 33*
Osteomyelitis, Pediatric *on page 33*
Pelvic Inflammatory Disease *on page 35*
Peritonitis *on page 36*
Pneumonia, Aspiration, Community-Acquired *on page 37*
Sinusitis, Community-Acquired, Chronic *on page 41*
Skin and Soft Tissue *on page 42*
Vaginosis, Bacterial *on page 46*

Organism(s)
Babesia microti on page 57
Bacteroides Species *on page 61*
Clostridium perfringens on page 86
Staphylococcus aureus, Methicillin-Susceptible *on page 198*
Staphylococcus epidermidis, Methicillin-Susceptible *on page 201*
Streptococcus-Related Gram-Positive Cocci *on page 212*
Toxoplasma gondii on page 217

Pregnancy Risk Factor B

Contraindications Hypersensitivity to clindamycin or any component

Warnings/Precautions Use with caution in patients with a history of pseudomembranous colitis; can cause severe and possibly fatal colitis characterized by severe persistent diarrhea, severe abdominal cramps and possibly, the passage of blood and mucus; discontinue drug if significant diarrhea occurs; dosage adjustment may be necessary in patients with severe hepatic dysfunction

Adverse Reactions
>10%: Diarrhea

1% to 10%: Pseudomembranous colitis, nausea, vomiting, skin rashes

<1%: Thrombophlebitis, hypotension, urticaria, Stevens-Johnson syndrome, eosinophilia, neutropenia, granulocytopenia, thrombocytopenia, elevation of liver enzymes, sterile abscess at I.M. injection site, rare renal dysfunction, polyarthritis

Drug Interactions Increased duration of neuromuscular blockade from tubocurarine, pancuronium

Stability Do **not** refrigerate the reconstituted oral solution because it will thicken; oral solution stable for 2 weeks at room temperature following reconstitution; I.V. infusion solution in NS or D$_5$W solution is stable for 24 hours at room temperature

Mechanism of Action Reversibly binds to 50S ribosomal subunits preventing peptide bond formation thus inhibiting bacterial protein synthesis; bacteriostatic or bactericidal depending on drug concentration, infection site, and organism

Pharmacokinetics

Absorption: ~10% of topically applied drug is absorbed systemically; 90% absorbed rapidly from GI tract following oral administration

Distribution: No significant levels are seen in CSF, even with inflamed meninges; crosses the placenta; distributes into breast milk; high concentrations in bone, bile, and urine

Metabolism: Hepatic metabolism

Half-life:

Neonates:

Premature: 8.7 hours

Full-term: 3.6 hours

Adults: 1.6-5.3 hours, average: 2-3 hours

Time to peak serum concentration:

Oral: Within 60 minutes

I.M.: Within 1-3 hours

Elimination: Most of drug eliminated by hepatic metabolism

Usual Dosage

Neonates: I.M., I.V.:

<7 days:

≤2000 g: 5 mg/kg/dose every 12 hours

>2000 g: 5 mg/kg/dose every 8 hours

>7 days:

<1200 g: 5 mg/kg/dose every 12 hours

1200-2000 g: 5 mg/kg/dose every 8 hours

>2000 g: 5 mg/kg/dose every 6 hours

Infants and Children:

Oral: 10-30 mg/kg/day in 4 divided doses

I.M., I.V.: 25-40 mg/kg/day in 3-4 divided doses

Adults:

Oral: 150-450 mg/dose every 6-8 hours; maximum dose: 1.8 g/day

I.M., I.V.: 600 mg every 6-8 hours or 900 mg every 8 hours; maximum dose: 4.8 g/day

Dosing adjustment in hepatic impairment: Adjustment recommended in patients with severe hepatic disease

Children and Adults: Topical: Apply a thin film twice daily

Monitoring Parameters Observe for changes in bowel frequency; during prolonged therapy monitor CBC, liver and renal function tests periodically

Patient Information Report any severe diarrhea immediately and do not take antidiarrheal medication; take each oral dose with a full glass of water; finish all medication; do not skip doses

Additional Information In adults, clindamycin injection can usually be dosed effectively on an every 8-hour basis

Dosage Forms

Capsule, as hydrochloride: 75 mg, 150 mg, 300 mg

Cream, vaginal: 2% (40 g)

Gel, topical, as phosphate: 1% (7.5 g, 30 g)

Granules for oral solution, as palmitate: 75 mg/5 mL (100 mL)

Infusion, as phosphate, in D$_5$W: 300 mg (50 mL); 600 mg (50 mL)

Injection, as phosphate: 150 mg/mL (2 mL, 4 mL, 6 mL, 50 mL, 60 mL)

Lotion: 1% (60 mL)

(Continued)

Clindamycin *(Continued)*

Solution, topical, as phosphate: 1% (30 mL, 60 mL, 480 mL)

Selected Readings

Smilack JD, Wilson WR, and Cockerill FR 3d, "Tetracyclines, Chloramphenicol, Erythromycin, Clindamycin, and Metronidazole," *Mayo Clin Proc*, 1991, 66(12):1270-80.

Clofazimine (kloe fa' zi meen)

Brand Names Lamprene®

Generic Available No

Use Treatment of dapsone-resistant leprosy; multibacillary dapsone-sensitive leprosy; erythema nodosum leprosum; *Mycobacterium avium* intracellular (MAI) infections

Drug of Choice or Alternative For

Organism(s)

Mycobacterium avium-intracellulare on page 152

Pregnancy Risk Factor C

Contraindications Hypersensitivity to clofazimine or any component

Adverse Reactions

>10%: Pink to brownish-black discoloration of the skin and conjunctiva, dry skin, abdominal pain, nausea, vomiting, diarrhea

1% to 10%: Rash and pruritus, irritation of the eyes; discoloration of urine, feces, sputum, sweat; elevated blood sugar

<1%: Phototoxicity, erythroderma, acneform eruptions, monilial cheilosis, bowel obstruction, GI bleeding, anorexia, constipation, weight loss, hepatitis, jaundice, eosinophilic enteritis, enlarged liver, diminished vision, dizziness, drowsiness, fatigue, headache, giddiness, neuralgia, taste disorder; elevated albumin, serum bilirubin and AST; eosinophilia, hypokalemia, anemia, cystitis, bone pain, edema, fever, lymphadenopathy, vascular pain

Mechanism of Action Binds preferentially to mycobacterial DNA to inhibit mycobacterial growth; also has some anti-inflammatory activity through an unknown mechanism

Pharmacokinetics

Absorption: Oral: 45% to 70% absorbed slowly

Distribution: Remains in tissues for prolonged periods; appears in breast milk; highly lipophilic; deposited primarily in fatty tissue and cells of the reticuloendothelial system; taken up by macrophages throughout the body; also distributed to breast milk, mesenteric lymph nodes, adrenal glands, subcutaneous fat, liver, bile, gallbladder, spleen, small intestine, muscles, bones, and skin; does not appear to cross blood-brain barrier

Metabolism: Partially in the liver to two metabolites

Half-life:

Terminal: 8 days

Tissue: 70 days

Time to peak serum concentration: 1-6 hours with chronic therapy

Elimination: Excreted mainly in feces; negligible amounts excreted unchanged in urine; small amounts excreted in sputum, saliva, and sweat

Usual Dosage Oral:

Children: Leprosy: 1 mg/kg/day every 24 hours in combination with dapsone and rifampin

Adults:

MAI: Combination therapy using clofazimine 100 mg/day in combination with other antimycobacterial agents

Dapsone-resistant leprosy: 50-100 mg/day in combination with one or more antileprosy drugs for 2 years; then alone 50-100 mg/day

Dapsone-sensitive multibacillary leprosy: 50-100 mg/day in combination with two or more antileprosy drugs for at least 2 years and continue until negative skin smears are obtained, then institute single drug therapy with appropriate agent

Erythema nodosum leprosum: 100-200 mg/day for up to 3 months or longer then taper dose to 100 mg/day when possible

Patient Information Drug may cause a pink to brownish-black discoloration of the skin, conjunctiva, tears, sweat, urine, feces, and nasal secretions; take with meals

Dosage Forms Capsule: 50 mg, 100 mg

Selected Readings

"Drugs for AIDS and Associated Infections," *Med Lett Drugs Ther*, 1993, 35(904):79-86.
"Effect of Combined Therapy with Ansamycin, Clofazimine, Ethambutol, and Isoniazid for *Mycobacterium avium* Infection in Patients With AIDS," *J Infect Dis*, 1989, 159(4):784-7.

Hoy J, Mijch A, Sandland M, et al, "Quadruple-Drug Therapy for *Mycobacterium avium-intracellulare* Bacteremia in AIDS Patients," *J Infect Dis*, 1990, 161(4):801-5.

Kemper CA, Meng TC, Nussbaum J, et al, "Treatment of *Mycobacterium avium* Complex Bacteremia in AIDS With a Four-Drug Oral Regimen. Rifampin, Ethambutol, Clofazimine, and Ciprofloxacin" *Ann Intern Med*, 1992, 116(6):466-72.

Clotrimazole (kloe trim' a zole)

Brand Names Gyne-Lotrimin® Vaginal [OTC]; Lotrimin AF® Topical [OTC]; Lotrimin® Topical; Mycelex®-G Topical; Mycelex®-G Vaginal [OTC]; Mycelex® Troche

Generic Available Yes

Use Treatment of susceptible fungal infections, including oropharyngeal candidiasis, dermatophytoses, superficial mycoses, and cutaneous candidiasis, as well as vulvovaginal candidiasis; limited data suggests that the use of clotrimazole troches may be effective for prophylaxis against oropharyngeal candidiasis in neutropenic patients

Pregnancy Risk Factor B; C (oral)

Contraindications Hypersensitivity to clotrimazole or any component

Adverse Reactions

>10%: Abnormal liver function tests

1% to 10%: Nausea, vomiting, mild burning, irritation, stinging to skin or vaginal area

Mechanism of Action Binds to phospholipids in the fungal cell membrane altering cell wall permeability resulting in loss of essential intracellular elements

Pharmacokinetics

Absorption: Through intact skin is negligible when administered topically

Time to peak serum concentration:

Oral topical administration: Salivary levels occur within 3 hours following 30 minutes of dissolution time in the mouth

Vaginal cream: High vaginal levels occur within 8-24 hours following administration

Vaginal tablet: High vaginal levels occur within 1-2 days following administration

Elimination: Eliminated as metabolites via bile

Usual Dosage

Children >3 years and Adults:

Oral: 10 mg troche dissolved slowly 5 times/day

Topical: Apply twice daily; if not improvement occurs after 4 weeks of therapy, re-evaluate diagnosis

Adults: Vaginal:

Cream: Insert 5 g (= 1 applicatorful) of 1% vaginal cream daily for 7-14 days

Tablets: Insert 100 mg/day for 7 days or 200 mg/day for 3 days or 500 mg single dose

Patients treated for 14 days had a significantly higher cure rate

Monitoring Parameters Periodic liver function tests during oral therapy with clotrimazole lozenges

Patient Information May cause irritation to the skin; lozenge (troche) must be dissolved slowly in the mouth

Dosage Forms

Cream:

Topical (Lotrimin®, Lotrimin® AF, Mycelex®, Mycelex® OTC): 1% (15 g, 30 g, 45 g, 90 g)

Vaginal (Gyne-Lotrimin®, Mycelex®-G): 1% (45 g, 90 g)

Lotion (Lotrimin®): 1% (30 mL)

Solution, topical (Lotrimin®, Lotrimin® AF, Mycelex®, Mycelex® OTC): 1% (10 mL, 30 mL)

Tablet, vaginal (Gyne-Lotrimin®, Mycelex®-G): 100 mg (7s); 500 mg (1s)

Troche (Mycelex®): 10 mg

Twin pack (Mycelex®): Tablet 500 mg (1's) and vaginal cream 1% (7 g)

Cloxacillin Sodium (klox a sill' in)

Related Information

Antimicrobial Activity Against Selected Organisms *on page 757-764*

Brand Names Cloxapen®; Tegopen®

Generic Available Yes

Use Treatment of susceptible bacterial infections, notably penicillinase-producing staphylococci causing respiratory tract, skin and skin structure, bone and joint, urinary tract infections

(Continued)

Cloxacillin Sodium *(Continued)*

Pregnancy Risk Factor B

Contraindications Hypersensitivity to cloxacillin or any component, or penicillins

Warnings/Precautions Use with caution in patients allergic to cephalosporins

Adverse Reactions

1% to 10%: Nausea, diarrhea

<1%: Fever, rash, vomiting, eosinophilia, leukopenia, neutropenia, thrombocytopenia, agranulocytosis, serum sickness-like reactions, hepatotoxicity, hematuria

Toxicology Many beta-lactam containing antibiotics have the potential to cause neuromuscular hyperirritability or convulsive seizures. Hemodialysis may be helpful to aid in the removal of the drug from the blood, otherwise most treatment is supportive or symptom directed.

Drug Interactions Increased levels with probenecid

Stability Refrigerate oral solution after reconstitution; discard after 14 days; stable for 3 days at room temperature

Mechanism of Action Inhibits bacterial cell wall synthesis by binding to one or more of the penicillin binding proteins (PBPs); which in turn inhibits the final transpeptidation step of peptidoglycan synthesis in bacterial cell walls, thus inhibiting cell wall biosynthesis. Bacteria eventually lyse due to ongoing activity of cell wall autolytic enzymes (autolysins and murein hydrolases) while cell wall assembly is arrested.

Pharmacokinetics

Absorption: Oral: ~50%

Distribution: Crosses the placenta; appears in breast milk; distributed widely to most body fluids and bone; penetration into cells, into the eye, and across normal meninges is poor; inflammation increased amount that crosses the blood-brain barrier

Metabolism: Significantly in the liver to active and inactive metabolites

Half-life: 30-90 minutes (prolonged with renal impairment and in neonates)

Time to peak serum concentration: Within 30 minutes to 2 hours

Elimination: Metabolites excreted in urine and through bile

Usual Dosage Oral:

Children >1 month (<20 kg): 50-100 mg/kg/day in divided doses every 6 hours; up to a maximum of 4 g/day

Children (>20 kg) and Adults: 250-500 mg every 6 hours

Not dialyzable (0% to 5%)

Overdosage Neuromuscular hypersensitivity, convulsions

Test Interactions May interfere with urinary glucose tests using cupric sulfate (Benedict's solution, Clinitest®); may inactivate aminoglycosides *in vitro*; false-positive urine and serum proteins; false-positive in uric acid, urinary steroids

Patient Information Take 1 hour before or 2 hours after meals; finish all medication; do not skip doses

Additional Information Sodium content of 250 mg capsule: 13.8 mg (0.6 mEq); 5 mL of 125 mg/5 mL: 11 mg (0.48 mEq)

Dosage Forms

Capsule: 250 mg, 500 mg

Powder for oral suspension: 125 mg/5 mL (100 mL, 200 mL)

Selected Readings

Donowitz GR and Mandell GL, "Beta-Lactam Antibiotics," *N Engl J Med*, 1988, 318(7):419-26 and 318(8):490-500.

Wright AJ and Wilkowske CJ, "The Penicillins," *Mayo Clin Proc*, 1991, 66(10):1047-63.

Cloxapen® *see* Cloxacillin Sodium *on previous page*

CMV-IGIV *see* Cytomegalovirus Immune Globulin Intravenous, Human *on page 549*

Colistimethate Sodium (koe lis ti meth' ate)

Brand Names Coly-Mycin® M Parenteral

Generic Available No

Use Treatment of infections due to sensitive strains of certain gram-negative bacilli which are resistant to other antibacterials or in patients allergic to other antibacterials

Pregnancy Risk Factor B

Contraindications Hypersensitivity to colistimethate or any component

Warnings/Precautions Use with caution in patients with pre-existing renal disease

Adverse Reactions 1% to 10%: Respiratory arrest, nephrotoxicity, GI upset, vertigo, slurring of speech, urticaria

Drug Interactions Other nephrotoxic drugs, neuromuscular blocking agents

Stability Freshly prepare any infusion and use for no longer than 24 hours

Mechanism of Action Hydrolyzed to colistin, which acts as a cationic detergent which damages the bacterial cytoplasmic membrane causing leaking of intracellular substances and cell death

Pharmacokinetics
Distribution: Widely distributed, except for CNS, synovial, pleural, and pericardial fluids
Half-life: 1.5-8 hours; may be as high as 2-3 days in anuric patients
Elimination: Excreted primarily unchanged in urine
Peak: About 2 hours

Usual Dosage Children and Adults: I.M., I.V.: 2.5-5 mg/kg/day in 2-4 divided doses

Dosing interval in renal impairment:
S_{cr} 1.3-1.5 mg/dL: Administer 2.5-3.8 mg/kg/day in 2 divided doses
S_{cr} 1.6-2.5 mg/dL: Administer 2.5 mg/kg/day
S_{cr} 2.6-4 mg/dL: Administer 1.5 mg/kg every 36 hours

Dosage Forms Powder for injection, lyophilized: 150 mg

Colistin Sulfate (koe lis' tin)

Brand Names Coly-Mycin® S Oral

Synonyms Polymyxin E

Generic Available No

Use Treatment of diarrhea in infants and children caused by susceptible organisms, especially *E. coli* and *Shigella*; however, other agents are preferred

Pregnancy Risk Factor C

Contraindications Known hypersensitivity to colistin

Warnings/Precautions Use with caution in patients with impaired renal function; some systemic absorption may occur; potential for renal toxicity exists; prolonged use may lead to superinfection

Adverse Reactions <1%: Neuromuscular blockade, nephrotoxicity, respiratory arrest, nausea, vomiting, hypersensitivity reactions, superinfections

Stability Stable for 2 weeks when refrigerated, shake well; discard after 14 days

Mechanism of Action Polypeptide antibiotic that binds to and damages the bacterial cell membrane

Pharmacokinetics
Absorption: Oral: Slightly absorbed from GI tract (adults); unpredictable absorption occurs in infants, can lead to significant serum levels
Half-life: 2.8-4.8 hours, prolonged in renal insufficiency; with anuria: 48-72 hours
Elimination: ~65% to 75% excreted unchanged in urine

Usual Dosage Diarrhea: Children: Oral: 5-15 mg/kg/day in 3 divided doses given every 8 hours

Dosage Forms Powder for oral suspension: 25 mg/5 mL (60 mL)

Coly-Mycin® M Parenteral *see* Colistimethate Sodium
on previous page

Coly-Mycin® S Oral *see* Colistin Sulfate *on this page*

Compound S *see* Zidovudine *on page 696*

Cotrim® *see* Co-trimoxazole *on this page*

Cotrim® DS *see* Co-trimoxazole *on this page*

Co-trimoxazole (ko-tri mox' a zole)

Related Information
Antimicrobial Activity Against Selected Organisms *on page 757-764*

Brand Names Bactrim™; Bactrim™ DS; Cotrim®; Cotrim® DS; Septra®; Septra® DS; Sulfamethoprim®; Sulfatrim®; Sulfatrim® DS; Sulfoxaprim®; Sulfoxaprim® DS; Trisulfam®; Uroplus® DS; Uroplus® SS

Synonyms SMX-TMP; Sulfamethoxazole and Trimethoprim; TMP-SMX; Trimethoprim and Sulfamethoxazole

(Continued)

Co-trimoxazole (Continued)

Generic Available Yes

Use

Oral treatment of urinary tract infections; acute otitis media in children; acute exacerbations of chronic bronchitis in adults; prophylaxis of *Pneumocystis carinii* pneumonitis (PCP)

I.V. treatment of documented PCP, treatment of PCP in immune compromised patients; treatment of documented or suspected shigellosis, typhoid fever, *Nocardia asteroides* infection, or other infections caused by susceptible bacterial

Drug of Choice or Alternative For

Disease/Syndrome(s)

Bronchitis *on page 19*

Otitis Media, Acute *on page 35*

Pneumonia, Community-Acquired *on page 37*

Prostatitis *on page 39*

Sinusitis, Community-Acquired, Acute *on page 41*

Urinary Tract Infection, Perinephric Abscess *on page 45*

Urinary Tract Infection, Pyelonephritis *on page 45*

Urinary Tract Infection, Uncomplicated *on page 45*

Organism(s)

Bartonella Species *on page 62*

Bordetella pertussis on page 65

Brucella Species *on page 69*

Calymmatobacterium granulomatis on page 71

Escherichia coli, Nonenterohemorrhagic *on page 113*

Haemophilus ducreyi on page 118

Haemophilus influenzae on page 119

Listeria monocytogenes on page 143

Moraxella catarrhalis on page 147

Nocardia Species *on page 164*

Pneumocystis carinii on page 172

Salmonella Species *on page 185*

Shigella Species *on page 191*

Staphylococcus aureus, Methicillin-Resistant *on page 195*

Staphylococcus epidermidis, Methicillin-Resistant *on page 200*

Staphylococcus saprophyticus on page 203

Vibrio cholerae on page 230

Xanthomonas maltophilia on page 231

Pregnancy Risk Factor C

Contraindications Hypersensitivity to any sulfa drug or any component; porphyria; megaloblastic anemia due to folate deficiency; infants <2 months of age

Warnings/Precautions Use with caution in patients with G-6-PD deficiency, impaired renal or hepatic function; adjust dosage in patients with renal impairment; injection vehicle contains benzyl alcohol and sodium metabisulfite; fatalities associated with sulfonamides, although rare, have occurred due to severe reactions including Stevens-Johnson syndrome, toxic epidermal necrolysis, hepatic necrosis, agranulocytosis, aplastic anemia and other blood dyscrasias; discontinue use at first sign of rash; elderly patients appear at greater risk for more severe adverse reactions

Adverse Reactions

>10%: Nausea, vomiting, anorexia, allergic skin reactions including rashes and urticaria, photosensitivity

1% to 10%: Blood dyscrasias, hepatitis, Stevens-Johnson syndrome, toxic epidermal necrolysis

<1%: Confusion, depression, hallucinations, seizures, fever, ataxia, erythema multiforme, stomatitis, diarrhea, pseudomembranous colitis, thrombocytopenia, megaloblastic anemia, granulocytopenia, aplastic anemia, hemolysis (with G-6-PD deficiency), serum sickness, hepatitis, kernicterus in neonates, interstitial nephritis

Drug Interactions

Decreased effect of cyclosporines

Increased effect of sulfonylureas and oral anticoagulants

Increased toxicity/levels of phenytoin

Increased toxicity by displacing methotrexate from protein binding sites
Increased nephrotoxicity of cyclosporines

Stability Do not refrigerate injection; is less soluble in more alkaline pH; protect from light; do not use NS as a diluent; injection vehicle contains benzyl alcohol and sodium metabisulfite

Stability of parenteral admixture at room temperature (25°C):
5 mL/125 mL D_5W: 6 hours
5 mL/100 mL D_5W: 4 hours
5 mL/75 mL D_5W: 2 hours

Mechanism of Action Sulfamethoxazole interferes with bacterial folic acid synthesis and growth via inhibition of dihydrofolic acid formation from para-aminobenzoic acid; trimethoprim inhibits dihydrofolic acid reduction to tetrahydrofolate resulting in sequential inhibition of enzymes of the folic acid pathway

Pharmacokinetics

Absorption: Oral: Almost completely (90% to 100%)

Distribution: Crosses the placenta; distributes widely into body tissues, breast milk, and fluids including middle ear fluid, prostatic fluid, bile, aqueous humor, and CSF

Metabolism: TMP is metabolized to oxide and hydroxylated metabolites, SMX is N-acetylated and glucuronidated by liver

Half-life:
Sulfamethoxazole: 9 hours
Trimethoprim: 6-17 hours, both are prolonged in renal failure

Time to peak serum concentration: Oral: Within 1-4 hours

Elimination: Both are excreted in urine as metabolites and unchanged drug

Usual Dosage Dosage recommendations are based on the trimethoprim component

Children >2 months:
Mild to moderate infections: Oral, I.V.: 8 mg TMP/kg/day in divided doses every 12 hours
Serious infection/*Pneumocystis*: I.V.: 20 mg TMP/kg/day in divided doses every 6 hours
Urinary tract infection prophylaxis: Oral: 2 mg TMP/kg/dose daily
Prophylaxis of *Pneumocystis*: Oral, I.V.: 10 mg TMP/kg/day or 150 mg TMP/m^2/day in divided doses every 12 hours for 3 days/week; dose should not exceed 320 mg trimethoprim and 1600 mg sulfamethoxazole 3 days/week

Adults:
Urinary tract infection/chronic bronchitis: Oral: 1 double strength tablet every 12 hours for 10-14 days
Sepsis: I.V.: 15-20 mg TMP/kg/day divided every 6 hours
Pneumocystis carinii:
Prophylaxis: Oral: 1 double strength tablet daily or every other day
Treatment: I.V.: 15-20 mg TMP/kg/day divided every 6 hours

Dosing adjustment in renal impairment:
Cl_{cr} 30-50 mL/minute: Administer every 12-18 hours or reduce dose by 25%
Cl_{cr} 15-30 mL/minute: Administer every 18-24 hours or reduce dose by 50%
Cl_{cr} <15 mL/minute: Not recommended

Monitoring Parameters CBC for patients on long-term or high-dose therapy

Patient Information Take oral medication with 8 oz of water on an empty stomach (1 hour before or 2 hours after meals) for best absorption; report any skin rashes immediately; finish all medication

Nursing Implications Infuse over 60-90 minutes, must dilute well before giving; not for I.M. injection; maintain adequate fluid intake to prevent crystalluria

Dosage Forms

Infusion: Sulfamethoxazole 80 mg and trimethoprim 16 mg per mL (5 mL, 10 mL, 20 mL, 30 mL, 50 mL)

Suspension, oral: Sulfamethoxazole 200 mg and trimethoprim 40 mg per 5 mL (20 mL, 100 mL, 150 mL, 200 mL, 480 mL)

Tablet: Sulfamethoxazole 400 mg and trimethoprim 80 mg

Tablet, double strength: Sulfamethoxazole 800 mg and trimethoprim 160 mg

Selected Readings
Cockerill FR and Edson RS, "Trimethoprim-Sulfamethoxazole," *Mayo Clin Proc*, 1991, 66(12):1260-9.
Fischl MA, Dickinson GM, and La Voie L, "Safety and Efficacy of Sulfamethoxazole and Trimethoprim Chemoprophylaxis for *Pneumocystis carinii* Pneumonia in AIDS," *JAMA*, 1988, 259(8):1185-9.

(Continued)

Co-trimoxazole *(Continued)*

Hughes W, Leoung G, Kramer F, et al, "Comparison of Atovaquone (566C80) With Trimetho-prim-Sulfamethoxazole to Treat *Pneumocystis carinii* Pneumonia in Patients With AIDS," *N Engl J Med*, 1993, 328(21):1521-7.

Masur H, "Prevention and Treatment of *Pneumocystis* Pneumonia," *N Engl J Med*, 1992, 327(26):1853-60.

Sattler FR, Cowan R, Nielsen DM, et al, " Trimethoprim-Sulfamethoxazole Compared With Pentamidine for Treatment of *Pneumocystis carinii* Pneumonia in the Acquired Immu-nodeficiency Syndrome," *Ann Intern Med*, 1988, 109(4):280-7.

Crystalline Penicillin *see* Penicillin G, Parenteral *on page 633*

Crystalline Penicillin *see* Penicillin G Potassium, Oral *on page 635*

Crystal Violet *see* Gentian Violet *on page 578*

Crysticillin® A.S. *see* Penicillin G Procaine, Aqueous *on page 636*

Cycloserine *(sye kloe ser' een)*

Brand Names Seromycin® Pulvules®

Generic Available No

Use Adjunctive treatment in pulmonary or extrapulmonary tuberculosis

Pregnancy Risk Factor C

Contraindications Known hypersensitivity to cycloserine

Adverse Reactions

1% to 10%: Drowsiness, headache

<1%: Cardiac arrhythmias, dizziness, tremor, vertigo, seizures, confusion, psy-chosis, coma, paresis, rash, elevated liver enzymes, vitamin B_{12} deficiency, folate deficiency

Toxicology Administer 100-300 mg/day of pyridoxine to reduce neurotoxic ef-fects

Drug Interactions Increased toxicity with alcohol, isoniazid, ethionamide; cy-closerine inhibits the hepatic metabolism of phenytoin

Mechanism of Action Inhibits bacterial cell wall synthesis by competing with amino acid (D-alanine) for incorporation into the bacterial cell wall; bacterio-static or bactericidal

Pharmacokinetics

Absorption: Oral: ~70% to 90% from the GI tract

Distribution: Crosses the placenta; appears in breast milk; distributed widely to most body fluids and tissues including CSF, breast milk, bile, sputum, lymph tissue, lungs, and ascitic, pleural, and synovial fluids

Half-life: 10 hours in patients with normal renal function

Metabolism: Extensive in liver

Time to peak serum concentration: Oral: Within 3-4 hours

Elimination: 60% to 70% of oral dose excreted unchanged in urine by glomeru-lar filtration within 72 hours, small amounts excreted in feces, remainder is metabolized

Usual Dosage Tuberculosis: Oral:

Children: 10-20 mg/kg/day in 2 divided doses up to 1000 mg/day

Adults: Initial: 250 mg every 12 hours for 14 days, then give 500 mg to 1 g/day in 2 divided doses (maximum daily dose: 1 g)

Dosing adjustment in renal impairment:

Cl_{cr} 10-50 mL/minute: Administer every 24 hours

Cl_{cr} <10 mL/minute: Administer every 24-48 hours

Monitoring Parameters Periodic renal, hepatic, hematological tests, and plas-ma cycloserine concentrations

Reference Range Toxicity is greatly increased at levels >30 µg/mL

Patient Information May cause drowsiness; notify physician if skin rash, men-tal confusion, dizziness, headache, or tremors occur

Dosage Forms Capsule: 250 mg

Selected Readings

Davidson PT and Le HQ, "Drug Treatment of Tuberculosis – 1992," *Drugs*, 1992, 43(5):651-73.

"Drugs for Tuberculosis," *Med Lett Drugs Ther*, 1993, 35(908):99-101.

Iseman MD, "Treatment of Multidrug-Resistant Tuberculosis," *N Engl J Med*, 1993, 329(11):784-91.

CytoGam™ *see* Cytomegalovirus Immune Globulin Intravenous, Human *on next page*

Cytomegalovirus Immune Globulin Intravenous, Human (sye toe meg a low vi' rus)

Brand Names CytoGam™

Synonyms CMV-IGIV

Generic Available No

Use Prevention of primary CMV disease associated with kidney transplantation

Pregnancy Risk Factor C

Contraindications Hypersensitivity to any component, patients with selective immunoglobulin A deficiency (↑ potential for anaphylaxis)

Warnings/Precautions Studies indicate that product carries little or no risk for transmission of HIV

Adverse Reactions
1% to 10%: Flushing of the face, diaphoresis, muscle cramps, back pain, nausea, vomiting, wheezing
<1%: Dizziness, fever, headache, tightness in the chest, hypersensitivity reactions, chills

Drug Interactions May inactivate live virus vaccines (eg, measles, mumps, rubella)

Stability Use reconstituted product within 6 hours

Mechanism of Action CMV-IGIV is a preparation of immunoglobulin G derived from pooled healthy blood donors with a high titer of CMV antibodies

Usual Dosage I.V.:
Dosing schedule:
Initial dose (within 72 hours after transplant): 150 mg/kg/dose
2 weeks after transplant: 100 mg/kg/dose
4, 6, 8 weeks after transplant: 100 mg/kg/dose
12 and 16 weeks after transplant: 50 mg/kg/dose

Administration rate: Administer at 15 mg/kg/hour initially, then increase to 30 mg/kg/hour after 30 minutes if no untoward reactions, then increase to 60 mg/kg/hour after another 30 minutes, volume not to exceed 75 mL/hour

Nursing Implications I.V. use only; administer as separate infusion if pre-existing line; must be used diluted no more than 1:2

Dosage Forms Powder for injection, lyophilized: 2500 mg ± 250 mg (50 mL)

Selected Readings
Levinson ML and Jacobson PA, "Treatment and Prophylaxis of Cytomegalovirus Disease," *Pharmacotherapy*, 1992, 12(4):300-18.
Snydman DR, "Cytomegalovirus Immunoglobulins in the Prevention and Treatment of Cytomegalovirus Disease," *Rev Infect Dis*, 1990, 12(Suppl 7):S839-48.

Cytovene® *see* Ganciclovir *on page 574*

d4T *see* Stavudine *on page 668*

Dapsone (dap' sone)

Brand Names Avlosulfon®

Synonyms Diaminodiphenylsulfone

Generic Available No

Use Treatment of leprosy and dermatitis herpetiformis; prophylaxis and treatment of *Pneumocystis carinii*

Pregnancy Risk Factor C

Contraindications Hypersensitivity to dapsone or any component

Warnings/Precautions Use with caution in patients with severe anemia, G-6-PD deficiency; hypersensitivity to other sulfonamides

Adverse Reactions
1% to 10%: Dose-related hemolysis, methemoglobinemia with cyanosis, reactional states
<1%: Peripheral neuropathy, insomnia, headache, exfoliative dermatitis, nausea, vomiting, hemolytic anemia, methemoglobinemia, leukopenia, agranulocytosis, hepatitis, cholestatic jaundice, blurred vision, tinnitus

Toxicology Symptoms of overdose include nausea, vomiting, hyperexcitability, methemoglobin-induced depression, seizures, cyanosis, hemolysis; following decontamination, methylene blue 1-2 mg/kg I.V. is treatment of choice; activated charcoal will increase elimination three- to five-fold

Drug Interactions
Decreased effect with para-aminobenzoic acid; decreased effect/levels with rifampin, didanosine
Increased toxicity with folic acid antagonists

Stability Protect from light

(Continued)

Dapsone *(Continued)*

Mechanism of Action Dapsone is a sulfone antimicrobial; the mechanism of action of the sulfones is similar to that of the sulfonamides; sulfonamides are competitive antagonists of para-aminobenzoic acid (PABA) and prevent normal bacterial utilization of PABA for the synthesis of folic acid

Pharmacokinetics

Absorption: Oral: Well absorbed

Distribution: Throughout total body water and present in all tissues, especially liver and kidney

Metabolism: In the liver

Half-life, elimination: 30 hours (range: 10-50 hours)

Elimination: Excreted in urine

Usual Dosage Oral:

Children: Leprosy: 1-2 mg/kg/24 hours; maximum: 100 mg/day

Adults:

Leprosy: 50-100 mg/day for 3-10 years

Dermatitis herpetiformis: Start at 50 mg/day, increase to 300 mg/day, or higher to achieve full control, reduce dosage to minimum level as soon as possible

PCP prophylaxis: 100 mg every other day or 50 mg/day

PCP treatment: 100 mg/day with trimethoprim 15-20 mg/kg/day in divided doses

Patient Information Frequent blood tests are required during early therapy; discontinue if rash develops and contact physician if persistent sore throat, fever, malaise, or fatigue occurs; may cause photosensitivity

Nursing Implications Monitor patient for signs of jaundice and hemolysis

Dosage Forms Tablet: 25 mg, 100 mg

Selected Readings

Medina I, Mills J, Leoung G, et al, "Oral Therapy for *Pneumocystis carinii* Pneumonia in the Acquired Immunodeficiency Syndrome. A Controlled Trial of Trimethoprim-Sulfamethoxazole Versus Trimethoprim-Dapsone," *N Engl J Med*, 1990, 323(12):776-82.

Daraprim® *see* Pyrimethamine *on page 653*

ddC *see* Zalcitabine *on page 695*

ddl *see* Didanosine *on page 552*

Declomycin® *see* Demeclocycline Hydrochloride *on this page*

Demeclocycline Hydrochloride *(dem e kloe sye' kleen)*

Brand Names Declomycin®

Synonyms Demethylchlortetracycline

Generic Available No

Use Treatment of susceptible bacterial infections (acne, gonorrhea, pertussis and urinary tract infections) caused by both gram-negative and gram-positive organisms (other agents are preferred); treatment of chronic syndrome of inappropriate secretion of antidiuretic hormone (SIADH)

Pregnancy Risk Factor D

Contraindications Hypersensitivity to demeclocycline, tetracyclines, or any component

Warnings/Precautions Do not administer to children <9 years of age; photosensitivity reactions occur frequently with this drug, avoid prolonged exposure to sunlight, do not use tanning equipment

Adverse Reactions

1% to 10%: Nausea, diarrhea, photosensitivity

<1%: Increased intracranial pressure, bulging fontanels in infants, paresthesia, dermatologic effects, diabetes insipidus syndrome, vomiting, esophagitis, anorexia, abdominal cramps, acute renal failure, azotemia, superinfections, pericarditis, anaphylaxis, pruritus, pigmentation of nails, exfoliative dermatitis

Toxicology Symptoms of overdose include diabetes insipidus, nausea, anorexia, diarrhea; following GI decontamination, treatment is supportive

Drug Interactions

Decreased effect with antacids (aluminum, calcium, zinc, or magnesium), bismuth salts, sodium bicarbonate, barbiturates, carbamazepine, hydantoins; decreased effect of oral contraceptives

Increased effect of warfarin

Mechanism of Action Inhibits protein synthesis by binding with the 30S and possibly the 50S ribosomal subunit(s) of susceptible bacteria; may also cause alterations in the cytoplasmic membrane

Pharmacokinetics
Onset of action for diuresis in SIADH: Several days
Absorption: ~50% to 80% from GI tract; food and dairy products reduce absorption
Metabolism: Small amounts metabolized in the liver to inactive metabolites; enterohepatically recycled
Time to peak serum concentration: Oral: Within 3-6 hours
Elimination: Excreted as unchanged drug (42% to 50%) in urine

Usual Dosage Oral:
Children ≥8 years: 8-12 mg/kg/day divided every 6-12 hours

Adults: 150 mg 4 times/day or 300 mg twice daily
SIADH: 900-1200 mg/day or 13-15 mg/kg/day divided every 6-8 hours initially, then decrease to 0.6-0.9 g/day

Dosing adjustment/comments in renal/hepatic impairment: Should be avoided in patients with renal/hepatic dysfunction

Monitoring Parameters CBC, renal and hepatic function

Test Interactions May interfere with tests for urinary glucose (false-negative urine glucose using Clinistix®, Tes-Tape®)

Patient Information Avoid prolonged exposure to sunlight or sunlamps; avoid taking antacids before tetracyclines

Nursing Implications Administer 1 hour before or 2 hours after food or milk with plenty of fluid

Dosage Forms
Capsule: 150 mg
Tablet: 150 mg, 300 mg

Selected Readings
Smilack JD, Wilson WR, and Cockerill FR 3d, "Tetracyclines, Chloramphenicol, Erythromycin, Clindamycin, and Metronidazole," *Mayo Clin Proc*, 1991, 66(12):1270-80.

Demethylchlortetracycline see Demeclocycline Hydrochloride *on previous page*

Devrom® [OTC] *see* Bismuth *on page 505*

Dey-Drop® Ophthalmic Solution *see* Silver Nitrate *on page 666*

DFMO *see* Eflornithine Hydrochloride *on page 559*

DHPG Sodium *see* Ganciclovir *on page 574*

Diaminodiphenylsulfone *see* Dapsone *on page 549*

Dicloxacillin Sodium (dye klox a sill' in)
Related Information
Antimicrobial Activity Against Selected Organisms *on page 757-764*
Brand Names Dycill®; Dynapen®; Pathocil®
Generic Available Yes
Use Treatment of systemic infections such as pneumonia, skin and soft tissue infections, and osteomyelitis caused by penicillinase-producing staphylococci
Pregnancy Risk Factor B
Contraindications Known hypersensitivity to dicloxacillin, other penicillins, or any components
Adverse Reactions
1% to 10%: Diarrhea
<1%: Fever, rash, nausea, vomiting, eosinophilia, neutropenia, leukopenia, thrombocytopenia, serum sickness-like reaction, elevation in liver enzymes
Toxicology Many beta-lactam containing antibiotics have the potential to cause neuromuscular hyperirritability or convulsive seizures. Hemodialysis may be helpful to aid in the removal of the drug from the blood, otherwise most treatment is supportive or symptom directed.
Drug Interactions
Decreased effect of warfarin
Increased effect with probenecid
Stability Refrigerate suspension after reconstitution; discard after 14 days if refrigerated or 7 days if kept at room temperature
Mechanism of Action Inhibits bacterial cell wall synthesis by binding to one or more of the penicillin binding proteins (PBPs); which in turn inhibits the final transpeptidation step of peptidoglycan synthesis in bacterial cell walls, thus
(Continued)

Dicloxacillin Sodium *(Continued)*

inhibiting cell wall biosynthesis. Bacteria eventually lyse due to ongoing activity of cell wall autolytic enzymes (autolysins and murein hydrolases) while cell wall assembly is arrested.

Pharmacokinetics
Absorption: 35% to 76% from GI tract

Distribution: Crosses the placenta; distributes into breast milk; distributed throughout body with highest concentrations in kidney and liver; CSF penetration is low

Metabolism: Partially eliminated by the liver

Half-life: 0.6-0.8 hour; elimination is prolonged in neonates

Time to peak serum concentration: Within 30 minutes to 2 hours

Elimination: Partially excreted in bile; metabolites of unchanged drug excreted in urine

Usual Dosage Oral:
Children <40 kg: 12.5-50 mg/kg/day divided every 6 hours; doses of 50-100 mg/kg/day in divided doses every 6 hours have been used for follow-up therapy of osteomyelitis

Children >40 kg and Adults: 125-500 mg every 6 hours

Not dialyzable (0% to 5%)

Overdosage Neuromuscular hypersensitivity, convulsions

Monitoring Parameters Periodic monitoring of CBC, UA, BUN, serum creatinine, and liver enzymes during prolonged therapy

Test Interactions False-positive urine and serum proteins; false-positive in uric acid, urinary steroids; may interfere with urinary glucose tests using cupric sulfate (Benedict's solution, Clinitest®); may inactivate aminoglycosides *in vitro*

Patient Information Take until all medication used; take 1 hour before or 2 hours after meals, do not skip doses

Additional Information
Sodium content of 250 mg capsule: 13 mg (0.6 mEq)

Sodium content of suspension 65 mg/5 mL: 27 mg (1.2 mEq)

Dosage Forms
Capsule: 125 mg, 250 mg, 500 mg

Powder for oral suspension: 62.5 mg/5 mL (80 mL, 100 mL, 200 mL)

Selected Readings
Donowitz GR and Mandell GL, "Beta-Lactam Antibiotics," *N Engl J Med*, 1988, 318(7):419-26 and 318(8):490-500.

Wright AJ and Wilkowske CJ, "The Penicillins," *Mayo Clin Proc*, 1991, 66(10):1047-63.

Didanosine (dye dan' oh seen)
Brand Names Videx® Oral

Synonyms ddl; Dideoxyinosine

Generic Available No

Use Treatment of advanced HIV infection in patients who are intolerant of zidovudine therapy or who have demonstrated significant clinical or immunologic deterioration during zidovudine therapy

Drug of Choice or Alternative For
Organism(s)
Human Immunodeficiency Virus *on page 133*

Pregnancy Risk Factor B

Contraindications Hypersensitivity to any component

Warnings/Precautions Didanosine is indicated for treatment of HIV infection only in patients intolerant of zidovudine or who have failed zidovudine. Patients receiving didanosine may still develop opportunistic infections. Peripheral neuropathy occurs in ~35% of patients receiving the drug; pancreatitis occurs in ~97% of patients receiving didanosine; patients should undergo retinal examination every 6 months to 1 year. Use with caution in patients with decreased renal or hepatic function; in high concentrations, didanosine is mutagenic; use with caution in patients with edema or congestive heart failure; use with caution in patients with hyperuricemia

Adverse Reactions
>10%: Peripheral neuropathy, anxiety, headache, irritability, insomnia, restlessness, abdominal pain, nausea, diarrhea

1% to 10%: Pancreatitis

<1%: Anemia, granulocytopenia, leukopenia, thrombocytopenia, hepatitis, hypersensitivity, retinal depigmentation, seizures

Toxicology Chronic overdose may cause pancreatitis, peripheral neuropathy, diarrhea, hyperuricemia, and hepatic impairment; there is no known antidote for didanosine overdose

Drug Interactions Decreased absorption of tetracyclines, ketoconazole, dapsone, and quinolones if given together; H_2 antagonists, antacids may increase absorption of didanosine

Stability Pediatric oral solution is stable 30 days under refrigeration

Mechanism of Action Didanosine, a purine nucleoside analogue and the deamination product of dideoxyadenosine (DDA), inhibits HIV replication *in vitro* in both T cells and monocytes. Didanosine is converted within the cell to the mono-, di-, and triphosphates of DDA. These DDA triphosphates act as substrate and inhibitor of HIV reverse transcriptase substrate and inhibitor of HIV reverse transcriptase thereby blocking viral DNA synthesis and suppressing HIV replication.

Usual Dosage Oral (administer on an empty stomach):
Children: Dosing is based on body surface area (m^2):
  <0.4: 25 mg tablets twice daily or 31 mg powder twice daily
  0.5-0.7: 50 mg tablets twice daily or 62 mg powder twice daily
  0.8-1: 75 mg tablets twice daily or 94 mg powder twice daily
  1.1-1.4: 100 mg tablets twice daily or 125 mg powder twice daily
Adults: Dosing is based on patient weight:
  35-49 kg: 125 mg tablets twice daily or 167 mg buffered powder twice daily
  50-74 kg: 200 mg tablets twice daily or 250 mg buffered powder twice daily
  ≥75 kg: 300 mg tablets twice daily or 375 mg buffered powder twice daily

Note: Children >1 year of age and Adults should receive 2 tablets per dose and children <1 year should receive 1 tablet per dose for adequate buffering and absorption; tablets should be chewed

Dosing adjustment in renal impairment: Should be considered in patients with Cl_{cr} <60 mL/minute

Dosing adjustment in hepatic impairment: Should be considered

Overdosage Chronic overdose may cause pancreatitis, peripheral neuropathy, diarrhea, hyperuricemia, and hepatic impairment

Monitoring Parameters Serum potassium, uric acid, creatinine; hemoglobin, CBC with neutrophil and platelet count, CD_4 cells; liver function tests, amylase; weight gain; perform dilated retinal exam every 6 months

Patient Information Thoroughly chew tablets or manually crush or disperse 2 tablets in 1 oz of water prior to taking; for powder, open packet and pour contents into 4 oz of liquid; do not mix with fruit juice or other acid containing liquid; stir until dissolved, drink immediately

Nursing Implications Administer liquified powder immediately after dissolving; avoid creating dust if powder spilled, use wet mop or damp sponge

Additional Information Sodium content of buffered tablets: 264.5 mg (11.5 mEq)

Dosage Forms
Powder for oral solution:
  Buffered (single dose packet): 100 mg, 167 mg, 250 mg, 375 mg
  Pediatric: 2 g, 4 g
Tablet, buffered, chewable (mint flavor): 25 mg, 50 mg, 100 mg, 150 mg

Selected Readings
Hirsch MS and D'Aquila RT, "Therapy for Human Immunodeficiency Virus Infection," *N Engl J Med*, 1993, 328(23):1686-95.
Rathbun RC and Martin ES 3d, "Didanosine Therapy in Patients Intolerant of or Failing Zidovudine Therapy," *Ann Pharmacother*, 1992, 26(11):1347-51.
Sande MA, Carpenter CC, Cobbs CG, et al, "Antiretroviral Therapy for Adult HIV-Infected Patients," *JAMA*, 1993, 270(21):2583-9.

Dideoxycytidine *see* Zalcitabine *on page 695*

Dideoxyinosine *see* Didanosine *on previous page*

Diflucan® *see* Fluconazole *on page 569*

Diiodohydroxyquin *see* Iodoquinol *on page 591*

Diloxanide Furoate (dye lox' a nide)
Brand Names Furamide®
Generic Available No
Use Treatment of amebiasis (asymptomatic cyst passers)
Drug of Choice or Alternative For
Organism(s)
  Entamoeba histolytica on page 102

Additional Information Available from:

The Centers for Disease Control Drug and Immunobiologic Service
1600 Clifton Road
Building 1
Room 1259
Atlanta, GA 30333
  Monday-Friday 8 AM to 4:30 PM
  (404) 639-3670
  Nonbusiness hours (emergencies only): (404) 639-2888

Selected Readings
  "Drugs for Parasitic Infections," *Med Lett Drugs Ther*, 1993, 35(911):111-22.

Dimethoxyphenyl Penicillin Sodium *see* Methicillin Sodium
  on page 608

Diphtheria and Tetanus Toxoid (dif theer' ee a)

Synonyms DT; Tetanus and Diphtheria Toxoid

Generic Available Yes

Use Active immunity against diphtheria and tetanus; tetanus prophylaxis in wound management

Pregnancy Risk Factor B

Contraindications Patients receiving immunosuppressive agents, prior anaphylactic, allergic, or systemic reactions; hypersensitivity to diphtheria and tetanus toxoid or any component

Warnings/Precautions Pregnancy is not a contraindication; however, waiting until the second trimester of pregnancy to administer tetanus and diphtheria toxoids is reasonable to minimize concern over teratogenicity. History of a neurologic reaction or immediate hypersensitivity reaction following a previous dose. History of severe local reaction (arthus-type) following previous dose; such individuals should not be given further routine or emergency doses of tetanus and diphtheria toxoids for 10 years.

Adverse Reactions All serious adverse reactions must be reported to the FDA.
  >10%: Fretfulness, drowsiness
  1% to 10%: Anorexia, vomiting, persistent crying
  <1%: Transient fever convulsions (rarely), tenderness, swelling, redness, pain, Arthus-type hypersensitivity reactions, tachycardia, hypotension, urticaria, pruritus

Drug Interactions Decreased effect with immunosuppressive agents, immunoglobulins if given within 1 month

Stability Refrigerate

Usual Dosage I.M.:

Infants and Children:

6 weeks to 1 year: Three 0.5 mL doses at least 4 weeks apart; give a reinforcing dose 6-12 months after the third injection

1-6 years: Two 0.5 mL doses at least 4 weeks apart; reinforcing dose 6-12 months after second injection; if final dose is given after seventh birthday, use adult preparation

4-6 years (booster immunization): 0.5 mL; not necessary if all 4 doses were given after fourth birthday – routinely give booster doses at 10-year intervals with the adult preparation

Children >7 years and Adults: Should receive T_d; 2 primary doses of 0.5 mL each, given at an interval of 4-6 weeks; third (reinforcing) dose of 0.5 mL 6-12 months later; boosters every 10 years

Patient Information A nodule may be palpable at the injection site for a few weeks

Nursing Implications Shake well before giving; do not inject the same site more than once

Additional Information Pediatric dosage form should only be used in patients ≤6 years of age. Federal law requires that the date of administration, the vaccine manufacturer, lot number of vaccine, and the administering person's name, title, and address be entered into the patient's permanent medical record.

Dosage Forms Injection:

Pediatric use:

Diphtheria 6.6 Lf units and tetanus 5 Lf units per 0.5 mL (5 mL)
Diphtheria 10 Lf units and tetanus 5 Lf units per 0.5 mL (0.5 mL, 5 mL)
Diphtheria 12.5 Lf units and tetanus 5 Lf units per 0.5 mL (5 mL)
Diphtheria 15 Lf units and tetanus 10 Lf units per 0.5 mL (5 mL)

Adult use:

Diphtheria 1.5 Lf units and tetanus 5 Lf units per 0.5 mL (0.5 mL, 5 mL)
Diphtheria 2 Lf units and tetanus 5 Lf units per 0.5 mL (5 mL)
Diphtheria 2 Lf units and tetanus 10 Lf units per 0.5 mL (5 mL)

Diphtheria and Tetanus Toxoids and Acellular Pertussis Vaccine (dif theer' ee a)

Related Information
Vaccines *on page 706-709*

Brand Names Acel-Immune®; Tripedia®

Synonyms DTaP

Therapeutic Class 80:08 Toxoids

Use Fourth or fifth immunization of children 15 months to 7 years of age (prior to seventh birthday) who have been previously immunized with 3 or 4 doses of whole-cell pertussis DTP vaccine

Pregnancy Risk Factor B

Contraindications Patients >7 years of age, patients with cancer, immunodeficiencies, an acute respiratory infection, or any other active infection; children with a history of neurologic disorders should not receive the pertussis or any component; history of any of the following effects from previous administration of pertussis vaccine precludes further use: >103°F fever (39.4°C), convulsions, focal neurologic signs, screaming episodes, shock, collapse, sleepiness or encephalopathy; known hypersensitivity to diphtheria and tetanus toxoids or pertussis vaccine; do not use for treatment of actual tetanus, diphtheria, or whooping cough infections

Warnings/Precautions DTaP should not be used in children <15 months of age and should not be used in children who have received fewer than 3 doses of DTP

Adverse Reactions All serious adverse reactions must be reported to the FDA.
<1%: Convulsions, screaming episodes, malaise sleepiness, focal neurological signs, shock, collapse, fever, erythema, swelling, induration, rash, urticaria, local tenderness, arthralgias, chills, all serious adverse reactions must be reported to FDA

Drug Interactions Decreased effect with Immunosuppressive agents, corticosteroids within 1 month

Stability Refrigerate

Mechanism of Action Promotes active immunity to diphtheria, tetanus, and pertussis by inducing production of specific antibodies and antitoxins.

Usual Dosage I.M.:
4th dose: 0.5 mL at 18 months of age, at least 6 months after 3rd DTwP dose
5th dose: 0.5 mL at 4-6 years of age

Patient Information A nodule may be palpable at the injection site for a few weeks

Nursing Implications Ensure that at least 3 doses of whole-cell DTwP vaccine have been previously given. Acetaminophen 10-15 mg/kg before and every 4 hours to 12-24 hours may reduce or prevent fever; shake well before administering; the child's medical record should document that the small risk of past vaccination seizure and the benefits of the pertussis vaccination were discussed with the patient.

Additional Information This preparation contains less endotoxin relative to DTP and, although immunogenic, it apparently is less reactogenic than DTP. Federal law requires that the date of administration, the vaccine manufacturer, lot number of vaccine, and the administering person's name, title, and address be entered into the patient's permanent medical record.

Dosage Forms Injection:
Acel-Immune®: Diphtheria 7.5 Lf units, tetanus 5 Lf units, and acellular pertussis vaccine 40 µg per 0.5 mL (7.5 mL)
Tripedia®: Diphtheria 6.7 Lf units, tetanus 5 Lf units, and acellular pertussis vaccine 46.8 µg per 0.5 mL (7.5 mL)

Diphtheria CRM$_{197}$ Protein Conjugate *see* Hemophilus b Conjugate Vaccine *on page 580*

Diphtheria, Tetanus Toxoids, and Whole-Cell Pertussis Vaccine (dif theer' ee a)

Related Information

Vaccines *on page 706-709*

Brand Names Tri-Immunol®

Synonyms DPT; DTP; DTwP

Generic Available Yes

Use Active immunization of infants and children through 6 years of age (between 2 months and the seventh birthday) against diphtheria, tetanus, and pertussis; recommended for both primary immunization and routine recall; start immunization at once if whooping cough or diphtheria is present in the community

Pregnancy Risk Factor B

Contraindications Patients >7 years of age, patients with cancer, immunodeficiencies, an acute respiratory infection, or any other active infection; children with a history of neurologic disorders should not receive the pertussis any component; history of any of the following effects from previous administration of pertussis vaccine precludes further use: fever >103°F (39.4°C), convulsions, focal neurologic signs, screaming episodes, shock, collapse, sleepiness or encephalopathy; known hypersensitivity to diphtheria and tetanus toxoids or pertussis vaccine; do not use DTP for treatment of actual tetanus, diphtheria or whooping cough infections

Warnings/Precautions If adverse reactions occurred with previous doses, immunization should be completed with diphtheria and tetanus toxoid absorbed (pediatric)

Adverse Reactions All serious adverse reactions must be reported to FDA

Convulsions, screaming episodes, malaise, sleepiness, focal neurological signs, shock, collapse, fever, chills, erythema, swelling, induration, rash, urticaria, local tenderness, arthralgias, warmth, increased risk of *Haemophilus* b infections in the week after vaccination, rarely allergic or anaphylactic reactions

Drug Interactions Immunosuppressive agents

Stability Refrigerate

Mechanism of Action Promotes active immunity to diphtheria, tetanus, and pertussis by inducing production of specific antibodies and antitoxins.

Usual Dosage The primary immunization for children 2 months to 6 years of age, ideally beginning at the age of 2-3 months or at 6-week check-up. Administer 0.5 mL I.M. on 3 occasions at 4- to 8-week intervals with a re-enforcing dose administered 1 year after the third injection. The booster doses are given when children are 4-6 years of age, 0.5 mL I.M.

Patient Information A nodule may be palpable at the injection site for a few weeks

Nursing Implications Acetaminophen 10-15 mg/kg before and every 4 hours to 12-24 hours may reduce or prevent fever; shake well before administering; federal law requires that the date of administration, the vaccine manufacturer, lot number of vaccine and the administering person's name, title and address be entered into the patient's permanent medical record; the child's medical record should document that the small risk of past vaccination seizure and the benefits of the pertussis vaccination were discussed with the patient

Additional Information Acellular pertussis vaccine indicated for fourth or fifth booster dose of the five-part DTP series for children, indicated specifically for children 15 months of age

Dosage Forms Injection:

Diphtheria 6.7 Lf units, tetanus 5 Lf units, and pertussis 4 protective units per 0.5 mL (7.5 mL)

Tri-Immunol®: Diphtheria 12.5 Lf units, tetanus 5 Lf units, and pertussis 4 protective units per 0.5 mL (7.5 mL)

Diphtheria, Tetanus Toxoids, and Whole-cell Pertussis Vaccine and Hemophilus b Conjugate Vaccine

Brand Names Tetramune®

Use Active immunization of infants and children through 5 years of age (between 2 months and the sixth birthday) against diphtheria, tetanus, and pertussis and Hemophilus b disease when indications for immunization with DTP vaccine and HIB vaccine coincide

Pregnancy Risk Factor B

Contraindications Children with any febrile illness or active infection, known hypersensitivity to *Haemophilus* b polysaccharide vaccine (thimerosal), children who are immunosuppressed or receiving immunosuppressive therapy; patients >7 years of age, patients with cancer, immunodeficiencies, an acute respiratory infection, or any other active infection; children with a history of neurologic disorders should not receive the pertussis any component; history of any of the following effects from previous administration of pertussis vaccine precludes further use: fever >103°F (39.4°C), convulsions, focal neurologic signs, screaming episodes, shock, collapse, sleepiness or encephalopathy; known hypersensitivity to diphtheria and tetanus toxoids or pertussis vaccine; do not use DTP for treatment of actual tetanus, diphtheria or whooping cough infections

Warnings/Precautions If adverse reactions occurred with previous doses, immunization should be completed with diphtheria and tetanus toxoid absorbed (pediatric); any febrile illness or active infection is reason for delaying use of *Haemophilus* b conjugate vaccine

Adverse Reactions All serious adverse reactions must be reported to the FDA.
>10%: Erythema, swelling, pain and warmth at injection site, fever, irritability, restlessness, drowsiness
1% to 10%: Rash, vomiting, diarrhea, loss of appetite

Drug Interactions Immunosuppressive agents; may interfere with antigen detection tests

Stability Keep in refrigerator, may be frozen (not diluent) without affecting potency

Mechanism of Action Promotes active immunity to diphtheria, tetanus, pertussis, and *H. influenzae* by inducing production of specific antibodies and antitoxins.

Usual Dosage The primary immunization for children 2 months to 5 years of age, ideally beginning at the age of 2-3 months or at 6-week check-up. Administer 0.5 mL I.M. on 3 occasions at ~2 month intervals, followed by a fourth 0.5 mL dose at ~15 months of age

Patient Information A nodule may be palpable at the injection site for a few weeks

Nursing Implications Acetaminophen 10-15 mg/kg before and every 4 hours to 12-24 hours may reduce or prevent fever; shake well before administering; federal law requires that the date of administration, the vaccine manufacturer, lot number of vaccine and the administering person's name, title and address be entered into the patient's permanent medical record; the child's medical record should document that the small risk of past vaccination seizure and the benefits of the pertussis vaccination were discussed with the patient

Dosage Forms Injection: 5 mL

Diphtheria Toxoid Conjugate *see* Hemophilus b Conjugate Vaccine *on page 580*

Doryx® *see* Doxycycline *on this page*

Doxy-200® *see* Doxycycline *on this page*

Doxy-Caps® *see* Doxycycline *on this page*

Doxychel® *see* Doxycycline *on this page*

Doxycycline (dox i sye' kleen)

Brand Names Doryx®; Doxy-200®; Doxy-Caps®; Doxychel®; Doxy-Tabs®; Vibramycin®; Vibra-Tabs®

Synonyms Doxycycline Hyclate; Doxycycline Monohydrate

Generic Available Yes

Use Principally in the treatment of infections caused by susceptible *Rickettsia*, *Chlamydia*, and *Mycoplasma* along with uncommon susceptible gram-negative and gram-positive organisms

Drug of Choice or Alternative For
Disease/Syndrome(s)
Bronchitis *on page 19*
Pelvic Inflammatory Disease *on page 35*
Urethritis, Nongonococcal *on page 44*
Organism(s)
Actinomyces Species *on page 51*

Pregnancy Risk Factor D

Contraindications Hypersensitivity to doxycycline, tetracycline or any component; severe hepatic dysfunction

Warnings/Precautions Use of tetracyclines during tooth development may cause permanent discoloration of the teeth and enamel hypoplasia; prolonged use may result in superinfection; photosensitivity reaction may occur with this drug; avoid prolonged exposure to sunlight or tanning equipment; do not administer to children ≤8 years of age

Adverse Reactions
>10%: Discoloration of teeth in children
1% to 10%: Esophagitis
<1%: Increased intracranial pressure, bulging fontanels in infants, phlebitis, rash, nausea, diarrhea, neutropenia, eosinophilia, hepatotoxicity, photosensitivity

Drug Interactions
Decreased effect with antacids (aluminum, calcium, zinc, or magnesium), bismuth salts, sodium bicarbonate, barbiturates, carbamazepine, hydantoins; decreased effect of oral contraceptives
Increased effect of warfarin

Stability Tetracyclines form toxic products when outdated or when exposed to light, heat, or humidity; reconstituted solution is stable for 72 hours (refrigerated); for I.V. infusion in NS or D_5W solution, complete infusion should be completed within 12 hours; discard remaining solution

Mechanism of Action Inhibits protein synthesis by binding with the 30S and possibly the 50S ribosomal subunit(s) of susceptible bacteria; may also cause alterations in the cytoplasmic membrane

Pharmacokinetics
Absorption: Almost completely from the GI tract; absorption can be reduced by food or milk by 20%
Distribution: Widely distributed into body tissues and fluids including synovial, pleural, prostatic, seminal fluids, and bronchial secretions; saliva, aqueous humor, and CSF penetration is poor; readily crosses placenta and appears in breast milk
Metabolism: Not metabolized in the liver, instead it is partially inactivated in the GI tract by chelate formation
Half-life: 12-15 hours (usually increases to 22-24 hours with multiple dosing)
Time to peak serum concentration: Within 1.5-4 hours
Elimination: Excreted in urine (23%) and feces (30%)

Usual Dosage Oral, I.V.:
Children ≥8 years (<45 kg): 2-4 mg/kg/day in 1-2 divided doses, not to exceed 200 mg/day

Children >8 years (>45 kg) and Adults: 100-200 mg/day in 1-2 divided doses

Sclerosing agent for pleural effusion injection: 500 mg as a single dose in 30-50 mL of NS or SWI

Not dialyzable (0% to 5%)

Overdosage Photosensitivity, nausea, anorexia, diarrhea

Test Interactions False-negative urine glucose using Clinistix®, Tes-Tape®

Patient Information Avoid unnecessary exposure to sunlight; do not take with antacids, iron products, or dairy products; finish all medication

Nursing Implications Infuse I.V. doxycycline over 1 hour
Additional Information
Doxycycline hyclate: Oral suspension
Doxycycline monohydrate: Capsule, tablet, and injection
Dosage Forms
Capsule, as hyclate: 50 mg, 100 mg
Capsule, coated pellets, as hyclate: 100 mg
Powder for injection, as hyclate: 100 mg, 200 mg
Powder for oral suspension, as monohydrate: 25 mg/5 mL (60 mL)
Syrup, as calcium: 50 mg/5 mL (30 mL, 473 mL)
Tablet, as hyclate: 50 mg, 100 mg
Selected Readings

Smilack JD, Wilson WR, and Cockerill FR 3d, "Tetracyclines, Chloramphenicol, Erythromy-cin, Clindamycin, and Metronidazole," *Mayo Clin Proc*, 1991, 66(12):1270-80.
US Department of Health and Human Services, "1993 Sexually Transmitted Diseases Treat-ment Guidelines," *MMWR Morb Mortal Wkly Rep*, 1993, 42(RR-14).
Wyler DJ, "Malaria: Overview and Update," *Clin Infect Dis*, 1993, 16(4):449-56.

Doxycycline Hyclate *see* Doxycycline *on page 557*

Doxycycline Monohydrate *see* Doxycycline *on page 557*

Doxy-Tabs® *see* Doxycycline *on page 557*

DPT *see* Diphtheria, Tetanus Toxoids, and Whole-Cell Pertussis Vaccine *on page 556*

DT *see* Diphtheria and Tetanus Toxoid *on page 554*

DTaP *see* Diphtheria and Tetanus Toxoids and Acellular Pertussis Vaccine *on page 555*

DTP *see* Diphtheria, Tetanus Toxoids, and Whole-Cell Pertussis Vaccine *on page 556*

DTwP *see* Diphtheria, Tetanus Toxoids, and Whole-Cell Pertussis Vaccine *on page 556*

Duricef® *see* Cefadroxil Monohydrate *on page 509*

Dycill® *see* Dicloxacillin Sodium *on page 551*

Dynapen® *see* Dicloxacillin Sodium *on page 551*

Econazole Nitrate (e kone' a zole)
Brand Names Spectazole™ Topical
Generic Available No
Use Topical treatment of tinea pedis, tinea cruris, tinea corporis, tinea versicolor, and cutaneous candidiasis
Pregnancy Risk Factor C
Contraindications Known hypersensitivity to econazole or any component
Warnings/Precautions Discontinue the drug if sensitivity or chemical irritation occurs; not for ophthalmic or intravaginal use
Adverse Reactions 1% to 10%: Pruritus, erythema, burning, stinging
Mechanism of Action Alters fungal cell wall membrane permeability; may in-terfere with RNA and protein synthesis, and lipid metabolism
Pharmacokinetics
Absorption: Topical: <10%
Metabolism: In the liver to >20 metabolites
Elimination: <1% of applied dose recovered in urine or feces
Usual Dosage Children and Adults: Topical: Apply a sufficient amount to cover affected areas once daily; for cutaneous candidiasis: apply twice daily; candid-al infections and tinea cruris, versicolor, and corporis should be treated for 2 weeks and tinea pedis for 1 month; occasionally, longer treatment periods may be required
Patient Information For external use only
Dosage Forms Cream: 1% (15 g, 30 g, 85 g)

Econochlor® *see* Chloramphenicol *on page 531*

E.E.S.® Oral *see* Erythromycin *on page 561*

Eflornithine Hydrochloride (ee flor' ni theen)
Brand Names Ornidyl® Injection
Synonyms DFMO
Generic Available No
Use Treatment of meningoencephalitic stage of *Trypanosoma brucei gambien-se* infection (sleeping sickness)

(Continued)

Eflornithine Hydrochloride *(Continued)*

Pregnancy Risk Factor C

Contraindications Hypersensitivity to eflornithine or any component

Warnings/Precautions Must be diluted before use; frequent monitoring for myelosuppression should be done; use with caution in patients with a history of seizures and in patients with renal impairment; serial audiograms should be obtained; due to the potential for relapse, patients should be followed up for at least 24 months

Adverse Reactions

>10%: Anemia, leukopenia, thrombocytopenia

1% to 10%: Diarrhea, seizures, hearing impairment, vomiting, alopecia, eosinophilia, dizziness

<1%: Abdominal pain, anorexia, headache, asthenia, facial edema

Toxicology No known antidote; treatment is supportive; in mice and rats, CNS depression, seizures, death have occurred

Stability Must be diluted before use and used within 24 hours of preparation

Mechanism of Action Eflornithine exerts antitumor and antiprotozoal effects through specific, irreversible ("suicide") inhibition of the enzyme ornithine decarboxylase (ODC). ODC is the rate-limiting enzyme in the biosynthesis of putrescine, spermine, and spermidine, the major polyamines in nucleated cells. Polyamines are necessary for the synthesis of DNA, RNA, and proteins and are, therefore, necessary for cell growth and differentiation. Although many microorganisms and higher plants are able to produce polyamines from alternate biochemical pathways, all mammalian cells depend on ornithine decarboxylase to produce polyamines. Eflornithine inhibits ODC and rapidly depletes animal cells of putrescine and spermidine; the concentration of spermine remains the same or may even increase. Rapidly dividing cells appear to most susceptible to the effects of eflornithine.

Usual Dosage Adults: I.V. infusion: 100 mg/kg/dose given every 6 hours (over at least 45 minutes) for 14 days

Dosing adjustment in renal impairment: Dose should be adjusted although no specific guidelines are available

Monitoring Parameters CBC with platelet counts

Patient Information Report any persistent or unusual fever, sore throat, fatigue, bleeding, or bruising; frequent blood tests are needed during therapy

Dosage Forms Injection: 200 mg/mL (100 mL)

Selected Readings

"Drugs for Parasitic Infections," *Med Lett Drugs Ther*, 1993, 35(911):111-22.

Elimite™ Cream *see* Permethrin *on page 640*

E-Mycin® Oral *see* Erythromycin *on next page*

End Lice® [OTC] *see* Pyrethrins *on page 653*

Engerix-B® *see* Hepatitis B Vaccine *on page 582*

Enhanced-potency Inactivated Poliovirus Vaccine *see* Poliovirus Vaccine, Inactivated *on page 645*

Enoxacin *(en ox' a sin)*

Brand Names Penetrex™ Oral

Generic Available No

Use Complicated and uncomplicated urinary tract infections caused by susceptible gram-negative and gram-positive bacteria

Pregnancy Risk Factor C

Contraindications Hypersensitivity to enoxacin, any component, or other quinolones

Adverse Reactions

1% to 10%: Nausea, vomiting

<1%: Tremor, restlessness, dizziness, confusion, seizures, headache, rash, diarrhea, GI bleeding, anemia, increased serum creatinine and BUN, increased liver enzymes, arthralgia, acute renal failure

Drug Interactions

Decreased effect with antacids (magnesium, aluminum), iron and zinc salts, sucralfate, bismuth salts

Increased toxicity/levels of warfarin, cyclosporine, digoxin, theophylline, caffeine; cimetidine increases enoxacin levels

Mechanism of Action Inhibits DNA-gyrase in susceptible organisms; inhibits relaxation of supercoiled DNA and promotes breakage of double-stranded DNA

Pharmacokinetics
Absorption: 98%
Distribution: Penetrates well into tissues and body secretions
Half-life: 3-6 hours (average)
Elimination: Primarily excreted in urine, however, significant drug concentrations are achieved in feces

Usual Dosage Adults: Oral: 400 mg twice daily

Dosing adjustment in renal impairment: Cl_{cr} <50 mL/minute: Administer 50% of dose

Monitoring Parameters Patients receiving concurrent enoxacin and theophylline should have serum levels of theophylline monitored

Patient Information May be taken with food to minimize upset stomach; avoid antacid use; drink fluid liberally

Dosage Forms Tablet: 200 mg, 400 mg

Selected Readings
Hooper DC and Wolfson JS, "Fluoroquinolone Antimicrobial Agents," *N Engl J Med*, 1991, 324(6):384-94.
Lomaestro BM and Bailie GR, "Quinolone-Cation Interactions: A Review," *DICP*, 1991, 25(11):1249-58.
Stein GE, "The 4-Quinolone Antibiotics: Past, Present, and Future," *Pharmacotherapy*, 1988, 8(6):301-14.
Walker RC and Wright AJ, "The Fluoroquinolones," *Mayo Clin Proc*, 1991, 66(12):1249-59.

E.P. Mycin® Oral *see* Oxytetracycline Hydrochloride *on page 629*

Eryc® Oral *see* Erythromycin *on this page*

EryPed® Oral *see* Erythromycin *on this page*

Ery-Tab® Oral *see* Erythromycin *on this page*

Erythrocin® Oral *see* Erythromycin *on this page*

Erythromycin (er ith roe mye' sin)
Related Information
Antimicrobial Activity Against Selected Organisms *on page 757-764*

Brand Names E.E.S.® Oral; E-Mycin® Oral; Eryc® Oral; EryPed® Oral; Ery-Tab® Oral; Erythrocin® Oral; Ilosone® Oral; PCE® Oral; Wyamycin® S Oral

Synonyms Erythromycin Base; Erythromycin Estolate; Erythromycin Ethylsuccinate; Erythromycin Gluceptate; Erythromycin Lactobionate; Erythromycin Stearate

Generic Available Yes

Use Treatment of susceptible bacterial infections including *M. pneumoniae*, *Legionella* pneumonia, diphtheria, pertussis, chancroid, *Chlamydia*, and *Campylobacter* gastroenteritis; used in conjunction with neomycin for decontaminating the bowel prior to colorectal surgical procedures; unlabeled use for gastroparesis

Drug of Choice or Alternative For
Disease/Syndrome(s)
Impetigo *on page 27*
Pharyngitis *on page 36*
Pneumonia, Community-Acquired *on page 37*
Urethritis, Nongonococcal *on page 44*

Organism(s)
Bartonella Species *on page 62*
Bordetella pertussis *on page 65*
Calymmatobacterium granulomatis *on page 71*
Campylobacter jejuni *on page 72*
Chlamydia pneumoniae *on page 76*
Chlamydia psittaci *on page 77*
Chlamydia trachomatis *on page 79*
Corynebacterium Species, Other than *C. jeikeium* *on page 91*
Haemophilus ducreyi *on page 118*
Legionella pneumophila *on page 139*
Mycoplasma pneumoniae *on page 159*
Streptococcus agalactiae *on page 203*
Streptococcus pneumoniae *on page 206*
Streptococcus pyogenes *on page 207*
Ureaplasma urealyticum *on page 225*

(Continued)

ANTIMICROBIAL THERAPY

Erythromycin *(Continued)*

Pregnancy Risk Factor B

Contraindications Known hypersensitivity to erythromycin or its any components

Warnings/Precautions Use with caution in patients with hepatic dysfunction; hepatic impairment with or without jaundice has occurred chiefly in older children and adults; it may be accompanied by malaise, nausea, vomiting, abdominal colic, and fever; discontinue use if these occur; avoid using erythromycin lactobionate in neonates since formulations may contain benzyl alcohol which is associated with toxicity in neonates

Adverse Reactions

>10%: Abdominal pain, cramping, nausea, vomiting

1% to 10%: Hypersensitivity reactions, cholestatic jaundice, phlebitis at the injection site, oral candidiasis

<1%: Thrombophlebitis, hypertrophic pyloric stenosis, ventricular arrhythmias, fever, skin rash, diarrhea, eosinophilia, allergic reactions

Drug Interactions Erythromycin decreases clearance of carbamazepine, cyclosporine, and triazolam; erythromycin decreases theophylline clearance and increases theophylline's half-life by up to 60% (patients on high-dose theophylline and erythromycin or who have received erythromycin for >5 days may be at higher risk); terfenadine or astemizole with concurrent erythromycin may cause life-threatening arrhythmias

Stability Erythromycin lactobionate should be reconstituted with sterile water for injection without preservatives to avoid gel formation; the reconstituted solution is stable for 2 weeks when refrigerated or 24 hours at room temperature. Erythromycin I.V. infusion solution is stable at pH 6-8. Do not use D_5W as a diluent unless sodium bicarbonate is added to solution.

Mechanism of Action Inhibits RNA-dependent protein synthesis at the chain elongation step; binds to the 50S ribosomal subunit resulting in blockage of transpeptidation

Pharmacokinetics

Absorption: Variable but better with salt forms than with base form; 18% to 45% absorbed orally

Distribution: Widely distributed to most body tissues and fluids except CSF where it appears only in low concentrations; crosses placenta and appears in breast milk

Metabolism: In the liver by demethylation

Half-life: 1.5-2 hours, prolonged with reduced renal function;

Time to peak serum concentration: 30 minutes to 4 hours depending on dosage form

Elimination: 2% to 15% unchanged drug in urine and major excretion in feces (via bile)

Usual Dosage

Neonates:

Oral:

Postnatal age <7 days: 20 mg/kg/day in divided doses every 12 hours

Postnatal age >7 days, <1200 g: 20 mg/kg/day in divided doses every 12 hours; ≥1200 g: 30 mg/kg/day in divided doses every 8 hours

Prophylaxis of neonatal gonococcal or chlamydial conjunctivitis: 0.5-1 cm ribbon of ointment should be instilled into each conjunctival sac

Infants and Children:

Oral: Do not exceed 2 g/day

Base and ethylsuccinate: 30-50 mg/kg/day divided every 6-8 hours

Estolate: 30-50 mg/kg/day divided every 8-12 hours

Stearate: 20-40 mg/kg/day divided every 6 hours

Pre-op bowel preparation: 20 mg/kg erythromycin base at 1, 2, and 11 PM on the day before surgery combined with mechanical cleansing of the large intestine and oral neomycin

I.V.: Lactobionate: 20-40 mg/kg/day divided every 6 hours, not to exceed 4 g/day

Children and Adults:

Ophthalmic: Instill one or more times daily depending on the severity of the infection

Topical: Apply 2% solution over the affected area twice daily after the skin has been thoroughly washed and patted dry

Adults:

Oral:

Base: 333 mg every 8 hours

Estolate, stearate or base: 250-500 mg every 6-12 hours

Ethylsuccinate: 400-800 mg every 6-12 hours

Pre-op bowel preparation: 1 g erythromycin base at 1, 2, and 11 PM on the day before surgery combined with mechanical cleansing of the large intestine and oral neomycin

I.V.: 15-20 mg/kg/day divided every 6 hours or given as a continuous infusion over 24 hours

Overdosage Nausea, vomiting, diarrhea, prostration

Monitoring Parameters Liver function tests

Test Interactions False-positive urinary catecholamines and steroids; false elevation of ALT and AST

Patient Information Take until gone, do not skip doses; chewable tablets should not be swallowed whole

Nursing Implications GI upset, including diarrhea, is common; can give with food to decrease GI upset; some formulations may contain benzyl alcohol as a preservative; use with extreme care in neonates; swallow tablets whole, do not crush or chew

Additional Information

Due to differences in absorption, 400 mg erythromycin ethylsuccinate produces the same serum levels as 250 mg erythromycin base, stearate, or estolate. Do not use D_5W as a diluent unless sodium bicarbonate is added to solution; infuse over 30 minutes.

Sodium content of oral suspension (ethylsuccinate) 200 mg/5 mL: 29 mg (1.3 mEq)

Sodium content of base Filmtab® 250 mg: 70 mg (3 mEq)

Dosage Forms

Erythromycin **base**:

Capsule, delayed release: 250 mg

Capsule, delayed release, enteric coated pellets (Eryc®): 250 mg

Tablet, delayed release: 333 mg

Tablet, enteric coated (E-Mycin®, Ery-Tab®, E-Base®): 250 mg, 333 mg, 500 mg

Tablet, film coated: 250 mg, 500 mg

Tablet, polymer coated particles (PCE®): 333 mg, 500 mg

Erythromycin **estolate**:

Capsule (Ilosone® Pulvules®): 250 mg

Suspension, oral (Ilosone®): 125 mg/5 mL (480 mL); 250 mg/mL (480 mL)

Tablet (Ilosone®): 500 mg

Erythromycin ethylsuccinate:

Granules for oral suspension (EryPed®): 400 mg/5 mL (60 mL, 100 mL, 200 mL)

Powder for oral suspension (E.E.S.®): 200 mg/5 mL (100 mL, 200 mL)

Suspension, oral (E.E.S.®, EryPed®): 200 mg/5 mL (5 mL, 100 mL, 200 mL, 480 mL); 400 mg/5 mL (5 mL, 60 mL, 100 mL, 200 mL, 480 mL)

Suspension, oral [drops] (EryPed®): 100 mg/2.5 mL (50 mL)

Tablet (E.E.S.®): 400 mg

Tablet, chewable (EryPed®): 200 mg

Erythromycin gluceptate:

Injection: 1000 mg (30 mL)

Erythromycin **lactobionate**:

Powder for injection, I.V.: 500 mg, 1000 mg

Erythromycin stearate:

Tablet, film coated (Eramycin®, Erythrocin®, Wyamycin® S): 250 mg, 500 mg

Selected Readings

Goldman MP and Longworth DL, "The Role of Azithromycin and Clarithromycin in Clinical Practice," *Cleve Clin J Med*, 1993, 60(5):359-64.

Smilack JD, Wilson WR, and Cockerill FR 3d, "Tetracyclines, Chloramphenicol, Erythromycin, Clindamycin, and Metronidazole," *Mayo Clin Proc*, 1991, 66(12):1270-80.

Erythromycin and Sulfisoxazole

(er ith roe mye' sin & sul fi sox' a zole)

Brand Names Eryzole®; Pediazole®

Synonyms Sulfisoxazole and Erythromycin

Generic Available Yes

Use Treatment of susceptible bacterial infections of the upper and lower respiratory tract, otitis media in children caused by susceptible strains of *Haemophilus influenzae*, and other infections in patients allergic to penicillin

Drug of Choice or Alternative For Disease/Syndrome(s)

Otitis Media, Acute *on page 35*

Pregnancy Risk Factor C

Contraindications Hepatic dysfunction, known hypersensitivity to erythromycin or sulfonamides; infants <2 months of age (sulfas compete with bilirubin for binding sites); patients with porphyria

Warnings/Precautions Use with caution in patients with impaired renal or hepatic function, G-6-PD deficiency (hemolysis may occur)

Adverse Reactions

>10%: Abdominal pain, cramping, nausea, vomiting

1% to 10%: Hypersensitivity reactions, cholestatic jaundice, phlebitis at the injection site, oral candidiasis

<1%: Thrombophlebitis, hypertrophic pyloric stenosis, ventricular arrhythmias, fever, skin rash, diarrhea, eosinophilia, headache, Stevens-Johnson syndrome, toxic epidermal necrolysis, agranulocytosis, aplastic anemia, hepatic necrosis, toxic nephrosis, crystalluria

Toxicology Symptoms of overdose include nausea, vomiting, diarrhea, prostration, reversible pancreatitis, hearing loss with or without tinnitus or vertigo; general and supportive care only; keep patient well hydrated

Drug Interactions Increased effect/toxicity/levels of alfentanil, anticoagulants, astemizole, terfenadine, loratadine, bromocriptine, carbamazepine, cyclosporine, digoxin, disopyramide, theophylline, triazolam, and warfarin

Stability Reconstituted suspension is stable for 14 days when refrigerated

Mechanism of Action Erythromycin inhibits bacterial protein synthesis; sulfisoxazole competitively inhibits bacterial synthesis of folic acid from para-aminobenzoic acid

Pharmacokinetics

Erythromycin ethylsuccinate:

Absorption: Well absorbed from GI tract

Distribution: Crosses the placenta; appears in breast milk

Metabolism: In the liver

Half-life: 1-1.5 hours

Elimination: Unchanged drug is excreted and concentrated in bile

Sulfisoxazole acetyl: Hydrolyzed in the GI tract to sulfisoxazole which has the following characteristics:

Absorption: Readily absorbed

Distribution: Crosses the placenta; appears in breast milk

Half-life: 6 hours, prolonged in renal impairment

Elimination: 50% excreted in urine as unchanged drug

Usual Dosage Oral (dosage recommendation is based on the product's erythromycin content):

Children ≥2 months: 50 mg/kg/day erythromycin and 150 mg/kg/day sulfisoxazole in divided doses every 6 hours; not to exceed 2 g erythromycin/day or 6 g sulfisoxazole/day for 10 days

Adults: 400 mg erythromycin and 1200 mg sulfisoxazole every 6 hours

Dosing adjustment in renal impairment (sulfisoxazole must be adjusted in renal impairment):

Cl_{cr} 10-50 mL/minute: Administer every 8-12 hours

Cl_{cr} <10 mL/minute: Administer every 12-24 hours

Monitoring Parameters CBC and periodic liver function test

Test Interactions False-positive urinary protein

Patient Information Maintain adequate fluid intake; avoid prolonged exposure to sunlight; discontinue if rash appears; take until gone, do not skip doses

Nursing Implications Shake well before use

Dosage Forms Suspension, oral: Erythromycin ethylsuccinate 200 mg and sulfisoxazole acetyl 600 mg per 5 mL (100 mL, 150 mL, 200 mL, 250 mL)

Erythromycin Base see Erythromycin on page 561

Erythromycin Estolate see Erythromycin on page 561

Erythromycin Ethylsuccinate see Erythromycin on page 561

Erythromycin Gluceptate see Erythromycin on page 561

Erythromycin Lactobionate see Erythromycin on page 561

Erythromycin Stearate see Erythromycin on page 561

Eryzole® see Erythromycin and Sulfisoxazole on previous page

Ethambutol Hydrochloride (e tham' byoo tole)

Brand Names Myambutol®

Generic Available No

Use Treatment of tuberculosis and other mycobacterial diseases in conjunction with other antimycobacterial agents

Drug of Choice or Alternative For
  Organism(s)
    Mycobacterium avium-intracellulare on page 152
    Mycobacterium kansasii on page 153
    Mycobacterium tuberculosis on page 155

Pregnancy Risk Factor B

Contraindications Hypersensitivity to ethambutol or any component

Adverse Reactions
  1% to 10%: Acute gout or hyperuricemia, abdominal pain, anorexia, nausea, vomiting, headache, confusion, and disorientation
  <1%: Malaise, peripheral neuritis, mental confusion, fever, rash, pruritus, abnormal liver function tests, optic neuritis, anaphylaxis

Toxicology Treatment is supportive

Drug Interactions Aluminum salts may decrease absorption

Mechanism of Action Suppresses mycobacteria multiplication by interfering with RNA synthesis

Pharmacokinetics
  Absorption: ~80%
  Distribution: Well distributed throughout the body with high concentrations in kidneys, lungs, saliva and red blood cells
  Metabolism: 20% by the liver to inactive metabolite
  Half-life: 2.5-3.6 hours (up to 7 hours or longer with renal impairment)
  Time to peak serum concentration: 2-4 hours
  Elimination: ~50% excreted in urine and 20% excreted in feces as unchanged drug

Usual Dosage Oral (not recommended in children <12 years of age):
  Children >12 years: 15 mg/kg/day once daily
  Adolescents and Adults: 15-25 mg/kg/day once daily, not to exceed 2.5 g/day

  Dosing adjustment in renal impairment:
    Cl_{cr} 10-50 mL/minute: Administer every 24-36 hours
    Cl_{cr} <10 mL/minute: Administer every 48 hours and/or reduce daily dose
  Slightly dialyzable (5% to 20%)

Overdosage Decrease in visual acuity, anorexia, joint pain, numbness of the extremities, toxic epidermal necrolysis

Monitoring Parameters Periodic visual testing in patients receiving more than 15 mg/kg/day as the incidence of optic neuritis increases significantly; periodic renal, hepatic, and hematopoietic tests

Patient Information Report any visual changes to physician; may cause stomach upset, take with food

Dosage Forms Tablet: 100 mg, 400 mg

Selected Readings
  Davidson PT and Le HQ, "Drug Treatment of Tuberculosis – 1992," *Drugs*, 1992, 43(5):651-73.
  "Drugs for Tuberculosis," *Med Lett Drugs Ther*, 1993, 35(908):99-101.
  Iseman MD, "Treatment of Multidrug-Resistant Tuberculosis," *N Engl J Med*, 1993, 329(11):784-91.
  Van Scoy RE and Wilkowske CJ, "Antituberculous Agents," *Mayo Clin Proc*, 1992, 67(2):179-87.

Ethionamide (e thye on am' ide)

Brand Names Trecator®-SC

Generic Available No

Use In conjunction with other antituberculosis agents in the treatment of tuberculosis and other mycobacterial diseases

Pregnancy Risk Factor C

Contraindications Contraindicated in patients with severe hepatic impairment or in patients who are sensitive to the drug

Warnings/Precautions Use with caution in patients receiving cycloserine or isoniazid, in diabetics

Adverse Reactions
  >10%: Anorexia, nausea, vomiting
  1% to 10%: Hepatitis, jaundice, peripheral neuritis, psychiatric disturbances, postural hypotension, metallic taste

(Continued)

Ethionamide *(Continued)*

<1%: Hypothyroidism or goiter, hypoglycemia, drowsiness, dizziness, optic neuritis, seizures, headache, rash, stomatitis, gynecomastia, abdominal pain, diarrhea, thrombocytopenia

Toxicology Treatment is supportive

Mechanism of Action Inhibits peptide synthesis

Pharmacokinetics

Absorption: Rapid from GI tract (~80%)

Distribution: Crosses the placenta; distributed widely to most tissues and fluids including liver, kidneys, and spleen

Metabolism: Probably hepatic; metabolized to sulfoxide which is active to inactive metabolites

Half-life: 2-3 hours

Time to peak serum concentration: Oral: Within 3 hours

Elimination: Excreted as metabolites (active and inactive) and parent drug in urine

Usual Dosage Oral:

Children: 15-20 mg/kg/day in 2 divided doses, not to exceed 1 g/day

Adults: 500-1000 mg/day in 1-3 divided doses

Dosing adjustment in renal impairment: Cl_{cr} <50 mL/minute: Administer 50% of dose

Overdosage Peripheral neuropathy, anorexia, joint pain

Monitoring Parameters Initial and periodic serum AST and ALT

Test Interactions Decreases thyroxine (S)

Patient Information Take with meals; notify physician of persistent or severe stomach upset, loss of appetite, or metallic taste; frequent blood tests are needed for monitoring

Additional Information Neurotoxic effects may be relieved by the administration of pyridoxine

Dosage Forms Tablet: 250 mg

Selected Readings

Davidson PT and Le HQ, "Drug Treatment of Tuberculosis – 1992," *Drugs*, 1992, 43(5):651-73.

"Drugs for Tuberculosis," *Med Lett Drugs Ther*, 1993, 35(908):99-101.

Iseman MD, "Treatment of Multidrug-Resistant Tuberculosis," *N Engl J Med*, 1993, 329(11):784-91.

Ethoxynaphthamido Penicillin Sodium *see* Nafcillin Sodium *on page 616*

Exelderm® *see* Sulconazole Nitrate *on page 670*

Exsel® *see* Selenium Sulfide *on page 665*

F₃T *see* Trifluridine *on page 687*

Famciclovir

Brand Names Famvir™

Generic Available No

Use Management of acute herpes zoster (shingles)

Pregnancy Risk Factor B

Contraindications Hypersensitivity to famciclovir

Warnings/Precautions Famciclovir has not been studied in immunocompromised patients or patients with ophthalmic or disseminated zoster. Dosage adjustment is required in patients with renal insufficiency. Safety and efficacy have not been established in children under 18 years of age.

Adverse Reactions

>10%: Headache, nausea

1% to 10%: Diarrhea, vomiting, fatigue, constipation, fever, rigors, anorexia, abdominal pain, dizziness, paresthesia, somnolence

Mechanism of Action Famciclovir is a prodrug which is rapidly metabolized to penciclovir. Penciclovir is triphosphorylated by viral and cellular kinases to its active form. This drug is active against herpes simplex and zoster.

Pharmacokinetics

Absorption: Food decreases the maximum peak concentration and delays the time to peak; AUC remains the same

Distribution: Vd_{ss}: 72-85 L; 0.98-1.08 L/kg

Protein binding: 20%

Metabolism: Rapidly metabolized to penciclovir (not by cytochrome p450)
Bioavailability: ~78%
Half-life: Penciclovir: 2-3 hours
Time to peak serum concentration: 0.9 hours
Elimination: >90% of penciclovir is eliminated unchanged in urine
Usual Dosage Adult: Oral: 500 mg every 8 hours for 7 days

Dosing interval in renal impairment:
Cl_{cr} ≥60 mL/minute: Administer 500 mg every 8 hours
Cl_{cr} 40-59 mL/minute: Administer 500 mg every 12 hours
Cl_{cr} 20-39 mL/minute: Administer 500 mg every 24 hours

Overdosage Appropriate symptomatic and supportive care should be administered. There is no information regarding the utility of hemodialysis.

Patient Information Patient may take medication with food or on an empty stomach.

Dosage Forms Tablet: 500 mg

Famvir™ *see* Famciclovir *on previous page*

Fansidar® *see* Sulfadoxine and Pyrimethamine *on page 673*

5-FC *see* Flucytosine *on page 570*

Filgrastim (fil gra' stim)
Brand Names Neupogen® Injection
Synonyms G-CSF; Granulocyte Colony Stimulating Factor
Generic Available No
Use Decreases the period of neutropenia and the associated risk of infection in patients with nonmyeloid malignancies receiving myelosuppressive chemotherapeutic regimens associated with a significant incidence of severe neutropenia with fever; it has also been used in AIDS patients on zidovudine and in patients with noncancer chemotherapy-induced neutropenia
Pregnancy Risk Factor C
Contraindications Hypersensitivity to *E. coli* derived proteins or G-CSF
Warnings/Precautions Complete blood count and platelet count should be obtained prior to chemotherapy. Do not use G-CSF in the period 24 hours before to 24 hours after administration of cytotoxic chemotherapy because of the potential sensitivity of rapidly dividing myeloid cells to cytotoxic chemotherapy. Precaution should be exercised in the usage of G-CSF in any malignancy with myeloid characteristics. G-CSF can potentially act as a growth factor for any tumor type, particularly myeloid malignancies. Tumors of nonhematopoietic origin may have surface receptors for G-CSF.
Adverse Reactions As this drug is indicated for patients receiving chemotherapeutic regiments, many of the adverse reactions listed below occurred in equal numbers in the placebo arms of clinical trials secondary to the chemotherapeutic agents. Included in the adverse effects associated with filgrastim alone is medullary bone pain which has been reported in up to 24% of patients.
>10%: Nausea, vomiting, skeletal pain, alopecia, diarrhea, neutropenic fever, mucositis, fever
1% to 10%: Anorexia, dyspnea, headache, cough, skin rash, chest pain, weakness, sore throat, stomatitis, constipation, pain at injection site, leukocytosis, fluid retention
<1%: Transient supraventricular arrhythmia, anaphylactic reaction, pericarditis, thrombophlebitis
Toxicology
Signs and symptoms: Leukocytosis which was not associated with any clinical adverse effects; after discontinuing the drug there is a 50% decrease in circulating levels of neutrophils within 1-2 days, return to pretreatment levels within 1-7 days. No clinical adverse effects seen with high-dose producing ANC >10,000/mm^3
Stability Store at 2°C to 8°C (36°F to 46°F); do not expose to freezing or dry ice. Prior to administration, filgrastim may be allowed to be at room temperature for a maximum of 24 hours. It may be diluted in dextrose 5% in water to a concentration of ≥15 µg/mL for I.V. infusion administration. Minimum concentration is 15 µg/mL; concentrations <15 µg/mL require addition of albumin (1 mL of 5%) to the bag to prevent absorption. This diluted solution is stable for 7 days under refrigeration or at room temperature. **Filgrastim is incompatible with 0.9% sodium chloride (normal saline).**
Standard diluent: ≥375 µg/25 mL D_5W
Mechanism of Action Stimulates the production, maturation, and activation of
(Continued)

Filgrastim *(Continued)*

neutrophils, G-CSF activates neutrophils to increase both their migration and cytotoxicity. Natural proteins which stimulate hematopoietic stem cells to proliferate, prolong cell survival, stimulate cell differentiation, and stimulate functional activity of mature cells. CSFs are produced by a wide variety of cell types. Specific mechanisms of action are not yet fully understood, but possibly work by a second-messenger pathway with resultant protein production. See table.

Proliferation/Differentiation	G–CSF (Filgrastim)	GM–CSF (Sargramostim)
Neutrophils	Yes	Yes
Eosinophils	No	Yes
Macrophages	No	Yes
Neutrophil migration	Enhanced	Inhibited

Pharmacokinetics

Onset of action: Rapid elevation in neutrophil counts within the first 24 hours, reaching a plateau in 3-5 days

Duration: ANC decreases by 50% within 2 days after discontinuing G-CSF; white counts return to the normal range in 4-7 days

Absorption: S.C.: 100%; peak plasma levels can be maintained for up to 12 hours

Distribution: V_d: 150 mL/kg; no evidence of drug accumulation over a 11- to 20-day period

Metabolism: Systemic

Bioavailability: Oral: Not bioavailable

Half-life: 1.8-3.5 hours

Time to peak serum concentration: S.C.: Within 2-6 hours

Usual Dosage Children and Adults:

Initial dosing recommendations: 5 μg/kg/day administered S.C. or I.V. as a single daily infusion over 20-30 minutes

Doses may be increased in increments of 5 μg/kg for each chemotherapy cycle, according to the duration and severity of the absolute neutrophil count (ANC) nadir. In phase III trials, efficacy was observed at doses of 4-6 μg/kg/day. Discontinue therapy if the ANC count is > 10,000/mm^3 after the ANC nadir has occurred.

Length of therapy:

Bone marrow transplant patients: G-CSF should be administered daily for up to 30 days, until the ANC has reached 1000/mm^3 for 3 consecutive days following the expected chemotherapy-induced neutrophil nadir.

Chemotherapy-treated patients: G-CSF may be administered daily for up to 2 weeks until the ANC has reached 10,000/mm^3 following the expected chemotherapy-induced neutrophil nadir. Duration of therapy needed to attenuate chemotherapy-induced neutropenia may be dependent on the myelosuppressive potential of the chemotherapy regimen employed. Duration of therapy in clinical studies has ranged from 2 weeks to 3 years. Safety and efficacy of chronic administration have not been established.

Premature discontinuation of G-CSF therapy prior to the time of recovery from the expected neutrophil is generally not recommended. A transient increase in neutrophil counts is typically seen 1-2 days after initiation of therapy.

Administration Infuse I.V. dose over 20-30 minutes

Monitoring Parameters Complete blood cell count and platelet count should be obtained twice weekly. Leukocytosis (white blood cell counts of $\geq$ 100,000/mm^3) has been observed in ~2% of patients receiving G-CSF at doses above 5 μg/kg/day. Monitor platelets and hematocrit regularly. Monitor patients with pre-existing cardiac conditions closely as cardiac events (myocardial infarctions, arrhythmias) have been reported in premarketing clinical studies.

Reference Range No clinical benefit seen with ANC > 10,000/mm^3

Patient Information Possible bone pain

Nursing Implications Do not mix with sodium chloride solutions

Additional Information Reimbursement hotline: 1-800-28-AMGEN

Dosage Forms Injection, preservative free: 300 μg/mL (1 mL, 1.6 mL)

Flagyl® Oral *see* Metronidazole *on page 610*

Floxin® Injection *see* Ofloxacin *on page 626*

Floxin® Oral *see* Ofloxacin *on page 626*

Fluconazole (floo koe' na zole)
Brand Names Diflucan®
Generic Available No
Use Treatment of susceptible fungal infections including oropharyngeal and esophageal candidiasis; treatment of systemic candidal infections including urinary tract infection, peritonitis, and pneumonia; treatment and suppression of cryptococcal meningitis; treatment for vaginal yeast infection
Drug of Choice or Alternative For
Organism(s)
Blastomyces dermatitidis *on page 63*
Candida *Species on page 73*
Cryptococcus neoformans *on page 94*
Pregnancy Risk Factor C
Contraindications Known hypersensitivity to fluconazole or other azoles
Warnings/Precautions Patients who develop abnormal liver function tests during fluconazole therapy should be monitored closely for the development of more severe hepatic injury; if clinical signs and symptoms consistent with liver disease develop that may be attributable to fluconazole, fluconazole should be discontinued
Adverse Reactions
1% to 10%: Nausea, headache, skin rash, vomiting, abdominal pain, diarrhea
<1%: Pallor, dizziness, hypokalemia; elevated AST, ALT, or alkaline phosphatase
Toxicology Supportive measures, a 3-hour hemodialysis will remove 50%
Drug Interactions
Decreased effect with rifampin
Increased effect of warfarin, oral sulfonylureas
Increased levels when high doses used; phenytoin, cyclosporine
Stability Parenteral admixture at room temperature (25°C): Manufacturer expiration dating; do not refrigerate
Mechanism of Action Fluconazole interferes with cytochrome P-450 activity decreasing ergosterol synthesis (principal sterol in fungal cell membrane) and inhibiting cell membrane formation
Pharmacokinetics
Absorption: Oral: Absorbed well
Distribution: Widely distributed throughout body with good penetration into CSF, eye, peritoneal fluid, sputum, skin, and urine
Bioavailability: Oral: >90%
Half-life: 25-30 hours with normal renal function
Time to peak serum concentration: Oral: 1-2 hours
Elimination: 80% of dose excreted unchanged in urine
Usual Dosage The daily dose of fluconazole is the same for oral and I.V. administration

Efficacy of fluconazole has not been established in children; a small number of patients from 3-13 years of age have been treated with fluconazole using doses of 3-6 mg/kg/day divided once daily. Doses as high as 12 mg/kg/day once daily have been used to treat candidiasis in immunocompromised children.

Adult doses of fluconazole: Oral, I.V.: See table for once daily dosing.

Indication	Day 1	Daily Therapy	Minimum Duration of Therapy
Oropharyngeal candidiasis	200 mg	100 mg	14 d
Esophageal candidiasis	200 mg	100 mg	21 d
Systemic candidiasis	400 mg	200 mg	28 d
Cryptococcal meningitis acute	400 mg	200 mg	10–12 wk after CSF culture becomes negative
relapse	200 mg	200 mg	

(Continued)

Fluconazole *(Continued)*
For vaginal yeast infection: 150 mg one time dose

Dosing adjustment in renal impairment: Give same loading dose:
Cl_{cr} 21-50 mL/minute: Administer 50% of recommended dose
Cl_{cr} <20 mL/minute: Administer 25% of recommended dose
50% removed by hemodialysis

Overdosage Decreased lacrimation, salivation, respiration and motility; urinary incontinence, cyanosis

Monitoring Parameters Periodic liver function and renal function tests

Nursing Implications Parenteral fluconazole must be administered by I.V. infusion over approximately 1-2 hours; do not exceed 200 mg/hour when giving I.V. infusion

Dosage Forms
Injection: 2 mg/mL (100 mL, 200 mL)
Tablet: 50 mg, 100 mg, 150 mg, 200 mg

Selected Readings
Como JA and Dismukes WE, "Oral Azole Drugs as Systemic Antifungal Therapy," *N Engl J Med*, 1993, 330(4):263-72.
Kowalsky SF and Dixon DM, "Fluconazole: A New Antifungal Agent," *Clin Pharm*, 1991, 10(3):179-94.
Lyman CA and Walsh TJ, "Systemically Administered Antifungal Agents. A Review of Their Clinical Pharmacology and Therapeutic Applications," *Drugs*, 1992, 44(1):9-35.
Terrell CL and Hughes CE, "Antifungal Agents Used for Deep-Seated Mycotic Infections," *Mayo Clin Proc*, 1992, 67(1):69-91.

Flucytosine (floo sye' toe seen)
Brand Names Ancobon®
Synonyms 5-FC; 5-Flurocytosine
Generic Available No
Use Treatment of susceptible fungal infections, usually strains of *Candida* or *Cryptococcus*
Drug of Choice or Alternative For Organism(s)
Cryptococcus neoformans on page 94
Pregnancy Risk Factor C
Contraindications Hypersensitivity to flucytosine or any component
Warnings/Precautions Use with extreme caution and modify dosage in patients with renal impairment; use caution in patients with bone marrow depression and patients with AIDS; monitor serum concentrations
Adverse Reactions
1% to 10%: Anemia, hepatitis, jaundice, skin rash, leukopenia, thrombocytopenia, abdominal pain, diarrhea, loss of appetite, nausea, vomiting
<1%: Confusion, hallucinations, photosensitivity, dizziness, drowsiness, headache, cardiac arrest, paresthesia, parkinsonism, psychosis, ataxia, temporary growth failure, hypoglycemia, hypokalemia, bone marrow depression, elevated liver enzymes, hearing loss, respiratory arrest
Drug Interactions Increased effect/toxicity with amphotericin
Stability Protect from light
Mechanism of Action Penetrates fungal cells and is converted to fluorouracil which competes with uracil interfering with fungal RNA and protein synthesis
Pharmacokinetics
Absorption: Oral: 75% to 90% from GI tract
Distribution: Widely distributed throughout the body; high concentrations in CSF; concentrations in liver, kidneys, spleen, heart, and lungs appear to equal those in serum; crosses the placenta
Metabolism: Minimal
Half-life: 3-8 hours (may be as long as 200 hours in anuria)
Time to peak serum concentration: 2-6 hours
Elimination: 75% to 90% excreted unchanged in urine by glomerular filtration
Usual Dosage Children and Adults: Oral: 50-150 mg/kg/day in divided doses every 6 hours

Dosing adjustment in renal impairment:
Cl_{cr} <50 mL/minute: Administer every 12 hours
Cl_{cr} <10 mL/minute: Administer every 24 hours
Dialyzable (50% to 100%)

Overdosage Nausea, vomiting, diarrhea, bone marrow suppression

Monitoring Parameters Serum creatinine, BUN, alkaline phosphatase, AST, ALT, CBC; serum flucytosine concentrations

Reference Range Therapeutic: 25-100 µg/mL (SI: 195-775 µmol/L)

Test Interactions Flucytosine causes markedly false elevations in serum creatinine values when the Ektachem® analyzer is used

Patient Information Take with food over a 15-minute period

Dosage Forms Capsule: 250 mg, 500 mg

Selected Readings
Lyman CA and Walsh TJ, "Systemically Administered Antifungal Agents. A Review of Their Clinical Pharmacology and Therapeutic Applications," *Drugs*, 1992, 44(1):9-35.
Terrell CL and Hughes CE, "Antifungal Agents Used for Deep-Seated Mycotic Infections," *Mayo Clin Proc*, 1992, 67(1):69-91.

Flu-Imune® *see* Influenza Virus Vaccine *on page 589*

Flumadine® *see* Rimantadine Hydrochloride *on page 664*

Fluogen® *see* Influenza Virus Vaccine *on page 589*

Fluoroquinolones
Refer To
Ciprofloxacin Hydrochloride *on page 537*
Enoxacin *on page 560*
Lomefloxacin Hydrochloride *on page 600*
Norfloxacin *on page 624*
Ofloxacin *on page 626*
Drug of Choice or Alternative For
Disease/Syndrome(s)
Prostatitis *on page 39*
Urinary Tract Infection, Pyelonephritis *on page 45*
Organism(s)
Campylobacter jejuni on page 72
Shigella Species *on page 191*
Staphylococcus saprophyticus on page 203
Xanthomonas maltophilia on page 231

5-Flurocytosine *see* Flucytosine *on previous page*

Fluzone® *see* Influenza Virus Vaccine *on page 589*

Footwork® [OTC] *see* Tolnaftate *on page 687*

Formula Q® [OTC] *see* Quinine Sulfate *on page 658*

Fortaz® *see* Ceftazidime *on page 520*

Foscarnet (fos kar' net)
Brand Names Foscavir®

Synonyms PFA; Phosphonoformic Acid

Generic Available No

Use Treatment of CMV retinitis and other CMV infections; alternative to acyclovir for treatment of acyclovir-resistant HSV infections; foscarnet also has antiretroviral activity

Drug of Choice or Alternative For
Organism(s)
Cytomegalovirus *on page 97*
Herpes Simplex Virus *on page 128*

Pregnancy Risk Factor C

Contraindications Hypersensitivity to foscarnet or any component

Adverse Reactions
>10%: Fever, nausea, anemia, diarrhea, abnormal renal function, decreased creatinine clearance, vomiting, headache, seizures
1% to 10%: Fatigue, rigors, asthenia, malaise, injection site pain, sepsis, paresthesia, dizziness, involuntary muscle contractions, hypoesthesia, neuropathy, anorexia, granulocytopenia, leukopenia, electrolyte imbalance, depression, confusion, anxiety, coughing, dyspnea, rash, increased sweating, decreased creatinine clearance, vision abnormalities
<1%: Hypothermia, leg edema, peripheral edema, syncope, ascites, substernal chest pain, abnormal crying, malignant hyperpyrexia, cardiac failure, bradycardia, arrhythmias, vertigo, coma, abnormal gait, hypertonia, dyskinesia, vocal cord paralysis, speech disorders, cerebral edema, nystagmus, decreased gonadotropins, gynecomastia

Drug Interactions Foscarnet may be additive to other nephrotoxic drugs, concomitant use of intravenous pentamidine has caused severe hypocalcemia
(Continued)

Foscarnet (Continued)

Mechanism of Action Pyrophosphate analogue which acts as a noncompetitive inhibitor of many viral RNA and DNA polymerases as well as HIV reverse transcriptase. Foscarnet is a virostatic agent; foscarnet does not require activation by thymidine kinase.

Pharmacokinetics

Distribution: In bone, cartilage, kidney, urine, and CSF

Metabolism: Biotransformation does not occur

Half-life: ~3 hours

Elimination: Up to 28% excreted unchanged in urine

Usual Dosage See tables.

Dose Adjustment for Renal Impairment

The induction dose of foscarnet should be adjusted according to creatinine clearance as follows:

Creatinine Clearance (mL/min/kg)	Foscarnet Induction Dose (mg/kg q8h)
1.6	60
1.5	57
1.4	53
1.3	49
1.2	46
1.1	42
1	39
0.9	35
0.8	32
0.7	28
0.6	25
0.5	21
0.4	18

The maintenance dose of foscarnet should be adjusted according to creatinine clearance as follows:

Creatinine Clearance (mL/min/kg)	Foscarnet Maintenance Dose (mg/kg/day)
1.4	90–120
1.2–1.4	78–104
1–1.2	75–100
0.8–1	71–94
0.6–0.8	63–84
0.4–0.6	57–75

Induction treatment: 60 mg/kg 3 times/day for 14-21 days

Maintenance therapy: 90-120 mg/kg/day

Monitoring Parameters Serum creatinine, BUN, calcium, phosphorus, potassium, magnesium; hemoglobin

Patient Information Foscarnet is not a cure for CMV retinitis; regular ophthalmologic examinations should be done. Tingling, numbness, or paresthesias should be reported to the physician, pharmacist, or nurse.

Nursing Implications Do not administer by rapid or bolus injection; limit concentration to 12 mg/mL when using a peripheral line

Dosage Forms Injection: 24 mg/mL (250 mL, 500 mL)

Selected Readings

Chrisp P and Clissold SP, "Foscarnet. A Review of Its Antiviral Activity, Pharmacokinetic Properties and Therapeutic Use in Immunocompromised Patients With Cytomegalovirus Retinitis," Drugs, 1991, 41(1):104-29.

"Drugs for Non-HIV Viral Infections," *Med Lett Drugs Ther*, 1994, 36(919):27.
Keating MR, "Antiviral Agents," *Mayo Clin Proc*, 1992, 67(2):160-78.

Foscavir® *see* Foscarnet *on page 571*

Fulvicin® P/G *see* Griseofulvin *on page 578*

Fulvicin-U/F® *see* Griseofulvin *on page 578*

Fungatin® [OTC] *see* Tolnaftate *on page 687*

Fungizone® *see* Amphotericin B *on page 493*

Furadantin® *see* Nitrofurantoin *on page 623*

Furalan® *see* Nitrofurantoin *on page 623*

Furamide® *see* Diloxanide Furoate *on page 553*

Furan® *see* Nitrofurantoin *on page 623*

Furanite® *see* Nitrofurantoin *on page 623*

Furazolidone (fur a zoe' li done)
Brand Names Furoxone®
Generic Available No
Use Treatment of bacterial or protozoal diarrhea and enteritis caused by suscep-tible organisms *Giardia lamblia* and *Vibrio cholerae*
Pregnancy Risk Factor C
Contraindications Known hypersensitivity to furazolidone; concurrent use of alcohol; patients <1 month of age because of the possibility of producing he-molytic anemia
Warnings/Precautions Use caution in patients with G-6-PD deficiency when administering large doses for prolonged periods; furazolidone inhibits mono-amine oxidase
Adverse Reactions
>10%: Dark yellow to brown discoloration of urine
1% to 10%: Abdominal pain, diarrhea, nausea, vomiting, headache
<1%: Leukopenia, skin rash, fever, joint pain, orthostatic hypotension, dizzi-ness, drowsiness, malaise, fever, hypoglycemia, disulfiram-like reaction after alcohol ingestion, agranulocytosis, hemolysis in patients with G-6-PD defi-ciency
Toxicology Symptoms of overdose include nausea, vomiting, serotonin crisis; supportive care only; serotonin crisis may require dantrolene/bromocriptine
Drug Interactions
Increased effect with sympathomimetic amines, tricyclic antidepressants, tyra-mine-containing foods, MAO inhibitors, meperidine, anorexiants, dextrome-thorphan, fluoxetine, paroxetine, sertraline, trazodone
Increased effect/toxicity of levodopa
Disulfiram-like reaction with alcohol
Mechanism of Action Inhibits several vital enzymatic reactions causing anti-bacterial and antiprotozoal action
Pharmacokinetics
Absorption: Oral: Poor
Elimination: Oral: $1/3$ of dose excreted in urine as active drug and metabolites
Usual Dosage Oral:
Children >1 month: 5-8 mg/kg/day in 4 divided doses, not to exceed 400 mg/day
Adults: 100 mg 4 times/day
Monitoring Parameters CBC
Test Interactions False-positive results for urine glucose with Clinitest®
Patient Information May discolor urine to a brown tint; avoid drinking alcohol during and for 4 days after therapy or eating tyramine-containing foods, con-sult with physician or pharmacist for a list of these foods. Do not take any pre-scription or nonprescription drugs without consulting the physician or pharma-cist.
Dosage Forms
Liquid: 50 mg/15 mL (60 mL, 473 mL)
Tablet: 100 mg
Selected Readings
"Drugs for Parasitic Infections," *Med Lett Drugs Ther*, 1993, 35(911):111-22.

Furoxone® *see* Furazolidone *on this page*

Gamastan® *see* Immune Globulin *on page 588*

Gamimune® N *see* Immune Globulin *on page 588*

Gamma Benzene Hexachloride *see* Lindane *on page 599*

Gammagard® *see* Immune Globulin *on page 588*

Gamma Globulin *see* Immune Globulin *on page 588*

Gammar® *see* Immune Globulin *on page 588*

Ganciclovir (gan sye' kloe vir)
Brand Names Cytovene®

Synonyms DHPG Sodium; GCV Sodium; Nordeoxyguanosine

Generic Available No

Use CMV retinitis in immunocompromised individuals including patients with acquired immunodeficiency syndrome; may be used in the treatment of other organ systems infected with CMV; also active against other herpes viruses; sometimes used as prophylaxis of CMV disease in solid organ and bone marrow transplants

Drug of Choice or Alternative For
Organism(s)
Cytomegalovirus *on page 97*
Herpes Simplex Virus *on page 128*

Pregnancy Risk Factor C

Contraindications Absolute neutrophil count <500/mm^3; platelet count <25,000/mm^3; known hypersensitivity to ganciclovir or acyclovir

Warnings/Precautions Dosage adjustment or interruption of ganciclovir therapy may be necessary in patients with neutropenia and/or thrombocytopenia and patients with impaired renal function. Use with extreme caution in children since long-term safety has not been determined and due to ganciclovir's potential for long-term carcinogenic and adverse reproductive effects; ganciclovir may adversely affect spermatogenesis and fertility; due to its mutagenic potential, contraceptive precautions for female and male patients need to be followed during and for at least 90 days after therapy with the drug; take care to administer only into veins with good blood flow

Adverse Reactions
>10%: Granulocytopenia, thrombocytopenia, headache
1% to 10%: Anemia, confusion, sepsis, rash, fever, abnormal liver function values
<1%: Eosinophilia, arrhythmia, hypertension, hypotension, ataxia, coma, dizziness, nervousness, paresthesia, psychosis, tremor, alopecia, pruritus, urticaria, nausea, vomiting, diarrhea, hemorrhage, abdominal pain, inflammation or pain at injection site, edema, malaise, dyspnea, retinal detachment

Toxicology Hemodialysis and hydration may be of some benefit

Drug Interactions
Increased effect/toxicity with probenecid, imipenem/cilastatin
Increased toxicity in rapidly dividing cells with cytotoxic drugs; increased hematologic toxicity with zidovudine

Stability Reconstituted solution is stable for 12 hours at room temperature; **do not refrigerate**; reconstitute with sterile water **not** bacteriostatic water because parabens may cause precipitation

Mechanism of Action Ganciclovir is phosphorylated to a substrate which competitively inhibits the binding of deoxyguanosine triphosphate to DNA polymerase resulting in inhibition of viral DNA synthesis

Pharmacokinetics
Distribution: Widely distributed to all tissues
Metabolism: Little to none
Half-life: 1.7-5.8 hours (half-life increases with impaired renal function)
Elimination: 94% to 99% excreted as unchanged drug in urine

Usual Dosage Slow I.V. infusion:
Retinitis: Children >3 months and Adults: Induction therapy: 5 mg/kg/dose every 12 hours for 14-21 days followed by maintenance therapy; maintenance therapy: 5 mg/kg/day as a single daily dose for 7 days/week or 6 mg/kg/day for 5 days/week

Other CMV infections: 5 mg/kg/dose every 12 hours for 14-21 days or 2.5 mg/kg/dose every 8 hours; maintenance therapy: 5 mg/kg/day as a single daily dose for 7 days/week or 6 mg/kg/day for 5 days/week

Dosing adjustment in renal impairment:
Cl$_{cr}$ 50-79 mL/minute per 1.73 m^2: Administer 2.5 mg/kg every 12 hours
Cl$_{cr}$ 25-49 mL/minute per 1.73 m^2: Administer 2.5 mg/kg every 24 hours
Cl$_{cr}$ <25 mL/minute per 1.73 m^2: Administer 1.25 mg/kg every 24 hours
40% to 50% removed by a 4-hour hemodialysis

Overdosage Vomiting, hypersalivation, bloody diarrhea, cytopenia, testicular atrophy

Monitoring Parameters CBC with differential and platelet count, serum creatinine

Patient Information Ganciclovir is not a cure for CMV retinitis; Regular ophthalmologic examinations should be done; close monitoring of blood counts should be done while on therapy

Nursing Implications Must be prepared in vertical flow hood; use chemotherapy precautions during administration; discard appropriately

Additional Information Sodium content of 500 mg vial: 46 mg (2 mEq)

Dosage Forms Powder for injection, lyophilized: 500 mg (10 mL)

Selected Readings
"Drugs for Non-HIV Viral Infections," *Med Lett Drugs Ther*, 1994, 36(919):27.
Keating MR, "Antiviral Agents," *Mayo Clin Proc*, 1992, 67(2):160-78.
Matthews T and Boehme R, "Antiviral Activity and Mechanism of Action of Ganciclovir," *Rev Infect Dis*, 1988, 10(Suppl 3):S490-4.

Gantanol® *see* Sulfamethoxazole *on page 674*

Gantrisin® *see* Sulfisoxazole *on page 675*

Garamycin® Injection *see* Gentamicin Sulfate *on this page*

Garamycin® Ophthalmic *see* Gentamicin Sulfate *on this page*

Garamycin® Topical *see* Gentamicin Sulfate *on this page*

G-CSF *see* Filgrastim *on page 567*

GCV Sodium *see* Ganciclovir *on previous page*

Genapax® *see* Gentian Violet *on page 578*

Genaspor® [OTC] *see* Tolnaftate *on page 687*

Genoptic® Ophthalmic *see* Gentamicin Sulfate *on this page*

Genoptic® S.O.P. Ophthalmic *see* Gentamicin Sulfate *on this page*

Gentacidin® Ophthalmic *see* Gentamicin Sulfate *on this page*

Gent-AK® Ophthalmic *see* Gentamicin Sulfate *on this page*

Gentamicin Sulfate (jen ta mye' sin)
Related Information
Aminoglycoside Dosing and Monitoring *on page 721-722*

Brand Names Garamycin® Injection; Garamycin® Ophthalmic; Garamycin® Topical; Genoptic® Ophthalmic; Genoptic® S.O.P. Ophthalmic; Gentacidin® Ophthalmic; Gent-AK® Ophthalmic; Gentrasul® Ophthalmic; G-myticin® Topical; Jenamicin® Injection

Generic Available Yes

Use Treatment of infections caused by susceptible bacterial infections (normally gram-negative organisms including *Pseudomonas*) including bone infections, CNS infections, respiratory tract infections, skin and soft tissue infections, as well as abdominal and urinary tract infections, endocarditis, and septicemia; used in combination for treatment of infections caused by specific gram-negative and gram-positive bacteria

Drug of Choice or Alternative For
Disease/Syndrome(s)
Catheter Infection, Intravascular *on page 20*
Endocarditis, Acute, I.V. Drug Abuse *on page 21*
Endocarditis, Acute Native Valve *on page 22*
Endocarditis, Prosthetic Valve, Early *on page 22*
Endocarditis, Prosthetic Valve, Late *on page 23*
Endocarditis, Subacute Native Valve *on page 23*
Meningitis, Neonatal (<2 months of age) *on page 29*
Otitis Externa, Severe (Malignant) *on page 34*
Pelvic Inflammatory Disease *on page 35*
Peritonitis *on page 36*

Pneumonia, Hospital-Acquired *on page 38*
Sinusitis, Hospital-Acquired *on page 41*
Urinary Tract Infection, Pyelonephritis *on page 45*
Organism(s)
Brucella Species *on page 69*
Calymmatobacterium granulomatis on page 71
Corynebacterium jeikeium on page 90
Enterococcus Species *on page 107*
HACEK Group *on page 117*
Listeria monocytogenes on page 143
Staphylococcus aureus, Methicillin-Resistant *on page 195*
Staphylococcus epidermidis, Methicillin-Resistant *on page 200*
Streptococcus, Viridans Group *on page 213*
Yersinia pestis on page 233
Pregnancy Risk Factor C
Contraindications Hypersensitivity to gentamicin or other aminoglycosides
Adverse Reactions
>10%: Nephrotoxicity, neurotoxicity, ototoxicity (auditory), ototoxicity (vestibular), decreased creatinine clearance
1% to 10%: Skin itching, redness, rash, swelling
<1%: Difficulty in breathing, drowsiness, weakness, headache, tremors, muscle cramps, pseudomotor cerebri, anorexia, nausea, vomiting, weight loss, increased salivation, enterocolitis, granulocytopenia, agranulocytosis, thrombocytopenia, photosensitivity, erythema, burning, stinging
Toxicology Because of the potential for toxicity, serum level monitoring is recommended for all patients. The treatment of choice following a single acute overdose appears to be the maintenance of good urine output of at least 3 mL/kg/hour. Dialysis is of questionable value in the enhancement of aminoglycoside elimination. If required, hemodialysis is preferred over peritoneal dialysis in patients with normal renal function. Careful hydration may be all that is required to promote diuresis and therefore the enhancement of the drug's elimination.
Drug Interactions
Increased/prolonged effect: Depolarizing and nondepolarizing neuromuscular blocking agents
Increased toxicity: Concurrent use of amphotericin may increase nephrotoxicity
Stability I.V. infusion solutions mixed in NS or D_5W solution are stable for 24 hours at room temperature; incompatible with penicillins
Mechanism of Action Interferes with bacterial protein synthesis by binding to 30S ribosomal subunits
Pharmacokinetics
Absorption: May be absorbed in minute quantities following topical application to eye
Distribution: Distributed to most body tissues; intraocular penetration is poor; CSF penetration is low even in patients with inflamed meninges; crosses the placenta
Metabolism: None
Half-life:
Infants <1 week: 3-11.5 hours
Infants 1 week to 6 months: 3-3.5 hours
Adults: 1.5-3 hours; anuria: 36-70 hours
Time to peak serum concentration: I.M.: Within 30-90 minutes
Elimination: Eliminated almost completely by glomerular filtration of unchanged drug with excretion into urine
Usual Dosage Individualization is critical because of the low therapeutic index. Use of ideal body weight (IBW) for determining the mg/kg/dose appears to be more accurate than dosing on the basis of total body weight (TBW). In morbid obesity, dosage requirement may best be estimated using a dosing weight of IBW + 0.4 (TBW - IBW). Peak and trough plasma drug levels should be determined, particularly in critically ill patients with serious infections or in disease states known to significantly alter aminoglycoside pharmacokinetics (eg, cystic fibrosis, burns, or major surgery).

Dosage should be based on an estimate of ideal body weight

Neonates: I.M., I.V.:
Postnatal age <7 days:
<1200 g, 0-4 weeks: 2.5 mg/kg/dose every 18-24 hours
>1200 g: 2.5 mg/kg/dose every 12 hours

Postnatal age >7 days, >1200 g: 2.5 mg/kg/dose every 8 hours

Newborns: Intrathecal: 1 mg every day

Infants and Children:
Intrathecal: >3 months: 1-2 mg/day
I.M., I.V.: 2.5 mg/kg/dose every 8 hours*
Cystic fibrosis: 2.5 mg/kg/dose every 6 hours
Topical: Apply 1-4 times/day to affected area
Ophthalmic:
Solution: Instill 1-2 drops every 2-4 hours, up to 2 drops every hour for severe infections
Ointment: Instill $\frac{1}{2}$" (1.25 cm) 2-3 times/day to every 3-4 hours

Adults:
Intrathecal: 4-8 mg/day
I.M., I.V.:
Severe life-threatening infections: 2-2.5 mg/kg/dose
Urinary tract infections: 1.5 mg/kg/dose
Synergy (for gram-positive infections): 1 mg/kg/dose

Some clinicians suggest a daily dose of 4-7 mg/kg for all patients with normal renal function. This dose is at least as efficacious with similar, if not less, toxicity than conventional dosing.

Dosing adjustment in renal impairment: Initial dosing:
All patients should receive a loading dose of at least 2 mg/kg (subsequent dosing should be based on serum concentrations)
Cl_{cr} ≥60 mL/minute: Administer every 8 hours
Cl_{cr} 40-60 mL/minute: Administer every 12 hours
Cl_{cr} 20-40 mL/minute: Administer every 24 hours
Dialyzable (50% to 100%)
* Some patients may require larger or more frequent doses (eg, every 6 hours) if serum levels document the need (ie, CF or febrile granulocytopenic patients)
** Two to three serum level measurements should be obtained after the initial dose to measure the half-life in order to determine the frequency of subsequent doses
Topical: Apply 1-4 times/day to affected area
Ophthalmic:
Solution: Instill 1-2 drops every 2-4 hours
Ointment: Instill $\frac{1}{2}$" (1.25 cm) 2-3 times/day to every 3-4 hours

Overdosage Ototoxicity, nephrotoxicity, and neuromuscular toxicity

Monitoring Parameters Urinalysis, urine output, BUN, serum creatinine, peak and trough plasma gentamicin levels

Reference Range Therapeutic: Peak: 4-10 μg/mL (SI: 8-21 μmol/L); Trough: <2 μg/mL (SI: 4 μmol/L); Toxic: Peak: >10 μg/mL (SI: >21 μmol/L); Trough: >2 μg/mL (SI: >4.2 μmol/L)

Test Interactions Penicillin may decrease aminoglycoside serum concentrations *in vitro*

Patient Information Report any dizziness or sensations of ringing or fullness in ears

Nursing Implications Peak levels are drawn 30 minutes after the end of a 30-minute infusion; trough levels are drawn within 30 minutes before the next dose; give other antibiotic drugs at least 1 hour before or after gentamicin, if possible.

Additional Information When injected into the muscles of paralyzed patients, there are slower absorption and lower peak concentrations probably due to poor circulation in the atrophic muscles, suggest I.V. route; aminoglycoside levels measured in blood taken from Silastic® central catheters can sometime give falsely high readings.

Dosage Forms
Cream, topical: 0.1% (15 g)
Injection: 40 mg/mL (1 mL, 2 mL, 10 mL, 20 mL)
Intrathecal: 2 mg/mL (2 mL)
Pediatric: 10 mg/mL (2 mL)
Ointment:
Ophthalmic: 0.3% (3.5 g)
Topical: 0.1% (15 g)
Solution, ophthalmic: 0.3% (1 mL, 5 mL, 15 mL)

Selected Readings
Cunha BA, "Aminoglycosides: Current Role in Antimicrobial Therapy," *Pharmacotherapy*, 1988, 8(6):334-50.

(Continued)

Gentamicin Sulfate *(Continued)*

Edson RS and Terrell CL, "The Aminoglycosides," *Mayo Clin Proc*, 1991, 66(11):1158-64.

Gilbert DN, "Once-Daily Aminoglycoside Therapy," *Antimicrob Agents Chemother*, 1991, 35(3):399-405.

Hustinx WN, and Hoepelman IM, "Aminoglycoside Dosage Regimens. Is Once a Day Enough?" *Clin Pharmacokinet*, 1993, 25(6):427-32.

Iseman MD, "Treatment of Multidrug-Resistant Tuberculosis," *N Engl J Med*, 1993, 329(11):784-91.

McCormack JP and Jewesson PJ, "A Critical Reevaluation of the "Therapeutic Range" of Aminoglycosides," *Clin Infect Dis*, 1992, 14(1):320-39.

Gentian Violet (jen' shun)

Brand Names Genapax®

Synonyms Crystal Violet; Methylrosaniline Chloride

Generic Available Yes

Use Treatment of cutaneous or mucocutaneous infections caused by *Candida albicans* and other superficial skin infections

Pregnancy Risk Factor C

Contraindications Known hypersensitivity to gentian violet; ulcerated areas; patients with porphyria

Warnings/Precautions Infants should be turned face down after application to minimize amount of drug swallowed; may result in tattooing of the skin when applied to granulation tissue; solution is for external use only; avoid contact with eyes

Adverse Reactions 1% to 10%: Esophagitis, burning, irritation, vesicle formation, sensitivity reactions, ulceration of mucous membranes, laryngitis, tracheitis, laryngeal obstruction

Toxicology Laryngeal obstruction

Mechanism of Action Topical antiseptic/germicide effective against some vegetative gram-positive bacteria, particularly *Staphylococcus* sp, and some yeast; it is much less effective against gram-negative bacteria and is ineffective against acid-fast bacteria

Usual Dosage

Children and Adults: Topical: Apply 0.5% to 2% locally with cotton to lesion 2-3 times/day for 3 days, do not swallow and avoid contact with eyes

Adults: Intravaginal: Insert one tampon for 3-4 hours once or twice daily for 12 days

Patient Information Drug stains skin and clothing purple; do not apply to an ulcerative lesion; may result in "tattooing" of the skin; when used for the treatment of vaginal candidiasis, coitus should be avoided; insert vaginal product high into vagina. Use condoms or refrain from sexual intercourse to avoid reinfection.

Dosage Forms

Solution, topical: 1% (30 mL); 2% (30 mL)

Tampons: 5 mg (12s)

Gentrasul® Ophthalmic *see* Gentamicin Sulfate *on page 575*

Geocillin® *see* Carbenicillin *on page 507*

German Measles Vaccine *see* Rubella Virus Vaccine, Live *on page 665*

G-myticin® Topical *see* Gentamicin Sulfate *on page 575*

Granulocyte Colony Stimulating Factor *see* Filgrastim *on page 567*

Grifulvin® V *see* Griseofulvin *on this page*

Grisactin® *see* Griseofulvin *on this page*

Grisactin® Ultra *see* Griseofulvin *on this page*

Griseofulvin (gri see oh ful' vin)

Brand Names Fulvicin® P/G; Fulvicin-U/F®; Grifulvin® V; Grisactin®; Grisactin® Ultra; Gris-PEG®

Synonyms Griseofulvin Microsize; Griseofulvin Ultramicrosize

Generic Available No

Use Treatment of susceptible tinea infections of the skin, hair, and nails

Drug of Choice or Alternative For

Organism(s)

Dermatophytes *on page 100*

Pregnancy Risk Factor C

Contraindications Hypersensitivity to griseofulvin or any component; severe liver disease, porphyria (interferes with porphyrin metabolism)

Warnings/Precautions Safe use in children <2 years of age has not been established; during long-term therapy, periodic assessment of hepatic, renal, and hematopoietic functions should be performed; may cause fetal harm when administered to pregnant women; avoid exposure to intense sunlight to prevent photosensitivity reactions; hypersensitivity cross reaction between penicillins and griseofulvin is possible

Adverse Reactions

>10%: Skin rash, urticaria

1% to 10%: Oral thrush, nausea, vomiting, epigastric distress, diarrhea, headache, fatigue, dizziness, insomnia, mental confusion

<1%: Proteinuria, nephrosis, leukopenia, hepatic toxicity, GI bleeding, menstrual toxicity, angioneurotic edema

Drug Interactions

Decreased effect of anticoagulants, oral contraceptives; decreased effect/levels with barbiturates

Disufiram-like reaction with alcohol

Mechanism of Action Inhibits fungal cell mitosis at metaphase; binds to human keratin making it resistant to fungal invasion

Pharmacokinetics

Absorption: Absorption of ultramicrosize griseofulvin is almost complete; absorption of microsize griseofulvin is variable (25% to 70% of an oral dose); absorption is enhanced by ingestion of a fatty meal

Distribution: Deposited in varying concentrations in the keratin layer of the skin, hair, and nails; can be detected in the stratum corneum of skin within a few hours following administration; only a very small fraction is distributed in the body fluids and tissues; crosses the placenta

Metabolism: Extensive in the liver

Half-life: 9-22 hours

Time to peak serum concentration: ~4 hours

Elimination: <1% excreted unchanged in urine; also excreted in feces and perspiration

Usual Dosage Oral:

Children:

Microsize: 10-15 mg/kg/day in single or divided doses;

Ultramicrosize: >2 months: 5.5-7.3 mg/kg/day in single or divided doses

Adults:

Microsize: 500-1000 mg/day in single or divided doses

Ultramicrosize: 330-375 mg/day in single or divided doses; doses up to 750 mg/day have been used for infections more difficult to eradicate such as tinea unguium

Duration of therapy depends on the site of infection:

Tinea corporis: 2-4 weeks

Tinea capitis: 4-6 weeks or longer

Tinea pedis: 4-8 weeks

Tinea unguium: 3-6 months

Overdosage Lethargy, vertigo, blurred vision, nausea, vomiting, diarrhea

Monitoring Parameters Periodic renal, hepatic, and hematopoietic function tests

Test Interactions False-positive urinary VMA levels

Patient Information Avoid exposure to sunlight, take with fatty meal; if patient gets headache, it usually goes away with continued therapy; may cause dizziness, drowsiness, and impair judgment; do not take if pregnant; if you become pregnant, discontinue immediately

Additional Information

Griseofulvin microsize: Fulvicin-U/F®, Grifulvin® V, Grisactin®

Griseofulvin ultramicrosize: Fulvicin® P/G, Grisactin® Ultra, Gris-PEG®

Dosage Forms

Griseofulvin Microsize:

Capsule (Grisactin®): 125 mg, 250 mg

Suspension, oral (Grifulvin® V): 125 mg/5 mL with alcohol 0.2% (120 mL)

Tablet:

Fulvicin-U/F®, Grifulvin® V: 250 mg

(Continued)

Griseofulvin *(Continued)*

Fulvicin-U/F®, Grifulvin® V, Grisactin-500®: 500 mg

Griseofulvin Ultramicrosize:
Tablet:
Fulvicin® P/G: 165 mg, 330 mg
Fulvicin® P/G, Grisactin® Ultra, Gris-PEG®: 125 mg, 250 mg
Grisactin® Ultra: 330 mg

Griseofulvin Microsize *see* Griseofulvin *on page 578*

Griseofulvin Ultramicrosize *see* Griseofulvin *on page 578*

Gris-PEG® *see* Griseofulvin *on page 578*

G-well® *see* Lindane *on page 599*

Gyne-Lotrimin® Vaginal [OTC] *see* Clotrimazole *on page 543*

Gyne-Sulf® *see* Sulfabenzamide, Sulfacetamide, and Sulfathiazole *on page 671*

***Haemophilus* b Conjugate Vaccine** *see* Hemophilus b Conjugate Vaccine *on this page*

***Haemophilus* b Oligosaccharide Conjugate Vaccine** *see* Hemophilus b Conjugate Vaccine *on this page*

***Haemophilus* b Polysaccharide Vaccine** *see* Hemophilus b Conjugate Vaccine *on this page*

Haloprogin (ha loe proe' jin)
Brand Names Halotex®
Generic Available No
Use Topical treatment of tinea pedis, tinea cruris, tinea corporis, tinea manuum caused by *Trichophyton rubrum*, *Trichophyton tonsurans*, *Trichophyton mentagrophytes*, *Microsporum canis*, or *Epidermophyton floccosum*
Pregnancy Risk Factor B
Contraindications Hypersensitivity to haloprogin or any component
Warnings/Precautions Safety and efficacy has not been established in children
Adverse Reactions <1%: Pruritus, folliculitis, irritation, burning sensation, vesicle formation, erythema
Mechanism of Action Interferes with fungal DNA replication
Pharmacokinetics
Absorption: Poorly through the skin (~11%)
Metabolism: To trichlorophenol
Elimination: Excretion in urine, 75% as unchanged drug
Usual Dosage Topical: Children and Adults: Apply twice daily for 2-3 weeks; intertriginous areas may require up to 4 weeks of treatment
Patient Information Avoid contact with eyes; for external use only; improvement should occur within 4 weeks
Dosage Forms
Cream: 1% (15 g, 30 g)
Solution, topical: 1% with alcohol 75% (10 mL, 30 mL)

Halotex® *see* Haloprogin *on this page*

HbCV *see* Hemophilus b Conjugate Vaccine *on this page*

HBIG *see* Hepatitis B Immune Globulin *on page 582*

H-BIG® *see* Hepatitis B Immune Globulin *on page 582*

HDCV *see* Rabies Virus Vaccine *on page 659*

Hemophilus b Conjugate Vaccine (hem off' fil us)
Related Information
Vaccines *on page 706-709*
Brand Names HibTITER®; PedvaxHIB™; ProHIBiT®
Synonyms Diphtheria CRM$_{197}$ Protein Conjugate; Diphtheria Toxoid Conjugate; *Haemophilus* b Conjugate Vaccine; *Haemophilus* b Oligosaccharide Conjugate Vaccine; *Haemophilus* b Polysaccharide Vaccine; HbCV; Hib Polysaccharide Conjugate; PRP-D
Generic Available No
Use Routine immunization of children 2 months to 5 years against invasive dis-

ease caused by hemophilus influenza b; hemophilus b conjugate vaccines are not indicated for prevention of bronchitis or other infections due to *H. influenzae* in adults; adults with specific dysfunction or certain complement deficiencies who are at especially high risk of *H. influenzae* type b infection may be considered for vaccination

Pregnancy Risk Factor C

Contraindications Children with any febrile illness or active infection, known hypersensitivity to *Haemophilus* b polysaccharide vaccine (thimerosal), children who are immunosuppressed or receiving immunosuppressive therapy

Warnings/Precautions Any febrile illness or active infection is reason for delaying use of *Haemophilus* b conjugate vaccine

Adverse Reactions

>10%: Acute febrile reactions

1% to 10%: Irritation at injection site, anorexia, diarrhea, fever (up to 102.2°F), irritability, lethargy

<1%: Allergic or anaphylactic reactions (difficulty in breathing, hives, itching, swelling of eyes, face, unusual tiredness or weakness), convulsions, vomiting, fever >102.2°F

Drug Interactions Decreased effect with immunosuppressive agents, immunoglobulins within 1 month may decrease antibody production; may interfere with antigen detection tests

Stability Keep in refrigerator, may be frozen (not diluent) without affecting potency; reconstituted Hib-Imune® remains stable for only 8 hours, whereas Hib-VAX® remain stable for 30 days when refrigerated

Mechanism of Action Stimulates production of anticapsular antibodies and provides active immunity to *Haemophilus influenzae*

Usual Dosage Children: I.M.: 0.5 mL as a single dose should be administered according to one of the following "brand-specific" schedules. Do not inject I.V.

Vaccination Schedule for *Haemophilus* b Conjugate Vaccines

Age at 1st Dose (mo)	HibTITER®		PedvaxHIB®		ProHIBiT®	
	Primary Series	Booster	Primary Series	Booster	Primary Series	Booster
2–6*	3 doses, 2 months apart	15 mo†	2 doses, 2 months apart	12 mo†		
7–11	2 doses, 2 months apart	15 mo†	2 doses, 2 months apart	15 mo†		
12–14	1 dose	15 mo†	1 dose	15 mo†		
15–60	1 dose	—	1 dose	—	1 dose	—

*It is not currently recommended that the various *Haemophilus* b conjugate vaccines be interchanged (ie, the same brand should be used throughout the entire vaccination series). If the health care provider does not know which vaccine was previously used, it is prudent that an infant, 2–6 months of age, be given a primary series of three doses.
†At least 2 months after previous dose.

Test Interactions May interfere with interpretation of antigen detection tests

Patient Information May use acetaminophen for post-dose fever

Nursing Implications Defer immunization if infection or febrile illness present. Do not give I.V.

Additional Information Federal law requires that the date of administration, the vaccine manufacturer, lot number of vaccine, and the administering person's name, title and address be entered into the patient's permanent medical record

Dosage Forms Injection:

HibTITER®: Capsular oligosaccharide 10 μg and diphtheria CRM$_{197}$ protein ~25 μg per 0.5 mL (0.5 mL, 2.5 mL, 5 mL)

PedvaxHIB™: Purified capsular polysaccharide 15 μg and *Neisseria meningitidis* OMPC 250 μg per dose (0.5 mL)

ProHIBiT®: Purified capsular polysaccharide 25 μg and conjugated diphtheria toxoid protein 18 μg per dose (0.5 mL, 2.5 mL, 5 mL)

Hepatitis B Immune Globulin (hep a tie' tiss)
Related Information
Postexposure Prophylaxis for Hepatitis B *on page 719-720*
Brand Names H-BIG®; Hep-B-Gammagee®; HyperHep®
Synonyms HBIG
Generic Available No
Use Provide prophylactic passive immunity to hepatitis B infection to those individuals exposed. Hepatitis B immune globulin is not indicated for treatment of active hepatitis B infections and is ineffective in the treatment of chronic active hepatitis B infection.
Pregnancy Risk Factor C
Contraindications Hypersensitivity to hepatitis B immune globulin or any component
Adverse Reactions
1% to 10%: Local pain and tenderness at injection site, urticaria, angioedema, dizziness, malaise, urticaria, rash, pain, tenderness, swelling erythema, joint pains
<1%: Anaphylaxis
Drug Interactions Interferes with immune response of live virus vaccines
Stability Refrigerate
Mechanism of Action Hepatitis B immune globulin (HBIG) is a nonpyrogenic sterile solution containing 10% to 18% protein of which at least 80% is monomeric immunoglobulin G (IgG). HBIG differs from immune globulin in the amount of anti-HBs. Immune globulin is prepared from plasma that is not preselected for anti-HBs content. HBIG is prepared from plasma preselected for high titer anti-HBs. In the U.S., HBIG has an anti-HBs high titer of higher than 1:100,000 by IRA. There is no evidence that the causative agent of AIDS (HTLV-III/LAV) is transmitted by HBIG.
Pharmacokinetics
Absorption: Slow
Time to peak serum concentration: 1-6 days
Usual Dosage I.M.:
Newborns: Hepatitis B: 0.5 mL as soon after birth as possible (within 12 hours)
Adults: Postexposure prophylaxis: 0.06 mL/kg; usual dose: 3-5 mL; maximum dose: 5 mL as soon as possible after exposure (within 7 days); repeat at 28-30 days after exposure
Nursing Implications I.M. injection only, do **not** administer I.V.; to prevent injury from injection, care should be taken when giving to patients with thrombocytopenia or bleeding disorders
Additional Information Hepatitis B immune globulin is not indicated for treatment of active hepatitis B infections and is ineffective in the treatment of chronic active hepatitis B infection
Dosage Forms Injection:
H-BIG®: 4 mL, 5 mL
Hep-B-Gammagee®: 5 mL
HyperHep®: 0.5 mL, 1 mL, 5 mL

Hepatitis B Inactivated Virus Vaccine (plasma derived) *see*
Hepatitis B Vaccine *on this page*

Hepatitis B Inactivated Virus Vaccine (recombinant DNA) *see*
Hepatitis B Vaccine *on this page*

Hepatitis B Vaccine
Related Information
Vaccines *on page 706-709*
Brand Names Engerix-B®; Recombivax HB®
Synonyms Hepatitis B Inactivated Virus Vaccine (plasma derived); Hepatitis B Inactivated Virus Vaccine (recombinant DNA)
Generic Available No
Use Immunization against infection caused by all known subtypes of hepatitis B virus in individuals considered at high risk of potential exposure to hepatitis B virus or HB$_s$Ag-positive materials; see chart
Pregnancy Risk Factor C
Contraindications Hypersensitivity to yeast, hypersensitivity to hepatitis B vaccine or any component

Pre−exposure Prophylaxis for Hepatitis B

Health care workers*

Special patient groups
    Hemodialysis patients†
    Recipients of certain blood products‡

Lifestyle factors
    Homosexual and bisexual men
    Intravenous drug abusers
    Heterosexually active persons with multiple sexual partners or recently
       acquired sexually transmitted diseases

Environmental factors
    Household and sexual contacts of HBV carriers
    Prison inmates
    Clients and staff of institutions for the mentally retarded
    Residents, immigrants and refugees from areas with endemic HBV infection
    International travelers at increased risk of acquiring HBV infection

---

*The risk of hepatitis B virus (HBV) infection for health care workers
varies both between hospitals and within hospitals. Hepatitis B
vaccination is recommended for all health care workers with blood
exposure.
†Hemodialysis patients often respond poorly to hepatitis B vaccination.
Patients with chronic renal disease should be vaccinated as early as
possible, ideally before they require hemodialysis. In addition, their anti−
HBs levels should be monitored at 6–12 month intervals to assess the
need for revaccination.
‡Patients with hemophilia should be immunized subcutaneously, not
intramuscularly.

Adverse Reactions
> >10%: Mild local tenderness, local inflammatory reaction, fever, malaise, fatigue, headache
> 1% to 10%: Nausea, diarrhea, pharyngitis
> <1%: Sweating, sensation of warmth, lightheadedness, chills, flushing, somnolence, insomnia, irritability, agitation, arthralgia, myalgia, stiffness in back/neck/arm or shoulder, vomiting, GI disturbances, constipation, abdominal cramps, dyspepsia, pruritus, anorexia, rash, erythema, urticaria, rhinitis, cough, nosebleed, earache, dysuria, tachycardia, hypotension

Drug Interactions Immunosuppressive agents

Stability Refrigerate, do not freeze

Mechanism of Action Recombinant hepatitis B vaccine is a noninfectious subunit viral vaccine. The vaccine is derived from hepatitis B surface antigen (HB_sAg) produced through recombinant DNA techniques from yeast cells. The portion of the hepatitis B gene which codes for HB_sAg is cloned into yeast which is then cultured to produce hepatitis B vaccine. The recombinant hepatitis B vaccine available from Merck Sharp & Dohme (Recombivax HB®) contains 10 μg/mL HB_sAg; the one available from SmithKline Beecham contains 20 μg/mL HB_sAg.

Pharmacokinetics Duration of action: Following all 3 doses of hepatitis B vaccine, immunity will last approximately 5-7 years

Usual Dosage See tables.

Recommended Dosage for Infants Born to HB_sAg Positive Mothers

Treatment	Birth	Within 7 d	1 mo	6 mo
Engerix-B® (pediatric dose 10 μg/0.5 mL)	*	0.5 mL*	0.5 mL	0.5 mL
Recombivax HB® (pediatric dose 5 μg/0.5 mL)	*	0.5 mL*	0.5 mL	0.5 mL
Hepatitis B immune globulin	0.5 mL	—	—	—

*The first dose may be given at birth at the same time as HBIG, but give in the opposite anterolateral thigh. This may better ensure vaccine absorption.

(Continued)

Hepatitis B Vaccine *(Continued)*

Immunization Regimen of Three I.M. Hepatitis B Vaccine Doses

Age	Initial		1 mo		6 mo	
	Recom-bivax HB® (mL)	En-gerix–B® (mL)	Recom-bivax HB® (mL)	En-gerix–B® (mL)	Recom-bivax HB® (mL)	En-gerix–B® (mL)
Birth*–10 y	0.25	0.5	0.25	0.5	0.25	0.5
11–19 y	0.5	1	0.5	1	0.5	1
≥20 y	1	1	1	1	1	1
Dialysis or immuno–compromised patients		2†		2†		2†

*Infants born of HB$_s$Ag negative mothers.
†Two 1 mL doses given at different sites.

Patient Information Must complete full course of injections for adequate immunization

Nursing Implications I.M. injection only; in adults, the deltoid muscle is the preferred site; the anterolateral thigh is the recommended site in infants and young children. Rare chance of anaphylactoid reaction; have epinephrine available.

Additional Information Inactivated virus vaccine; federal law requires that the date of administration, the vaccine manufacturer, lot number of vaccine, and the administering person's name, title and address be entered into the patient's permanent medical record

Dosage Forms Injection:
Recombinant DNA (Engerix-B®): Hepatitis B surface antigen 20 µg/mL (1 mL)
Recombinant DNA, Pediatric, (Engerix-B®): Hepatitis B surface antigen 10 µg/ 0.5 mL (0.5 mL)
Recombinant DNA (Recombivax HB®): Hepatitis B surface antigen 10 µg/mL (1 mL, 3 mL)
Dialysis formulation, recombinant DNA (Recombivax HB®): Hepatitis B surface antigen 40 µg/mL (1 mL)

Hep-B-Gammagee® *see* Hepatitis B Immune Globulin *on page 582*

Herplex® *see* Idoxuridine *on page 586*

Hexachlorocyclohexane *see* Lindane *on page 599*

Hexamethylenetetramine *see* Methenamine *on page 607*

Hib Polysaccharide Conjugate *see* Hemophilus b Conjugate Vaccine *on page 580*

HibTITER® *see* Hemophilus b Conjugate Vaccine *on page 580*

Hiprex® *see* Methenamine *on page 607*

Hivid® *see* Zalcitabine *on page 695*

Human Diploid Cell Cultures Rabies Vaccine *see* Rabies Virus Vaccine *on page 659*

Human Diploid Cell Cultures Rabies Vaccine (Intradermal use) *see* Rabies Virus Vaccine *on page 659*

Humatin® *see* Paromomycin Sulfate *on page 630*

Hydroxychloroquine Sulfate *(hye drox ee klor' oh kwin)*
Brand Names Plaquenil®
Generic Available No
Use Suppresses and treats acute attacks of malaria; treatment of systemic lupus erythematosus (SLE) and rheumatoid arthritis (RA)
Pregnancy Risk Factor C
Contraindications Retinal or visual field changes attributable to 4-

aminoquinolines; hypersensitivity to hydroxychloroquine, 4-aminoquinoline derivatives, or any component

Warnings/Precautions Use with caution in patients with hepatic disease, G-6-PD deficiency, psoriasis, and porphyria; long-term use in children is not recommended; perform baseline and periodic (6 months) ophthalmologic examinations; test periodically for muscle weakness

Adverse Reactions

> 10%: Ciliary muscle dysfunction, diarrhea, loss of appetite, nausea, stomach cramps, vomiting, headache, itching

1% to 10%: Ocular toxicity, keratopathy, retinopathy, bleaching of hair, blueblack discoloration of skin, dizziness, lightheadedness, nervousness, restlessness, skin rash

<1%: Agranulocytosis, aplastic anemia, neutropenia, thrombocytopenia, emotional changes, neuromyopathy, ototoxicity, seizures

Toxicology Symptoms of overdose include headache, drowsiness, visual changes, cardiovascular collapse, and seizures followed by respiratory and cardiac arrest; treatment is symptomatic; activated charcoal will bind the drug following GI decontamination; urinary alkalinization will enhance renal elimination; seizures can be treated with diazepam 0.01 mg/kg; shock and hypotension should be treated with fluids and pressors if needed

Mechanism of Action Interferes with digestive vacuole function within sensitive malarial parasites by increasing the pH and interfering with lysosomal degradation of hemoglobin; inhibits locomotion of neutrophils and chemotaxis of eosinophils; impairs complement-dependent antigen-antibody reactions

Pharmacokinetics

Absorption: Oral: Complete

Metabolism: In the liver

Elimination: Metabolites and unchanged drug slowly excreted in urine, may be enhanced by urinary acidification

Usual Dosage Oral:

Children:

Chemoprophylaxis of malaria: 5 mg/kg (base) once weekly; should not exceed the recommended adult dose; begin 2 weeks before exposure; continue for 4-6 weeks after leaving endemic area

Acute attack: 10 mg/kg (base) initial dose; followed by 5 mg/kg in 6 hours on day 1; 5 mg/kg in 1 dose on day 2 and on day 3

RA or SLE: 3-5 mg/kg/day divided 1-2 times/day to a maximum of 400 mg/day; not to exceed 7 mg/kg/day

Adults:

Chemoprophylaxis of malaria: 2 tablets weekly on same day each week; begin 2 weeks before exposure; continue for 4-6 weeks after leaving endemic area

Acute attack: 4 tablets first dose day 1; 2 tablets in 6 hours day 1; 2 tablets in 1 dose day 2; and 2 tablets in 1 dose on day 3

Rheumatoid arthritis: 2-3 tablets/day to start taken with food or milk; increase dose until optimum response level is reached; usually after 4-12 weeks dose should be reduced by $\frac{1}{2}$ and a maintenance dose of 1-2 tablets/day given

Lupus erythematosus: 2 tablets every day or twice daily for several weeks depending on response; 1-2 tablets/day for prolonged maintenance therapy

Monitoring Parameters Ophthalmologic exam, CBC

Patient Information Take with food or milk; complete full course of therapy; wear sunglasses in bright sunlight; notify physician if blurring or other vision changes, ringing in the ears, or hearing loss occurs

Nursing Implications Periodic blood counts and eye examinations are recommended when patient is on chronic therapy

Dosage Forms Tablet: 200 mg [base 155 mg]

Selected Readings

"Drugs for Parasitic Infections," *Med Lett Drugs Ther*, 1993, 35(911):111-22.

Panisko DM and Keystone JS, "Treatment of Malaria – 1990," *Drugs*, 1990, 39(2):160-89.

HyperHep® *see* Hepatitis B Immune Globulin *on page 582*

Hyper-Tet® *see* Tetanus Immune Globulin, Human *on page 677*

I-Chlor® *see* Chloramphenicol *on page 531*

Idoxuridine (eye dox yoor' i deen)

Brand Names Herplex®

Synonyms IDU; IUDR

Generic Available No

Use Treatment of herpes simplex keratitis

Pregnancy Risk Factor C

Contraindications Hypersensitivity to idoxuridine or any component; concurrent use in patients receiving corticosteroids with superficial dendritic keratitis

Warnings/Precautions Use with caution in patients with corneal ulceration or patients receiving corticosteroid applications; if no response in epithelial infections within 14 days, consider a second form of therapy

Adverse Reactions
1% to 10%: Pruritus, follicular conjunctivitis, irritation, pain, inflammation, mild edema of the eyelids and cornea, visual haze, corneal clouding, photophobia
<1%: Small punctate defects on the corneal epithelium

Toxicology Due to frequent dosing, small defects on the epithelium may result. Mutagenic and cytotoxic and should be considered as being potentially carcinogenic; no treatment is indicated for accidental ingestion

Drug Interactions Increased toxicity (initiation): Do not coadminister with boric acid containing solutions

Stability Store in tight, light-resistant containers at 2 °C to 8°C until dispensed; do not mix with other medications; solution must be refrigerated

Mechanism of Action Incorporated into viral DNA in place of thymidine resulting in mutations and inhibition of viral replication

Pharmacokinetics
Absorption: Ophthalmic: Poor following instillation; tissue uptake is a function of cellular metabolism, which is inhibited by high concentrations of the drug (absorption decreases as the concentration of drug increases)
Distribution: Crosses the placenta
Metabolism: To iodouracil, uracil, and iodide
Elimination: Unchanged drug and metabolites excreted in urine

Usual Dosage Adults: Ophthalmic:
Ointment: Instill 5 times/day (every 4 hours) in the conjunctival sac with last dose at bedtime; continue therapy for 5-7 days after healing appears complete
Solution: Instill 1 drop in eye(s) every hour during day and every 2 hours at night, continue until definite improvement is noted, then reduce daytime dose to 1 drop every 2 hours and every 4 hours at night; continue for 5-7 days after healing appears complete

Patient Information May cause sensitivity to bright light; minimize by wearing sunglasses; notify physician if improvement is not seen in 7-8 days, if condition worsens, or if pain, decreased vision, itching, or swelling of the eye occur; do not exceed recommended dose

Dosage Forms Ophthalmic:
Ointment: 0.5% (4 g)
Solution: 0.1% (15 mL)

IDU see Idoxuridine *on this page*

IFN-alpha 2 see Interferon Alfa-2b *on page 590*

IG see Immune Globulin *on page 588*

IGIM see Immune Globulin *on page 588*

IGIV see Immune Globulin *on page 588*

Ilosone® Oral see Erythromycin *on page 561*

Imipemide see Imipenem/Cilastatin *on this page*

Imipenem/Cilastatin (i mi pen' em)

Related Information
Antimicrobial Activity Against Selected Organisms *on page 757-764*

Brand Names Primaxin®

Synonyms Imipemide

Generic Available No

Use Treatment of documented multidrug-resistant gram-negative infection due to organisms proven or suspected to be susceptible to imipenem/cilastatin; treatment of multiple organism infection in which other agents have an insufficient spectrum of activity or are contraindicated due to toxic potential

Drug of Choice or Alternative For
Disease/Syndrome(s)
Osteomyelitis, Diabetic Foot *on page 32*

Organism(s)
   Acinetobacter Species *on page 50*
   Citrobacter Species *on page 82*
   Clostridium perfringens on page 86
   Enterobacter Species *on page 104*
   Klebsiella Species *on page 137*
   Mycobacterium avium-intracellulare on page 152
   Proteus Species *on page 176*
   Pseudomonas aeruginosa on page 177
   Serratia Species *on page 190*

Pregnancy Risk Factor C

Contraindications Hypersensitivity to imipenem/cilastatin or any component

Warnings/Precautions Dosage adjustment required in patients with impaired renal function; safety and efficacy in children <12 years of age have not yet been established; prolonged use may result in superinfection; use with caution in patients with a history of seizures or allergy to any beta-lactams

Adverse Reactions
   1% to 10%: Phlebitis, nausea, diarrhea, vomiting
   <1%: Pain at injection site, hypotension, palpitations, seizures, rash, pseudomembranous colitis, neutropenia, eosinophilia, emergence of resistant strains of *P. aeruginosa*

Toxicology Hemodialysis may be helpful to aid in the removal of the drug from the blood, otherwise most treatment is supportive or symptom directed; diazepam 0.01 mg/kg can be used for seizures

Drug Interactions Increased effect/toxicity with probenecid; ganciclovir may potentiate seizures; aminoglycosides (synergy)

Stability Stable for 10 hours at room temperature following reconstitution with 100 mL of 0.9% sodium chloride injection; up to 48 hours when refrigerated at 5°C. If reconstituted with 5% or 10% dextrose injection, 5% dextrose and sodium bicarbonate, 5% dextrose and 0.9% sodium chloride, is stable for 4 hours at room temperature and 24 hours when refrigerated.

Mechanism of Action Inhibits bacterial cell wall synthesis by binding to one or more of the penicillin binding proteins (PBPs); which in turn inhibits the final transpeptidation step of peptidoglycan synthesis in bacterial cell walls, thus inhibiting cell wall biosynthesis. Bacteria eventually lyse due to ongoing activity of cell wall autolytic enzymes (autolysins and murein hydrolases) while cell wall assembly is arrested.

Pharmacokinetics
   Distribution: Imipenem appears in breast milk; crosses the placenta; distributed rapidly and widely to most tissues and fluids including sputum, pleural fluid, peritoneal fluid, interstitial fluid, bile, aqueous humor, reproductive organs, and bone; highest concentrations in pleural fluid, interstitial fluid, peritoneal fluid, and reproductive organs; low concentrations in cerebrospinal fluid
   Metabolism: Imipenem is metabolized in the kidney by dehydropeptidase, this activity is blocked by cilastatin; cilastatin is partially metabolized in the kidneys
   Half-life: Both: 60 minutes, extended with renal insufficiency
   Elimination: Both: ~70% excreted unchanged in urine

Usual Dosage I.V. infusion (dosage recommendation based on imipenem component):

   Children: 60-100 mg/kg/day in 4 divided doses (up to 2 g)

   Adults: 500 mg every 6 hours; if organism causing infection is only moderately susceptible to imipenem, may increase dose to 1 g every 6 hours

   Dosing adjustment in renal impairment: Imipenem doses should be reduced in patients with a Cl_{cr} <30-70 mL/minute/1.73m². See table.

Creatinine Clearance mL/min/1.73 m²	Frequency	Dose (mg)
30–70	q8h	500
20–30	q12h	500
5–20	q12h	250

Imipenem/Cilastatin *(Continued)*

Moderately dialyzable (20% to 50%)

Overdosage Many beta-lactam containing antibiotics have the potential to cause neuromuscular hyperirritability or convulsive seizures

Monitoring Parameters Periodic renal, hepatic, and hematologic function tests

Test Interactions Interferes with urinary glucose determination using Clinitest®

Nursing Implications Not for direct infusion; vial contents must be transferred to 100 mL of infusion solution; final concentration should not exceed 5 mg/mL; infuse over 30-60 minutes; watch for convulsions; do not mix with or physically add to other antibiotics; however, may administer concomitantly

Additional Information Sodium content of 1 g injection:

I.M.: 64.4 mg (2.8 mEq)

I.V.: 73.6 mg (3.2 mEq)

Dosage Forms Powder for injection:

I.M.:

Imipenem 500 mg and cilastatin 500 mg

Imipenem 750 mg and cilastatin 750 mg

I.V.:

Imipenem 250 mg and cilastatin 250 mg (13 mL)

Imipenem 500 mg and cilastatin 500 mg (13 mL)

Selected Readings

Barza M, "Imipenem: First of a New Class of Beta-Lactam Antibiotics," *Ann Intern Med*, 1985, 103(4):552-60.

Donowitz GR and Mandell GL, "Beta-Lactam Antibiotics," *N Engl J Med*, 1988, 318(7):419-26 and 318(8):490-500.

Hellinger WC and Brewer NS, "Imipenem," *Mayo Clin Proc*, 1991, 66(10):1074-81.

Immune Globulin *(im myoon' glob' yoo lin)*

Brand Names Gamastan®; Gamimune® N; Gammagard®; Gammar®; Sandoglobulin®; Venoglobulin®-I

Synonyms Gamma Globulin; IG; IGIM; IGIV; Immune Globulin Intramuscular; Immune Globulin Intravenous; Immune Serum Globulin; ISG

Generic Available No

Use Prophylaxis against hepatitis A, measles, varicella, and possibly rubella and immunoglobulin deficiency, idiopathic thrombocytopenia purpura, Kawasaki syndrome, lymphocytic leukemia

Drug of Choice or Alternative For

Organism(s)

Hepatitis A Virus *on page 122*

Measles Virus *on page 145*

Pregnancy Risk Factor C

Contraindications Hypersensitivity to immune globulin or thimerosal; patients with selective IgA deficiencies

Adverse Reactions

>10%: Pain, tenderness, muscle stiffness at I.M. site

1% to 10%: Nausea, flushing, chills

<1%: Lethargy, fever, urticaria, angioedema, emesis, erythema, myalgia, hypersensitivity reactions

Drug Interactions Decreased antibody response with immune globulin administered within 1-3 months of live virus vaccines (measles, mumps, rubella)

Stability Keep in refrigerator; do not freeze

Mechanism of Action Provides passive immunity by increasing the antibody titer and antigen-antibody reaction potential

Pharmacokinetics

Distribution: Evenly to intravascular and extravascular fluid compartments

Half-life: 23 days

Duration of immune effects: Usually 3-4 weeks

Usual Dosage

Hepatitis A: I.M.:

Pre-exposure prophylaxis: One I.M. dose of 0.02 mL/kg for anticipated risk of ≤3 months; I.M. dose of 0.06 mL/kg for anticipated risk of >3 months; repeat approximate dose at above intervals if exposure continues

Postexposure prophylaxis: One I.M. dose of 0.02 mL/kg given within 2 weeks of exposure

Measles: Prophylaxis: I.M.: 0.25 mL/kg/dose (maximum dose: 15 mL) given within 6 days of exposure followed by live attenuated measles vaccine in 3 months or at 15 months of age (whichever is later); for patients with leukemia, lymphoma, immunodeficiency disorders, generalized malignancy, or receiving immunosuppressive therapy: 0.5 mL/kg (maximum dose: 15 mL)

Poliomyelitis: Prophylaxis: I.M.: 0.3 mL/kg/dose as a single dose

Rubella: Prophylaxis: I.M.: 0.55 mL/kg/dose during pregnancy

Varicella: Prophylaxis: I.M.: 0.6-1.2 mL/kg (Varicella zoster immune globulin preferred)

Hepatitis B: Prophylaxis: I.M.: 0.06 mL/kg/dose (HBIG preferred)

Primary immunodeficiency diseases: Children and Adults: I.V.: 100-400 mg/kg every month

Idiopathic thrombocytopenia purpura: Children and Adults: I.V.: 400-500 mg/kg/day every 2-7 days

Test Interactions Skin tests should **not** be done

Nursing Implications I.M. injection dosage forms cannot be given I.V.; do not mix with other medications; skin testing should not be performed as local irritation can occur and be misinterpreted as a positive reaction

Additional Information

Immune globulin intramuscular: Gamastan®, Gammar®
Immune globulin intravenous: Gamimune® N, Gammagard®, Sandoglobulin®, Venoglobulin®-I

Epidemiologic and laboratory data indicate current IMIG products do not have a discernible risk of transmitting HIV

Dosage Forms

Injection: I.M.: 165 ± 15 mg (of protein)/mL (2 mL, 10 mL)
Injection: I.V.:
  0.5 g, 1 g, 2.5 g, 3 g, 5 g, 6 g, 10 g
  5% (10 mL, 50 mL, 100 mL)

Selected Readings

ASHP Commission on Therapeutics, "ASHP Therapeutic Guidelines for Intravenous Immune Globulin," *Clin Pharm,* 1992, 11(2):117-36.
Berkman SA, Lee ML, and Gale RP, "Clinical Uses of Intravenous Immunoglobulins," *Ann Intern Med,* 1990, 112(4):278-92.

Immune Globulin Intramuscular *see* Immune Globulin *on previous page*

Immune Globulin Intravenous *see* Immune Globulin *on previous page*

Immune Serum Globulin *see* Immune Globulin *on previous page*

Imovax® Rabies I.D. Vaccine *see* Rabies Virus Vaccine *on page 659*

Imovax® Rabies Vaccine *see* Rabies Virus Vaccine *on page 659*

Indanyl Sodium *see* Carbenicillin *on page 507*

Influenza Virus Vaccine (in floo en' za)

Related Information

Vaccines *on page 706-709*

Brand Names Flu-Imune®; Fluogen®; Fluzone®

Synonyms Influenza Virus Vaccine (inactivated whole-virus); Influenza Virus Vaccine (purified surface antigen); Influenza Virus Vaccine (split-virus)

Generic Available No

Use Provides active immunity for adults with high-risk conditions, residents of nursing homes or other chronic-care facilities, health care personnel, healthy persons ≥65 years of age

Pregnancy Risk Factor C

Contraindications History of anaphylactic hypersensitivity to egg ingestion

Warnings/Precautions Although there is no evidence of maternal or fetal risk when vaccine is given in pregnancy, waiting until the second or third trimester to vaccinate the pregnant woman with a high-risk condition may be reasonable. Antigenic response may not be as great as expected in patients requiring immunosuppressive drug; hypersensitivity reactions may occur; because of potential for febrile reactions, risks and benefits must carefully be considered in patients with history of febrile convulsions; influenza vaccines from previous seasons must not be used; patients with sulfite sensitivity may be affected by this product.

(Continued)

Influenza Virus Vaccine *(Continued)*

Adverse Reactions
1% to 10%: Tenderness, redness, or induration at the site of injection, fever, malaise
<1%: Anaphylactoid reactions (most likely to residual egg protein), allergic reactions, fever, hives, angioedema, myalgia, Guillain-Barré syndrome (rare), asthma

Drug Interactions
Decreased effect with immunosuppressive agents; do not administer within 7 days after administration of diphtheria and tetanus toxoids and pertussis vaccine adsorbed (DTP)
Increased effect/toxicity of theophylline and warfarin

Stability Refrigerate

Mechanism of Action Promotes immunity to influenza virus by inducing specific antibody production. Each year the formulation is standardized according to the U.S. Public Health Service. Preparations from previous seasons must not be used.

Usual Dosage Annual vaccination with current vaccine; either whole- or split-virus vaccine may be used

Nursing Implications Inspect for particulate matter and discoloration prior to administration; for I.M. administration only

Additional Information Federal law requires that the date of administration, the vaccine manufacturer, lot number of vaccine, and the administering person's name, title and address be entered into the patient's permanent medical record. Target groups for annual vaccinations can be found in the appendix.

Dosage Forms Injection:
Purified surface antigen (Flu-Imune®): 5 mL
Split-virus (Fluogen®, Fluzone®): 0.5 mL, 5 mL
Whole-virus (Fluzone®): 5 mL

Influenza Virus Vaccine (inactivated whole-virus) *see* Influenza Virus Vaccine *on previous page*

Influenza Virus Vaccine (purified surface antigen) *see* Influenza Virus Vaccine *on previous page*

Influenza Virus Vaccine (split-virus) *see* Influenza Virus Vaccine *on previous page*

INH *see* Isoniazid *on page 592*

α-2-interferon *see* Interferon Alfa-2b *on this page*

Interferon Alfa-2b (in ter feer' on)

Brand Names Intron® A
Synonyms IFN-alpha 2; α-2-interferon; rLFN-α2
Generic Available No
Use Induce hairy cell leukemia remission; treatment of AIDS-related Kaposi's sarcoma; condylomata acuminata; chronic hepatitis C

Drug of Choice or Alternative For
Organism(s)
Hepatitis B Virus *on page 122*
Hepatitis C Virus *on page 124*

Pregnancy Risk Factor C

Contraindications Known hypersensitivity to interferon alfa-2b or any component

Warnings/Precautions Use with caution in patients with seizure disorders, brain metastases, compromised CNS, multiple sclerosis, and patients with pre-existing cardiac disease, severe renal or hepatic impairment, or myelosuppression; safety and efficacy in children <18 years of age have not been established. The US Food and Drug Administration (FDA) currently recommends that procedures for proper handling and disposal of antineoplastic agents be considered. Higher doses in the elderly or in malignancies other than hairy cell leukemia may result in severe obtundation.

Adverse Reactions
>10%: Anemia, leukopenia, flu-like syndrome, skin rash, diarrhea, dizziness, tiredness, dry mouth, thrombocytopenia, metallic taste, anorexia, nausea, vomiting
1% to 10%: Hepatotoxicity, dry skin, diaphoresis, leg cramps, blurred vision, neurotoxicity, peripheral neuropathy, stomatitis, alopecia

<1%: Cardiotoxicity, hypothyroidism, weight loss, arrhythmias, hypotension, nasal congestion, edema, EEG abnormalities, confusion, sensory neuropathy, fever, headache, decreased hemoglobin, hematocrit, platelets, increased ALT and AST, myalgia, arthralgia, rigors, proteinuria, increased uric acid level, increased Cr, increased BUN, coughing, chest pain, chills, neutralizing antibodies

Toxicology Treatment is supportive

Drug Interactions

Increased effect: Cimetidine: May augment the antitumor effects of interferon in melanoma

Increased toxicity: Vinblastine: Enhances interferon toxicity in several patients; increased incidence of paresthesia has also been noted

Theophylline: Clearance has been reported to be decreased in hepatitis patients receiving interferon

Stability Refrigerate; reconstituted solution is stable for 1 month when refrigerated

Mechanism of Action Inhibits cellular growth, alters the state of cellular differentiation, interferes with oncogene expression, alters cell surface antigen expression, increases phagocytic activity of macrophages and augments cytotoxicity of lymphocytes for target cells

Pharmacokinetics

Metabolism: Majority of dose is thought to be metabolized in the kidney, filtered and absorbed at the renal tubule

Half-life: 2-3.5 hours

Time to peak serum concentration: I.M., S.C.: Within 6-8 hours

Usual Dosage Adults:

Hairy cell leukemia: I.M., S.C.: 2 million units/m^2 3 times/week

AIDS-related Kaposi's sarcoma: I.M., S.C.: 30 million units/m^2 3 times/week or 50 million units/m^2 I.V. 5 days/week every other week

Condylomata acuminata: Intralesionally: 1 million units/lesion 3 times/week for 3 weeks; not to exceed 5 million units per treatment (maximum: 5 lesions at one time)

Chronic hepatitis C: I.M., S.C.: 3 million units 3 times/week for approximately a 6-month course

Overdosage CNS depression, obtundation, flu-like symptoms, myelosuppression

Monitoring Parameters Baseline chest x-ray, EKG, CBC with differential, liver function tests, electrolytes, platelets, weight

Patient Information Do not change brands of interferon as changes in dosage may result; do not operate heavy machinery while on therapy since changes in mental status may occur; report to physician any persistent or severe sore throat, fever, fatigue, unusual bleeding, or bruising

Nursing Implications Do not use 3, 5, and 25 million unit strengths intralesionally, solutions are hypertonic; 50 million unit strength is not for use in condylomata

Dosage Forms Powder for injection, lyophilized: 3 million units, 5 million units, 10 million units, 18 million units, 25 million units, 50 million units

Selected Readings
"Drugs for Non-HIV Viral Infections," *Med Lett Drugs Ther*, 1994, 36(919):27.

Intron® A *see* Interferon Alfa-2b *on previous page*

Iodoquinol (eye oh doe kwin' ole)
Brand Names Sebaquin® [OTC]; Yodoxin®
Synonyms Diiodohydroxyquin
Generic Available No
Use Treatment of acute and chronic intestinal amebiasis; asymptomatic cyst passers; *Blastocystis hominis* infections; ineffective for amebic hepatitis or hepatic abscess
Pregnancy Risk Factor C
Contraindications Known hypersensitivity to iodine or iodoquinol; hepatic damage; pre-existing optic neuropathy
Warnings/Precautions Use with caution in patients with thyroid disease or neurological disorders
Adverse Reactions
>10%: Diarrhea, nausea, vomiting, stomach pain
(Continued)

Iodoquinol (Continued)

1% to 10%: Fever, chills, skin rash, hives, thyroid gland enlargement, headache, itching of rectal area, peripheral neuropathy, agitation, retrograde amnesia, weakness, optic neuritis, optic atrophy, visual impairment

Toxicology

Chronic overdose can result in vomiting, diarrhea, abdominal pain, metallic taste, paresthesias, paraplegia, and loss of vision; can lead to destruction of the long fibers of the spinal cord and optic nerve

Acute overdose: Delirium, stupor, coma, amnesia

Following GI decontamination, treatment is symptomatic

Mechanism of Action Contact amebicide that works in the lumen of the intestine by an unknown mechanism

Pharmacokinetics

Absorption: Oral: Poor and irregular

Metabolism: In the liver

Elimination: High percentage of dose excreted in feces

Usual Dosage Oral:

Children: 30-40 mg/kg/day (maximum: 650 mg/dose) in 3 divided doses for 20 days; not to exceed 1.95 g/day

Adults: 650 mg 3 times/day after meals for 20 days; not to exceed 1.95 g/day

Monitoring Parameters Ophthalmologic exam

Test Interactions May increase protein-bound serum iodine concentrations reflecting a decrease in ^{131}I uptake; false-positive ferric chloride test for phenylketonuria

Patient Information May take with food or milk to reduce stomach upset

Nursing Implications Tablets may be crushed and mixed with applesauce or chocolate syrup

Dosage Forms

Powder: 25 g

Tablet: 210 mg, 650 mg

Selected Readings

"Drugs for Parasitic Infections," *Med Lett Drugs Ther*, 1993, 35(911):111-22.

IPOL™ *see* Poliovirus Vaccine, Inactivated *on page 645*

IPV *see* Poliovirus Vaccine, Inactivated *on page 645*

ISG *see* Immune Globulin *on page 588*

Isoniazid (eye soe nye' a zid)

Brand Names Laniazid® Oral; Nydrazid® Injection

Synonyms INH; Isonicotinic Acid Hydrazide

Generic Available Yes

Use Treatment of susceptible tuberculosis infections and prophylaxis in those individuals exposed to tuberculosis

Drug of Choice or Alternative For

Organism(s)

Mycobacterium kansasii *on page 153*

Mycobacterium tuberculosis *on page 155*

Pregnancy Risk Factor C

Contraindications Acute liver disease; hypersensitivity to isoniazid or any component; previous history of hepatic damage during isoniazid therapy

Warnings/Precautions Use with caution in patients with renal impairment and chronic liver disease. Severe and sometimes fatal hepatitis may occur or develop even after many months of treatment; patients must report any prodromal symptoms of hepatitis, such as fatigue, weakness, malaise, anorexia, nausea, or vomiting. Children with low milk and low meat intake should receive concomitant pyridoxine therapy. Periodic ophthalmic examinations are recommended even when usual symptoms do not occur; pyridoxine (10-50 mg/day) is recommended in individuals likely to develop peripheral neuropathies

Adverse Reactions

>10%: Peripheral neuritis, loss of appetite, nausea, vomiting, stomach pain, weakness, hepatitis

1% to 10%: Dizziness, slurred speech, lethargy, hyperreflexia

<1%: Blood dyscrasias, fever, skin rash, arthralgia, seizures, mental depression, psychosis, blurred vision, loss of vision

Toxicology Because of the severe morbidity and high mortality rates with isoniazid overdose, patients who are asymptomatic after an overdose should be monitored for 4-6 hours. Pyridoxine has been shown to be effective in the treatment of intoxication, especially when seizures occur. Pyridoxine I.V. is administered on a milligram to milligram dose. If the amount of isoniazid ingested is unknown, 5 g of pyridoxine should be given over 3-5 minutes and may be followed by an additional 5 g in 30 minutes.

Drug Interactions
Decreased effect/levels of isoniazid with aluminum salts
Increased toxicity/levels of oral anticoagulants, carbamazepines, cycloserine, hydantoins, hepatically metabolized benzodiazepines; reaction with disulfiram

Stability Protect oral dosage forms from light

Mechanism of Action Inhibits myocolic acid synthesis resulting in disruption of the bacterial cell wall

Pharmacokinetics
Absorption: Oral, I.M.: Rapid and complete; rate of absorption can be slowed when administered with food
Distribution: Crosses the placenta; appears in breast milk; distributes into all body tissues and fluids including the CSF
Metabolism: By the liver with decay rate determined genetically by acetylation phenotype
Half-life:
Fast acetylators: 30-100 minutes
Slow acetylators: 2-5 hours; half-life may be prolonged in patients with impaired hepatic function or severe renal impairment
Time to peak serum concentration: Within 1-2 hours
Elimination: Metabolite as unchanged drug excreted in urine (75% to 95%), feces, and saliva

Usual Dosage Oral, I.M., I.V.:
Children: 10-20 mg/kg/day in 1-2 divided doses (maximum: 300 mg total dose)
Prophylaxis: 10 mg/kg/day given daily (up to 300 mg total dose) for 12 months

Adults: 5 mg/kg/day given daily (usual dose is 300 mg)
Disseminated disease: 10 mg/kg/day in 1-2 divided doses
Treatment should be continued for 9 months with rifampin or for 6 months with rifampin and pyrazinamide
Prophylaxis: 300 mg/day given daily for 12 months

American Thoracic Society and CDC currently recommend twice weekly therapy as part of a short-course regimen which includes 1-2 months of daily treatment for uncomplicated pulmonary tuberculosis in compliant patients
Children: 20-40 mg/kg/dose (up to 900 mg) twice weekly
Adults: 15 mg/kg/dose (up to 900 mg) twice weekly

Dosing adjustment in hepatic impairment: Dose should be reduced in severe hepatic disease
Dialyzable (50% to 100%)

Overdosage Nausea, vomiting, slurred speech, dizziness, blurred vision, hallucinations, stupor, coma, intractable seizures

Monitoring Parameters Periodic liver function tests; monitoring for prodromal signs of hepatitis

Test Interactions False-positive urinary glucose with Clinitest® or Benedict's solution

Patient Information Report any prodromal symptoms of hepatitis (fatigue, weakness, nausea, vomiting, dark urine, or yellowing of eyes) or any burning, tingling, or numbness in the extremities

Dosage Forms
Injection: 100 mg/mL (10 mL)
Syrup (orange flavor): 50 mg/5 mL (473 mL)
Tablet: 50 mg, 100 mg, 300 mg

Selected Readings
Davidson PT and Le HQ, "Drug Treatment of Tuberculosis – 1992," *Drugs*, 1992, 43(5):651-73.
"Drugs for Tuberculosis," *Med Lett Drugs Ther*, 1993, 35(908):99-101.
Iseman MD, "Treatment of Multidrug-Resistant Tuberculosis," *N Engl J Med*, 1993, 329(11):784-91.
Van Scoy RE and Wilkowske CJ, "Antituberculosis Agents," *Mayo Clin Proc*, 1992, 67(2):179-87.

Isonicotinic Acid Hydrazide *see* Isoniazid *on previous page*

Isoxazolyl Penicillin *see* Oxacillin Sodium *on page 627*

Itraconazole (i tra koe' na zole)
Brand Names Sporanox®
Generic Available No
Use Treatment of susceptible fungal infections in immunocompromised and nonimmunocompromised patients including blastomycosis and histoplasmosis; itraconazole is also indicated for aspergillosis in patients who are intolerant of or are refractory to amphotericin B
Drug of Choice or Alternative For
Organism(s)
  Blastomyces dermatitidis on page 63
  Candida Species *on page 73*
  Histoplasma capsulatum on page 130
Pregnancy Risk Factor C
Contraindications Known hypersensitivity to itraconazole or other azoles
Warnings/Precautions Coadministration with terfenadine is contraindicated; rare cases of serious cardiovascular adverse event, including death, ventricular tachycardia and torsade de pointes have been observed due to increased terfenadine concentrations induced by itraconazole; patients who develop abnormal liver function tests during fluconazole therapy should be monitored closely for the development of more severe hepatic injury; if clinical signs and symptoms consistent with liver disease develop that may be attributable to itraconazole, itraconazole should be discontinued
Adverse Reactions
  >10%: Nausea
  1% to 10%: Rash, abdominal pain, headache, vomiting
  <1%: Diarrhea, anorexia, edema, fatigue, fever, malaise, pruritus, dizziness, decreased libido, somnolence, hypertension, abnormal hepatic function, hypokalemia, albuminuria, impotence
Toxicology Overdoses are well tolerated; supportive measures and gastric decontamination with ipecac or sodium bicarbonate lavage should be employed
Drug Interactions
  Decreased effect: Rifampin, isoniazid, phenytoin; antacids, H_2 antagonists, and omeprazole may decrease absorption of itraconazole
  Increased effect: May increase cyclosporine levels when high doses used; phenytoin levels, effect of warfarin and sulfonylureas
  Increased toxicity of astemizole, terfenadine (cardiotoxicity)
Pharmacokinetics
  Absorption: Rapid and complete
  Metabolism: Hepatic, >97%
  Elimination: 85% renally excreted, 40% as inactive metabolites
Usual Dosage Adults: Oral:
  Blastomycosis and histoplasmosis: 200 mg once daily, if no obvious improvement or there is evidence of progressive fungal disease, increase the dose in 100 mg increments to a maximum of 400 mg/day

  Aspergillosis: 200-400 mg/day

  Life-threatening: Loading dose: 200 mg 3 times/day (600 mg/day) should be given for the first 3 days
Patient Information Take with food
Nursing Implications Do not administer with antacids
Dosage Forms Capsule: 100 mg
Selected Readings
  Cleary JD, Taylor JW, and Chapman SW, "Itraconazole in Antifungal Therapy," *Ann Pharmacother*, 1992, 26(4):502-9.
  Grant SM and Clissold SP, "Itraconazole. A Review of Its Pharmacodynamic and Pharmacokinetic Properties, and Therapeutic Use in Superficial and Systemic Mycoses," *Drugs*, 1989, 37(3):310-44.
  Jennings TS and Hardin TC, "Treatment of Aspergillosis With Itraconazole," *Ann Pharmacother*, 1993, 27(10):1206-11.
  Lyman CA and Walsh TJ, "Systemically Administered Antifungal Agents. A Review of Their Clinical Pharmacology and Therapeutic Applications," *Drugs*, 1992, 44(1):9-35.
  Terrell CL and Hughes CE, "Antifungal Agents Used for Deep-Seated Mycotic Infections," *Mayo Clin Proc*, 1992, 67(1):69-91.

IUDR *see* Idoxuridine *on page 586*

Ivermectin (eye ver mek' tin)

Brand Names Mectizan®
Generic Available No
Drug of Choice or Alternative For
Organism(s)
  Strongyloides stercoralis on page 215
Pharmacokinetics
  Distribution: Does not cross the blood-brain barrier
  Half life: 22-28 hours
  Metabolism: Hepatic, >97%
  Elimination: <2% excreted in urine, the remainder in feces
Usual Dosage Oral:
  Children >5 years of age and older: 150 µg/kg as a single dose once every 12 months
  Adults: 150 µg/kg as a single dose; may be repeated every 6-12 **months**
Additional Information Available from:
  The Centers for Disease Control Drug and Immunobiologic Service
  1600 Clifton Road
  Building 1
  Room 1259
  Atlanta, GA 30333
    Monday-Friday 8 AM to 4:30 PM
    (404) 639-3670
    Nonbusiness hours (emergencies only): (404) 639-2888
Dosage Forms Tablet: 6 mg
Selected Readings
  "Drugs for Parasitic Infections," *Med Lett Drugs Ther*, 1993, 35(911):111-22.

Japanese Encephalitis Virus Vaccine, Inactivated

Brand Names JE-VAX®
Use Active immunization against Japanese encephalitis for persons 1 year of age and older who plan to spend 1 month or more in endemic areas in Asia, especially persons traveling during the transmission season or visiting rural areas; consider vaccination for shorter trips to epidemic areas or extensive outdoor activities in rural endemic areas; elderly (>55 years of age) individuals should be considered for vaccination, since they have increased risk of developing symptomatic illness after infection; **those planning travel to or residence in endemic areas should consult the Travel Advisory Service (Central Campus) for specific advice (see Restrictions)**
Pregnancy Risk Factor C
Contraindications Serious adverse reaction (generalized urticaria or angioedema) to a prior dose of this vaccine; proven or suspected hypersensitivity to proteins or rodent or neural origin; hypersensitivity to thimerosal (used as a preservative). *CDC recommends that the following should not generally receive the vaccine, unless benefit to the individual clearly outweighs the risk*:
  * those acutely ill or with active infections
  * persons with heart, kidney, or liver disorders
  * persons with generalized malignancies such as leukemia or lymphoma
  * persons with a history of multiple allergies or hypersensitivity to components of the vaccine
  * pregnant women, unless there is a very high risk of Japanese encephalitis during the woman's stay in Asia
Warnings/Precautions Severe adverse reactions manifesting as generalized urticaria or angioedema may occur within minutes following vaccination, or up to 17 days later; most reactions occur within 10 days, with the majority within 48 hours; observe vaccinees for 30 minutes after vaccination; warn them of the possibility of delayed generalized urticaria and to remain where medical care is readily available for 10 days following any dose of the vaccine; because of the potential for severe adverse reactions, Japanese encephalitis vaccine is **not** recommended for all persons traveling to or residing in Asia; safety and efficacy in infants <1 year of age have not been established; therefore, immunization of infants should be deferred whenever possible; it is not known whether the vaccine is excreted in breast milk
Adverse Reactions Commonly, tenderness, redness, and swelling at injection site; systemic side effects include fever, headache, malaise, rash, chills, dizziness, myalgia, nausea, vomiting, abdominal pain, urticaria, itching with or without accompanying rash, and hypotension; rarely, anaphylactic reaction, en-
(Continued)

Japanese Encephalitis Virus Vaccine, Inactivated
(Continued)

cephalitis, encephalopathy, seizure, peripheral neuropathy, erythema multiforme, erythema nodosum, angioedema, dyspnea, and joint swelling; report allergic or unusual adverse reactions to the Vaccine Adverse Event Reporting System (VAERS 1-800-822-7967)

Drug Interactions Simultaneous administration of DTP vaccine and Japanese encephalitis vaccine does not compromise the immunogenicity of either vaccine; data on administration with other vaccines, chloroquine, or mefloquine are lacking

Stability Refrigerate, discard 8 hours after reconstitution

Usual Dosage US recommended primary immunization schedule:

Children >3 years and Adults: S.C.: Three 1 mL doses given on days 0, 7, and 30. Give third dose on day 14 when time does not permit waiting; 2 doses a week apart produce immunity in about 80% of vaccines; the longest regimen yields highest titers after 6 months

Children 1-3 years: S.C.: Three 0.5 mL doses given on days 0, 7, and 30; abbreviated schedules should be used only when necessary due to time constraints

Booster dose: Give after 2 years, or according to current recommendation

Note: Travel should not commence for at least 10 days after the last dose of vaccine, to allow adequate antibody formation and recognition of any delayed adverse reaction

Advise concurrent use of other means to reduce the risk of mosquito exposure when possible, including bed nets, insect repellents, protective clothing, avoidance of travel in endemic areas, and avoidance of outdoor activity during twilight and evening periods

Patient Information Adverse reactions may occur shortly after vaccination or up to 17 days (usually within 10 days) after vaccination

Additional Information Japanese encephalitis vaccine is currently available only from the Centers for Disease Control. Contact Centers for Disease Control at (404) 639-6370 (Mon-Fri) or (404) 639-2888 (nights, weekends, or holidays).

Dosage Forms Powder for injection, lyophilized: 1 mL, 10 mL

Jenamicin® Injection see Gentamicin Sulfate on page 575

JE-VAX® see Japanese Encephalitis Virus Vaccine, Inactivated on previous page

Kanamycin Sulfate (kan a mye' sin)
Brand Names Kantrex®
Generic Available Yes
Use Orally for preoperative bowel preparation in the prophylaxis of infections and adjunctive treatment of hepatic coma (oral kanamycin is not indicated in the treatment of systemic infections); parenterally is indicated for initial therapy of severe infections where the strain is only susceptible to kanamycin; other aminoglycosides are preferred

Pregnancy Risk Factor D

Contraindications Hypersensitivity to kanamycin or any component

Warnings/Precautions

I.V. therapy is not intended for long-term therapy due to toxic hazards associated with extended administration; pre-existing renal insufficiency, vestibular or cochlear impairment, myasthenia gravis, hypocalcemia, conditions which depress neuromuscular transmission

Parenteral aminoglycosides are associated with significant nephrotoxicity or ototoxicity; the ototoxicity is directly proportional to the amount of drug given and the duration of treatment; tinnitus or vertigo are indications of vestibular injury and impending irreversible bilateral deafness; renal damage is usually reversible

Adverse Reactions

>10%: Nephrotoxicity

1% to 10%: Skin itching, redness, rash, swelling, neurotoxicity, ototoxicity (auditory), ototoxicity (vestibular)

<1%: Difficulty in breathing, drowsiness, weakness, headache, tremors, muscle cramps, pseudomotor cerebri, anorexia, nausea, vomiting, weight loss, increased salivation, enterocolitis, granulocytopenia, agranulocytosis, thrombocytopenia, photosensitivity, erythema, burning, stinging

Toxicology The treatment of choice following a single acute overdose appears to be the maintenance of good urine output of at least 3 mL/kg/hour. Dialysis is of questionable value in the enhancement of aminoglycoside elimination. If required, hemodialysis is preferred over peritoneal dialysis in patients with normal renal function. Careful hydration may be all that is required to promote diuresis and therefore the enhancement of the drug's elimination.

Stability Darkening of vials does not indicate loss of potency

Mechanism of Action Interferes with protein synthesis in bacterial cell by binding to ribosomal subunit

Pharmacokinetics

Absorption: Oral: Poor; completely absorbed after I.M. injection

Distribution: Widely distributed after parenteral administration; intraocular penetration is poor; CSF penetration is low even in patients with inflamed meninges; intraventricular administration produces high concentrations throughout CNS; crosses the placenta and appears in breast milk

Half-life: 2-4 hours, increases in anuria to 80 hours

Elimination: Excreted entirely in the kidney, principally by glomerular filtration

Usual Dosage

Neonates: I.M., I.V.:

<7 days:

<2000 g: 7.5 mg/kg/dose every 12 hours

>2000 g: 10 mg/kg/dose every 12 hours

>7 days:

<2000 g: 7 mg/kg/dose every 8 hours

>2000 g: 10 mg/kg/dose every 8 hours

Children:

Infections: I.M., I.V.: 15-30 mg/kg/day in divided doses every 8 hours

Suppression of bowel flora: Oral: 150-250 mg/kg/day in divided doses administered every 1-6 hours

Adults:

Infections: I.M., I.V.: 15 mg/kg/day in divided doses every 8-12 hours

Preoperative intestinal antisepsis: Oral: 1 g every 4-6 hours for 36-72 hours

Hepatic coma: Oral: 8-12 g/day in divided doses

Dosing adjustment in renal impairment:

Cl_{cr} 50-80 mL/minute: Administer 60% to 90% of dose or administer every 8-12 hours

Cl_{cr} 10-50 mL/minute: Administer 30% to 70% of dose or administer every 12 hours

Cl_{cr} <10 mL/minute: Administer 20% to 30% of dose or administer every 24-48 hours

Dialyzable (50% to 100%)

Overdosage Ototoxicity, nephrotoxicity, and neuromuscular toxicity

Monitoring Parameters Urinalysis, urine output, BUN, serum creatinine, peak and trough, kanamycin serum concentrations

Reference Range Therapeutic: Peak: 25-35 μg/mL (SI: 52-72 μmol/L); Trough: 4-8 μg/mL (SI: 8-16 μmol/L); Toxic: Peak: >35 μg/mL (SI: >72 μmol/L); Trough: >10 μg/mL (SI: >21 μmol/L)

Test Interactions Penicillin may decrease aminoglycoside serum concentrations *in vitro*

Patient Information Report any dizziness or sensations of ringing or fullness in ears

Dosage Forms

Capsule: 500 mg

Injection:

Pediatric: 75 mg (2 mL)

Adults: 500 mg (2 mL); 1 g (3 mL)

Selected Readings

Cunha BA, "Aminoglycosides: Current Role in Antimicrobial Therapy," *Pharmacotherapy*, 1988, 8(6):334-50.

"Drugs for Tuberculosis," *Med Lett Drugs Ther*, 1993, 35(908):99-101.

Iseman MD, "Treatment of Multidrug-Resistant Tuberculosis," *N Engl J Med*, 1993, 329(11):784-91.

Kantrex® *see* Kanamycin Sulfate *on previous page*

Keflet® *see* Cephalexin Monohydrate *on page 526*

Keflex® *see* Cephalexin Monohydrate *on page 526*

ANTIMICROBIAL THERAPY

Keflin® Neutral *see* Cephalothin Sodium *on page 528*
Keftab® *see* Cephalexin Monohydrate *on page 526*
Kefurox® Injection *see* Cefuroxime *on page 524*
Kefzol® *see* Cefazolin Sodium *on page 511*

Ketoconazole (kee toe koe' na zole)
Brand Names Nizoral®
Generic Available No
Use Treatment of susceptible fungal infections, including candidiasis, oral thrush, blastomycosis, histoplasmosis, paracoccidioidomycosis, chronic mucocutaneous candidiasis, as well as certain recalcitrant cutaneous dermatophytoses; used topically for treatment of tinea corporis, tinea cruris, tinea versicolor and cutaneous candidiasis
Drug of Choice or Alternative For
Organism(s)
Blastomyces dermatitidis *on page 63*
Candida Species *on page 73*
Coccidioides immitis *on page 89*
Histoplasma capsulatum *on page 130*
Pregnancy Risk Factor C
Contraindications Hypersensitivity to ketoconazole or any component
Warnings/Precautions Gastric acidity is necessary for the dissolution and absorption of ketoconazole; avoid concomitant (within 2 hours) administration of antacids, H$_2$-blockers, anticholinergics; use with caution in patients with impaired hepatic function; has been associated with hepatotoxicity, including some fatalities; perform periodic liver function tests; high doses of ketoconazole may depress adrenocortical function
Adverse Reactions
1% to 10%: Nausea, vomiting, pruritus, abdominal pain
<1%: Headache, dizziness, somnolence, fever, chills, photophobia, diarrhea, gynecomastia, impotence, thrombocytopenia, leukopenia, hemolytic anemia, bulging fontanelles
Drug Interactions
Decreased effect/toxicity of theophylline; antacids, H$_2$ receptor antagonists, and omeprazole decrease absorption; isoniazid and rifampin decrease serum levels
Increased effect/toxicity/serum levels of warfarin, terfenadine, astemizole, cyclosporine
Mechanism of Action Alters the permeability of the cell wall; inhibits biosynthesis of triglycerides and phospholipids by fungi; inhibits several fungal enzymes that results in a build-up of toxic concentrations of hydrogen peroxide
Pharmacokinetics
Absorption: Oral: Rapid (~75%)
Distribution: Well distributed to inflamed joint fluid, saliva, bile, urine, breast milk, sebum, cerumen, feces, tendons, skin and soft tissues, and testes; crosses blood-brain barrier poorly; only negligible amounts reach CSF
Metabolism: Partially in the liver by enzymes to inactive compounds
Half-life: biphasic:
Initial: 2 hours
Terminal: 8 hours
Time to peak serum concentration: Within 1-4 hours
Elimination: Excreted primarily in feces (57%) with smaller amounts excreted in urine (13%)
Usual Dosage
Children: Oral: 5-10 mg/kg/day divided every 12-24 hours
Adults:
Oral: 200-400 mg/day as a single daily dose
Topical: Rub gently into the affected area once daily to twice daily for 2 weeks
Dosing adjustment in hepatic impairment: Dose reductions should be considered in patients with severe liver disease
Not dialyzable (0% to 5%)
Overdosage Dizziness, headache, nausea, vomiting, diarrhea
Monitoring Parameters Liver function tests
Patient Information Cream is for topical application to the skin only; avoid con-

tact with the eye; avoid taking antacids or H_2 antagonists at the same time as ketoconazole. May cause drowsiness, impair judgment, or coordination. Notify physician of unusual fatigue, anorexia, vomiting, dark urine, or pale stools.

Nursing Implications Administer 2 hours prior to antacids H_2-receptor antagonist to prevent decreased absorption due to the high pH of gastric contents

Dosage Forms
Cream: 2% (15 g, 30 g, 60 g)
Shampoo: 2% (120 mL)
Suspension, oral: 100 mg/5 mL (120 mL)
Tablet: 200 mg

Selected Readings
Como JA and Dismukes WE, "Oral Azole Drugs as Systemic Antifungal Therapy," *N Engl J Med*, 1993, 330(4):263-72.
Lyman CA and Walsh TJ, "Systemically Administered Antifungal Agents. A Review of Their Clinical Pharmacology and Therapeutic Applications," *Drugs*, 1992, 44(1):9-35.
Terrell CL and Hughes CE, "Antifungal Agents Used for Deep-Seated Mycotic Infections," *Mayo Clin Proc*, 1992, 67(1):69-91.

KI *see* Potassium Iodide *on page 648*

Kwell® *see* Lindane *on this page*

Lamprene® *see* Clofazimine *on page 542*

Laniazid® Oral *see* Isoniazid *on page 592*

Lariam® *see* Mefloquine Hydrochloride *on page 605*

Larotid® *see* Amoxicillin Trihydrate *on page 491*

Ledercillin® VK *see* Penicillin V Potassium *on page 638*

Legatrin® [OTC] *see* Quinine Sulfate *on page 658*

Lice-Enz® [OTC] *see* Pyrethrins *on page 653*

Lindane (lin' dane)
Brand Names G-well®; Kwell®; Scabene®
Synonyms Benzene Hexachloride; Gamma Benzene Hexachloride; Hexachlorocyclohexane
Generic Available Yes
Use Treatment of scabies (*Sarcoptes scabiei*) and pediculosis (*Pediculus capitis* – head lice, *Pediculus pubis* – crab lice)
Drug of Choice or Alternative For
Organism(s)
Lice *on page 142*
Sarcoptes scabiei on page 188
Pregnancy Risk Factor B
Contraindications Hypersensitivity to lindane or any component; premature neonates; acutely inflamed skin or raw, weeping surfaces
Adverse Reactions <1%: Dizziness, restlessness, ataxia, seizures, headache, eczematous eruptions, contact dermatitis, nausea, vomiting, aplastic anemia, hepatitis, hematuria, pulmonary edema, skin and adipose tissue may act as repositories
Toxicology Absorbed through skin and mucous membranes and GI tract, has occasionally caused serious CNS, hepatic and renal toxicity when used excessively for prolonged periods, or when accidental ingestion has occurred; diazepam 0.01 mg/kg can be used to control seizures
Drug Interactions Increased toxicity: Oil-based hair dressing → ↑ toxic potential
Mechanism of Action Directly absorbed by parasites and ova through the exoskeleton; stimulates the nervous system resulting in seizures and death of parasitic arthropods
Pharmacokinetics
Absorption: Systemic absorption up to 13% may occur
Distribution: Stored in body fat
Metabolism: By the liver
Half-life: Children: 17-22 hours
Time to peak serum concentration: In children, occurs 6 hours after topical application
Elimination: Excreted in urine and feces
Usual Dosage Children and Adults: Topical:
Pediculosis/Scabies: Apply a thin layer of lotion or cream and massage it on skin from the neck to the toes. For children, wash off 6 hours after applica-
(Continued)

Lindane *(Continued)*

tion; for adults, bathe and remove the drug after 8-12 hours; repeat treatment in 7 days if lice or nits are still present

Pediculosis, capitis and pubis: 15-30 mL of shampoo is applied and lathered for 4-5 minutes; rinse hair thoroughly and comb with a fine tooth comb to remove nits; repeat treatment in 7 days if lice or nits are still present

Overdosage Vomiting, restlessness, ataxia, seizures, arrhythmia, pulmonary edema, hematuria, hepatitis

Patient Information For topical use only; do not apply to face, avoid getting in eyes; notify if condition worsens; treat sexual contact simultaneously

Nursing Implications Drug should not be administered orally

Dosage Forms
Cream: 1% (60 g)
Lotion: 1% (30 mL, 60 mL, 473 mL, 4000 mL)
Shampoo: 1% (30 mL, 60 mL, 473 mL, 4000 mL)

Lomefloxacin Hydrochloride *(loe me flox' a sin)*

Related Information
Antimicrobial Activity Against Selected Organisms *on page 757-764*

Brand Names Maxaquin®

Generic Available No

Use Quinolone antibiotic for skin and skin structure, lower respiratory and urinary tract infections, and sexually transmitted diseases

Pregnancy Risk Factor C

Contraindications Hypersensitivity to lomefloxacin or other members of the quinolone group such as nalidixic acid, norfloxacin, and ciprofloxacin; avoid use in children <18 years of age due to association of other quinolones with transient arthropathies

Warnings/Precautions Use with caution in patients with epilepsy or other CNS diseases which could predispose them to seizures

Adverse Reactions
1% to 10%: Nausea, headache, photosensitivity, dizziness, diarrhea
<1%: Dry mouth, flushing, increased sweating, fatigue, back pain, malaise, asthenia, chest pain, chills, allergic reaction, face edema, flu-like symptoms, decreased heat tolerance, hypotension, hypertension, edema, syncope, tachycardia, bradycardia, arrhythmia, extrasystoles, cyanosis, cardiac failure, angina pectoris, myocardial infarction, convulsions, coma, hyperkinesia, tremor, vertigo, paresthesias, abdominal pain, vomiting, flatulence, constipation, tongue discoloration, earache, thrombocytopenia, purpura, increased fibrinolysis, thirst, gout, hypoglycemia, leg cramps, myalgia, dyspnea, epistaxis, cough, rash, taste perversion, dysuria, hematuria, micturition disorder, anuria

Toxicology Symptoms of overdose include acute renal failure, seizures; GI decontamination and supportive care; diazepam for seizures; not removed by peritoneal or hemodialysis

Drug Interactions
Decreased lomefloxacin effect with bismuth subsalicylate, antacids (aluminum, magnesium), iron salts, zinc salts, sucralfate
Increased lomefloxacin levels with probenecid, cimetidine
Increased levels/effect/toxicity of warfarin, cyclosporine, NSAIDs (↑ seizures)

Mechanism of Action Inhibits DNA-gyrase in susceptible organisms; inhibits relaxation of supercoiled DNA and promotes breakage of double-stranded DNA

Pharmacokinetics
Absorption: Well absorbed
Half-life, elimination: 5-7.5 hours
Elimination: Excreted primarily unchanged in urine

Usual Dosage Adults: Oral: 400 mg once daily for 10-14 days

Patient Information Take 1 hour before or 2 hours after meals

Dosage Forms Tablet: 400 mg

Selected Readings
Hooper DC and Wolfson JS, "Fluoroquinolone Antimicrobial Agents," *N Engl J Med*, 1991, 324(6):384-94.
Lomaestro BM and Bailie GR, "Quinolone-Cation Interactions: A Review," *DICP*, 1991, 25(11):1249-58.
Stein GE, "The 4-Quinolone Antibiotics: Past, Present, and Future," *Pharmacotherapy*, 1988, 8(6):301-14.
Walker RC and Wright AJ, "The Fluoroquinolones," *Mayo Clin Proc*, 1991, 66(12):1249-59.

Loprox® *see Ciclopirox Olamine on page 536*

Lorabid™ *see Loracarbef on this page*

Loracarbef (loe ra kar' bef)

Related Information
Antimicrobial Activity Against Selected Organisms *on page 757-764*

Brand Names Lorabid™

Generic Available No

Use Infections caused by susceptible organisms involving the respiratory tract, acute otitis media, sinusitis, skin and skin structure, bone and joint, and urinary tract and gynecologic

Pregnancy Risk Factor B

Contraindications Patients with a history of hypersensitivity to loracarbef or cephalosporins

Warnings/Precautions Use with caution in patients with a previous history of hypersensitivity to other beta-lactam antibiotics (eg, penicillins, cephalosporins)

Adverse Reactions
1% to 10%: Diarrhea, nausea, vomiting, headache, abdominal pain, anorexia, skin rashes, vaginitis, vaginal moniliasis

<1%: Somnolence, nervousness, dizziness, transient thrombocytopenia, leukopenia, and eosinophilia, transient elevations of ALT, AST, alkaline phosphatase and BUN, creatinine, vasodilation

Toxicology Symptoms of overdose include abdominal discomfort, diarrhea; supportive care only

Drug Interactions Increased serum levels with probenecid

Stability Suspension may be kept at room temperature for 14 days

Mechanism of Action Inhibits bacterial cell wall synthesis by binding to one or more of the penicillin binding proteins (PBPs); which in turn inhibits the final transpeptidation step of peptidoglycan synthesis in bacterial cell walls, thus inhibiting cell wall biosynthesis. Bacteria eventually lyse due to ongoing activity of cell wall autolytic enzymes (autolysins and murein hydrolases) while cell wall assembly is arrested.

Pharmacokinetics
Absorption: Oral: Rapid
Half-life, elimination: ~1 hour
Time to peak serum concentration: Oral: Within 1 hour
Elimination: Plasma clearance: ~200-300 mL/minute

Usual Dosage Oral:
Children:
Acute otitis media: 15 mg/kg twice daily for 10 days
Pharyngitis: 7.5-15 mg/kg twice daily for 10 days
Adults: Female:
Uncomplicated urinary tract infections: 200 mg once daily for 7 days
Skin and soft tissue: 200-400 mg every 12-24 hours
Uncomplicated pyelonephritis: 400 mg every 12 hours for 14 days

Dosing comments in renal impairment:
Cl$_{cr}$ ≥50 mL/minute: Give usual dose
Cl$_{cr}$ 10-49 mL/minute: 50% of usual dose at usual interval or usual dose given half as often
Cl$_{cr}$ <10 mL/minute: Give usual dose every 3-5 days
Hemodialysis: Doses should be administered after dialysis sessions

Patient Information Take on an empty stomach at least 1 hour before or 2 hours after meals; finish all medication

Dosage Forms
Capsule: 200 mg
Suspension, oral: 100 mg/5 mL; 200 mg/5 mL

Selected Readings
Force RW and Nahata MC, "Loracarbef: A New Orally Administered Carbacephem Antibiotic," *Ann Pharmacother*, 1993, 27(3):321-9.

Lotrimin AF® Topical [OTC] *see Clotrimazole on page 543*

Lotrimin® Topical *see Clotrimazole on page 543*

Lugol's Solution *see Potassium Iodide on page 648*

Macrobid® *see Nitrofurantoin on page 623*

Macrodantin® *see* Nitrofurantoin *on page 623*

Malathion (mal a thye' on)
Brand Names Ovide™
Generic Available No
Use Treatment of head lice and their ova
Drug of Choice or Alternative For
Organism(s)
Lice *on page 142*
Pregnancy Risk Factor B
Contraindications Known hypersensitivity to malathion
Usual Dosage Sprinkle Ovide™ lotion on dry hair and rub gently until the scalp is thoroughly moistened; pay special attention to the back of the head and neck. Allow to dry naturally – use no heat and leave uncovered. After 8-12 hours, the hair should be washed with a nonmedicated shampoo; rinse and use a fine-toothed comb to remove dead lice and eggs. If required, repeat with second application in 7-9 days. Further treatment is generally not necessary. Other family members should be evaluated to determine if infested and if so, receive treatment.
Patient Information Topical use only
Dosage Forms Lotion: 0.5% (59 mL)
Selected Readings
"Drugs for Parasitic Infections," *Med Lett Drugs Ther*, 1993, 35(911):111-22.

Mandelamine® *see* Methenamine *on page 607*

Mandol® *see* Cefamandole Nafate *on page 510*

Marcillin® *see* Ampicillin *on page 495*

Maxaquin® *see* Lomefloxacin Hydrochloride *on page 600*

Measles and Rubella Vaccines, Combined
Related Information
Vaccines *on page 706-709*
Brand Names M-R-VAX® II
Synonyms Rubella and Measles Vaccines, Combined
Generic Available No
Use Simultaneous immunization against measles and rubella Adults born before 1957 are generally considered to be immune to measles; all born in or after 1957 without documentation of live vaccine on or after first birthday, physician-diagnosed measles, or laboratory evidence of immunity should be vaccinated with two doses separated by or less than 1 month. For those previously vaccinated with one dose of measles vaccine, revaccination is indicated for students entering institutions of higher learning, for health care workers at time of employment, and for travelers to endemic areas. Guidelines for rubella vaccination are the same with the exception of birth year. All adults should be vaccinated against rubella. A booster dose of rubella vaccine is not necessary. Women who are pregnant when vaccinated or become pregnant within 3 months of vaccination should be consulted on the risks to the fetus; although the risks appear negligible. MMR is the vaccine of choice if recipients are likely to be susceptible to mumps as well as measles and rubella.
Pregnancy Risk Factor X
Contraindications Immune deficiency condition, pregnancy
Warnings/Precautions Pregnancy, immunocompromised persons, history of anaphylactic reaction following receipt of neomycin
Adverse Reactions All serious adverse reactions must be reported to the FDA.
> 10%: Fever <100°F, burning at injection site, arthralgias, local tenderness and erythema, urticaria, rash
1% to 10%: Fever between 100°F and 103°F, allergic reaction (delayed type), malaise, headache, sore throat, lymphadenopathy
<1%: Difficulty of breathing, hives, itching, reddening of skin (especially around ears and eyes), tiredness, convulsions, encephalitis, confusion, severe headache, stiff neck, vomiting, diplopia, thrombocytopenic purpura, fever >103°F (prolonged), lymphadenopathy, optic neuritis, hypersensitivity
Drug Interactions Whole blood, immune globulin, immunosuppressive drugs should not be given within 1 month of other live virus vaccines except monovalent or trivalent polio vaccine; may temporarily depress tuberculin skin test sensitivity; decreased effect when immune globulin is given within 3 months

and with concurrent use of corticosteroids and other immunosuppressant agents

Stability Refrigerate prior to use, use as soon as possible; discard if not used within 8 hours of reconstitution

Mechanism of Action Promotes active immunity to measles and rubella by inducing specific antibodies including measles-specific IgG and IgM and rubella hemagglutination-inhibiting antibodies.

Usual Dosage Children at 15 months and Adults: S.C.: Inject 0.5 mL into outer aspect of upper arm; no routine booster for rubella

Patient Information Parents should monitor children closely for fever 5-11 days after vaccination; pregnancy should be avoided for 3 months; burning or stinging may occur along with joint pain 1-10 weeks after vaccination and persist for 1-3 days

Nursing Implications Not for I.V. administration

Additional Information Federal law requires that the date of administration, the vaccine manufacturer, lot number of vaccine, and the administering person's name, title and address be entered into the patient's permanent medical record

Dosage Forms Injection: 1000 $TCID_{50}$ each of live attenuated measles virus vaccine and live rubella virus vaccine

Measles, Mumps, and Rubella Vaccines, Combined

Related Information

Vaccines *on page 706-709*

Brand Names M-M-R® II

Synonyms MMR; Mumps, Measles and Rubella Vaccines, Combined; Rubella, Measles and Mumps Vaccines, Combined

Generic Available No

Use Measles, mumps, and rubella prophylaxis

Adults born before 1957 are generally considered to be immune to measles and mumps; all born in or after 1957 without documentation of live vaccine on or after first birthday, physician-diagnosed measles or mumps, or laboratory evidence of immunity should be vaccine with two doses separated by no less than one month; for those previously vaccinated with one dose of measles vaccine, revaccination is indicated for students entering institutions of higher learning, health care workers at time of employment, and for travelers to endemic areas. Guidelines for rubella vaccination are the same with the exception of birth year; all adults should be vaccinated against rubella. Booster doses of mumps and rubella are not necessary; women who are pregnant when vaccinated or become pregnant within 3 months should be counseled on the risks to the fetus; although the risks appear negligible.

Pregnancy Risk Factor X

Contraindications Blood dyscrasias, cancers affecting the bone marrow or lymphatic systems, known hypersensitivity to measles, mumps, and rubella vaccine

Warnings/Precautions Females should not become pregnant within 3 months of vaccination

Adverse Reactions All serious adverse reactions must be reported to the FDA.

1% to 10%: Transient rash, tenderness erythema and swelling, sore throat, allergic reactions

<1%: Seizures, malaise, fever

Drug Interactions Decreased effect when immune globulin is given within 3 months and with concurrent use of corticosteroids and other immunosuppressant agents; decreased effect with concurrent infection, immunoglobulin within 1 month, other live vaccines with the exception of attenuated measles, rubella, or polio

Stability Refrigerate, protect from light prior to reconstitution; use as soon as possible; discard 8 hours after reconstitution

Mechanism of Action Promotes active immunity to measles, mumps, and rubella by inducing specific antibodies including measles-specific IgG and IgM and rubella hemagglutination-inhibiting antibodies.

Usual Dosage Children >15 months and Adults: S.C.: Inject 0.5 mL in outer aspect of the upper arm; revaccination with a booster is recommended to the primary dose given after 12 months of age; revaccination is recommended upon entry into either kindergarten/first grade or middle school/junior high school

Test Interactions Temporary suppression of TB skin test reactivity with onset approximately 3 days after administration

(Continued)

Measles, Mumps, and Rubella Vaccines, Combined
(Continued)

Patient Information Pregnancy should be avoided for 3 months following vaccination

Nursing Implications Not for I.V. administration

Additional Information Federal law requires that the date of administration, the vaccine manufacturer, lot number of vaccine, and the administering person's name, title and address be entered into the patient's permanent medical record

Dosage Forms Injection: 1000 TCID$_{50}$ each of measles virus vaccine and rubella virus vaccine, 5000 TCID$_{50}$ mumps virus vaccine

Measles Virus Vaccine, Live
Related Information
Vaccines *on page 706-709*
Brand Names Attenuvax®
Synonyms More Attenuated Enders Strain; Rubeola vaccine
Generic Available No

Use Adults born before 1957 are generally considered to be immune. All those born in or after 1957 without documentation of live vaccine on or after first birthday, physician-diagnosed measles, or laboratory evidence of immunity should be vaccinated, ideally with two doses of vaccine separated by no less than 1 month. For those previously vaccinated with one dose of measles vaccine, revaccination is recommended for students entering colleges and other institutions of higher education, for health care workers at the time of employment, and for international travelers who visit endemic areas.

MMR is the vaccine of choice if recipients are likely to be susceptible to rubella and/or mumps as well as to measles. Persons vaccinated between 1963 and 1967 with a killed measles vaccine, followed by live vaccine within 3 months, or with a vaccine of unknown type should be revaccinated with live measles virus vaccine.

Pregnancy Risk Factor X

Contraindications Pregnant females, known hypersensitivity to eggs, known hypersensitivity to neomycin

Warnings/Precautions Immunocompromised persons

Adverse Reactions All serious adverse reactions must be reported to the FDA.
>10%: Fever <100°F, burning at injection site
1% to 10%: Fever between 100°F and 103°F, allergic reaction (delayed type)
<1%: Difficulty of breathing, hives, itching, reddening of skin (especially around ears and eyes), tiredness, convulsions, encephalitis, confusion, severe headache, stiff neck, vomiting, diplopia, thrombocytopenic purpura, fever >103°F (prolonged), lymphadenopathy

Drug Interactions Whole blood, immune globulin, immunosuppressive drugs should not be given within 1 month of other live virus vaccines except monovalent or trivalent polio vaccine; may temporarily depress tuberculin skin test sensitivity

Stability Refrigerate

Mechanism of Action Promotes active immunity to measles virus by inducing specific measles IgG and IgM antibodies.

Usual Dosage Children >15 months and Adults: S.C.: 0.5 mL in outer aspect of the upper arm, no routine boosters

Test Interactions May temporarily depress tuberculin skin test sensitivity

Patient Information Parents should monitor children closely for fever for 5-11 days after vaccination

Nursing Implications Vaccine should not be given I.V.; S.C. injection preferred

Additional Information Federal law requires that the date of administration, the vaccine manufacturer, lot number of vaccine, and the administering person's name, title and address be entered into the patient's permanent medical record

Dosage Forms Injection: 1000 TCID$_{50}$ per dose

Mebendazole (me ben' da zole)
Brand Names Vermox®
Generic Available No

Use Treatment of pinworms (*Enterobius vermicularis*), whipworms (*Trichuris trichiura*), roundworms (*Ascaris lumbricoides*), and hookworms (*Ancylostoma duodenale*)

Drug of Choice or Alternative For
  Organism(s)
    Ancylostoma duodenale on page 54
    Ascaris on page 55
    Enterobius vermicularis on page 106
    Trichinella spiralis on page 222
Pregnancy Risk Factor C
Contraindications Hypersensitivity to mebendazole or any component
Warnings/Precautions Pregnancy and children <2 years of age are relative contraindications since safety has not been established; not effective for hydatid disease
Adverse Reactions
  1% to 10%: Abdominal pain, diarrhea, nausea, vomiting
  <1%: Fever, skin rash, itching, neutropenia (sore throat, unusual tiredness and weakness), alopecia (with high doses), dizziness, headache
Drug Interactions Increased metabolism with anticonvulsants such as carbamazepine and phenytoin
Mechanism of Action Selectively and irreversibly blocks glucose uptake and other nutrients in susceptible adult intestine-dwelling helminths
Pharmacokinetics
  Absorption: Oral: 2% to 10%
  Distribution: Distributed to serum, cyst fluid, liver, omental fat, and pelvic, pulmonary, and hepatic cysts; highest concentrations found in liver; relatively high concentrations also found in muscle-encysted *Trichinella spiralis* larvae; crosses placenta
  Metabolism: Extensive in the liver
  Half-life: 1-11.5 hours
  Time to peak serum concentration: Within 2-4 hours
  Elimination: Primarily excreted in feces with 2% to 10% eliminated in urine
Usual Dosage Children and Adults: Oral:
  Pinworms: Single chewable tablet; may need to repeat after 2 weeks

  Whipworms, roundworms, hookworms: 1 tablet twice daily, morning and evening on 3 consecutive days; if patient is not cured within 3-4 weeks, a second course of treatment may be administered

  Dosing adjustment in hepatic impairment: Dosage reduction may be necessary in patients with liver dysfunction
  Not dialyzable (0% to 5%)
Overdosage Abdominal pain, altered mental status
Monitoring Parameters For treatment of trichuriasis, ascariasis, hookworm or mixed infections, check for helminth ova in the feces within 3-4 weeks following the initial therapy
Patient Information Tablets may be chewed, swallowed whole, or crushed and mixed with food; hygienic precautions to prevent reinfection such as wearing shoes, washing hands
Dosage Forms Tablet, chewable: 100 mg
Selected Readings
  "Drugs for Parasitic Infections," *Med Lett Drugs Ther*, 1993, 35(911):111-22.

Mectizan® *see* Ivermectin *on page 595*

Mefloquine Hydrochloride (me' floe kwin)
Brand Names Lariam®
Generic Available No
Use Treatment of acute malarial infections and prevention of malaria
Drug of Choice or Alternative For
  Organism(s)
    Plasmodium Species *on page 172*
Pregnancy Risk Factor C
Contraindications Hypersensitivity to mefloquine or any of its components
Warnings/Precautions If mefloquine is to be used for a prolonged period, periodic evaluations including liver function tests should be performed. Retinal abnormalities have not been observed with mefloquine in humans; however, long-term administration of mefloquine to rats has resulted in dose-related ocular lesions (retinal degeneration, retinal edema, and lenticular opacity at 12 mg/kg/day and higher). Therefore, periodic ophthalmic examinations are recommended. In cases of life-threatening, serious, or overwhelming malaria infec-
(Continued)

Mefloquine Hydrochloride *(Continued)*

tions due to *Plasmodium falciparum*, patients should be treated with an intravenous antimalarial drug. Mefloquine may be given orally to complete the course. Caution should be exercised with regard to driving, piloting airplanes, and operating machines since dizziness, disturbed sense of balance; neuropsychiatric reactions have been reported with mefloquine.

Adverse Reactions

1% to 10%: Vomiting, difficulty concentrating, headache, insomnia, lightheadedness, vertigo, diarrhea, stomach pain, nausea, visual disturbances

<1%: Bradycardia, extrasystoles, anxiety, dizziness, syncope, confusion, seizures, hallucinations, mental depression, psychosis

Drug Interactions

Decreased effect of valproic acid

Increased toxicity with beta-blockers; increased toxicity/levels of chloroquine, quinine, quinidine (hold treatment until at least 12 hours after these drugs)

Mechanism of Action Mefloquine's effectiveness in the treatment and prophylaxis of malaria is due to the destruction of the asexual blood forms of the malarial pathogens that affect humans, *Plasmodium falciparum, P. vivax, P. malariae, P. ovale*

Pharmacokinetics

Absorption: Oral: Well absorbed

Distribution: Appears in breast milk; distributed to blood, urine, CSF, and tissues; concentrates in erythrocytes

Half-life: 21-22 days

Time to peak serum concentration: 7-24 hours

Elimination: ~1.5% to 9% of dose excreted unchanged in urine

Usual Dosage Oral:

Children: Malaria prophylaxis:

15-19 kg: $\frac{1}{4}$ tablet

20-30 kg: $\frac{1}{2}$ tablet

31-45 kg: $\frac{3}{4}$ tablet

>45 kg: 1 tablet

Administer weekly starting 1 week before travel, continuing weekly during travel and for 4 weeks after leaving endemic area

Adults:

Treatment of mild to moderate malaria infection: 5 tablets (1250 mg) as a single dose with at least 8 oz of water

Malaria prophylaxis: 1 tablet (250 mg) once weekly for 4 weeks, then 1 tablet every other week; start treatment 1 week prior to departure to an endemic area; to avoid development of malaria after return from an endemic area, continue prophylaxis for 4 additional weeks; for prolonged stays in an endemic area this prophylaxis be achieved by continuing the recommended dosage schedule, once weekly for 4 weeks, then once every other week, until traveler has taken 3 doses following return to a malaria-free area

Overdosage Vomiting, diarrhea

Monitoring Parameters LFTS; ocular examination

Patient Information Begin therapy before trip and continue after; take drug of empty stomach; women of childbearing age should use reliable contraception during prophylaxis treatment and for 2 months after the last dose; be aware of signs and symptoms of malaria when traveling to an endemic area

Dosage Forms Tablet: 250 mg

Selected Readings

Panisko DM and Keystone JS, "Treatment of Malaria – 1990," *Drugs*, 1990, 39(2):160-89.

Wyler DJ, "Malaria Chemoprophylaxis for the Traveler," *N Engl J Med*, 1993, 329(1):31-7.

Mefoxin® *see* Cefoxitin Sodium *on page 518*

Meningococcal Polysaccharide Vaccine, Groups A, C, Y, and W-135

Related Information

Vaccines *on page 706-709*

Brand Names Menomune®-A/C/Y/W-135

Generic Available No

Use Immunization of persons 2 years of age and above in epidemic or endemic areas as might be determined in a population delineated by neighborhood, school, dormitory, or other reasonable boundary. The prevalent serogroup in such a situation should match a serogroup in the vaccine. Individuals at particular high-risk to include persons with terminal component complement deficiencies and those with anatomic or functional asplenia. Travelers visiting areas of a country that are recognized as having hyperendemic or epidemic meningococcal disease. Some countries experiencing epidemic meningococcal disease may require meningococcal vaccination of foreign travelers before arrival. Vaccinations also should be considered for household or institutional contacts of persons with meningococcal disease as as adjunct to appropriate antibiotic chemoprophylaxis as well as medical and laboratory personnel at risk of exposure to meningococcal disease.

Pregnancy Risk Factor C

Contraindications Children under 2 years of age

Warnings/Precautions Patients who undergo splenectomy secondary to trauma or nonlymphoid tumors respond well; however, those asplenic patients with lymphoid tumors who receive either chemotherapy or irradiation respond poorly; pregnancy, unless there is substantial risk of infection.

Adverse Reactions
>10%: Tenderness, pain, erythema and induration (local)
1% to 10%: Headache, malaise, fever, chills

Drug Interactions Decreased effect with administration of immunoglobulin within 1 month

Stability Discard remainder of vaccine within 5 days after reconstitution; store reconstituted vaccine in refrigerator

Usual Dosage One dose I.M. (0.5 mL); the need for booster is unknown

Nursing Implications Epinephrine 1:1000 should be available to control allergic reaction

Dosage Forms Injection: 10 dose, 50 dose

Menomune®-A/C/Y/W-135 see Meningococcal Polysaccharide Vaccine, Groups A, C, Y, and W-135 on previous page

Mepacrine Hydrochloride see Quinacrine Hydrochloride on page 655

Mepron™ see Atovaquone on page 499

Meruvax® II see Rubella Virus Vaccine, Live on page 665

Methacycline Hydrochloride (meth a sye' kleen)
Brand Names Rondomycin®
Generic Available No
Use Treatment of susceptible bacterial infections of both gram-negative and gram-positive organisms
Pregnancy Risk Factor D
Contraindications Hypersensitivity to methacycline or any component, children <8 years of age
Usual Dosage Oral:
Children >8 years: 6-12 mg/kg/day into 2-4 divided doses
Adults: 150 mg 4 times/day or 30 mg twice daily
Test Interactions Increases catecholamines (U), uric acid (S); decreases urea nitrogen (B)
Dosage Forms Capsule: 150 mg [base 140 mg]

Methenamine (meth en' a meen)
Brand Names Hiprex®; Mandelamine®; Urex®; Urised®
Synonyms Hexamethylenetetramine
Generic Available Yes
Use Prophylaxis or suppression of recurrent urinary tract infections; urinary tract discomfort secondary to hypermotility
Pregnancy Risk Factor C
Contraindications Severe dehydration, renal insufficiency, hepatic insufficiency in patients receiving hippurate salt, hypersensitivity to methenamine or any component
Warnings/Precautions Use with caution in patients with hepatic disease, gout, and the elderly; doses of 8 g/day may cause bladder irritation, some products may contain tartrazine; methenamine should not be used to treat infections outside of the lower urinary tract
Adverse Reactions
1% to 10%: Skin rash, nausea, vomiting, diarrhea, anorexia, abdominal cramping
(Continued)

607

Methenamine *(Continued)*

<1%: Headache, elevation in AST and ALT, hematuria, bladder irritation, dysuria, crystalluria

Toxicology Well tolerated GI decontamination and supportive care

Drug Interactions Decreased effect with sodium bicarbonate and acetazolamide; sulfonamides may cause a urinary precipitate

Stability Protect from excessive heat

Mechanism of Action Methenamine is hydrolyzed to formaldehyde and ammonia in acidic urine; formaldehyde has nonspecific bactericidal action

Pharmacokinetics

Absorption: Readily absorbed from GI tract

Metabolism: 10% to 30% of drug will be hydrolyzed by gastric juices unless it is protected by an enteric coating; ~10% to 25% metabolized in the liver

Half-life: 3-6 hours

Elimination: Excretion occurs via glomerular filtration and tubular secretion with ~70% to 90% of dose excreted unchanged in urine within 24 hours

Usual Dosage Oral:

Children: 6-12 years:

Hippurate: 25-50 mg/kg/day divided every 12 hours

Mandelate: 50-75 mg/kg/day divided every 6 hours

Children >12 years and Adults:

Hippurate: 1 g twice daily

Mandelate: 1 g 4 times/day after meals and at bedtime

Dosing adjustment/comments in renal impairment: Cl_{cr} <50 mL/minute: Avoid use

Monitoring Parameters Urinalysis, periodic liver function tests in patients

Test Interactions ↑ catecholamines and VMA (U); ↓ HIAA (U)

Patient Information Take with food to minimize GI upset; drink plenty of fluids to ensure adequate urine flow; notify physician if skin rash, painful urination, or intolerable GI upset occurs

Additional Information Should not be used to treat infections outside of the lower urinary tract; methenamine has little, if any, role in the treatment or prevention of infections in patients with indwelling urinary (Foley) catheters; furthermore, in noncatheterized patients, more effective antibiotics are available for the prevention or treatment of urinary tract infections; the influence of decreased renal function on the pharmacologic effects of methenamine results are unknown

Dosage Forms

Granules (orange flavor): 1 g (56s)

Suspension, oral, as mandelate (Mandelamine®): 250 mg/5 mL (coconut flavor), 500 mg/5 mL (cherry flavor)

Tablet, as hippurate (Hiprex®, Urex®): 1 g (Hiprex® contains tartrazine dye)

Tablet, as mandelate, enteric coated (Mandelamine®): 250 mg, 500 mg, 1 g

Methicillin Sodium *(meth i sill' in)*

Related Information

Antimicrobial Activity Against Selected Organisms *on page 757-764*

Brand Names Staphcillin®

Synonyms Dimethoxyphenyl Penicillin Sodium; Sodium Methicillin

Generic Available No

Use Treatment of susceptible bacterial infections such as osteomyelitis, septicemia, endocarditis, and CNS infections due to susceptible strains of staphylococcal species; other antistaphylococcal penicillins are usually preferred

Pregnancy Risk Factor B

Contraindications Known hypersensitivity to methicillin or any penicillin

Warnings/Precautions Elimination rate will be slow in neonates; modify dosage in patients with renal impairment and in the elderly; use with caution in patients with cephalosporin hypersensitivity

Adverse Reactions

1% to 10%: Skin rash, acute interstitial nephritis

<1%: Phlebitis, fever, rash, eosinophilia, anemia, leukopenia, neutropenia, thrombocytopenia, serum sickness-like reactions, hemorrhagic cystitis

Toxicology Many beta-lactam containing antibiotics have the potential to cause neuromuscular hyperirritability or convulsive seizures. Hemodialysis may be helpful to aid in the removal of the drug from the blood, otherwise most treatment is supportive or symptom directed. Seizures can be treated with diazepam 0.1 mg/kg; in patients with renal failure, penicillin can be removed by dialysis

Drug Interactions Probenecid decreases warfarin effect; aminoglycosides (synergy), probenecid may increase dicloxacillin levels

Stability Reconstituted solution is stable for 24 hours at room temperature and 4 days when refrigerated; discard solutions if it has a distinctive hydrogen sulfide odor and/or color turns to a deep orange; incompatible with aminoglycosides and tetracyclines

Mechanism of Action Inhibits bacterial cell wall synthesis by binding to one or more of the penicillin binding proteins (PBPs); which in turn inhibits the final transpeptidation step of peptidoglycan synthesis in bacterial cell walls, thus inhibiting cell wall biosynthesis. Bacteria eventually lyse due to ongoing activity of cell wall autolytic enzymes (autolysins and murein hydrolases) while cell wall assembly is arrested.

Pharmacokinetics
Distribution: Well into various body tissues and fluids; crosses the placenta and appears in breast milk

Metabolism: Only partially

Half-life:
Neonates:
<2 weeks: 2-3.9 hours
>2 weeks: 0.9-3.3 hours
Children 2-16 years: 0.8 hour
Adults: 0.4-0.5 hour with normal renal function
Time to peak serum concentration: I.M.: Within 30-60 minutes
Elimination: ~60% to 70% of dose eliminated unchanged in urine within 4 hours, by tubular secretion and glomerular filtration

Usual Dosage I.M., I.V.:
Neonates:
0-4 weeks, <1200 g: 25 mg/kg/dose every 12 hours; meningitis: 50 mg/kg/dose every 12 hours
<7 days:
1200-2000 g: 25 mg/kg/dose every 12 hours; meningitis: 50 mg/kg/dose every 12 hours
>2000 g: 25 mg/kg/dose every 8 hours; meningitis: 50 mg/kg/dose every 8 hours
>7 days:
1200-2000 g: 25 mg/kg/dose every 8 hours; meningitis: 50 mg/kg/dose every 8 hours
>2000 g: 25 mg/kg/dose every 6 hours; meningitis: 50 mg/kg/dose every 6 hours

Children: 150-200 mg/kg/day divided every 6 hours; 200-400 mg/kg/day divided every 4-6 hours has been used for treatment of severe infections; maximum dose: 12 g/day

Adults: 4-12 g/day in divided doses every 4-6 hours

Dosing adjustment in renal impairment:
Cl_{cr} 10-50 mL/minute: Administer every 6-8 hours
Cl_{cr} <10 mL/minute: Administer every 8-12 hours
Not dialyzable (0% to 5%)

Overdosage Neuromuscular hypersensitivity, seizure

Test Interactions Interferes with tests for urinary and serum proteins, uric acid, urinary steroids; may cause false-positive Coombs' test; may inactivate aminoglycosides *in vitro*

Nursing Implications Can be administered IVP at a rate not to exceed 200 mg/minute or intermittent infusion over 20-30 minutes; final concentration for administration should not exceed 20 mg/mL

Additional Information Sodium content of 1 g injection: 59.8-71.3 mg (2.6-3.1 mEq)

Dosage Forms Powder for injection: 1 g, 4 g, 6 g, 10 g

Selected Readings
Donowitz GR and Mandell GL, "Beta-Lactam Antibiotics," *N Engl J Med*, 1988, 318(7):419-26 and 318(8):490-500.
Wright AJ and Wilkowske CJ, "The Penicillins," *Mayo Clin Proc*, 1991, 66(10):1047-63.

Methylphenyl *see* Oxacillin Sodium *on page 627*

Methylrosaniline Chloride *see* Gentian Violet *on page 578*

Metizol® Oral *see* Metronidazole *on this page*

MetroGel® Topical *see* Metronidazole *on this page*

MetroGel®-Vaginal *see* Metronidazole *on this page*

Metro I.V.® Injection *see* Metronidazole *on this page*

Metronidazole (me troe ni' da zole)

Related Information
Antimicrobial Activity Against Selected Organisms *on page 757-764*

Brand Names Flagyl® Oral; Metizol® Oral; MetroGel® Topical; Metro-Gel®-Vaginal; Metro I.V.® Injection; Protostat® Oral

Generic Available Yes

Use Treatment of susceptible anaerobic bacterial and protozoal infections in the following conditions: amebiasis, symptomatic and asymptomatic trichomoniasis; skin and skin structure infections; CNS infections; intra-abdominal infections; systemic anaerobic infections; topically for the treatment of acne rosacea; treatment of antibiotic-associated pseudomembranous colitis (AAPC) caused by *C. difficile*; bacterial vaginosis

Drug of Choice or Alternative For
Disease/Syndrome(s)
Peritonitis *on page 36*
Vaginosis, Bacterial *on page 46*

Organism(s)
Bacteroides Species *on page 61*
Clostridium difficile on page 85*
Clostridium perfringens on page 86*
Clostridium tetani on page 88*
Entamoeba histolytica on page 102*
Gardnerella vaginalis on page 114*
Giardia lamblia on page 116*
Helicobacter pylori on page 121*
Microsporidia *on page 146*
Trichomonas vaginalis on page 224*

Pregnancy Risk Factor B

Contraindications Hypersensitivity to metronidazole or any component; contraindicated in the 1st trimester of pregnancy

Warnings/Precautions Use with caution in patients with liver impairment, blood dyscrasias; history of seizures, congestive heart failure, or other sodium-retaining states; reduce dosage in patients with severe liver impairment, CNS disease, and severe renal failure (Cl_{cr} <10 mL/minute). Has been shown to be carcinogenic in rodents.

Adverse Reactions
>10%: Nausea, dizziness, headache, diarrhea, loss of appetite, vomiting

1% to 10%: Peripheral neuropathy, seizures

<1%: Ataxia, hypersensitivity, leukopenia, pancreatitis, thrombophlebitis, vaginal candidiasis, change in taste sensation, dry mouth, metallic taste, disulfiram-type reaction with alcohol, furry tongue, dark urine

Toxicology Treatment is symptomatic and supportive

Drug Interactions
Decreased effect with barbiturates
Increased toxicity/levels of phenytoin, lithium, and warfarin
Disulfiram-like reaction with alcohol

Stability Reconstituted solution is stable for 96 hours when refrigerated; for I.V. infusion in NS or D_5W and neutralized (with sodium bicarbonate), solution is stable for 24 hours at room temperature; do not refrigerate neutralized solution because a precipitate will occur

Mechanism of Action Reduced to a product which interacts with DNA to cause a loss of helical DNA structure and strand breakage resulting in inhibition of protein synthesis and cell death in susceptible organisms

Pharmacokinetics
Absorption: Oral: Well absorbed

Distribution: To saliva, bile, seminal fluid, breast milk, bone, liver, and liver abscesses, lung and vaginal secretions; crosses placenta and blood-brain barrier; appears in breast milk

Metabolism: Metabolized 30% to 60% in the liver

Half-life:
  Neonates: 25-75 hours
  Others: 6-8 hours (half-life increases with hepatic impairment)
Time to peak serum concentration: Within 1-2 hours
Elimination: Via urine (20% as unchanged drug) and feces (6% to 15%); removed by hemodialysis and peritoneal dialysis

Usual Dosage
Neonates: Anaerobic infections: Oral, I.V.:
  0-4 weeks: <1200 g: 7.5 mg/kg every 48 hours
  Postnatal age <7 days:
    1200-2000 g: 7.5 mg/kg/day given every 24 hours
    >2000 g: 15 mg/kg/day in divided doses every 12 hours
  Postnatal age >7 days:
    1200-2000 g: 15 mg/kg/day in divided doses every 12 hours
    >2000 g: 30 mg/kg/day in divided doses every 12 hours

Infants and Children:
  Amebiasis: Oral: 35-50 mg/kg/day in divided doses every 8 hours
  Other parasitic infections: Oral: 15-30 mg/kg/day in divided doses every 8 hours
  Anaerobic infections: Oral, I.V.: 30 mg/kg/day in divided doses every 6 hours
  Clostridium difficile (antibiotic-associated colitis): Oral: 20 mg/kg/day divided every 6 hours
  Maximum dose: 2 g/day

Adults:
  Amebiasis: Oral: 500-750 mg every 8 hours
  Other parasitic infections: Oral: 250 mg every 8 hours or 2 g as a single dose
  Anaerobic infections: Oral, I.V.: 500 mg every 6 hours
  Antibiotic-associated pseudomembranous colitis: Oral: 250-500 mg 3-4 times/day for 10-14 days
  Topical: Apply a thin film twice daily to affected areas
  Vaginal: One applicatorful in vagina each morning and evening, as needed

Dosing adjustment in renal impairment: Cl_{cr} <10 mL/minute: Administer at 50% of dose
Dialyzable (50% to 100%)

Dosing adjustment/comments in hepatic disease: Unchanged in mild liver disease; reduce dosage in severe liver disease

Overdosage Nausea, vomiting, ataxia, seizures, peripheral neuropathy

Test Interactions May interfere with AST, ALT, triglycerides, glucose, and LDH testing

Patient Information Urine may be discolored to a dark or reddish-brown; do not take alcohol for at least 24 hours after the last dose; avoid beverage alcohol during therapy; may cause metallic taste; may be taken with food to minimize stomach upset; notify physician if numbness or tingling of extremities occur

Nursing Implications Avoid contact between the drug and aluminum in the infusion set

Additional Information Sodium content of 500 mg (I.V.): 322 mg (14 mEq)

Dosage Forms
Gel:
  Topical: 0.75% (30 g)
  Vaginal: 0.75% (70 g)
Injection, ready to use: 5 mg/mL (100 mL)
Powder for injection, as hydrochloride: 500 mg
Tablet: 250 mg, 500 mg

Selected Readings
Fekety R and Shah AB, "Diagnosis and Treatment of Clostridium difficile Colitis," JAMA, 1993, 269(1):71-5.

Kelly CP, Pothoulakis C, and LaMont JT, "Clostridium difficile Colitis," N Engl J Med, 1994, 330(4):257-62.

Smilack JD, Wilson WR, and Cockerill FR 3d, "Tetracyclines, Chloramphenicol, Erythromycin, Clindamycin, and Metronidazole," Mayo Clin Proc, 1991, 66(12):1270-80.

Mezlocillin Sodium (mez loe sill' in)
Related Information
Antimicrobial Activity Against Selected Organisms *on page 757-764*
Brand Names Mezlin®
Generic Available No
(Continued)

Mezlocillin Sodium *(Continued)*

Use Treatment of infections caused by susceptible organisms involving the skin and skin structure, bone and joint, respiratory tract, urinary tract, gastrointestinal tract, as well as septicemia

Pregnancy Risk Factor B

Contraindications Hypersensitivity to mezlocillin or any component or penicillins

Warnings/Precautions If bleeding occurs during therapy, mezlocillin should be discontinued; dosage modification required in patients with impaired renal function; use with caution in patients with renal impairment or biliary obstruction, or history of allergy to cephalosporins

Adverse Reactions

1% to 10%: Nausea, diarrhea

<1%: Fever, rash, vomiting, eosinophilia, leukopenia, neutropenia, thrombocytopenia, agranulocytosis, serum sickness-like reactions, hepatotoxicity, hematuria, seizures, dizziness, headache, exfoliative dermatitis, hypokalemia, hypernatremia, hemolytic anemia, prolonged bleeding time, positive Coombs' [direct], elevated liver enzymes, elevated serum creatinine and BUN, interstitial nephritis

Toxicology Many beta-lactam containing antibiotics have the potential to cause neuromuscular hyperirritability or convulsive seizures. Hemodialysis may be helpful to aid in the removal of the drug from the blood, otherwise most treatment is supportive or symptom directed.

Drug Interactions

Increased duration of neuromuscular blockers

Increased/prolonged levels with probenecid

Stability Reconstituted solution is stable for 48 hours at room temperature and 7 days when refrigerated; for I.V. infusion in NS or D_5W solution is stable for 48 hours at room temperature, 7 days when refrigerated or 28 days when frozen; after freezing, thawed solution is stable for 48 hours at room temperature or 7 days when refrigerated; if precipitation occurs under refrigeration, warm in water bath (37°C) for 20 minutes and shake well

Mechanism of Action Inhibits bacterial cell wall synthesis by binding to one or more of the penicillin binding proteins (PBPs); which in turn inhibits the final transpeptidation step of peptidoglycan synthesis in bacterial cell walls, thus inhibiting cell wall biosynthesis. Bacteria eventually lyse due to ongoing activity of cell wall autolytic enzymes (autolysins and murein hydrolases) while cell wall assembly is arrested.

Pharmacokinetics

Absorption: I.M.: 63%

Distribution: Into bile, heart, peritoneal fluid, sputum, bone; does not cross the blood-brain barrier well unless meninges are inflamed; crosses the placenta; distributes into breast milk at low concentrations

Metabolism: Minimal

Half-life:

Neonates:

<7 days: 3.7-4.4 hours

>7 days: 2.5 hours

Children 2-19 years: 0.9 hour

Adults: 50-70 minutes (dose dependent); half-life increases in renal impairment

Time to peak serum concentration: I.M.: 45-90 minutes

Elimination: Principally excreted as unchanged drug in urine, also excreted via bile

Usual Dosage I.M., I.V.:

Neonates:

Postnatal age <7 days: 150 mg/kg/day divided every 12 hours

Postnatal age >7 days: 225 mg/kg/day divided every 8 hours

Children: 200-300 mg/kg/day divided every 4-6 hours; maximum: 24 g/day

Adults:

For uncomplicated urinary tract infection: 1.5-2 g every 6 hours; serious infections: 3 g every 4 hours, or 4 g every 6 hours, or 5 g every 8 hours

Dosing adjustment in renal impairment:

Cl_{cr} 10-30 mL/minute: Administer every 6-8 hours

Cl_{cr} <10 mL/minute: Administer every 8 hours

Moderately dialyzable (20% to 50%)

Overdosage Neuromuscular hypersensitivity, seizure

Test Interactions False-positive direct Coombs'; false-positive urinary or serum protein; may inactivate aminoglycosides *in vitro*

Nursing Implications Administer at least 1 hour prior to aminoglycosides

Additional Information Minimum volume: 50 mL D$_5$W (concentration should not exceed 1 g/10 mL); sodium content of 1 g: 42.6 mg (1.85 mEq)

Dosage Forms Powder for injection: 1 g, 2 g, 3 g, 4 g, 20 g

Selected Readings

Donowitz GR and Mandell GL, "Beta-Lactam Antibiotics," *N Engl J Med*, 1988, 318(7):419-26 and 318(8):490-500.

Wright AJ and Wilkowske CJ, "The Penicillins," *Mayo Clin Proc*, 1991, 66(10):1047-63.

Micatin® Topical [OTC] *see* Miconazole *on this page*

Miconazole (mi kon' a zole)

Brand Names Micatin® Topical [OTC]; Monistat-Derm™ Topical; Monistat i.v.™ Injection; Monistat™ Vaginal

Synonyms Miconazole Nitrate

Generic Available Yes

Use

I.V.: Treatment of severe systemic fungal infections and fungal meningitis that are refractory to standard treatment

Topical: Treatment of vulvovaginal candidiasis and a variety of skin and mucous membrane fungal infections

Pregnancy Risk Factor C

Contraindications Hypersensitivity to miconazole or polyoxyl 35 castor oil or any component

Adverse Reactions

>10%: Fever, chills, skin rash, itching, pain at injection site, anorexia, diarrhea, nausea, vomiting

1% to 10%: Anemia, thrombocytopenia

<1%: Drowsiness, flushing of face or skin

Drug Interactions Increases warfarin effects; increases effect of oral sulfonylureas

Stability Protect from heat; darkening of solution indicates deterioration

Stability of parenteral admixture at room temperature (25°C): 2 days

Mechanism of Action Inhibits biosynthesis of ergosterol, damaging the fungal cell wall membrane, which increases permeability causing leaking of nutrients

Pharmacokinetics

Distribution: Appears to be widely distributed to body tissues; penetrates well into inflamed joints, vitreous humor of eye, and peritoneal cavity, but poorly into saliva and sputum; crosses blood-brain barrier but only to a small extent

Metabolism: Multiphasic degradation; metabolized in the liver

Half-life:

Initial: 40 minutes

Secondary: 126 minutes

Terminal: 24 hours

Elimination: ~50% excreted in feces and <1% in urine as unchanged drug

Usual Dosage

Children:

I.V.: 20-40 mg/kg/day divided every 8 hours

Topical: Apply twice daily for up to 1 month

Adults:

I.T.: 20 mg every 1-2 days

I.V.: Initial: 200 mg, then 1.2-3.6 g/day divided every 8 hours for up to 20 weeks

Topical: Apply twice daily for up to 1 month

Vaginal: Insert contents of 1 applicator of vaginal cream (100 mg) or 100 mg suppository at bedtime for 7 days, or 200 mg suppository at bedtime for 3 days

Not dialyzable (0% to 5%)

Overdosage Nausea, vomiting, drowsiness

Patient Information Avoid contact with the eyes; vaginal: insert high into vagina, complete full course of therapy; notify physician if itching or burning occurs; refrain from intercourse to prevent reinfection

Nursing Implications Administer I.V. dose over 2 hours; observe patient closely during first I.V. dose for allergic reactions

(Continued)

Miconazole *(Continued)*

Additional Information
Miconazole: Monistat i.v.™
Miconazole nitrate: Micatin®, Monistat™, Monistat-Derm™

Dosage Forms
Cream:
Topical, as nitrate: 2% [20 mg/g] (15 g, 30 g, 85 g)
Vaginal, as nitrate: 2% [20 mg/g] (45 g is equivalent to 7 doses)
Injection: 1% [10 mg/mL] (20 mL)
Lotion, as nitrate: 2% [20 mg/g] (30 mL, 60 mL)
Powder, topical: 2% [20 mg/g] (45 g, 90 g)
Spray, topical: 2% [20 mg/g] (105 mL)
Suppository, vaginal, as nitrate: 100 mg (7s); 200 mg (3s)

Miconazole Nitrate *see Miconazole on previous page*

Microsulfon® *see Sulfadiazine on page 671*

Minocin® *see Minocycline Hydrochloride on this page*

Minocin® IV *see Minocycline Hydrochloride on this page*

Minocycline Hydrochloride (mi noe sye' kleen)

Brand Names Minocin®; Minocin® IV
Generic Available No
Use Treatment of susceptible bacterial infections of both gram-negative and gram-positive organisms; acne, meningococcal carrier state
Drug of Choice or Alternative For
Organism(s)
Nocardia Species *on page 164*
Pregnancy Risk Factor D
Contraindications Hypersensitivity to minocycline, other tetracyclines, or any component; children <8 years of age
Warnings/Precautions Should be avoided in renal insufficiency, children ≤8 years of age, pregnant and nursing women; photosensitivity reactions can occur with minocycline
Adverse Reactions
>10%: Discoloration of teeth in children
1% to 10%: Nausea, diarrhea, photosensitivity
<1%: Increased intracranial pressure, bulging fontanels in infants, paresthesia, dermatologic effects, diabetes insipidus syndrome, vomiting, esophagitis, anorexia, abdominal cramps, acute renal failure, azotemia, superinfections, pericarditis, anaphylaxis, pruritus, pigmentation of nails, exfoliative dermatitis rash
Toxicology Symptoms of overdose include diabetes insipidus, nausea, anorexia, diarrhea; following GI decontamination, supportive care only; fluid support may be required
Drug Interactions
Decreased effect with antacids (aluminum, calcium, zinc, or magnesium), bismuth salts, sodium bicarbonate, barbiturates, carbamazepine, hydantoins; decreased effect of oral contraceptives
Increased effect of warfarin
Mechanism of Action Inhibits bacterial protein synthesis by binding with the 30S and possibly the 50S ribosomal subunit(s) of susceptible bacteria; cell wall synthesis is not affected
Pharmacokinetics
Absorption: Well absorbed
Distribution: Crosses placenta; appears in breast milk; majority of a dose deposits for extended periods in fat
Half-life: 15 hours
Elimination: Eventually cleared renally
Usual Dosage
Children >8 years: Oral, I.V.: Initial: 4 mg/kg followed by 2 mg/kg/dose every 12 hours

Adults:
Infection: Oral, I.V.: 200 mg stat, 100 mg every 12 hours not to exceed 400 mg/24 hours
Acne: Oral: 50 mg 1-3 times/day

Not dialyzable (0% to 5%)
Patient Information Avoid unnecessary exposure to sunlight; do not take with

antacids, iron products, or dairy products; finish all medication; do not skip doses; take 1 hour before or 2 hours after meals

Nursing Implications Infuse I.V. minocycline over 1 hour

Dosage Forms
Capsule, pellet-filled: 50 mg, 100 mg
Injection: 100 mg
Suspension, oral: 50 mg/5 mL (60 mL)

Selected Readings
Smilack JD, Wilson WR, and Cockerill FR 3d, "Tetracyclines, Chloramphenicol, Erythromycin, Clindamycin, and Metronidazole," *Mayo Clin Proc*, 1991, 66(12):1270-80.

Mintezol® *see* Thiabendazole *on page 681*

M-KYA® [OTC] *see* Quinine Sulfate *on page 658*

MMR *see* Measles, Mumps, and Rubella Vaccines, Combined *on page 603*

M-M-R® II *see* Measles, Mumps, and Rubella Vaccines, Combined *on page 603*

Monistat-Derm™ Topical *see* Miconazole *on page 613*

Monistat i.v.™ Injection *see* Miconazole *on page 613*

Monistat™ Vaginal *see* Miconazole *on page 613*

Monocid® *see* Cefonicid Sodium *on page 514*

More Attenuated Enders Strain *see* Measles Virus Vaccine, Live *on page 604*

M-R-VAX® II *see* Measles and Rubella Vaccines, Combined *on page 602*

Multiple Sulfonamides *see* Sulfadiazine, Sulfamethazine, and Sulfamerazine *on page 672*

Mumps, Measles and Rubella Vaccines, Combined *see* Measles, Mumps, and Rubella Vaccines, Combined *on page 603*

Mumpsvax® *see* Mumps Virus Vaccine, Live, Attenuated *on this page*

Mumps Virus Vaccine, Live, Attenuated

Related Information
Vaccines *on page 706-709*

Brand Names Mumpsvax®

Generic Available No

Use All adults without documentation of live vaccine on or after first birthdays, or physician-diagnosed mumps, or laboratory evidence of immunity (particularly males and young adults who work in or congregate in hospitals, colleges, and on military bases) should be vaccinated. It is reasonable to consider persons persons born before 1957 immune, but there is no contraindications to vaccination of older persons. Susceptible travelers should be vaccinated.

Pregnancy Risk Factor X

Warnings/Precautions Pregnancy, immunocompromised persons, history of anaphylactic reaction following egg ingestion or receipt of neomycin

Adverse Reactions All serious adverse reactions must be reported to the FDA.
>10%: Burning or stinging at injection site
1% to 10%: Fever ≤100°F, parotitis, skin rash
<1%: Anaphylactic reactions, convulsions, confusion, severe or continuing headache, fever >103°F, orchitis in postpubescent and adult males, thrombocytopenic purpura

Drug Interactions Decreased effect with concurrent infection, immunoglobulin with in 1 month, other live vaccines with the exception of attenuated measles, rubella, or polio

Stability Refrigerate

Mechanism of Action Promotes active immunity to mumps virus by inducing specific antibodies.

Usual Dosage 1 vial (5000 units) S.C. in outer aspect of the upper arm, no booster

Test Interactions Temporary suppression of tuberculosis skin test

Patient Information Pregnancy should be avoided for 3 months following vaccination

(Continued)

Mumps Virus Vaccine, Live, Attenuated *(Continued)*

Nursing Implications Reconstitute only with diluent provided; administer only S.C. on outer aspect of upper arm

Additional Information Federal law requires that the date of administration, the vaccine manufacturer, lot number of vaccine, and the administering person's name, title and address be entered into the patient's permanent medical record

Dosage Forms Injection: Single dose

Mupirocin *(myoo peer' oh sin)*

Brand Names Bactroban® Topical

Synonyms Pseudomonic Acid A

Generic Available No

Use Topical treatment of impetigo due to *Staphylococcus aureus*, beta-hemolytic *Streptococcus*, and *S. pyogenes*

Drug of Choice or Alternative For
Disease/Syndrome(s)
Impetigo *on page 27*

Pregnancy Risk Factor B

Contraindications Known hypersensitivity to mupirocin or polyethylene glycol

Warnings/Precautions Potentially toxic amounts of polyethylene glycol contained in the vehicle may be absorbed percutaneously in patients with extensive burns or open wounds; prolonged use may result in overgrowth of non-susceptible organisms; for external use only

Adverse Reactions 1% to 10%: Swelling, pruritus, rash, erythema, dry skin, burning, stinging, pain, tenderness

Stability Do not mix with Aquaphor®, coal tar solution, or salicylic acid

Mechanism of Action Binds to bacterial isoleucyl transfer-RNA synthetase resulting in the inhibition of protein and RNA synthesis

Pharmacokinetics
Absorption: Topical: Penetrates the outer layers of the skin; systemic absorption minimal through intact skin
Protein binding: 95%
Metabolism: Extensively to monic acid, principally in the liver and skin
Half-life: 17-36 minutes
Elimination: Excreted in urine

Usual Dosage Children and Adults: Topical: Apply small amount to affected area 2-5 times/day for 5-14 days

Patient Information For topical use only; do not apply into the eye; discontinue if rash, itching, or irritation occurs; improvement should be seen in 5 days

Nursing Implications Improvement should be seen in 5 days

Additional Information Not for treatment of pressure sores in elderly; contains polyethylene glycol vehicle

Dosage Forms Ointment, topical: 2% (15 g)

Myambutol® *see* Ethambutol Hydrochloride *on page 565*

Mycelex®-G Topical *see* Clotrimazole *on page 543*

Mycelex®-G Vaginal [OTC] *see* Clotrimazole *on page 543*

Mycelex® Troche *see* Clotrimazole *on page 543*

Mycifradin® Sulfate *see* Neomycin Sulfate *on page 619*

Mycobutin® *see* Rifabutin *on page 661*

Mycostatin® Oral *see* Nystatin *on page 625*

Mycostatin® Topical *see* Nystatin *on page 625*

Mycostatin® Vaginal *see* Nystatin *on page 625*

Nafcil™ *see* Nafcillin Sodium *on this page*

Nafcillin Sodium *(naf sill' in)*

Related Information
Antimicrobial Activity Against Selected Organisms *on page 757-764*

Brand Names Nafcil™; Nallpen®; Unipen®

Synonyms Ethoxynaphthamido Penicillin Sodium; Sodium Nafcillin

Generic Available Yes

Use Treatment of susceptible infections such as osteomyelitis, septicemia, endocarditis, and CNS infections due to susceptible strains of staphylococcal species

Pregnancy Risk Factor B

Contraindications Hypersensitivity to nafcillin or any component or penicillins

Warnings/Precautions Extravasation of I.V. infusions should be avoided; modification of dosage is necessary in patients with both severe renal and hepatic impairment; elimination rate will be slow in neonates; use with caution in patients with cephalosporin hypersensitivity

Adverse Reactions <1%: Thrombophlebitis, fever, skin rash, nausea, diarrhea, neutropenia, pain, acute interstitial nephritis, hypersensitivity reactions

Toxicology Many beta-lactam containing antibiotics have the potential to cause neuromuscular hyperirritability or convulsive seizures. Hemodialysis may be helpful to aid in the removal of the drug from the blood, otherwise most treatment is supportive or symptom directed.

Drug Interactions Probenecid decreases warfarin effect; may increase heparin anticoagulation effect

Stability Refrigerate oral suspension after reconstitution; discard after 7 days; reconstituted parenteral solution is stable for 3 days at room temperature and 7 days when refrigerated or 12 weeks when frozen; for I.V. infusion in NS or D_5W, solution is stable for 24 hours at room temperature and 96 hours when refrigerated

Mechanism of Action Inhibits bacterial cell wall synthesis by binding to one or more of the penicillin binding proteins (PBPs); which in turn inhibits the final transpeptidation step of peptidoglycan synthesis in bacterial cell walls, thus inhibiting cell wall biosynthesis. Bacteria eventually lyse due to ongoing activity of cell wall autolytic enzymes (autolysins and murein hydrolases) while cell wall assembly is arrested.

Pharmacokinetics

Absorption: Oral: Poor and erratic

Distribution: Widely distributed; CSF penetration is poor but enhanced by meningeal inflammation; crosses the placenta

Metabolism: Primarily in the liver; it undergoes enterohepatic circulation

Half-life:

Neonates:

<3 weeks: 2.2-5.5 hours

4-9 weeks: 1.2-2.3 hours

Children 3 months to 14 years: 0.75-1.9 hours

Adults: 30 minutes to 1.5 hours, with normal renal and hepatic function

Time to peak serum concentration:

Oral: Within 2 hours

I.M.: Within 30-60 minutes

Elimination: Primarily eliminated in bile, 10% to 30% in urine as unchanged drug; undergoes enterohepatic recycling

Usual Dosage

Neonates: I.V.:

0-4 weeks: <1200 g: 25 mg/kg/dose every 12 hours

<7 days:

1200-2000 g: 25 mg/kg/dose every 12 hours

>2000 g: 20 mg/kg/dose every 8 hours

>7 days:

1200-2000 g: 25 mg/kg/dose every 8 hours

>2000 g: 37.5 mg/kg/dose every 6 hours

Children:

Mild to moderate infections: I.M., I.V.: 50-100 mg/kg/day in divided doses every 6 hours

Severe infections: I.M., I.V.: 100-200 mg/kg/day in divided doses every 4-6 hours

Maximum dose: 12 g/day

Oral: 50-100 mg/kg/day divided every 6 hours

Adults:

Oral: 250-500 mg every 4-6 hours, up to 1 g every 4-6 hours for more severe infections

I.M.: 500 mg every 4-6 hours

I.V.: 500-2000 mg every 4-6 hours

Dosing adjustment in concomitant renal/hepatic impairment: Reduce dose to 33% to 50% of normal dose

Not dialyzable (0% to 5%)

Overdosage Neuromuscular hypersensitivity, seizure

(Continued)

Nafcillin Sodium *(Continued)*

Monitoring Parameters Periodic CBC, urinalysis, BUN, serum creatinine, AST and ALT

Test Interactions False-positive urinary and serum proteins; may inactivate aminoglycosides *in vitro*

Nursing Implications If extravasation occurs, use cold packs and/or Hyaluronidase (Wydase®): Add 1 mL NS to 150 unit vial to make 150 units/mL of concentration; mix 0.1 mL of above with 0.9 mL NS in 1 mL syringe to make final concentration = 15 units/mL

Additional Information Sodium content of 1 g: 66.7 mg (2.9 mEq); other penicillinase-resistant penicillins (ie, dicloxacillin or cloxacillin) are preferred for oral therapy

Dosage Forms
Capsule: 250 mg
Powder for injection: 500 mg, 1 g, 2 g, 4 g, 10 g
Solution: 250 mg/5 mL (100 mL)
Tablet: 500 mg

Selected Readings
Donowitz GR and Mandell GL, "Beta-Lactam Antibiotics," *N Engl J Med*, 1988, 318(7):419-26 and 318(8):490-500.
Wright AJ and Wilkowske CJ, "The Penicillins," *Mayo Clin Proc*, 1991, 66(10):1047-63.

Naftifine Hydrochloride (naf' ti feen)

Brand Names Naftin®
Generic Available No
Use Topical treatment of tinea cruris and tinea corporis
Pregnancy Risk Factor B
Warnings/Precautions For external use only
Adverse Reactions
>10%: Burning, stinging
1% to 10%: Dryness, erythema, itching, irritation

Mechanism of Action Naftifine is a synthetic, broad-spectrum antifungal agent in the allylamine class. This is the first agent of a new class of topical antifungals that are totally unrelated to the imidazole compounds. As with all allylamine derivatives, naftifine is most active when the allylamine double bond has the transorientation; the corresponding cis-isomer is much less active. The drug appears to have both fungistatic and fungicidal activity with no systemic adverse effects. Naftifine exhibits antifungal activity by selectively inhibiting the enzyme squalene epoxidase in a dose-dependent manner. As a result of this inhibitor, the primary sterol, ergosterol, within the fungal membrane is not synthesized.

Usual Dosage Adults: Topical: Apply twice daily
Patient Information For external use only; avoid eyes, mouth, and other mucous membranes; do not use occlusive dressings unless directed to do so; discontinue if irritation or sensitivity develops

Dosage Forms
Cream: 1% (15 g, 30 g, 60 g)
Gel, topical: 1% (20 g, 40 g, 60 g)

Naftin® *see* Naftifine Hydrochloride *on this page*

Nalidixic Acid (nal i dix' ik)

Brand Names NegGram®
Synonyms Nalidixinic Acid
Generic Available Yes
Use Treatment of urinary tract infections
Pregnancy Risk Factor B
Contraindications Hypersensitivity to nalidixic acid or any component; infants <3 months of age
Warnings/Precautions Use with caution in patients with impaired hepatic or renal function and prepubertal children; has been shown to cause cartilage degeneration in immature animals; may induce hemolysis in patients with G-6-PD deficiency

Adverse Reactions
>10%: Dizziness, drowsiness, headache
1% to 10%: Nausea, vomiting
<1%: Increased intracranial pressure, malaise, vertigo, confusion, toxic psychosis, convulsions, fever, rash, urticaria, metabolic acidosis, leukopenia,

thrombocytopenia, hepatotoxicity, visual disturbances, photosensitivity reactions, chills

Toxicology Symptoms of overdose include nausea, vomiting, toxic psychosis, convulsions, increased intracranial pressure, metabolic acidosis; severe overdose, intracranial hypertension, increased pressure, and seizures have occurred; after GI decontamination, treatment is symptomatic

Drug Interactions
Decreased effect with antacids
Increased effect of warfarin

Mechanism of Action Inhibits DNA polymerase in late stages of chromosomal replication

Pharmacokinetics
Distribution: Crosses the placenta; appears in breast milk; achieves significant antibacterial concentrations only in the urinary tract
Metabolism: Partly in the liver
Half-life: 6-7 hours; increases significantly with renal impairment
Time to peak serum concentration: Oral: Within 1-2 hours
Elimination: Excreted in urine as unchanged drug and 80% as metabolites; small amounts appear in feces

Usual Dosage Oral:
Children 3 months to 12 years: 55 mg/kg/day divided every 6 hours; suppressive therapy is 33 mg/kg/day divided every 6 hours

Adults: 1 g 4 times/day for 2 weeks; then suppressive therapy of 500 mg 4 times/day

Dosing comments in renal impairment: Cl_{cr} <50 mL/minute: Avoid use

Test Interactions False-positive urine glucose with Clinitest®, false increase in urinary VMA

Patient Information Avoid undue exposure to direct sunlight or use a sunscreen; take 1 hour before meals, but can take with food to decrease GI upset, finish all medication, do not skip doses; if persistent cough occurs, notify physician

Dosage Forms
Suspension, oral (raspberry flavor): 250 mg/5 mL (473 mL)
Tablet: 250 mg, 500 mg, 1 g

Nalidixinic Acid *see* Nalidixic Acid *on previous page*

Nallpen® *see* Nafcillin Sodium *on page 616*

Nebcin® Injection *see* Tobramycin *on page 685*

NebuPent™ Inhalation *see* Pentamidine Isethionate *on page 639*

NegGram® *see* Nalidixic Acid *on previous page*

Neomycin Sulfate (nee oh mye' sin)

Brand Names Mycifradin® Sulfate; Neo-Tabs®
Generic Available Yes
Use Orally to prepare GI tract for surgery; topically to treat minor skin infections; treat diarrhea caused by *E. coli*; adjunct in the treatment of hepatic encephalopathy
Drug of Choice or Alternative For
Disease/Syndrome(s)
Otitis Externa, Mild *on page 34*
Pregnancy Risk Factor C
Contraindications Hypersensitivity to neomycin or any component or other aminoglycosides; patients with intestinal obstruction
Warnings/Precautions Use with caution in patients with renal impairment, pre-existing hearing impairment, neuromuscular disorders; modify dosage in patients with renal impairment; neomycin is more toxic than other aminoglycosides when given parenterally; **do not administer parenterally**; topical neomycin is a contact sensitizer with sensitivity occurring in 5% to 15% of patients treated with the drug, symptoms include itching, reddening, edema, and failure to heal; systemic absorption can occur when utilized as irrigating solution
Adverse Reactions
1% to 10%: Dermatitis, burning, erythema, rash, urticaria, contact conjunctivitis
<1%: Nausea, vomiting, diarrhea, neuromuscular blockade, ototoxicity, nephrotoxicity
(Continued)

Neomycin Sulfate *(Continued)*

Toxicology The treatment of choice following a single acute overdose appears to be the maintenance of good urine output of at least 3 mL/kg/hour. Dialysis is of questionable value in the enhancement of aminoglycoside elimination. If required, hemodialysis is preferred over peritoneal dialysis in patients with normal renal function. Careful hydration may be all that is required to promote diuresis and therefore the enhancement of the drug's elimination.

Drug Interactions

Decreased effect/levels of digoxin and methotrexate, vitamin K

Increased effect of oral anticoagulants; increased adverse effects with other neurotoxic, ototoxic or nephrotoxic drugs

Mechanism of Action Interferes with bacterial protein synthesis by binding to 30S ribosomal subunits

Pharmacokinetics

Absorption: May be absorbed through ear, eye, denuded or inflamed skin, and body cavities; poorly absorbed orally (3%) or percutaneously

Distribution: Widely distributed in body tissues and fluids; crosses placenta

Metabolism: Slight hepatic metabolism

Half-life: 3 hours (age and renal function dependent)

Time to peak serum concentration: Oral: 1-4 hours

Elimination: In urine (30% to 50% as unchanged drug); 97% of an oral dose is eliminated unchanged in feces

Usual Dosage

Neonates: Oral: Necrotizing enterocolitis: 50-100 mg/kg/day divided every 6 hours

Children: Oral:

Preoperative intestinal antisepsis: 90 mg/kg/day divided every 4 hours for 2 days; or 25 mg/kg at 1 PM, 2 PM, and 11 PM on the day preceding surgery as an adjunct to mechanical cleansing of the intestine and in combination with erythromycin base

Hepatic coma: 50-100 mg/kg/day in divided doses every 6-8 hours or 2.5-7 g/m²/day divided every 4-6 hours for 5-6 days not to exceed 12 g/day

Children and Adults: Topical: Apply ointment 1-4 times/day; topical solutions containing 0.1% to 1% neomycin have been used for irrigation

Adults: Oral:

Preoperative intestinal antisepsis: 1 g each hour for 4 doses then 1 g every 4 hours for 5 doses; or 1 g at 1 PM, 2 PM, and 11 PM on day preceding surgery as an adjunct to mechanical cleansing of the bowel and oral erythromycin; or 6 g/day divided every 4 hours for 2-3 days

Hepatic coma: 500-2000 mg every 6-8 hours or 4-12 g/day divided every 4-6 hours for 5-6 days

Chronic hepatic insufficiency: 4 g/day

Dialyzable (50% to 100%)

Overdosage Ototoxicity, nephrotoxicity, and neuromuscular toxicity

Monitoring Parameters Renal function tests, audiometry in symptomatic patients

Patient Information Notify physician if ringing in the ears, hearing impairment, or dizziness occurs

Dosage Forms Also available in topical creams/ointments with a combination of other agents

Cream: 0.5% (15 g)

Ointment, topical: 0.5% (15 g, 30 g, 120 g)

Solution, oral: 125 mg/5 mL (480 mL)

Tablet: 500 mg

Selected Readings

Edson RS and Terrell CL, "The Aminoglycosides," *Mayo Clin Proc*, 1991, 66(11):1158-64.

Neo-Tabs® *see* Neomycin Sulfate *on previous page*

1-*N*-Ethyl Sisomicin *see* Netilmicin Sulfate *on this page*

Netilmicin Sulfate *(ne til mye' sin)*

Related Information

Aminoglycoside Dosing and Monitoring *on page 721-722*

Antimicrobial Activity Against Selected Organisms *on page 757-764*

Brand Names Netromycin®

Synonyms 1-*N*-Ethyl Sisomicin

Generic Available No

Use Short-term treatment of serious or life-threatening infections including septicemia, peritonitis, intra-abdominal abscess, lower respiratory tract infections, urinary tract infections, skin, bone and joint infections caused by susceptible organisms

Pregnancy Risk Factor D

Contraindications Known hypersensitivity to netilmicin (aminoglycosides, bisulfites)

Adverse Reactions
>10%: Nephrotoxicity, neurotoxicity, ototoxicity (auditory), ototoxicity (vestibular), decreased creatinine clearance

1% to 10%: Skin itching, redness, rash, swelling

<1%: Difficulty in breathing, drowsiness, weakness, headache, tremors, muscle cramps, pseudomotor cerebri, anorexia, nausea, vomiting, weight loss, increased salivation, enterocolitis, granulocytopenia, agranulocytosis, thrombocytopenia, photosensitivity, erythema, burning, stinging

Toxicology Potential for toxicity, serum level monitoring is recommended for all patients. The treatment of choice following a single acute overdose appears to be the maintenance of good urine output of at least 3 mL/kg/hour. Dialysis is of questionable value in the enhancement of aminoglycoside elimination. If required, hemodialysis is preferred over peritoneal dialysis in patients with normal renal function. Careful hydration may be all that is required to promote diuresis and therefore the enhancement of the drug's elimination. Chelation with penicillins is experimental.

Drug Interactions
Increased/prolonged effect of depolarizing and nondepolarizing neuromuscular blocking agents

Increased toxicity: Concurrent use of amphotericin, vancomycin, ethacrynic acid, or furosemide may increase nephrotoxicity

Mechanism of Action Interferes with protein synthesis in bacterial cell by binding to 30S ribosomal subunits

Pharmacokinetics
Absorption: I.M.: Well absorbed

Distribution: To extracellular fluid including serum, abscesses, ascitic, pericardial, pleural, synovial, lymphatic, and peritoneal fluids; high concentrations in urine; crosses placenta

Half-life: 2-3 hours (age and renal function dependent)

Time to peak serum concentration: I.M.: Within 30-60 minutes

Elimination: Excreted by glomerular filtration

Usual Dosage Individualization is critical because of the low therapeutic index. Use of ideal body weight (IBW) for determining the mg/kg/dose appears to be more accurate than dosing on the basis of total body weight (TBW). In morbid obesity, dosage requirement may best be estimated using a dosing weight of IBW + 0.4 (TBW - IBW). Peak and trough plasma drug levels should be determined, particularly in critically ill patients with serious infections or in disease states known to significantly alter aminoglycoside pharmacokinetics (eg, cystic fibrosis, burns, or major surgery).

I.M., I.V.:
Neonates <6 weeks: 2-3.25 mg/kg/dose every 12 hours
Children 6 weeks to 12 years: 1-2.5 mg/kg/dose every 8 hours
Children >12 years and Adults: 1.5-2 mg/kg/dose every 8-12 hours

Some clinicians suggest a daily dose of 4-7 mg/kg for all patients with normal renal function. This dose is at least as efficacious with similar, if not less, toxicity than conventional dosing.

Dosing adjustment in renal impairment: Initial dose:
All patients should receive a loading dose of at least 2 mg/kg (subsequent dosing should be base on serum concentrations)
Cl_{cr} ≥60 mL/minute: Administer every 8 hours
Cl_{cr} 40-60 mL/minute: Administer every 12 hours
Cl_{cr} 20-40 mL/minute: Administer every 24 hours

Overdosage Ototoxicity, nephrotoxicity, and neuromuscular toxicity

Reference Range Therapeutic: Peak: 4-10 μg/mL (SI: 8-21 μmol/L); Trough: <2 μg/mL (SI: 4 μmol/L); Toxic: Peak: >10 μg/mL (SI: >21 μmol/L); Trough: >2 μg/mL (SI: >4.2 μmol/L)

Test Interactions Penicillins may decrease aminoglycoside serum concentrations *in vitro*

(Continued)

Netilmicin Sulfate (Continued)

Patient Information Report any dizziness or sensations of ringing or fullness in ears

Nursing Implications Peak levels are drawn 30 minutes after the end of a 30-minute infusion; trough levels are drawn within 30 minutes before the next dose; give other antibiotic drugs at least 1 hour before or after gentamicin, if possible.

Dosage Forms
Injection: 100 mg/mL (1.5 mL)
Injection:
Neonatal: 10 mg/mL (2 mL)
Pediatric: 25 mg/mL (2 mL)

Selected Readings

Blaser J, König C, Simmen HP, et al, "Monitoring Serum Concentrations for Once-Daily Netilmicin Dosing Regimens," *J Antimicrob Chemother*, 1994, 33:341-8.

Cunha BA, "Aminoglycosides: Current Role in Antimicrobial Therapy," *Pharmacotherapy*, 1988, 8(6):334-50.

Edson RS and Terrell CL, "The Aminoglycosides," *Mayo Clin Proc*, 1991, 66(11):1158-64.

McCormack JP and Jewesson PJ, "A Critical Reevaluation of the "Therapeutic Range" of Aminoglycosides," *Clin Infect Dis*, 1992, 14(1):320-39.

Rozdzinski E, Kern WV, Reichle A, et al, "Once-Daily Versus Trice-Daily Dosing of Netilmicin in Combination With β-lactam Antibiotics as Empirical Therapy for Febrile Neutropenic Patients," *J Antimicrob Chemother*, 1993, 31:585-98.

Netromycin® see Netilmicin Sulfate *on page 620*

Neupogen® Injection see Filgrastim *on page 567*

Neutrexin™ see Trimetrexate Glucuronate *on page 689*

Niclocide® see Niclosamide *on this page*

Niclosamide (ni kloe' sa mide)

Brand Names Niclocide®

Generic Available No

Use Treatment of intestinal beef, fish, and dwarf tapeworm infections

Drug of Choice or Alternative For
Organism(s)
Cestodes *on page 75*

Pregnancy Risk Factor B

Contraindications Known hypersensitivity to niclosamide

Warnings/Precautions Affects cestodes of the intestine only; it is without effect in cysticercosis

Adverse Reactions
1% to 10%: Nausea, vomiting, loss of appetite, diarrhea, drowsiness, dizziness, headache
<1%: Rash, pruritus ani, oral irritation, fever, rectal bleeding, weakness, bad taste in mouth, sweating, palpitations, constipation, alopecia, edema in the arm, backache

Toxicology In the event of an overdose, do not administer ipecac

Mechanism of Action Inhibits the synthesis of ATP through inhibition of oxidative phosphorylation in the mitochondria of cestodes

Pharmacokinetics
Absorption: Oral: Not significantly absorbed
Metabolism: Not appreciably metabolized by mammalian host, but may be metabolized in GI tract by the worm
Elimination: Excreted in feces

Usual Dosage Oral:
Beef and fish tapeworm:
Children:
11-34 kg: 1 g (2 tablets) as a single dose
>34 kg: 1.5 g (3 tablets) as a single dose
Adults: 2 g (4 tablets) in a single dose
May require a second course of treatment 7 days later

Dwarf tapeworm:
Children:
11-34 g: 1 g (2 tablets) chewed thoroughly in a single dose the first day, then 500 mg/day (1 tablet) for next 6 days
>34 g: 1.5 g (3 tablets) in a single dose the first day, then 1 g/day for 6 days

Adults: 2 g (4 tablets) in a single daily dose for 7 days

Overdosage Nausea, vomiting, anorexia

Monitoring Parameters Stool cultures

Patient Information Chew tablets thoroughly; tablets can be pulverized and mixed with water to form a paste for administration to children; can be taken with food; a mild laxative can be used for constipation

Nursing Implications Administer a laxative 2-3 hours after the niclosamide dose if treating *Taenia solium* infections to prevent the development of cysticercosis

Dosage Forms Tablet, chewable (vanilla flavor): 500 mg

Selected Readings
"Drugs for Parasitic Infections," *Med Lett Drugs Ther*, 1993, 35(911):111-22.

Nilstat® Oral *see* Nystatin *on page 625*

Nilstat® Topical *see* Nystatin *on page 625*

Nilstat® Vaginal *see* Nystatin *on page 625*

Nitrofurantoin (nye troe fyoor an' toyn)

Related Information
Antimicrobial Activity Against Selected Organisms *on page 757-764*

Brand Names Furadantin®; Furalan®; Furan®; Furanite®; Macrobid®; Macrodantin®

Generic Available Yes: Tablet and suspension

Use Prevention and treatment of urinary tract infections caused by susceptible gram-negative and some gram-positive organisms; *Pseudomonas, Serratia*, and most species of *Proteus* are generally resistant to nitrofurantoin

Drug of Choice or Alternative For
Organism(s)
Staphylococcus saprophyticus on page 203

Pregnancy Risk Factor B

Contraindications Hypersensitivity to nitrofurantoin or any component; renal impairment; infants <1 month of age (due to the possibility of hemolytic anemia)

Warnings/Precautions Use with caution in patients with G-6-PD deficiency, patients with anemia, vitamin B deficiency, diabetes mellitus or electrolyte abnormalities; therapeutic concentrations of nitrofurantoin are not attained in urine of patients with Cl_{cr} <40 mL/minute; use with caution if prolonged therapy is anticipated due to possible pulmonary toxicity

Adverse Reactions
>10%: Chest pains, chills, cough, fever, difficult breathing, stomach upset, diarrhea, loss of appetite, vomiting
1% to 10%: Sore throat, tiredness, weakness, drowsiness, headache, dizziness, numbness, tingling
<1%: Hemolytic anemia, hepatitis, skin rash, itching, arthralgia

Toxicology Symptoms of overdose include vomiting; supportive care only

Drug Interactions
Decreased effect with antacids
Increased effect/levels with probenecid

Mechanism of Action Inhibits several bacterial enzyme systems including acetyl coenzyme A interfering with metabolism and possibly cell wall synthesis

Pharmacokinetics
Absorption: Well absorbed from GI tract; the macrocrystalline form is absorbed more slowly due to slower dissolution, but causes less GI distress; absorption is increased by presence of food
Distribution: Crosses the placenta; appears in breast milk
Metabolism: 60% of drug metabolized by body tissues throughout the body, with exception of plasma, to inactive metabolites
Half-life: 20-60 minutes; prolonged with renal impairment
Elimination: Excreted as metabolites and unchanged drug (40%) in urine and small amounts in bile; renal excretion via glomerular filtration and tubular secretion

Usual Dosage Oral:
Children >1 month: 5-7 mg/kg/day divided every 6 hours; maximum: 400 mg/day
Chronic therapy: 1-2 mg/kg/day in divided doses every 12-24 hours; maximum dose: 400 mg/day

(Continued)

Nitrofurantoin *(Continued)*

Adults: 50-100 mg/dose every 6 hours (not to exceed 400 mg/24 hours); extended release: 100 mg every 12 hours with meals for 7 days
Prophylaxis: 50-100 mg/dose at bedtime

Dosing adjustment/comments in renal impairment: Cl$_{cr}$ <50 mL/minute: Avoid use

Monitoring Parameters Signs of pulmonary reaction, signs of numbness or tingling of the extremities, periodic liver function tests

Test Interactions Causes false-positive urine glucose with Clinitest®

Patient Information Take with food or milk; may discolor urine to a dark yellow or brown color; notify physician if fever, chest pain, persistent, nonproductive cough, or difficulty breathing occurs

Nursing Implications Higher peak serum levels may cause increased GI upset; give with meals to slow the rate of absorption and thus decrease adverse effects

Dosage Forms
Capsule: 50 mg, 100 mg
Capsule:
Extended release: 100 mg
Macrocrystal: 25 mg, 50 mg, 100 mg
Macrocrystal/monohydrate: 100 mg
Suspension, oral: 25 mg/5 mL (470 mL)
Tablet: 50 mg, 100 mg

Nix™ Creme Rinse *see* Permethrin *on page 640*

Nizoral® *see* Ketoconazole *on page 598*

Nordeoxyguanosine *see* Ganciclovir *on page 574*

Norfloxacin (nor flox' a sin)

Related Information
Antimicrobial Activity Against Selected Organisms *on page 757-764*

Brand Names Chibroxin™ Ophthalmic; Noroxin® Oral

Generic Available No

Use Complicated and uncomplicated urinary tract infections caused by susceptible gram-negative and gram-positive bacteria; ophthalmic solution for conjunctivitis

Pregnancy Risk Factor C

Contraindications Known hypersensitivity to quinolones

Warnings/Precautions Not recommended in children <18 years of age; other quinolones have caused transient arthropathy in children; CNS stimulation may occur which may lead to tremor, restlessness, confusion, and very rarely to hallucinations or convulsive seizures. Use with caution in patients with known or suspected CNS disorders.

Adverse Reactions
1% to 10%: Nausea, headache, dizziness, fatigue
<1%: Rash, abdominal pain, dyspepsia, somnolence, depression, insomnia, constipation, flatulence, heartburn, dry mouth, diarrhea, fever, vomiting, pruritus, loose stools, back pain, hyperhidrosis, erythema, anorexia, bitter taste, asthenia, GI bleeding, increased serum creatinine and BUN, increased liver enzymes, acute renal failure

Toxicology Symptoms of overdose include acute renal failure, seizures; following GI decontamination, use supportive measures

Drug Interactions
Decreased absorption with antacids, bismuth salts, iron and zinc salts, sucralfate by up to 98% if given at the same time
Increased effect/levels of warfarin, theophylline, cyclosporine

Mechanism of Action Norfloxacin is a DNA gyrase inhibitor. DNA gyrase is an essential bacterial enzyme that maintains the superhelical structure of DNA. DNA gyrase is required for DNA replication and transcription, DNA repair, recombination, and transposition; bactericidal

Pharmacokinetics
Absorption: Oral: Rapid, up to 40%
Distribution: Crosses the placenta; small amounts appear in breast milk
Metabolism: In the liver
Half-life: 4.8 hours (can be higher with reduced glomerular filtration rates)
Time to peak serum concentration: Within 1-2 hours

Elimination: Excreted in urine and feces (30%)

Usual Dosage
Oral: Adults: 400 mg twice daily for 7-21 days depending on infection; maximum: 800 mg/day

Ophthalmic: Children >1 year and Adults: Instill 1-2 drops in affected eye(s) 4 times/day for up to 7 days

Dosing interval in renal impairment:
Cl_{cr} 10-30 mL/minute: Administer every 24 hours
Cl_{cr} <10 mL/minute: Do not use

Patient Information Do not take with antacids; finish all the medication
Nursing Implications Hold antacids, sucralfate for 3-4 hours after giving
Dosage Forms
Solution, ophthalmic: 0.3% [3 mg/mL] (5 mL)
Tablet: 400 mg

Selected Readings
Hooper DC and Wolfson JS, "Fluoroquinolone Antimicrobial Agents," *N Engl J Med*, 1991, 324(6):384-94.
Lomaestro BM and Bailie GR, "Quinolone-Cation Interactions: A Review," *DICP*, 1991, 25(11):1249-58.
Stein GE, "The 4-Quinolone Antibiotics: Past, Present, and Future," *Pharmacotherapy*, 1988, 8(6):301-14.
Walker RC and Wright AJ, "The Fluoroquinolones," *Mayo Clin Proc*, 1991, 66(12):1249-59.

Noroxin® Oral *see* Norfloxacin *on previous page*
Nor-tet® *see* Tetracycline *on page 679*
NP-27® [OTC] *see* Tolnaftate *on page 687*
Nydrazid® Injection *see* Isoniazid *on page 592*

Nystatin (nye stat' in)
Brand Names Mycostatin® Oral; Mycostatin® Topical; Mycostatin® Vaginal; Nilstat® Oral; Nilstat® Topical; Nilstat® Vaginal; Nystat-Rx®; Nystex® Oral; Nystex® Topical; O-V Staticin® Oral/Vaginal
Generic Available Yes
Use Treatment of susceptible cutaneous, mucocutaneous, oral cavity, and vaginal fungal infections normally caused by the *Candida* species
Pregnancy Risk Factor B
Contraindications Hypersensitivity to nystatin or any component
Adverse Reactions
1% to 10%: Nausea, vomiting, diarrhea, stomach pain
<1%: Hypersensitivity reactions
Stability Keep vaginal inserts in refrigerator; protect from temperature extremes, moisture and light
Mechanism of Action Binds to sterols in fungal cell membrane, changing the cell wall permeability allowing for leakage of cellular contents
Pharmacokinetics
Absorption: Not absorbed through mucous membranes or intact skin; poorly absorbed from the GI tract
Elimination: Excreted in feces as unchanged drug after oral administration
Usual Dosage
Oral candidiasis: Suspension (swish and swallow orally):
Neonates: 100,000 units 4 times/day or 50,000 units to each side of mouth 4 times/day
Infants: 200,000 units 4 times/day or 100,000 units to each side of mouth 4 times/day
Children and Adults: 500,000 units 4 times/day

Mucocutaneous infections: Children and Adults: Topical: Apply 2-3 times/day to affected areas; very moist topical lesions are treated best with powder

Intestinal infections: Adults: Oral tablets: 500,000-1,000,000 units every 8 hours

Vaginal infections: Adults: Vaginal tablets: Insert 1 tablet/day at bedtime for 2 weeks
Overdosage Nausea, vomiting, diarrhea
Patient Information The oral suspension should be swished about the mouth and retained in the mouth for as long as possible (several minutes) before swallowing. For neonates and infants, paint nystatin suspension into recesses of the mouth. If topical irritation occurs, discontinue; for external use only; do not discontinue therapy even if symptoms are gone
(Continued)

Nystatin *(Continued)*

Dosage Forms
Cream: 100,000 units/g (15 g, 30 g)

Ointment, topical: 100,000 units/g (15 g, 30 g)

Powder, for preparation of oral suspension: 50 million units, 1 billion units, 2 billion units, 5 billion units

Powder, topical: 100,000 units/g (15 g)

Suspension, oral: 100,000 units/mL (5 mL, 60 mL, 480 mL)

Tablet:
Oral: 500,000 units
Vaginal: 100,000 units (15 and 30/box with applicator)

Troche: 200,000 units

Nystat-Rx® *see Nystatin on previous page*

Nystex® Oral *see Nystatin on previous page*

Nystex® Topical *see Nystatin on previous page*

Ocu-Chlor® *see Chloramphenicol on page 531*

Ocuflox™ Ophthalmic *see Ofloxacin on this page*

Ofloxacin *(oh floks' a sin)*

Related Information
Antimicrobial Activity Against Selected Organisms *on page 757-764*

Brand Names Floxin® Injection; Floxin® Oral; Ocuflox™ Ophthalmic

Generic Available No

Use Quinolone antibiotic used in the treatment of skin and skin structure, lower respiratory and urinary tract infections, and sexually transmitted diseases

Drug of Choice or Alternative For
Organism(s)
Neisseria gonorrhoeae on page 161

Pregnancy Risk Factor C

Contraindications Hypersensitivity to ofloxacin or other members of the quinolone group such as nalidixic acid, oxolinic acid, cinoxacin, norfloxacin, and ciprofloxacin

Adverse Reactions
>10%: Nausea

1% to 10%: Headache, insomnia, external genital pruritus in women, dizziness, vaginitis, diarrhea, vomiting, GI distress, pain and cramps, abdominal cramps, flatulence, dysgeusia, dry mouth, decreased appetite, fatigue, somnolence, sleep disorders, visual disturbances, nervousness, rash, pruritus, pyrexia, chest pain, trunk pain, superinfection (ophthalmic), photophobia, lacrimation, dry eyes, stinging

<1%: Asthenia, chills, malaise, extremity pain, thirst, weight loss, decreased hearing acuity, tinnitus, photophobia, anxiety, cognitive change, depression, dream abnormality, euphoria, hallucinations, paresthesia, syncope, vertigo, edema, hypertension, palpitations, vasodilation, cough

Toxicology Treatment is supportive, ofloxacin is not removed by dialysis

Drug Interactions
Decreased effect/levels with bismuth salts, antacids (magnesium, calcium, aluminum), iron, zinc salts, sucralfate

Increased effect/levels of warfarin, cyclosporine, theophylline

Mechanism of Action Ofloxacin is a DNA gyrase inhibitor. DNA gyrase is an essential bacterial enzyme that maintains the superhelical structure of DNA. DNA gyrase is required for DNA replication and transcription, DNA repair, recombination, and transposition; bactericidal

Pharmacokinetics
Absorption: Well absorbed; administration with food causes only minor alterations in absorption

Distribution: Widely distributed into body tissues

Half-life, elimination: 5-7.5 hours

Elimination: Excreted primarily unchanged in urine

Usual Dosage Adults: Oral: 200-400 mg every 12 hours for 7-10 days for most infections or for 6 weeks for prostatitis

Dosing adjustment in renal impairment:
Cl_{cr} 10-50 mL/minute: Administer 50% of normal dose or administer every 24 hours

Cl$_{cr}$ <10 mL/minute: Administer 25% of normal dose or administer 50% of normal dose every 24 hours

Overdosage Nausea, vomiting, seizures

Patient Information Report any skin rash or other allergic reactions; avoid excessive sunlight; do not take with food; do not take within 2 hours of any products including antacids which contain zinc, magnesium, or aluminum

Dosage Forms
Injection: 200 mg (50 mL); 400 mg (10 mL, 20 mL, 100 mL)
Solution, ophthalmic: 0.3% (5 mL)
Tablet: 200 mg, 300 mg, 400 mg

Selected Readings
Hooper DC and Wolfson JS, "Fluoroquinolone Antimicrobial Agents," *N Engl J Med*, 1991, 324(6):384-94.
Lomaestro BM and Bailie GR, "Quinolone-Cation Interactions: A Review," *DICP*, 1991, 25(11):1249-58.
Monk JP and Campoli-Richards DM, "Ofloxacin. A Review of Its Antibacterial Activity, Pharmacokinetic Properties and Therapeutic Use," *Drugs*, 1987, 33(4):346-91.
Stein GE, "The 4-Quinolone Antibiotics: Past, Present, and Future," *Pharmacotherapy*, 1988, 8(6):301-14.
US Department of Health and Human Services, "1993 Sexually Transmitted Diseases Treatment Guidelines," *MMWR Morb Mortal Wkly Rep*, 1993, 42(RR-14).
Walker RC and Wright AJ, "The Fluoroquinolones," *Mayo Clin Proc*, 1991, 66(12):1249-59.

Omnipen® *see* Ampicillin *on page 495*

Omnipen®-N *see* Ampicillin *on page 495*

Ophthochlor® *see* Chloramphenicol *on page 531*

OPV *see* Poliovirus Vaccine, Live, Trivalent, Oral *on page 646*

Orimune® *see* Poliovirus Vaccine, Live, Trivalent, Oral *on page 646*

Ornidyl® Injection *see* Eflornithine Hydrochloride *on page 559*

Otobiotic® *see* Polymyxin B Sulfate *on page 647*

Ovide™ *see* Malathion *on page 602*

O-V Staticin® Oral/Vaginal *see* Nystatin *on page 625*

Oxacillin Sodium (ox a sill' in)

Related Information
Antimicrobial Activity Against Selected Organisms *on page 757-764*

Brand Names Bactocill® Injection; Bactocill® Oral; Prostaphlin® Injection; Prostaphlin® Oral

Synonyms Isoxazolyl Penicillin; Methylphenyl

Generic Available Yes

Use Treatment of susceptible bacterial infections such as osteomyelitis, septicemia, endocarditis, and CNS infections due to susceptible strains of *Staphylococcus*

Drug of Choice or Alternative For Disease/Syndrome(s)
Arthritis, Septic *on page 18*

Pregnancy Risk Factor B

Contraindications Hypersensitivity to oxacillin or other penicillins or any component

Adverse Reactions
1% to 10%: Nausea, diarrhea
<1%: Fever, rash, vomiting, eosinophilia, leukopenia, neutropenia, thrombocytopenia, agranulocytosis, serum sickness-like reactions, hepatotoxicity, hematuria, mild leukopenia, agranulocytosis, elevated AST, acute interstitial nephritis

Toxicology Many beta-lactam containing antibiotics have the potential to cause neuromuscular hyperirritability or convulsive seizures. Hemodialysis may be helpful to aid in the removal of the drug from the blood, otherwise most treatment is supportive or symptom directed.

Drug Interactions Increased effect with probenecid; aminoglycosides (synergy)

Stability Reconstituted parenteral solution is stable for 3 days at room temperature and 7 days when refrigerated; for I.V. infusion in NS or D$_5$W, solution is stable for 6 hours at room temperature

Mechanism of Action Inhibits bacterial cell wall synthesis by binding to one or more of the penicillin binding proteins (PBPs); which in turn inhibits the final

(Continued)

Oxacillin Sodium *(Continued)*

transpeptidation step of peptidoglycan synthesis in bacterial cell walls, thus inhibiting cell wall biosynthesis. Bacteria eventually lyse due to ongoing activity of cell wall autolytic enzymes (autolysins and murein hydrolases) while cell wall assembly is arrested.

Pharmacokinetics

Absorption: Oral: 35% to 67%

Distribution: Into bile, synovial and pleural fluids, bronchial secretions; also distributes to peritoneal and pericardial fluids; crosses the placenta and appears in breast milk; penetrates the blood-brain barrier only when meninges are inflamed

Metabolism: In the liver to active metabolites

Half-life:

Children 1 week to 2 years: 0.9-1.8 hours

Adults: 23-60 minutes (prolonged with reduced renal function and in neonates)

Time to peak serum concentration:

Oral: Within 2 hours

I.M.: Within 30-60 minutes

Elimination: Excreted by kidneys and to small degree the bile as parent drug and metabolites

Usual Dosage

Neonates: I.M., I.V.:

Postnatal age <7 days:

<2000 g: 25 mg/kg/dose every 12 hours

>2000 g: 25 mg/kg/dose every 8 hours

Postnatal age >7 days:

<1200 g: 25 mg/kg/dose every 12 hours

1200-2000 g: 30 mg/kg/dose every 8 hours

>2000 g: 37.5 mg/kg/dose every 6 hours

Infants and Children:

I.M., I.V.: 150-200 mg/kg/day in divided doses every 6 hours; maximum dose: 12 g/day

Oral: 50-100 mg/kg/day divided every 6 hours

Adults:

I.M., I.V.: 1 mg to 2 g/dose every 4-6 hours

Oral: 500-1000 mg every 4-6 hours for at least 5 days

Dosing adjustment in renal impairment: Cl_{cr} <10 mL/minute: Use lower range of the usual dosage

Not dialyzable (0% to 5%)

Overdosage Neuromuscular hypersensitivity, seizure

Monitoring Parameters Periodic CBC, urinalysis, BUN, serum creatinine, AST and ALT

Test Interactions May interfere with urinary glucose tests using cupric sulfate (Benedict's solution, Clinitest®); may inactivate aminoglycosides *in vitro*; false-positive urinary and serum proteins

Patient Information Take on an empty stomach 1 hour before meals or 2 hours after meals

Additional Information Sodium content of 1 g: 64.4-71.3 mg (2.8-3.1 mEq)

Dosage Forms

Capsule: 250 mg, 500 mg

Powder for injection: 250 mg, 500 mg, 1 g, 2 g, 4 g, 10 g

Powder for oral solution: 250 mg/5 mL (100 mL)

Selected Readings

Donowitz GR and Mandell GL, "Beta-Lactam Antibiotics," *N Engl J Med*, 1988, 318(7):419-26 and 318(8):490-500.

Wright AJ and Wilkowske CJ, "The Penicillins," *Mayo Clin Proc*, 1991, 66(10):1047-63.

Oxamniquine *(ox am' ni kwin)*

Brand Names Vansil™

Generic Available No

Use Treat all stages of *Schistosoma mansoni* infection

Drug of Choice or Alternative For

Organism(s)

Schistosoma mansoni on page 189

Pregnancy Risk Factor C

Warnings/Precautions Rare epileptiform convulsions have been observed within the first few hours of administration, especially in patients with a history of CNS pathology

Adverse Reactions
>10%: Dizziness, drowsiness, headache
<10%: Insomnia, malaise, hallucinations, behavior changes, GI effects, orange/red discoloration of urine, elevated LFTs, rash, urticaria, pruritus, proteinuria

Drug Interactions May be synergistic with praziquantel

Mechanism of Action Not fully elucidated; causes worms to dislodge from their usual site of residence (mesenteric veins to the liver) by paralysis and contraction of musculature and subsequently phagocytized

Pharmacokinetics
Absorption: Oral: Well absorbed
Metabolism: Extensive in the GI tract via oxidation
Half-life: 1-2.5 hours
Time to peak: 1-3 hours
Elimination: <2% unchanged in urine; up to 75% of metabolites excreted in urine

Usual Dosage Oral:
Children <30 kg: 20 mg/kg in 2 divided doses of 10 mg/kg at 2- to 8-hour intervals

Adults: 12-15 mg/kg as a single dose

Test Interactions May interfere with spectrometric or color reaction urinalysis

Patient Information Take with food

Additional Information Strains other than from the western hemisphere may require higher doses

Dosage Forms Capsule: 250 mg

Selected Readings
"Drugs for Parasitic Infections," *Med Lett Drugs Ther*, 1993, 35(911):111-22.

Oxiconazole Nitrate (ox i kon' a zole)

Brand Names Oxistat®

Generic Available No

Use Treatment of tinea pedis, tinea cruris, and tinea corporis

Pregnancy Risk Factor B

Contraindications Sensitivity to this agent; not for ophthalmic use

Warnings/Precautions May cause irritation during therapy; if a sensitivity to oxiconazole occurs, therapy should be discontinued

Adverse Reactions 1% to 10%: Itching, transient burning, local irritation, stinging, erythema, dryness

Mechanism of Action The cytoplasmic membrane integrity of fungi is destroyed by oxiconazole which exerts a fungicidal activity through inhibition of ergosterol synthesis

Pharmacokinetics
Absorption: In each layer of the dermis; very little is absorbed systemically after one topical dose
Distribution: To each layer of the dermis
Elimination: <0.3% excreted in urine; excreted in breast milk

Usual Dosage Topical: Apply once daily to affected areas for 2 weeks to 1 month

Patient Information For external use only; discontinue if sensitivity or chemical irritation occurs, contact physician if condition fails to improve in 3-4 days

Dosage Forms
Cream: 1% (15 g, 30 g, 60 g)
Lotion: 1% (30 mL)

Oxistat® *see* Oxiconazole Nitrate *on this page*

Oxytetracycline Hydrochloride (ox i tet ra sye' kleen)

Brand Names E.P. Mycin® Oral; Terramycin® I.M. Injection; Terramycin® Oral; Uri-Tet® Oral

Generic Available Yes

Use Treatment of susceptible bacterial infections; both gram-positive and gram-negative, as well as, *Rickettsia* and *Mycoplasma* organisms

Pregnancy Risk Factor D

Contraindications Hypersensitivity to tetracycline or any component

(Continued)

Oxytetracycline Hydrochloride *(Continued)*

Warnings/Precautions Avoid in children ≤8 years of age, pregnant and nursing women; photosensitivity can occur with oxytetracycline

Adverse Reactions

>10%: Discoloration of teeth and enamel hypoplasia (infants)

1% to 10%: Nausea, diarrhea, photosensitivity

<1%: Increased intracranial pressure, bulging fontanels in infants, paresthesia, dermatologic effects, diabetes insipidus syndrome, vomiting, esophagitis, anorexia, abdominal cramps, acute renal failure, azotemia, superinfections, pericarditis, anaphylaxis, pruritus, pigmentation of nails, exfoliative dermatitis, thrombophlebitis, pseudotumor cerebri, antibiotic-associated pseudomembranous colitis, staphylococcal enterocolitis, hepatotoxicity, renal damage, hypersensitivity reactions, candidal superinfection

Toxicology Symptoms of overdose include nausea, anorexia, diarrhea; following GI decontamination, supportive care only

Drug Interactions

Decreased effect with antacids (aluminum, calcium, zinc, or magnesium), bismuth salts, sodium bicarbonate, barbiturates, carbamazepine, hydantoins; decreased effect of oral contraceptives

Increased effect of warfarin

Mechanism of Action Inhibits bacterial protein synthesis by binding with the 30S and possibly the 50S ribosomal subunit(s) of susceptible bacteria, cell wall synthesis is not affected

Pharmacokinetics

Absorption:

Oral: Adequate (~75%)

I.M.: Poor

Distribution: Crosses the placenta

Metabolism: Small amounts in the liver

Half-life: 8.5-9.6 hours (increases with renal impairment)

Time to peak serum concentration: Within 2-4 hours

Elimination: Excreted in urine, while much higher amounts can be found in bile

Usual Dosage

Oral:

Children: 40-50 mg/kg/day in divided doses every 6 hours (maximum: 2 g/24 hours)

Adults: 250-500 mg/dose every 6 hours

I.M.:

Children >8 years: 15-25 mg/kg/day (maximum: 250 mg/dose) in divided doses every 8-12 hours

Adults: 250-500 mg every 24 hours or 300 mg/day divided every 8-12 hours

Dosing interval in renal impairment: Cl_{cr} <10 mL/minute: Administer every 24 hours or avoid use if possible

Dosing adjustment/comments in hepatic impairment: Avoid use in patients with severe liver disease

Patient Information Avoid unnecessary exposure to sunlight; do not take with antacids, iron products, or dairy products; finish all medication; do not skip doses; take 1 hour before or 2 hours after meals

Nursing Implications Injection for intramuscular use only

Dosage Forms

Capsule: 250 mg

Injection, with lidocaine 2%: 5% [50 mg/mL] (2 mL, 10 mL); 12.5% [125 mg/mL] (2 mL)

Panmycin® *see* Tetracycline *on page 679*

Paromomycin Sulfate *(par oh moe mye' sin)*

Brand Names Humatin®

Generic Available No

Use Treatment of acute and chronic intestinal amebiasis; preoperatively to suppress intestinal flora; tapeworm infestations; has also been used in the treatment of *Cryptosporidium*

Drug of Choice or Alternative For

Organism(s)

Entamoeba histolytica on page 102

Pregnancy Risk Factor C

Contraindications Intestinal obstruction, impaired renal function, known hypersensitivity to paromomycin

Warnings/Precautions Use with caution in patients with impaired renal function or possible or proven ulcerative bowel lesions

Adverse Reactions

1% to 10%: Diarrhea, abdominal cramps, nausea, vomiting, heartburn

<1%: Headache, vertigo, steatorrhea, secondary enterocolitis, exanthema, rash, pruritus, ototoxicity, eosinophilia

Mechanism of Action Acts directly on ameba; has antibacterial activity against normal and pathogenic organisms in the GI tract

Pharmacokinetics

Absorption: Hardly absorbed in the systemic circulation

Elimination: 100% excreted unchanged in feces

Usual Dosage Oral:

Intestinal amebiasis: Children and Adults: 25-35 mg/kg/day in 3 divided doses for 5-10 days

Tapeworm (fish, dog, bovine, porcine):

Children: 11 mg/kg every 15 minutes for 4 doses

Adults: 1 g every 15 minutes for 4 doses

Hepatic coma: Adults: 4 g/day in 2-4 divided doses for 5-6 days

Dwarf tapeworm: Children and Adults: 45 mg/kg/dose every day for 5-7 days

Overdosage Nausea, vomiting, diarrhea

Patient Information Take full course of therapy; do not skip doses; notify physician if ringing in ears, hearing loss, or dizziness occurs

Dosage Forms Capsule: 250 mg

Selected Readings

Danziger LH, Kanyok TP, and Novak RM, "Treatment of Cryptosporidial Diarrhea in an AIDS Patient With Paromomycin," *Ann Pharmacother*, 1993, 27(12):1460-2.

"Drugs for Parasitic Infections," *Med Lett Drugs Ther*, 1993, 35(911):111-22.

Penicillin G Benzathine and Procaine Combined

Brand Names Bicillin® C-R; Bicillin® C-R 900/300

Synonyms Penicillin G Procaine and Benzathine Combined

Generic Available No

Use May be used in specific situations in the treatment of streptococcal infections

Pregnancy Risk Factor B

Contraindications Known hypersensitivity to penicillin or any component

Warnings/Precautions Use with caution in patients with impaired renal function, impaired cardiac function or seizure disorder

Toxicology Many beta-lactam containing antibiotics have the potential to cause neuromuscular hyperirritability or convulsive seizures; hemodialysis may be helpful to aid in the removal of the drug from the blood, otherwise most treatment is supportive or symptom directed

Drug Interactions Probenecid, tetracyclines, methotrexate, aminoglycosides

Stability Store in the refrigerator

Mechanism of Action Inhibits bacterial cell wall synthesis by binding to one or more of the penicillin binding proteins (PBPs); which in turn inhibits the final transpeptidation step of peptidoglycan synthesis in bacterial cell walls, thus inhibiting cell wall biosynthesis. Bacteria eventually lyse due to ongoing activity of cell wall autolytic enzymes (autolysins and murein hydrolases) while cell wall assembly is arrested.

Usual Dosage I.M.:

Children:

<30 lb: 600,000 units in a single dose

30-60 lb: 900,000 units to 1.2 million units in a single dose

(Continued)

Penicillin G Benzathine and Procaine Combined
(Continued)
Children >60 lb and Adults: 2.4 million units in a single dose

Overdosage Neuromuscular hypersensitivity, seizure

Test Interactions May interfere with urinary glucose tests using cupric sulfate (Benedict's solution, Clinitest®); may inactivate aminoglycosides *in vitro*; positive Coombs' [direct], increased protein

Nursing Implications Administer by deep I.M. injection in the upper outer quadrant of the buttock

Dosage Forms
Injection:
300,000 units [150,000 units each of penicillin G benzathine and penicillin G procaine] (10 mL)
600,000 units [300,000 units each penicillin G benzathine and penicillin G procaine] (1 mL)
1,200,000 units [600,000 units each penicillin G benzathine and penicillin G procaine] (2 mL)
2,400,000 units [1,200,000 units each penicillin G benzathine and penicillin G procaine] (4 mL)
Penicillin G benzathine 900,000 units and penicillin G procaine 300,000 units per dose (2 mL)

Penicillin G Benzathine, Parenteral
Brand Names Bicillin® L-A; Permapen®

Synonyms Benzathine Benzylpenicillin; Benzathine Penicillin G; Benzylpenicillin Benzathine

Generic Available No

Use Treatment of mild to moderate infections caused by organisms susceptible to low concentrations of penicillin G, or for prophylaxis of infections caused by these organisms; used in the treatment of syphilis

Drug of Choice or Alternative For
Organism(s)
Treponema pallidum on page 218

Pregnancy Risk Factor B

Contraindications Known hypersensitivity to penicillin or any component

Warnings/Precautions Use with caution in patients with impaired renal function, seizure disorder, or history of hypersensitivity to other beta-lactams

Adverse Reactions
1% to 10%: Local pain
<1%: Thrombophlebitis, convulsions, confusion, drowsiness, fever, rash, electrolyte imbalance, hemolytic anemia, positive Coombs' reaction, myoclonus, acute interstitial nephritis, Jarisch-Herxheimer reaction, hypersensitivity reactions, anaphylaxis

Toxicology Many beta-lactam containing antibiotics have the potential to cause neuromuscular hyperirritability or convulsive seizures. Hemodialysis may be helpful to aid in the removal of the drug from the blood, otherwise most treatment is supportive or symptom directed.

Drug Interactions Increased levels with probenecid; aminoglycosides (synergy); tetracyclines decrease penicillin activity

Stability Store in the refrigerator

Mechanism of Action Inhibits bacterial cell wall synthesis by binding to one or more of the penicillin binding proteins (PBPs); which in turn inhibits the final transpeptidation step of peptidoglycan synthesis in bacterial cell walls, thus inhibiting cell wall biosynthesis. Bacteria eventually lyse due to ongoing activity of cell wall autolytic enzymes (autolysins and murein hydrolases) while cell wall assembly is arrested.

Pharmacokinetics
Absorption: I.M.: Slowly absorbed
Time to peak serum concentration: Within 12-24 hours; serum levels are usually detectable for 1-4 weeks depending on the dose; larger doses result in more sustained levels rather than higher levels

Usual Dosage I.M.: Give undiluted injection, very slowly released from site of injection, providing uniform levels over 2-4 weeks; higher doses result in more sustained rather than higher levels. Use a penicillin G benzathine-penicillin G procaine combination to achieve early peak levels in acute infections

Neonates >1200 g: 50,000 units as a single dose

Infants and Children:

Group A streptococcal upper respiratory infection: 25,000 units/kg as a single dose; maximum: 1.2 million units

Prophylaxis of recurrent rheumatic fever: 25,000 units/kg every 3-4 weeks; maximum: 1.2 million units/dose

Early syphilis: 50,000 units/kg as a single injection; maximum: 2.4 million units

Syphilis of more than 1-year duration: 50,000 units/kg every week for 3 doses; maximum: 2.4 million units/dose

Adults:

Group A streptococcal upper respiratory infection: 1.2 million units as a single dose

Prophylaxis of recurrent rheumatic fever: 1.2 million units every 3-4 weeks or 600,000 units twice monthly; a single dose of 600,000 to 1,2000,000 units is effective in the prevention of rheumatic fever secondary to streptococcal pharyngitis

Early syphilis: 2.4 million units as a single dose

Syphilis of more than 1-year duration: 2.4 million units once weekly for 3 doses

Overdosage Neuromuscular hypersensitivity, seizure

Test Interactions May interfere with urinary glucose tests using cupric sulfate (Benedict's solution, Clinitest®); may inactivate aminoglycosides *in vitro*; positive Coombs' [direct], false-positive urinary and/or serum proteins

Patient Information Report any rash

Nursing Implications Administer by deep I.M. injection in the upper outer quadrant of the buttock; do **not** give I.V., intra-arterially, or S.C.; in children, I.M. injections should be made into the midlateral muscle of the thigh

Dosage Forms Injection: 300,000 units/mL (10 mL); 600,000 units/mL (1 mL, 2 mL, 4 mL)

Selected Readings

US Department of Health and Human Services, "1993 Sexually Transmitted Diseases Treatment Guidelines," *MMWR Morb Mortal Wkly Rep*, 1993, 42(RR-14).

Wright AJ and Wilkowske CJ, "The Penicillins," *Mayo Clin Proc*, 1991, 66(10):1047-63.

Penicillin G, Parenteral

Related Information

Antimicrobial Activity Against Selected Organisms *on page 757-764*

Brand Names Pfizerpen®

Synonyms Benzylpenicillin Potassium; Benzylpenicillin Sodium; Crystalline Penicillin; Penicillin G Potassium; Penicillin G Sodium

Generic Available Yes

Use Active against most gram-positive organisms including streptococci, enterococci, and rarely staphylococci; *Neisseria meningitidis*, and some anaerobes and spirochetes

Drug of Choice or Alternative For

Disease/Syndrome(s)

Endocarditis, Subacute Native Valve *on page 23*

Meningitis, Community Acquired, Adult *on page 29*

Pneumonia, Aspiration, Community-Acquired *on page 37*

Organism(s)

Actinomyces Species *on page 51*

Bacillus anthracis on page 58

Borrelia burgdorferi on page 68

Clostridium perfringens on page 86

Clostridium tetani on page 88

Corynebacterium jeikeium on page 90

Corynebacterium Species, Other than *C. jeikeium on page 91*

Enterococcus Species *on page 107*

Leptospira interrogans on page 140

Listeria monocytogenes on page 143

Neisseria meningitidis on page 163

Pasteurella multocida on page 170

Streptococcus agalactiae on page 203

Streptococcus bovis on page 205

Streptococcus pneumoniae on page 206

Streptococcus pyogenes on page 207
Streptococcus-Related Gram-Positive Cocci *on page 212*
Streptococcus, Viridans Group *on page 213*
Treponema pallidum on page 218

Pregnancy Risk Factor B

Contraindications Known hypersensitivity to penicillin or any component

Warnings/Precautions Avoid intravascular or intra-arterial administration or injection into or near major peripheral nerves or blood vessels since such injections may cause severe and/or permanent neurovascular damage; use with caution in patients with renal impairment, pre-existing seizure disorders, or with a history of hypersensitivity to cephalosporins

Adverse Reactions <1%: Thrombophlebitis, convulsions, confusion, drowsiness, fever, rash, electrolyte imbalance, hemolytic anemia, positive Coombs' reaction, myoclonus, acute interstitial nephritis, Jarisch-Herxheimer reaction, hypersensitivity reactions, anaphylaxis

Toxicology Many beta-lactam containing antibiotics have the potential to cause neuromuscular hyperirritability or convulsive seizures. Hemodialysis may be helpful to aid in the removal of the drug from the blood, otherwise most treatment is supportive or symptom directed.

Drug Interactions Increased levels with probenecid; aminoglycosides (synergy); tetracyclines decrease penicillin activity

Stability Reconstituted parenteral solution is stable for 7 days when refrigerated; for I.V. infusion in NS or D_5W, solution is stable for 24 hours at room temperature

Mechanism of Action Inhibits bacterial cell wall synthesis by binding to one or more of the penicillin binding proteins (PBPs); which in turn inhibits the final transpeptidation step of peptidoglycan synthesis in bacterial cell walls, thus inhibiting cell wall biosynthesis. Bacteria eventually lyse due to ongoing activity of cell wall autolytic enzymes (autolysins and murein hydrolases) while cell wall assembly is arrested.

Pharmacokinetics

Distribution: Penetration across the blood-brain barrier is poor, somewhat increased with inflamed meninges; crosses the placenta and appears in breast milk

Metabolism: In the liver (30%) to penicilloic acid

Half-life: 20-50 minutes

Elimination: Excreted in urine

Usual Dosage I.M., I.V.:

Neonates:

Postnatal age <7 days:

<2000 g: 25,000 units/kg/dose every 12 hours; meningitis: 50,000 units/kg/dose every 12 hours

>2000 g: 20,000 units/kg/dose every 8 hours; meningitis: 50,000 units/kg/dose every 8 hours

Postnatal age >7 days:

<1200 g: 25,000 units/kg/dose every 12 hours; meningitis: 50,000 units/kg/dose every 12 hours

1200-2000 g: 25,000 units/kg/dose every 8 hours; meningitis: 75,000 units/kg/dose every 8 hours

>2000 g: 25,000 units/kg/dose every 6 hours; meningitis: 50,000 units/kg/dose every 6 hours

Infants and Children (sodium salt is preferred in children): 100,000-250,000 units/kg/day in divided doses every 4 hours; maximum: 4.8 million units/24 hours

Severe infections: Up to 400,000 units/kg/day in divided doses every 4 hours; maximum dose: 24 million units/day

Adults: 2-24 million units/day in divided doses every 4 hours

Dosing adjustment in renal impairment:

Cl_{cr} 30-50 mL/minute: Administer every 6 hours

Cl_{cr} 10-30 mL/minute: Administer every 8 hours

Cl_{cr} <10 mL/minute: Administer every 12 hours

Moderately dialyzable (20% to 50%)

Overdosage Neuromuscular hypersensitivity, seizure

Test Interactions May interfere with urinary glucose tests using cupric sulfate (Benedict's solution, Clinitest®); may inactivate aminoglycosides *in vitro*; positive Coombs' [direct]; false-positive urinary and/or serum proteins

Patient Information Report any rash or shortness of breath

Nursing Implications Administer by deep I.M. injection in the upper outer quadrant of the buttock

Additional Information 1 million units is approximately equal to 625 mg

Penicillin G potassium: 1.7 mEq of potassium and 0.3 mEq of sodium per 1 million units of penicillin G

Penicillin G sodium: 2 mEq of sodium per 1 million units of penicillin G

Dosage Forms

Injection, as sodium: 5 million units

Injection:

Frozen premixed, as potassium: 1 million units, 2 million units, 3 million units

Powder, as potassium: 1 million units, 5 million units, 10 million units, 20 million units

Selected Readings

Donowitz GR and Mandell GL, "Beta-Lactam Antibiotics," *N Engl J Med*, 1988, 318(7):419-26 and 318(8):490-500.

Wright AJ and Wilkowske CJ, "The Penicillins," *Mayo Clin Proc*, 1991, 66(10):1047-63.

Penicillin G Potassium *see* Penicillin G, Parenteral *on page 633*

Penicillin G Potassium, Oral

Related Information

Antimicrobial Activity Against Selected Organisms *on page 757-764*

Synonyms Crystalline Penicillin; Pen G

Generic Available Yes

Use Treatment of susceptible bacterial infections including most gram-positive organisms (except *Staphylococcus aureus*) and some anaerobes and spirochetes

Pregnancy Risk Factor B

Contraindications Known hypersensitivity to penicillin or any component

Warnings/Precautions Use with caution in patients with renal impairment, history of hypersensitivity to cephalosporins

Adverse Reactions <1%: Thrombophlebitis, convulsions, confusion, drowsiness, fever, rash, electrolyte imbalance, hemolytic anemia, positive Coombs' reaction, myoclonus, acute interstitial nephritis, Jarisch-Herxheimer reaction, hypersensitivity reactions, anaphylaxis

Toxicology Symptoms of overdose include neuromuscular hypersensitivity, seizures. Many beta-lactam containing antibiotics have the potential to cause neuromuscular hyperirritability or convulsive seizures. Hemodialysis may be helpful to aid in the removal of the drug from the blood, otherwise most treatment is supportive or symptom directed.

Drug Interactions Increased levels with probenecid

Stability Reconstituted parenteral solution is stable for 7 days when refrigerated; **incompatible** with aminoglycosides; inactivated in acidic or alkaline solutions; reconstituted oral solution is stable for 14 days when refrigerated

Mechanism of Action Inhibits bacterial cell wall synthesis by binding to one or more of the penicillin binding proteins (PBPs); which in turn inhibits the final transpeptidation step of peptidoglycan synthesis in bacterial cell walls, thus inhibiting cell wall biosynthesis. Bacteria eventually lyse due to ongoing activity of cell wall autolytic enzymes (autolysins and murein hydrolases) while cell wall assembly is arrested.

Pharmacokinetics

Absorption: Oral: <30%

Distribution: Crosses the placenta; appears in breast milk; penetration across the blood-brain barrier is poor with uninflamed meninges

Metabolism: In the liver (30%) to penicilloic acid

Time to peak serum concentration: Oral: Within 0.5-1 hour

Elimination: Penicillin G and its metabolites are excreted in urine mainly by tubular secretion

Usual Dosage Oral:

Infants and Children: 25-50 mg/kg/day or 40,000-80,000 units/kg/day divided every 6-8 hours hours

Adults: 125-500 mg every 6-8 hours

Dosing interval in renal impairment:

Cl_{cr} 10-30 mL/minute: Administer every 8-12 hours

Cl_{cr} <10 mL/minute: Administer every 12-18 hours

(Continued)

Penicillin G Potassium, Oral *(Continued)*

Moderately dialyzable (20% to 50%)

Monitoring Parameters Periodic serum electrolytes, renal and hematologic function tests

Test Interactions May interfere with urinary glucose tests using cupric sulfate (Benedict's solution, Clinitest®); may inactivate aminoglycosides *in vitro*; positive Coombs' [direct]; false-positive urinary and/or serum proteins

Patient Information Take until gone, do not skip doses, notify physician if rash develops, take 1 hour before or 2 hours after meals

Additional Information Penicillin V potassium is preferred for oral therapy

Dosage Forms

Powder for oral solution, as potassium: 400,000 units/5 mL (100 mL, 200 mL); 400,000 units = 250 mg

Tablet, as potassium: 200,000 units, 250,000 units, 400,000 units, 500,000 units, 800,000 units; 400,000 units = 250 mg

Penicillin G Procaine and Benzathine Combined *see* Penicillin G
Benzathine and Procaine Combined *on page 631*

Penicillin G Procaine, Aqueous

Related Information

Antimicrobial Activity Against Selected Organisms *on page 757-764*

Brand Names Crysticillin® A.S.; Pfizerpen®-AS; Wycillin®

Synonyms APPG; Aqueous Procaine Penicillin G; Procaine Benzylpenicillin; Procaine Penicillin G

Generic Available Yes

Use Moderately severe infections due to *Treponema pallidum* and other penicillin G-sensitive microorganisms

Drug of Choice or Alternative For

Disease/Syndrome(s)

Pharyngitis *on page 36*

Organism(s)

Treponema pallidum on page 218

Pregnancy Risk Factor B

Contraindications Known hypersensitivity to penicillin or any component; also contraindicated in patients hypersensitive to procaine

Adverse Reactions

>10%: Pain at injection site

<1%: CNS stimulation, seizures, myocardial depression, vasodilation, conduction disturbances, confusion, drowsiness, hemolytic anemia, positive Coombs' reaction, sterile abscess at injection site, myoclonus, interstitial nephritis, pseudoanaphylactic reactions, Jarisch-Herxheimer reaction, hypersensitivity reactions

Toxicology Many beta-lactam containing antibiotics have the potential to cause neuromuscular hyperirritability or convulsive seizures. Hemodialysis may be helpful to aid in the removal of the drug from the blood, otherwise most treatment is supportive or symptom directed.

Drug Interactions Increased levels with probenecid; aminoglycosides (synergy); tetracyclines decrease penicillin activity

Stability Store in refrigerator

Mechanism of Action Inhibits bacterial cell wall synthesis by binding to one or more of the penicillin binding proteins (PBPs); which in turn inhibits the final transpeptidation step of peptidoglycan synthesis in bacterial cell walls, thus inhibiting cell wall biosynthesis. Bacteria eventually lyse due to ongoing activity of cell wall autolytic enzymes (autolysins and murein hydrolases) while cell wall assembly is arrested.

Pharmacokinetics

Absorption: I.M.: Slowly absorbed

Distribution: Penetration across the blood-brain barrier is poor; appears in breast milk; distributed widely in body; highest concentrations in kidneys and to a lesser extent in liver, skin, intestines, and CSF

Metabolism: ~30% of dose is inactivated by the liver

Half-life: 20-50 minutes

Time to peak serum concentration: Within 1-4 hours

Elimination: Renal clearance is delayed in neonates, young infants, and patients with impaired renal function; 60% to 90% of drug excreted unchanged via renal tubular excretion

Usual Dosage I.M.:

Newborns: 50,000 units/kg/day given every 24 hours (avoid using in this age group since sterile abscesses and procaine toxicity occur more frequently with neonates than older patients)

Children: 25,000-50,000 units/kg/day in divided doses 1-2 times/day; not to exceed 4.8 million units/24 hours
Congenital syphilis: 50,000 units/kg/day for 10-14 days

Adults: 0.6-4.8 million units/day in divided doses 1-2 times/day
Primary, secondary syphilis: 600,000 units/day for 18 days for a total of 4.8 million units
Neurosyphilis: 2.4 million units/day for 10-14 days with probenecid
Moderately dialyzable (20% to 50%)

Overdosage Neuromuscular hypersensitivity, seizure

Monitoring Parameters Periodic renal and hematologic function tests with prolonged therapy

Test Interactions May interfere with urinary glucose tests using cupric sulfate (Benedict's solution, Clinitest®); may inactivate aminoglycosides *in vitro*; positive Coombs' [direct]; false-positive urinary and/or serum proteins

Patient Information Notify physician if skin rash, itching, hives or severe diarrhea occurs

Nursing Implications Procaine suspension for deep I.M. injection only; when doses are repeated, rotate the injection site; avoid I.V., intravascular, or intra-arterial administration of penicillin G procaine since severe and/or permanent neurovascular damage may occur

Dosage Forms Injection, suspension: 300,000 units/mL (10 mL); 500,000 units/mL (1.2 mL); 600,000 units/mL (1 mL, 2 mL, 4 mL)

Selected Readings
Donowitz GR and Mandell GL, "Beta-Lactam Antibiotics," *N Engl J Med*, 1988, 318(7):419-26 and 318(8):490-500.
Wright AJ and Wilkowske CJ, "The Penicillins," *Mayo Clin Proc*, 1991, 66(10):1047-63.

Penicillin G Sodium *see* Penicillin G, Parenteral *on page 633*

Penicillins, Extended Spectrum
Refer To
Mezlocillin Sodium *on page 611*
Piperacillin Sodium *on page 641*
Piperacillin Sodium and Tazobactam Sodium *on page 642*
Ticarcillin and Clavulanate Potassium *on page 682*
Ticarcillin Disodium *on page 683*

Drug of Choice or Alternative For
Disease/Syndrome(s)
Fever, Neutropenic *on page 25*
Meningitis, Postsurgical *on page 31*
Meningitis, Post-Traumatic *on page 31*
Otitis Externa, Severe (Malignant) *on page 34*
Pneumonia, Hospital-Acquired *on page 38*
Sepsis *on page 40*
Sinusitis, Hospital-Acquired *on page 41*

Organism(s)
Acinetobacter Species *on page 50*
Citrobacter Species *on page 82*
Enterobacter Species *on page 104*
Klebsiella Species *on page 137*
Proteus Species *on page 176*
Pseudomonas aeruginosa on page 177
Serratia Species *on page 190*

Penicillins, Penicillinase-Resistant
Refer To
Cloxacillin Sodium *on page 543*
Dicloxacillin Sodium *on page 551*
Methicillin Sodium *on page 608*
Nafcillin Sodium *on page 616*
Oxacillin Sodium *on page 627*

Drug of Choice or Alternative For
Disease/Syndrome(s)
Endocarditis, Acute Native Valve *on page 22*

Organism(s)

Penicillin V Potassium

Related Information

Brand Names Beepen-VK®; Betapen®-VK; Ledercillin® VK; Pen.Vee® K; Robicillin® VK; V-Cillin K®; Veetids®

Synonyms Pen VK; Phenoxymethyl Penicillin

Generic Available Yes

Use Treatment of infections caused by susceptible organisms involving the respiratory tract, otitis media, sinusitis, skin, and urinary tract; prophylaxis in rheumatic fever

Drug of Choice or Alternative For
Disease/Syndrome(s)

Pregnancy Risk Factor B

Contraindications Known hypersensitivity to penicillin or any component

Warnings/Precautions Use with caution in patients with severe renal impairment, history of seizures, or hypersensitivity to cephalosporins

Adverse Reactions
>10%: Mild diarrhea, vomiting, nausea, oral candidiasis
<1%: Convulsions, fever, hemolytic anemia, positive Coombs' reaction, acute interstitial nephritis, hypersensitivity reactions, anaphylaxis

Toxicology Symptoms of overdose include neuromuscular hypersensitivity, seizures. Many beta-lactam containing antibiotics have the potential to cause neuromuscular hyperirritability or convulsive seizures. Hemodialysis may be helpful to aid in the removal of the drug from the blood, otherwise most treatment is supportive or symptom directed.

Drug Interactions Increased levels with probenecid

Stability Refrigerate suspension after reconstitution; discard after 14 days

Mechanism of Action Inhibits bacterial cell wall synthesis by binding to one or more of the penicillin binding proteins (PBPs); which in turn inhibits the final transpeptidation step of peptidoglycan synthesis in bacterial cell walls, thus inhibiting cell wall biosynthesis. Bacteria eventually lyse due to ongoing activity of cell wall autolytic enzymes (autolysins and murein hydrolases) while cell wall assembly is arrested.

Pharmacokinetics
Absorption: Oral: 60% to 73% from GI tract
Distribution: Appears in breast milk
Half-life: 0.5 hour; prolonged in patients with renal impairment
Time to peak serum concentration: Oral: Within 0.5-1 hour
Elimination: Penicillin V and its metabolites are excreted in urine mainly by tubular secretion

Usual Dosage Oral:
Systemic infections:
Children <12 years: 25-50 mg/kg/day in divided doses every 6-8 hours; maximum dose: 3 g/day
Children ≥12 years and Adults: 125-500 mg every 6-8 hours

Prophylaxis of pneumococcal infections:
Children <5 years: 125 mg twice daily
Children ≥5 years and Adults: 250 mg twice daily

Prophylaxis of recurrent rheumatic fever:
Children <5 years: 125 mg twice daily
Children ≥5 years and Adults: 250 mg twice daily

Dosing interval in renal impairment:
Cl_{cr} 10-50 mL/minute: Administer every 8-12 hours

Cl_{cr} <10 mL/minute: Administer every 12-16 hours

Monitoring Parameters Periodic renal and hematologic function tests during prolonged therapy

Test Interactions May interfere with urinary glucose tests using cupric sulfate (Benedict's solution, Clinitest®); may inactivate aminoglycosides *in vitro*; positive Coombs' [direct]; false-positive urinary and/or serum proteins

Patient Information Take until gone, do not skip doses; report any rash or shortness of breath; shake liquid well before use

Additional Information 0.7 mEq of potassium per 250 mg penicillin V; 250 mg equals 400,000 units of penicillin

Dosage Forms

Powder for oral solution: 125 mg/5 mL (3 mL, 100 mL, 150 mL, 200 mL); 250 mg/5 mL (100 mL, 150 mL, 200 mL)

Tablet: 125 mg, 250 mg, 500 mg

Pentacef™ *see* Ceftazidime *on page 520*

Pentam-300® Injection *see* Pentamidine Isethionate *on this page*

Pentamidine Isethionate (pen tam' i deen)

Brand Names NebuPent™ Inhalation; Pentam-300® Injection

Generic Available No

Use Treatment and prevention of pneumonia caused by *Pneumocystis carinii*; treatment of trypanosomiasis

Drug of Choice or Alternative For

Organism(s)

Pneumocystis carinii on page 172

Pregnancy Risk Factor C

Contraindications Hypersensitivity to pentamidine isethionate or any component (inhalation and injection)

Adverse Reactions

>10%: Chest pain, skin rash, wheezing, dyspnea, coughing, pharyngitis, hyperkalemia, local reactions at injection site

1% to 10%: Bitter or metallic taste

<1%: Extrapulmonary pneumocystosis, pancreatitis, pneumothorax, hyperglycemia or hypoglycemia, renal insufficiency, hypotension, tachycardia, dizziness, fever, Jarisch-Herxheimer-like reaction, hypocalcemia, vomiting, megaloblastic anemia, granulocytopenia, leukopenia, thrombocytopenia, mild renal or hepatic injury, irritation of the airway, fatigue

Stability Reconstituted solution is stable for 24 hours at room temperature; do not refrigerate due to the possibility of crystallization

Mechanism of Action Interferes with RNA/DNA, phospholipids and protein synthesis, through inhibition of oxidative phosphorylation and/or interference with incorporation of nucleotides and nucleic acids into RNA and DNA, in protozoa

Pharmacokinetics

Absorption: I.M.: Well absorbed

Distribution: Well distributed to tissues including liver, kidneys, spleen, lung, and pancreas. Systemic accumulation of pentamidine does not appear to occur following inhalation therapy.

Metabolism: Unknown

Half-life: 6.4-9.4 hours; half-life may be prolonged in patients with severe renal impairment

Elimination: 33% to 66% excreted in urine as unchanged drug

Usual Dosage

Children:

Treatment: I.M., I.V. (I.V. preferred): 4 mg/kg/day once daily for 14-21 days

Prevention:

I.M., I.V.: 4 mg/kg monthly or biweekly

Inhalation (aerosolized pentamidine in children ≥5 years): 300 mg/dose given every 3 weeks or monthly via Respirgard® II inhaler (8 mg/kg dose has also been used in children <5 years)

Adults:

Treatment: I.M., I.V. (I.V. preferred): 4 mg/kg/day once daily for 21 days

Prevention: Inhalation: 300 mg every 4 weeks via Respirgard® II nebulizer

Dosing adjustment in renal impairment:

Cl_{cr} 10-50 mL/minute: Administer every 24-36 hours

(Continued)

Pentamidine Isethionate *(Continued)*

Cl_{cr} <10 mL/minute: Administer every 48 hours

Overdosage Hypotension, hypoglycemia, cardiac arrhythmias

Monitoring Parameters Liver function tests, renal function tests, blood glucose, serum potassium and calcium, CBC with differential and platelet count, EKG, blood pressure

Patient Information PCP pneumonia may still occur despite pentamidine prophylaxis; notify physician of fever, shortness of breath, or coughing up blood

Nursing Implications Infuse I.V. slowly over a period of at least 60 minutes or administer deep I.M.; patients receiving I.V. or I.M. pentamidine should be lying down and blood pressure should be monitored closely during administration of drug and several times thereafter until it is stable; virtually indetectable amounts are transferred to healthcare personnel during aerosol administration; do not use NS as a diluent, NS is incompatible with pentamidine

Dosage Forms

Inhalation: 300 mg

Powder for injection, lyophilized: 300 mg

Selected Readings

Goa KL and Campoli-Richards DM, "Pentamidine Isethionate. A Review of Its Antiprotozoal Activity, Pharmacokinetic Properties and Therapeutic Use in *Pneumocystis carinii* Pneumonia," *Drugs*, 1987, 33(3):242-58.

Masur H, "Prevention and Treatment of *Pneumocystis* Pneumonia," *N Engl J Med*, 1992, 327(26):1853-60.

Monk JP and Benfield P, "Inhaled Pentamidine. An Overview of Its Pharmacological Properties and a Review of Its Therapeutic Use in *Pneumocystis carinii* Pneumonia," *Drugs*, 1990, 39(5):741-56.

Sattler FR, Cowan R, Nielsen DM, et al, " Trimethoprim-Sulfamethoxazole Compared With Pentamidine for Treatment of *Pneumocystis carinii* Pneumonia in the Acquired Immunodeficiency Syndrome," *Ann Intern Med*, 1988, 109(4):280-7.

Pen.Vee® K *see* Penicillin V Potassium *on page 638*

Pen VK *see* Penicillin V Potassium *on page 638*

Pepto-Bismol® [OTC] *see* Bismuth *on page 505*

Permapen® *see* Penicillin G Benzathine, Parenteral *on page 632*

Permethrin (per meth' rin)

Brand Names Elimite™ Cream; Nix™ Creme Rinse

Generic Available No

Use Single application treatment of infestation with *Pediculus humanus capitis* (head louse) and its nits, or *Sarcoptes scabiei* (scabies)

Drug of Choice or Alternative For

Organism(s)

Lice *on page 142*

Sarcoptes scabiei on page 188

Pregnancy Risk Factor B

Contraindications Known hypersensitivity to pyrethyroid, pyrethrin or to chrysanthemums

Warnings/Precautions Treatment with Nix™ may temporarily exacerbate the symptoms of itching, redness, swelling; for external use only; use during pregnancy only if clearly needed

Adverse Reactions 1% to 10%: Edema, pruritus, numbness or scalp discomfort, erythema, rash of the scalp, burning, stinging, tingling

Mechanism of Action Inhibits sodium ion influx through nerve cell membrane channels in parasites resulting in delayed repolarization and thus paralysis of the pest

Pharmacokinetics

Absorption: Topical: Minimal (<2%)

Metabolism: In the liver

Elimination: Excreted in urine

Usual Dosage

Head lice: Children >2 months and Adults: After hair has been washed with shampoo, rinsed with water and towel dried, apply a sufficient volume to saturate the hair and scalp. Leave on hair for 10 minutes before rinsing off with water; remove remaining nits.

Scabies: Apply cream from head to toe; leave on for 8-14 hours before washing off with water; a single application is usually adequate

Patient Information Avoid contact with eyes and mucous membranes during application; shake well before using; for topical use only; notify physician of persistent irritation

Dosage Forms

Cream: 5% (60 g)

Liquid, topical: 1% (60 mL)

Selected Readings

"Drugs for Parasitic Infections," *Med Lett Drugs Ther*, 1993, 35(911):111-22.

PFA *see* Foscarnet *on page 571*

Pfizerpen® *see* Penicillin G, Parenteral *on page 633*

Pfizerpen®-AS *see* Penicillin G Procaine, Aqueous *on page 636*

Phenoxymethyl Penicillin *see* Penicillin V Potassium *on page 638*

Phosphonoformic Acid *see* Foscarnet *on page 571*

***p*-Hydroxyampicillin** *see* Amoxicillin Trihydrate *on page 491*

Pima® *see* Potassium Iodide *on page 648*

Pin-Rid® [OTC] *see* Pyrantel Pamoate *on page 651*

Pin-X® [OTC] *see* Pyrantel Pamoate *on page 651*

Piperacillin Sodium (pi per' a sill in)

Related Information

Antimicrobial Activity Against Selected Organisms *on page 757-764*

Brand Names Pipracil®

Generic Available No

Use Treatment of infections caused by susceptible gram-negative bacilli including *Pseudomonas aeruginosa* infections in combination with an aminoglycoside; also useful in the treatment of susceptible streptococcal and anaerobic organisms

Pregnancy Risk Factor B

Contraindications Hypersensitivity to piperacillin or any component or penicillins

Adverse Reactions <1%: Thrombophlebitis, convulsions, confusion, drowsiness, fever, rash, electrolyte imbalance, hemolytic anemia, positive Coombs' reaction, myoclonus, acute interstitial nephritis, Jarisch-Herxheimer reaction, hypersensitivity reactions, anaphylaxis, abnormal platelet aggregation and prolonged prothrombin time (high doses)

Toxicology Many beta-lactam containing antibiotics have the potential to cause neuromuscular hyperirritability or convulsive seizures. Hemodialysis may be helpful to aid in the removal of the drug from the blood, otherwise most treatment is supportive or symptom directed.

Drug Interactions

Decreased effect if administration is within 1 hour prior to or 4 hours after aminoglycosides in patients with renal impairment

Increased levels with probenecid

Stability Reconstituted solution is stable (I.V. infusion) in NS or D_5W for 24 hours at room temperature, 7 days when refrigerated or 4 weeks when frozen; after freezing, thawed solution is stable for 24 hours at room temperature or 48 hours when refrigerated; 40 g bulk vial should **not** be frozen after reconstitution; incompatible with aminoglycosides

Mechanism of Action Inhibits bacterial cell wall synthesis by binding to one or more of the penicillin binding proteins (PBPs); which in turn inhibits the final transpeptidation step of peptidoglycan synthesis in bacterial cell walls, thus inhibiting cell wall biosynthesis. Bacteria eventually lyse due to ongoing activity of cell wall autolytic enzymes (autolysins and murein hydrolases) while cell wall assembly is arrested.

Pharmacokinetics

Absorption: I.M.: 70% to 80%

Distribution: Into pleural, peritoneal, wound and synovial fluids, sputum, and bone; minimal CSF unless meninges are inflamed; crosses the placenta; distributes into milk at low concentrations

Metabolism: Not appreciably metabolized except in gut; inactive metabolites formed by bacterial hydrolysis

Half-life:

Neonates:

1-5 days: 3.6 hours

(Continued)

Piperacillin Sodium *(Continued)*

>6 days: 2.1-2.7 hours
Children:
  1-6 months: 0.79 hour
  6 months to 12 years: 0.39-0.5 hour
Adults: 36-80 minutes (dose-dependent)
Time to peak serum concentration: I.M.: Within 30-50 minutes
Elimination: Excreted principally in urine and partially in feces (via bile)

Usual Dosage
Neonates: I.M., I.V.: 100 mg/kg/dose every 12 hours

Infants and Children: I.M., I.V.: 200-300 mg/kg/day in divided doses every 4-6 hours; maximum dose: 24 g/day
  Higher doses have been used in cystic fibrosis: 350-500 mg/kg/day in divided doses every 4 hours

Adults:
  I.M.: 2-3 g/dose every 6-12 hours; maximum: 24 g/day
  I.V.: 3-4 g/dose every 4-6 hours; maximum: 24 g/day

Dosing adjustment in renal impairment:
  Cl_{cr} 10-50 mL/minute: Administer every 6-8 hours
  Cl_{cr} <10 mL/minute: Administer every 8 hours
Moderately dialyzable (20% to 50%)

Overdosage Neuromuscular hypersensitivity, seizure

Monitoring Parameters Serum electrolytes, bleeding time especially in patients with renal impairment, periodic tests of renal, hepatic and hematologic function

Test Interactions May interfere with urinary glucose tests using cupric sulfate (Benedict's solution, Clinitest®); may inactivate aminoglycosides *in vitro*; false-positive urinary and serum proteins, positive Coombs' test [direct]

Nursing Implications Administer 1 hour apart from aminoglycosides

Additional Information Sodium content of 1 g: 42.6 mg (1.85 mEq)

Dosage Forms Powder for injection: 2 g, 3 g, 4 g, 40 g

Selected Readings
Donowitz GR and Mandell GL, "Beta-Lactam Antibiotics," *N Engl J Med*, 1988, 318(7):419-26 and 318(8):490-500.
Wright AJ and Wilkowske CJ, "The Penicillins," *Mayo Clin Proc*, 1991, 66(10):1047-63.

Piperacillin Sodium and Tazobactam Sodium

(pi per' a sill in) and (ta zoe bak' tam)

Related Information
Antimicrobial Activity Against Selected Organisms *on page 757-764*

Brand Names Zosyn™

Generic Available No

Use Treatment of infections of lower respiratory tract, urinary tract, skin and skin structures, gynecologic, bone and joint infections, and septicemia caused by susceptible organisms. Tazobactam expands activity of piperacillin to include beta-lactamase producing strains of *S. aureus*, *H. influenzae*, *Bacteroides*, and some other gram-negative organisms

Drug of Choice or Alternative For
Disease/Syndrome(s)
  Peritonitis *on page 36*

Pregnancy Risk Factor B

Contraindications Hypersensitivity to piperacillin, tazobactam, other penicillins, or any component

Warnings/Precautions Use with caution in patients with known hypersensitivity to cephalosporins or other beta-lactamase inhibitors; not approved for use in patients <12 years of age; use with caution in patients with a history of seizures and in patients with renal function impairment

Adverse Reactions
>10%: Diarrhea
1% to 10%: Constipation, nausea, vomiting, insomnia, headache, rash, dyspepsia, leukopenia
<1%: Hypertension, hypotension, edema, dizziness, *Pseudomonas* colitis, agitation, confusion, bronchospasm

Toxicology Symptoms of overdose include neuromuscular hypersensitivity, seizures; many beta-lactam containing antibiotics have the potential to cause neuromuscular hyperirritability or convulsive seizures. Hemodialysis may be helpful to aid in the removal of the drug from the blood, otherwise most treatment is supportive or symptom directed.

Drug Interactions
Increased duration of neuromuscular blockers
Increased/prolonged levels with probenecid

Stability Store at controlled room temperature; after reconstitution, stable for 24 hours at room temperature and 1 week when refrigerated; unused portions should be discarded after 24 hours at room temperature and 48 hours when refrigerated

Mechanism of Action Inhibits bacterial cell wall synthesis by binding to one or more of the penicillin binding proteins (PBPs); which in turn inhibits the final transpeptidation step of peptidoglycan synthesis in bacterial cell walls, thus inhibiting cell wall biosynthesis. Bacteria eventually lyse due to ongoing activity of cell wall autolytic enzymes (autolysins and murein hydrolases) while cell wall assembly is arrested.

Pharmacokinetics Both AUC and peak concentrations are dose proportional
Distribution: Distributes well into lungs, intestinal mucosa, skin, muscle, uterus, ovary, prostate, gallbladder, and bile; penetration into CSF is low in subject with noninflamed meninges
Metabolism:
Piperacillin: 6% to 9%
Tazobactam: ~26%
Half-life:
Piperacillin: 1 hour
Metabolite: 1-1.5 hours
Tazobactam: 0.7-0.9 hour
Elimination: Both piperacillin and tazobactam are directly proportional to renal function
Piperacillin: 50% to 70% eliminated unchanged in urine, 10% to 20% excreted in bile
Tazobactam: Found in urine at 24 hours, with 26% as the inactive metabolite
Hemodialysis removes 30% to 40% of piperacillin and tazobactam; peritoneal dialysis removes 11% to 21% of tazobactam and 6% of piperacillin; hepatic impairment does not affect the kinetics of piperacillin or tazobactam significantly

Usual Dosage Adults: I.V.: 3.375 g (3 g piperacillin/0.375 g tazobactam) every 6 hours

Dosing interval in renal impairment:
Cl_{cr} 20-40 mL/minute: Administer 2.25 g every 6 hours
Cl_{cr} <20 mL/minute: Administer 2.25 g every 8 hours

Hemodialysis: Administer 2.25 g every 8 hours with an additional dose of 0.75 g after each dialysis

Test Interactions May interfere with urinary glucose tests using cupric sulfate (Benedict's solution, Clinitest®); may inactivate aminoglycosides *in vitro*; positive Coombs' [direct] test, ↑ ALT, ↑ AST

Nursing Implications Administer 1 hour apart from aminoglycosides

Additional Information Sodium content of 1 g injection: 54 mg (2.35 mEq)

Dosage Forms Injection:
Piperacillin sodium 2 g and tazobactam sodium 0.25 g
Piperacillin sodium 3 g and tazobactam sodium 0.375 g
Piperacillin sodium 4 g and tazobactam sodium 0.5 g

Selected Readings
"Piperacillin/Tazobactam," *Med Lett Drugs Ther*, 1994, 36(914):7-9.

Piperazine Citrate (pi' per a zeen)

Brand Names Vermizine®
Generic Available Yes
Use Treatment of pinworm and roundworm infections (used as an alternative to first-line agents, mebendazole, or pyrantel pamoate)
Pregnancy Risk Factor B
Contraindications Seizure disorders, liver or kidney impairment, hypersensitivity to piperazine or any component
Warnings/Precautions Use with caution in patients with anemia or malnutrition; avoid prolonged use especially in children
Adverse Reactions <1%: Dizziness, vertigo, weakness, seizures, EEG changes, headache, nausea, vomiting, diarrhea, hemolytic anemia, visual impairment, hypersensitivity reactions, bronchospasms
(Continued)

Piperazine Citrate *(Continued)*

Drug Interactions Pyrantel pamoate (antagonistic mode of action)

Mechanism of Action Causes muscle paralysis of the roundworm by blocking the effects of acetylcholine at the neuromuscular junction

Pharmacokinetics

Absorption: Well absorbed from GI tract

Time to peak serum concentration: 1 hour

Elimination: Excreted in urine as metabolites and unchanged drug

Usual Dosage Oral:

Pinworms: Children and Adults: 65 mg/kg/day (not to exceed 2.5 g/day) as a single daily dose for 7 days; in severe infections, repeat course after a 1-week interval

Roundworms:

Children: 75 mg/kg/day as a single daily dose for 2 days; maximum: 3.5 g/day

Adults: 3.5 g/day for 2 days (in severe infections, repeat course, after a 1-week interval)

Monitoring Parameters Stool exam for worms and ova

Patient Information Take on empty stomach; if severe or persistent headache, loss of balance or coordination, dizziness, vomiting, diarrhea, or rash occurs, contact physician. If used for pinworm infections, all members of the family should be treated.

Dosage Forms

Syrup: 500 mg/5 mL (473 mL, 4000 mL)

Tablet: 250 mg

Selected Readings

"Drugs for Parasitic Infections," *Med Lett Drugs Ther*, 1993, 35(911):111-22.

Pipracil® *see* Piperacillin Sodium *on page 641*

Plague Vaccine

Generic Available No

Use Selected travelers to countries reporting cases for whom avoidance of rodents and fleas is impossible; all laboratory and field personnel working with *Yersinia pestis* organisms possibly resistant to antimicrobials; those engaged in *Yersinia pestis* aerosol experiments or in field operations in areas with enzootic plague where regular exposure to potentially infected wild rodents, rabbits, or their fleas cannot be prevented. Prophylactic antibiotics may be indicated following definite exposure, whether or not the exposed persons have been vaccinated.

Pregnancy Risk Factor C

Contraindications Persons with known hypersensitivity to any of the vaccine constituents (see manufacturer's label); patients who have had severe local or systemic reactions to a previous dose; defer immunization in patients with a febrile illness until resolved

Warnings/Precautions Pregnancy, unless there is substantial and unavoidable risk of exposure

Adverse Reactions

1% to 10%: Local erythema, malaise, fever, headache

<1%: Sterile abscess, nausea, vomiting, tachycardia

Drug Interactions Decreased effect with immunoglobulin, other live vaccine used within 1 month

Mechanism of Action Promotes active immunity to plague in high-risk individuals.

Usual Dosage Three I.M. doses: First dose 1 mL, second dose (0.2 mL) 1 month later, third dose (0.2 mL) 5 months after the second dose; booster doses (0.2 mL) at 1- to 2-year intervals if exposure continues

Test Interactions Temporary suppression of tuberculosis skin test

Additional Information Federal law requires that the date of administration, the vaccine manufacturer, lot number of vaccine, and the administering person's name, title and address be entered into the patient's permanent medical record

Dosage Forms Injection: 2 mL, 20 mL

Plaquenil® *see* Hydroxychloroquine Sulfate *on page 584*

Pneumococcal Polysaccharide Vaccine, Polyvalent

Related Information

Vaccines *on page 706-709*

Brand Names Pneumovax® 23; Pnu-Imune® 23

Generic Available No

Use Children >2 years of age and adults who are at increased risk of pneumococcal disease and its complications because of underlying health conditions; older adults, including all those ≥65 years of age; pneumococcal and influenza vaccines can be administered simultaneously at separate sites

Pregnancy Risk Factor C

Contraindications Active infections, Hodgkin's disease patients, <2 years of age, pregnancy, hypersensitivity to pneumococcal vaccine or any component. Epinephrine injection (1:1,000) must be immediately available in the case of anaphylaxis. Pregnant patients and patients <5 years of age should not receive pneumococcal vaccine. Children <5 years of age do not respond satisfactorily to the capsular types of 23 capsular pneumococcal vaccine.

Warnings/Precautions The safety of vaccine in pregnant women has not been evaluated; it should not be given during pregnancy unless the risk of infection is high; have epinephrine available; should be administered with caution in individuals who have had episodes of pneumococcal infection within the preceding 3 years; pre-existing pneumococcal antibodies may result in increased reactions to vaccine; may cause relapse in patients with stable idiopathic thrombocytopenia purpura

Adverse Reactions

>10%: Induration and soreness at the injection site (2-3 days)

<1%: Paresthesias, Guillain-Barré syndrome, low-grade fever, erythema, rash, myalgia, arthralgia, anaphylaxis

Drug Interactions Decreased effect with immunosuppressive agents, immunoglobulin, other live vaccines within 1 month

Stability Refrigerate

Mechanism of Action Although there are more than 80 known pneumococcal capsular types, pneumococcal disease is mainly caused by only a few types of pneumococci. Pneumococcal vaccine contains capsular polysaccharides of 23 pneumococcal types which represent at least 98% of pneumococcal disease isolates in the United States and Europe. The pneumococcal vaccine with 23 pneumococcal capsular polysaccharide types became available in 1983. The 23 capsular pneumococcal vaccine contains purified capsular polysaccharides of pneumococcal types 1, 2, 3, 4, 5, 8, 9, 12, 14, 17, 19, 20, 22, 23, 26, 34, 43, 51, 56, 57, 67, 70 (American Classification). These are the main pneumococcal types associated with serious infections in the United States.

Usual Dosage Children >2 years and Adults: I.M., S.C.: 0.5 mL

Revaccination should be considered if 6 or more years since initial vaccination; revaccination is recommended in patients who received 14-valent pneumococcal vaccine and are at highest risk (asplenic) for fatal infection, or at 6 or more years in patients with nephrotic syndrome, renal failure, or transplant recipients, or 3-5 years in children with nephrotic syndrome, asplenia, or sickle cell disease

Nursing Implications Do not inject I.V., avoid intradermal, administer S.C. or I.M. (deltoid muscle or lateral midthigh)

Additional Information Federal law requires that the date of administration, the vaccine manufacturer, lot number of vaccine, and the administering person's name, title and address be entered into the patient's permanent medical record; inactivated bacteria vaccine

Dosage Forms Injection: 25 μg each of 23 polysaccharide isolates/0.5 mL dose (0.5 mL, 1 mL, 5 mL)

Pneumovax® 23 *see* Pneumococcal Polysaccharide Vaccine, Polyvalent *on this page*

Pnu-Imune® 23 *see* Pneumococcal Polysaccharide Vaccine, Polyvalent *on this page*

Poliovirus Vaccine, Inactivated

Related Information

Vaccines *on page 706-709*

Brand Names IPOL™

Synonyms Enhanced-potency Inactivated Poliovirus Vaccine; IPV; Salk Vaccine

(Continued)

Poliovirus Vaccine, Inactivated *(Continued)*

Generic Available No

Use Although a protective immune response to IPV cannot be assured in the immunocompromised individual, IPV is recommended because the vaccine is safe and some protection may result from its administration.

Pregnancy Risk Factor C

Contraindications Hypersensitivity to any component including neomycin, streptomycin, or polymyxin B; defer vaccination for persons with acute febrile illness until recovery

Warnings/Precautions Although there is no convincing evidence documenting adverse effects of either OPV or E-IPV on the pregnant woman or developing fetus, it is prudent on theoretical grounds to avoid vaccinating pregnant women. However, if immediate protection against poliomyelitis is needed, OPV is recommended. OPV should not be given to immunocompromised individuals or to persons with known or possibly immunocompromised family members; E-IPV is recommended in such situations.

Adverse Reactions All serious adverse reactions must be reported to the FDA.
1% to 10%: Skin rash, fever >101.3°F, tenderness or pain at injection site
<1%: Difficulty in breathing, reddening of skin, tiredness, weakness, Guillain-Barré, erythema, fussiness, sleepiness, crying, decreased appetite

Drug Interactions Decreased effect with immunosuppressive agents, immune globulin, other live vaccines within 1 month; may temporarily suppress tuberculin skin test sensitivity (4-6 weeks)

Mechanism of Action Immunization with poliovirus vaccine produces active immunity to the three types of polio virus.

Usual Dosage Subcutaneous: IPV is preferred for primary vaccination of adults, two doses S.C. 4-8 weeks apart, a third dose 6-12 months after the second. For adults with a completed primary series and for whom a booster is indicated, either OPV or E-IPV can be given. If immediate protection is needed, either OPV or E-IPV is recommended.

Nursing Implications Do not administer I.V.

Additional Information Federal law requires that the date of administration, the vaccine manufacturer, lot number of vaccine, and the administering person's name, title and address be entered into the patient's permanent medical record

Dosage Forms Injection:
Mixture (Poliovax®): Three types of poliovirus (Types 1, 2 and 3) grown in human diploid cell cultures (0.5 mL)
Suspension (IPOL™): Three types of poliovirus (Types 1, 2, and 3) grown in monkey kidney cell cultures (0.5 mL)

Poliovirus Vaccine, Live, Trivalent, Oral

(poe lee oh vye' russ)

Related Information

Vaccines *on page 706-709*

Brand Names Orimune®

Synonyms OPV; Sabin Vaccine; TOPV

Generic Available No

Use Poliovirus immunization

Pregnancy Risk Factor C

Contraindications Persistent vomiting or diarrhea, patients allergic to sorbitol, streptomycin, or neomycin, known hypersensitivity to poliovirus vaccine

Warnings/Precautions The vaccine will not modify or prevent cases of existing or incubating poliomyelitis

Adverse Reactions All serious adverse reactions must be reported to the FDA.

Drug Interactions May temporarily suppress tuberculin skin test sensitivity (4-6 weeks), immunosuppressive agents, immune globulin

Stability Keep in freezer; vaccine must remain frozen to retain potency

Mechanism of Action Immunization with poliovirus vaccine produces active immunity to the three types of polio virus.

Usual Dosage Oral:
Infants: 0.5 mL dose at age 2 months, 4 months, and 18 months; optional dose may be given at 6 months in areas where poliomyelitis is endemic

Older Children, Adolescents, and Adults: Two 0.5 mL doses 8 weeks apart; third dose of 0.5 mL 6-12 months after second dose; a reinforcing dose of 0.5 mL should be given before entry to school, in children who received the third primary dose before their fourth birthday

Patient Information Because of the risk of vaccine-associated paralysis, unvaccinated family members and close personal contacts should be vaccinated prior to the child

Nursing Implications Reconstitute only with diluent provided; federal law requires that the date of administration, the vaccine manufacturer, lot number of vaccine, and the administering person's name, title and address be entered into the patient's permanent medical record

Dosage Forms Oral: Mixture of type 1, 2, and 3 viruses in monkey kidney tissue (0.5 mL)

Polycillin® *see* Ampicillin *on page 495*

Polycillin-N® *see* Ampicillin *on page 495*

Polymox® *see* Amoxicillin Trihydrate *on page 491*

Polymyxin B Sulfate (pol i mix' in)
Brand Names Aerosporin® Injection; Otobiotic®; PediOtic®
Generic Available Yes
Use
Topical: Treatment of mild, uncomplicated otitis externa. Empiric therapy of bacterial conjunctivitis. Wound irrigation and bladder instillation against *Pseudomonas aeruginosa*; used occasionally for gut decontamination

Parenteral use of polymyxin B has mainly been replaced by less toxic antibiotics; it is reserved for life-threatening infections caused by organisms resistant to the preferred drugs.

Drug of Choice or Alternative For
Disease/Syndrome(s)
Otitis Externa, Mild *on page 34*
Pregnancy Risk Factor B
Contraindications Concurrent use of neuromuscular blockers
Warnings/Precautions Use with caution in patients with impaired renal function, modify dosage in patients with renal impairment if given I.M. or I.V.; neurotoxic reactions may be manifested by irritability, weakness, drowsiness, ataxia, perioral paresthesia, numbness of the extremities, and blurring of vision. These are usually associated with high serum levels found in patients with impaired renal function or nephrotoxicity. Avoid concurrent or sequential use of other nephrotoxic and neurotoxic drugs, particularly bacitracin, kanamycin, streptomycin, paromomycin, colistin, tobramycin, neomycin, gentamicin, and amikacin. The drug's neurotoxicity can result in respiratory paralysis from neuromuscular blockade, especially when the drug is given soon after anesthesia or muscle relaxants. Polymyxin B sulfate is toxic when given parenterally; avoid parenteral use whenever possible.

Adverse Reactions <1%: Drug fever, urticarial rash, anaphylactoid reaction, neurotoxicity, hypocalcemia, hyponatremia, hypokalemia, hypochloremia, neuromuscular blockade, nephrotoxicity, respiratory arrest, facial flushing, meningeal irritation with intrathecal administration

Toxicology Symptoms of overdose include respiratory paralysis, ototoxicity, nephrotoxicity; supportive care, ventilatory support may be necessary

Drug Interactions Increased/prolonged effect of neuromuscular blocking agents

Stability Parenteral solutions stable for 7 days when refrigerated; discard any unused portion after 72 hours. **Incompatible** with calcium, magnesium, cephalothin, chloramphenicol, heparin, penicillins; aqueous solutions remain stable for 6-12 months under refrigeration

Mechanism of Action Binds to phospholipids, alters permeability, and damages the bacterial cytoplasmic membrane permitting leakage of intracellular constituents

Pharmacokinetics
Absorption: Well absorbed from the peritoneum; minimal absorption from the GI tract (except in neonates) from mucous membranes or intact skin
Distribution: Minimal distribution into the CSF; crosses the placenta
Half-life: 4.5-6 hours, increased with reduced renal function
Time to peak serum concentration: I.M.: Within 2 hours
Elimination: Excreted primarily as unchanged drug (>60%) in urine via glomerular filtration

Usual Dosage
Otic: 1-2 drops, 3-4 times daily. Should be used sparingly to avoid accumulation of excess debris.

(Continued)

Polymyxin B Sulfate *(Continued)*

Infants <2 years:
I.M.: 25,000-30,000 units/kg/day divided every 6 hours
I.V.: 30,000-45,000 units/kg/day by continuous I.V. infusion
Intrathecal: 20,000 units/day for 3-4 days, then 25,000 units every other day for at least 2 weeks

Children ≥2 years and Adults:
I.M.: 25,000-30,000 units/kg/day divided every 4-6 hours
I.V.: 15,000-25,000 units/kg/day divided every 12 hours or by continuous infusion
Intrathecal: 50,000 units/day for 3-4 days, then every other day for at least 2 weeks
Total daily dose should not exceed 2,000,000 units/day

Dosing adjustment/interval in renal impairment:
Cl_{cr} 50-20 mL/minute: Administer 75% to 100% of normal dose every 12 hours
Cl_{cr} 5-20 mL/minute: Administer 50% of normal dose every 12 hours
Cl_{cr} <5 mL/minute: Administer 15% of normal dose every 12 hours

Bladder irrigation: Continuous irrigant or rinse in the urinary bladder for up to 10 days using 20 mg (equal to 200,000 units) added to 1 L of normal saline; usually no more than 1 L of irrigant is used per day unless urine flow rate is high; administration rate is adjusted to patient's urine output

Topical irrigation or topical solution: 500,000 units/L of normal saline; topical irrigation should not exceed 2 million units/day in adults
Gut sterilization: Oral: 15,000-25,000 units/kg/day in divided doses every 6 hours

Clostridium difficile enteritis: Oral: 25,000 units every 6 hours for 10 days

Ophthalmic: A concentration of 0.1% to 0.25% is administered as 1-3 drops every hour, then increasing the interval as response indicates to 1-2 drops 4-6 times/day

Monitoring Parameters WBC, serum electrolytes, renal function tests, serum drug concentration, urine output

Reference Range Serum concentrations >5 μg/mL are toxic in adults

Patient Information Report any dizziness or sensations of ringing in the ear, loss of hearing, or any muscle weakness

Nursing Implications Parenteral use is indicated only in life-threatening infections caused by organisms not susceptible to other agents

Additional Information 1 mg = 10,000 units

Dosage Forms
Injection: 500,000 units (20 mL)
Solution (otic): 10,000 units of polymyxin B per mL in combination with hydrocortisone 0.5% solution (eg, Otobiotic®)
Suspension (otic): 10,000 units of polymixin B per mL in combination with hydrocortisone 1% and neomycin sulfate 0.5% (eg, PediOtic®)
Also available in a variety of other combination products for ophthalmic and otic use.

Polymyxin E *see* Colistin Sulfate *on page 545*

Postexposure Prophylaxis for Hepatitis B *see page 719*

Potassium Iodide

Brand Names Pima®; Potassium Iodide Enseals®; SSKI®; Thyro-Block®
Synonyms KI; Lugol's Solution; Strong Iodine Solution
Generic Available Yes
Use Used in the treatment of cutaneous sporotrichosis; facilitate bronchial drainage and cough; reduce thyroid vascularity prior to thyroidectomy and management of thyrotoxic crisis; block thyroidal uptake of radioactive isotopes of iodine in a radiation emergency
Drug of Choice or Alternative For
Organism(s)
Sporothrix schenckii on page 193
Pregnancy Risk Factor D
Contraindications Known hypersensitivity to iodine; hyperkalemia, pulmonary tuberculosis, pulmonary edema, bronchitis
Warnings/Precautions Prolonged use can lead to hypothyroidism; cystic fibrosis patients have an exaggerated response; can cause acne flare-ups, can

cause dermatitis, some preparations may contain sodium bisulfite (allergy); use with caution in patients with a history of thyroid disease, patients with renal failure, or GI obstruction

Adverse Reactions 1% to 10%: Angioedema, fever, headache, urticaria, acne, goiter with hypothyroidism, metallic taste, GI upset, cutaneous and mucosal hemorrhage, eosinophilia, arthralgia, lymph node enlargement, soreness of teeth and gums, rhinitis

Toxicology

Signs and symptoms: Angioedema, laryngeal edema in patients with hypersensitivity; muscle weakness, paralysis, peaked T waves, flattened P waves, prolongation of QRS complex, ventricular arrhythmias

Treatment: Removal of potassium can be accomplished by various means; removal through the GI tract with Kayexalate® administration; by way of the kidney through diuresis, mineralocorticoid administration or increased sodium intake; by hemodialysis or peritoneal dialysis; or by shifting potassium back into the cells by insulin and glucose infusion

Drug Interactions Increased effect/toxicity: Lithium → additive hypothyroid effect

Stability Store in tight, light-resistant containers at temperature <40°C; freezing should be avoided

Mechanism of Action Reduces viscosity of mucus by increasing respiratory tract secretions; inhibits secretion of thyroid hormone, fosters colloid accumulation in thyroid follicles

Pharmacokinetics

Onset of action: 24-48 hours

Peak effect: 10-15 days after continuous therapy

Elimination: In euthyroid patient, renal clearance rate is 2 times that of the thyroid

Usual Dosage Oral:

Sporotrichosis:

Oral: Initial:

Preschool: 50 mg/dose 3 times/day

Children: 250 mg/dose 3 times/day

Adults: 500 mg/dose 3 times/day

Oral increase 50 mg/dose daily

Maximum dose:

Preschool: 500 mg/dose 3 times/day

Children and Adults: 1-2 g/dose 3 times/day

Continue treatment for 4-6 weeks after lesions have completely healed

Adults: RDA: 130 μg

Expectorant:

Children: 60-250 mg every 6-8 hours; maximum single dose: 500 mg

Adults: 300-650 mg 3-4 times/day

Preoperative thyroidectomy:

Children and Adults: 50-250 mg (1-5 drops SSKI®) 3 times/day **or** 0.1-0.3 mL (3-5 drops) of strong iodine (Lugol's solution) 3 times/day; give for 10 days before surgery

Thyrotoxic crisis:

Infants <1 year: 150-250 mg (3-5 drops SSKI®) 3 times/day

Children and Adults: 300-500 mg (6-10 drops SSKI®) 3 times/day or 1 mL strong iodine (Lugol's solution) 3 times/day

Graves' disease in neonates: 1 drop of strong iodine (Lugol's solution) 3 times/day

Monitoring Parameters Thyroid function tests

Patient Information Take after meals with food or milk or dilute with a large quantity of water, fruit juice, milk, or broth; discontinue use if stomach pain, skin rash, metallic taste, or nausea and vomiting occurs

Nursing Implications Must be diluted before administration of 240 mL of water, fruit juice, milk, or broth

Additional Information 10 drops of SSKI® = potassium iodide 500 mg

Dosage Forms

Solution, oral:

SSKI®: 1 g/mL (30 mL, 240 mL)

Lugol's Solution, strong iodine: Potassium iodide 100 mg and iodine 50 mg per mL (120 mL, 473 mL, 4000 mL)

Syrup: 325 mg/5 mL (473 mL, 4000 mL)

Tablet: 130 mg

Potassium Iodide Enseals® *see* Potassium Iodide *on page 648*

Praziquantel (pray zi kwon' tel)
Brand Names Biltricide®
Generic Available No
Use Treatment of all stages of schistosomiasis caused by all *Schistosoma* species pathogenic to humans; also active in the treatment of clonorchiasis, opisthorchiasis, cysticercosis, and many intestinal tapeworms
Drug of Choice or Alternative For
 Organism(s)
  Cestodes *on page 75*
  Schistosoma mansoni on page 189
Pregnancy Risk Factor B
Contraindications Ocular cysticercosis, known hypersensitivity to praziquantel
Warnings/Precautions Use caution in patients with severe hepatic disease, patients with cerebral cysticercosis require hospitalization
Adverse Reactions
 1% to 10%: Dizziness, drowsiness, headache, malaise, abdominal pain, loss of appetite, nausea, vomiting, sweating
 <1%: Skin rash, hives, itching, CSF reaction syndrome in patients being treated for neurocysticercosis, fever, diarrhea
Toxicology Treatment is supportive following GI decontamination
Mechanism of Action Increases the cell permeability to calcium in schistosomes, causing strong contractions and paralysis of worm musculature leading to detachment of suckers from the blood vessel walls and to dislodgment
Pharmacokinetics
 Absorption: Oral: ~80%
 Distribution: CSF concentration is 14% to 20% of plasma concentration; appears in breast milk
 Metabolism: Extensive first-pass
 Half-life: 0.8-1.5 hours
 Time to peak serum concentration: Within 1-3 hours
 Elimination: Urinary excretion (99% as metabolites)
Usual Dosage Children >4 years and Adults: Oral:
 Schistosomiasis: 20 mg/kg/dose 2-3 times/day for 1 day at 4- to 6-hour intervals
 Flukes: 25 mg/kg/dose every 8 hours for 1-2 days
 Cysticercosis: 50 mg/kg/day divided every 8 hours for 14 days
 Tapeworms: 10-20 mg/kg as a single dose (25 mg/kg for *Hymenolepis nana*)
Overdosage Dizziness, drowsiness, headache, liver function impairment
Patient Information Do not chew tablets due to bitter taste; take with food; caution should be used when performing tasks requiring mental alertness, may impair judgment and coordination; tablets can be halved or quartered
Dosage Forms Tablet, tri-scored: 600 mg
Selected Readings
 "Drugs for Parasitic Infections," *Med Lett Drugs Ther*, 1993, 35(911):111-22.

Primaquine and Chloroquine *see* Chloroquine and Primaquine
on page 533

Primaquine Phosphate (prim' a kween)
Synonyms Prymaccone
Generic Available No
Use Provides radical cure of *P. vivax* or *P. ovale* malaria after a clinical attack has been confirmed by blood smear or serologic titer and postexposure prophylaxis
Pregnancy Risk Factor C
Contraindications Patients receiving quinacrine
Warnings/Precautions Use with caution in patients with G-6-PD deficiency, NADH methemoglobin reductase deficiency, acutely ill patients who have a tendency to develop granulocytopenia; patients receiving other drugs capable of depressing the bone marrow; do not exceed recommended dosage
Adverse Reactions
 >10%: Hemolytic anemia, abdominal pain, nausea, vomiting

1% to 10%: Methemoglobinemia

<1%: Leukopenia, agranulocytosis, arrhythmias, headache, pruritus, leukocytosis, interference with visual accommodation

Toxicology Symptoms of overdose include abdominal cramps, vomiting, cyanosis, methemoglobinemia, leukopenia, acute hemolytic anemia, granulocytopenia; following GI decontamination, treatment is supportive

Drug Interactions Increased toxicity/levels with quinacrine

Mechanism of Action Eliminates the primary tissue exoerythrocytic forms of *P. falciparum*; disrupts mitochondria and binds to DNA

Pharmacokinetics

Absorption: Oral: Well absorbed

Metabolism: Liver metabolism to carboxyprimaquine, an active metabolite

Half-life: 3.7-9.6 hours

Time to peak serum concentration: Within 1-2 hours

Elimination: Only a small amount of unchanged drug excreted in urine

Usual Dosage Oral:

Children: 0.3 mg base/kg/day once daily for 14 days (not to exceed 15 mg/day) or 0.9 mg base/kg once weekly for 8 weeks not to exceed 45 mg base/week

Adults: 15 mg/day (base) once daily for 14 days or 45 mg base once weekly for 8 weeks

Monitoring Parameters Periodic CBC, visual color check of urine

Patient Information Take with meals to decrease adverse GI effects; drug has a bitter taste; notify physician if a darkening of urine occurs; complete full course of therapy

Dosage Forms Tablet: 26.3 mg [15 mg base]

Selected Readings

Panisko DM and Keystone JS, "Treatment of Malaria – 1990," *Drugs*, 1990, 39(2):160-89.

Wyler DJ, "Malaria Chemoprophylaxis for the Traveler," *N Engl J Med*, 1993, 329(1):31-7.

Primaxin® *see* Imipenem/Cilastatin *on page 586*

Principen® *see* Ampicillin *on page 495*

Procaine Benzylpenicillin *see* Penicillin G Procaine, Aqueous *on page 636*

Procaine Penicillin G *see* Penicillin G Procaine, Aqueous *on page 636*

ProHIBiT® *see* Hemophilus b Conjugate Vaccine *on page 580*

Proloprim® *see* Trimethoprim *on page 688*

Prostaphlin® Injection *see* Oxacillin Sodium *on page 627*

Prostaphlin® Oral *see* Oxacillin Sodium *on page 627*

Protostat® Oral *see* Metronidazole *on page 610*

PRP-D *see* Hemophilus b Conjugate Vaccine *on page 580*

Prymaccone *see* Primaquine Phosphate *on previous page*

Pseudomonic Acid A *see* Mupirocin *on page 616*

Pyrantel Pamoate (pi ran' tel)

Brand Names Antiminth® [OTC]; Pin-Rid® [OTC]; Pin-X® [OTC]; Reese's® Pinworm Medicine [OTC]

Generic Available No

Use Treatment of pinworms (*Enterobius vermicularis*), whipworms (*Trichuris trichiura*), roundworms (*Ascaris lumbricoides*), and hookworms (*Ancylostoma duodenale*)

Drug of Choice or Alternative For

Organism(s)

Ancylostoma duodenale on page 54

Ascaris on page 55

Enterobius vermicularis on page 106

Pregnancy Risk Factor C

Contraindications Known hypersensitivity to pyrantel pamoate

Adverse Reactions

1% to 10%: Anorexia, nausea, vomiting, abdominal cramps, diarrhea

<1%: Dizziness, weakness, drowsiness, insomnia, headache, rash, elevated liver enzymes, tenesmus

Drug Interactions Decreased effect with piperazine

Stability Protect from light

(Continued)

Pyrantel Pamoate *(Continued)*

Mechanism of Action Causes the release of acetylcholine and inhibits cholinesterases, like a depolarizing neuromuscular blocker, paralyzing the worm

Pharmacokinetics
Absorption: Oral: Poor
Metabolism: Undergoes partial hepatic metabolism
Time to peak serum concentration: Within 1-3 hours
Elimination: Excreted in feces (50% as unchanged drug) and urine (7% as unchanged drug)

Usual Dosage Children and Adults: (Purgation is not required prior to use) Oral: Hookworm, roundworm, pinworm, or trichostrongyliasis: 11 mg/kg administered as a single dose; maximum dose: 1 g; dosage should be repeated in 2 weeks and all family members should be treated for pinworm infection

Overdosage Anorexia, nausea, vomiting, cramps, diarrhea, ataxia

Monitoring Parameters Stool for presence of eggs, worms, and occult blood, serum AST AND ALT

Patient Information May mix drug with milk or fruit juice; strict hygiene is essential to prevent reinfection

Nursing Implications Shake well before pouring to assure accurate dosage

Dosage Forms
Capsule: 180 mg
Liquid: 50 mg/mL (30 mL); 144 mg/mL (30 mL)
Suspension, oral (caramel-currant flavor): 50 mg/mL (60 mL)

Selected Readings
"Drugs for Parasitic Infections," *Med Lett Drugs Ther*, 1993, 35(911):111-22.

Pyrazinamide *(peer a zin' a mide)*

Synonyms Pyrazinoic Acid Amide

Generic Available No

Use Adjunctive treatment of tuberculosis as part of a multidrug regimen

Drug of Choice or Alternative For
Organism(s)
Mycobacterium tuberculosis on page 155

Pregnancy Risk Factor C

Contraindications Severe hepatic damage; hypersensitivity to pyrazinamide or any component

Warnings/Precautions Use with caution in patients with renal failure, gout, diabetes mellitus, or porphyria; administer with at least one other effective agent for tuberculosis

Adverse Reactions
1% to 10%: Arthralgia, myalgia, nausea, vomiting, anorexia
<1%: Skin rash, itching, gout, hepatotoxicity, fever, acne, photosensitivity, porphyria, dysuria, interstitial nephritis, thrombocytopenia

Drug Interactions Decreases INH serum levels

Mechanism of Action Converted to pyrazinoic acid in susceptible strains of *Mycobacterium* which lowers the pH of the environment; exact mechanism of action has not been elucidated

Pharmacokinetics
Absorption: Oral: Well absorbed
Distribution: Widely distributed into body tissues and fluids including the liver, lung, and CSF
Metabolism: In the liver
Half-life: 9-10 hours, increased with reduced renal or hepatic function
Time to peak serum concentration: Within 2 hours
Elimination: Excreted in urine (4% as unchanged drug)

Usual Dosage Oral (Calculate dose on ideal body weight rather than total body weight):
Children: 15-30 mg/kg/day in divided doses every 12-24 hours; daily dose not to exceed 2 g

Adults: 15-30 mg/kg/day in 3-4 divided doses; maximum daily dose: 3 g/day

Dosing adjustment in renal impairment: Cl_{cr} <50 mL/minute: Avoid use or reduce dose to 12-20 mg/kg/day

Dosing adjustment in hepatic impairment: Reduce dose

Overdosage Gout, gastric upset, hepatic damage

Monitoring Parameters Periodic liver function tests, serum uric acid

Patient Information Notify physician if fever, loss of appetite, malaise, nausea, vomiting, darkened urine occur

Dosage Forms Tablet: 500 mg

Selected Readings

Davidson PT and Le HQ, "Drug Treatment of Tuberculosis – 1992," *Drugs*, 1992, 43(5):651-73.

"Drugs for Tuberculosis," *Med Lett Drugs Ther*, 1993, 35(908):99-101.

Iseman MD, "Treatment of Multidrug-Resistant Tuberculosis," *N Engl J Med*, 1993, 329(11):784-91.

Van Scoy RE and Wilkowske CJ, "Antituberculosis Agents," *Mayo Clin Proc*, 1992, 67(2):179-87.

Pyrazinoic Acid Amide *see* Pyrazinamide *on previous page*

Pyrethrins (pye ree' thrins)

Brand Names A-200™ Pyrinate [OTC]; End Lice® [OTC]; Lice-Enz® [OTC]; Pyrinyl II® [OTC]; RID® [OTC]; Tisit® [OTC]

Generic Available Yes

Use Treatment of *Pediculus humanus* infestations

Drug of Choice or Alternative For

Organism(s)

Lice *on page 142*

Pregnancy Risk Factor C

Contraindications Known hypersensitivity to pyrethrins

Warnings/Precautions For external use only

Adverse Reactions 1% to 10%: Pruritus, burning, stinging, irritation with repeat use

Mechanism of Action The mechanism of action on the neuronal membranes of lice is similar to that of DDT. Piperonyl butoxide is usually added to pyrethrin to enhance the product's activity by decreasing the metabolism of pyrethrins in arthropods.

Pharmacokinetics

Absorption: Topical: Minimal

Metabolism: By ester hydrolysis and hydroxylation

Usual Dosage Application of pyrethrins:

Apply enough solution to completely wet infested area, including hair

Allow to remain on area for 10 minutes

Wash and rinse with large amounts of warm water

Use fine-toothed comb to remove lice and eggs from hair

Shampoo hair to restore body and luster

Treatment may be repeated if necessary once in a 24-hour period

Repeat treatment in 7-10 days to kill newly hatched lice

Patient Information Avoid touching eyes, mouth, or other mucous membranes; contact physician if irritation occurs or if condition does not improve in 2-3 days

Dosage Forms

Gel, topical: 0.3% (30 g, 480 g)

Liquid, topical: 0.18% (60 mL); 0.2% (60 mL, 120 mL); 0.3% (60 mL, 120 mL, 240 mL)

Shampoo: 0.3% (60 mL, 118 mL); 0.33% (60 mL, 120 mL)

Selected Readings

"Drugs for Parasitic Infections," *Med Lett Drugs Ther*, 1993, 35(911):111-22.

Pyrimethamine (peer i meth' a meen)

Brand Names Daraprim®

Generic Available No

Use Prophylaxis of malaria due to susceptible strains of plasmodia; used in conjunction with quinine and sulfadiazine for the treatment of uncomplicated attacks of chloroquine-resistant *P. falciparum* malaria; used in conjunction with fast-acting schizonticide to initiate transmission control and suppression cure; synergistic combination with sulfadiazine in treatment of toxoplasmosis

Drug of Choice or Alternative For

Organism(s)

Toxoplasma gondii on page 217

Pregnancy Risk Factor C

Contraindications Megaloblastic anemia; known hypersensitivity to pyrimethamine, chloroguanide; resistant malaria

Warnings/Precautions When used for more than 3-4 days, it may be advisable to give leucovorin to prevent hematologic complications; monitor CBC and platelet counts every 2 weeks; use with caution in patients with impaired renal or hepatic function or with possible G-6-PD

(Continued)

Pyrimethamine *(Continued)*

Adverse Reactions

1% to 10%: Megaloblastic anemia, leukopenia, thrombocytopenia, agranulocytosis

<1%: Skin rash, insomnia, diarrhea, lightheadedness, dry mouth, fever, malaise, dermatitis, abnormal skin pigmentation, depression, seizures, pulmonary eosinophilia, atrophic glossitis

Toxicology Leucovorin should be administered in a dosage of 5-15 mg/day for 3 days or as required to reverse symptoms of folic acid deficiency; diazepam 0.1-0.25 mg/kg can be used to treat seizures

Drug Interactions

Decreased effect by acid, sulfonamides

Increased toxicity with methotrexate, co-trimoxazole

Stability Pyrimethamine tablets may be crushed to prepare oral suspensions of the drug in water, cherry syrup, or sucrose-containing solutions at a concentration of 1 mg/mL; stable at room temperature for 5-7 days

Mechanism of Action Inhibits parasitic dihydrofolate reductase, resulting in inhibition of tetrahydrofolic acid synthesis

Pharmacokinetics

Absorption: Oral: Well absorbed

Distribution: Widely distributed ; mainly concentrated in blood cells, kidneys, lungs, liver, and spleen; crosses into CSF; crosses placenta; appears in breast milk

Metabolism: Hepatic

Half-life: 80-95 hours

Time to peak serum concentration: Within 1.5-8 hours

Elimination: 20% to 30% excreted unchanged in urine

Usual Dosage Oral:

Malaria chemoprophylaxis:

Children: 0.5 mg/kg once weekly; not to exceed 25 mg/dose **or**

Children:

<4 years: 6.25 mg once weekly

4-10 years: 12.5 mg once weekly

Children >10 years and Adults: 25 mg once weekly

Dosage should begin 1 day before entering endemic area and be continued for all age groups for at least 6-10 weeks after leaving endemic areas

Chloroquine-resistant *P. falciparum* malaria (when used in conjunction with quinine and sulfadiazine): Oral:

Children 4-10 years: 25 mg/day once daily for 2 days

Children >10 years and Adults: 25 mg twice daily for 2 days

Toxoplasmosis (with sulfadiazine or trisulfapyrimidines):

Children: 1 mg/kg/day divided into 2 equal daily doses; decrease dose after 2-4 days by $^1/_2$, continue for about 1 month; used with 100 mg sulfadiazine/kg/day divided every 6 hours; **or** 2 mg/kg/day divided every 12 hours for 3 days followed by 1 mg/kg/day (maximum: 25 mg/day) once daily for 4 weeks

Adults: 50-75 mg/day together with 2-8 g of sulfadiazine for 1-3 weeks depending on patient's tolerance and response then reduce both drug dosages to $^1/_2$ and continue for additional 4-5 weeks; leucovorin should be given to prevent hematologic problems due to folic acid deficiency

In HIV, life-long suppression is necessary to prevent relapse; leucovorin (5-10 mg/day) is given concurrently

Overdosage Megaloblastic anemia, leukopenia, thrombocytopenia, anorexia, vomiting, CNS stimulation, seizures, nausea

Monitoring Parameters CBC, including platelet counts

Patient Information Take with meals to minimize vomiting; begin malaria prophylaxis at least 1 week prior to departure

Dosage Forms Tablet: 25 mg

Selected Readings

"Drugs for Parasitic Infections," *Med Lett Drugs Ther*, 1993, 35(911):111-22.

Porter SB and Sande MA, "Toxoplasmosis of the Central Nervous System in the Acquired Immunodeficiency Syndrome," *N Engl J Med*, 1992, 327(23):1643-8.

Pyrinyl II® [OTC] *see* Pyrethrins *on previous page*

Quinacrine Hydrochloride (kwin' a kreen)

Brand Names Atabrine®

Synonyms Mepacrine Hydrochloride

Generic Available No

Use Treatment of giardiasis and cestodiasis (tapeworm); reserve agent for suppression and chemoprophylaxis of malaria

Drug of Choice or Alternative For
Organism(s)
  Giardia lamblia on page 116

Pregnancy Risk Factor C

Contraindications Hypersensitivity to quinacrine or any component; patients receiving primaquine

Warnings/Precautions Use with caution in patients with hepatic disease, G-6-PD deficiency, history of psychosis, patients >60 years or <1 year of age; patients with psoriasis or porphyria; complete blood counts and periodic ophthalmic exams are necessary with prolonged therapy

Adverse Reactions
  >10%: Yellow discoloration of skin and urine
  1% to 10%: Diarrhea, anorexia, nausea, abdominal cramps, nervousness, vertigo, irritability, emotional change, nightmares
  <1%: Vomiting, convulsions, transient toxic psychosis, aplastic anemia, hepatitis, lichen planus-like eruptions, dermatitis, urticaria, black skin and nail pigmentation, blood dyscrasias, retinopathy, corneal deposits

Toxicology No specific therapy is indicated after GI decontamination; therapy is supportive in nature

Drug Interactions
  Increased concentration with primaquine
  Disulfiram-like reaction with alcohol

Mechanism of Action Binds to parasite's DNA by intercalation between adjacent base pairs inhibiting replication and protein synthesis

Pharmacokinetics
  Absorption: Oral: Well absorbed
  Distribution: Widely distributed; concentrates in liver, spleen, lungs, and adrenal glands; also deposited in skin, fingernails, and hair; CSF concentrations are 1% to 5% of corresponding plasma levels; lowest concentration in brain, heart, skeletal muscles, and breast milk; crosses the placenta and appears in breast milk
  Half-life: 120 hours
  Time to peak serum concentration: Within 1-3 hours
  Elimination: Slowly excreted principally in urine with secondary elimination in saliva, bile, sweat, and milk; 11% of dose excreted unchanged in urine

Usual Dosage Normally an enema is given before treatment to reduce amount of stool that requires examination after treatment. Oral:
  Children:
    Dwarf tapeworm:
      4-8 years: 200 mg stat, 100 mg before breakfast for 3 days
      8-10 years: 300 mg stat, 100 mg twice daily for 3 days
      11-14 years: 400 mg stat, 100 mg 3 times/day for 3 days
    Tapeworm (beef, pork, or fish):
      5-10 years: 100 mg every 10 minutes for 4 doses, give 300 mg sodium bicarbonate with each dose
      11-14 years: 200 mg every 10 minutes for 3 doses, give 300 mg sodium bicarbonate with each dose
    Giardiasis: 7 mg/kg/day in 3 divided doses for 5-7 days; maximum dose: 300 mg/day
    Malaria treatment:
      1-4 years: 100 mg 3 times/day for one day then 100 mg/day for 6 days
      4-8 years: 200 mg 3 times/day for one day then 100 mg 2 times/day for 6 days
      >8 years: 200 mg and 1 g sodium bicarbonate every 6 hours for 5 doses, then 100 mg 3 times/day for 6 days
    Malaria suppression: 50 mg/day for 1-3 months
  Adults:
    Dwarf tapeworm: 900 mg in 3 portions 20 minutes apart, then 100 mg 3 times/day for 3 days
    Tapeworm (beef, pork, or fish): 200 mg every 10 minutes for 4 doses with 600 mg sodium bicarbonate with each dose

(Continued)

Quinacrine Hydrochloride *(Continued)*

Giardiasis: 100 mg 3 times/day for 5-7 days
Malaria:
Treatment: 200 mg and 1 g sodium bicarbonate every 6 hours for 5 doses, then 100 mg 3 times/day for 6 days
Suppression: 100 mg/day, continue for 1-3 months; for endemic areas, drug therapy should be started 2 weeks before arrival and continued for 3-4 weeks after departure

Dosing adjustment in renal impairment: Dose should be reduced

Overdosage CNS excitation with restlessness, insomnia, psychic stimulation, seizures, nausea, vomiting, abdominal cramps, diarrhea, hypotension, cardiac arrhythmias or arrest

Monitoring Parameters CBC, periodic ophthalmologic examinations, liver function tests

Patient Information May discolor urine and skin; take after meals; report to physician any visual disturbances, skin rash, or mental aberrations during therapy

Nursing Implications For tapeworms use cathartic 1-2 hours after quinacrine administered in order to expel the worms for examination; collect and examine all stool for 48 hours after treatment for worm's attachment organ (stained yellow).

Dosage Forms Tablet: 100 mg

Selected Readings
"Drugs for Parasitic Infections," *Med Lett Drugs Ther*, 1993, 35(911):111-22.

Quinaglute® Dura-Tabs® *see* Quinidine *on this page*

Quinalan® *see* Quinidine *on this page*

Quin-Amino® *see* Quinine Sulfate *on page 658*

Quinaminoph® *see* Quinine Sulfate *on page 658*

Quinamm® *see* Quinine Sulfate *on page 658*

Quindan® *see* Quinine Sulfate *on page 658*

Quine® [OTC] *see* Quinine Sulfate *on page 658*

Quinidex® Extentabs® *see* Quinidine *on this page*

Quinidine *(kwin' i deen)*

Brand Names Cardioquin®; Quinaglute® Dura-Tabs®; Quinalan®; Quinidex® Extentabs®; Quinora®

Synonyms Quinidine Gluconate; Quinidine Polygalacturonate; Quinidine Sulfate
Generic Available Yes

Use Active against *Plasmodium falciparum* malaria (used as I.V.); prophylaxis after cardioversion of atrial fibrillation and/or flutter to maintain normal sinus rhythm; also used to prevent reoccurrence of paroxysmal supraventricular tachycardia, paroxysmal A-V junctional rhythm, paroxysmal ventricular tachycardia, paroxysmal atrial fibrillation, and atrial or ventricular premature contractions

Drug of Choice or Alternative For
Organism(s)
Plasmodium Species *on page 172*
Pregnancy Risk Factor C

Contraindications Patients with complete A-V block with an A-V junctional or idioventricular pacemaker; patients with intraventricular conduction defects (marked widening of QRS complex); patients with cardiac-glycoside induced A-V conduction disorders; hypersensitivity to the drug or cinchona derivatives

Warnings/Precautions Use with caution in patients with myocardial depression, sick sinus syndrome, incomplete A-V block, hepatic and/or renal insufficiency, myasthenia gravis; hemolysis may occur in patients with G-6-PD (glucose-6-phosphate dehydrogenase) deficiency; quinidine-induced hepatotoxicity, including granulomatous hepatitis can occur, increased serum AST and alkaline phosphatase concentrations, and jaundice may occur; use with caution in nursing women.

Adverse Reactions
>10%: Bitter taste, diarrhea, anorexia, nausea, vomiting, stomach cramping
1% to 10%: Skin rash, wheezing, blurred vision, lightheadedness, severe headache, tinnitus, hypotension, syncope

<1%: Anemia, tachycardia, thrombocytopenic purpura, heart block, ventricular fibrillation, vascular collapse, vertigo, confusion, delirium, fever, angioedema, blood dyscrasias, impaired hearing, respiratory depression

Toxicology Electrolyte balance should be monitored and treated, especially when refractory arrhythmias develop. Sodium bicarbonate 1-2 mEq/kg I.V. (or 0.5-1 mEq/kg in children) may decrease drug toxicity. Phenytoin or lidocaine are often effective at controlling drug-induced arrhythmias

Drug Interactions

Decreased serum concentrations with phenobarbital, phenytoin, and rifampin

Increased effect of nondepolarizing/depolarizing muscle relaxants and anticoagulants

Increased serum concentrations with verapamil, amiodarone, alkalinizing agents, and cimetidine

Increased plasma concentration of digoxin, closely monitor digoxin concentrations, digoxin dosage may need to be reduced (50%) when quinidine is initiated, new steady-state digoxin plasma concentrations occur in 5-7 days

Stability Do not use discolored parenteral solution

Mechanism of Action The drug probably interferes with *Plasmodium* DNA; depresses phase O of the action potential; decreases myocardial excitability and conduction velocity, and myocardial contractility by decreasing sodium influx during depolarization and potassium efflux in repolarization; also reduces calcium transport across cell membrane

Pharmacokinetics

Absorption: Well from GI tract

Distribution: All tissues except brain; concentrates in heart, liver, kidneys, and skeletal muscle; crosses the placenta and appears in breast milk

Metabolism: Extensively in the liver

Bioavailability: 80% (sulfate), 70% (gluconate)

Half-life:

Adults: 6-8 hours

Children: 2.5-6.7 hours

Increased half-life with elderly, cirrhosis, and congestive heart failure

Elimination: Excretion in urine (15% to 25% as unchanged drug)

Usual Dosage Malaria:

Continuous infusion (preferred): Children and Adults: Loading dose: 10 mg/kg (in 250 mL NS) over 1-2 hours; then 20 µg/kg/minute for 72 hours or until patient can take orally, or until parasitemia is <1%

or

Intermittent infusion: Adults: Loading dose: 24 mg/kg (in 250 mL NS) over 4 hours, then 12 mg/kg every 8 hours (over 4 hours) until patient can take orally

Oral: Therapy with quinine is preferred over quinidine

Overdosage Ataxia, lethargy, respiratory distress, apnea, severe hypotension, anuria, absence of P waves, broadening QRS complex, P-R and Q-T intervals, ventricular arrhythmias, hallucinations, and seizures

Monitoring Parameters Complete blood counts, liver and renal function tests, should be routinely performed during long-term administration; monitor EKG during I.V. infusion; decrease infusion rate if Q-T interval is >0.6 seconds, if QRS increases to >25% of baseline, or if significant hypotension is present

Reference Range Therapeutic: 2-5 µg/mL (SI: 6.2-15.4 µmol/L). Patient dependent therapeutic response occurs at levels of 3-6 µg/mL (SI: 9.2-18.5 µmol/L). Optimal therapeutic level is method dependent

Patient Information Patients should notify their physician if rash, fever, unusual bleeding or bruising, ringing in the ears, or visual disturbances occur. Complete blood counts, liver and renal function tests should be routinely performed during long-term administration. Do not crush sustained release products

Nursing Implications When injecting I.M., aspirate carefully to avoid injection into a vessel

Additional Information If serum concentration is >6 µg/mL, may reduce infusion rate

Dosage Forms

Injection, as gluconate (*GENERIC*): 80 mg/mL (10 mL)

Also comes in oral dosage forms for therapy of dysrhythmias

Selected Readings

Panisko DM and Keystone JS, "Treatment of Malaria – 1990," *Drugs*, 1990, 39(2):160-89.

Wyler DJ, "Malaria Chemoprophylaxis for the Traveler," *N Engl J Med*, 1993, 329(1):31-7.

Wyler DJ, "Malaria: Overview and Update," *Clin Infect Dis*, 1993, 16(4):449-56.

Quinidine Gluconate *see* Quinidine *on previous page*

Quinidine Polygalacturonate *see* Quinidine *on page 656*

Quinidine Sulfate *see* Quinidine *on page 656*

Quinine Sulfate (kwye' nine)

Brand Names Formula Q® [OTC]; Legatrin® [OTC]; M-KYA® [OTC]; Quin-Amino®; Quinaminoph®; Quinamm®; Quindan®; Quine® [OTC]; Quiphile®; Q-vel® [OTC]

Generic Available Yes

Use Suppression or treatment of chloroquine-resistant *P. falciparum* malaria; treatment of *Babesia microti* infection; prevention and treatment of nocturnal recumbency leg muscle cramps

Drug of Choice or Alternative For
Organism(s)
Babesia microti on page 57

Pregnancy Risk Factor X

Contraindications Tinnitus, optic neuritis, G-6-PD deficiency, hypersensitivity to quinine or any component, history of black water fever

Adverse Reactions
>10%: Nausea, vomiting, diarrhea, blurred vision, severe headache, tinnitus
<1%: Flushing of the skin, anginal symptoms, fever, rash, pruritus, hypoglycemia, epigastric pain, hemolysis, thrombocytopenia, hepatitis, night blindness, diplopia, optic atrophy, impaired hearing, hypersensitivity reactions

Toxicology Hypotension will respond to I.V. fluids and Trendelenburg position; if pressors are required, pure alpha agonists such as norepinephrine should be used; ventricular arrhythmias may respond to lidocaine; torsade de pointes may be reversed with magnesium administration

Drug Interactions
Decreased serum concentrations with phenobarbital, phenytoin, and rifampin
Increased effect of nondepolarizing/depolarizing muscle relaxants and coumarin anticoagulants
Increased serum concentrations with verapamil, amiodarone, alkalinizing agents, and cimetidine
Increased plasma concentration of digoxin, closely monitor digoxin concentrations, digoxin dosage may need to be reduced (by one-half) when quinine is initiated, new steady-state digoxin plasma concentrations occur in 5-7 days

Stability Protect from light

Mechanism of Action Intercalates into DNA, disrupting the parasite's replication and transcription; affects calcium distribution within muscle fibers and decreases the excitability of the motor end-plate region

Pharmacokinetics
Absorption: Oral: Readily absorbed, mainly from the upper small intestine
Distribution: All tissues except brain; concentrates in heart, liver, kidneys, and skeletal muscle
Metabolism: Primarily in the liver
Half-life:
Children: 6-12 hours
Adults: 8-14 hours
Time to peak serum concentration: Within 1-3 hours
Elimination: Excreted in bile and saliva with <5% excreted unchanged in urine

Usual Dosage Parenteral dosage form is no longer available in the US; if parenteral therapy is needed, see quinidine

Children: Chloroquine-resistant malaria and babesiosis: 25 mg/kg/day in divided doses every 8 hours for 7 days; maximum: 650 mg/dose

Adults:
Chloroquine-resistant malaria: 650 mg every 8 hours for 7 days in conjunction with another agent
Babesiosis: 650 mg every 6-8 hours for 7 days
Leg cramps: 200-300 mg at bedtime

Dosing adjustment in renal impairment:
Cl_{cr} 10-50 mL/minute: Administer every 8-12 hours or 75% of normal dose
Cl_{cr} <10 mL/minute: Administer every 24 hours or 30% to 50% of normal dose
Not effectively removed by peritoneal dialysis, removed by hemodialysis

Overdosage Cinchonism (tinnitus, headache, nausea, abdominal pain, visual disturbance) blood dyscrasias, photosensitivity, cardiac arrhythmias, hypotension, renal injury, hemolysis, hypoprothrombinemia

Reference Range Toxic: >10 μg/mL

Test Interactions False elevation of urinary steroids and catecholamines

Patient Information Avoid use of aluminum-containing antacids because of drug absorption problems; swallow dose whole to avoid bitter taste; report any unusual bleeding or bruising, may cause night blindness

Dosage Forms
Capsule: 64.8 mg, 65 mg, 200 mg, 300 mg, 325 mg
Tablet: 162.5 mg, 260 mg

Selected Readings
Panisko DM and Keystone JS, "Treatment of Malaria – 1990," *Drugs*, 1990, 39(2):160-89.
Wyler DJ, "Malaria Chemoprophylaxis for the Traveler," *N Engl J Med*, 1993, 329(1):31-7.
Wyler DJ, "Malaria: Overview and Update," *Clin Infect Dis*, 1993, 16(4):449-56.

Quinora® *see* Quinidine *on page 656*

Quinsana Plus® [OTC] *see* Tolnaftate *on page 687*

Quiphile® *see* Quinine Sulfate *on previous page*

Q-vel® [OTC] *see* Quinine Sulfate *on previous page*

Rabies Virus Vaccine

Related Information
Vaccines *on page 706-709*

Brand Names Imovax® Rabies I.D. Vaccine; Imovax® Rabies Vaccine

Synonyms HDCV; Human Diploid Cell Cultures Rabies Vaccine; Human Diploid Cell Cultures Rabies Vaccine (Intradermal use)

Generic Available No

Use Veterinarians, animal handlers, certain laboratory workers, and persons living in or visiting countries for longer than 1 month where rabies is a constant threat.

Complete pre-exposure prophylaxis does not eliminate the need for additional therapy with rabies vaccine after a rabies exposure. The Food and Drug Administration has not approved the I.D. use of rabies vaccine for postexposure prophylaxis. Recommendations for I.D. use of HDCV are currently being discussed. The decision for postexposure rabies vaccination depends on the species of biting animal, the circumstances of biting incident, and the type of exposure (bite, saliva contamination of wound, and so on). The type of and schedule for postexposure prophylaxis depends upon the person's previous rabies vaccination status or the result of a previous or current serologic test for rabies antibody. For postexposure prophylaxis, rabies vaccine should always be administered I.M., **not** I.D.

Pregnancy Risk Factor C

Contraindications Developing febrile illness (pre-exposure treatment only)

Adverse Reactions >10%: Swelling, erythema, itching, pain, local discomfort, nausea, headache, abdominal pain, muscle aches, dizziness, malaise, neuroparalytic reactions

Drug Interactions Decreased effect with immunosuppressive agents, corticosteroids, antimalarial drugs (ie, chloroquine); persons on these drugs should receive RIG (3 doses/1 mL each) by the I.M. route

Stability Refrigerate; reconstituted vaccine should be used immediately

Mechanism of Action Rabies vaccine is an inactivated virus vaccine which promotes immunity by inducing an active immune response. The production of specific antibodies requires about 7-10 days to develop. Rabies immune globulin or antirabies serum, equine (ARS) is given in conjunction with rabies vaccine to provide immune protection until an antibody response can occur.

Pharmacokinetics
Onset of effect: I.M.: Rabies antibody appears in the serum within 7-10 days
Peak effect: Within 30-60 days and persists for at least 1 year

Usual Dosage
Pre-exposure prophylaxis: Series of 3 doses given I.D. (0.1 mL dose) in deltoid area on days 0, 7, and 28; or series of 3 doses given I.M. (1 mL dose) in deltoid area on days 0, 7, and 21 (or 0, 7, and 28). If exposure continues, booster doses can be given every 2 years, or an antibody titer determined and a booster dose given if the titer is inadequate.

Postexposure prophylaxis: All postexposure treatment should begin with immediate cleansing of the wound with soap and water. Persons not previously immunized as above: Rabies immune globulin 20 units/kg body weight, ½ infiltrated at bite site if possible, remainder I.M.; and 5 doses of rabies vaccine, 1 mL I.M., one each on days 0, 3, 7, 14, 28.

(Continued)

Rabies Virus Vaccine (Continued)

Persons who have previously received postexposure prophylaxis with rabies vaccine, received a recommended I.M. or I.D. pre-exposure series of rabies vaccine, or have a previously documented rabies antibody titer considered adequate: 2 doses of rabies vaccine, 1 mL I.M., one each on days 0 and 3

Reference Range Antibody titers of ≥115 as determined by rapid fluorescent-focus inhibition test are indicative of adequate response

Nursing Implications Federal law requires that the date of administration, the vaccine manufacturer, lot number of vaccine, and the administering person's name, title and address be entered into the patient's permanent medical record

Dosage Forms Injection:
I.M. (HDCV): Rabies antigen 2.5 units/mL (1 mL)
Intradermal: Rabies antigen 0.25 units/mL (1 mL)

Recombivax HB® see Hepatitis B Vaccine on page 582

Reese's® Pinworm Medicine [OTC] see Pyrantel Pamoate on page 651

Retrovir® see Zidovudine on page 696

Ribavirin (rye ba vye' rin)

Brand Names Virazole®
Synonyms RTCA; Tribavirin
Generic Available No
Use Treatment of patients with respiratory syncytial virus (RSV) infections; may also be used in other viral infections including influenza A and B and adenovirus; specially indicated for treatment of severe lower respiratory tract RSV infections in patients with an underlying compromising condition (prematurity, bronchopulmonary dysplasia, congenital heart disease, immunodeficiency, and immunosuppression)
Drug of Choice or Alternative For
Organism(s)
Respiratory Syncytial Virus on page 181
Pregnancy Risk Factor X
Contraindications Females of childbearing age
Warnings/Precautions Use with caution in patients requiring assisted ventilation because precipitation of the drug in the respiratory equipment may interfere with safe and effective patient ventilation; also monitor carefully in patients with COPD and asthma for deterioration of respiratory function. Ribavirin is potentially mutagenic, tumor-promoting, and gonadotoxic; there is evidence that ribavirin is teratogenic in small animals. Health care workers who are pregnant or may become pregnant should be advised of the potential risks of exposure and counseled about risk reduction strategies including alternate job responsibilities; virus resistance does not appear to develop; incubation period for RSV is 4-8 days.
Adverse Reactions
1% to 10%: Fatigue, headache, insomnia, nausea, anorexia, anemia
<1%: Hypotension, cardiac arrest, digitalis toxicity, rash, skin irritation, conjunctivitis, mild bronchospasm, worsening of respiratory function, apnea, accumulation of fluid in ventilator tubing
Drug Interactions Decreased effect of zidovudine
Stability Do not use any water containing antimicrobial agent to reconstitute drug; reconstituted solution is stable for 24 hours at room temperature
Mechanism of Action Inhibits replication of RNA and DNA viruses; inhibits influenza virus RNA polymerase activity and inhibits the initiation and elongation of RNA fragments resulting in inhibition of viral protein synthesis
Pharmacokinetics
Absorption: Absorbed systemically from the respiratory tract following nasal and oral administration; absorption is dependent upon respiratory factors and method of drug delivery; maximal absorption occurs with the use of the aerosol generator via an endotracheal tube
Distribution: Highest concentrations are found in the respiratory tract and erythrocytes; crosses placenta and breast milk; does not cross blood-brain barrier
Metabolism: Occurs intracellularly and may be necessary for drug action; hepatic metabolism is the major route of elimination

Half-life: Plasma:
Children: 6.5-11 hours
Adults: 24 hours; half-life is much longer in the erythrocyte (16-40 days), which can be used as a marker for intracellular metabolism
Time to peak serum concentration: Inhalation: Within 60-90 minutes
Elimination: 40% cleared renally as unchanged drug and metabolites

Usual Dosage Infants, Children, and Adults: Aerosol inhalation:
Use with Viratek® small particle aerosol generator (SPAG-2) at a concentration of 20 mg/mL (6 g reconstituted with 300 mL of sterile water without preservatives)

Aerosol only: 12-18 hours/day for 3 days, up to 7 days in length

Monitoring Parameters Respiratory function

Nursing Implications Keep accurate I & O record, discard solutions placed in the SPAG-2 unit at least every 24 hours and before adding additional fluid

Dosage Forms Powder for aerosol: 6 g (100 mL)

Selected Readings
"Drugs for Non-HIV Viral Infections," *Med Lett Drugs Ther*, 1994, 36(919):27.
Keating MR, "Antiviral Agents," *Mayo Clin Proc*, 1992, 67(2):160-78.

RID® [OTC] *see* Pyrethrins *on page 653*

Rifabutin (rif a bu' tin)
Brand Names Mycobutin®
Synonyms Ansamycin
Generic Available No
Use Prevention of disseminated *Mycobacterium avium* complex (MAC) in patients with advanced HIV infection; also utilized in multiple drug regimens for treatment of MAC
Drug of Choice or Alternative For
Organism(s)
Mycobacterium avium-intracellulare on page 152
Pregnancy Risk Factor B
Contraindications Hypersensitivity to rifabutin or any other rifamycins; rifabutin is contraindicated in patients with a WBC <1000/mm³ or a platelet count <50,000/mm³
Warnings/Precautions Rifabutin as a single agent must not be administered to patients with active tuberculosis since its use may lead to the development of tuberculosis that is resistant to both rifabutin and rifampin; rifabutin should be discontinued in patients with AST >500 units/L or if total bilirubin is >3.0 mg/dL. Use with caution in patients with liver impairment; modification of dosage should be considered in patients with renal impairment.
Adverse Reactions
>10%: Discolored urine, neutropenia, leukopenia, rash
1% to 10%: Anemia, nausea, thrombocytopenia, vomiting, abdominal pain, headache, diarrhea, anorexia, myalgia, flatulence, eructation
<1%: Chest pain, fever, insomnia, dyspepsia, flatulence, nausea, vomiting, taste perversion
Toxicology Symptoms of overdose include nausea, vomiting, hepatotoxicity, lethargy, CNS depression; treatment is supportive; lavage with activated charcoal is preferred to ipecac as emesis is frequently present with overdose; hemodialysis will remove rifabutin, its effect on outcome is unknown
Drug Interactions Decreased plasma concentration (because of induced liver enzymes) of verapamil, methadone, digoxin, cyclosporine, corticosteroids, oral anticoagulants, theophylline, barbiturates, chloramphenicol, ketoconazole, oral contraceptives, quinidine, halothane
Mechanism of Action Inhibits DNA-dependent RNA polymerase at the beta subunit which prevents chain initiation
Pharmacokinetics
Absorption: Oral: ~53%
Distribution: To body tissues including the lungs, liver, spleen, eyes, and kidneys
Metabolism: To active and inactive metabolites
Half life, terminal: 45 hours (range: 16-69 hours)
Peak serum level: Within 2-4 hours
Elimination: Renal and biliary clearance of unchanged drugs is 10%; 30% excreted in feces; 53% in urine unchanged
(Continued)

Rifabutin *(Continued)*

Usual Dosage Oral:

Children: Efficacy and safety of rifabutin have not been established in children; a limited number of HIV-positive children with MAC (n=22) have been given rifabutin for MAC prophylaxis; doses of 5 mg/kg/day have been useful

Adults: 300 mg once daily; for patients who experience gastrointestinal upset, rifabutin can be administered 150 mg twice daily with food

Monitoring Parameters Periodic liver function tests, CBC with differential, platelet count, hemoglobin, hematocrit

Patient Information May discolor urine, tears, sweat, or other body fluids to a red-orange color; soft contact lenses may be permanently stained; report to physician any severe or persistent flu-like symptoms, nausea, vomiting, dark urine or pale stools, or unusual bleeding or bruising; can be taken with meals or sprinkled on applesauce

Additional Information Can be administered without regard to meals; rifabutin is insoluble in water and ethanol; prepare powder packets or compound with a suspending agent and shake well before using

Dosage Forms Capsule: 150 mg

Selected Readings

Agins BD, Berman DS, Spicehandler D, et al, "Effect of Combined Therapy with Ansamycin, Clofazimine, Ethambutol, and Isoniazid for *Mycobacterium avium* Infection in Patients With AIDS," *J Infect Dis*, 1989, 159(4):784-7.

"Drugs for AIDS and Associated Infections," *Med Lett Drugs Ther*, 1993, 35(904):79-86.

Hoy J, Mijch A, Sandland M, et al, "Quadruple-Drug Therapy for *Mycobacterium avium-intracellulare* Bacteremia in AIDS Patients," *J Infect Dis*, 1990, 161(4):801-5.

Nightingale SD, Cameron DW, Gordin FM, et al, "Two Controlled Trials of Rifabutin Prophylaxis Against *Mycobacterium avium* Complex Infection in AIDS," *N Engl J Med*, 1993, 329(12):828-33.

Rifadin® *see* Rifampin *on this page*

Rifampicin *see* Rifampin *on this page*

Rifampin (rif′ am pin)

Related Information

Antimicrobial Activity Against Selected Organisms *on page 757-764*

Brand Names Rifadin®; Rimactane®

Synonyms Rifampicin

Generic Available No

Use Management of active tuberculosis (in combination with other agents); eliminate meningococci from asymptomatic carriers; prophylaxis of *Haemophilus influenzae* type B infection; part of a regimen in the treatment of staphylococcal infections

Drug of Choice or Alternative For
Organism(s)

Brucella Species *on page 69*

Legionella pneumophila on page 139

Mycobacterium avium-intracellulare on page 152

Mycobacterium kansasii on page 153

Mycobacterium tuberculosis on page 155

Staphylococcus aureus, Methicillin-Resistant *on page 195*

Staphylococcus epidermidis, Methicillin-Resistant *on page 200*

Pregnancy Risk Factor C

Contraindications Hypersensitivity to rifampin or any component

Adverse Reactions

1% to 10%: Diarrhea, stomach cramps; discoloration of urine, feces, saliva, sputum, sweat, and tears (reddish orange); fungal overgrowth

<1%: Drowsiness, fatigue, ataxia, confusion, fever, headache, rash, pruritus, nausea, vomiting, stomatitis, eosinophilia, blood dyscrasias (leukopenia, thrombocytopenia), hepatitis, irritation at the I.V. site, renal failure, flu-like syndrome

Toxicology Treatment is supportive; lavage with activated charcoal is preferred to ipecac as emesis is frequently present with overdose; hemodialysis will remove rifampin, its effect on outcome is unknown

Drug Interactions Decreased plasma concentration (because of induced liver enzymes) of verapamil, methadone, digoxin, cyclosporine, corticosteroids, oral anticoagulants, theophylline, barbiturates, chloramphenicol, ketoconazole, oral contraceptives, quinidine, halothane

Stability Reconstituted I.V. solution is stable for 24 hours at room temperature; rifampin oral suspension can be compounded with simple syrup or wild cherry syrup at a concentration of 10 mg/mL; the suspension is stable for 4 weeks at room temperature or in a refrigerator when stored in a glass amber prescription bottle

Mechanism of Action Inhibits bacterial RNA synthesis by binding to the beta subunit of DNA-dependent RNA polymerase, blocking RNA transcription

Pharmacokinetics
Absorption: Oral: Well absorbed
Distribution: Well to most body tissues and fluids including CSF, where concentrations are increased if meninges are inflamed; concentrations in liver, gallbladder, bile, and urine are higher than those found in blood; crosses the blood-brain barrier well; highly lipophilic
Metabolism: In the liver; undergoes enterohepatic recycling
Half-life: 3-4 hours, prolonged with hepatic impairment
Time to peak serum concentration: Within 2-4 hours
Elimination: Undergoes enterohepatic recycling; principally excreted in feces (60% to 65%) and urine (~30%); plasma rifampin concentrations are not significantly affected by hemodialysis or peritoneal dialysis

Usual Dosage I.V. infusion dose is the same as for the oral route
Tuberculosis: Oral:
Children: 10-20 mg/kg/day in divided doses every 12-24 hours
Adults: 10 mg/kg/day; maximum: 600 mg/day

American Thoracic Society and CDC currently recommend twice weekly therapy as part of a short-course regimen which follows 1-2 months of daily treatment of uncomplicated pulmonary tuberculosis **in the compliant patient**
Children: 10-20 mg/kg/dose (up to 600 mg) twice weekly under supervision to ensure compliance
Adults: 10 mg/kg (up to 600 mg) twice weekly

H. influenza prophylaxis:
Infants and Children: 20 mg/kg/day every 24 hours for 4 days
Adults: 600 mg every 24 hours for 4 days

Meningococcal prophylaxis:
<1 month: 10 mg/kg/day in divided doses every 12 hours
Infants and Children: 20 mg/kg/day in divided doses every 12 hours for 2 days
Adults: 600 mg every 12 hours for 2 days

Nasal carriers of *Staphylococcus aureus*: Adults: 600 mg/day for 5-10 days in combination with other antibiotics

Synergy for *Staphylococcus aureus* infections: Oral, I.V.: Adults: 300-600 mg twice daily with other antibiotics

Dosing adjustment in hepatic impairment: Dose reductions may be necessary to reduce hepatotoxicity

Overdosage Nausea, vomiting, hepatotoxicity

Monitoring Parameters Periodic monitoring of liver function (AST, ALT), CBC

Test Interactions Increases bilirubin (S) in overdose; interferes with microbiologic assays for B_{12} and folate

Patient Information May discolor urine, tears, sweat, or other body fluids to a red-orange color; soft contact lenses may be permanently stained; report to physician any severe or persistent flu-like symptoms, nausea, vomiting, dark urine or pale stools, or unusual bleeding or bruising; take 1 hour before or 2 hours after a meal on an empty stomach

Dosage Forms
Capsule: 150 mg, 300 mg
Powder for injection: 600 mg

Selected Readings
Davidson PT and Le HQ, "Drug Treatment of Tuberculosis – 1992," *Drugs*, 1992, 43(5):651-73.
"Drugs for Tuberculosis," *Med Lett Drugs Ther*, 1993, 35(908):99-101.
Iseman MD, "Treatment of Multidrug-Resistant Tuberculosis," *N Engl J Med*, 1993, 329(11):784-91.
Van Scoy RE and Wilkowske CJ, "Antituberculosis Agents," *Mayo Clin Proc*, 1992, 67(2):179-87.

Rimactane® *see* Rifampin *on previous page*

Rimantadine Hydrochloride (ri man' to deen)

Brand Names Flumadine®

Generic Available No

Use Prophylaxis (adults and children) and treatment (adults) of influenza A viral infection

Pregnancy Risk Factor C

Contraindications Hypersensitivity to drugs of the adamantine class (rimantadine or amantadine)

Warnings/Precautions Use with caution in patients with liver disease, a history of recurrent and eczematoid dermatitis, uncontrolled psychosis or severe psychoneurosis, seizures in those receiving CNS stimulant drugs

Adverse Reactions 1% to 10%: Orthostatic hypotension, edema, dizziness, confusion, headache, insomnia, difficulty in concentrating, anxiety, restlessness, irritability, hallucinations, nausea, vomiting, dry mouth, urinary retention

Mechanism of Action Blocks the uncoating of influenza A virus preventing penetration of virus into host and inhibiting viral growth

Pharmacokinetics

Absorption: Oral: Well absorbed

Metabolism: In the liver (hydroxylation and conjugation)

Half-life: 13-65 kg: 25 hours

Elimination: 25% as unchanged drug

Usual Dosage Oral:

Prophylaxis:

Children <10 years: 5 mg/kg give once daily

Children >10 years and Adults: 100 mg twice/day

Treatment: Adults: 100 mg twice/day

Dosing interval in renal/hepatic impairment: Cl_{cr} <10 mL/minute: 100 mg every 24 hours

Elderly nursing home patients should receive 100 mg every 24 hours

Dosage Forms

Syrup: 50 mg/5 mL (60 mL, 240 mL, 480 mL)

Tablet: 100 mg

Selected Readings

Dolin R, Reichman RC, Madore HP, et al, "A Controlled Trial of Amantadine and Rimantadine in the Prophylaxis of Influenza A Infection," *N Engl J Med*, 1982, 307(10):580-4.

"Drugs for Non-HIV Viral Infections," *Med Lett Drugs Ther*, 1994, 36(919):27.

Keating MR, "Antiviral Agents," *Mayo Clin Proc*, 1992, 67(2):160-78.

rLFN-α2 *see* Interferon Alfa-2b *on page 590*

Robicillin® VK *see* Penicillin V Potassium *on page 638*

Robitet® *see* Tetracycline *on page 679*

Rocephin® *see* Ceftriaxone Sodium *on page 523*

Rondomycin® *see* Methacycline Hydrochloride *on page 607*

RTCA *see* Ribavirin *on page 660*

Rubella and Measles Vaccines, Combined *see* Measles and Rubella Vaccines, Combined *on page 602*

Rubella and Mumps Vaccines, Combined (rue bell' a)

Brand Names Biavax®₁₁

Generic Available No

Use Promote active immunity to rubella and mumps by inducing production of antibodies

Pregnancy Risk Factor X

Contraindications Known hypersensitivity to neomycin, eggs, children <1 year

Warnings/Precautions Women planning on becoming pregnant in the next 3 months should not be vaccinated

Adverse Reactions All serious adverse reactions must be reported to the FDA.

1% to 10%: Febrile seizures, fever, soreness, burning, stinging, allergic reactions

Drug Interactions Immune globulin, whole blood

Stability Refrigerate, discard unused portion within 8 hours, protect from light

Mechanism of Action Promotes active immunity by inducing specific antibodies to rubella and mumps viruses.

Usual Dosage Children >12 months and Adults: 1 vial in outer aspect of the upper arm

Test Interactions Temporary suppression of TB skin test

Nursing Implications Children immunized before 12 months of age should be reimmunized

Additional Information Federal law requires that the date of administration, the vaccine manufacturer, lot number of vaccine, and the administering person's name, title and address be entered into the patient's permanent medical record

Dosage Forms Injection (mixture of 2 viruses):
1. Wistar RA 27/3 strain of rubella virus
2. Jeryl Lynn (B level) mumps strain grown cell cultures of chick embryo

Rubella, Measles and Mumps Vaccines, Combined *see* Measles, Mumps, and Rubella Vaccines, Combined *on page 603*

Rubella Virus Vaccine, Live (rue bell' a)

Brand Names Meruvax® II

Synonyms German Measles Vaccine

Generic Available No

Use All adults, both male and female, lacking documentation of live vaccine on or after first birthday, or laboratory evidence of immunity (particularly women of childbearing age and young adults who work in or congregate in hospitals, colleges, and on military bases) should be vaccinated. Susceptible travelers should be vaccinated.

Women who are pregnant when vaccinated or who become pregnant within 3 months of vaccination should be counseled on the theoretical risks to the fetus. The risk of rubella-associated malformations in these women is so small as to be negligible. MMR is the vaccine of choice if recipients are likely to be susceptible to measles or mumps as well as to rubella.

Pregnancy Risk Factor X

Warnings/Precautions Pregnancy, immunocompromised persons, history of anaphylactic reaction following receipt of neomycin

Adverse Reactions All serious adverse reactions must be reported to the FDA.
>10%: Arthralgias, local tenderness and erythema, urticaria, rash
1% to 10%: Malaise, fever, headache, sore throat, lymphadenopathy
<1%: Hypersensitivity, allergic reactions to the vaccine, optic neuritis

Drug Interactions Decreased effect when immune globulin is given within 3 months and with concurrent use of corticosteroids and other immunosuppressant agents

Stability Refrigerate, discard reconstituted vaccine after 8 hours

Mechanism of Action Promotes active immunity by inducing rubella hemagglutination-inhibiting antibodies

Usual Dosage One dose S.C., no booster

Test Interactions May depress tuberculin skin test sensitivity

Patient Information Patient may experience burning or stinging at the injection site; joint pain usually occurs 1-10 weeks after vaccination and persists 1-3 days

Nursing Implications Reconstituted vaccine should be used within 8 hours; S.C. injection only

Additional Information Federal law requires that the date of administration, the vaccine manufacturer, lot number of vaccine, and the administering person's name, title and address be entered into the patient's permanent record

Dosage Forms Injection, single dose: 1000 $TCID_{50}$ (Wistar RA 27/3 Strain)

Rubeola vaccine *see* Measles Virus Vaccine, Live *on page 604*

Sabin Vaccine *see* Poliovirus Vaccine, Live, Trivalent, Oral *on page 646*

Salk Vaccine *see* Poliovirus Vaccine, Inactivated *on page 645*

Sandoglobulin® *see* Immune Globulin *on page 588*

Scabene® *see* Lindane *on page 599*

Sebaquin® [OTC] *see* Iodoquinol *on page 591*

Selenium Sulfide (se lee' nee um)

Brand Names Exsel®; Selsun®; Selsun Blue® [OTC]

Generic Available Yes

Use Treatment of itching and flaking of the scalp associated with dandruff, to control scalp seborrheic dermatitis; treatment of tinea versicolor

(Continued)

Selenium Sulfide *(Continued)*

Pregnancy Risk Factor C

Contraindications Known hypersensitivity to selenium or any component

Warnings/Precautions Do not use on damaged skin to avoid any systemic toxicity; avoid topical use in very young children; safety of topical in infants has not been established

Adverse Reactions

>10%: Unusual dryness or oiliness of scalp

1% to 10%: Perspiration, tremors, lethargy, hair loss or discoloration, vomiting following long-term use on damaged skin, abdominal pain, garlic breath, local irritation

Toxicology Nausea, vomiting, diarrhea

Mechanism of Action May block the enzymes involved in growth of epithelial tissue

Pharmacokinetics

Absorption: Topical: Not absorbed through intact skin, but can be absorbed through damaged skin

Elimination: Urine, feces, lungs, skin

Usual Dosage Topical:

Dandruff, seborrhea: Massage 5-10 mL into wet scalp, leave on scalp 2-3 minutes, rinse thoroughly, and repeat application; shampoo twice weekly for 2 weeks initially, then use once every 1-4 weeks as indicated depending upon control

Tinea versicolor: Apply the 2.5% lotion to affected area and lather with small amounts of water; leave on skin for 10 minutes, then rinse thoroughly; apply every day for 7 days

Patient Information Topical formulations are for external use only; notify physician if condition persists or worsens; avoid contact with eyes; thoroughly rinse after application

Dosage Forms Lotion, shampoo; 1% (120 mL, 210 mL, 240 mL, 330 mL); 2.5% (120 mL)

Selsun® *see* Selenium Sulfide *on previous page*

Selsun Blue® [OTC] *see* Selenium Sulfide *on previous page*

Septra® *see* Co-trimoxazole *on page 545*

Septra® DS *see* Co-trimoxazole *on page 545*

Seromycin® Pulvules® *see* Cycloserine *on page 548*

Silver Nitrate

Brand Names Dey-Drop® Ophthalmic Solution

Synonyms AgNO$_3$

Generic Available Yes

Use Prevention of gonococcal ophthalmia neonatorum; cauterization of wounds and sluggish ulcers, removal of granulation tissue and warts; aseptic prophylaxis of burns

Pregnancy Risk Factor C

Contraindications Not for use on broken skin or cuts; hypersensitivity to silver nitrate or any component

Warnings/Precautions Do not use applicator sticks on the eyes; repeated applications of the ophthalmic solution into the eye can cause cauterization of the cornea and blindness

Adverse Reactions

>10%: Chemical conjunctivitis, burning and skin irritation,

1% to 10%: Staining of the skin, methemoglobinemia, cauterization of the cornea, blindness

Toxicology Symptoms of overdose include pain and burning of mouth, salivation, vomiting, diarrhea, shock, coma, convulsions, death; blackening of skin and mucous membranes; absorbed nitrate can cause methemoglobinemia. Fatal dose is as low as 2 g; administer sodium chloride in water (10 g/L) to cause precipitation of silver

Drug Interactions Decreased effect: Sulfacetamide preparations are incompatible

Stability Must be stored in a dry place; exposure to light causes silver to oxidize and turn brown, dipping in water causes oxidized film to readily dissolve

Mechanism of Action Free silver ions precipitate bacterial proteins by combining with chloride in tissue forming silver chloride; coagulates cellular protein to form an eschar; silver ions or salts or colloidal silver preparations can inhibit the growth of both gram-positive and gram-negative bacteria. This germicidal action is attributed to the precipitation of bacterial proteins by liberated silver ions. Silver nitrate coagulates cellular protein to form an eschar, and this mode of action is the postulated mechanism for control of benign hematuria, rhinitis, and recurrent pneumothorax.

Pharmacokinetics

Absorption: Because silver ions readily combine with protein, there is minimal GI and cutaneous absorption of the 0.5% and 1% preparations

Elimination: Although the highest amounts of silver noted on autopsy have been in the kidneys, excretion in urine is minimal

Usual Dosage

Neonates: Ophthalmic: Instill 2 drops immediately after birth (no later than 1 hour after delivery) into conjunctival sac of each eye as a single dose, allow to sit for ≥30 seconds; do not irrigate eyes following instillation of eye drops

Children and Adults:

Ointment: Apply in an apertured pad on affected area or lesion for approximately 5 days

Sticks: Apply to mucous membranes and other moist skin surfaces only on area to be treated 2-3 times/week for 2-3 weeks

Topical solution: Apply a cotton applicator dipped in solution on the affected area 2-3 times/week for 2-3 weeks

Monitoring Parameters With prolonged use, monitor methemoglobin levels

Patient Information Discontinue topical preparation if redness or irritation develop

Nursing Implications Silver nitrate solutions stain skin and utensils

Additional Information Applicators are **not** for ophthalmic use

Dosage Forms

Applicator sticks: 75% with potassium nitrate 25% (6")

Ointment: 10% (30 g)

Solution:

Ophthalmic: 1% (wax ampuls)

Topical: 10% (30 mL); 25% (30 mL); 50% (30 mL)

Selected Readings

US Department of Health and Human Services, "1993 Sexually Transmitted Diseases Treatment Guidelines," *MMWR Morb Mortal Wkly Rep*, 1993, 42(RR-14).

Smallpox Vaccine

Use There are no indications for the use of smallpox vaccine in the general civilian population. Laboratory workers involved with Orthopoxvirus or in the production and testing of smallpox vaccines should receive regular smallpox vaccinations. For advice on vaccine administration and contraindications, contact the Division of Immunization, CDC, Atlanta, GA 30333 (404-639-3356).

Pregnancy Risk Factor X

SMX-TMP *see* Co-trimoxazole *on page 545*

Sodium Methicillin *see* Methicillin Sodium *on page 608*

Sodium Nafcillin *see* Nafcillin Sodium *on page 616*

Sodium P.A.S. *see* Aminosalicylate Sodium *on page 489*

Spectam® Injection *see* Spectinomycin Hydrochloride *on this page*

Spectazole™ Topical *see* Econazole Nitrate *on page 559*

Spectinomycin Hydrochloride (spek ti noe mye' sin)

Brand Names Spectam® Injection; Trobicin® Injection

Generic Available No

Use Treatment of uncomplicated gonorrhea

Drug of Choice or Alternative For Organism(s)

Neisseria gonorrhoeae on page 161

Pregnancy Risk Factor B

Contraindications Hypersensitivity to spectinomycin or any component

Adverse Reactions <1%: Dizziness, headache, urticaria, rash, pruritus, nausea, vomiting, pain at injection site, chills

Stability Use reconstituted solutions within 24 hours; reconstitute with supplied diluent only

(Continued)

Spectinomycin Hydrochloride *(Continued)*

Mechanism of Action A bacteriostatic antibiotic that selectively binds to the 30s subunits of ribosomes and thereby inhibiting bacterial protein synthesis

Pharmacokinetics

Absorption: I.M.: Rapid and almost completely

Distribution: Concentrates in urine; does not distribute well into the saliva

Half-life: 1.7 hours

Time to peak serum concentration: I.M.: Within 60 minutes

Elimination: Excreted almost entirely as unchanged drug in urine (70% to 100%)

Usual Dosage I.M.:

Children:

<45 kg: 40 mg/kg/dose 1 time

≥45 kg: See adult dose

Children >8 years who are allergic to PCNS/cephalosporins may be treated with oral tetracycline

Adults:

Uncomplicated urethral endocervical or rectal gonorrhea: 2 g deep I.M. or 4 g where antibiotic resistance is prevalent 1 time; 4 g (10 mL) dose should be given as two 5 mL injections, followed by doxycycline 100 mg twice daily for 7 days

Disseminated gonococcal infection: 2 g every 12 hours

50% removed by hemodialysis

Overdosage Paresthesia, dizziness, blurring of vision, ototoxicity, renal damage, nausea, sleeplessness, decrease in hemoglobin

Nursing Implications For I.M. use only

Additional Information Ineffective against syphilis

Dosage Forms Powder for injection: 2 g, 4 g

Selected Readings

US Department of Health and Human Services, "1993 Sexually Transmitted Diseases Treatment Guidelines," *MMWR Morb Mortal Wkly Rep*, 1993, 42(RR-14).

Spectro-Chlor® *see* Chloramphenicol *on page 531*

Sporanox® *see* Itraconazole *on page 594*

SSKI® *see* Potassium Iodide *on page 648*

Staphcillin® *see* Methicillin Sodium *on page 608*

Stavudine

Brand Names Zerit®

Synonyms d4T

Use For the treatment of adults with advanced HIV infection who are intolerant to approved therapies with proven clinical benefit or who have experienced significant clinical or immunologic deterioration while receiving these therapies, or for whom such therapies are contraindicated

Pregnancy Risk Factor C

Contraindications Hypersensitivity to stavudine

Warnings/Precautions Use with caution in patients who demonstrate previous hypersensitivity to zidovudine, didanosine, zalcitamine, pre-existing bone marrow suppression, or renal insufficiency, peripheral neuropathy, folic acid or vitamin B_{12} deficiency. Peripheral neuropathy may be the dose limiting side effect.

Adverse Reactions

>10%: peripheral neuropathy

1% to 10%: Headache, chills/fever, abdominal or back pain, malaise, asthenia, nausea, vomiting, diarrhea, myalgia, insomnia, anxiety, depression, pancreatitis

Mechanism of Action Inhibits reverse transcriptase of the human immunodeficiency virus (HIV)

Pharmacokinetics

Distribution: V_d: 0.5 L/kg

Peak serum level: 1 hour after administration

Bioavailability: 82%

Half-life: 1-1.6 hours

Elimination: Renal (40%)

Usual Dosage Adults: Oral:

≥60 kg: 40 mg every 12 hours

<60 kg: 30 mg every 12 hours
Dose may be cut in half if symptoms of peripheral neuropathy occur.

Dosing adjustment in renal impairment:
Cl_{cr} >50 mL/minute: ≥60 kg: 40 mg every 12 hours
Cl_{cr} >50 mL/minute: <60 kg: 30 mg every 12 hours
Cl_{cr} 26-50 mL/minute: ≥60 kg: 20 mg every 12 hours
Cl_{cr} 26-50 mL/minute: <60 kg: 15 mg every 12 hours
Cl_{cr} 10-25 mL/minute: ≥60 kg: 20 mg every 24 hours
Cl_{cr} 10-25 mL/minute: <60 kg: 15 mg every 24 hours

Monitoring Parameters Monitor liver function tests and signs and symptoms of peripheral neuropathy.

Patient Information Contact physician at first signs or symptoms of peripheral neuropathy

Dosage Forms Capsule: 15 mg, 20 mg, 30 mg, 40 mg

Streptomycin Sulfate (strep toe mye' sin)
Related Information
Antimicrobial Activity Against Selected Organisms *on page 757-764*
Generic Available Yes
Use Part of combination therapy of active tuberculosis; used in combination with other agents for treatment of streptococcal or enterococcal endocarditis, mycobacterial infections, plague, tularemia, and brucellosis
Drug of Choice or Alternative For
Organism(s)
Enterococcus Species *on page 107*
Mycobacterium tuberculosis on page 155
Yersinia pestis on page 233
Pregnancy Risk Factor D
Contraindications Hypersensitivity to streptomycin or any component
Warnings/Precautions Use with caution in patients with pre-existing vertigo, tinnitus, hearing loss, neuromuscular disorders, or renal impairment; modify dosage in patients with renal impairment; aminoglycosides are associated with significant nephrotoxicity or ototoxicity; the ototoxicity is directly proportional to the amount of drug given and the duration of treatment; tinnitus or vertigo are indications of vestibular injury and impending bilateral irreversible damage; renal damage is usually reversible
Adverse Reactions
1% to 10%: Nephrotoxicity, neurotoxicity, ototoxicity (auditory), ototoxicity (vestibular)
<1%: Skin rash, drug fever, headache, paresthesia, tremor, nausea, vomiting, eosinophilia, arthralgia, anemia, hypotension, difficulty in breathing, drowsiness, weakness
Toxicology The treatment of choice following a single acute overdose appears to be the maintenance of good urine output of at least 3 mL/kg/hour. Dialysis is of questionable value in the enhancement of aminoglycoside elimination. If required, hemodialysis is preferred over peritoneal dialysis in patients with normal renal function. Careful hydration may be all that is required to promote diuresis and therefore the enhancement of the drug's elimination.
Drug Interactions
Increased/prolonged effect: Depolarizing and nondepolarizing neuromuscular blocking agents
Increased toxicity: Concurrent use of amphotericin may increase nephrotoxicity
Stability Depending upon manufacturer, reconstituted solution remains stable for 2-4 weeks when refrigerated; exposure to light causes darkening of solution without apparent loss of potency
Mechanism of Action Inhibits bacterial protein synthesis by binding directly to the 30S ribosomal subunits causing faulty peptide sequence to form in the protein chain
Pharmacokinetics
Absorption: I.M.: Absorbed well
Distribution: To extracellular fluid including serum, abscesses, ascitic, pericardial, pleural, synovial, lymphatic, and peritoneal fluids; crosses the placenta; small amounts appear in breast milk
Half-life:
Newborns: 4-10 hours
(Continued)

Streptomycin Sulfate *(Continued)*

Adults: 2-4.7 hours and is prolonged with renal impairment

Time to peak serum concentration: I.M.: Within 1 hour

Elimination: Almost completely (90%) excreted as unchanged drug in urine, with small amounts (1%) excreted in bile, saliva, sweat, and tears

Usual Dosage I.M.:

Infants: 20-30 mg/kg/day in divided doses every 12 hours

Children: Tuberculosis: 20-40 mg/kg/day in divided doses every 12-24 hours, not to exceed 2 g/day; usually discontinued after 2-3 months of therapy or sooner

Adults:

Tuberculosis: 15 mg/kg/day in divided doses every 12 hours, not to exceed 2 g/day

Enterococcal endocarditis: 1 g every 12 hours for 2 weeks, 500 mg every 12 hours for 4 weeks in combination with penicillin

Streptococcal endocarditis: 1 g every 12 hours for 1 week, 500 mg every 12 hours for 1 week

Tularemia: 1-2 g/day in divided doses for 7-10 days or until patient is afebrile for 5-7 days

Plague: 2-4 g/day in divided doses until the patient is afebrile for at least 3 days

Dosing adjustment in renal impairment:

Cl_{cr} 10-50 mL/minute: Administer every 24-72 hours

Cl_{cr} <10 mL/minute: Administer every 72-96 hours

Overdosage Ototoxicity, nephrotoxicity, and neuromuscular toxicity

Monitoring Parameters Hearing (audiogram), BUN, creatinine; serum concentration of the drug should be monitored in all patients; eighth cranial nerve damage is usually preceded by high-pitched tinnitus, roaring noises, sense of fullness in ears, or impaired hearing and may persist for weeks after drug is discontinued

Reference Range Therapeutic: Peak: 20-30 μg/mL; Trough: <5 μg/mL; Toxic: Peak: >50 μg/mL; Trough: >10 μg/mL

Test Interactions False-positive urine glucose with Benedict's solution or Clinitest®; penicillin may decrease aminoglycoside serum concentrations *in vitro*

Patient Information Report any unusual symptom of hearing loss, dizziness, roaring noises, or fullness in ears

Nursing Implications Inject deep I.M. into large muscle mass

Additional Information Due to the critical supply of streptomycin, the drug is being released on a per patient basis at no cost; patient specific information will be required to obtain the drug from Pfizer Inc. For more information, call 1-800-254-4445.

Dosage Forms Injection: 1 g vials

Selected Readings

Cunha BA, "Aminoglycosides: Current Role in Antimicrobial Therapy," *Pharmacotherapy*, 1988, 8(6):334-50.

Davidson PT and Le HQ, "Drug Treatment of Tuberculosis – 1992," *Drugs*, 1992, 43(5):651-73.

"Drugs for Tuberculosis," *Med Lett Drugs Ther*, 1993, 35(908):99-101.

Edson RS and Terrell CL, "The Aminoglycosides," *Mayo Clin Proc*, 1991, 66(11):1158-64.

Iseman MD, "Treatment of Multidrug-Resistant Tuberculosis," *N Engl J Med*, 1993, 329(11):784-91.

Van Scoy RE and Wilkowske CJ, "Antituberculosis Agents," *Mayo Clin Proc*, 1992, 67(2):179-87.

Strong Iodine Solution *see* Potassium Iodide *on page 648*

Sulbactam and Ampicillin *see* Ampicillin Sodium and Sulbactam Sodium *on page 497*

Sulconazole Nitrate *(sul kon' a zole)*

Brand Names Exelderm®; Sulcosyn®

Generic Available No

Use Treatment of superficial fungal infections of the skin, including tinea cruris, tinea corporis, tinea versicolor and possibly tinea pedis

Pregnancy Risk Factor C

Contraindications Known hypersensitivity to sulconazole

Adverse Reactions 1% to 10%: Itching, burning, stinging, redness

Mechanism of Action Sulconazole is a substituted imidazole derivative similar in structure to other antifungal agents such as miconazole and econazole. The exact mechanism of sulconazole's antifungal effects is not known; however, the primary site of action appears to be at the fungal cell membrane. Imidazole antifungal agents inhibit metabolic reactions necessary for the synthesis of ergosterol, an essential membrane component. The end result is usually fungistatic; however, sulconazole may act as a fungicide in *Candida albicans* and parapsilosis during certain growth phases.

Pharmacokinetics
Absorption: Topical: ~8.7% absorbed percutaneously
Elimination: Most excreted in urine

Usual Dosage Topical: Apply once or twice daily for 4-6 weeks

Patient Information For external use only; avoid contact with eyes, if burning or irritation develop, notify physician

Dosage Forms
Cream: 1% (15 g, 30 g, 60 g)
Solution, topical: 1% (30 mL)

Sulcosyn® *see* Sulconazole Nitrate *on previous page*

Sulfabenzamide, Sulfacetamide, and Sulfathiazole
(sul fa benz' a mide, sul fa see' ta mide, and sul fa thye' a zole)
Brand Names Gyne-Sulf®; Sultrin™; Trysul®; Vagilia®; V.V.S.®
Synonyms Triple Sulfa
Generic Available Yes
Use Treatment of *Gardnerella vaginalis* vaginitis, although other agents are preferred
Pregnancy Risk Factor C
Contraindications Hypersensitivity to sulfabenzamide, sulfacetamide, sulfathiazole or any component
Warnings/Precautions If local irritation develops, discontinue therapy
Adverse Reactions
>10%: Local irritation, pruritus, urticaria
<1%: Allergic reactions, Stevens-Johnson syndrome
Mechanism of Action Interferes with microbial folic acid synthesis and growth via inhibition of para-aminobenzoic acid metabolism
Pharmacokinetics
Absorption: From the vagina is variable and unreliable
Metabolism: Primarily by acetylation
Elimination: Excreted by glomerular filtration into urine
Usual Dosage Adults:
Cream: Insert one applicatorful in vagina twice daily for 4-6 days; dosage may then be decreased to $\frac{1}{2}$ to $\frac{1}{4}$ of an applicatorful twice daily
Tablet: Insert one intravaginally twice daily for 10 days
Patient Information Complete full course of therapy; notify physician if burning, irritation, or signs of a systemic allergic reaction occur
Dosage Forms
Cream, vaginal: Sulfabenzamide 3.7%, sulfacetamide 2.86%, and sulfathiazole 3.42% (78 g with applicator, 90 g, 120 g)
Tablet, vaginal: Sulfabenzamide 184 mg, sulfacetamide 143.75 mg, and sulfathiazole 172.5 mg (20 tablets/box with vaginal applicator)

Sulfadiazine (sul fa dye' a zeen)
Brand Names Microsulfon®
Generic Available Yes
Use Treatment of urinary tract infections and nocardiosis, rheumatic fever prophylaxis; part of combination regimen in the treatment of toxoplasmosis; uncomplicated attack of malaria
Drug of Choice or Alternative For Organism(s)
Nocardia Species *on page 164*
Toxoplasma gondii on page 217
Pregnancy Risk Factor B (D at term)
Contraindications Porphyria, hypersensitivity to any sulfa drug or any component, children <2 months of age unless indicated for the treatment of congenital toxoplasmosis
Warnings/Precautions Use with caution in patients with impaired hepatic function or impaired renal function, G-6-PD deficiency; fluid intake should be
(Continued)
671

Sulfadiazine *(Continued)*

maintained ≥1500 mL/day, or give sodium bicarbonate to keep urine alkaline; more likely to cause crystalluria because it is less soluble than other sulfonamides

Adverse Reactions

>10%: Fever, itching, skin rash, photosensitivity, dizziness, headache, anorexia, nausea, vomiting, diarrhea

1% to 10%: Granulocytopenia, leukopenia, thrombocytopenia, aplastic anemia, hemolytic anemia, hepatitis, Lyell's syndrome, Stevens-Johnson syndrome

<1%: Crystalluria, hematuria, thyroid function disturbance, interstitial nephritis, serum sickness-like reactions, jaundice, acute nephropathy

Toxicology Doses of as little as 2-5 g/day may produce toxicity; the aniline radical is responsible for hematologic toxicity; high volume diuresis may aid in elimination and prevention of renal failure

Drug Interactions Decreased effect with PABA or PABA metabolites of drugs (ie, procaine, proparacaine, tetracaine); decreased effect of oral anticoagulants and oral hypoglycemic agents

Stability Tablets may be crushed to prepare oral suspension of the drug in water or with a sucrose-containing solution; aqueous suspension with concentrations of 100 mg/mL should be stored in the refrigerator and used within 7 days

Mechanism of Action Interferes with bacterial growth by inhibiting bacterial folic acid synthesis through competitive antagonism of PABA

Pharmacokinetics

Absorption: Oral: Well absorbed

Distribution: Throughout body tissues and fluids including pleural, peritoneal, synovial, and ocular fluids; distributed throughout total body water; readily diffused into CSF; appears in breast milk

Metabolism: By N-acetylation

Half-life: 10 hours

Time to peak serum concentration: Within 3-6 hours

Elimination: Excreted in urine as metabolites (15% to 40%) and as unchanged drug (43% to 60%)

Usual Dosage Oral:

Congenital toxoplasmosis:

Newborns and Children <2 months: 100 mg/kg/day divided every 6 hours in conjunction with pyrimethamine 1 mg/kg/day once daily and supplemental folinic acid 5 mg every 3 days for 6 months

Children >2 months: 25-50 mg/kg/dose 4 times/day

Toxoplasmosis:

Children: 120-150 mg/kg/day, maximum dose: 6 g/day; divided every 6 hours in conjunction with pyrimethamine 2 mg/kg/day divided every 12 hours for 3 days followed by 1 mg/kg/day once daily (maximum: 25 mg/day) with supplemental folinic acid

Adults: 2-8 g/day divided every 6 hours in conjunction with pyrimethamine and with supplemental folinic acid

Overdosage Drowsiness, dizziness, anorexia, abdominal pain, nausea, vomiting, hemolytic anemia, acidosis, jaundice

Monitoring Parameters CBC, renal function tests, urinalysis

Patient Information Drink plenty of fluids; avoid prolonged exposure to sunlight or wear protective clothing and sunscreen; notify physician if rash, difficulty breathing, severe or persistent fever, or sore throat occurs

Nursing Implications Maintain adequate hydration and monitor urine output

Additional Information Due to critical supplies, sulfadiazine is being released on a per patient basis at no cost from the Centers for Disease Control; for more information call (404) 488-4928

Dosage Forms Tablet: 500 mg

Selected Readings

Porter SB and Sande MA, "Toxoplasmosis of the Central Nervous System in the Acquired Immunodeficiency Syndrome," *N Engl J Med*, 1992, 327(23):1643-8.

Sulfadiazine, Sulfamethazine, and Sulfamerazine

(sul fa dye' a zeen, sul fa meth' a zeen, and sul fa mer' a zeen)

Synonyms Multiple Sulfonamides; Trisulfapyrimidines

Generic Available No

Use Treatment of toxoplasmosis and other susceptible organisms, however, other agents are preferred

Pregnancy Risk Factor B (D at term)

Contraindications Porphyria, known hypersensitivity to any sulfa drug or any component

Mechanism of Action Interferes with microbial folic acid synthesis and growth via inhibition of para-aminobenzoic acid metabolism

Pharmacokinetics
Metabolism: By acetylation
Elimination: Excreted in urine via glomerular filtration

Usual Dosage Adults: Oral: 2-4 g to start, then 2-4 g/day in 3-6 divided doses

Test Interactions Increases cholesterol (S), protein, uric acid (S)

Patient Information Drink plenty of fluids

Dosage Forms Tablet: Sulfadiazine 167 mg, sulfamethazine 167 mg, and sulfamerazine 167 mg

Sulfadoxine and Pyrimethamine

(sul fa dox' een and peer i meth' a meen)

Brand Names Fansidar®

Generic Available No

Use Treatment of *Plasmodium falciparum* malaria in patients in whom chloroquine resistance is suspected; malaria prophylaxis for travelers to areas where chloroquine-resistant malaria is endemic

Drug of Choice or Alternative For
Organism(s)
Plasmodium Species *on page 172*

Pregnancy Risk Factor C

Contraindications Known hypersensitivity to any sulfa drug, pyrimethamine, or any component; porphyria, megaloblastic anemia, severe renal insufficiency; children <2 months of age due to competition with bilirubin for protein binding sites

Warnings/Precautions Use with caution in patients with renal or hepatic impairment, patients with possible folate deficiency, and patients with seizure disorders, increased adverse reactions are seen in patients also receiving chloroquine; fatalities associated with sulfonamides, although rare, have occurred due to severe reactions including Stevens-Johnson syndrome, toxic epidermal necrolysis, hepatic necrosis, agranulocytosis, aplastic anemia and other blood dyscrasias; discontinue use at first sign of rash or any sign of adverse reaction; hemolysis occurs in patients with G-6-PD deficiency; leucovorin should be administered to reverse signs and symptoms of folic acid deficiency

Adverse Reactions
>10%: Megaloblastic anemia, leukopenia, thrombocytopenia, pancytopenia, photosensitivity, hypersensitivity, atrophic glossitis, ataxia, tremors, seizures, headache, vomiting, gastritis
1% to 10%: Stevens-Johnson syndrome, hepatitis
<1%: Crystalluria, thyroid dysfunction, erythema multiforme, toxic epidermal necrolysis, rash, anorexia, glossitis, hepatic necrosis, respiratory failure

Toxicology Leucovorin should be administered in a dosage of 3-9 mg/day for 3 days or as required to reverse symptoms of folic acid deficiency; doses of as little as 2-5 g/day may produce toxicity; the aniline radical is responsible for hematologic toxicity; high volume diuresis may aid in elimination and prevention of renal failure; diazepam can be used to control seizures

Drug Interactions
Decreased effect with PABA or PABA metabolites of local anesthetics
Increased toxicity with methotrexate, other sulfonamides, co-trimoxazole

Mechanism of Action Sulfadoxine interferes with bacterial folic acid synthesis and growth via competitive inhibition of para-aminiobenzoic acid; pyrimethamine inhibits microbial dihydrofolate reductase, resulting in inhibition of tetrahydrofolic acid synthesis

Pharmacokinetics
Absorption: Oral: Well absorbed
Distribution:
Pyrimethamine: Widely distributed; mainly concentrated in blood cells, kidneys, lungs, liver, and spleen
Sulfadoxine: Well distributed like other sulfonamides
Metabolism:
Pyrimethamine: Hepatic
Sulfadoxine: None

(Continued)

673

Sulfadoxine and Pyrimethamine *(Continued)*

Half-life:
Pyrimethamine: 80-95 hours
Sulfadoxine: 5-8 days

Time to peak serum concentration: Within 2-8 hours

Elimination: Excreted in urine as parent compounds and several unidentified metabolites

Usual Dosage Children and Adults: Oral:

Treatment of acute attack of malaria: A single dose of the following number of Fansidar™ tablets is used in sequence with quinine or alone:

2-11 months: $^1/_4$ tablet
1-3 years: $^1/_2$ tablet
4-8 years: 1 tablet
9-14 years: 2 tablets
>14 years: 2-3 tablets

Malaria prophylaxis:

The first dose of Fansidar® should be taken 1-2 days before departure to an endemic area (CDC recommends that therapy be initiated 1-2 weeks before such travel), administration should be continued during the stay and for 4-6 weeks after return. Dose = pyrimethamine 0.5 mg/kg/dose and sulfadoxine 10 mg/kg/dose up to a maximum of 25 mg pyrimethamine and 500 mg sulfadoxine/dose weekly.

2-11 months: $^1/_8$ tablet weekly **or** $^1/_4$ tablet once every 2 weeks
1-3 years: $^1/_4$ tablet once weekly **or** $^1/_2$ tablet once every 2 weeks
4-8 years: $^1/_2$ tablet once weekly **or** 1 tablet once every 2 weeks
9-14 years: $^3/_4$ tablet once weekly **or** $1^1/_2$ tablets once every 2 weeks
>14 years: 1 tablet once weekly **or** 2 tablets once every 2 weeks

Overdosage Anorexia, vomiting, CNS stimulation including seizures, megaloblastic anemia, leukopenia, thrombocytopenia, crystalluria

Monitoring Parameters CBC, including platelet counts, and urinalysis should be performed periodically

Patient Information Begin prophylaxis at least 2 days before departure; drink plenty of fluids; avoid prolonged exposure to the sun; notify physician if rash, sore throat, pallor, or glossitis occurs

Dosage Forms Tablet: Sulfadoxine 500 mg and pyrimethamine 25 mg

Selected Readings
Panisko DM and Keystone JS, "Treatment of Malaria – 1990," *Drugs*, 1990, 39(2):160-89.
Wyler DJ, "Malaria Chemoprophylaxis for the Traveler," *N Engl J Med*, 1993, 329(1):31-7.
Wyler DJ, "Malaria: Overview and Update," *Clin Infect Dis*, 1993, 16(4):449-56.

Sulfamethoprim® *see* Co-trimoxazole *on page 545*

Sulfamethoxazole (sul fa meth ox' a zole)

Brand Names Gantanol®; Urobak®

Generic Available Yes: Tablet

Use Treatment of urinary tract infections, nocardiosis, toxoplasmosis, acute otitis media, and acute exacerbations of chronic bronchitis due to susceptible organisms

Pregnancy Risk Factor B (D at term)

Contraindications Porphyria, hypersensitivity to any sulfa drug or any component, pregnancy at term, children <2 months of age unless indicated for the treatment of congenital toxoplasmosis, sunscreens containing PABA

Warnings/Precautions Maintain adequate fluid intake to prevent crystalluria; use with caution in patients with renal or hepatic impairment, and patients with G-6-PD deficiency; should not be used for group A beta-hemolytic streptococcal infections

Adverse Reactions

>10%: Fever, itching, skin rash, photosensitivity, dizziness, headache, anorexia, nausea, vomiting, diarrhea

1% to 10%: Granulocytopenia, leukopenia, thrombocytopenia, aplastic anemia, hemolytic anemia, hepatitis, Lyell's syndrome, Stevens-Johnson syndrome

<1%: Crystalluria, hematuria, thyroid function disturbance, interstitial nephritis, serum sickness-like reactions, jaundice, acute nephropathy

Toxicology Symptoms of overdose include drowsiness, dizziness, anorexia, abdominal pain, nausea, vomiting, hemolytic anemia, acidosis, jaundice, fever, agranulocytosis; doses of as little as 2-5 g/day may produce toxicity; the aniline radical is responsible for hematologic toxicity; high volume diuresis may aid in elimination and prevention of renal failure

Drug Interactions
Decreased effect with PABA or PABA metabolites of drugs (ie, procaine, proparacaine, tetracaine)
Increased effect of oral anticoagulants and oral sulfonylureas

Stability Protect from light

Mechanism of Action Interferes with bacterial growth by inhibiting bacterial folic acid synthesis through competitive antagonism of PABA

Pharmacokinetics
Absorption: Oral: 90%
Distribution: Crosses the placenta; readily enters the CSF
Metabolism: Primarily in the liver, with 10% to 20% as the N-acetylated form in the plasma
Half-life: 9-12 hours, prolonged with renal impairment
Time to peak serum concentration: Within 3-4 hours
Elimination: Unchanged drug (20%) and its metabolites are excreted in urine

Usual Dosage Oral:
Children >2 months: 50-60 mg/kg/day divided every 12 hours; maximum: 3 g/24 hours or 75 mg/kg/day
Adults: 2 g stat, 1 g 2-3 times/day; maximum: 3 g/24 hours

Dosing adjustment/interval in renal impairment:
Cl_{cr} 10-50 mL/minute: Administer every 18 hours
Cl_{cr} <10 mL/minute: Administer every 24 hours
Moderately dialyzable (20% to 50%)

Test Interactions Decreased effect with PABA or PABA metabolites of drugs (ie, procaine, proparacaine, tetracaine)

Patient Information Drink plenty of fluids; avoid prolonged exposure to sunlight or wear protective clothing and sunscreen; notify physician if rash, difficulty breathing, severe or persistent fever, or sore throat occurs

Nursing Implications Maintain adequate hydration and monitor urine output; give around-the-clock to promote less variation in peak and trough serum levels

Dosage Forms
Suspension, oral (cherry flavor): 500 mg/5 mL (480 mL)
Tablet: 500 mg

Sulfamethoxazole and Trimethoprim *see* Co-trimoxazole *on page 545*

Sulfatrim® *see* Co-trimoxazole *on page 545*

Sulfatrim® DS *see* Co-trimoxazole *on page 545*

Sulfisoxazole (sul fi sox' a zole)

Brand Names Gantrisin®
Synonyms Sulfisoxazole Acetyl; Sulphafurazole
Generic Available Yes
Use Treatment of urinary tract infections, otitis media, *Chlamydia*; nocardiosis
Drug of Choice or Alternative For
Organism(s)
Nocardia Species *on page 164*
Pregnancy Risk Factor B (D at term)
Contraindications Hypersensitivity to any sulfa drug or any component, porphyria, pregnancy at term, infants <2 months of age (sulfas compete with bilirubin for protein binding sites), patients with urinary obstruction, sunscreens containing PABA
Warnings/Precautions Use with caution in patients with G-6-PD deficiency (hemolysis may occur), hepatic or renal impairment; dosage modification required in patients with renal impairment; risk of crystalluria should be considered in patients with impaired renal function
Adverse Reactions
>10%: Fever, itching, skin rash, photosensitivity, dizziness, headache, anorexia, nausea, vomiting, diarrhea
1% to 10%: Granulocytopenia, leukopenia, thrombocytopenia, aplastic anemia, hemolytic anemia, hepatitis, Lyell's syndrome, Stevens-Johnson syndrome
<1%: Crystalluria, hematuria, thyroid function disturbance, interstitial nephritis, serum sickness-like reactions, jaundice, acute nephropathy

(Continued)

Sulfisoxazole *(Continued)*

Toxicology Symptoms of overdose include drowsiness, dizziness, anorexia, abdominal pain, nausea, vomiting, hemolytic anemia, acidosis, jaundice, fever, agranulocytosis; doses of as little as 2-5 g/day may produce toxicity; the aniline radical is responsible for hematologic toxicity; high volume diuresis may aid in elimination and prevention of renal failure

Drug Interactions
Decreased effect with PABA or PABA metabolites of drugs (ie, procaine, proparacaine, tetracaine)
Increased effect of oral anticoagulants and oral sulfonylureas

Stability Protect from light

Mechanism of Action Interferes with bacterial growth by inhibiting bacterial folic acid synthesis through competitive antagonism of PABA

Pharmacokinetics
Absorption: Sulfisoxazole acetyl is hydrolyzed in the GI tract to sulfisoxazole which is readily absorbed
Distribution: Crosses the placenta; excreted into breast milk
Metabolized: In the liver by acetylation and glucuronide conjugation to inactive compounds
Half-life: 4-7 hours, prolonged with renal impairment
Time to peak serum concentration: Within 2-3 hours
Elimination: Primarily excreted in urine (95% within 24 hours), 40% to 60% as unchanged drug

Usual Dosage Not for use in patients <2 months of age
Children >2 months: Oral: 75 mg/kg stat, 120-150 mg/kg/day in divided doses every 4-6 hours; not to exceed 6 g/day

Adults: Oral: 2-4 g stat, 4-8 g/day in divided doses every 4-6 hours

Dosing interval in renal impairment:
Cl_{cr} 10-50 mL/minutes: Administer every 8-12 hours
Cl_{cr} <10 mL/minute: Administer every 12-24 hours
>50% removed by hemodialysis

Children and Adults: Ophthalmic:
Solution: Instill 1-2 drops to affected eye every 2-3 hours
Ointment: Apply small amount to affected eye 1-3 times/day and at bedtime

Monitoring Parameters CBC, urinalysis, renal function tests

Test Interactions False-positive protein in urine; false-positive urine glucose with Clinitest®

Patient Information Take with a glass of water on an empty stomach; avoid prolonged exposure to sunlight; report to physician any sore throat, mouth sores, rash, unusual bleeding, or fever

Nursing Implications Maintain adequate fluid intake

Additional Information
Sulfisoxazole: Gantrisin® tablet
Sulfisoxazole acetyl: Gantrisin® pediatric syrup/suspension

Dosage Forms
Ointment, ophthalmic, as diolamine: 4% [40 mg/mL] (3.75 g)
Solution, ophthalmic, as diolamine: 4% [40 mg/mL] (15 mL)
Suspension, oral, pediatric, as acetyl (raspberry flavor): 500 mg/5 mL (480 mL)
Syrup, as acetyl (chocolate flavor): 500 mg/5 mL (480 mL)
Tablet: 500 mg

Sulfisoxazole Acetyl *see* Sulfisoxazole *on previous page*

Sulfisoxazole and Erythromycin *see* Erythromycin and Sulfisoxazole *on page 563*

Sulfoxaprim® *see* Co-trimoxazole *on page 545*

Sulfoxaprim® DS *see* Co-trimoxazole *on page 545*

Sulphafurazole *see* Sulfisoxazole *on previous page*

Sultrin™ *see* Sulfabenzamide, Sulfacetamide, and Sulfathiazole *on page 671*

Sumycin® *see* Tetracycline *on page 679*

Suprax® *see* Cefixime *on page 512*

Symadine® *see* Amantadine Hydrochloride *on page 486*

Symmetrel® *see* Amantadine Hydrochloride *on page 486*

Tao® *see* Troleandomycin *on page 690*

Tazicef® *see* Ceftazidime *on page 520*

Tazidime® *see* Ceftazidime *on page 520*

TCN *see* Tetracycline *on page 679*

Tegopen® *see* Cloxacillin Sodium *on page 543*

Teline® *see* Tetracycline *on page 679*

Terramycin® I.M. Injection *see* Oxytetracycline Hydrochloride *on page 629*

Terramycin® Oral *see* Oxytetracycline Hydrochloride *on page 629*

Tetanus and Diphtheria Toxoid *see* Diphtheria and Tetanus Toxoid *on page 554*

Tetanus Immune Globulin, Human

Brand Names Hyper-Tet®
Synonyms TIG
Generic Available No
Use Passive immunization against tetanus; tetanus immune globulin is preferred over tetanus antitoxin for treatment of active tetanus; part of the management of an unclean, nonminor wound in a person whose history of previous receipt of tetanus toxoid is unknown or who has received less than three doses of tetanus toxoid
Drug of Choice or Alternative For Organism(s)
   Clostridium tetani on page 88
Pregnancy Risk Factor C
Contraindications Hypersensitivity to tetanus immune globulin or any component; I.V. administration
Warnings/Precautions Have epinephrine 1:1000 available for anaphylactic reactions
Adverse Reactions
   >10%: Pain, tenderness, erythema at injection site
   1% to 10%: Fever (mild), hives, angioedema, muscle stiffness, anaphylaxis reaction
   <1%: Sensitization to repeated injections
Drug Interactions Never administer tetanus toxoid and TIG in same syringe (toxoid will be neutralized)
Stability Refrigerate
Mechanism of Action Tetanus immune globulin (TIG) must not contain <50 units/mL. Protein makes up 10% to 18% of TIG preparations. The great majority of this (≥90%) is IgG. TIG has almost no color or odor and it is a sterile, nonpyrogenic, concentrated preparation of immunoglobulins that has been derived from the plasma of adults hyperimmunized with tetanus toxoid. The pooled material from which the immunoglobulin is derived may be from fewer than 1000 donors. This plasma has been shown to be free of hepatitis B surface antigen.
Pharmacokinetics Absorption: Well absorbed
Usual Dosage I.M.:
   Prophylaxis of tetanus:
      Children: 4 units/kg; some recommend administering 250 units to small children
      Adults: 250 units

   Treatment of tetanus:
      Children: 500-3000 units; some should infiltrate locally around the wound
      Adults: 3000-6000 units
Nursing Implications Do not administer I.V.; I.M. use only
Dosage Forms Injection: 250 units/mL

Tetanus Toxoid, Adsorbed

Generic Available No
Use Active immunity against tetanus
Pregnancy Risk Factor C
Contraindications Hypersensitivity to tetanus toxoid or any component; neurological signs or symptoms after prior administration
   (Continued)

677

Tetanus Toxoid, Adsorbed *(Continued)*

Warnings/Precautions Not equivalent to tetanus toxoid fluid; the tetanus toxoid adsorbed is the preferred toxoid for immunization; avoid injection into a blood vessel; have epinephrine (1:100) available

Adverse Reactions All serious adverse reactions must be reported to the FDA.
>10%: Induration/redness at injection site
1% to 10%: Allergic reaction, chills, fever, sterile abscess at injection site
<1%: Fever >103°F, blistering at injection site, malaise, neurological disturbances, Arthus-type hypersensitivity reactions

Drug Interactions If primary immunization is started in individuals receiving an immunosuppressive agent or corticosteroids, serologic testing may be needed to ensure adequate antibody response

Stability Refrigerate, do not freeze

Mechanism of Action Tetanus toxoid preparations contain the toxin produced by virulent tetanus bacilli (detoxified growth products of *Clostridium tetani*). The toxin has been modified by treatment with formaldehyde so that is has lost toxicity but still retains ability to act as antigen and produce active immunity.

Pharmacokinetics Duration of immunization following primary immunization: ~12 years

Usual Dosage Adults: I.M.:
Primary immunization: 0.5 mL; repeat 0.5 mL at 4-8 weeks after first dose and at 6-12 months after second dose
Routine booster doses are recommended only every 5-10 years
Routine wound management: See table.

Tetanus Prophylaxis in Wound Management

Number of Prior Tetanus Toxoid Doses	Clean, Minor Wounds		All Other Wounds	
	Td*	TIG†	Td*	TIG†
Unknown or fewer than 3	Yes	No	Yes	Yes
3 or more‡	No#	No	No¶	No

Adapted from Report of the Committee on Infectious Diseases, American Academy of Pediatrics, Elk Grove Village, IL: © American Academy of Pediatrics, 1986.
*Adult tetanus and diphtheria toxoids; use pediatric preparations (DT or DTP) if the patient is less than 7 years old.
†Tetanus immune globulin.
‡If only three doses of fluid tetanus toxoid have been received, a fourth dose of toxoid, preferably an adsorbed toxoid, should be given.
#Yes, if more than 10 years since last dose.
¶Yes, if more than 5 years since last dose.

Patient Information A nodule may be palpable at the injection site for a few weeks

Nursing Implications Inject intramuscularly in the area of the vastus lateralis (midthigh laterally) or deltoid

Additional Information Tetanus is a rare disease in U.S. with <100 cases annually; 66% of cases occur in persons >50 years of age; protective tetanus and diphtheria antibodies decline with age; it is estimated that <50% of elderly are protected.

Elderly are at risk because:
Many lack proper immunization maintenance
Higher case fatality ratio
Immunizations are not available from childhood
Indications for vaccination:
Primary series with combined tetanus-diphtheria (Td) should be given to all elderly lacking a clean history of vaccination
Boosters should be given at 10-year intervals; earlier for wounds
Elderly are more likely to require tetanus immune globulin with infection of tetanus due to lower antibody titer

Dosage Forms Injection, adsorbed:
Tetanus 5 Lf units per 0.5 mL dose (0.5 mL, 5 mL)
Tetanus 10 Lf units per 2.5 mL dose (5 mL)

Tetanus Toxoid, Fluid

Synonyms Tetanus Toxoid Plain

Generic Available No

Use Active immunization against tetanus in adults and children

Pregnancy Risk Factor C

Contraindications Prior hypersensitivity reactions, neurological signs or symptoms after prior administrations

Warnings/Precautions For primary immunization, tetanus toxoid, adsorbed is preferred; in concomitant administration of immunosuppressive therapy, allergic reactions may occur; epinephrine 1:1000 must be available; use in pediatrics should be deferred until >1 year of age when a history of a CNS disorder is present

Adverse Reactions

>10%: Induration/redness at injection site

1% to 10%: Allergic reaction, chills, fever, sterile abscess at injection site

<1%: Fever >103°F, blistering at injection site, malaise, neurological disturbances, Arthus-type hypersensitivity reactions

Drug Interactions If primary immunization is started in individuals receiving an immunosuppressive agent or corticosteroids, serologic testing may be needed to ensure adequate antibody response

Stability Refrigerate

Mechanism of Action Tetanus toxoid preparations contain the toxin produced by virulent tetanus bacilli (detoxified growth products of *Clostridium tetani*). The toxin has been modified by treatment with formaldehyde so that is has lost toxicity but still retains ability to act as antigen and produce active immunity.

Pharmacokinetics Duration of immunization following primary immunization: ~12 years

Usual Dosage Adults:

Primary immunization: Inject 3 doses of 0.5 mL I.M. or S.C. at 4- to 8-week intervals with fourth dose given only 6-12 months after third dose

Booster doses: I.M., S.C.: 0.5 mL every 10 years

Anergy testing: Intradermal: 0.1 mL

Patient Information A nodule may be palpable at the injection site for a few weeks

Nursing Implications Must not be used I.V.

Additional Information Tetanus is a rare disease in U.S. with <100 cases annually; 66% of cases occur in persons >50 years of age; protective tetanus and diphtheria antibodies decline with age; it is estimated that <50% of elderly are protected

Elderly are at risk because:

Many lack proper immunization maintenance

Higher case fatality ratio

Immunizations are not available from childhood

Indications for vaccination:

Primary series with combined tetanus-diphtheria (Td) should be given to all elderly lacking a clean history of vaccination

Boosters should be given at 10-year intervals; earlier for wounds

Elderly are more likely to require tetanus immune globulin with infection of tetanus due to lower antibody titer

Dosage Forms Injection, fluid:

Tetanus 4 Lf units per 0.5 mL dose (7.5 mL)

Tetanus 5 Lf units per 0.5 mL dose (0.5 mL, 7.5 mL)

Tetanus Toxoid Plain *see* Tetanus Toxoid, Fluid *on this page*

Tetracycline (tet ra sye' kleen)

Brand Names Achromycin®; Achromycin® V; Nor-tet®; Panmycin®; Robitet®; Sumycin®; Teline®; Tetracyn®; Tetralan®; Topicycline®

Synonyms TCN; Tetracycline Hydrochloride

Generic Available Yes

Use Treatment of susceptible bacterial infections of both gram-positive and gram-negative organisms; also *Mycoplasma*, *Chlamydia*, and *Rickettsia*; may also be used for acne, exacerbations of chronic bronchitis, and treatment of gonorrhea and syphilis in patients that are allergic to penicillin

Drug of Choice or Alternative For

Disease/Syndrome(s)

Urethritis, Nongonococcal *on page 44*

Organism(s)

Bacillus anthracis on page 58

Bordetella pertussis on page 65
Calymmatobacterium granulomatis on page 71
Chlamydia pneumoniae on page 76
Chlamydia trachomatis on page 79
Coxiella burnetii on page 93
Ehrlichia Species *on page 101*
Helicobacter pylori on page 121
Leptospira interrogans on page 140
Mycoplasma pneumoniae on page 159
Rickettsia rickettsii on page 183
Ureaplasma urealyticum on page 225
Vibrio cholerae on page 230
Yersinia pestis on page 233

Pregnancy Risk Factor D; B (topical)

Contraindications Hypersensitivity to tetracycline or any component; do not administer to children ≤ 8 years of age

Warnings/Precautions Use of tetracyclines during tooth development may cause permanent discoloration of the teeth and enamel, hypoplasia and retardation of skeletal development and bone growth; use with caution in patients with renal or hepatic impairment and in pregnancy; pseudomotor cerebri has been reported with tetracycline use

Adverse Reactions
> 10%: Discoloration of teeth and enamel hypoplasia (infants)

1% to 10%: Nausea, diarrhea, photosensitivity

< 1%: Increased intracranial pressure, bulging fontanels in infants, paresthesia, dermatologic effects, diabetes insipidus syndrome, vomiting, esophagitis, anorexia, abdominal cramps, acute renal failure, azotemia, superinfections, pericarditis, anaphylaxis, pruritus, pigmentation of nails, exfoliative dermatitis, thrombophlebitis, pseudotumor cerebri, antibiotic-associated pseudomembranous colitis, staphylococcal enterocolitis, hepatotoxicity, renal damage, hypersensitivity reactions, candidal superinfection

Toxicology Treatment is supportive only

Drug Interactions
Decreased effect with antacids (aluminum, calcium, zinc, or magnesium), bismuth salts, sodium bicarbonate, barbiturates, carbamazepine, hydantoins; decreased effect of oral contraceptives
Increased effect of warfarin

Stability Outdated tetracyclines have caused a Fanconi-like syndrome

Mechanism of Action Inhibits bacterial protein synthesis by binding with the 30S and possibly the 50S ribosomal subunit(s) of susceptible bacteria; may also cause alterations in the cytoplasmic membrane; usually bacteriostatic, may be bactericidal

Pharmacokinetics
Absorption: Oral: 75%

Distribution: Readily to most body fluids including bile, sinus secretions, and synovial, pleural, ascitic, and gingival crevicular fluids; tends to localize in bone, liver, spleen, tumors, and teeth; crosses placenta and is excreted in breast milk; small amount appears in the bile

Half-life, normal renal function: 6-11 hours

Time to peak serum concentration: Within 2-4 hours

Elimination: Primary route of elimination is the kidney, with 60% of dose excreted as unchanged drug in urine

Usual Dosage
Children >8 years:
Oral: 25-50 mg/kg/day in divided doses every 6 hours; not to exceed 3 g/day
Ophthalmic:
Suspension: Instill 1-2 drops 2-4 times/day or more often as needed
Ointment: Instill every 2-12 hours

Adults:
Oral: 250-500 mg/dose every 6 hours
Ophthalmic:
Suspension: Instill 1-2 drops 2-4 times/day or more often as needed
Ointment: Instill every 2-12 hours
Topical: Apply to affected areas 1-4 times/day

Dosing adjustment in renal impairment:
Cl$_{cr}$ 50-80 mL/minute: Administer every 8-12 hours
Cl$_{cr}$ 10-50 mL/minute: Administer every 12-24 hours

Cl$_{cr}$ <10 mL/minute: Administer every 24 hours
Slightly dialyzable (5% to 20%)

Dosing adjustment in hepatic impairment: Avoid use or maximum dose is 1 g/day

Overdosage Photosensitivity, nausea, anorexia, diarrhea

Monitoring Parameters Renal, hepatic and hematologic function test

Test Interactions False-negative urine glucose with Clinistix®

Patient Information Take 1 hour before or 2 hours after meals with adequate amounts of fluid; avoid prolonged exposure to sunlight or sunlamps; avoid taking antacids, iron, or dairy products before tetracyclines

Additional Information Use of tetracycline in animal feed has caused emergence of resistant organisms

Tetracycline: Achromycin® V oral suspension, Sumycin® syrup, Tetralan® syrup

Tetracycline hydrochloride: Achromycin® injection, Achromycin® V capsule, Nor-tet® capsule, Panmycin® capsule, Robitet® capsule, Sumycin® capsule and tablet, Teline® capsule, Tetracyn® capsule, Tetralan® capsule

Dosage Forms
Capsule: 100 mg, 250 mg, 500 mg
Ointment:
  Ophthalmic: 1% [10 mg/mL] (3.5 g)
  Topical: 3% [30 mg/mL] (14.2 g, 30 g)
Solution, topical: 2.2 mg/mL (70 mL)
Suspension:
  Ophthalmic: 1% [10 mg/mL] (0.5 mL, 1 mL, 4 mL)
  Oral: 125 mg/5 mL (60 mL, 480 mL)
Tablet: 250 mg, 500 mg

Selected Readings
Smilack JD, Wilson WR, and Cockerill FR 3d, "Tetracyclines, Chloramphenicol, Erythromycin, Clindamycin, and Metronidazole," Mayo Clin Proc, 1991, 66(12):1270-80.

Tetracycline Hydrochloride see Tetracycline on page 679

Tetracyn® see Tetracycline on page 679

Tetralan® see Tetracycline on page 679

Tetramune® see Diphtheria, Tetanus Toxoids, and Whole-cell Pertussis Vaccine and Hemophilus b Conjugate Vaccine on page 556

TheraCys® see Bacillus Calmette-Guérin (BCG) Live on page 502

Thiabendazole (thye a ben' da zole)

Brand Names Mintezol®

Synonyms Tiabendazole

Generic Available No

Use Treatment of strongyloidiasis, cutaneous larva migrans, visceral larva migrans, dracunculiasis, trichinosis, and mixed helminthic infections

Drug of Choice or Alternative For
Organism(s)
Ancylostoma duodenale on page 54
Strongyloides stercoralis on page 215
Trichinella spiralis on page 222

Pregnancy Risk Factor C

Contraindications Known hypersensitivity to thiabendazole

Adverse Reactions
>10%: Numbness, seizures, anorexia, diarrhea, nausea, vomiting, hallucinations, delirium, dizziness, drowsiness, headache, tinnitus, drying of mucous membranes

1% to 10%: Skin rash, Stevens-Johnson syndrome

<1%: Leukopenia, hepatotoxicity, lymphadenopathy, nephrotoxicity, malodor of urine, hypersensitivity reactions, chills, blurred or yellow vision

Toxicology Supportive care only following GI decontamination

Drug Interactions Increased levels of theophylline and other xanthines

Mechanism of Action Inhibits helminth-specific mitochondrial fumarate reductase

Pharmacokinetics
Absorption: Rapid and well from GI tract
Metabolism: Rapid
Half-life: 1.2 hours
Time to peak serum concentration: Within 1-2 hours

(Continued)

Thiabendazole *(Continued)*

Elimination: Excreted in feces (5%) and urine (87%), primarily as conjugated metabolites

Usual Dosage Purgation is not required prior to use; drinking of fruit juice aids in expulsion of worms by removing the mucous the intestinal tapeworms attach themselves.

Children and Adults: Oral: 50 mg/kg/day divided every 12 hours; maximum dose: 3 g/day
Strongyloidiasis: For 2 consecutive days
Cutaneous larva migrans: For 2-5 consecutive days
Visceral larva migrans: For 5-7 consecutive days
Trichinosis: For 2-4 consecutive days
Dracunculosis: 50-75 mg/kg/day divided every 12 hours for 3 days
Dosing comments in renal/hepatic impairment: Use with caution

Overdosage Altered mental status, visual problems

Patient Information Take after meals, chew tablet well; may decrease alertness, avoid driving or operating machinery; drinking of fruit juice aids in expulsion of worms by removing the mucous to which the intestinal tapeworms attach themselves

Dosage Forms
Suspension, oral: 500 mg/5 mL (120 mL)
Tablet, chewable (orange flavor): 500 mg

Selected Readings
"Drugs for Parasitic Infections," *Med Lett Drugs Ther*, 1993, 35(911):111-22.

Thyro-Block® *see* Potassium Iodide *on page 648*

Tiabendazole *see* Thiabendazole *on previous page*

Ticar® *see* Ticarcillin Disodium *on next page*

Ticarcillin and Clavulanate Potassium

(tye kar sill' in and klav' yoo la nate)
Related Information
Antimicrobial Activity Against Selected Organisms *on page 757-764*
Brand Names Timentin®
Synonyms Ticarcillin and Clavulanic Acid
Generic Available No
Use Treat infections of lower respiratory tract, urinary tract, skin and skin structures, bone and joint, and septicemia caused by susceptible organisms. Clavulanate expands activity of ticarcillin to include beta-lactamase producing strains of *S. aureus, H. influenzae, Bacteroides* species, and some other gram-negative bacilli
Drug of Choice or Alternative For
Disease/Syndrome(s)
Osteomyelitis, Diabetic Foot *on page 32*
Peritonitis *on page 36*
Organism(s)
Xanthomonas maltophilia on page 231
Pregnancy Risk Factor B
Contraindications Known hypersensitivity to ticarcillin, clavulanate, and any penicillin
Warnings/Precautions Not approved for use in children <12 years of age; use with caution and modify dosage in patients with renal impairment; use with caution in patients with a history of allergy to cephalosporins and in patients with CHF due to high sodium load
Adverse Reactions <1%: Thrombophlebitis, convulsions, confusion, drowsiness, fever, rash, electrolyte imbalance, hemolytic anemia, positive Coombs' reaction, myoclonus, acute interstitial nephritis, Jarisch-Herxheimer reaction, hypersensitivity reactions, anaphylaxis
Toxicology Many beta-lactam containing antibiotics have the potential to cause neuromuscular hyperirritability or convulsive seizures. Hemodialysis may be helpful to aid in the removal of the drug from the blood, otherwise most treatment is supportive or symptom directed.
Drug Interactions
Increased duration of neuromuscular blockers
Increased/prolonged levels with probenecid
Stability Reconstituted solution is stable for 6 hours at room temperature and

72 hours when refrigerated; for I.V. infusion in NS is stable for 24 hours at room temperature, 7 days when refrigerated or 30 days when frozen; after freezing, thawed solution is stable for 8 hours at room temperature; for I.V. infusion in D_5W solution is stable for 24 hours at room temperature, 3 days when refrigerated or 7 days when frozen; after freezing, thawed solution is stable for 8 hours at room temperature; darkening of drug indicates loss of potency of clavulanate potassium; incompatible with sodium bicarbonate, aminoglycosides

Mechanism of Action Inhibits bacterial cell wall synthesis by binding to one or more of the penicillin binding proteins (PBPs); which in turn inhibits the final transpeptidation step of peptidoglycan synthesis in bacterial cell walls, thus inhibiting cell wall biosynthesis. Bacteria eventually lyse due to ongoing activity of cell wall autolytic enzymes (autolysins and murein hydrolases) while cell wall assembly is arrested.

Pharmacokinetics
Distribution: Low concentrations of ticarcillin distribute into the CSF and increase when meninges are inflamed, otherwise, widely distributed
Metabolism: Clavulanic acid is metabolized in the liver
Half-life:
Clavulanate: 66-90 minutes
Ticarcillin: 66-72 minutes in patients with normal renal function
Clavulanic acid does not affect the clearance of ticarcillin
Elimination: 45% of clavulanate excreted unchanged in urine, whereas 60% to 90% of ticarcillin excreted unchanged in urine

Usual Dosage I.V.:
Children <60 kg: 200-300 mg of ticarcillin/kg/day in divided doses every 4-6 hours
Children >60 kg and Adults: 3.1 g (ticarcillin 3 g plus clavulanic acid 0.1 g) every 4-6 hours; maximum: 24 g/day; for urinary tract infections: 3.1 g every 6-8 hours

Dosing adjustment in renal impairment:
Cl_{cr} 30-60 mL/minute: Administer 2 g every 4 hours or 3.1 g every 8 hours
Cl_{cr} 10-30 mL/minute: Administer 2 g every 8 hours or 3 g every 12 hours
Cl_{cr} <10 mL/minute: Administer 2 g every 12 hours
Moderately dialyzable (20% to 50%)

Overdosage Neuromuscular hypersensitivity, seizures

Test Interactions May interfere with urinary glucose tests using cupric sulfate (Benedict's solution, Clinitest®); may inactivate aminoglycosides *in vitro*; positive Coombs' test, false-positive urinary proteins

Nursing Implications Infuse over 30 minutes

Additional Information Sodium content of 1 g: 109.3 mg (4.75 mEq)

Dosage Forms
Infusion, premixed (frozen): Ticarcillin disodium 3 g and clavulanic acid 0.1 g (100 mL)
Powder for injection: Ticarcillin disodium 3 g and clavulanic acid 0.1 g (3.1 g, 31 g)

Selected Readings
Donowitz GR and Mandell GL, "Beta-Lactam Antibiotics," *N Engl J Med*, 1988, 318(7):419-26 and 318(8):490-500.
Itokazu GS and Danziger LH, "Ampicillin-Sulbactam and Ticarcillin-Clavulanic Acid: A Comparison of Their *In Vitro* Activity and Review of Their Clinical Efficacy," *Pharmacotherapy*, 1991, 11(5):382-414.
Wright AJ and Wilkowske CJ, "The Penicillins," *Mayo Clin Proc*, 1991, 66(10):1047-63.

Ticarcillin and Clavulanic Acid *see* Ticarcillin and Clavulanate Potassium *on previous page*

Ticarcillin Disodium (tye kar sill' in)
Related Information
Antimicrobial Activity Against Selected Organisms *on page 757-764*
Brand Names Ticar®
Generic Available No
Use Treatment of susceptible infections such as septicemia, respiratory tract infections, skin and soft tissue infections, and urinary tract infections due to susceptible organisms
Pregnancy Risk Factor B
Contraindications Hypersensitivity to ticarcillin or any component or penicillins
Warnings/Precautions Use with caution in patients with a history of allergy to cephalosporins and in patients with CHF due to high sodium load
(Continued)

Ticarcillin Disodium *(Continued)*

Adverse Reactions <1%: Thrombophlebitis, convulsions, confusion, drowsiness, fever, rash, electrolyte imbalance, hemolytic anemia, positive Coombs' reaction, myoclonus, acute interstitial nephritis, Jarisch-Herxheimer reaction, hypersensitivity reactions, anaphylaxis

Toxicology Many beta-lactam containing antibiotics have the potential to cause neuromuscular hyperirritability or convulsive seizures. Hemodialysis may be helpful to aid in the removal of the drug from the blood, otherwise most treatment is supportive or symptom directed.

Drug Interactions
Increased duration of neuromuscular blockers
Increased/prolonged levels with probenecid

Stability Reconstituted solution is stable for 72 hours at room temperature and 14 days when refrigerated; for I.V. infusion in NS or D_5W solution is stable for 72 hours at room temperature, 14 days when refrigerated or 30 days when frozen; after freezing, thawed solution is stable for 72 hours at room temperature or 14 days when refrigerated; incompatible with aminoglycosides

Mechanism of Action Inhibits bacterial cell wall synthesis by binding to one or more of the penicillin binding proteins (PBPs); which in turn inhibits the final transpeptidation step of peptidoglycan synthesis in bacterial cell walls, thus inhibiting cell wall biosynthesis. Bacteria eventually lyse due to ongoing activity of cell wall autolytic enzymes (autolysins and murein hydrolases) while cell wall assembly is arrested.

Pharmacokinetics
Absorption: I.M.: 86%
Distribution: In blister fluid, lymph tissue, and gallbladder; crosses placenta; distributed into milk at low concentrations
Half-life:
Neonates:
<1 week: 3.5-5.6 hours
1-8 weeks: 1.3-2.2 hours
Children 5-13 years: 0.9 hour
Adults: 66-72 minutes, prolonged with renal impairment and/or hepatic impairment
Time to peak serum concentration: Within 30-75 minutes
Elimination: Excreted almost entirely in urine as unchanged drug and its metabolites with small amounts excreted in feces (3.5%)

Usual Dosage Ticarcillin is generally given I.V., I.M. injection is only for the treatment of uncomplicated urinary tract infections and dose should not exceed 2 g/injection when administered I.M.

Neonates: I.M., I.V.:
Postnatal age <7 days:
<2000 g: 75 mg/kg/dose every 12 hours
>2000 g: 75 mg/kg/dose every 8 hours
Postnatal age >7 days:
<1200 g: 75 mg/kg/dose every 12 hours
1200-2000 g: 75 mg/kg/dose every 8 hours
>2000 g: 75 mg/kg/dose every 6 hours

Infants and Children:
Systemic infections: I.V.: 200-300 mg/kg/day in divided doses every 4-6 hours
Urinary tract infections: I.M., I.V.: 50-100 mg/kg/day in divided doses every 6-8 hours
Maximum dose: 24 g/day

Adults: I.M., I.V.: 1-4 g every 4-6 hours, usual dose: 3 g I.V. every 4-6 hours

Dosing adjustment in renal impairment:
Cl_{cr} 30-60 mL/minute: Administer 2 g every 4 hours or 3.1 g every 8 hours
Cl_{cr} 10-30 mL/minute: Administer 2 g every 8 hours or 3 g every 12 hours
Cl_{cr} <10 mL/minute: Administer 2 g every 12 hours
Moderately dialyzable (20% to 50%)

Overdosage Neuromuscular hypersensitivity, seizure

Monitoring Parameters Serum electrolytes, bleeding time, and periodic tests of renal, hepatic, and hematologic function

Test Interactions May interfere with urinary glucose tests using cupric sulfate (Benedict's solution, Clinitest®); may inactivate aminoglycosides *in vitro*; false-positive urinary or serum protein

Additional Information Sodium content of 1 g: 119.6-149.5 mg (5.2-6.5 mEq)
Dosage Forms Powder for injection: 1 g, 3 g, 6 g, 20 g, 30 g
Selected Readings
Donowitz GR and Mandell GL, "Beta-Lactam Antibiotics," *N Engl J Med*, 1988, 318(7):419-26 and 318(8):490-500.
Wright AJ and Wilkowske CJ, "The Penicillins," *Mayo Clin Proc*, 1991, 66(10):1047-63.

TICE® BCG *see* Bacillus Calmette-Guérin (BCG) Live *on page 502*

TIG *see* Tetanus Immune Globulin, Human *on page 677*

Timentin® *see* Ticarcillin and Clavulanate Potassium *on page 682*

Tinactin® [OTC] *see* Tolnaftate *on page 687*

Ting® [OTC] *see* Tolnaftate *on page 687*

Tisit® [OTC] *see* Pyrethrins *on page 653*

TMP *see* Trimethoprim *on page 688*

TMP-SMX *see* Co-trimoxazole *on page 545*

Tobramycin (toe bra mye' sin)
Related Information
Aminoglycoside Dosing and Monitoring *on page 721-722*
Antimicrobial Activity Against Selected Organisms *on page 757-764*
Brand Names Nebcin® Injection; Tobrex® Ophthalmic
Generic Available Yes
Use Treatment of documented or suspected infections caused by susceptible gram-negative bacilli including *Pseudomonas aeruginosa*
Drug of Choice or Alternative For
Disease/Syndrome(s)
Meningitis, Postsurgical *on page 31*
Pregnancy Risk Factor C
Contraindications Hypersensitivity to tobramycin or other aminoglycosides
Warnings/Precautions Use with caution in patients with renal impairment; pre-existing auditory or vestibular impairment; and in patients with neuromuscular disorders; dosage modification required in patients with impaired renal function; (I.M. & I.V.) Aminoglycosides are associated with significant nephrotoxicity or ototoxicity; the ototoxicity is directly proportional to the amount of drug given and the duration of treatment; tinnitus or vertigo are indications of vestibular injury; ototoxicity is often irreversible; renal damage is usually reversible
Adverse Reactions
1% to 10%: Nephrotoxicity, neurotoxicity, ototoxicity (auditory), ototoxicity (vestibular)
<1%: Skin rash, drug fever, headache, paresthesia, tremor, nausea, vomiting, eosinophilia, arthralgia, anemia, hypotension, difficulty in breathing, drowsiness, weakness, lacrimation, itching, edema of the eyelid, keratitis
Toxicology The treatment of choice following a single acute overdose appears to be the maintenance of good urine output of at least 3 mL/kg/hour. Dialysis is of questionable value in the enhancement of aminoglycoside elimination. If required, hemodialysis is preferred over peritoneal dialysis in patients with normal renal function. Careful hydration may be all that is required to promote diuresis and therefore the enhancement of the drug's elimination.
Drug Interactions
Increased/prolonged effect: Depolarizing and nondepolarizing neuromuscular blocking agents
Increased toxicity: Concurrent use of amphotericin, vancomycin, or loop diuretics may increase nephrotoxicity
Stability Reconstituted solution is stable for 24 hours at room temperature and 96 hours when refrigerated; incompatible with penicillins
Mechanism of Action Interferes with bacterial protein synthesis by binding to 30S and 50S ribosomal subunits resulting in a defective bacterial cell membrane
Pharmacokinetics
Absorption: I.M.: Rapid and complete
Distribution: To extracellular fluid including serum, abscesses; ascitic, pericardial, pleural, synovial, lymphatic, and peritoneal fluids; crosses the placenta
(Continued)

Tobramycin (Continued)

Half-life:
  Neonates:
    ≤1200 g: 11 hours
    >1200 g: 2-9 hours
  Adults: 2-3 hours, directly dependent upon glomerular filtration rate
Time to peak serum concentration: I.M.: Within 30-60 minutes
Elimination: With normal renal function, ~90% to 95% of dose excreted in urine within 24 hours

Usual Dosage Individualization is critical because of the low therapeutic index. Use of ideal body weight (IBW) for determining the mg/kg/dose appears to be more accurate than dosing on the basis of total body weight (TBW) (see Appendix). In morbid obesity, dosage requirement may best be estimated using a dosing weight of IBW + 0.4 (TBW - IBW). Peak and trough plasma drug levels should be determined, particularly in critically ill patients with serious infections or in disease states known to significantly alter aminoglycoside pharmacokinetics (eg, cystic fibrosis, burns, or major surgery).

Neonates: I.M., I.V.:
  Postnatal age <7 days:
    <1000 g, <28 weeks gestational age: 3 mg/kg/dose every 24 hours
    <1500 g, <34 weeks gestational age: 2.5 mg/kg/dose every 18 hours
    >1500 g, >34 weeks gestational age: 2.5 mg/kg/dose every 12 hours
  Postnatal age >7 days:
    <2000 g: 2.5 mg/kg/dose every 12 hours
    >2000 g: 2.5 mg/kg/dose every 8 hours

Infants and Children: I.M., I.V.: 2.5 mg/kg/dose every 8 hours

Adults: I.M., I.V.:
  Severe life-threatening infections: 2-2.5 mg/kg/dose
  Urinary tract infection: 1.5 mg/kg/dose

Some clinicians suggest a daily dose of 4-7 mg/kg for all patients with normal renal function. This dose is at least as efficacious with similar, if not less, toxicity than conventional dosing.

Dosing adjustment in renal impairment: Initial dose:
  All patients should receive a loading dose of at least 2 mg/kg (subsequent dosing should be base on serum concentrations)
  Cl_{cr} >60 mL/minute: Administer every 8 hours
  Cl_{cr} 40-60 mL/minute: Administer every 12 hours
  Cl_{cr} 20-40 mL/minute: Administer every 24 hours
Dialyzable (50% to 100%)

Children and Adults: Ophthalmic: Instill 1-2 drops of solution every 4 hours; apply ointment 2-3 times/day; for severe infections apply ointment every 3-4 hours, or solution 2 drops every 30-60 minutes initially, then reduce to less frequent intervals

Overdosage Ototoxicity, nephrotoxicity, and neuromuscular toxicity

Monitoring Parameters Urinalysis, urine output, BUN, serum creatinine, peak and trough plasma tobramycin levels; be alert to ototoxicity; hearing may be tested before or during treatment

Reference Range Therapeutic: Peak: 5-10 µg/mL (SI: 11-21 µmol/L); Trough: <2 µg/mL (SI: <2-3 µmol/L); Toxic: Peak: >10 µg/mL (SI: >21 µmol/L); Trough: >2 µg/mL (SI: >4 µmol/L)

Test Interactions Penicillin may decrease aminoglycoside serum concentrations *in vitro*

Patient Information Do not use any other eye drops 5-10 minutes before or after tobramycin; report any dizziness or sensations of ringing or fullness in ears

Nursing Implications Eye solutions: Allow 5 minutes between application of "multiple-drop" therapy

Additional Information Should not be mixed with other drugs

Dosage Forms
Injection, as sulfate: 10 mg/mL (2 mL); 40 mg/mL (1.5 mL, 2 mL, 30 mL)
Ointment, ophthalmic: 0.3% (3.5 g)
Powder for injection: 1.2 g
Solution, ophthalmic: 0.3% (5 mL)

Selected Readings
Cunha BA, "Aminoglycosides: Current Role in Antimicrobial Therapy," *Pharmacotherapy*, 1988, 8(6):334-50.

Edson RS and Terrell CL, "The Aminoglycosides," *Mayo Clin Proc*, 1991, 66(11):1158-64.

Gilbert DN, "Once-Daily Aminoglycoside Therapy," *Antimicrob Agents Chemother*, 1991, 35(3):399-405.

Hustinx WN, and Hoepelman IM, "Aminoglycoside Dosage Regimens. Is Once a Day Enough?" *Clin Pharmacokinet*, 1993, 25(6):427-32.

McCormack JP and Jewesson PJ, "A Critical Reevaluation of the "Therapeutic Range" of Aminoglycosides," *Clin Infect Dis*, 1992, 14(1):320-39.

Tobrex® Ophthalmic *see* Tobramycin *on page 685*

Tolnaftate (tole naf' tate)

Brand Names Aftate® [OTC]; Footwork® [OTC]; Fungatin® [OTC]; Genaspor® [OTC]; NP-27® [OTC]; Quinsana Plus® [OTC]; Tinactin® [OTC]; Ting® [OTC]; Zeasorb-AF® [OTC]

Generic Available Yes

Use Treatment of tinea pedis, tinea cruris, tinea corporis, tinea manuum, tinea versicolor infections

Pregnancy Risk Factor C

Contraindications Known hypersensitivity to tolnaftate; nail and scalp infections

Warnings/Precautions Cream is not recommended for nail or scalp infections; keep from eyes; if no improvement within 4 weeks treatment should be discontinued

Adverse Reactions 1% to 10%: Pruritus, contact dermatitis, irritation, stinging

Mechanism of Action Distorts the hyphae and stunts mycelial growth in susceptible fungi

Usual Dosage Children and Adults: Topical: Wash and dry affected area; apply 1-2 drops of solution or a small amount of cream or powder and rub into the affected areas twice daily for 2-4 weeks

Patient Information Avoid contact with the eyes; apply to clean dry area; consult the physician if a skin irritation develops or if the skin infection worsens or does not improve after 10 days of therapy; does not stain skin or clothing

Nursing Implications Itching, burning soreness usually relieved within 24-72 hours

Dosage Forms

Aerosol:
  Topical:
    Liquid: 1% (90 mL, 120 mL)
    Powder: 1% (90 g, 100 g, 105 g, 150 g)
Cream: 1% (0.7 g, 15 g, 30 g)
Gel, topical: 1% (15 g)
Powder, topical: 1% (45 g, 67.5 g, 90 g)
Solution, topical: 1% (10 mL, 15 mL)

Topicycline® *see* Tetracycline *on page 679*

TOPV *see* Poliovirus Vaccine, Live, Trivalent, Oral *on page 646*

Totacillin® *see* Ampicillin *on page 495*

Totacillin®-N *see* Ampicillin *on page 495*

Trecator®-SC *see* Ethionamide *on page 565*

Triacetyloleandomycin *see* Troleandomycin *on page 690*

Tribavirin *see* Ribavirin *on page 660*

Trifluorothymidine *see* Trifluridine *on this page*

Trifluridine (trye flure' i deen)

Brand Names Viroptic®

Synonyms F_3T; Trifluorothymidine

Generic Available No

Use Treatment of primary keratoconjunctivitis and recurrent epithelial keratitis caused by herpes simplex virus types I and II

Pregnancy Risk Factor C

Contraindications Known hypersensitivity to trifluridine or any component

Warnings/Precautions Mild local irritation of conjunctival and cornea may occur when instilled but usually transient effects

Adverse Reactions

1% to 10%: Burning, stinging

(Continued)

Trifluridine *(Continued)*

<1%: Palpebral edema, epithelial keratopathy, keratitis, stromal edema, increased intraocular pressure, hyperemia, hypersensitivity reactions

Stability Refrigerate at 2°C to 8°C (36°F to 46°F); storage at room temperature may result in a solution altered pH which could result in ocular discomfort upon administration and/or decreased potency

Mechanism of Action Interferes with viral replication by incorporating into viral DNA in place of thymidine, inhibiting thymidylate synthetase resulting in the formation of defective proteins

Pharmacokinetics Absorption: Ophthalmic instillation: Systemic absorption is negligible, while corneal penetration is adequate

Usual Dosage Adults: Instill 1 drop into affected eye every 2 hours while awake, to a maximum of 9 drops/day, until re-epithelialization of corneal ulcer occurs; then use 1 drop every 4 hours for another 7 days; do **not** exceed 21 days of treatment; if improvement has not taken place in 7-14 days, consider another form of therapy

Patient Information Notify physician if improvement is not seen after 7 days, condition worsens, or if irritation occurs; do not discontinue without notifying the physician, do not exceed recommended dosage

Dosage Forms Solution, ophthalmic: 1% (7.5 mL)

Tri-Immunol® *see* Diphtheria, Tetanus Toxoids, and Whole-Cell Pertussis Vaccine *on page 556*

Trimethoprim *(trye meth' oh prim)*

Brand Names Proloprim®; Trimpex®

Synonyms TMP

Generic Available Yes

Use Treatment of urinary tract infections; acute otitis media in children; acute exacerbations of chronic bronchitis in adults; in combination with other agents for treatment of *Pneumocystis carinii*

Pregnancy Risk Factor C

Contraindications Hypersensitivity to trimethoprim or any component, megaloblastic anemia due to folate deficiency

Warnings/Precautions Use with caution in patients with impaired renal or hepatic function or with possible folate deficiency

Adverse Reactions

>10%: Rash, pruritus

1% to 10%: Megaloblastic anemia

<1%: Fever, exfoliative dermatitis, nausea, vomiting, epigastric distress, cholestatic jaundice, thrombocytopenia, neutropenia, leukopenia; increased LFTS, BUN, and serum creatinine

Toxicology

Acute: Nausea, vomiting, confusion, dizziness

Chronic: Bone marrow depression

Treatment of acute overdose is supportive following GI decontamination; in chronic overdose, bone marrow suppression should be treated with oral leucovorin 5-15 mg/day

Drug Interactions Increased effect/toxicity/levels of phenytoin

Mechanism of Action Inhibits folic acid reduction to tetrahydrofolate, and thereby inhibits microbial growth

Pharmacokinetics

Absorption: Oral: Readily and extensive

Metabolism: Partially in the liver

Half-life: 8-14 hours, prolonged with renal impairment

Time to peak serum concentration: Within 1-4 hours

Elimination: Significantly excreted in urine (60% to 80% as unchanged drug)

Usual Dosage Oral:

Children: 4 mg/kg/day in divided doses every 12 hours

Adults: 100 mg every 12 hours or 200 mg every 24 hours; in the treatment of *Pneumocystis carinii* pneumonia; dose may be as high as 15-20 mg/kg/day in 3-4 divided doses

Dosing interval in renal impairment:

Cl$_{cr}$ 15-30 mL/minute: Administer 100 mg every 18 hours or 50 mg every 12 hours

Cl$_{cr}$ <15 mL/minute: Administer 100 mg every 24 hours or avoid use

Moderately dialyzable (20% to 50%)

Reference Range Therapeutic: Peak: 5-15 mg/L; Trough: 2-8 mg/L

Patient Information Take with milk or food; report any skin rash, persistent or severe fatigue, fever, sore throat, or unusual bleeding or bruising; complete full course of therapy

Dosage Forms Tablet: 100 mg, 200 mg

Trimethoprim and Sulfamethoxazole *see* Co-trimoxazole *on page 545*

Trimetrexate Glucuronate (tri me trex' ate)

Brand Names Neutrexin™

Generic Available No

Use Alternative therapy for the treatment of moderate-to-severe *Pneumocystis carinii* pneumonia (PCP) in immunocompromised patients, including patients with acquired immunodeficiency syndrome (AIDS), who are intolerant of, or are refractory to, co-trimoxazole therapy or for whom co-trimoxazole and pentamidine are contraindicated (concurrent folinic acid (leucovorin) must always be administered)

Pregnancy Risk Factor D

Contraindications Previous hypersensitivity to trimetrexate or methotrexate, severe existing myelosuppression

Warnings/Precautions Must be administered with concurrent leucovorin to avoid potentially serious or life-threatening toxicities; leucovorin therapy must extend for 72 hours past the last dose of trimetrexate; use with caution in patients with mild myelosuppression, severe hepatic or renal dysfunction, hypoproteinemia, hypoalbuminemia, or previous extensive myelosuppressive therapies

Adverse Reactions 1% to 10%: Peripheral neuropathy, seizures, rash, neutropenia, thrombocytopenia, anemia, stomatitis, nausea, vomiting, elevated liver function tests, increased serum creatinine, fever, flu-like illness, hypersensitivity reactions

Drug Interactions
Decreased effect of pneumococcal vaccine
Increased toxicity (infection rates) of yellow fever vaccine

Stability Reconstituted I.V. solution is stable for 24 hours at room temperature or 7 days when refrigerated; intact vials should be refrigerated at 2°C to 8°C

Mechanism of Action Exerts an antimicrobial effect through potent inhibition of the enzyme dihydrofolate reductase (DHFR)

Pharmacokinetics
Metabolism: Extensive in the liver
Half-life: 15-17 hours

Usual Dosage Adults: I.V.: 45 mg/m^2 once daily over 60 minutes for 21 days; it is necessary to reduce the dose in patients with liver dysfunction, although no specific recommendations exist; concurrent folinic acid 20 mg/m^2 every 6 hours orally or I.V. for 24 days

Monitoring Parameters Check and record patient's temperature daily
Lab tests:
Hematology (absolute neutrophil counts (ANC)), platelets
Renal functions (serum creatinine, BUN)
Hepatic function (ALT, AST, alkaline phosphatase)

Patient Information Report promptly any fever, rash, flu-like symptoms, numbness or tingling in the extremities, nausea, vomiting, abdominal pain, mouth sores, increased bruising or bleeding, black tarry stools

Nursing Implications Must administer folinic acid 20 mg/m^2 orally or I.V. every 6 hours for 24 days

Additional Information Not a vesicant; methotrexate derivative

Dosage Forms Injection: 25 mg

Selected Readings
Marshall JL and De Lap RJ, "Clinical Pharmacokinetics and Pharmacology of Trimetrexate," *Clin Pharmacokinet*, 1994, 26(3):190-200.
Masur H, "Prevention and Treatment of *Pneumocystis* Pneumonia," *N Engl J Med*, 1992, 327(26):1853-60.

Trimox® *see* Amoxicillin Trihydrate *on page 491*

Trimpex® *see* Trimethoprim *on previous page*

Tripedia® *see* Diphtheria and Tetanus Toxoids and Acellular Pertussis Vaccine *on page 555*

Triple Sulfa *see* Sulfabenzamide, Sulfacetamide, and Sulfathiazole *on page 671*

Trisulfam® *see* Co-trimoxazole *on page 545*

Trisulfapyrimidines *see* Sulfadiazine, Sulfamethazine, and Sulfamerazine *on page 672*

Trobicin® Injection *see* Spectinomycin Hydrochloride *on page 667*

Troleandomycin (troe lee an doe mye' sin)

Brand Names Tao®

Synonyms Triacetyloleandomycin

Generic Available No

Use Adjunct in the treatment of corticosteroid-dependent asthma due to its steroid-sparing properties; antibiotic with spectrum of activity similar to erythromycin

Pregnancy Risk Factor C

Contraindications Hypersensitivity to troleandomycin, other macrolides, or any component

Warnings/Precautions Use with caution in patients with impaired hepatic function

Adverse Reactions
>10%: Abdominal cramping and discomfort
1% to 10%: Nausea, vomiting, diarrhea, urticaria, skin rashes
<1%: Rectal burning, cholestatic jaundice

Toxicology Symptoms of overdose include nausea, vomiting, diarrhea, hearing loss; following GI decontamination, treatment is supportive

Drug Interactions Increased effect/toxicity/levels of carbamazepine, ergot alkaloids, methylprednisolone, theophylline, and triazolam

Mechanism of Action Decreases methylprednisolone clearance from a linear first order decline to a nonlinear decline in plasma concentration. Troleandomycin also has an undefined action independent of its effects on steroid elimination. Inhibits RNA-dependent protein synthesis at the chain elongation step; binds to the 50S ribosomal subunit resulting in blockage of transpeptidation.

Pharmacokinetics
Time to peak serum concentration: Within 2 hours
Elimination: 10% to 25% excreted in urine as active drug; also excreted in feces via bile

Usual Dosage Oral:
Children 7-13 years: 25-40 mg/kg/day divided every 6 hours (125-250 mg every 6 hours)
Adjunct in corticosteroid-dependent asthma: 14 mg/kg/day in divided doses every 6-12 hours not to exceed 250 mg every 6 hours; dose is tapered to once daily then alternate day dosing

Adults: 250-500 mg 4 times/day
Monitoring Parameters Hepatic function tests
Patient Information Complete full course of therapy; notify physician if persistent or severe abdominal pain, nausea, vomiting, or fever occurs
Dosage Forms Capsule: 250 mg

Trysul® *see* Sulfabenzamide, Sulfacetamide, and Sulfathiazole *on page 671*

Ultracef® *see* Cefadroxil Monohydrate *on page 509*

Unasyn® *see* Ampicillin Sodium and Sulbactam Sodium *on page 497*

Unipen® *see* Nafcillin Sodium *on page 616*

Urex® *see* Methenamine *on page 607*

Urised® *see* Methenamine *on page 607*

Uri-Tet® Oral *see* Oxytetracycline Hydrochloride *on page 629*

Urobak® *see* Sulfamethoxazole *on page 674*

Uroplus® DS *see* Co-trimoxazole *on page 545*

Uroplus® SS *see* Co-trimoxazole *on page 545*

Utimox® *see* Amoxicillin Trihydrate *on page 491*

Vaccines *see page 706*

Vagilia® *see* Sulfabenzamide, Sulfacetamide, and Sulfathiazole *on page 671*

Vancocin® *see* Vancomycin Hydrochloride *on this page*

Vancoled® *see* Vancomycin Hydrochloride *on this page*

Vancomycin Hydrochloride (van koe mye' sin)

Related Information

Antimicrobial Activity Against Selected Organisms *on page 757-764*

Brand Names Vancocin®; Vancoled®

Generic Available Yes

Use Treatment of patients with infections caused by staphylococcal species and streptococcal species; used orally for staphylococcal enterocolitis or for antibiotic-associated pseudomembranous colitis produced by *C. difficile*

Drug of Choice or Alternative For

Disease/Syndrome(s)

Catheter Infection, Intravascular *on page 20*

Endocarditis, Acute, I.V. Drug Abuse *on page 21*

Endocarditis, Acute Native Valve *on page 22*

Endocarditis, Prosthetic Valve, Early *on page 22*

Endocarditis, Prosthetic Valve, Late *on page 23*

Endocarditis, Subacute Native Valve *on page 23*

Fever, Neutropenic *on page 25*

Joint Replacement, Early Infection *on page 27*

Joint Replacement, Late Infection *on page 27*

Meningitis, Pediatric (>2 months of age) *on page 30*

Meningitis, Postsurgical *on page 31*

Meningitis, Neonatal (<2 months of age) *on page 29*

Meningitis, Post-Traumatic *on page 31*

Osteomyelitis, Healthy Adult *on page 33*

Osteomyelitis, Pediatric *on page 33*

Pneumonia, Hospital-Acquired *on page 38*

Sepsis *on page 40*

Sinusitis, Hospital-Acquired *on page 41*

Skin and Soft Tissue *on page 42*

Thrombophlebitis, Suppurative *on page 43*

Toxic Shock Syndrome *on page 43*

Urinary Tract Infection, Catheter-Associated *on page 44*

Wound Infection, Surgical *on page 46*

Organism(s)

Bacillus cereus on page 60

Clostridium difficile on page 85

Corynebacterium jeikeium on page 90

Enterococcus Species on page 107

Staphylococcus aureus, Methicillin-Resistant *on page 195*

Staphylococcus aureus, Methicillin-Susceptible *on page 198*

Staphylococcus epidermidis, Methicillin-Resistant *on page 200*

Staphylococcus epidermidis, Methicillin-Susceptible *on page 201*

Streptococcus agalactiae on page 203

Streptococcus bovis on page 205

Streptococcus pneumoniae on page 206

Streptococcus pyogenes on page 207

Streptococcus-Related Gram-Positive Cocci *on page 212*

Streptococcus, Viridans Group *on page 213*

Pregnancy Risk Factor C

Contraindications Hypersensitivity to vancomycin or any component; avoid in patients with previous hearing loss

Adverse Reactions

Oral:

>10%: Bitter taste, nausea, vomiting

1% to 10%: Drug fever, chills, eosinophilia

<1%: Ototoxicity, renal failure, interstitial nephritis, thrombocytopenia, vasculitis

Parenteral:

>10%: Hypotension accompanied by flushing and erythematous rash on face and upper body (red neck or red man syndrome)

(Continued)

Vancomycin Hydrochloride *(Continued)*

1% to 10%: Drug fever, chills, eosinophilia

<1%: Renal failure, ototoxicity, thrombocytopenia, vasculitis

Toxicology There is no specific therapy for an overdosage with vancomycin. Care is symptomatic and supportive in nature. Peritoneal filtration and hemofiltration have been shown to reduce the serum concentration of vancomycin.

Drug Interactions Ototoxic or nephrotoxic agents

Stability After the oral or parenteral solution is reconstituted, refrigerate and discard after 14 days; after further dilution, the parenteral solution is stable, at room temperature, for 24 hours

Mechanism of Action Inhibits bacterial cell wall synthesis by blocking glycopeptide polymerization through binding tightly to D-alanyl-D-alanine portion of cell wall precursor

Pharmacokinetics

Absorption: Oral: Poor

Distribution: To pleural, ascitic, pericardial, and synovial fluids; penetrates into CSF when meninges are inflamed

Half-life, terminal (biphasic):

Newborns: 6-10 hours

3 months to 4 years: 4 hours

>3 years: 2.2-3 hours

Adults: 5-11 hours, half-life prolonged significantly with reduced renal function

Elimination: Excreted as unchanged drug in urine (80% to 90%); oral doses are excreted primarily in feces

Usual Dosage Initial dosage recommendation: I.V.:

Neonates:

Postnatal age <7 days:

<1200 g: 15 mg/kg/dose given every 24 hours

1200-2000 g: 10 mg/kg/dose divided every 12 hours

>2000 g: 15 mg/kg/dose divided every 12 hours

Postnatal age >7 days:

<1200 g: 15 mg/kg/dose given every 24 hours

≥1200 g: 10 mg/kg/dose divided every 8 hours

Infants >1 month and Children: 40 mg/kg/day in divided doses every 6 hours

Infants >1 month and Children with staphylococcal central nervous system infection: 60 mg/kg/day in divided doses every 6 hours

Adults: With normal renal function: 1 g every 12 hours

Dosing interval in renal impairment (vancomycin levels **should** be monitored in patients with any renal impairment):

Cl_{cr} >60 mL/minute: Start with 1 g every 12 hours

Cl_{cr} 40-60 mL/minute: Start with 1 g every 24 hours

Cl_{cr} <40 mL minute: Will need longer intervals; determine by serum concentration monitoring

Not dialyzable (0% to 5%)

Intrathecal:

Neonates: 5-10 mg/day

Children: 5-20 mg/day

Adults: Up to 20 mg/day

Oral:

Pseudomembranous colitis produced by *C. difficile*:

Neonates: 10 mg/kg/day in divided doses

Children: 40 mg/kg/day in divided doses, added to fluids

Adults: 500 mg to 2 g/day given in 3 or 4 divided doses for 7-10 days

Monitoring Parameters Periodic renal function tests, urinalysis, serum vancomycin concentrations, WBC

Reference Range Therapeutic: Depends on MIC of organism being treated, usually peak: 20-35 μg/mL (SI: 20-35 mg/L); Trough: 5-10 μg/mL (SI: 5-10 mg/L); Toxic: >80-100 μg/mL (SI: >80-100 mg /L)

Patient Information Report pain at infusion site, dizziness, fullness or ringing in ears with I.V. use; nausea or vomiting with oral use

Dosage Forms

Capsule: 125 mg, 250 mg

Powder for oral solution: 1 g, 10 g

Powder for injection: 500 mg, 1 g, 2 g, 5 g, 10 g

Selected Readings

Cantú TG, Yamanaka-Yuen NA, and Lietman PS, "Serum Vancomycin Concentrations: Reappraisal of Their Clinical Value," *Clin Infect Dis*, 1994, 18:533-43.

Kelly CP, Pothoulakis C, and LaMont JT, "*Clostridium difficile* colitis," *N Engl J Med*, 1994, 330(4):257-62.

Wilhelm MP, "Vancomycin," *Mayo Clin Proc*, 1991, 66(11):1165-70.

Vansil™ *see* Oxamniquine *on page 628*

Vantin® *see* Cefpodoxime Proxetil *on page 519*

Varicella-Zoster Immune Globulin (Human)

(veer i sel' a - zos' ter)

Synonyms VZIG

Generic Available No

Use Passive immunization of susceptible immunodeficient patients after exposure to varicella; most effective if begun within 96 hours of exposure

VZIG supplies are limited, restrict administration to those meeting the following criteria:

One of the following underlying illnesses or conditions:

Neoplastic disease (eg, leukemia or lymphoma)

Congenital or acquired immunodeficiency

Immunosuppressive therapy with steroids, antimetabolites or other immunosuppressive treatment regimens

Newborn of mother who had onset of chickenpox within 5 days before delivery or within 48 hours after delivery

Premature (≥28 weeks gestation) whose mother has no history of chickenpox

Premature (<28 weeks gestation or ≤1000 g VZIG) regardless of maternal history

One of the following types of exposure to chickenpox or zoster patient(s):

Continuous household contact

Playmate contact (>1 hour play indoors)

Hospital contact (in same 2-4 bedroom or adjacent beds in a large ward or prolonged face-to-face contact with an infectious staff member or patient)

Susceptible to varicella-zoster

Age of <15 years; administer to immunocompromised adolescents and adults and to other older patients on an individual basis

An acceptable alternative to VZIG prophylaxis is to treat varicella, if it occurs, with high-dose I.V. acyclovir

Pregnancy Risk Factor C

Contraindications Not for prophylactic use in immunodeficient patients with history of varicella, unless patient's immunosuppression is associated with bone marrow transplantation; **not** recommended for nonimmunodeficient patients, including pregnant women, because the severity of chickenpox is much less than in immunosuppressed patients

Adverse Reactions

1% to 10%: Local discomfort at the site of injection (pain, redness, swelling)

<1%: GI symptoms, malaise, headache, rash, respiratory symptoms, angioedema, anaphylactic shock

Drug Interactions Interferes with immune response of live virus vaccines (do not administer within 3 months of immune globulin administration)

Stability Refrigerate

Mechanism of Action The exact mechanism has not been clarified but the antibodies in varicella-zoster immune globulin most likely neutralize the varicella-zoster virus and prevent its pathological actions.

Usual Dosage High risk susceptible patients who are exposed again more than 3 weeks after a prior dose of VZIG should receive another full dose; there is no evidence VZIG modifies established varicella-zoster infections.

I.M.: Administer by deep injection in the gluteal muscle or in another large muscle mass. Inject 125 units/10 kg (22 lb); maximum dose: 625 units (5 vials); minimum dose: 125 units; do not give fractional doses. Do not inject I.V. See table.

Nursing Implications Administer deep I.M. into the gluteal muscle or other large muscle mass. For patients ≤10 kg, administer 1.25 mL at a single site. For patients >10 kg, give no more than 2.5 mL at a single site.

Dosage Forms Injection: 125 units of antibody in single dose vials

VZIG Dose Based on Weight

Weight of Patient		Dose	
kg	lb	Units	No. of Vials
0–10	0–22	125	1
10.1–20	22.1–44	250	2
20.1–30	44.1–66	375	3
30.1–40	66.1–88	500	4
>40	>88	625	5

V-Cillin K® *see* Penicillin V Potassium *on page 638*
Veetids® *see* Penicillin V Potassium *on page 638*
Velosef® *see* Cephradine *on page 530*
Venoglobulin®-I *see* Immune Globulin *on page 588*
Vermizine® *see* Piperazine Citrate *on page 643*
Vermox® *see* Mebendazole *on page 604*
Vibramycin® *see* Doxycycline *on page 557*
Vibra-Tabs® *see* Doxycycline *on page 557*

Vidarabine (vye dare' a been)
Brand Names Vira-A®
Synonyms Adenine Arabinoside; Ara-A; Arabinofuranosyladenine
Generic Available No
Use Treatment of acute keratoconjunctivitis and epithelial keratitis due to herpes simplex virus; herpes simplex encephalitis (acyclovir is the preferred agent); neonatal herpes simplex virus infections; herpes zoster in immunosuppressed patients; definitive diagnosis of herpes simplex conjunctivitis should be made before instituting ophthalmic therapy
Pregnancy Risk Factor C
Contraindications Hypersensitivity to vidarabine or any component
Warnings/Precautions Vidarabine must be administered slow I.V. to neonates; administration requires dilution in large fluid volumes; use with caution in patients at risk of fluid overload (cerebral edema) and in patients with impaired renal function; reduce dosage in patients with severe renal insufficiency
Adverse Reactions
   1% to 10%: Nausea, vomiting, anorexia, diarrhea, weight loss, elevated bilirubin and AST
   <1%: Thrombophlebitis, weakness, ataxia, disorientation, depression, agitation, rash, hypokalemia, decreased WBC and platelets, burning, lacrimation, pain, myoclonus, keratitis, photophobia, foreign body sensation, uveitis, stromal edema, SIADH
Toxicology Symptoms of overdose include bone marrow depression, thrombocytopenia, leukopenia with doses >20 mg/kg/day; treatment is supportive only
Drug Interactions Increased toxicity with allopurinol
Stability Do **not** refrigerate diluted I.V. solution; constituted solutions remain stable for 2 weeks at room temperature; however, should be diluted just prior to administration and used within 48 hours
   Stability of parenteral admixture at room temperature (25°C): 2 days
Mechanism of Action Inhibits viral DNA synthesis by blocking DNA polymerase
Pharmacokinetics
   Absorption: Not to be administered oral, I.V., or S.C.
   Distribution: Crosses into the CNS
   Metabolism: Following administration rapidly deaminated to ara-hypoxanthine (active)
   Half-life:
      Infants: 2.4-3.1 hours
      Children: 2.8 hours
      Adults: 1.5 hours

Ara-hypoxanthine: Normal renal function: 3.3 hours
Elimination: Excreted in urine as unchanged drug (1% to 3%) and the active metabolite (40% to 53%)

Usual Dosage Administer through an in-line 0.22 or 0.45 micron filter
Neonates: I.V.: 15-30 mg/kg/day as an 18- to 24-hour infusion for 10-14 days

Children and Adults:
I.V.: 15 mg/kg/day as a 12-hour or longer infusion for 10 days

Dosing adjustment in renal impairment: Cl_{cr} <10 mL/minute: Administer 75% of normal dose

Ophthalmic: Keratoconjunctivitis: Instill $1/2$" of ointment in lower conjunctival sac 5 times/day every 3 hours while awake until complete re-epithelialization has occurred, then twice daily for an additional 7 days

Patient Information Do not use eye make-up when on this medication for ophthalmic infection; use sunglasses if photophobic reaction occurs; may cause blurred vision; notify physician if improvement not seen after 7 days or if condition worsens

Nursing Implications Do not give I.M. or S.C.; administer I.V. solution through an in-line 0.22 or 0.45 micron filter; administer by slow I.V. infusion over 12-24 hours

Dosage Forms
Injection, suspension: 200 mg/mL [base 187.4 mg] (5 mL)
Ointment, ophthalmic, as monohydrate: 3% [30 mg/g = 28 mg/g base] (3.5 g)

Selected Readings
"Drugs for Non-HIV Viral Infections," *Med Lett Drugs Ther*, 1994, 36(919):27.

Videx® Oral *see* Didanosine *on page 552*

Vira-A® *see* Vidarabine *on previous page*

Virazole® *see* Ribavirin *on page 660*

Viroptic® *see* Trifluridine *on page 687*

V.V.S.® *see* Sulfabenzamide, Sulfacetamide, and Sulfathiazole *on page 671*

VZIG *see* Varicella-Zoster Immune Globulin (Human) *on page 693*

Wyamycin® S Oral *see* Erythromycin *on page 561*

Wycillin® *see* Penicillin G Procaine, Aqueous *on page 636*

Wymox® *see* Amoxicillin Trihydrate *on page 491*

Yodoxin® *see* Iodoquinol *on page 591*

Zalcitabine (zal site' a been)
Brand Names Hivid®
Synonyms ddC; Dideoxycytidine
Generic Available No
Use The FDA has approved zalcitabine for use in the treatment of HIV infections only in combination with zidovudine in adult patients with advanced HIV disease demonstrating a significant clinical or immunological deterioration
Drug of Choice or Alternative For
Organism(s)
Human Immunodeficiency Virus *on page 133*
Pregnancy Risk Factor C
Warnings/Precautions Approved for use only in combination with zidovudine for the treatment of adult patients with advanced HIV infection who have severe clinical and immunological deterioration in their health status. Major side effect is peripheral neuropathy and to a lesser extent pancreatitis; cases of severe to moderate peripheral neuropathy have been reported which were clinically disabling for patients; since side effects associated with zidovudine are likely to occur in patients treated with combined zalcitabine and zidovudine therapy, it is recommended that warnings and precautions associated with zidovudine should be observed.

Complete blood counts and clinical chemistry tests should be performed prior to initiating combination therapy with zalcitabine and zidovudine and at appropriate intervals thereafter. Baseline testing of serum amylase and triglyceride levels should be performed in individuals with a prior history of pancreatitis, increased amylase, those on parenteral nutrition, or with a history of ethanol abuse.

(Continued)

Zalcitabine *(Continued)*

Zalcitabine could possibly exacerbate existing liver dysfunction in patients with a previous history of liver disease or alcohol abuse. An increase in liver function tests was observed in patients on zalcitabine therapy; caution should be exercised in patients with hepatic impairment

Adverse Reactions

>10%: Oral ulcers

1% to 10%: Nausea, dysphagia, anorexia, abdominal pain, vomiting, diarrhea, rash, pruritus, headache, dizziness, myalgia, foot pain, fatigue, pharyngitis, chest pain, weight decrease

<1%: Constipation, night sweats, fever, pain, malaise, asthenia, edema, hypertension, palpitations, syncope, atrial fibrillation, tachycardia, heart racing, epistaxis, hyperglycemia, hypocalcemia, jaundice, hepatitis, myositis

Drug Interactions Amphotericin, foscarnet, and aminoglycosides may potentiate the risk of developing peripheral neuropathy or other toxicities associated with zalcitabine by interfering with the renal elimination of zalcitabine. Other drugs associated with peripheral neuropathy include chloramphenicol, cisplatin, dapsone, disulfiram, ethionamide, glutethimide, gold, hydralazine, iodoquinol, isoniazid, metronidazole, nitrofurantoin, phenytoin, ribavirin, and vincristine; concomitant use of zalcitabine with didanosine is not recommended. One case of fulminant pancreatitis associated with concomitant zalcitabine and pentamidine use has been reported. If I.V. pentamidine is required to treat *Pneumocystis carinii* pneumonia, treatment with zalcitabine should be interrupted.

Stability Tablets should be stored in tightly closed bottles at 59°F to 86°F

Usual Dosage

Children <13 years: Safety and efficacy have not been established

Adults: Oral (dosed in combination with zidovudine): Daily dose: 0.750 mg every 8 hours, given together with 200 mg of zidovudine (ie, total daily dose: 2.25 mg of zalcitabine and 600 mg of zidovudine)

Dosing adjustment in renal impairment:

Cl_{cr} between 10-40 mL/minute: Administer 0.750 mg every 12 hours

Cl_{cr} <10 mL/minute: Administer 0.750 mg every 24 hours

Dosage Forms Tablet: 0.375 mg, 0.75 mg

Selected Readings

"Drugs for AIDS and Associated Infections," *Med Lett Drugs Ther*, 1993, 35(904):79-86.

Hirsch MS and D'Aquila RT, "Therapy for Human Immunodeficiency Virus Infection," *N Engl J Med*, 1993, 328(23):1686-95.

Shelton MJ, O'Donnell AM, and Morse GD, "Zalcitabine," *Ann Pharmacother*, 1993, 27(4):480-9.

Skowron G, Bozzette SA, Lim L, et al, "Alternating and Intermittent Regimens of Zidovudine and Dideoxycytidine in Patients With AIDS or AIDS-Related Complex," *Ann Intern Med*, 1993, 118(5):321-30.

Zeasorb-AF® [OTC] *see* Tolnaftate *on page 687*

Zefazone® *see* Cefmetazole Sodium *on page 513*

Zerit® *see* Stavudine *on page 668*

Zidovudine *(zye doe' vue deen)*

Brand Names Retrovir®

Synonyms Azidothymidine; AZT; Compound S

Generic Available No

Use Management of patients with HIV infections who have CD4 cell counts of ≤500/mm³; patients who have HIV-related symptoms or who are asymptomatic with abnormal laboratory values indicating HIV-related immunosuppression

Drug of Choice or Alternative For

Organism(s)

Human Immunodeficiency Virus *on page 133*

Pregnancy Risk Factor C

Contraindications Life-threatening hypersensitivity to zidovudine or any component

Warnings/Precautions Often associated with hematologic toxicity including granulocytopenia and severe anemia requiring transfusions; zidovudine has been shown to be carcinogenic in rats and mice

Adverse Reactions

>10%: Anemia, leukopenia, neutropenia, severe headache, insomnia, nausea

1% to 10%: Changes in platelet count, hyperpigmentation of nails (bluish-brown)

<1%: Hepatotoxicity, anorexia, myopathy, weakness, tenderness, neurotoxicity, confusion, mania, seizures, bone marrow depression, granulocytopenia, thrombocytopenia, pancytopenia, cholestatic hepatitis

Toxicology Erythropoietin, thymidine and cyanocobalamin have been used experimentally to treat zidovudine-induced hematopoietic toxicity, yet none are presently specified as the agent of choice.

Drug Interactions
Dapsone, pentamidine, amphotericin B, flucytosine, vincristine, vinblastine, doxorubicin, interferon
Increased toxicity: Coadministration with drugs that are nephrotoxic, cytotoxic, or interfere with RBC/WBC number or function

Mechanism of Action Zidovudine is a thymidine analog which interferes with the HIV viral RNA dependent DNA polymerase resulting in inhibition of viral replication; reverse transcriptase inhibitor

Pharmacokinetics
Absorption: Oral: Well absorbed (66% to 70%) from GI tract
Distribution: Significant penetration into the CSF; crosses the placenta
Metabolism: Extensive first-pass; metabolized in the liver via glucuronidation to inactive metabolites
Half-life, terminal: 60 minutes
Time to peak serum concentration: Within 30-90 minutes
Elimination: Urinary excretion (63% to 95%); following oral administration, 72% to 74% of the drug excreted in urine as metabolites and 14% to 18% as unchanged drug; following I.V. administration, 45% to 60% excreted in urine as metabolites and 18% to 29% as unchanged drug

Usual Dosage
Children 3 months to 12 years:
Oral: 90-180 mg/m^2/dose every 6 hours; maximum: 200 mg every 6 hours
I.V. continuous infusion: 0.5-1.8 mg/kg/hour
I.V. intermittent infusion: 100 mg/m^2/dose every 6 hours

Adults:
Oral: 100 mg 5 times/day (500 mg/day)
I.V.: 1-2 mg/kg/dose every 4 hours

Overdosage Nausea, vomiting, ataxia, granulocytopenia

Monitoring Parameters CBC with platelet count at least every 2 weeks; MCV, serum creatinine kinase

Patient Information Take 30 minutes before or 1 hour after a meal with a glass of water

Additional Information Does not reduce risk of transmitting HIV infections

Dosage Forms
Capsule: 100 mg
Injection: 10 mg/mL (20 mL)
Syrup (strawberry flavor): 50 mg/5 mL (240 mL)

Selected Readings

"Drugs for AIDS and Associated Infections," *Med Lett Drugs Ther*, 1993, 35(904):79-86.
Hirsch MS and D'Aquila RT, "Therapy for Human Immunodeficiency Virus Infection," *N Engl J Med*, 1993, 328(23):1686-95.
McLeod GX and Hammer SM, "Zidovudine: Five Years Later," *Ann Intern Med*, 1992, 117(6):487-501.
Skowron G, Bozzette SA, Lim L, et al, "Alternating and Intermittent Regimens of Zidovudine and Dideoxycytidine in Patients With AIDS or AIDS-Related Complex," *Ann Intern Med*, 1993, 118(5):321-30.

Zinacef® Injection see Cefuroxime *on page 524*

Zithromax™ see Azithromycin Dihydrate *on page 500*

Zolicef® see Cefazolin Sodium *on page 511*

Zosyn™ see Piperacillin Sodium and Tazobactam Sodium *on page 642*

Zovirax® see Acyclovir *on page 484*

APPENDIX

Pharmaceutical Measurements

Immunizations

Infectious Disease Information

Antimicrobial Activity Against Selected Organisms

**U.S. Department of Health and Human Services
Clinical Practice Guidelines**

Parenteral Nutrition Information

BODY SURFACE AREA OF ADULTS AND CHILDREN

Calculating Body Surface Area in Children

In a child of average size, find weight and corresponding surface area on the boxed scale to the left. Or, use the nomogram to the right. Lay a straightedge on the correct height and weight points for the child, then read the intersecting point on the surface area scale.

FOR CHILDREN OF
NORMAL HEIGHT AND WEIGHT

NOMOGRAM

BODY SURFACE AREA FORMULA
(Adult and Pediatric)

$$BSA\ (m^2) = \sqrt{\frac{Ht\ (in)\ x\ Wt\ (lb)}{3131}} \quad \text{or, in metric:} \quad BSA\ (m^2) = \sqrt{\frac{Ht\ (cm)\ x\ Wt\ (kg)}{3600}}$$

AVERAGE WEIGHTS AND SURFACE AREAS

Average Weight and Surface Area of Preterm Infants, Term Infants and Children

Age	Average Weight (kg)*	Approximate Surface Area (m²)
Weeks Gestation		
26	0.9-1	0.1
30	1.3-1.5	0.12
32	1.6-2	0.15
38	2.9-3	0.2
40	3.1-4	0.25
(term infant at birth)		
Months		
3	5	0.29
6	7	0.38
9	8	0.42
Year		
1	10	0.49
2	12	0.55
3	15	0.64
4	17	0.74
5	18	0.76
6	20	0.82
7	23	0.90
8	25	0.95
9	28	1.06
10	33	1.18
11	35	1.23
12	40	1.34
Adult	70	1.73

*Weights from age 3 months and over are rounded off to the nearest kilogram.

IDEAL BODY WEIGHT CALCULATION

Adults   (18 years and older)

IBW (male)   = 50 + (2.3 x height in inches over 5 feet)
IBW (female) = 45.5 + (2.3 x height in inches over 5 feet)
*IBW is in kg.

Children

a.   1-18 years

$$IBW = \frac{(height^2 \times 1.65)}{1000}$$

*IBW is in kg.
Height is in cm.

b.   5 feet and taller

IBW (male)   = 39 + (2.27 x height in inches over 5 feet)
IBW (female) = 42.2 + (2.27 x height in inches over 5 feet)
*IBW is in kg.

CREATININE CLEARANCE ESTIMATING METHODS
IN PATIENTS WITH STABLE RENAL FUNCTION

The following formulas provide an acceptable estimate of the patient's creatinine clearance except when:

   a.   patient's serum creatinine is changing rapidly (either up or down)

   b.   patients are markedly emaciated

In these situations (a and b above), certain assumptions have to be made.

   a.   In patients with rapidly rising serum creatinines (ie, $>0.5\text{-}0.7$ mg/dL/day), it is best to assume that the patient's creatinine clearance is probably <10 mL/minute.

   b.   In emaciated patients, although their actual creatinine clearance is less than their calculated creatinine clearance (because of decreased creatinine production), it is not possible to easily predict how much less.

Adults   (18 years and older)

Method 1: (Cockroft DW and Gault MH, *Nephron*, 1976, 16:31-41)

Estimated creatinine clearance (Cl_{cr}):
         (mL/min)

$$\text{Male} = \frac{(140 - \text{age})\ \text{IBW (kg)}}{72 \times S_{cr}}$$

$$\text{Female} = \text{Estimated } Cl_{cr} \text{ male} \times 0.85$$

Note: The use of the patient's ideal body weight (IBW) is recommended for the above formula except when the patient's actual body weight is less than ideal. Use of the IBW is especially important in obese patients.

Method 2: (Jelliffe RW, *Ann Intern Med*, 1973, 79:604)

Estimated creatinine clearance (Cl_{cr}):
         (mL/min/1.73 m^2)

$$\text{Male} = \frac{98 - 0.8\ (\text{age} - 20)}{S_{cr}}$$

$$\text{Female} = \text{Estimated } Cl_{cr} \text{ male} \times 0.90$$

Children   (1-18 years)

Method 1: (Traub SL, Johnson CE, *Am J Hosp Pharm*, 1980, 37:195-201)

$$Cl_{cr} = \frac{0.48 \times (\text{height}) \times \text{BSA}}{S_{cr} \times 1.73}$$

where

BSA	=	body surface area in m^2
Cl_{cr}	=	creatinine clearance in mL/min
S_{cr}	=	serum creatinine in mg/dL
Height	=	in cm

Method 2: Nomogram (Traub SL and Johnson CE, *Am J Hosp Pharm*, 1980, 37:195-201)

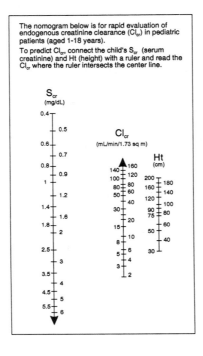

The nomogram below is for rapid evaluation of endogenous creatinine clearance (Cl_{cr}) in pediatric patients (aged 1-18 years).

To predict Cl_{cr}, connect the child's S_{cr} (serum creatinine) and Ht (height) with a ruler and read the Cl_{cr} where the ruler intersects the center line.

TEMPERATURE CONVERSION

Centigrade to Fahrenheit = (°C x 9/5) + 32 = °F
Fahrenheit to Centigrade = (°F - 32) x 5/9 = °C

°C	=	°F	°C	=	°F	°C	=	°F
100.0		212.0	39.0		102.2	36.8		98.2
50.0		122.0	38.8		101.8	36.6		97.9
41.0		105.8	38.6		101.5	36.4		97.5
40.8		105.4	38.4		101.1	36.2		97.2
40.6		105.1	38.2		100.8	36.0		96.8
40.4		104.7	38.0		100.4	35.8		96.4
40.2		104.4	37.8		100.1	35.6		96.1
40.0		104.0	37.6		99.7	35.4		95.7
39.8		103.6	37.4		99.3	35.2		95.4
39.6		103.3	37.2		99.0	35.0		95.0
39.4		102.9	37.0		98.6	0		32.0
39.2		102.6						

VACCINES

Table 1. **Vaccines To Be Considered for Patient Groups***

Patient Group	Major Vaccines†	Other Considerations‡
Healthy adults		
Adolescents and young adults	Td, MMR	
25-64 y	Td, rubella (women only), polio	
65 y and older	Td, influenza, pneumococcal	
Pregnant women	MMR is contraindicated; test for rubella antibody and hepatitis B surface antigen	
Environmental situations		
Nursing home residents	Influenza, pneumococcal	Tuberculin test
Institutionalized mentally retarded	Hepatitis B	
Prison inmates	Hepatitis B	
Homeless persons	Review all vaccines	Tuberculin test
Occupational groups		
College students	MMR; consider hepatitis B, polio, influenza	
Health care workers	Hepatitis B, influenza, MMR	
Essential community services	Influenza	
Day care center personnel	MMR, polio, influenza	IG (hepatitis A)
Laboratory personnel	Hepatitis B	Consider individually
Veterinarians, animal handlers, rural workers, other field personnel		Rabies, plague, anthrax
Immigrants and refugees	Review all vaccines, test for hepatitis B surface antigen	Tuberculin test
Lifestyles		
Homosexual and bisexual men	Hepatitis B	
Intravenous drug abusers	Hepatitis B, Td	
Prostitutes, persons with multiple sexual partners or sexually transmitted diseases	Hepatitis B	
Accidents		
Wounds	Td	TIG
Animal bites	Td	Rabies vaccine, RIG
Snake and spider bites	Td	Specific antivenins
Immunocompromised		
HIV infection and AIDS	Pneumococcal, influenza, hepatitis B	IG (measles), VZIG
Splenic disorders	Pneumococcal	*Haemophilus influenzae* type b, meningococcal
Diabetes	Pneumococcal, influenza	
Renal failure and dialysis	Pneumococcal, influenza Hepatitis B	
Alcoholism, cirrhosis	Pneumococcal, influenza	
Organ transplantation, immunosuppressive therapy	Pneumococcal, influenza	
Malignant diseases	Consider individually	

(continued)

Patient Group	Major Vaccines†	Other Considerations‡
Congenital immunodeficiency diseases		IG, IVIG
International travel	Review Td, MMR, polio; consider influenza, pneumococcal, hepatitis B	Yellow fever, IG, meningococcal, typhoid, cholera, rabies, Japanese encephalitis, antimalarial prophylaxis

From *Guide for Adult Immunization*, 2nd ed, American College of Physicians, 1990.

*See text for specific details on indications, administration, adverse reactions, precautions, contraindications, and special considerations for each vaccine, toxoid, and immune globulin preparation.

†Major vaccines include combined tetanus and diphtheria (Td) toxoids; measles, mumps, and rubella (MMR) vaccines; oral polio vaccine and enhanced-potency inactivated polio vaccine; influenza vaccine; pneumococcal vaccine; and hepatitis B vaccine.

‡Other considerations include immune globulin (IG), tetanus immune globulin (TIG), rabies immune globulin (RIG), varicella-zoster immune globulin (VZIG), and intravenous immune globulin (IVIG).

Table 2. **Reporting of Events Occurring After Vaccination**

	Vaccine Purchased With Public Money	Vaccine Purchased With Private Money
Who reports	Healthcare provider who administered the vaccine	Healthcare provider who administered the vaccine
What products to report	DTP, P, measles, mumps, rubella, DT, Td, T, OPV, IPV, and DTP/polio combined	DTP, P, measles, mumps, rubella, DT, Td, T, OPV, IPV, and DTP/polio combined
What reactions to report	Events listed in Table 3, including contraindicating reactions specified in manufacturers' package inserts	Events listed in Table 3, including contraindicating reactions specified in manufacturers' package inserts
How to report	Initial report taken by local, county, or state health department. State health department completes CDC form 71.19	Healthcare provider completes Adverse Reaction Report — FDA form 1639 (include interval from vaccination, manufacturer, and lot number on form)
Where to report	State health departments send CDC form 71.19 to: MSAEFI/IM (E05) Centers for Disease Control Atlanta, GA 30333	Completed FDA form 1639 is sent to: Food and Drug Administration (HFN-730) Rockville, MD 20857
Where to obtain forms	State health departments	FDA and publications such as *FDA Drug Bulletin*

MMWR, 1988, 37:197-200.

Table 3. **Reportable Events After Vaccination**

Vaccine/Toxoid	Event	Interval From Vaccination
DTP, P, DTP/polio combined	• Anaphylaxis or anaphylactic shock	24 h
	• Encephalopathy (or encephalitis)*	7 d
	• Shock-collapse or hypotonic-hyporesponsive collapse*	7 d
	• Residual seizure disorder*	See Aids to Interpretation*
	• Any acute complication or sequela (including death) of above events	No limit
	• Events in vaccines described in manufacturer's package insert as contraindications to additional doses of vaccine† (such as convulsions)	See package insert
Measles, mumps, and rubella; DT, Td, tetanus toxoid	• Anaphylaxis or anaphylactic shock	24 h
	• Encephalopathy (or encephalitis)*	15 d for measles, mumps, and rubella vaccines; 7 d for DT, Td, and T toxoids
	• Residual seizure disorder*	See Aids to Interpretation*
	• Any acute complication or sequela (including death) of above events	No limit
	• Events in vaccines described in manufacturer's package insert as contraindications to additional doses of vaccine†	See package insert
Oral polio vaccine	• Paralytic poliomyelitis	
	– in a nonimmunodeficient recipient	30 d
	– in an immunodeficient recipient	6 mo
	– in a vaccine-associated community case	No limit
	• Any acute complication or sequela (including death) of above events	No limit
	• Events in vaccines described in manufacturer's package insert as contraindications to additional doses of vaccine†	See package insert
Inactivated polio vaccine	• Anaphylaxis or anaphylactic shock	24 h
	• Any acute complication or sequela (including death) of above events	No limit
	• Events in vaccines described in manufacturer's package insert as contraindications to additional doses of vaccine†	See package insert

ˑAids to Interpretation:
Shock-collapse or hypotonic-hyporesponsive collapse may be evidenced by signs or symptoms such as decrease in or loss of muscle tone, paralysis (partial or complete), hemiplegia, hemiparesis, loss of color or turning pale white or blue, unresponsiveness to environmental stimuli, depression of or loss of consciousness, prolonged sleeping with difficulty arousing, or cardiovascular or respiratory arrest.

Residual seizure disorder may be considered to have occurred if no other seizure or convulsion, unaccompanied by fever or accompanied by a fever of less than 102°F, occurred before the first seizure or convulsion after the administration of the vaccine involved;

and if in the case of measles-, mumps-, or rubella-containing vaccines, the first seizure or convulsion occurred within 15 days after vaccination **or**, in the case of any other vaccine, the first seizure or convulsion occurred within 3 days after vaccination;

and if two or more seizures or convulsions unaccompanied by fever or accompanied by a fever of less than 102°F occurred within 1 year after vaccination.

The terms seizure and convulsion include grand mal, petit mal, absence, myoclonic, tonic-clonic, and focal motor seizures and signs. Encephalopathy means any significant, acquired abnormality, injury to or impairment of function of the brain. Among the frequent manifestations of encephalopathy are focal and diffuse neurologic signs, increased intracranial pressure, or changes lasting at least 6 hours in level of consciousness (with or without convulsions). The neurologic signs and symptoms of encephalopathy may be temporary with complete recovery, or they may result in various degrees of permanent impairment. Signs and symptoms such as high-pitched and unusual screaming, persistent unconsolable crying, and bulging fontanelle are compatible with an encephalopathy, but in and of themselves are not conclusive evidence of encephalopathy. Encephalopathy usually can be documented by slow wave activity on an electroencephalogram.

†The healthcare provider must refer to the **Contraindication** section of the manufacturer's package insert for each vaccine.

Adapted from *MMWR Morb Mortal Wkly Rep*, 1988, 37:197-200.

IMMUNIZATION GUIDELINES

Table 1. **Dosage and Administration Guidelines for Vaccines Available in the United States**

Vaccine	Dosage	Route of Administration	Type
DT*	0.5 mL	I.M.	Toxoids
Td*	0.5 mL	I.M.	Toxoids
DTP*	0.5 mL	I.M.	Diphtheria and tetanus toxoids with killed *B. pertussis* organisms
DTaP (Acel-Imune™)‖	0.5 mL	I.M.	Diphtheria and tetanus toxoids with acellular pertussis
DTP-HbOC (Tetramune™)+	0.5 mL	I.M.	Diphtheria and tetanus toxoids with killed *B pertussis* organisms and *Haemophilus* b conjugate (diphtheria CRM_{197} protein conjugate)
Haemophilus B conjugate vaccine	0.5 mL	I.M.	
ProHIBit™ (PRP-D), manufactured by Connaught Laboratories	0.5 mL	I.M.	Polysaccharide (diphtheria toxoid conjugate)
HibTITER™ (HbOC),† manufactured by Praxis Biologicals	0.5 mL	I.M.	Oligosaccharide (diphtheria CRM_{197} protein conjugate)
PedvaxHIB™ (PRP-OMP),‡ manufactured by MSD	0.5 mL	I.M.	Polysaccharide (meningococcal protein conjugate)
Hepatitis B§		I.M. in the anterolateral thigh or in the upper arm; S.C. in individuals at risk of hemorrhage	Yeast recombinant-derived inactivated viral antigen
Infants born to HB_sAg-negative mothers and children <11 y■			
Recombivax HB™ (MSD)	2.5 µg (0.25 mL)		
Engerix-B™ (SKF)	10 µg (0.5 mL)		

Infants born to HB_sAg-positive mothers (immunization and administration of 0.5 mL hepatitis B immune globulin is recommended for **infants** born to HB_sAg^+ mothers using different administration sites) within 12 hours of birth; administer vaccine at birth; repeat vaccine dose at 1 and 6 months following the initial dose

Recombivax HB™ (MSD)	5 µg (0.5 mL)		
Engerix-B™ (SKF)	10 µg (0.5 mL)		
Children 11-19 y			
Recombivax HB™ (MSD)	5 µg (0.5 mL)		
Engerix-B™ (SKF)	20 µg (1 mL)		
Adults >19 y			
Recombivax HB™ (MSD)	10 µg (1 mL)		
Engerix-B™ (SKF)	20 µg (1 mL)		
Dialysis patients and immunosuppressed patients			

(continued)

Vaccine	Dosage	Route of Administration	Type
Recombivax HB™ (MSD)	<11 y, 20 μg (0.5 mL); ≥11 y, 40 μg (1 mL) using special dialysis formulation		
Engerix-B™ (SKF)¶	<11 y, 20 μg (1 mL); ≥11 y, 40 μg (2 mL), give as two 1 mL doses at different sites		
Influenza split virus only in pediatric patients		I.M. (2 doses 4+ weeks apart in children <9 years of age not previously immunized; only 1 dose needed for annual updates)	Inactivated virus subvirion (split) (contraindicated in patients allergic to chicken eggs)
6-35 mo	0.25 mL (1 or 2 doses)		
3-8 y	0.5 mL (1 or 2 doses)		
≥9 y	0.5 mL (1 dose)		
Measles	0.5 mL	S.C.	Live virus (contraindicated in patients with anaphylactic allergy to neomycin)

Most areas: Two doses (1st dose at 15 months with MMR; 2nd dose at 4-6 years or 11-12 years, depending on local school entry requirements)

High-risk area: Two doses (1st dose at 12 months with MMR; 2nd dose as above)

Children 6-15 months in epidemic situations: Dose is given at the time of first contact with a health care provider; children <1 year of age should receive single antigen measles vaccine. If vaccinated before 1 year, revaccinate at 15 months with MMR. A 3rd dose is administered at 4-6 years or 11-12 years, depending on local school entry requirements.

Vaccine	Dosage	Route of Administration	Type
Meningococcal	0.5 mL#	S.C.	Polysaccharide
MMR•	0.5 mL	S.C.	Live virus
MR	0.5 mL	S.C.	Live virus
Mumps	0.5 mL	S.C.	Live virus
Pneumococcal polyvalent♦	0.5 mL (≥2 y)	I.M. or S.C. (I.M. preferred)	Polysaccharide
Poliovirus (OPV) trivalent	0.5 mL	Oral	Live virus
Poliovirus (IPV)**·†† trivalent	0.5 mL	S.C.	Inactivated virus
Rabies	1 mL	I.M.‡‡, ID§§	Inactivated virus
Rubella	0.5 mL (≥12 mo)¶¶	S.C.	Live virus
Tetanus (adsorbed)##	0.5 mL	I.M.	Toxoid
Tetanus (fluid)	0.5 mL	I.M., S.C.	Toxoid
Yellow fever	0.5 mL➥	S.C.	Live attenuated virus

*DT & DTP for use in children <7 years of age. Td contains same amount of tetanus toxoid as DT & DTP, but a reduced dose of diphtheria toxoid. Td for use in children ≥7 years of age.

‖DTaP (Acel-Imune™) may be used only for the 4th and 5th doses for children >15 months and <7 years of age. The occurrence of fever and local reactions is lower with acellular pertussis vaccine than with whole-cell DTP.

*DTP-HbOC may be substituted for DTP and *Haemophilus* B conjugate vaccines which are administered separately, whenever recommended schedules for use of these 2 vaccines coincide. Initiate at 2 months of age for 3 doses (2 months, 4 months, and 6 months), followed by a 4th dose at 15-18 months of age. DTaP and *Haemophilus* B conjugate vaccine may be administered separately as an alternative to DTP-HbOC at 15-18 months of age.

†The conjugate (HbCV) vaccine is preferred over the polysaccharide (HbPV) vaccine. In children with a high risk for *Haemophilus influenzae* type b disease and HbCV is unavailable, an acceptable alternate is to give HbPV at 18 months of age with a 2nd dose at 24 months of age. Children <5 years of age who were previously vaccinated with HbPV between 18-23 months of age should be revaccinated with a single dose of HbCV at least 2 months after the initial dose of HbPV. Either HbCV or HbPV can be administered up to the 5th birthday. However they are generally not recommended for children >5 years of age.

‡PRP-OMP (PedvaxHIB®) manufactured by Merck, Sharp & Dohme is initiated at 2 months of age for 3 doses (2 months, 4 months and 12 months). If initiated at 7-11 months of age, 3 doses are administered (initial 2 doses at 2-month intervals, 3rd dose at 15-18 months of age); initiated at 12-14 months of age, 2 doses are administered at 2- to 3-month intervals between doses; initiated at 15-59 months of age, 1 dose is administered.

§Hepatitis B vaccine can be given at the same time with DTP, HbOC, polio, and/or MMR; administer 3 doses at 0, 1, and 6 months).

■Administer to newborns at 0-2 days of age before hospital discharge; repeat at 1-2 months and 6-18 months following the initial dose. If not vaccinated at birth, administer at 2, 4, and 6-18 months of age.

¶Engerix-B® — an alternate schedule for postexposure prophylaxis or more rapid induction using 4 doses at 0, 1, 2, and 12 months of age is recommended.

#Indicated in children ≥2 years of age at risk in epidemic or highly endemic areas.

•See measles.

♦Indicated for children with sickle cell disease; asplenia; nephrotic syndrome or chronic renal failure; conditions associated with immunosuppression; CSF leaks; HIV infection.

**The primary series consists of 3 doses. The first 2 doses should be administered at an interval of 8 weeks. The 3rd dose should be given at least 6 and preferably 12 months after the 2nd dose. A booster dose of 0.5 mL should be given to all children who have completed the primary series, before entering school. However, if the 3rd dose of the primary series is given on or after the 4th birthday, a 4th dose is not required before entering school. When polio vaccine is given to persons >18 years of age, IPV should be given.

††IPV is indicated for unimmunized or partially immunized patients with compromised immunity; HIV infection; unimmunized adults (>18 years of age) or adults at future risk of exposure to poliomyelitis; household contacts of an immunodeficient individual.

‡‡In infants and small children, I.M. injection can be given into the midlateral aspect of the thigh; in older children and adults, I.M. injection can be given into the deltoid muscle. Repeat doses are given on days 3, 7, 14, and 28 postexposure.

§§For pre-exposure prophylaxis against rabies for high-risk individuals, 1 mL I.M. or 0.1 mL intradermal is administered on days 0, 7, and 21 (or 28). Both I.M. and I.D. dosage forms are available.

¶¶As MMR in a 2-dose schedule.

##Adsorbed preferred to fluid toxoid because of longer lasting immunity.

➡≥9 months of age living in or traveling to endemic areas. Contraindicated in infants <4 months of age and in patients who have had an anaphylactic reaction to eggs. Increased risk of encephalitis associated with use of yellow fever vaccine in infants <9 months of age.

Note: For each vaccine, check the manufacturer's package insert for specific product information since preparations may change from time to time.

References:

ACIP, General Recommendations on Immunization, MMWR 1989, 38:205-14, 219-27.

ACIP, Measles Prevention, Recommendations of the Immunization Practices Advisory Committee, MMWR 1989, 38(5-9):1-18.

American Academy of Pediatrics, Report of the Committee on Infectious Diseases (Red Book), 22nd ed. 1991.

American Academy of Pediatrics, Committee on Infectious Diseases, "Acellular Pertussis Vaccines: Recommendations for Use as the Fourth and Fifth Doses," *Pediatrics*, 1992, 90:121-3.

American Academy of Pediatrics, Committee on Infectious Diseases, "Universal Hepatitis B Immunization," *Pediatrics*, 1992, 89:795-800.

Table 2. **Recommended Schedule for Active Immunization
of Normal Infants and Children****

Recommended Age	Vaccine(s)	Comments
2 mo	DTP1,* OPV1, HbCV1†	OPV and DTP can be given earlier in areas of high endemicity or during epidemics; DTP-HbOC can be given in place of DTP1 and HbCV1
4 mo	DTP2, OPV2, HbCV2†	6 weeks to 2 months interval desired between OPV doses; DTP-HbOC can be given in place of DTP2 and HbCV2
6 mo	DTP3, HbOC3	An additional dose of OPV is optional in high risk areas; DTP-HbOC can be given in place of DTP3 and HbOC3
12 mo	PRP-OMP	
15 mo	MMR,‡ DTP4,¶ OPV3, HbCV3, or HbCV4§	Completion of primary series of DTP and OPV; DTP-HbOC can be given in place of DTP4 and HbCV
4-6 y	DTP5,¶ OPV4, measles	At or before school entry
11-12 y	MMR	At entry to middle school unless 2nd dose was given at 4-6 years at time of school entry
14-16 y	Td	Repeat every 10 years throughout life

**Please also refer to Hepatitis B Vaccine Guidelines in Table 1.

*DTP may be used up to the 7th birthday. The 1st dose can be given at 6th week of age, and the 2nd and 3rd doses given 4-8 weeks after the preceding dose.

†HbCV — can use either HbOC or PRP-OMP.

‡Can be given at 12 months of age in high-risk areas.

§HbCV — can use either PRP-OMP, PRP-D, or HbOC for children ≥15 months of age.

¶DTaP may be used in place of whole cell DTP only for the 4th and 5th doses for children >15 months and <7 years of age. DTaP can be given at the same time with OPV, IPV, MMR, *Haemophilus influenzae* type b conjugate vaccine, and/or hepatitis B vaccine.

References:

Centers for Disease Control, "Protection Against Viral Hepatitis: Recommendations of the Immunization Practices Advisory Committee (ACIP)," *MMWR Morb Mortal Wkly Rep*, 1990, 39:11.

American Academy of Pediatrics Committee on Infectious Diseases, "*Haemophilus influenzae* Type B Conjugate Vaccines: Recommendations for Immunization of Infants and Children 2 Months of Age and Older," *Pediatrics*, 1991, 88(1):169-72.

Table 3. **Recommended Immunization Schedule for Infants and Children up to the 7th Birthday Not Immunized at the Recommended Time in Early Infancy**

Timing	Vaccine(s)	Comments
First visit	DTP1, OPV1 MMR* (if child ≥15 months)	DTP, OPV and MMR should be administered simultaneously to children ≥15 months of age
	HbCV† ‡	DTP, OPV, MMR and HbCV may be given simultaneously to children aged 15 months to 5 years at separate sites
2 mo after DTP1, OPV1	DTP2, OPV2 (HbCV)‡	Second HbCV for children whose 1st dose was received when <15 months of age
2 mo after DTP2	DTP3	An additional dose of OPV is optional in high-risk areas
6-12 mo after DTP3	DTP4§ (OPV3)	OPV is given if 3rd dose was not given earlier
4-6 y	DTP5,§ OPV4 (MMR2)	Preferably at or before school entry. OTP5 and OPV4 are not needed if DTP4 and OPV3 were given after the 4th birthday. Local public health regulations may require MMR2 at school entry.
11-12 y	MMR2	MMR2 is given if 2nd dose was not given earlier
14-16 y	Td	Repeat every 10 years throughout life

*Can be given at 12 months of age to children residing in areas at high-risk for measles transmission.

†Only HbOC or PRP-OMP are licensed for use in children <15 months of age.

‡DTP-HbOC may be substituted for DTP and *Haemophilus* B conjugate vaccines which are administered separately, whenever recommended schedules for use of these 2 vaccines coincide. Initiate at 2 months of age for 3 doses (2 months, 4 months, and 6 months), followed by a 4th dose at 15-18 months of age. DTaP and *Haemophilus* B conjugate vaccine may be administered separately as an alternative to DTP-HbOC at 15-18 months.

§DTaP may be used in place of whole cell DTP only for the 4th and 5th doses for children >15 months and <7 years of age.

Table 4. **Recommended Immunization Schedule for Children >7 Years of Age Not Immunized at the Recommended Time in Early Infancy**

Timing	Vaccine(s)	Comments
First visit	Td1, OPV1, MMR, HbCV*	OPV not routinely recommended for persons ≥18 years of age
2 mo after Td1, OPV1	Td2, OPV2	OPV may be given as soon as 6 weeks after OPV1
6-12 mo after Td2, OPV2	Td3, OPV3	OPV3 may be given as soon as 6 weeks after OPV2
10 y after Td3	Td	Repeat every 10 years throughout life
11-12 y	MMR	

*Indicated only in children with a chronic illness associated with increased risk of *Haemophilus influenzae* type B disease.

Table 5. **High-Risk Groups Who Should Receive Hepatitis B Immunization Regardless of Age***

- Hemophiliac patients and other recipients of certain blood products
- Intravenous drug abusers
- Heterosexual persons who have had more than one sex partner in the previous 6 months and/or those with a recent episode of a sexually transmitted disease
- Sexually active homosexual and bisexual males
- Household and sexual contacts of hepatitis B virus (HBV) carriers
- Members of households with adoptees from HBV-endemic, high-risk countries who are hepatitis B surface antigen-positive
- Children and other household contacts in populations of high HBV endemnicity
- Staff and residents of institutions for the developmentally disabled
- Staff of nonresidential day care and school programs for developmentally disabled if attended by known HBV carrier; other attendees in certain circumstances
- Hemodialysis patients
- Health care workers and others with occupational risk
- International travelers who will live for more than 6 months in areas of high HBV endemnicity and who otherwise will be at risk
- Inmates of long-term correctional facilities

*Adapted from Report of the Committee on Infectious Disease, 1991, 246-9.

Table 6. **Guidelines for Spacing Live and Killed Antigen Administration**

Antigen Combinations	Recommended Minimum Interval Between Doses
≥2 killed antigens	None. May be given simultaneously or at any interval between doses.
Killed and live antigens	None. May be given simultaneously or at any interval between doses. (Exception: Concurrent administration of cholera and yellow fever vaccines should be avoided. Separate these vaccines by at least 3 weeks.)
≥2 live antigens	4 weeks minimum interval if not administered simultaneously. (Recent receipt of OPV is not a contraindication to MMR.) Vaccines associated with systemic reactions (cholera and parenteral typhoid or influenza and DTP in young children) should be given on separate occasions.

Table 7. **Passive Immunization Agents — Immune Globulins**

Immune Globulin	Dosage	Route
Hepatitis B (H-BIG")		I.M.
percutaneous inoculation	0.06 mL/kg/dose (within 24 hours) (5 mL max)	
perinatal	0.5 mL/dose (within 12 hours of birth)	
sexual exposure	0.06 mL/kg/dose (within 14 days of contact) (5 mL max)	
Immune globulin (IG)		I.M.*
hepatitis A prophylaxis	0.02 mL/kg/dose (as soon as possible or within 2 weeks after exposure) (single exposure)	
	0.06 mL/kg/dose (>3 months or continuous exposure) repeat every 4-6 months	
hepatitis B	0.06 mL/kg/dose (H-BIG® should be used)	
hepatitis C	0.06 mL/kg/dose (percutaneous exposure)	
measles†	0.25 mL/kg/dose (max 15 mL/dose) (within 6 days of exposure)	
	0.5 mL/kg/dose (max 15 mL/dose) (immunocompromised children)	
Rabies‡	20 IU/kg/dose (within 3 days)	
Tetanus (serious, contaminated, wounds; <3 previous tetanus vaccine doses)	250-500 units/dose	I.M.
Varicella-zoster§ (VZIG)	Within 48 hours but not later than 96 hours after exposure	I.M.¶
	0-10 kg 125 units = 1 vial	
	10.1-20 kg 250 units = 2 vials	
	20.1-30 kg 375 units = 3 vials	
	30.1-40 kg 500 units = 4 vials	
	>40 kg 625 units = 5 vials	

*Deep I.M. in the gluteal region for large doses only. Deltoid muscle or the anterolateral aspect of the thigh are preferred sites for injection. No greater than 5 mL/site in adults or large children; 1-3 mL/site in small children and infants. Maximum dose: 20 mL at one time.

†IG prophylaxis may not be indicated in a patient who has received IGIV within 3 weeks of exposure.

‡½ of dose used to infiltrate the wound with the remaining ½ of dose given I.M. Rabies immune globulin is not recommended in previously HDCV immunized patients.

§Infants born to women who develop varicella within 5 days before or 48 hours after delivery should receive 125 units I.M. as a single dose.

¶No greater than 2.5 mL of VZIG/one injection site. Doses >2.5 mL should be divided and administered at different sites.

Table 8. **Guidelines for Spacing the Administration of Immune Globulin (IG) Preparations and Vaccines**

Immunobiologic Combinations	Recommended Minimum Interval Between Doses
Simultaneous Administration	
IG and killed antigen	None. May be given simultaneously at different sites or at any time between doses.
IG and live antigen	Should generally not be given simultaneously. If unavoidable to do so, give at different sites and revaccinate or test for seroconversion in 3 months. Example: MMR should not be given to patients who have received immune globulin within the previous 3 months.

Nonsimultaneous Administration

First	Second	
IG	Killed antigen	None
Killed antigen	IG	None
IG	Live antigen	6 weeks, and preferably 3 months
Live antigen	IG	2 weeks

*The live virus vaccines, OPV, and yellow fever are exceptions to these recommendations. Either vaccine may be administered simultaneously or any time before or after IG without significantly decreasing antibody response.

Table 9. **Recommended for Routine Immunization of HIV-Infected Children — United States**

Vaccine	Known HIV Infection	
	Asymptomatic	Symptomatic
DTP	Yes	Yes
OPV	No	No
IPV	Yes	Yes
MMR	Yes	Yes
HbCV	Yes	Yes
Pneumococcal	Yes	Yes
Influenza	No*	Yes

*Not contraindicated.

INFLUENZA VACCINE*

Target Groups for Special Vaccination Programs

To maximize protection of high-risk persons, they and their close contacts should be targeted for organized vaccination programs.

Groups at Increased Risk for Influenza-Related Complications:

- Persons ≥65 years of age
- Residents of nursing homes and other chronic-care facilities that house persons of any age with chronic medical conditions
- Adults and children with chronic disorders of the pulmonary or cardiovascular systems, including children with asthma
- Adults and children who have required regular medical follow-up or hospitalization during the preceding year because of chronic metabolic diseases (including diabetes mellitus), renal dysfunction, hemoglobinopathies, or immunosuppression (including immunosuppression caused by medications)
- Children and teenagers (6 months to 18 years of age) who are receiving long-term aspirin therapy and therefore, may be at risk for developing Reye syndrome after influenza

Influenza Vaccine* Dosage by Age Group — United States, 1994-95 Season

Age	Product†	Dosage	No. Doses
6-35 mo	Split virus only	0.25 mL	1 or 2‡
3-8 y	Split virus only	0.50 mL	1 or 2‡
9-12 y	Split virus only	0.50 mL	1
>12 y	Whole or split virus	0.50 mL	1

Vaccine given I.M.; the recommended site of vaccination is the deltoid muscle for adults and older children. The preferred site for infants and young children is the anterolateral aspect of the thigh.

*Contains 15 μg each of A/Texas/36/91-like (H1N1), A/Shangdong/9/93-like (H3N2), and B/Panama/45/90-like hemagglutinin antigens in each 0.5 mL. Manufacturers include: Connaught Laboratories, Inc (Fluzone® whole or split); Evans Medical Ltd (distributed by Adams Laboratories, Inc) (Fluviron™ purified surface antigen vaccine); Parke-Davis (Flugen™ split); and Wyeth-Ayerst Laboratories (Flushield™ split). For further product information call Connaught, (800) 822-2463; Adams, (800) 932-1950; Parke-Davis, (800) 223-0432; Wyeth-Ayerst, (800) FLU-SHIELD.

†Because of the lower potential for causing febrile reactions, only split-virus vaccines should be used for children. They may be labeled as "split," "subvirion," or "purified-surface-antigen" vaccine. Immunogenicity and side effects of split- and whole-virus vaccines are similar among adults when vaccines are administered at the recommended dosage.

‡Two doses administered at least 1 month apart are recommended for children <9 years of age who are receiving influenza vaccine for the first time.

Groups That Can Transmit Influenza to Persons at High Risk

Persons who are clinically or subclinically infected and who care for or live with members of high-risk groups can transmit influenza virus to them. Some persons at high risk (eg, the elderly, transplant recipients, and persons with AIDS) can have low antibody responses to influenza vaccine. Efforts to protect these members of high-risk groups against influenza may be improved by reducing the likelihood of influenza exposure from their care givers. The following groups should be vaccinated:

- Physicians, nurses, and other personnel in both hospital and outpatient-care settings
- Employees of nursing homes and chronic-care facilities who have contact with patients or residents
- Providers of home care to persons at high risk (eg, visiting nurses and volunteer workers)
- Household members (including children) of persons in high-risk groups

*From *MMWR Morb Mortal Wkly Rep*, 1994, 43(RR9):4-5.

POSTEXPOSURE PROPHYLAXIS FOR HEPATITIS B*

Exposure	Hepatitis B Immune Globulin	Hepatitis B Vaccine
Perinatal	0.5 mL I.M. within 12 h of birth	0.5 mL† I.M. within 12 h of birth (no later than 7 d), and at 1 and 6 mo‡; test for HB_sAg and anti-HB_s at 12-15 mo
Sexual	0.06 mL/kg I.M. within 14 d of sexual contact; a second dose should be given if the index patient remains HB_sAg-positive after 3 mo and hepatitis B vaccine was not given initially	1 mL I.M. at 0, 1, and 6 mo for homosexual and bisexual men and regular sexual contacts of persons with acute and chronic hepatitis B
Percutaneous; exposed person unvaccinated		
Source known HB_sAg-positive	0.06 mL/kg I.M. within 24 h	1 mL I.M. within 7 d, and at 1 and 6 mo§
Source known, HB_sAg status not known	Test source for HB_sAg; if source is positive, give exposed person 0.06 mL/kg I.M. once within 7 d	1 mL I.M. within 7 d, and at 1 and 6 mo§
Source not tested or unknown	Nothing required	1 mL I.M. within 7 d, and at 1 and 6 mo
Percutaneous; exposed person vaccinated		
Source known HB_sAg-positive	Test exposed person for anti-HB_s¶. If titer is protective, nothing is required; if titer is not protective, give 0.06 mL/kg within 24 h	Review vaccination status#
Source known, HB_sAg status not known	Test source for HB_sAg and exposed person for anti-HB_s. If source is HB_sAg-negative, or if source is HB_sAg-positive but anti-HB_s titer is protective, nothing is required. If source is HB_sAg-positive and anti-HB_s titer is not protective or if exposed person is a known nonresponder, give 0.06 mL/kg I.M. within 24 h. A second dose of hepatitis B immune globulin can be given 1 mo later if a booster dose of hepatitis B vaccine is not given.	Review vaccination status#
Source not tested or unknown	Test exposed person for anti-HB_s. If anti-HB_s titer is protective, nothing is required. If anti-HB_s titer is not protective, 0.06 mL/kg may be given along with a booster dose of hepatitis B vaccine	Review vaccination status#

*HB_sAg = hepatitis B surface antigen; anti-HB_s = antibody to hepatitis B surface antigen; I.M. = intramuscularly; SRU = standard ratio units.

†Each 0.5 mL dose of plasma-derived hepatitis B vaccine contains 10 μg of HB$_s$Ag; each 0.5 mL dose of recombinant hepatitis B vaccine contains 5 μg (Merck Sharp & Dohme) or 10 μg (SmithKline Beecham) of HB$_s$Ag.

‡If hepatitis B immune globulin and hepatitis B vaccine are given simultaneously, they should be given at separate sites.

§If hepatitis B vaccine is not given, a second dose of hepatitis B immune globulin should be given 1 month later.

¶Anti-HB$_s$ titers <10 SRU by radioimmunoassay or negative by enzyme immunoassay indicate lack of protection. Testing the exposed person for anti-HB$_s$ is not necessary if a protective level of antibody has been shown within the previous 24 months.

#If the exposed person has not completed a three-dose series of hepatitis B vaccine, the series should be completed. Test the exposed person for anti-HB$_s$. If the antibody level is protective, nothing is required. If an adequate antibody response in the past is shown on retesting to have declined to an inadequate level, a booster dose (1 mL) of hepatitis B vaccine should be given. If the exposed person has inadequate antibody or is a known nonresponder to vaccination, a booster dose can be given along with one dose of hepatitis B immune globulin.

AMINOGLYCOSIDE DOSING AND MONITORING

All aminoglycoside therapy should be individualized for specific patients in specific clinical situation. The following are guidelines for initiating therapy.

1. Loading dose based on estimated ideal body weight (IBW). **All patients require a loading dose independent of renal function**.

Agent	Dose
Gentamicin	2 mg/kg
Tobramycin	2 mg/kg
Amikacin	7.5 mg/kg

Significantly higher loading doses may be required in severely ill intensive care unit patients.

2. Initial maintenance doses as a percent of loading dose according to desired dosing interval and creatinine clearance (Cl_{cr}):

$$\text{Male } Cl_{cr} \text{ (mL/min)} = \frac{(140 - \text{age}) \times IBW}{72 \times \text{serum creatinine}}$$

$$\text{Female} = 0.85 \times Cl_{cr} \text{ males}$$

Cl_{cr} (mL/min)	Dosing Interval (h) 8	12	24
90	84%	—	—
80	80%	—	—
70	76%	88%	—
60	—	84%	—
50	—	79%	—
40	—	72%	92%
30	—	—	86%
25	—	—	81%
20	—	—	75%

Patients older than 65 years of age should not receive initial aminoglycoside maintenance dosing more often than every 12 hours.

3. Serum concentration monitoring

   a. Serum concentration monitoring is necessary for **safe** and **effective** therapy, particularly in patients with serious infections and those with risk factors for toxicity.

   b. Peak serum concentrations should be drawn 30 minutes after the completion of a 30-minute infusion. Trough serum concentrations should be drawn within 30 minutes prior to the administered dose.

   c. Serum concentrations should be drawn after 5 half-lives, usually around the third dose or thereafter.

4. Desired measured serum concentrations

	Peak (μg/mL)	Trough (μg/mL)
Gentamicin	6-10	0.5-2
Tobramycin	6-10	0.5-2
Amikacin	20-30	<5
Netilmycin	4-10	<2

5. For patients receiving hemodialysis:

- administer the **same** loading dose
- administer ⅔ of the loading dose after each dialysis
- **serum concentrations must be monitored**
- watch for ototoxicity from accumulation of drug

6. For individual clinical situations the prescribing physician should feel free to consult Infectious Disease, the Pharmacology Service, or the Pharmacy.

AMINOGLYCOSIDE PENETRATION INTO VARIOUS TISSUES

Site	Extent of Distribution
Eye	Poor
CNS	Poor (<25%)
Pleural	Excellent
Bronchial secretions	Poor
Sputum	Fair (10%-50%)
Pulmonary tissue	Excellent
Ascitic fluid	Variable (43%-132%)
Peritoneal fluid	Poor
Bile	Variable (25%-90%)
Bile with obstruction	Poor
Synovial fluid	Excellent
Bone	Poor
Prostate	Poor
Urine	Excellent
Renal tissue	Excellent

From Neu HC, "Pharmacology of Aminoglycosides," *The Aminoglycosides*, Whelton E, Neu HC, eds, New York, NY: Marcel Dekker, Inc, 1981.

TIMING OF FOOD POISONING

Symptoms	Time from Ingestion			
	<2 h	2-7 h	8-14 h	>14 h
Nausea/vomiting	—	*S. aureus* *B. cereus*	—	—
Diarrhea	—	—	*C. perfringens* *B. cereus*	*V. cholerae* Enterotoxic or invasive *E. coli* *Shigella* sp *Vibrio* sp
Both upper and lower gastrointestinal	—	—	—	*Salmonella* *Vibrio* sp
Extragastrointestinal (ie, some gastrointestinal plus other symptoms, usually paresthesias or other abnormal sensory complaints)	Scombrotoxin Shellfish toxin Mushroom toxin	Ciguatoxin	Mushroom toxin	*C. botulinum*

From Altman DF, "Food Poisoning," *Cecil's Textbook of Medicine*, 19th ed, chapter 110, Wyngaarden JB, Smith LH Jr, and Bennett JC, eds, Philadelphia, PA: WB Saunders Co, 1992.

INTERPRETATION OF GRAM STAIN RESULTS GUIDELINES

These guidelines are not definitive but presumptive for the identification of organisms on Gram stain. Treatment will depend on the quality of the specimen and appropriate clinical evaluation.

Gram-Negative Bacilli (GNB)	**Example**
Enterobacteriaceae	*E coli* *Serratia* sp *Klebsiella* sp *Enterobacter* sp *Citrobacter* sp
Pseudomonas aeruginosa	
Xanthomonas maltophilia	
Nonfermentative GNB	
Haemophilus influenzae	
Bacteroides fragilis group	
If fusiform (long and pointed)	*Fusobacterium* sp *Capnocytophaga* sp

Gram-Negative Cocci (GNC)	
Diplococci, pairs	*Neisseria meningitidis* *Neisseria gonorrhoeae* *Moraxella (Branhamella)* *catarrhalis*
Coccobacilli	*Acinetobacter* sp

Gram-Positive Bacilli (GPB)	
Diphtheroids (small pleomorphic)	*Corynebacterium* sp *Propionibacterium*
Large, with spores	*Clostridium* sp *Bacillus* sp
Branching, beaded, rods	*Nocardia* sp *Actinomyces* sp
Other	*Listeria* sp *Lactobacillus* sp

Gram-Positive Cocci (GPC)	
Pairs, chains, clusters	*Staphylococcus* sp *Streptococcus* sp *Enterococcus* sp
Pairs, lancet-shaped	*S pneumoniae*

KEY CHARACTERISTICS OF SELECTED BACTERIA

Gram-Negative Bacilli (GNB)

Lactose-positive	*Escherichia coli* *Klebsiella pneumoniae* *Enterobacter* sp* *Citrobacter* sp*
Lactose-negative/ oxidase-negative	*Proteus mirabilis:* indole negative *Proteus vulgaris:* indole positive *Providencia* sp *Morganella morganii* *Serratia* sp† *Salmonella* sp *Shigella* sp *Acinetobacter* sp *Xanthomonas maltophilia*
Lactose-negative/ oxidase-positive	*Pseudomonas aeruginosa* *Aeromonas hydrophila* (may be lactose positive) Other *Pseudomonas* sp *Moraxella* sp‡ *Alcaligenes* sp *Flavobacterium* sp
Other	*Haemophilus influenzae* (coccobacillus)

Gram-Positive Bacilli (GPB)

Often blood culture contaminants	Diphtheroids (may be *Corynebacterium* sp)
Resistant to many agents except vancomycin	*C. jeikeium*
Anaerobic diphtheroids	*Propionibacterium acnes*
Bacillus sp	*B cereus, B subtilis*
CSF, blood	*Listeria monocytogenes*
Vaginal flora, rarely blood	*Lactobacillus* sp
Branching, beaded; partial acid-fast positive	*Nocardia* sp
Rapidly growing mycobacteria	*M fortuitum* *M chelonei*

Gram-Positive Cocci (GPC)

Catalase-positive	*Staphylococcus* sp
Catalase-negative	*Streptococcus* sp (chains) *Micrococcus* sp (usually insignificant)
Coagulase-positive	*S aureus*
Coagulase-negative	Coagulase-negative staphylococci (CNS)
Bloods	*S epidermidis* or CNS
Urine	*S saprophyticus* (CNS)

INFECTIOUS DISEASE INFORMATION

Fungi	Example
Yeast	*Candida* sp (germ tube positive = *C albicans*)
	Cryptococcus sp (no pseudohyphae)
	C neoformans
	Torulopsis glabrata
	Trichosporon sp
	Rhodotorula, Saccharomyces sp
Molds	
Sparsely septate hyphae	Zygomycetes (eg, *Rhizopus* sp and *Mucor*)
Septate hyphae brown pigment	Phaeohyphomycetes, for example,
	Bipolaris sp
	Exserohilum sp
	Alternaria sp
	Curvularia sp
Nonpigmented (hyaline)	Hyalophomycetes, for example
	Aspergillus sp (*A fumigatus, A flavus*)
	Fusarium sp
	Penicillium sp
	Paecilomyces sp
	Dermatophytes
Thermally dimorphic (yeast in tissue; mold *in vitro*)	*Histoplasma capsulatum* (slow growing)
	Blastomyces dermatitidis
	Coccidioides immitis
	Sporothrix schenckii
	Paracoccidioides brasiliensis

Anaerobes	
Gram-positive bacilli	*Propionibacterium acnes*
	Clostridium sp (spores)
	Actinomyces sp (branching, filamentous)
	Lactobacillus sp
	Eubacterium sp
	Bifidobacterium sp
Gram-positive cocci	*Peptostreptococcus* sp
Gram-negative bacilli	*Bacteroides* sp (*B fragilis*)
	Fusobacterium sp
Gram-negative cocci	*Veillonella* sp

Most Common Blood Culture Contaminants

Coagulase-negative staphylococci

Alpha-hemolytic streptococci

Diphtheroids

Micrococcus sp

Lactobacilli

Propionibacterium sp

Bacillus sp

---

*May be lactose-negative.
†May produce red pigment and appear lactose-positive initially.
‡May be either bacillary or coccoid.

PREVENTION OF BACTERIAL ENDOCARDITIS

Recommendations by the American Heart Association
(*JAMA*, December 12, 1990, 264:22)

Table 1. **Cardiac Conditions***

Endocarditis Prophylaxis Recommended

Prosthetic cardiac valves, including bioprosthetic and homograft valves
Previous bacterial endocarditis, even in the absence of heart disease
Most congenital cardiac malformations
Rheumatic and other acquired valvular dysfunction, even after valvular
  surgery
Hypertrophic cardiomyopathy
Mitral valve prolapse with valvular regurgitation

Endocarditis Prophylaxis Not Recommended

Isolated secundum atrial septal defect
Surgical repair without residua beyond 6 months of secundum atrial
  septal defect, ventricular septal defect, or patent ductus arteriosus
Previous coronary artery bypass graft surgery
Mitral valve prolapse without valvular regurgitation†
Physiologic, functional, or innocent heart murmurs
Previous Kawasaki disease without valvular dysfunction
Previous rheumatic fever without valvular dysfunction
Cardiac pacemakers and implanted defibrillators

*This table lists selected conditions but is not meant to be all-inclusive.
†Individuals who have a mitral valve prolapse associated with thickening
  and/or redundancy of the valve leaflets may be at increased risk for
  bacterial endocarditis, particularly men who are 45 years of age or older.

Table 2. **Dental or Surgical Procedures***

Endocarditis Prophylaxis Recommended

Dental procedures known to induce gingival or mucosal bleeding, including professional cleaning

Tonsillectomy and/or adenoidectomy

Surgical operations that involve intestinal or respiratory mucosa

Bronchoscopy with a rigid bronchoscope

Sclerotherapy for esophageal varices

Esophageal dilatation

Gallbladder surgery

Cystoscopy

Urethral dilatation

Urethral catheterization if urinary tract infection is present†

Urinary tract surgery if urinary tract infection is present†

Prostatic surgery

Incision and drainage of infected tissue†

Vaginal hysterectomy

Vaginal delivery in the presence of infection†

Endocarditis Prophylaxis Not Recommended‡

Dental procedures not likely to induce gingival bleeding, such as simple adjustment of orthodontic appliances or fillings above the gum line

Injection of local intraoral anesthetic (except intraligamentary injections)

Shedding of primary teeth

Tympanostomy tube insertion

Endotracheal intubation

Bronchoscopy with a flexible bronchoscope, with or without biopsy

Cardiac catheterization

Endoscopy with or without gastrointestinal biopsy

Cesarean section

In the absence of infection (for urethral catheterization, dilatation and curettage, uncomplicated vaginal delivery, therapeutic abortion, sterilization procedures, or insertion or removal of intrauterine devices

---

*This table lists selected conditions but is not meant to be all-inclusive.

†In addition to prophylactic regimen for genitourinary procedures, antibiotic therapy should be directed against the most likely bacterial pathogen.

‡In patients who have prosthetic heart valves, a previous history of endocarditis, or surgically constructed systemic-pulmonary shunts or conduits, physicians may choose to administer prophylactic antibiotics even for low-risk procedures that involve the lower respiratory, genitourinary, or gastrointestinal tracts.

Table 3. **Recommended Standard Prophylactic Regimen for Dental, Oral, or Upper Respiratory Tract Procedures in Patients Who Are at Risk***

Drug	Dosing Regimen†
Standard Regimen	
Amoxicillin	3 g orally 1 hour before procedure; then 1.5 g 6 hours after initial dose
Amoxicillin/Penicillin-Allergic Patients	
Erythromycin	Erythromycin ethylsuccinate, 800 mg, or erythromycin stearate, 1 g, orally 2 hours before procedure; then half the dose 6 hours after initial dose
or	
Clindamycin	300 mg orally 1 hour before procedure and 150 mg 6 hours after initial dose

*Includes those with prosthetic heart valves and other high-risk patients.

†Initial pediatric doses are as follows: amoxicillin, 50 mg/kg; erythromycin ethylsuccinate or erythromycin stearate, 20 mg/kg; and clindamycin, 10 mg/kg. Follow-up doses should be half the initial dose. **Total pediatric dose should not exceed total adult dose**. The following weight ranges may also be used for the initial pediatric dose of amoxicillin: <15 kg, 750 mg; 15-30 kg, 1500 mg; and >30 kg, 3000 mg (full adult dose).

Table 4. **Alternate Prophylactic Regimens for Dental, Oral, or Upper Respiratory Tract Procedures in Patients Who Are at Risk**

Drug	Dosing Regimen*
Patients Unable to Take Oral Medications	
Ampicillin	Intravenous or intramuscular administration of ampicillin, 2 g, 30 minutes before procedure; then intravenous or intramuscular administration of ampicillin, 1 g or oral administration of amoxicillin, 1.5 g, 6 hours after initial dose
Ampicillin/Amoxicillin/Penicillin-Allergic Patients Unable to Take Oral Medications	
Clindamycin	Intravenous administration of 300 mg 30 minutes before procedure and an intravenous or oral administration of 150 mg 6 hours after initial dose
Patients Considered High Risk and Not Candidates for Standard Regimen	
Ampicillin, gentamicin, and amoxicillin	Intravenous or intramuscular administration of ampicillin, 2 g, plus gentamicin, 1.5 mg/kg (not to exceed 80 mg), 30 minutes before procedure; followed by amoxicillin, 1.5 g, orally 6 hours after initial dose; alternatively, the parenteral regimen may be repeated 8 hours after initial dose
Ampicillin/Amoxicillin/Penicillin-Allergic Patients Considered High Risk	
Vancomycin	Intravenous administration of 1 g over 1 hour, starting 1 hour before procedure; no repeated dose necessary

*Initial pediatric doses are as follows: ampicillin, 50 mg/kg; clindamycin, 10 mg/kg; gentamicin, 2 mg/kg; and vancomycin, 20 mg/kg. Follow-up doses should be half the initial dose. **Total pediatric dose should not exceed total adult dose**. No initial dose is recommended in this table for amoxicillin (25 mg/kg is the follow-up dose).

Table 5. **Regimens for Genitourinary/Gastrointestinal Procedures**

Drug	Dosing Regimen*
Standard Regimen	
Ampicillin, gentamicin, and amoxicillin	Intravenous or intramuscular administration of ampicillin, 2 g plus gentamicin, 1.5 mg/kg (not to exceed 80 mg), 30 minutes before procedure; followed by amoxicillin, 1.5 g orally 6 hours after initial dose; alternatively, the parenteral regimen may be repeated once 8 hours after initial dose
Ampicillin/Amoxicillin/Penicillin-Allergic Patient Regimen	
Vancomycin and gentamicin	Intravenous administration of vancomycin, 1 g over 1 hour plus intravenous or intramuscular administration of gentamicin, 1.5 mg/kg (not to exceed 80 mg), 1 hour before procedure; may be repeated once 8 hours after initial dose
Alternate Low-Risk Patient Regimen	
Amoxicillin	3 g orally 1 hour before procedure: then 1.5 g 6 hours after initial dose

*Initial pediatric doses are as follows: ampicillin, 50 mg/kg; amoxicillin, 50 mg/kg; gentamicin, 2 mg/kg; and vancomycin, 20 mg/kg. Follow-up doses should be half the initial dose. **Total pediatric dose should not exceed total adult dose**.

PREVENTION OF WOUND INFECTION AND SEPSIS IN SURGICAL PATIENTS

Nature of Operation	Likely Pathogens	Recommended Drugs	Adult Dosage Before Surgery*
CLEAN			
Cardiac			
Prosthetic valve and other open-heart surgery	*S. epidermidis, S. aureus, Corynebacterium*, enteric gram-negative bacilli	Cefazolin **or** vancomycin‡	1 g I.V.
Vascular			
Arterial surgery involving the abdominal aorta, a prosthesis, or a groin incision	*S. aureus, S. epidermidis*, enteric gram-negative bacilli	Cefazolin **or** vancomycin‡	1 g I.V.
Lower extremity amputation for ischemia	*S. aureus, S. epidermidis*, enteric gram-negative bacilli, clostridia	Cefazolin **or** vancomycin‡	1 g I.V.
Neurosurgery			
Craniotomy	*S. aureus, S. epidermidis*	Cefazolin **or** vancomycin‡	1 g I.V.
Orthopedic			
Total joint replacement, internal fixation of fractures	*S. aureus, S. epidermidis*	Cefazolin **or** vancomycin‡	1 g I.V.
Ocular§	*S. aureus, S. epidermidis*, streptococci, enteric gram-negative bacilli, *Pseudomonas*	Gentamicin **or** tobramycin **or** combination of neomycin, gramicidin, and polymyxin B, cefazolin	Multiple drops topically over 2-24 h; 100 mg subconjunctivally at end of procedure
CLEAN-CONTAMINATED			
Head and neck			
Entering oral cavity or pharynx	*S. aureus*, streptococci, oral anaerobes	Cefazolin **or** clindamycin	2 g I.V.¶; 600 mg I.V.
Gastroduodenal			
High risk, gastric bypass, or percutaneous endoscopic gastrostomy only	Enteric gram-negative bacilli, gram-positive cocci	Cefazolin	1 g I.V.
Biliary tract			
High risk only	Enteric gram-negative bacilli, enterococci, clostridia	Cefazolin	1 g I.V.
Colorectal	Enteric gram-negative bacilli, anaerobes	Oral: Neomycin plus erythromycin base	1 g of each at 1 PM, 2 PM, and 11 PM the day before the operation#
		Parenteral: Cefoxitin **or** cefotetan	1 g I.V.¶; 1 g I.V.
Appendectomy	Enteric gram-negative bacilli, anaerobes		

(continued)

Nature of Operation	Likely Pathogens	Recommended Drugs	Adult Dosage Before Surgery*
		Cefoxitin **or**	1 g I.V.¶
		cefotetan	1 g I.V.
Vaginal or abdominal hysterectomy	Enteric gram-negative bacilli, anaerobes, group B streptococci, enterococci	Cefazolin **or** Cefoxitin **or**	1 g I.V.¶
		cefotetan	1 g I.V.
Cesarean section	Same as for hysterectomy	High risk only: Cefazolin	1 g I.V. after cord clamping
Abortion	Same as for hysterectomy	First trimester in patients with previous pelvic inflammatory disease:	
		Aqueous penicillin G **or**	1 million units I.V.
		doxycycline	100 mg P.O. 1 hour before abortion, then 200 mg P.O. 30 minutes after abortion
		Second trimester: Cefazolin	1 g I.V.

DIRTY

Nature of Operation	Likely Pathogens	Recommended Drugs	Adult Dosage Before Surgery*
Ruptured viscus	Enteric gram-negative bacilli, anaerobes, enterococci	Cefoxitin **or**	1 g I.V.
		cefotetan with or without gentamicin **or**	1 g I.V. 1.5 mg/kg q8h I.V.
		clindamycin plus gentamicin	600 mg I.V. q6h 1.5 mg/kg q8h I.V.
Traumatic wound•	*S. aureus*, group A streptococci, clostridia	Cefazolin	1 g q8h I.V.

*Parenteral prophylactic antimicrobials for clean and clean-contaminated surgery can be given as a single intravenous dose just before the operation. Cefazolin can also be given intramuscularly. For prolonged operations, additional intraoperative doses should be given every 4-8 hours for the duration of the procedure. For "dirty" surgery, therapy should usually be continued for 5-10 days.

‡For hospitals in which methicillin-resistant *S. aureus* and *S. epidermidis* frequently cause wound infection, or for patients allergic to penicillins or cephalosporin.

§In addition, at the end of the operation many ophthalmologists give a subconjunctival injection of an aminoglycoside such as gentamicin (10-20 mg), with or without a cephalosporin such as cefazolin (100 mg).

¶In controlled studies, 2 g were effective, while 0.5 g was not (JT Johnson and VL Yu, *Ann Surg*, 1988, 207:108).

#After appropriate diet and catharsis.

•For bite wounds, in which likely pathogens may also include oral anaerobes, *Eikenella corrodens* (humans), and *Pasteurella multocida* (dog and cat), some *Medical Letter* consultants recommend use of amoxicillin-clavulanic acid (Augmentin") or ampicillin/sulbactam (Unasyn").

PROPHYLAXIS FOR PATIENTS EXPOSED TO COMMON COMMUNICABLE DISEASES

Disease	Exposure	Prophylaxis/Management
Invasive *Haemophilus influenza* disease	Close contact with an infected child for more than 4 hours	Give rifampin 20 mg/kg orally once daily for 4 days (600 mg maximum daily dose) to entire family with at least one household contact less than 48 months old. Contraindication: Pregnant contacts.
Hepatitis A	Direct contact with an infected child, or sharing of food or utensils	Give 0.02 mL/kg immune globulin (IG) within 7 days of exposure.
Hepatitis B	• Needlestick (used needle) • Mucous membrane exposure with blood or body fluid • Direct inoculation of blood or body fluid into open cut, lesion, or laceration	**Known source and employee status unknown: test patient for HB$_s$Ag and employee for anti-HB$_s$.** • If patient is HB$_s$Ag negative and the patient does not have non-A, non-B hepatitis, do nothing. • If patient is HB$_s$Ag negative and has non-A, non-B hepatitis, **offer** ISG (optional). • If patient is HB$_s$Ag positive, give HBIG and hepatitis B vaccine within 48 hours of exposure. Employee antibody status may not be available for up to a week, so the above should be given as soon as patient's antigen status is known. Occasionally, the patient's antigen status will be unavailable for more than 24 hours. In these cases, HBIG should be given if the patient is high risk (ie, Asian immigrants, institutionalized patients, homosexuals, intravenous drug abusers, hemodialysis patients, patients with a history of hepatitis). • If the employee is anti-HB$_s$ negative, give the second and third doses of hepatitis B vaccine. **Known source if employee documented anti-HB$_s$ positive:** • If source has non-A, non-B hepatitis, offer ISG (optional). • If employee is believed to be anti-HB$_s$ positive due to vaccination, has received 3 doses of vaccine, and has not had an anti-HB$_s$ test done, draw serum for anti-HB$_s$.

(continued)

Disease	Exposure	Prophylaxis/Management
Measles	15 minutes or more in the same room with a child with measles from 2 days before the onset of symptoms to 4 days after the appearance of the rash	Children who have not been vaccinated and have not had natural infection should be isolated from the 7th through the 18th day after exposure and/or for 4 days after the rash appears. Those who have not been vaccinated should be vaccinated within 72 hours of exposure if no contraindication exists, or receive immune globulin (IG) 0.25 mL/kg I.M. for immunocompetent individuals and 0.5 mL/kg (maximum 15 mL) for immunosuppressed individuals.

Children who are younger than 15 months of age should be revaccinated at 15 months of age but at least 3 months after receipt of vaccine or IG. Older individuals who have received IG should be vaccinated 3 months later. |
| Tuberculosis | Housed in the same room with a child with contagious tuberculosis (tuberculosis is contagious if the child has a cough plus AFB seen on smear plus cavitation on CXR) | Place PPD immediately and 10 weeks after exposure. Start on INH. Consult Infectious Diseases if seroconversion occurs. |
| Meningococcal disease | Household contact or direct contact with secretions | Household, day care center, and nursery school children should receive rifampin prophylaxis for 2 days. Dosages are given every 12 hours for a total of 4 doses. Dosage is 10 mg/kg/dose for children ages 1 month to 12 years (maximum 600 mg/dose), 5 mg/kg/dose for infants less than 1 month of age, and 600 mg/dose for adults. Contraindication: Pregnant contacts

Because prophylaxis is not always effective, exposed children should be monitored for symptoms.

Employee exposure: Anyone who develops a febrile illness should receive prompt medical evaluation. If indicated, antimicrobial therapy should be administered. |

(continued)

Disease	Exposure	Prophylaxis/Management
Pertussis	Housed in the same room with an infected child or spent 15 minutes in the playroom with the infected child	**Prophylaxis:** Contacts less than 7 years old who have had at least 4 doses of pertussis vaccine should receive a booster dose of DTP, unless a dose has been given within the past 3 years, and should receive erythromycin 40-50 mg/kg/day orally for 14 days. Contacts less than 7 years old who are not immunized or who have received less than 4 doses of DTP should have DTP immunization initiated or continued according to the recommended schedule. Children who have received their third dose 6 months or more before exposure should be given their fourth dose at this time. Erythromycin should also be given for 14 days. Contacts 7 years of age and above should receive prophylactic erythromycin (maximum of 1 g/day) for 10-14 days. All exposed patients should be watched closely for respiratory symptoms for 14 days after exposure has stopped because immunity conferred by the vaccine is not absolute and the efficacy of erythromycin in prophylaxis has not been established.
Varicella-zoster	1 hour or more in the same room with a contagious child from 24 hours before vesicles appear to when all vesicles are crusted, which is usually 5 to 7 days after vesicles appear. In household exposure, communicability is 48 hours before vesicles appear.	**Immunocompetent** children who have not been vaccinated or had natural infection, should have titers drawn only if they will still be hospitalized for more than 10 days after exposure. If titers are negative, they should be isolated from 10 to 21 days after exposure and/or until all lesions are crusted and dry. If VZIG was given the child should be isolated from 10 to 28 days after exposure. **Immunocompromised** children who have not been vaccinated or had natural infection should first have titers drawn, and then receive VZIG (varicella-zoster immune globulin) **1 vial/10 kg I.M.** up to a maximum of 5 vials as soon as possible but at most 96 hours after exposure. Fractional doses are not recommended. If titers are positive, nothing further need be done. If titers are negative, the child should be isolated from 10 to 28 days after exposure and should be monitored very carefully for tite appearance of vesicles so that treatment can be initiated. VZIG is available from the Blood Bank.

ANIMAL AND HUMAN BITES GUIDELINES

Wound Management

Irrigation: Critically important; irrigate all penetration wounds using 20 mL syringe, 19 gauge needle and >250 mL 1% povidone iodine solution. This method will reduce wound infection by a factor of 20. When there is high risk of rabies, use viricidal 1% benzalkonium chloride in addition to the 1% povidone iodine. Irrigate wound with normal saline after antiseptic irrigation.

Debridement: Remove all crushed or devitalized tissue remaining after irrigation; minimize removal on face and over thin skin areas or anywhere you would create a worse situation than the bite itself already has; do not extend puncture wounds surgically — rather, manage them with irrigation and antibiotics.

Suturing: Close most dog bites if <8 hours (<12 hours on face); do not routinely close puncture wounds, or deep or severe bites on the hands or feet, as these are at highest risk for infection. Cat and human bites should not be sutured unless cosmetically important. Wound edge freshening, where feasible, reduces infection; minimize sutures in the wound and use monofilament on the surface.

Immobilization: Critical in all hand wounds; important for infected extremities.

Hospitalization/I.V. Antibiotics: Admit for I.V. antibiotics all significant human bites to the hand, especially closed fist injuries, and bites involving penetration of the bone or joint (a high index of suspicion is needed). Consider I.V. antibiotics for significant established wound infections with cellulitis or lymphangitis, any infected bite on the hand, any infected cat bite, and any infection in an immunocompromised or asplenic patient. Outpatient treatment with I.V. antibiotics may be possible in selected cases by consulting with infectious disease.

Laboratory Assessment

Gram Stain: Not useful prior to onset of clinically apparent infection; examination of purulent material may show a predominant organism in established infection, aiding antibiotic selection; not warranted unless results will change your treatment.

Culture: Not useful or cost effective prior to onset of clinically apparent infection.

X-Ray: Whenever you suspect bony involvement, especially in craniofacial dog bites in very small children or severe bite/crush in an extremity; cat bites with their long needle like teeth may cause osteomyelitis or a septic joint, especially in the hand or wrist.

Immunizations

Tetanus: All bite wounds are contaminated. If not immunized in last 5 years, or if not current in a child, give DPT, DT, Td, or TT as indicated. For absent or incomplete primary immunization, give 250 units tetanus immune globulin (TIG) in addition.

Rabies: In the U.S. 30,000 persons are treated each year in an attempt to prevent 1-5 cases. Domestic animals should be quarantined for 10 days to prove need for prophylaxis. High risk animal bites (85% of cases = bat >>skunk >racoon) usually receive treatment consisting of:

• human rabies immune globulin (HRIG): 20 units/kg I.M. (unless previously immunized with HDCV)

- human diploid cell vaccine (HDCV): 1 mL I.M. on days 0, 3, 7, 14 and 28 (unless previously immunized with HDCV — then give only first 2 doses)

Consult with Infectious Disease before ordering rabies prophylaxis.

Bite Wounds and Prophylactic Antibiotics

Parenteral vs Oral: If warranted, consider an initial I.V. dose to rapidly establish effective serum levels, especially if high risk, delayed treatment, or if patient reliability is poor.

Dog Bite:

1. Rarely get infected (~5%)
2. Infecting organisms: Staph coag negative, staph coag positive, alpha strep, diphtheroids, beta strep, *pseudomonas aeruginosa*, gamma strep, *pasteurella multocida*
3. Prophylactic antibiotics are seldom indicated. Consider for high risk wounds such as distal extremity puncture wounds, severe crush injury, bites occurring in cosmetically sensitive areas (eg, face), or in immunocompromised or asplenic patients.

Cat Bite:

1. Often get infected (~25% to 50%)
2. Infecting organisms: *Pasteurella multocida* (first 24 hours), coag positive staph, anaerobic cocci (after first 24 hours)
3. Prophylactic antibiotics are indicated in all cases.

Human Bite:

1. Intermediate infection rate (~15% to 20%)
2. Infecting organisms: Coag positive staph α, β, γ strep, *Haemophilus*, *Eikenella corrodens*, anaerobic streptococci, *Fusobacterium*, *Veillonella*, bacteroides.
3. Prophylactic antibiotics are indicated in almost all cases except superficial injuries.

See attached table for prophylactic antibiotic summary.

Bite Wound Antibiotic Regimens

	Dog Bite	Cat Bite	Human Bite
Prophylactic Antibiotics			
Prophylaxis	No routine prophylaxis, consider if involves face or hand, or immunosuppressed or asplenic patients	Routine prophylaxis	Routine prophylaxis
Prophylactic antibiotic	Amoxicillin	Amoxicillin	Amoxicillin
Penicillin allergy	Doxycycline if >10 y or co-trimoxazole	Doxycycline if >10 y or co-trimoxazole	Doxycycline if >10 y or erythromycin and cephalexin*
Outpatient Oral Antibiotic Treatment (mild to moderate infection)			
Established infection	Amoxicillin and clavulanic acid	Amoxicillin and clavulanic acid	Amoxicillin and clavulanic acid
Penicillin allergy (mild infection only)	Doxycycline if >10 y	Doxycycline if >10 y	Cephalexin* or clindamycin
Outpatient Parenteral Antibiotic Treatment (moderate infections — single drug regimens)			
	Ceftriaxone	Ceftriaxone	Cefotetan

INFECTIOUS DISEASE INFORMATION

Inpatient Parenteral Antibiotic Treatment

Established infection	Ampicillin + cefazolin	Ampicillin + cefazolin	Ampicillin + clindamycin
Penicillin allergy	Cefazolin*	Ceftriaxone*	Cefotetan* or imipenem

*Contraindicated if history of immediate hypersensitivity reaction (anaphylaxis) to penicillin.

Duration of Prophylactic and Treatment Regimens

Prophylaxis: 5 days
Treatment: 10-14 days

Antibiotic Dosages

Antibiotic	Adult Dosage	Pediatric Dosage
Oral regimens		
Amoxicillin	500 mg P.O. tid	50 mg/kg/d with tid dosing
Amoxicillin/clavulanate	500/125 P.O. tid (750 mg P.O. qid if > 180 lb)	50 mg/kg/d based on amoxicillin content with tid dosing
Cephalexin	500 mg P.O. qid (750 mg P.O. qid if > 180 lb)	50 mg/kg/d with qid dosing
Clindamycin	450 mg P.O. tid	25-30 mg/kg/d with tid-qid dosing
Co-trimoxazole	2 tabs P.O. bid	8 mg/kg/d based on trimethoprim content with bid dosing
Dicloxacillin	500 mg P.O. qid	50 mg/kg/d with qid dosing
Doxycycline	100 mg P.O. bid	5 mg/kg/d with bid dosing
Erythromycin	500 mg P.O. qid	50 mg/kg/d with qid dosing
Penicillin VK	500 mg P.O. qid	75-100 mg/kg/d with qid dosing
Parenteral Regimens		
Ampicillin	2 g I.V. q4-6h	250-300 mg/kg/d I.V. given q6h
Ampicillin/sulbactam	2 g I.V. q6h based on ampicillin component	250-300 mg/kg/d I.V. based on ampicillin component given q6h
Cefazolin	2 g I.V. q8h	100 mg/kg/d I.V. given q8h
Cefotetan	2 g I.V. q12h	60-80 mg/kg/d I.V. given q12h
Ceftriaxone	2 g I.V. or I.M. q24h	75 mg/kg/d I.M./I.V. given q24h
Clindamycin	900 mg I.V. q8h	25-30 mg/kg/d I.V. given q8h
Imipenem	500 mg I.V. q6h	

IMPAIRED RENAL FUNCTION DOSING, ADULTS

Drug	Cl_{cr} (mL/min)	Suggested Dosage Regimen	Supplement for Dialysis	
			Hemo-dialysis	Peritoneal Dialysis
Acyclovir (I.V.)	>50	5–10 mg/kg q8h	Yes	—
	25–50	5–10 mg/kg q12h		
	10–25	5–10 mg/kg q24h		
Amantadine (P.O.)	>80	100 mg bid	No	No
	60–80	200 mg/100 mg alternating daily		
	40–60	100 mg/d		
	30–40	200 mg 2 times/wk		
	20–30	100 mg 3 times/wk		
	10–20	200 mg/100 mg alternating weekly		
Amikacin (I.M., I.V.)	Individualize regimen with serum concentrations.		Yes	Yes
Aminosalicylic acid (P.O.)	>50	150 mg/kg/day in 2–3 divided doses	—	—
	10–50	50%–70%		
	<10	50% of dose		
Amoxicillin (P.O.)	>50	250–500 mg q8h	Yes	No
	10–50	250–500 mg q8-12h		
	<10	250–500 mg q12h		
Amoxicillin clavulanate (P.O.)	>30	250–500 mg q6h	Yes	No
	15–30	250–500 mg q8-12h		
	5–15	250–500 mg q24h		
Amphotericin B (I.V.)	Usual dose: 0.3–0.7 mg/kg q24h; a 1 mg test dose may be administered over 30 minutes with vital sign monitoring over the next hour to assure no anaphylactoid reaction; then remaining full dose may be administered.			
Ampicillin (I.V.)	>50	1–2 g q4-6h	Yes	No
	10–50	1–2 g q6-12h		
	<10	1–2 g q8-12h		
Ampicillin/sulbactam (I.V.)	≥30	1.5–3 g q6-8h	Yes	—
	15–29	1.5–3 g q12h		
	5–14	1.5–3 g q24h		
Atovaquone* (P.O.)	—	750 mg tid	—	—
Azithromycin* (P.O.)	—	500 mg day 1 then 250 mg daily	—	—
Aztreonam (I.V.)	>50	500 mg-2 g q6-8h	Yes	Yes
	10–50	50%–75% of usual dosage		
	10	25% of usual dosage		
Bismuth (P.O.)	See specific indication. Avoid use in renal failure.			
Capreomycin sulfate (I.M.)	>100	13–15 mg/kg q24h	—	—
	80–100	10–13 mg/kg q24h		
	60–80	7–10 mg/kg q24h		
	40–60	11–14 mg/kg q48h		
	20–40	10–14 mg/kg q72h		
	<20	4–7 mg/kg q72h		

*No renal dose adjustment necessary.

(continued)

Drug	Cl_{cr} (mL/min)	Suggested Dosage Regimen	Supplement for Dialysis	
			Hemo-dialysis	Peritoneal Dialysis
Carbenicillin (P.O.)	>50	382–764 mg q8–12h	Yes	—
	10–50	382–764 mg q12–24h		
	10	382–764 mg q24–48h		
Cefaclor (P.O.)	>50	250–500 mg q8h	Yes	Yes
	10–50	125–500 mg q8h		
Cefadroxil monohydrate (P.O.)	>50	500 mg–1 g q12h	Yes	No
	10–50	500 mg q24h		
	<10	500 mg q36h		
Cefamandole nafate (I.V.)	>50	1–2 g q4h	Yes	—
	25–50	1–2 g q8h		
	10–25	1 g q8h		
	<10	1 g q12h		
Cefazolin (I.V.)	>30	1–2 g q8h	Yes	No
	10–30	1 g q12h		
	<10	1 g q24h		
Cefixime (P.O.)	>60	400 mg q24h	—	—
	21–60	300 mg q24h		
	≤20	200 mg q24h		
Cefmetazole sodium (I.V.)	>50	1–2 g q12h	—	—
	30–49	1–2 g q16h		
	10–29	1–2 g q24h		
	<10	1–2 g q48h		
Cefonicid sodium (I.M., I.V.)	>20	1 g q24h	No	No
	10–20	500 mg–1 g q48h		
	<10	250 mg–1 g q72h		
Cefoperazone sodium* (I.M., I.V.)	—	1–2 g q8–12h	No	No
Cefotaxime sodium (I.M., I.V.)	>50	1–2 g q6–8h	Yes	No
	10–50	1–2 g q8–12h		
	<10	1–2 g q24h		
Cefotetan disodium (I.M., I.V.)	>30	1–2 g q12h	Yes	No
	10–30	1–2 g q24h		
	<10	1–2 g q48h		
Cefoxitin sodium (I.M., I.V.)	>50	1–2 g q6–8h	Yes	No
	30–50	1–2 g q8–12h		
	10–30	1–2 g q12–24h		
	<10	500 mg–1 g q24–48h		
Cefpodoxime proxetil (P.O.)	>30	100–200 mg q12h	Yes	—
	<30	100–200 mg q24h		
Cefprozil (P.O.)	≥30	250–500 mg q12–24h	Yes	—
	<30	125–250 mg q12–24h		

*No renal dose adjustment necessary.

(continued)

Drug	Cl_{cr} (mL/min)	Suggested Dosage Regimen	Supplement for Dialysis	
			Hemo–dialysis	Peritoneal Dialysis
Ceftazidime (I.V.)	>50	1 g q8–12h	Yes	Yes
	30–50	1 g q12h		
	15–30	1 g q24h		
	<15	500 mg–1 g q24h		
Ceftizoxime (I.V.)	>30	1–2 g q8–12h	Yes	—
	10–30	1 g q12h		
	<10	1 g q24h		
Ceftriaxone sodium (I.M., I.V.)*	—	1–2 g q24h	—	—
Cefuroxime (I.V.)	>20	750 mg–1.5 g q8h	Yes	No
	10–20	750 mg q12h		
	<10	750 mg q24h		
Cephalexin (P.O.)	>40	250–500 mg q6h	Yes	Yes
	10–40	250–500 mg q8–12h		
	<10	250 mg q12–24h		
Cephalothin sodium (I.M., I.V.)	>50	500 mg–2 g q4–6h	Yes	No
	10–50	500 mg–1 g q6–8h		
	<10	500 mg–1 g q12h		
Cephapirin sodium (I.M., I.V.)	>50	1 g q6h	Yes	No
	10–50	1 g q6–8h		
	<10	1 g q12h		
Cephradine (P.O.)	>50	500 mg q6h	Yes	Yes
	10–50	250 mg q6h		
	<10	250 mg q12h		
Chloramphenicol (I.V.)*	—	0.5–1 g q6h	No	No
Chloroquine (P.O.)	See monograph for dosing information.		No	—
Cinoxacin (P.O.)	>50	250 mg q6–12h	—	—
	20–50	250 mg bid		
	<20	250 mg/d		
Ciprofloxacin (P.O.)	>30	250 mg q12h, 500 mg q12h, or 750 mg q12h	No	No
	<30	500 mg q24h or 750 mg q24h		
Clarithromycin (P.O.)	>30	250–500 mg bid	—	—
	<30	500 mg loading dose, then 250 mg once daily or bid		

*No renal dose adjustment necessary.

(continued)

Drug	Cl$_{cr}$ (mL/min)	Suggested Dosage Regimen	Supplement for Dialysis	
			Hemo–dialysis	Peritoneal Dialysis
Clindamycin (I.V.)*	—	900 mg q8h	No	No
Clindamycin (P.O.)*	—	150–450 mg q6h	No	No
Cloxacillin sodium (P.O.)*	—	250–500 mg q6h	—	—
Colistimethate (I.M., I.V.)	S$_{cr}$ (mg/dL) 0.7–1.2	100–125 mg bid–qid	—	—
	1.3–1.5	75–115 mg bid		
	1.6–2.5	66–150 mg bid or once daily		
	2.6–4	100–150 mg q36h		
Co-trimoxazole† (P.O., I.V.)	>30	5 mg/kg q6–8h	Yes	No
	15–30	2.5–5 mg/kg q12h		
	<15	2.5–5 mg/kg q24h		
Cycloserine (P.O.)	>50	250 mg q12h	—	—
	10–50	250 mg q24h		
	<10	250 mg q36h–48h		
Dapsone (P.O.)*	—	100 mg q24h	No	No
Demeclocycline (P.O.)	—	300 mg bid (do not use in renal impairment)		
Dicloxacillin (P.O.)*	—	500 mg q6h	No	—
Didanosine (P.O.)	>60	See individual dosing per body weight range.	—	—
	<60	Consider dosage reduction.		
Doxycycline (P.O., I.V.)	>10	100 mg q12h	No	—
	<10	100 mg q24h		
Eflornithine (P.O.)	>60	100 mg/kg q6h	—	—
	<60	Consider dosage reduction.		
Enoxacin (P.O.)	>30	400 mg bid	—	—
	<30	200 mg bid		
Erythromycin (I.V.)	>10	0.5–1 g q6h	No	No
	<10	250–500 mg q6h		
Erythromycin (P.O.)*	—	250–500 mg q6h	No	No
Ethambutol (P.O.)	>50	15–25 mg/kg q24h	Yes	Yes
	10–50	15 mg/kg q24–36h		
	<10	15 mg/kg q48h		
	—	Maximum dose: 2.5 g/d		
Ethionamide (P.O.)	>50	250–500 mg q12h	—	—
	<50	125–250 mg q12h		
Fluconazole (P.O., I.V.)	>50	100–400 mg loading dose x 1 then ½ loading dose q24h	Yes	—
	20–50	Loading dose then 50% of recommended dose		
	<20	Loading dose then 25% of recommended dose		

*No renal dose adjustment necessary.
†All doses based on trimethoprim.

(continued)

Drug	Cl$_{cr}$ (mL/min)	Suggested Dosage Regimen	Supplement for Dialysis	
			Hemo-dialysis	Peritoneal Dialysis
Flucytosine (P.O.)	>40	12.5–37.5 mg/kg q6h	Yes	—
	20–40	12.5–37.5 mg/kg q12h		
	<20	12.5–37.5 mg/kg q24h		
Foscarnet (I.V.)# (induction)	(mL/min/kg)		—	—
	≥1.6	60 mg/kg q8h		
	1.5	57 mg/kg q8h		
	1.4	53 mg/kg q8h		
	1.3	49 mg/kg q8h		
	1.2	46 mg/kg q8h		
	1.1	42 mg/kg q8h		
	1.0	39 mg/kg q8h		
	0.9	35 mg/kg q8h		
	0.8	32 mg/kg q8h		
	0.7	28 mg/kg q8h		
	0.6	25 mg/kg q8h		
	0.5	21 mg/kg q8h		
	0.4	18 mg/kg q8h		
Ganciclovir (I.V.)	>80	5 mg/kg q12h	—	—
	50–80	2.5 mg/kg q12h		
	25–50	2.5 mg/kg q24h		
	<25	1.25 mg/kg q24h		
Gentamicin (I.M., I.V.)	Individualize regimen with serum concentrations.		Yes	Yes
Imipenem/cilastatin (I.V.)	>70	500 mg q6h	Yes	—
	30–70	500 mg q8h		
	20–30	500 mg q12h		
	0–20	250–500 mg q12h		
Isoniazid (P.O., I.V.)*	—	300 mg q24h	Yes	Yes
Itraconazole (P.O.)	—	200 mg once daily	—	—
Kanamycin	Avoid I.V. administration.		—	—
Ketoconazole (P.O.)*	—	200 mg q24h	No	No
Lomefloxacin (P.O.)	>40	400 mg q24h	—	—
	≤40	400 mg 1st dose, then 200 mg once a day		
Loracarbef (P.O.)	>50	200–400 mg q12h	—	—
	10–49	200–400 mg q24h		
	<10	200–400 mg q3–5d		
Mefloquine* (P.O.)	—	See individual dosing for prophylaxis vs treatment.	—	—
Methicillin sodium (I.M., I.V.)	>50	1–2 g q4–6h	No	No
	10–50	1–2 g q6–8h		
	<10	1–2 g q8–12h		
Metronidazole (P.O., I.V.)	>10	250–500 mg q6–8h	Yes	—
	<10	250–500 mg q8–12h		

*No renal dose adjustment necessary.
#See monograph for maintenance dosing.

(continued)

Drug	Cl_{cr} (mL/min)	Suggested Dosage Regimen	Supplement for Dialysis	
			Hemo-dialysis	Peritoneal Dialysis
Mezlocillin sodium (I.M., I.V.)	>30	3–4 g q4–6h	No	No
	10–30	1.5–3 g q6–8h		
	<10	3 g q8h		
Miconazole (I.V.)*	—	400–1200 mg q8h	No	No
Nafcillin sodium (I.M., I.V.)*	—	1–2 g q4–6h	No	No
Neomycin sulfate (P.O.)	Avoid I.V. administration.		—	—
Netilmicin sulfate (I.M., I.V.)	Individualize regimen with serum concentrations.		Yes	Yes
Nitrofurantoin (P.O.)	>50	50–100 mg q6h	—	—
	<50	Avoid use		
Norfloxacin (P.O.)	>30	400 mg q12h	No	—
	<30	400 mg q24h		
Ofloxacin (P.O., I.V.)	>50	200–400 mg q12h	—	—
	10–50	200–400 mg q24h		
	<10	100–200 mg q24h		
Oxacillin (I.V.)*	—	1–2 g q4–6h	No	—
Oxytetracycline (P.O.)	>10	250–500 mg q6h	—	—
	<10	Avoid use		
Penicillin G (I.V.)	>50	2–4 million units q2–4h	Yes	—
	10–50	1–2 million units q4–6h		
	<10	1–2 million units q8–12h or 0.5–1 million units q4–6h		
Penicillin V potassium (P.O.)	>10	250–500 mg q6h	Yes	—
	<10	250 mg q6h		
Pentamidine (I.V.)	>50	4 mg/kg q24h	—	—
	10–50	4 mg/kg q24–36h		
	<10	4 mg/kg q48h		
Piperacillin (I.V.)	>40	3–4 g q4–6h	Yes	—
	20–40	3–4 g q8h		
	<20	3–4 g q12h		
Piperacillin/tazobactam (I.V.)	>40	3.375 g q6h	Yes	Yes
	20–40	2.25 g q6h		
	<20	2.25 g q8h		
Polymyxin B	Avoid I.V. administration.		—	—
Pyrazinamide (P.O.)	—	15–30 mg/kg q24h	—	—
	—	Maximum dose: 2 g/d		
Pyrimethamine (P.O.)*	—	100 mg q24h	—	—
Quinacrine (P.O.)	—	See individual dosing per disease.	—	—
Quinidine*	—	See monograph.	Yes	Yes

*No renal dose adjustment necessary.

(continued)

Drug	Cl$_{cr}$ (mL/min)	Suggested Dosage Regimen	Supplement for Dialysis	
			Hemo–dialysis	Peritoneal Dialysis
Quinine sulfate (P.O.)	>50	650 mg q6–8h	Yes	No
	10–50	650 mg q8–12h		
	<10	650 mg q24h		
Rifampin (P.O., I.V.)*	—	600 mg/d	No	—
Rimantadine (P.O.)	>10	100 mg q12h	—	—
	<10	100 mg q24h		
Spectinomycin hydrochloride (I.M.)*	—	2–4 g q24h	Yes	Yes
Streptomycin sulfate (I.M.)	—	See individual dosing per disease.	Yes	—
Sulfadiazine (P.O.)*	—	1–2 g q6h	—	—
Sulfamethoxazole (P.O.)	>50	1 g q12h	Yes	No
	10–50	1 g q12–24h		
	<10	1 g q24h		
Sulfisoxazole (P.O.)	>50	1–2 g q6h	Yes	No
	10–50	1 g q8–12h		
	<10	1 g q12–24h		
Tetracycline hydrochloride (P.O.)	>50	250–500 mg q6–12h	No	No
	10–50	250–500 mg q12–24h		
	<10	250–500 mg q24h		
Thiabendazole (P.O.)	—	See individual dosing per disease.	—	—
Ticarcillin/clavulanate (I.V.)	>60	3.1 g q4–6h	Yes	Yes
	30–60	3.1 g q8h		
	10–30	3.1 g q12h		
Ticarcillin disodium (I.M., I.V.)	>60	3 g q4h	Yes	No
	30–60	2 g q4h		
	10–30	2 g q8h		
	<10	2 g q12h		
Tobramycin	Individualize regimen with serum concentrations.		Yes	Yes
Trimethoprim (P.O.)	>50	100–200 mg q6h	Yes	—
	10–50	100 mg q12–24h		
	<10	50–100 mg q24h		
Vancomycin (I.V.)	Individualize dosing with serum concentrations; 1 g q12h is usual starting dose in patients with normal renal function.			
Vancomycin (P.O.)*	—	125–250 mg q6h	—	—
Vidarabine (I.V.)	>10	15 mg/kg/d	Yes	—
	<10	75% of usual dosage		
Zalcitabine (P.O.)	>40	0.75 mg q8h	—	—
	10–40	0.75 mg q12h		
	<10	0.75 mg q24h		
Zidovudine	—	100 mg 5 times/d	—	—

*No renal dose adjustment necessary.

PHARMACOKINETICS, ADULTS

Drug	Half-life (h) Normal Renal Function	Half-life (h) Impaired Renal Function	V_d (L/kg)	Protein Binding (%)	Time to Peak (h)	Bioavail-ability (%)
Acyclovir	3	20	0.7-0.8	15-30	P.O.: 1.7	20
Amantadine hydrochloride	10-28	7-10 d	4-5	60	1-4	90
Amikacin sulfate	1.6-96	17-150	0.22-0.29	<5	I.M.: 0.75-2	
Amoxicillin trihydrate	0.7-1.4	7-21	0.26	15-25	2	85
Amphotericin B	15-48		4	90		
Ampicillin	1-1.8	7-20	0.17-0.31	8-20	I.M.: 1 P.O.: 2	50
Ampicillin/sulbactam	1	5-9		20-40		
Atovaquone	2.9 d			>99.9	1-8	~30
Azithromycin dihydrate	35-40		31.1	7-51	3-4	37
Aztreonam	1.3-2.6	6-8	0.1-0.2	50-60	I.M.: 0.6-1.3	
Capreomycin sulfate	4-6	55			I.M.: 1-2	
Carbenicillin	1.5	10-20	0.12-0.2	30-60	1-3	30-50
Cefaclor	0.5-1	3	0.34-0.35	25	0.5-1	95
Cefadroxil sodium	1-2	20-24	0.31	20	1.2-1.5	95
Cefamandole nafate	0.5-1	3-18	0.16-0.25	75		
Cefazolin sodium	1.5-2.4	40-70	0.13-0.22	80		
Cefixime	3-4	11.5	0.11	65-70	2-6	45
Cefonicid sodium	3.5-4.5	17-56	0.09-0.15	96		
Cefoperazone sodium	1.6-2.5	2.9	0.14-0.2	90		
Cefotaxime sodium	1-1.5	15	0.15-0.55	37		
Cefotetan disodium	3-5	13-25	0.15	85		
Cefoxitin sodium	0.75-1	13-25	0.13-0.39	41-75		
Cefpodoxime proxetil	2-3	9.8	0.46	21-29	1	40-60
Cefprozil	1-2	5.2		36	1-2	95
Ceftazidime	1-2	13-25	0.28	17		
Ceftizoxime sodium	1.6	25	0.26-0.42	28-50		
Ceftriaxone sodium	5-9	12-24	0.12-0.14	85-95		
Cefuroxime	1-2	17	0.13-1.8	33	P.O.: 3	52
Cephalexin monohydrate	0.5-1.2	20-40	0.26	10-15	1	95
Cephalothin sodium	0.5-1	20-40	0.18-0.33	15		
Cephapirin sodium	0.5-1	2.4-2.7	45-60	0.5		
Cephradine	1-2	6-15	0.25-0.33	10	1-2	95
Chloramphenicol	1.6-3.3	3-7	0.6-1	60	P.O.: 0.5-3	80
Chloroquine phosphate	3-5 d	5-50 d	800*	50-65	1-2	89
Cinoxacin	1.5	>10	0.24-0.26	60-80	2-3	30-40
Ciprofloxacin hydrochloride	3-5	6-9	2.1	40	P.O.: 0.5-2	70-80
Clarithromycin	3-7	22		65-75	2-4	55
Clindamycin	2-3	3-5	0.6-1.2	60-95	P.O.: 1-3	90
Clofazimine	70 d				1-6	45-62
Cloxacillin sodium	0.5-1.5	1	0.15-0.2	85-94	0.5-2	

*In plasma

(continued)

Drug	Half-life (h) Normal Renal Function	Half-life (h) Impaired Renal Function	V$_d$ (L/kg)	Protein Binding (%)	Time to Peak (h)	Bioavail-ability (%)
Co-trimoxazole SMZ	9	20-50	0.21	60-70	P.O.: 2-4	90-100
TMP	6-17	20-40	1.2-2	40-70	P.O.: 1-4	90-100
Cycloserine	10		0.11-0.26		3-4	
Demeclocycline	10-17	40-60	1.79	91	3-6	41-50
Dicloxacillin sodium	0.6-0.8	1-2	0.13-0.19	91-98	0.5-2	80
Didanosine	0.8-2.7		0.7-1		0.5-1	33
Doxycycline	12-15	24	22-24	80-93	P.O.: 1.5-4	90-100
Eflornithine	3.2-3.6		0.3-0.43			50
Enoxacin	3-6	9.4		40	1-2	90
Erythromycin	1.5-2	5-6	0.72	75-90	P.O.: 1-4	Variable
Ethambutol	2.5-3.6	7-15	1.6-2.3	10-30	2-4	75-80
Ethionamide	3		2-8	10	1.8	100
Fluconazole	25-30		0.7-1	11	P.O.: 1-2	<90
Flucytosine	2.5-6	12-250	0.6	2-4	1-2	78-90
Foscarnet	3.3-6.8		0.3-0.7	14-17		
Ganciclovir	1.7-5.8	5-28	0.15-0.31	1-2		
Gentamicin sulfate	1.5-3	36-70	0.23-0.26	0.5-1.5		
Griseofulvin	9-22				4	25-70
Imipenem/cilastatin imipenem	1	4	0.26	20		
cilastatin	1	17		40	1	
Interferon alfa-2b	6-8				3.8	
Isoniazide fast acetylizers	0.5-1.5		0.6	<10	1.2	
slow acetylizers	2-5	22-28				
Itraconazole	21		796	99	3-4	
Ivermectin	22-28		46.8	93	3.6	
Kanamycin	2-4	40-96	0.23-0.29	<5	3.6	
Ketoconazole	1.5-3		0.36	99	1-4	37-97
Lomefloxacin	7-8	21-45	1.8-2.5	10	1.5	95-98
Loracarbef	1	≤32		25	1.2	
Mebendazole	1-11.5	35		90-95	2-4	
Mefloquine hydrochloride	21-22		20	98	7-24	85
Methenamine	3-6		0.56		2-8	
Methicillin sodium	0.4-0.5	4	0.43	35-60		
Metronidazole	6-8	21	0.25-0.85	20	P.O.: 1-2	80
Mezlocillin sodium	0.8-1.2	2.6-5.4	0.17-0.2	20-46		
Miconazole	0.8-2.1	20-24	2.1	90		
Minocycline	15	11-23	0.14-0.7	70-75	2-4	
Moxalactam disodium	2-3	18-23	0.18-0.4	35-50		
Nafcillin sodium	0.5-1.5	1.2	0.31-0.38	80-90		
Nalidixic acid	6-7	21	0.25-0.35	90	1-2	90
Neomycin sulfate	2-4	40-96	0.23-0.29	<5	3.6	
Netilmicin sulfate	2-3	24-52	0.6-1.3	<5		

(continued)

Drug	Half-life (h) Normal Renal Function	Half-life (h) Impaired Renal Function	V_d (L/kg)	Protein Binding (%)	Time to Peak (h)	Bioavail-ability (%)
Nitrofurantoin	0.3-0.6	1	0.8	40		60
Norfloxacin	4.8	6-9	3.2	10-15	1-2	30-70
Ofloxacin	5-7.5	30	0.9-1.8	20-25	P.O.: 1.2-2	95-100
Oxacillin sodium	0.5-0.7	1-3	0.2	90-93		
Oxamniquine	1-2.5				1-1.5	50
Oxytetracycline	8.5-9.6	47-66	0.9-1.6	35	2-4	
Penicillin G benzathine, parenteral	0.5	6-20	0.2	40-60	12-24	
Penicillin G, parenteral	0.3-0.9	6-20	0.2	40-60		
Penicillin G procaine, aqueous	0.3-0.9	6-20	0.2	40-60	1-4	
Pentamidine isethionate	6.4-9.4†	48	3	69		
Piperacillin sodium	0.5-1.2	3.3-5.1	0.18-0.3	20-40	0.5-0.9	
Polymyxin B	4.6-6				I.M.: <2	
Praziquantel	0.8-1.5			80	1-3	80
Primaquine	3.7-9.6		3.5		<6	
Pyrazinamide	9-10	26	0.57-0.74	10-20	1-2	~100
Pyrimethamine	111		3	87	2	
Quinacrine hydrochloride	5-14 d			80-90	8-12	
Quinidine	6			70-80	I.M.: 1	
Quinine sulfate	8-14	8-14	0.7-3.7	70	1-3	
Rifabutin	16-69		9.32	85	2-4	20
Ribavirin	24	1-40 d		0	1-1.5	45
Rifampin	3-4	1.8-11	1.6	89	P.O.: 1.5-4	
Spectinomycin hydrochloride	1.7	16-29	0.25	5-20	1-2	
Stavudine	1-1.6		0.5		1	82
Streptomycin sulfate	2-4.7	100	0.26	35	I.M.: 1	
Sulfadiazine	10	34	0.29	45	3-6	
Sulfadoxine	169			90	2.5-6	
Sulfamethoxazole	9-12	20-50	0.15	70	3-4	
Sulfisoxazole	4-7	6-12	0.14-0.28	85-88	2-3	
Tetracycline	6-11	57-108	1.3-1.6	65	2-3 d	
Thiabendazole	1.2				1-2	
Ticarcillin disodium	1.1-1.2	16	0.18-0.21	45-60		
Tobramycin	2.5	27-60	0.22-0.33	<5	I.M.: 0.5-1	
Trimetrexate	15-17		0.62	86-94	1.8	42
Vancomycin hydrochloride	6-8	200-250	0.47-1.25	55		
Vidarabine	1.5		0.7	20-30		
Zalcitabine	1-3	8.5	0.54	<4	1-2	80
Zidovudine	0.8-1.2		1.4-1.7	30-38	0.5-1.5	

†Multiphasic elimination.

SODIUM CONTENT

Drug Name and Dosage Unit	Sodium	
	mg	mEq
Acyclovir, 1 g	96.6	4.2
Amikacin sulfate, 1 g	29.9	1.3
Aminosalicylate sodium, 1 g	108.1	4.7
Ampicillin, 1 g	66.7	3
Ampicillin sodium & sulbactam sodium, 1.5 g	115	5
Ampicillin, suspension 250 mg/5 mL, 5 mL	10	0.4
Carbenicillin, 382 mg, tablet	23	1
Cefamandole nafate, 1 g	76	3.3
Cefazolin sodium, 1 g	47	2
Cefmetazole sodium, 1 g	47	2
Cefonicid sodium, 1 g	85.1	3.7
Cefoperazone sodium, 1 g	34.5	1.5
Cefotaxime sodium, 1 g	50.6	2.2
Cefotetan disodium, 1 g	80.5	3.5
Cefoxitin sodium, 1 g	53	2.3
Ceftazidime, 1 g	54	2.3
Ceftizoxime sodium, 1 g	59.8	2.6
Ceftriaxone sodium, 1 g	59.8	2.6
Cefuroxime, 1 g	55.2	2.4
Cephalothin sodium, 1 g	64.4	2.8
Cephapirin sodium, 1 g	55.2	2.4
Chloramphenicol, 1 g	51.8	2.25
Cloxacillin sodium, 125 mg/5 mL	11	0.48
Cloxacillin sodium, 250 mg, capsule	13.8	0.6
Colistimethate sodium, 150 mg	22.9	1
Dicloxacillin, 250 mg (capsule)	13	0.6
Dicloxacillin, suspension 65 mg/5 mL	27	1.2
Didanosine, buffered tablets	264.5	11.5
Erythromycin base Filmtab™, 250 mg	70	3
Erythromycin, ethyl succinate, suspension 200 mg/5 mL	29	1.3
Ganciclovir, 500 mg vial	46	2
Imipenem/cilastatin, injection, 1 g, I.V.	73.6	3.2
Imipenem/cilastatin, injection, 1 g, I.M.	64.4	2.8
Methicillin sodium, 1 g	59.8-71.3	2.6-3.1
Metronidazole, 500 mg I.V.	322	14
Mezlocillin sodium, 1 g	42.6	1.85
Nafcillin sodium, 1 g	66.7	2.9
Oxacillin sodium, 1 g	64.4-71.3	2.8-3.1
Penicillin G potassium, 1 million units parenteral	7	0.3
Penicillin G sodium, 1 million units parenteral	46	2
Piperacillin sodium, 1 g	42.6	1.85
Piperacillin sodium & tazobactam sodium	54 mg	2.35
Ticarcillin and clavulanate potassium, 1 g	109.3	4.75
Ticarcillin disodium, 1 g	119.6-149.5	5.2-6.5

OCCUPATIONAL EXPOSURE TO BLOODBORNE PATHOGENS (UNIVERSAL PRECAUTIONS)

Overview and Regulatory Considerations

Every healthcare employee, from nurse to housekeeper, has some (albeit small) risk of exposure to HIV and other viral agents such as hepatitis B and Jakob-Creutzfeldt agent. The incidence of HIV-1 transmission associated with a percutaneous exposure to blood from an HIV-1 infected patient is approximately 0.3% per exposure.[1] In 1989, it was estimated that 12,000 United States healthcare workers acquired hepatitis B annually.[2] An understanding of the appropriate procedures, responsibilities, and risks inherent in the collection and handling of patient specimens is necessary for safe practice and is required by Occupational Safety and Health Administration (OSHA) regulations.

The Occupational Safety and Health Administration published its "Final Rule on Occupational Exposure to Bloodborne Pathogens" in the Federal Register on December 6, 1991. OSHA has chosen to follow the Center for Disease Control (CDC) definition of universal precautions. The Final Rule provides full legal force to universal precautions and requires employers and employees to treat blood and certain body fluids as if they were infectious. The Final Rule mandates that healthcare workers must avoid parenteral contact and must avoid splattering blood or other potentially infectious material on their skin, hair, eyes, mouth, mucous membranes, or on their personal clothing. Hazard abatement strategies must be used to protect the workers. Such plans typically include, but are not limited to, the following:

- safe handling of sharp items ("sharps") and disposal of such into puncture resistant containers

- gloves required for employees handling items soiled with blood or equipment contaminated by blood or other body fluids

- provisions of protective clothing when more extensive contact with blood or body fluids may be anticipated (eg, surgery, autopsy, or deliveries)

- resuscitation equipment to reduce necessity for mouth to mouth resuscitation

- restriction of HIV- or hepatitis B-exposed employees to noninvasive procedures

OSHA has specifically defined the following terms: **Occupational exposure** means reasonably anticipated skin, eye mucous membrane, or parenteral contact with blood or other potentially infectious materials that may result from the performance of an employee's duties. **Other potentially infectious materials** are human body fluids including semen, vaginal secretions, cerebrospinal fluid, synovial fluid, pleural fluid, pericardial fluid, peritoneal fluid, amniotic fluid, saliva in dental procedures, and body fluids that are visibly contaminated with blood, and all body fluids in situations where it is difficult or impossible to differentiate between body fluids; any unfixed tissue or organ (other than intact skin) from a human (living or dead); and HIV-containing cell or tissue cultures, organ cultures,

---

[1] Henderson DK, Fahey BJ, Willy M, et al, "Risk for Occupational Transmission of Human Immunodeficiency Virus Type 1 (HIV-1) Associated With Clinical Exposures. A Prospective Evaluation," *Ann Intern Med*, 1990, 113(10):740-6.

[2] Niu MT and Margolis HS, "Moving Into a New Era of Government Regulation: Provisions for Hepatitis B Vaccine in the Workplace, *Clin Lab Manage Rev*, 1989, 3:336-40.

and HIV- or HBV-containing culture medium or other solutions, and blood, organs, or other tissues from experimental animals infected with HIV or HBV. An **exposure incident** involves specific eye, mouth, other mucous membrane, nonintact skin, or parenteral contact with blood or other potentially infectious materials that results from the performance of an employee's duties.[3] It is important to understand that some exposures may go unrecognized despite the strictest precautions.

A written Exposure Control Plan is required. Employers must provide copies of the plan to employees and to OSHA upon request. Compliance with OSHA rules may be accomplished by the following methods.

- **Universal precautions (UPs)** means that all human blood and certain body fluids are treated as if known to be infectious for HIV, HBV, and other bloodborne pathogens. UPs do not apply to feces, nasal secretions, saliva, sputum, sweat, tears, urine, or vomitus unless they contain visible blood.

- **Engineering controls (ECs)** are physical devices which reduce or remove hazards from the workplace by eliminating or minimizing hazards or by isolating the worker from exposure. Engineering control devices include sharps disposal containers, self-resheathing syringes, etc.

- **Work practice controls (WPCs)** are practices and procedures that reduce the likelihood of exposure to hazards by altering the way in which a task is performed. Specific examples are the prohibition of two-handed recapping of needles, prohibition of storing food alongside potentially contaminated material, discouragement of pipetting fluids by mouth, encouraging handwashing after removal of gloves, safe handling of contaminated sharps, and appropriate use of sharps containers.

- **Personal protective equipment (PPE)** is specialized clothing or equipment worn to provide protection from occupational exposure. PPE includes gloves, gowns, laboratory coats (the type and characteristics will depend upon the task and degree of exposure anticipated), face shields or masks, and eye protection. Surgical caps or hoods and/or shoe covers or boots are required in instances in which gross contamination can reasonably be anticipated (eg, autopsies, orthopedic surgery). If PPE is penetrated by blood or any contaminated material, the item must be removed immediately or as soon as feasible. **The employer must provide and launder or dispose of all PPE at no cost to the employee.** Gloves must be worn when there is a reasonable anticipation of hand contact with potentially infectious material, including a patient's mucous membranes or nonintact skin. Disposable gloves must be changed as soon as possible after they become torn or punctured. Hands must be washed after gloves are removed. OSHA has revised the PPE standards, effective July 5, 1994, to include the requirement that the employer certify in writing that it has conducted a hazard assessment of the workplace to determine whether hazzards are present that will necessitate the use of PPE. Also, verification that the employee has received and understood the PPE training is required.[4]

Housekeeping protocols: OSHA requires that all bins, cans, and similar receptacles, intended for reuse which have a reasonable likelihood for becoming contaminated, be inspected and decontaminated immediately

---

[3] Bruning LM, "The Bloodborne Pathogens Final Rule — Understanding the Regulation," *AORN Journal*, 1993, 57(2):439-40.

[4] "Rules and Regulations," *Federal Register*, 1994, 59(66):16360-3.

or as soon as feasible upon visible contamination and on a regularly scheduled basis. Broken glass that may be contaminated must not be picked up directly with the hands. Mechanical means (eg, brush, dust pan, tongs, or forceps) must be used. Broken glass must be placed in a proper sharps container.

Employers are responsible for teaching appropriate clean-up procedures for the work area and personal protective equipment. A 1:10 dilution of household bleach is a popular and effective disinfectant. It is prudent for employers to maintain signatures or initials of employees who have been properly educated. If one does not have written proof of education of universal precautions teaching, then by OSHA standards, such education never happened.

Pre-exposure and postexposure protocols: OSHA's Final Rule includes the provision that employees, who are exposed to contamination, be offered the hepatitis B vaccine at no cost to the employee. Employees may decline; however, a declination form must be signed. The employee must be offered free vaccine if he/she changes his/her mind. Vaccination to prevent the transmission of hepatitis B in the healthcare setting is widely regarded as sound practice.[5] In the event of exposure, a confidential medical evaluation and follow-up must be offered at no cost to the employee. Follow-up must include collection and testing of blood from the source individual for HBV and HIV if permitted by state law if a blood sample is available. If a postexposure specimen must be specially drawn, the individual's consent is usually required. Some states may not require consent for testing of patient blood after accidental exposure. One must refer to state and/or local guidelines for proper guidance.

The employee follow-up must also include appropriate postexposure prophylaxis, counseling, and evaluation of reported illnesses. The employee has the right to decline baseline blood collection and/or testing. If the employee gives consent for the collection but not the testing, the sample must be preserved for 90 days in the event that the employee changes his/her mind within that time. Confidentiality related to blood testing must be ensured. **The employer does not have the right to know the results** of the testing of either the source individual or the exposed employee.[3]

The Management of Occupational Exposure to HIV in the Workplace[3]

1. Likelyhood of transmission of HIV-1 from occupational exposure is 0.2% per parenteral exposure (eg, needlestick) to blood from HIV infected patients.

2. Factors that increase risk for occupational transmission include advanced stages of HIV in source patient, hollow bore needle puncture, a poor state of health or inexperience of healthcare worker (HCW).

3. Immediate actions an exposed healthcare worker should take include aggressive first aid at the puncture site (eg, scrubbing site with povodone-iodine solution for 10 minutes) or at mucus membrane site (eg, saline irrigation of eye for 15 minutes). Then immediate reporting to the hospital's occupational medical service. The authors indicate that there is no direct evidence for the efficacy of

[5] Schaffner W, Gardner P, and Gross PA, "Hepatitis B Immunization Strategies: Expanding the Target," *Ann Intern Med*, 1993, 118(4):308-9.

[3] Fahey BJ, Beekmann SE, Schmitt JM, et al, "Managing Occupational Exposures to HIV-1 in the Healthcare Workplace," *Infect Control Hosp Epidemiol*, 1993, 14(7):405-12.

their recommendations. Other institutions suggest rigorous scrubbing with soap.

4. After first aid is initiated, the healthcare worker should report exposure to a supervisor and to the institution's occupational medical service for evaluation.

5. Occupational medicine should perform a thorough investigation including identifying the HIV and hepatitis B status of the source, type of exposure, volume of innoculum, timing of exposure, extent of injury, appropriateness of first aid, as well as psychological status of the healthcare worker. HIV serologies should be performed on the healthcare worker. HIV risk counselling should begin at this point.

6. All parenteral exposures should be treated equally until they can be evaluated by the occupational medicine service, who will then determine the actual risk of exposure. Follow-up counselling sessions may be necessary.

7. Although the data are not clear, antiviral prophylaxis may be offered to healthcare workers who are parenterally or mucous membrane exposed. If used, antiretroviral prophylaxis should be initiated within 1-2 hours after exposure.

8. Counselling regarding risk of exposure, antiviral prophylaxis, plans for follow up, exposure prevention, sexual activity, and providing emotional support and response to concerns are necessary to support the exposed healthcare worker. Follow-up should consist of periodic serologic evaluation and blood chemistries and counts if antiretroviral prophylaxis is initiated. Additional information should be provided to healthcare workers who are pregnant or planning to become pregnant.

See also Postexposure Prophylaxis for Hepatitis B in the Appendix.

Hazardous Communication

Communication regarding the dangers of bloodborne infections through the use of labels, signs, information, and education is required. Storage locations (eg, refrigerators and freezers, waste containers) that are used to store, dispose of, transport, or ship blood or other potentially infectious materials require labels. The label background must be red or bright orange with the biohazard design and the word biohazard in a contrasting color. The label must be part of the container or affixed to the container by permanent means.

Education provided by a qualified and knowledgeable instructor is mandated. The sessions for employees must include:[4]

-   accessible copies of the regulation

-   general epidemiology of bloodborne diseases

-   modes of bloodborne pathogen transmission

-   an explanation of the exposure control plan and a means to obtain copies of the written plan

-   an explanation of the tasks and activities that may involve exposure

-   the use of exposure prevention methods and their limitations (eg, engineering controls, work practices, personal protective equipment)

- information on the types, proper use, location, removal, handling, decontamination, and disposal of personal protective equipment)

- an explanation of the basis for selection of personal protective equipment

- information on the HBV vaccine, including information on its efficacy, safety, and method of administration and the benefits of being vaccinated (ie, the employee must understand that the vaccine and vaccination will be offered free of charge)

- information on the appropriate actions to take and persons to contact in an emergency involving exposure to blood or other potentially infectious materials

- an explanation of the procedure to follow if an exposure incident occurs, including the method of reporting the incident

- information on the postexposure evaluation and follow-up that the employer is required to provide for the employee following an exposure incident

- an explanation of the signs, labels, and color coding

- an interactive question-and-answer period

Record Keeping

The OSHA Final Rule requires that the employer maintain both education and medical records. The medical records must be kept confidential and be maintained for the duration of employment plus 30 years. They must contain a copy of the employee's HBV vaccination status and postexposure incident information. Education records must be maintained for 3 years from the date the program was given.

OSHA has the authority to conduct inspections without notice. Penalties for cited violation may be assessed as follows.[3]

Serious violations. In this situation, there is a substantial probability of death or serious physical harm, and the employer knew, or should have known, of the hazard. A violation of this type carries a mandatory penalty of up to $7000 for each violation.

Other-than-serious violations. The violation is unlikely to result in death or serious physical harm. This type of violation carries a discretionary penalty of up to $7000 for each violation.

Willful violations. These are violations committed knowingly or intentionally by the employer and have penalties of up to $70,000 per violation with a minimum of $5000 per violation. If an employee dies as a result of a willful violation, the responsible party, if convicted, may receive a personal fine of up to $250,000 and/or a 6-month jail term. A corporation may be fined $500,000.

Large fines frequently follow visits to laboratories, physicians' offices, and healthcare facilities by OSHA Compliance Safety and Health Offices (CSHOS). Regulations are vigorously enforced. A working knowledge of the final rule and implementation of appropriate policies and practices is imperative for all those involved in the collection and analysis of medical specimens.

Effectiveness of universal precautions in averting exposure to potentially infectious materials has been documented.[5] Compliance with appropriate rules, procedures, and policies, including reporting exposure incidents, is a matter of personal professionalism and prudent self-preservation.

References

Buehler JW and Ward JW, "A New Definition for AIDS Surveillance," *Ann Intern Med*, 1993, 118(5):390-2.

Brown JW and Blackwell H, "Complying With the New OSHA Regs, Part 1: Teaching Your Staff About Biosafety," *MLO*, 1992, 24(4)24-8. Part 2: "Safety Protocols No Lab Can Ignore," 1992, 24(5):27-9. Part 3: "Compiling Employee Safety Records That Will Satisfy OSHA," 1992, 24(6):45-8.

Department of Labor, Occupational Safety and Health Administration, "Occupational Exposure to Bloodborne Pathogens; Final Rule (29 CFR Part 1910.1030)," *Federal Register*, December 6, 1991, 64004-182.

Gold JW, "HIV-1 Infection: Diagnosis and Management," *Med Clin North Am*, 1992, 76(1):1-18.

"Hepatitis B Virus: A Comprehensive Strategy for Eliminating Transmission in the United States Through Universal Childhood Vaccination," *MMWR Morb Mortal Wkly Rep*, 1991, 40(RR-13):1-25.

"Mortality Attributable to HIV Infection/AIDS — United States", *MMWR Morb Mortal Wkly Rep*, 1991, 40(3):41-4.

National Committee for Clinical Laboratory Standards, "Protection of Laboratory Workers From Infectious Disease Transmitted by Blood, Body Fluids, and Tissue," NCCLS Document M29-T, Villanova, PA: NCCLS, 1989, 9(1).

"Nosocomial Transmission of Hepatitis B Virus Associated With a Spring-Loaded Fingerstick Device — California," *MMWR Morb Mortal Wkly Rep*, 1990, 39(35):610-3.

Polish LB, Shapiro CN, Bauer F, et al, "Nosocomial Transmission of Hepatitis B Virus Associated With the Use of a Spring-Loaded Fingerstick Device," *N Engl J Med*, 1992, 326(11):721-5.

"Recommendations for Preventing Transmission of Human Immunodeficiency Virus and Hepatitis B Virus to Patients During Exposure-Prone Invasive Procedures," *MMWR Morb Mortal Wkly Rep*, 1991, 40(RR-8):1-9.

"Update: Acquired Immunodeficiency Syndrome — United States," *MMWR Morb Mortal Wkly Rep*, 1992, 41(26):463-8.

"Update: Transmission of HIV Infection During an Invasive Dental Procedure — Florida," *MMWR Morb Mortal Wkly Rep*, 1991, 40(2):21-7, 33.

"Update: Universal Precautions for Prevention of Transmission of Human Immunodeficiency Virus, Hepatitis B Virus, and Other Bloodborne Pathogens in Healthcare Settings," *MMWR Morb Mortal Wkly Rep*, 1988, 37(24):377-82, 387-8.

---

[5] Wong ES, Stotka JL, Chinchilli VM, et al, "Are Universal Precautions Effective in Reducing the Number of Occupational Exposures Among Healthcare Workers?" *JAMA*, 1991, 265:1123-8.

Penicillins, Penicillin-Related Antibiotics & Other Antibiotics

KEY TO TABLE

- **A** Recommended drug therapy
- **B** Alternate drug therapy
- **C** Organism is usually or always sensitive to this agent
- **D** Organism portrays variable sensitivity to this agent
- (Blank) This drug should not be used for this organism or insufficient data is available

		Listeria monocytogenes	Corynebacterium jeikeium	Corynebacterium sp.	Streptococcus, Viridans Group	Streptococcus pneumoniae	Streptococcus bovis (Group D)	Enterococcus sp. (Group D)	Streptococcus agalactiae (Group B)	Streptococcus pyogenes (Group A)	Staph. epidermidis: Methicillin-Resistant	Staph. epidermidis: Methicillin-Susceptible	Staph. aureus: Methicillin-Resistant	Staph. aureus: Methicillin-Susceptible
Penicillins	Amoxicillin				C	C	C		C	C				
	Ampicillin	A			C	C	C	A	C	C				
	Penicillin G	A	B	B	A	A	A	A	A	A				
	Penicillin V			C	C	C	C	C	C	C				
	Azlocillin													
	Mezlocillin				D	C	D	D	C	C				
	Piperacillin				D	C	D	C	C	C				
	Ticarcillin				D	C	D		C	C				
	Cloxacillin				D					D		A		A
	Dicloxacillin				D					D		A		A
	Methicillin				D					D		A		A
	Nafcillin				D					D		A		A
	Oxacillin				D					D		A		A
Penicillin-Related Antibiotics	Amoxicillin/Clavulanate	C			C	C	C	C	C	C		C		C
	Ampicillin/Sulbactam	C			C	C	C	C	C	C		C		C
	Ticarcillin/Clavulanate				C	C	C	D	C	C		C		C
	Aztreonam													
	Imipenem/Cilastatin				C	C	C	D	C	C		C		C
	Piperacillin/Tazobactam				C	C	C	C	C	C		C		C
Other Antibiotics	Chloramphenicol	C				B		D						
	Clindamycin			D	D	C	D		C	C		B		B
	Co-trimoxazole	B				C					B	C	B	C
	Metronidazole													
	Rifampin			D							A	C	A	C
	Sulfonamides													
	Tetracyclines	C			C	C			C				A	D
	Vancomycin	D	A		B	B	B	B	B	B	B	A	B	A
UTI Agents	Indanyl Carbenicillin							D						
	Nitrofurantoin							D						

Penicillins, Penicillin-Related Antibiotics & Other Antibiotics

KEY TO TABLE

- **A** Recommended drug therapy
- **B** Alternate drug therapy
- **C** Organism is usually or always sensitive to this agent
- **D** Organism portrays variable sensitivity to this agent
- (Blank) This drug should not be used for this organism or insufficient data is available

GRAM-NEGATIVE AEROBES

Class	Drug	Yersinia enterocolitica	Shigella sp.	Serratia sp.	Salmonella sp.	Proteus sp.	Proteus mirabilis	Klebsiella pneumoniae	Escherichia coli	Enterobacter sp.[1]	Citrobacter sp.[1]	Neisseria meningitidis	Neisseria gonorrhoeae	Moraxella (Branhamella) catarrhalis
Penicillin	Amoxicillin						B		A		C		C	D
Penicillin	Ampicillin	A					B		A		A		C	D
Penicillin	Penicillin G												A	D
Penicillin	Penicillin V													D
Penicillin	Azlocillin													
Penicillin	Mezlocillin			A		B	C	B	C	A	A		D	
Penicillin	Piperacillin			A		B	C	B	C	A	A		D	
Penicillin	Ticarcillin			A		B	C	D	C	A	A		D	
Penicillin	Cloxacillin													
Penicillin	Dicloxacillin													
Penicillin	Methicillin													
Penicillin	Nafcillin													
Penicillin	Oxacillin													
Penicillin-Related Antibiotics	Amoxicillin/Clavulanate					C		C	C	C		C	C	A
Penicillin-Related Antibiotics	Ampicillin/Sulbactam		C			C		C	C	C		C	C	C
Penicillin-Related Antibiotics	Ticarcillin/Clavulanate			A	C	B	C	B	C	A	A	C	C	C
Penicillin-Related Antibiotics	Aztreonam			B	C	C	C	B	C	A	C		C	C
Penicillin-Related Antibiotics	Imipenem/Cilastatin			B	C	B	C	B	C	B	B	D	C	C
Penicillin-Related Antibiotics	Piperacillin/Tazobactam			A	C	B	C	B	C	A	A	C	C	C
Other Antibiotics	Chloramphenicol		C		B				C			B		
Other Antibiotics	Clindamycin													
Other Antibiotics	Co-trimoxazole	C	A	C	B	C	B	C	A	C	C			A
Other Antibiotics	Metronidazole													
Other Antibiotics	Rifampin											D		
Other Antibiotics	Sulfonamides		C		C			C	C	C		D		
Other Antibiotics	Tetracyclines	C	C					C	C		D	C	B	C
Other Antibiotics	Vancomycin													
UTI Agents	Indanyl Carbenicillin			C		C	C	C	C	C	C			
UTI Agents	Nitrofurantoin							C	C	C	C			

[1] Citrobacter freundii, Citrobacter diversus, Enterobacter cloacae and Enterobacter aerogenes often have significantly different antibiotic sensitivity patterns. Speciation and susceptibility testing are particularly important

Penicillins, Penicillin-Related Antibiotics & Other Antibiotics

KEY TO TABLE

- **A** Recommended drug therapy
- **B** Alternate drug therapy
- **C** Organism is usually or always sensitive to this agent
- **D** Organism portrays variable sensitivity to this agent
- (Blank) This drug should not be used for this organism or insufficient data is available

		\multicolumn{12}{c}{GRAM-NEGATIVE AEROBES — Other bacilli}											
		Vibrio cholerae	Xanthomonas maltophilia	Pseudomonas aeruginosa	Pasteurella multocida	Legionella pneumophila	Haemophilus influenzae	Haemophilus ducreyi	Gardnerella vaginalis	Campylobacter jejuni	Brucella sp.	Bordetella pertussis	Acinetobacter sp.
Penicillin	Amoxicillin				C		B			C			
	Ampicillin				C		B			B	D		
	Penicillin G				A								
	Penicillin V				C								
	Azlocillin												
	Mezlocillin			A	C		D						A
	Piperacillin			A	C		D						A
	Ticarcillin			A	C		D						A
	Cloxacillin												
	Dicloxacillin												
	Methicillin												
	Nafcillin												
	Oxacillin												
Penicillin-Related Antibiotics	Amoxicillin/Clavulanate				B		B	B	C				C
	Ampicillin/Sulbactam				B		C	C	C				C
	Ticarcillin/Clavulanate		B	A	C		C						A
	Aztreonam			C			C						B
	Imipenem/Cilastatin			A			C						B
	Piperacillin/Tazobactam			A	C		C						A
Other Antibiotics	Chloramphenicol		C		C		B			C	C		
	Clindamycin									C	C		
	Co-trimoxazole	A	A				A	B			B	A	
	Metronidazole									A			
	Rifampin					A	D				A		
	Sulfonamides				C			C			C		
	Tetracyclines	A			C		C	C			A	C	
	Vancomycin												
UTI Agents	Indanyl Carbenicillin			D									C
	Nitrofurantoin												

Penicillins, Penicillin-Related Antibiotics & Other Antibiotics

KEY TO TABLE

- **A** Recommended drug therapy
- **B** Alternate drug therapy
- **C** Organism is usually or always sensitive to this agent
- **D** Organism portrays variable sensitivity to this agent
- (Blank) This drug should not be used for this organism or insufficient data is available

Class	Drug	Treponema pallidum	Leptospira sp.	Borrelia burgdorferi (Lyme disease)	Rickettsia sp.	Ureaplasma urealyticum	Mycoplasma pneumoniae	Chlamydia trachomatis	Chlamydia pneumoniae (TWAR)	Chlamydia psittaci	Bacteroides sp. (Gram −)	Streptococcus, anaerobic (Gram +)	Clostridium perfringens (Gram +)	Clostridium difficile [2] (Gram +)
Penicillin	Amoxicillin			B							D	C	D	
	Ampicillin			B							C	C	D	
	Penicillin G	A	A	B							C	A	A	
	Penicillin V	C	C	B							C	C	C	
	Azlocillin													
	Mezlocillin										C	C	C	
	Piperacillin										C	C	C	
	Ticarcillin										C	C	C	
	Cloxacillin													
	Dicloxacillin													
	Methicillin													
	Nafcillin													
	Oxacillin													
Penicillin-Related Antibiotics	Amoxicillin/Clavulanate										C	C	C	
	Ampicillin/Sulbactam										C	C	C	
	Ticarcillin/Clavulanate										C	C	C	
	Aztreonam													
	Imipenem/Cilastatin										C	C	B	
	Piperacillin/Tazobactam										C	C	C	
Other Antibiotics	Chloramphenicol				A						C	C	C	D
	Clindamycin										A	B	B	
	Co-trimoxazole													
	Metronidazole										A	D	A	A
	Rifampin													
	Sulfonamides								D					
	Tetracyclines	B	B	A	A	A	A	A	B	B	B	D	C	C
	Vancomycin											B		B
UTI Agents	Indanyl Carbenicillin													
	Nitrofurantoin													

[2] Vancomycin is effective orally only.

Cephalosporins, Aminoglycosides, Macrolides & Quinolones

KEY TO TABLE

- **A** — Recommended drug therapy
- **B** — Alternate drug therapy
- **C** — Organism is usually or always sensitive to this agent
- **D** — Organism portrays variable sensitivity to this agent
- (Blank) — This drug should not be used for this organism or insufficient data is available

GRAM-POSITIVE AEROBES

Column key — Bacilli: L.m = *Listeria monocytogenes*[d]; C.j = *Corynebacterium jeikeium*; C.sp = *Corynebacterium* sp. Cocci: Vir = *Streptococcus*, Viridans Group; Pn = *Streptococcus pneumoniae*; Bov = *Streptococcus bovis* (Group D); Ent = *Enterococcus* sp. (Group D); Agal = *Streptococcus agalactiae* (Group B); Pyo = *Streptococcus pyogenes* (Group A); SE-MR = *Staphylococcus epidermidis*: Methicillin-Resistant[a]; SE-MS = *Staphylococcus epidermidis*: Methicillin-Susceptible; SA-MR = *Staphylococcus aureus*: Methicillin-Resistant[a]; SA-MS = *Staphylococcus aureus*: Methicillin-Susceptible.

Class	Drug	L.m[d]	C.j	C.sp	Vir	Pn	Bov	Ent	Agal	Pyo	SE-MR[a]	SE-MS	SA-MR[a]	SA-MS
1st Generation	Cefadroxil				B	B	C		B	B		B		B
1st Generation	Cefazolin				B	B	C		B	B		B		B
1st Generation	Cephalexin				B	B	C		B	B		B		B
1st Generation	Cephalothin				B	B	C		B	B		B		B
1st Generation	Cephapirin				B	B	C		B	B		B		B
1st Generation	Cephradine				B	B	C		B	B		B		B
2nd Generation and others	Cefaclor				C	C	C		C	C		D		D
2nd Generation and others	Cefamandole				C	C	C		C	C		C		C
2nd Generation and others	Cefmetazole				C	C	C		C	C		D		D
2nd Generation and others	Cefonicid				C	C	C		C	C		D		D
2nd Generation and others	Cefotetan				C	C	C		C	C		D		D
2nd Generation and others	Cefoxitin				C	C	C		C	C		D		D
2nd Generation and others	Cefpodoxime Proxetil				C	C	C		C	C		D		D
2nd Generation and others	Cefprozil				C	C	D		C	C				D
2nd Generation and others	Cefuroxime				C	C	C		C	C		D		D
2nd Generation and others	Cefuroxime Axetil				C	C			C	C		C		C
2nd Generation and others	Loracarbef				C	C	D		C	C		C		C
3rd Generation	Cefixime				D	D			C	C				
3rd Generation	Cefoperazone				D	D	C		C	C		D		D
3rd Generation	Cefotaxime				D	D	C		C	C		D		D
3rd Generation	Ceftazidime				D		D		D	D				
3rd Generation	Ceftizoxime				D	D	C		C	C		D		D
3rd Generation	Ceftriaxone				C	C	C		C	C		D		D
Aminoglycosides	Amikacin	C	C				D	D						
Aminoglycosides	Gentamicin	A	B		A		D	A			A	D	A	D
Aminoglycosides	Netilmicin	C	C					C						
Aminoglycosides	Streptomycin						D	C						
Aminoglycosides	Tobramycin	C	C					D						D
Macrolides	Azithromycin	C			C	C			C	C				C
Macrolides	Clarithromycin	C			C	C			C	C				C
Macrolides	Erythromycin	C	C	A	C	B			B	B				C
Quinolones	Lomefloxacin		D		D	D	D	D	D	D	D	D	D	D
Quinolones	Ciprofloxacin		D		D	D	D	D	D	D	D	D	D	D
Quinolones	Norfloxacin										D	D		
Quinolones	Ofloxacin		D		D	D	D	D	D	D	D	D	D	D

Cephalosporins, Aminoglycosides, Macrolides & Quinolones

KEY TO TABLE

- **A** — Recommended drug therapy
- **B** — Alternate drug therapy
- **C** — Organism is usually or always sensitive to this agent
- **D** — Organism portrays variable sensitivity to this agent
- (Blank) This drug should not be used for this organism or insufficient data is available

GRAM-NEGATIVE AEROBES

		Enteric bacilli									Cocci		
		Yersinia enterocolitica	Shigella sp.	Serratia sp.	Salmonella sp.	Proteus mirabilis	Klebsiella pneumoniae	Escherichia coli	Enterobacter sp.[1]	Citrobacter sp.[1]	Neisseria meningitidis	Neisseria gonorrhoeae	Moraxella (Branhamella) catarrhalis
1st Generation	Cefadroxil					A	A	B					D
	Cefazolin					A	A	B					D
	Cephalexin					A	A	B					D
	Cephalothin					A	A	B					D
	Cephapirin					A	A	B					D
	Cephradine					A	A	B					D
2nd Generation and others	Cefaclor						C	A	B			C	B
	Cefamandole					D	C	A	B			C	B
	Cefmetazole	D	C	C		D	C	A	B			C	B
	Cefonicid						C	A	B			C	B
	Cefotetan	C	C	C		D	C	A	B			C	B
	Cefoxitin				D	D	C	A	B			C	B
	Cefpodoxime Proxetil						C	A	B			C	B
	Cefprozil		C				C	D	B			C	B
	Cefuroxime	C	C			D	C	A	B			C	B
	Cefuroxime Axetil						C	A	B		C	C	B
	Loracarbef						C	C	B			C	B
3rd Generation	Cefixime		C	C		C	C	A	A			C	B
	Cefoperazone		B	A	A	A	C	A	A	A			B
	Cefotaxime	A	B	A	A	A	C	A	A	A	B	C	B
	Ceftazidime		B	A		A	C	A	A	A			B
	Ceftizoxime	A	B	A	A	A	C	A	A	A	B	C	B
	Ceftriaxone	A	B	A	A	A	C	A	A	A	B	A	B
Aminoglycosides	Amikacin	A		C		C	C	C	C	C			
	Gentamicin	A	D	C	D	C	C	C	C	C			
	Netilmicin	A	D	C	D	C	C	C	C	C			
	Streptomycin												
	Tobramycin	A		C	D	C	C	C	C	C			
Macrolides	Azithromycin											C	C
	Clarithromycin											C	C
	Erythromycin											D	C
Quinolones	Lomefloxacin	C	C	C	C	C	C	C	C	C	D	C	C
	Ciprofloxacin	C	B	C	B	C	C	C	C	C	C	A	C
	Norfloxacin	C	C	C	C	C	C	C	C	C		C	
	Ofloxacin	C	C	C	C	C	C	C	C	C	C	A	C

[1] Citrobacter freundii, Citrobacter diversus, Enterobacter cloacae and Enterobacter aerogenes often have significantly different antibiotic sensitivity patterns. Speciation and susceptibility testing are particularly important

Cephalosporins, Aminoglycosides, Macrolides & Quinolones

KEY TO TABLE

A	Recommended drug therapy
B	Alternate drug therapy
C	Organism is usually or always sensitive to this agent
D	Organism portrays variable sensitivity to this agent
(Blank)	This drug should not be used for this organism or insufficient data is available

GRAM-NEGATIVE AEROBES — Other bacilli

Generation	Drug	Vibrio cholerae	Xanthomonas maltophilia	Pseudomonas aeruginosa	Pasteurella multocida	Legionella pneumophila	Haemophilus influenzae	Haemophilus ducreyi	Gardnerella vaginalis	Campylobacter jejuni	Brucella sp.	Bordetella pertussis	Acinetobacter sp.
1st Generation	Cefadroxil						D						
1st Generation	Cefazolin						D						
1st Generation	Cephalexin						D						
1st Generation	Cephalothin						D						
1st Generation	Cephapirin						D						
1st Generation	Cephradine						D						
2nd Generation and others	Cefaclor						B						
2nd Generation and others	Cefamandole				C		B						
2nd Generation and others	Cefmetazole				D		C						
2nd Generation and others	Cefonicid						C						
2nd Generation and others	Cefotetan				D		C						
2nd Generation and others	Cefoxitin				D		C						
2nd Generation and others	Cefpodoxime Proxetil						B						
2nd Generation and others	Cefprozil						B						
2nd Generation and others	Cefuroxime						B						
2nd Generation and others	Cefuroxime Axetil				D		B						
2nd Generation and others	Loracarbef						B						
3rd Generation	Cefixime						A						D
3rd Generation	Cefoperazone		D	D	C		A	C					D
3rd Generation	Cefotaxime		D		C			C					A
3rd Generation	Ceftazidime		D	A				C					A
3rd Generation	Ceftizoxime		D		C			C					A
3rd Generation	Ceftriaxone		D		C			A					A
Aminoglycosides	Amikacin		C	A				C		C			C
Aminoglycosides	Gentamicin		C	A				C		C	C		C
Aminoglycosides	Netilmicin		C	A				C		C			C
Aminoglycosides	Streptomycin										C		
Aminoglycosides	Tobramycin		C	A				C		C			C
Macrolides	Azithromycin				D	B	C	C		C		C	
Macrolides	Clarithromycin				D	B	C			C		C	
Macrolides	Erythromycin				D	A		C		A		A	
Quinolones	Lomefloxacin	C	C	D	C		C	C	D	B	C		D
Quinolones	Ciprofloxacin	C	B	A	C	B	C	B	C	B	C		C
Quinolones	Norfloxacin			C							B		D
Quinolones	Ofloxacin	C	B	D	C	C	C	C	C	C	B		C

Cephalosporins, Aminoglycosides, Macrolides & Quinolones

KEY TO TABLE

A	Recommended drug therapy
B	Alternate drug therapy
C	Organism is usually or always sensitive to this agent
D	Organism portrays variable sensitivity to this agent
(Blank)	This drug should not be used for this organism or insufficient data is available

	Drug	Treponema pallidum	Leptospira sp.	Borrelia burgdorferi (Lyme disease)	Rickettsia sp.	Ureaplasma urealyticum	Mycoplasma pneumoniae	Chlamydia trachomatis	Chlamydia pneumoniae (TWAR)	Chlamydia psittaci	Bacteroides sp. (Gram −)	Streptococcus, anaerobic (Gram +)	Clostridium perfringens (Gram +)	Clostridium difficile [2] (Gram +)
1st Generation	Cefadroxil											B		
	Cefazolin											B		
	Cephalexin											B		
	Cephalothin											B		
	Cephapirin											B		
	Cephradine											B		
2nd Generation and others	Cefaclor													
	Cefamandole													
	Cefmetazole										C	C	C	
	Cefonicid													
	Cefotetan										B	C	C	
	Cefoxitin										B	C	C	
	Cefpodoxime Proxetil													
	Cefprozil													
	Cefuroxime											C	C	
	Cefuroxime Axetil													
	Loracarbef													
3rd Generation	Cefixime													
	Cefoperazone												D	
	Cefotaxime		C								D	C	C	
	Ceftazidime												D	
	Ceftizoxime		C								D	C	C	
	Ceftriaxone	C	A									C		
Aminoglycosides	Amikacin													
	Gentamicin													
	Netilmicin													
	Streptomycin													
	Tobramycin													
Macrolides	Azithromycin	D		C		B	C	C	C	C		D	D	
	Clarithromycin	D		D		B	C	C	C	C		D	D	
	Erythromycin	D		C		A	A	A	A	A		D	D	
Quinolones	Lomefloxacin						D	D	D					
	Ciprofloxacin					D	D	D	D					
	Norfloxacin													
	Ofloxacin					D	D	D	C					

[2] Vancomycin is effective orally only.

ALGORITHM 1.

SELECTED ELEMENTS OF THE INITIAL AND ONGOING EVALUATION OF ADULTS WITH EARLY HIV INFECTION

[1]Provider should review and evaluate the adequacy of HIV diagnostic tests.

[2]Appropriate immunizations should be provided (this topic was not reviewed by the HIV panel).

[3]Schedule followup appropriate for patient's condition.

[4]Many other screening tests were not reviewed by this panel, including toxoplasmosis, hepatitis serology, and routine laboratory tests.

Note: The algorithm presents recommendations only for the items reviewed by the HIV panel.

From U.S. Department of Health and Human Services, *Evaluation and Management of Early HIV Infection,* Clinical Practice Guideline, Number 7, 1994; 167-76.

ALGORITHM 2.

EVALUATION FOR INITIATION OF ANTIRETROVIRAL THERAPY AND PCP PROPHYLAXIS; MEN AND NONPREGNANT WOMEN WITH EARLY HIV INFECTION

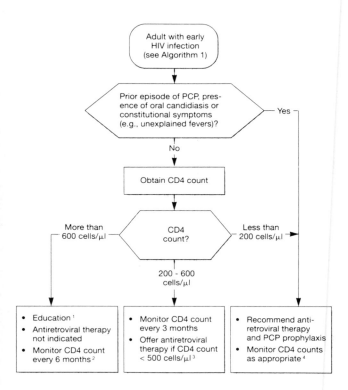

[1]Education should include a discussion of enrollment into relevant investigational drug trials for asymptomatic persons.

[2]If CD4 count has shown great variability or is rapidly declining, repeat the CD4 within 3 months.

[3]If patient develops symptoms, recommend antiretroviral therapy.

[4]If CD4 count <200 cells/μL, continued monitoring of CD4 count may be needed to determine eligibility for clinical trials, and prophylaxis for opportunistic infections other than PCP and to guide antiretroviral therapy.

Note: The algorithm presents recommendations only for the items reviewed by the HIV panel.

From U.S. Department of Health and Human Services, *Evaluation and Management of Early HIV Infection.* Clinical Practice Guideline. Number 7. 1994. 167-76.

ALGORITHM 3.

EVALUATION FOR INITIATION OF ANTIRETROVIRAL THERAPY AND PCP PROPHYLAXIS; PREGNANT WOMEN WITH EARLY HIV INFECTION

[1]CD4 count should be obtained on presentation for prenatal care; women who have received no prenatal care should have CD4 counts taken at delivery.

[2]Unless indicated by the presence of clinical symptoms.

[3]The possible benefits and risks of antiretroviral therapy to both mother and fetus should be discussed fully with the patient.

Note: The algorithm presents recommendations only for the items reviewed by the HIV panel.

From U.S. Department of Health and Human Services, *Evaluation and Management of Early HIV Infection*, Clinical Practice Guideline, Number 7. 1994, 167-76.

ALGORITHM 4.

EVALUATION FOR *MYCOBACTERIUM* TUBERCULOSIS INFECTION IN ADULTS AND ADOLESCENTS WITH EARLY HIV INFECTION

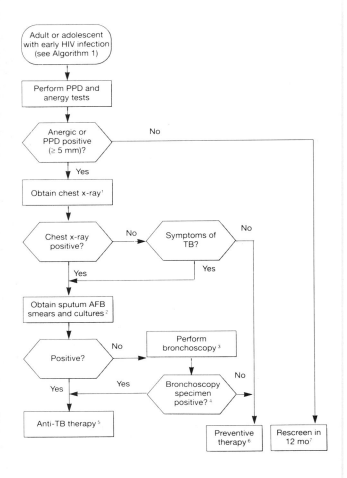

[1]Chest x-ray can be performed, using a lead apron shield, after the first trimester in pregnant women asymptomatic for TB or at any stage of pregnancy in women symptomatic for TB.

[2]At least three sputum smears and cultures should be obtained.

[3]If there is no other etiology for the abnormal chest x-ray.

[4]Both AFB smears and cultures should be obtained at bronchoscopy.

[5]Anti-TB therapy should be guided by local susceptibility patterns and modified appropriately when isolated susceptibilities become available.

[6]Preventive therapy is indicated for PPD-positive patients and should be strongly considered for anergic patients who are known contacts of patients with tuberculosis and for anergic patients belonging to groups in which the prevalence of tuberculosis is at least 10% (eg, injection drug users, prisoners, homeless persons, persons in congregate housing, migrant laborers, and persons born in foreign countries with high rates of TB).

[7]Individuals who reside in settings where TB prevalence is high should be retested in 6 months; individuals who are exposed acutely to others with suspected or confirmed TB should be retested in 3 months; anergic individuals need not be retested, except in special circumstances.

Note: The algorithm presents recommendations only for the items reviewed by the HIV panel.

From U.S. Department of Health and Human Services, *Evaluation and Management of Early HIV Infection*, Clinical Practice Guideline, Number 7, 1994, 167-76.

ALGORITHM 5.

EVALUATION FOR SYPHILIS IN ADULTS AND SEXUALLY ACTIVE ADOLESCENTS WITH EARLY HIV INFECTION

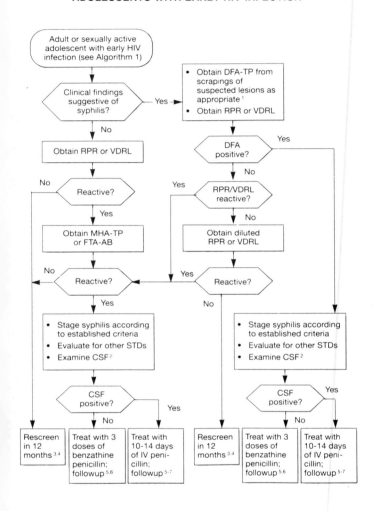

[1]If dark-field exam cannot be performed and primary syphilis is suspected, empiric treatment should be instituted.

[2]Treatment for neurosyphilis recommended if the CSF cannot be evaluated (See *Guideline for Evaluation and Management of Early HIV Infection* for recommended followup).

[3]Or after exposure to or diagnosis of any sexually transmitted disease.

[4]Pregnant women should be screened for syphilis at entry to prenatal care, during the third trimester, or at delivery.

[5]See *Guideline for Evaluation and Management of Early HIV Infection* for recommended followup.

[6]For issues specific to pregnant women, see *Guideline for Evaluation and Management of Early HIV Infection* for recommended followup.

[7]Alternative treatments include 10 days of I.M. procaine penicillin or 10-14 days of 1-2 g of I.M. ceftriaxone.

Note: The algorithm presents recommendations only for the items reviewed by the HIV panel.

From U.S. Department of Health and Human Services, *Evaluation and Management of Early HIV Infection*, Clinical Practice Guideline, Number 7, 1994, 167-76.

ALGORITHM 6.

PAP SMEARS IN WOMEN WITH EARLY HIV INFECTION

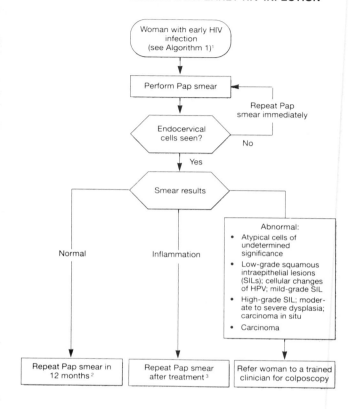

¹Pap smears should be performed at entry to prenatal care for pregnant women and prior to discharge for women who present for delivery without prenatal care.

²HIV-infected women with a history of human papilloma virus (HPV) or with previous Pap smears showing squamous intraepithelial lesions should have their Pap smears repeated every 6 months.

³Treatment should be guided by diagnosis of the cause of inflammation.

Note: The algorithm presents recommendations only for the items reviewed by the HIV panel.

From U.S. Department of Health and Human Services, *Evaluation and Management of Early HIV Infection*, Clinical Practice Guideline, Number 7, 1994, 167-76.

ALGORITHM 7.

EVALUATION FOR INITIATION OF ANTIRETROVIRAL THERAPY AND PCP PROPHYLAXIS; INFANTS AND CHILDREN WITH EARLY HIV INFECTION

Infants and children with early HIV infection

Obtain CD4 count and percentage

- Initiate antiretroviral therapy as indicated by either CD4 count (Table A) or CD4 percentage (Table B)
- Initiate PCP prophylaxis as indicated by either CD4 count (Figure A) or CD4 percentage (Figure B)[1]
- Infants and children receiving neither antiretroviral therapy nor PCP prophylaxis should have their CD4 counts and percentages monitored[2]

Figure A

	CD4 count (cells/mL)						
Age	200	300	500	750	1000	1500	1750
<12 mo[1]							
12-24 mo[2]							
2-6 yr[2]							
≥ 6 yr[2]							

▨ Initiate PCP prophylaxis
■ Initiate antiretroviral therapy

Figure B

	CD4 percentage		
Age	20	25	30
<12 mo			
12-24 mo			
>24 mo			

▨ Initiate PCP prophylaxis
■ Initiate antiretroviral therapy

Source: Figure A adapted from Centers for Disease Control, 1991

[1]Patients with prior episode of PCP should receive PCP prophylaxis regardless of CD4 count and percentage.

[2]Obtain CD4 count and percentage at 1 month of age, 3 months of age, and then at 3-month intervals through 24 months of age; thereafter obtain CD4 count and percentage every 6 months, unless values reach an age-related threshold where testing should be repeated monthly.

Note: The algorithm presents recommendations only for the items reviewed by the HIV panel.

From U.S. Department of Health and Human Services, *Evaluation and Management of Early HIV Infection,* Clinical Practice Guideline, Number 7, 1994, 167-76.

ALGORITHM 8.

NEUROLOGIC EVALUATION OF INFANTS AND CHILDREN WITH EARLY HIV INFECTION

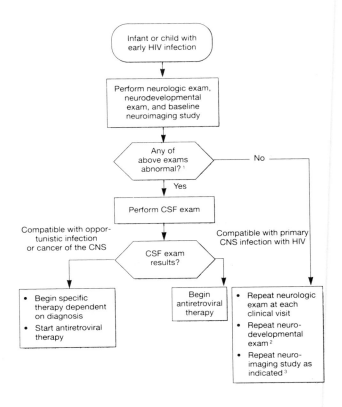

[1]Abnormal exam is defined as focal pathology, obstructive lesion, atypical CNS manifestations, or evidence of progressive neurologic disease (see *Guideline for Evaluation and Management of Early HIV Infection*),

[2]Neurodevelopmental exams should be performed at 3-month intervals up to 24 months of age, then every 6 months thereafter.

[3]Neuroimaging studies should be performed if CNS symptoms occur; such studies should be performed in conjunction with CSF analysis.

Note: The algorithm presents recommendations only for the items reviewed by the HIV panel.

From U.S. Department of Health and Human Services, *Evaluation and Management of Early HIV Infection*, Clinical Practice Guideline, Number 7, 1994, 167-76.

COMPATIBILITY OF MEDICATIONS
WITH HYPERALIMENTATION SOLUTIONS

The following is a list to be used as a quick reference guide. Drug compatibility is dependent on several factors such as drug concentration, the type, pH and volume of solutions used, and duration of mixing. These variations make it impossible to determine the compatibility of various medications at all times.

Antibiotics — Compatible	**References**
‡ Amikacin sulfate	1,2,4
Azlocillin sodium	1,2,4
Aztreonam	7
Carbenicillin disodium	1,2
Cefamandole nafate	1,2,4
Cefazolin sodium	1,2
Cefoperazone sodium	1,2
Cefotaxime sodium	1,2
Cefoxitin sodium	1,2
Ceftazidime	7
Ceftriaxone sodium	7
Cefuroxime sodium	7
Cephalothin sodium	1,2,4
Chloramphenicol sodium succinate	1,2
Clindamycin phosphate	1,2
Dopamine	
* Doxycycline hyclate	1,2
*‡ Erythromycin gluceptate	2
*‡ Erythromycin lactobionate	1,2
‡ Gentamicin sulfate	1,2
†‡ Kanamycin sulfate	1,2
Methicillin sodium	1,2
Mezlocillin sodium	1,2,4
* Miconazole	1,2
Morphine	
Moxalactam disodium	1,2,4
Nafcillin sodium	1,2,4
‡ Netilmicin sulfate	1,2
Oxacillin sodium	1,2,4
Penicillin G potassium	1,2,4
Piperacillin sodium	1,2,4
Polymyxin B sulfate	1,2
*§ Tetracycline hydrochloride	1,2,5
‡ Tobramycin sulfate	1,2,4
Ticarcillin disodium	1,2,4
‡ Vancomycin hydrochloride	1,2,3

*Physically compatible — no chemical compatibility data.
†Reported physical compatibility with conflicting chemical compatibility data.
‡Heparin in various concentrations is incompatible with amikacin, erythromycin, gentamicin, kanamycin, netilmicin, tobramycin, and vancomycin at usual dosages.[1] The interaction may be drug concentration dependent and less likely to occur in more dilute concentrations. A TPN solution containing 1 unit/mL of heparin was physically compatible with vancomycin, tobramycin, gentamicin, and amikacin.[6]
§Chelation with magnesium and calcium ions has been documented. The degree of chelation is influenced by the concentration of magnesium and calcium ions as well as pH of the solution.

Ampicillin sodium was reported physically compatible and physically incompatible with precipitate formation in different studies (1,2). Reference number 4 states incompatible.

Antibiotics — Incompatible	**References**
Acyclovir	
Amphotericin B	1,5
Metronidazole	1,5
Trimethoprim-sulfamethoxazole	5

Other Medications — Compatible	
* Albumin	2,8
¶ Aminophylline	1,2,9
Cimetidine HCl	1,2,9
* Cyanocobalamin	1
* Cyclophosphamide	1
* Cytarabine	1,9

Digoxin physically compatible for 4 h (Y-site)	1
Dobutamine physically compatible for 4 h (Y-site)	1
*Dopamine HCl	1,2
*Famotidine	9
*Fluorouracil	1,9
*Folic acid	1,2
*Furosemide	1,2
*Heparin sodium	1,2
*Hydrocortisone sodium succinate	9
Isoproterenol HCl	1,2
*Levarterenol bitartrate	2,9
*Lidocaine HCl	1,2
*Meperidine HCl	1,9
*Metaraminol bitartrate	1,2
*Methotrexate sodium	1
*Methyldopate HCl	1,2
*Methylprednisolone sodium succinate	1,2
Metoclopramide HCl	1,2
*Morphine sulfate	1,9
*Nizatidine	9
Norepinephrine bitartrate	1,2
*Ranitidine HCl	1,9
Urokinase (no loss of urokinase activity when assayed immediately after mixing)	1

*Physically compatible — no chemical compatibility data.

¶Precipitation is more likely to be seen in neonatal TPN solutions upon the addition of aminophylline, than adult solutions because of the lesser concentrations of amino acids and greater concentrations of calcium and phosphate. The high pH of aminophylline also contributes to the problem. With the administration of aminophylline by retrograde injection, TPN solutions of Travasol® 1% and dextrose 10% will show precipitation at levels of 10 mEq/L calcium and 10 mmol/L phosphorus. Solutions of Travasol® 2% and dextrose were compatible with the same levels of electrolytes.[4]

Other Medications — Incompatible

Bleomycin sulfate	1
Blood (possible pseudoagglutination)	1

COMPATIBILITY OF MEDICATIONS WITH FAT EMULSIONS

Antibiotics — Compatible	References
Ampicillin sodium	1
Cefamandole nafate	1
Cefazolin sodium	1
Cefoxitin sodium	1
Clindamycin phosphate	1
Erythromycin lactobionate	1
Gentamicin sulfate	1
Kanamycin sulfate	1
Penicillin G potassium	1
Ticarcillin sodium	1
Tobramycin sulfate	1

Above antibiotics are physically compatible via Y-site (1:1 mixture) for 4 hours at 25°C by visual observation.

Antibiotics — Incompatible

Tetracycline hydrochloride	1

Other Medications — Compatible

Aminophylline	
physically compatible for 48 h	4
conflicting data — states compatible and incompatible	1
Cimetidine HCl	1
physically compatible	
Digoxin	1,4
physically compatible for 4 h (Y-site only)	
Diphenhydramine HCl	1,4
physically compatible	
Dopamine HCl	1,4
physically compatible for 4 h (Y-site only)	
Furosemide	1,4
physically compatible for 4 h (Y-site only)	
Heparin	1,4
physically compatible	
Hydrocortisone sodium succinate	1
physically compatible	
Isoproterenol HCl	1,4
physically compatible for 4 h (Y-site only)	
Lidocaine HCl	1,4
physically compatible for 4 h (Y-site only)	
Methyldopate HCl	1
compatible when diluted with sodium chloride 0.9%; incompatible when diluted with dextrose 5% water	
Norepinephrine bitartrate	1,4
physically compatible for 4 h (Y-site only)	

Other Medications — Incompatible

Calcium gluconate	1,4
Phenytoin sodium	1

References

1. Trissel LA, *Handbook on Injectable Drugs*, Bethesda, MD: American Society of Hospital Pharmacists, Inc, 1988.

2. Frey AM, "Taking the Confusion Out of Multiple Infusion: I.V. Medications and TPN," *NITA*, 1986, 9(6):460-3.

3. Schilling CG, Watson DM, McCoy HG, et al, "Stability and Delivery of Vancomycin Hydrochloride When Admixed in a Total Parenteral Nutrition Solution," *JPEN J Parenter Enteral Nutr*, 1989, 13(1):63-4.

4. Kamen BA, Gunther N, Sowinsky N, et al, "Analysis of Antibiotic Stability in a Parenteral Nutrition Solution," *Pediatr Infect Dis*, 1985, 4(4):387-9.

5. Stranz MH and Barfoot KS, "Total Parenteral Nutrition. Compatibility of Antibiotic Admixtures," *J Intraven Nurs*, 1988, 11(1):43-8.

6. Schilling CG, "Compatibility of Drugs With a Heparin-Containing Neonatal Total Parenteral Nutrient Solution," *Am J Hosp Pharm*, 1988, 45(2):313-4.

7. Fox AS, Boyer KM, and Sweeney HM, "Antibiotic Stability in a Pediatric Parenteral Alimentation Solution," *J Pediatr*, 1988, 112(5):813-7.

8. Niemiec PW Jr and Vanderveen TW, "Compatibility Considerations in Parenteral Nutrient Solutions," *Am J Hosp Pharm*, 1984, 41(5):893-911.

9. King J, *Guide to Parenteral Admixtures*, St Louis, MO: Pacemarq, Inc, 1989.

CLASSIFICATION OF ORGANISMS

CLASSIFICATION OF ORGANISMS

ANAEROBES

CHLAMYDIA

DNA VIRUSES

FUNGI

GRAM-NEGATIVE BACILLI

GRAM-NEGATIVE COCCI

GRAM-POSITIVE BACILLI

(Continued)

CLASSIFICATION OF ORGANISMS

ALPHABETICAL INDEX

ALPHABETICAL INDEX

ALPHABETICAL INDEX

ALPHABETICAL INDEX

ALPHABETICAL INDEX

ALPHABETICAL INDEX

ALPHABETICAL INDEX

ALPHABETICAL INDEX

ALPHABETICAL INDEX

NOTES